PRINCIPLES OF NEURO-ONCOLOGY

Notice

PRINCIPLES OF NEURO-ONCOLOGY

Editors

David Schiff, MD
Associate Professor of Neurology, Neurosurgery, and Medicine
Co-Director, Neuro-Oncology Center
University of Virginia Health System
Charlottesville, Virginia

Brian Patrick O'Neill, MD
Professor of Neurology
Mayo Clinic College of Medicine
Mayo Medical School
Director, Neuro-Oncology Program
Mayo Clinic Cancer Center
Rochester, Minnesota

McGraw-Hill
Medical Publishing Division

New York Chicago San Francisco Lisbon London Madrid Mexico City Milan
New Delhi San Juan Seoul Singapore Sydney Toronto

The McGraw-Hill Companies

Principles of Neuro-Oncology

1 2 3 4 5 6 7 8 9 0 KGP/KGP 0 9 8 7 6 5

ISBN: 0-07-142515-2

This book was set in Garamond by International Typesetting and Composition.
The editors were Marc Strauss, Nicky Fernando, and Lester Sheinis.
The production manager was Philip Galea.
The cover designer was Pehrsson Design.
The indexer was Jerry Ralya.
Quebecor-World Kingsport was printer and binder.

This book is printed on acid-free paper.

Library of Congress Cataloging-in-Publication Data

Schiff, David, 1959-
Principles of neuro-oncology/David Schiff, Brian O'Neill.
p. ; cm.
Includes bibliographical references and index.
ISBN 0-07-142515-2 (alk. paper)
1. Nervous system—Cancer. I. O'Neill, Brian, M.D. II. Title.
[DNLM: 1. Neoplasms, Nerve Tissue. 2. Nervous System Neoplasms. WL 160 S333p 2005]
RC 280.N4S32 2005
616.99'48—dc22

2004058192

This book is dedicated to our patients and their families who struggle with the most dreadful of human cancers.

CONTENTS

Contributors . . . . *ix*
Foreword . . . . *xv*
Preface . . . . *xvii*
Acknowledgments . . . . *xviii*

PART I Overview and Principles

1 Epidemiology of Brain Cancer 3
Melissa L. Bondy, Randa El-Zein, & Margaret Wrensch

2 Translational Applications of Molecular Biology in Neuro-Oncology 17
Joon H. Uhm

3 Presentation and Approach to Patient 37
Patrick Y. Wen, Siew Koon Teoh, Debra C. Gigas, & Lisa MacDonald

4 Neuroimaging 53
L. Burt Nabors

5 Neuropathology 81
M. Beatriz S. Lopes

6 Surgical Management 121
Michael D. Taylor & Mark Bernstein

7 Principles of Radiotherapy and Radiosurgery . . . 143
Paul D. Brown & Bruce E. Pollock

8 Principles of Chemotherapy 163
Sanjay P. Ahuja & Regina I. Jakacki

9 Supportive Care 183
Herbert B. Newton

10 Neuropsychological Issues 201
Elana Farace & Mark E. Shaffrey

11 Clinical Trial Design in Neuro-Oncology 217
Judith R. O'Fallon & Jan C. Buckner

12 The Phakomatoses 233
David H. Gutmann, Cynthia Wetmore, & Brian Patrick O'Neill

PART II Specific Tumors

13 High-Grade Astrocytomas 259
John F. de Groot, Kenneth D. Aldape, & Howard Colman

14 Low-Grade Astrocytomas 289
Warren P. Mason

15 Oligodendroglioma and Mixed Gliomas 311
Martin J. van den Bent & Johan M. Kros

16 Brainstem Gliomas 333
Bruce H. Cohen & Cameron L. Nicholson

17 Primary Central Nervous System Lymphoma . . . 343
Brian Patrick O'Neill & David Schiff

18 Primary Meningeal Neoplasms 369
John K. Park & Peter McL. Black

19 Pituitary Adenomas and Sellar Lesions: Multidisciplinary Management 381
John A. Jane, Jr., Aaron S. Dumont, Mary Lee Vance, & Edward R. Laws, Jr.

20 Primitive Neuroectodermal Tumors 415
Corey Raffel & Cormac O. Maher

21 Ependymomas and Intraventricular Tumors. . . . 431
Joao Siffert & George Jallo

22 Primary Tumors of the Cranial Nerves and Skull Base 447
L. Gerard Toussaint III & Michael J. Link

23 Intracranial Germ Cell Tumors 481
Patricia L. Robertson

24 Primary Spinal Tumors 501
Volker W. Stieber, Stephen B. Tatter, Mark E. Shaffrey, & Edward G. Shaw

25 Spinal Root and Peripheral Nerve Tumors 533
Asis Kumar Bhattacharyya & Abhijit Guha

PART III Metastatic Disease

26 The Management of Brain Metastases 553
American College of Surgical Oncology CNS Working Group

27 Spinal Metastases 581
Tali Siegal & Tzony Siegal

28 Leptomeningeal Metastases and Dural/Skull Metastases 607
Susan M. Blaney & David G. Poplack

29 Cancer Metastasis to the Peripheral Nervous System 629
Naganand Sripathi & Lisa R. Rogers

PART IV Indirect Complications of Cancer

30 Paraneoplasia 649
Setareh Shams'ili & Peter Sillevis Smitt

31 Neurologic Complications of Chemotherapy and Biologic Therapies 679
Julie E. Hammack

32 Neurologic Complications of Radiation Therapy 711
Lauren E. Abrey & Denise D. Correa

Color Plates appear between pages 110 and 111 and pages 398 and 399.

Index 729

CONTRIBUTORS

Lauren E. Abrey, MD *(Chapter 32)*
Assistant Attending
Memorial Sloan-Kettering Cancer Center
Department of Neurology
New York, New York

Sanjay P. Ahuja, MD *(Chapter 8)*
Fellow, Pediatric Hematology/Oncology
Children's Hospital of Pittsburgh
Pittsburgh, Pennsylvania

Kenneth D. Aldape, MD *(Chapter 13)*
Department of Pathology
Brain Tumor Center
University of Texas M. D. Anderson Cancer Center
Houston, Texas

Anthony L. Asher, MD, FACS *(Chapter 26)*
Director, Brain Tumor Program
Carolinas Medical Center
Charlotte, North Carolina

Mark A. Bernstein, MD, FRCSC *(Chapter 6)*
Professor, Department of Surgery
University of Toronto
Division of Neurosurgery
Toronto Western Hospital
Toronto, Ontario, Canada

Asis Kumar Bhattacharyya, MBBS, MS, MCh *(Chapter 25)*
Clinical Fellow
Division of Neurosurgery
Toronto Western Hospital
University Health Network
University of Toronto
Toronto, Ontario, Canada

Peter McL. Black, MD, PhD *(Chapter 18)*
Chief, Department of Neurosurgery
Brigham & Women's Hospital
Harvard Medical School
Boston, Massachussetts

Susan M. Blaney, MD *(Chapter 28)*
Associate Professor of Pediatrics
Baylor College of Medicine
Head, Neuro-Oncology Program
Texas Children's Cancer Center
Texas Children's Hospital
Houston, Texas

Melissa L. Bondy, PhD *(Chapter 1)*
University of Texas M. D. Anderson Cancer Center
Department of Epidemiology
Houston, Texas

Paul D. Brown, MD *(Chapter 7)*
Assistant Professor
Division of Radiation Oncology
Mayo Clinic and Foundation
Rochester, Minnesota

Jan C. Buckner, MD *(Chapter 11)*
Professor of Oncology
Division of Medical Oncology
Mayo Clinic
Rochester, Minnesota

Stuart H. Burri, MD *(Chapter 26)*
Co-Director, Radiosurgery Program
Carolinas Medical Center
Charlotte, North Carolina

A. Chahlavi, MD *(Chapter 26)*
Cleveland Clinic
Cleveland, Ohio

S. M. Chang, MD *(Chapter 26)*
Department of Neurosurgery
University of California, San Fransisco
San Francisco, California

Bruce H. Cohen, MD *(Chapter 16)*
Cleveland Clinic
Cleveland, Ohio

Howard Colman, MD, PhD *(Chapter 13)*
Assistant Professor, Department of Neuro-Oncology
Brain Tumor Center
University of Texas M. D. Anderson Cancer Center
Houston, Texas

Denise D. Correa, PhD *(Chapter 32)*
Memorial Sloan-Kettering Cancer Center
Department of Neurology
New York, New York

John F. de Groot, MD *(Chapter 13)*
Assistant Professor
Department of Neuro-Oncology
Brain Tumor Center
University of Texas M. D. Anderson Cancer Center
Houston, Texas

Aaron S. Dumont, MD *(Chapter 19)*
Resident
Department of Neurosurgery
University of Virginia Health System
Charlottesville, Virginia

Randa El-Zein, MD *(Chapter 1)*
University of Texas M. D. Anderson Cancer Center
Houston, Texas

Elana Farace, PhD *(Chapters 10, 26)*
Assistant Professor of Neurosurgery, Psychology, and Health Evaluation Sciences
Department of Neurosurgery
University of Virginia Health System
Charlottesville, Virginia

John B. Fiveash, MD *(Chapter 26)*
Department of Radiation Oncology
University of Alabama
Birmingham, Alabama

Debra C. Gigas, RN, OCN *(Chapter 3)*
Center for Neuro-Oncology
Dana Farber Cancer Institute
Boston, Massachusetts

Abhijit Guha, MD, MSc, FRCS, FACS *(Chapter 25)*
Professor of Surgery
Alan & Susan Hudson Chair in Neurooncology
Toronto Western Hospital, University Health Network
Co-Director, Arthur & Sonia Labatts Brain Tumor Center
Hospital for Sick Children's Research Institute
University of Toronto
Toronto, Ontario, Canada

David H. Gutmann, MD, PhD *(Chapter 12)*
Department of Neurology
Washington University School of Medicine
Saint Louis, Missouri

Julie E. Hammack, MD *(Chapter 31)*
Assistant Professor
Neurology
Mayo Clinic and Foundation
Rochester, Minnesota

Regina I. Jakacki, MD *(Chapter 8)*
Associate Professor of Pediatrics
Director, Neuro-Oncology Program
Pediatric Hematology/Oncology
Children's Hospital of Pittsburgh
Pittsburgh, Pennsylvania

George I. Jallo, MD *(Chapter 21)*
Assistant Professor of Neurosurgery
Division of Pediatric Neurosurgery
Johns Hopkins School of Medicine
Baltimore, Maryland

John A. Jane, Jr., MD *(Chapter 19)*
Assistant Professor of Neurosurgery
University of Virginia Health System
Charlottesville, Virginia

Johan M. Kros, MD *(Chapter 14)*
Department of Pathology
Erasmus University Hospital Rotterdam
Rotterdam, The Netherlands

F. F. Lang, MD *(Chapter 26)*
Department of Neurosurgery
M. D. Anderson Cancer Center
Charlottesville, Virginia

Edward R. Laws, Jr., MD *(Chapter 19)*
Professor of Neurosurgery
University of Virginia Health System
Charlottesville, Virginia

Michael J. Link, MD *(Chapter 22)*
Associate Professor
Department of Neurosurgery
Mayo Clinic
Rochester, Minnesota

M. Beatriz S. Lopes, MD *(Chapter 5)*
Associate Professor of Pathology
University of Virginia School of Medicine
Charlottesville, Virginia

Lisa MacDonald, NP, OCN *(Chapter 3)*
Center for Neuro-Oncology
Dana Farber Cancer Institute
Boston, Massachusetts

Cormac O. Maher, MD *(Chapter 20)*
Department of Neurosurgery
Childrens Hospital
Boston, Massachusetts

James M. Markert, MD *(Chapter 26)*
Departmentof Neurosurgery
University of Alabama
Birmingham, Alabama

Warren P. Mason, MD, FRCPC *(Chapter 14)*
Staff Physician, Princess Margaret Hospital
Assistant Professor, Department of Medicine
University of Toronto
Toronto, Ontario, Canada

M. Mut, MD *(Chapter 26)*
Department of Neurosurgery
University of Virginia Health System
Charlottesville, Virginia

L. Burt Nabors, MD *(Chapter 4)*
Brain Tumor Treatment and Research Program
University of Alabama at Birmingham
Birmingham, Alabama

Herbert B. Newton, MD, FAAN *(Chapter 9)*
Associate Professor of Neurology and Pediatrics
Dardinger Neuro-Oncology Center
Department of Neurology
The Ohio State University Hospitals
Columbus, Ohio

Cameron L. Nicholson, MD *(Chapter 16)*
Cleveland Clinic
Cleveland, Ohio

Judith R. O'Fallon, PhD *(Chapter 11)*
Department of Statistics
Mayo Clinic
Rochester, Minnesota

Brian Patrick O'Neill, MD *(Chapters 12, 17)*
Professor of Neurology
Mayo Clinic
College of Medicine
Mayo Medical School
Director, Neuro-Oncology Program
Mayo Clinic Cancer Center
Rochester, Minnesota

John K. Park, MD, PhD *(Chapter 18)*
Head, Surgical and Molecular
Neuro-Oncology Unit
National Institute of Neurological Disorders
and Stroke
National Institutes of Health
Bethesda, Maryland

Bruce E. Pollock, MD *(Chapter 7)*
Professor
Department of Neurological Surgery and Division
of Radiation Oncology
Mayo Clinic and Foundation
Rochester, Minnesota

David G. Poplack, MD *(Chapter 28)*
Elise C. Young Professor of Pediatric Oncology
Chief, Hematology-Oncology Section
Department of Pediatrics
Baylor College of Medicine
Director, Texas Children's Cancer Center
Texas Children's Hospital
Houston, Texas

Corey Raffel, MD, PhD *(Chapter 20)*
Professor of Neurosurgery
Mayo Clinic
Rochester, Minnesota

Patricia L. Robertson, MD *(Chapter 23)*
Associate Professor of Neurology
and Pediatrics
University of Michigan School of Medicine
Ann Arbor, Michigan

Lisa R. Rogers, DO *(Chapter 29)*
Co-Director, Clinical Neuro-Oncology
Program
Henry Ford Hospital, Neurology
Detroit, Michigan

David Schiff, MD *(Chapters 17, 26)*
Associate Professor of Neurology, Neurosurgery,
and Medicine
Co-Director, Neuro-Oncology Center
University of Virginia Health System
Charlottesville, Virginia

Mark E. Shaffrey, MD, FACS *(Chapters 10, 24, 26)*
Professor, Vice-Chairman of the Department
of Neurological Surgery
Co-Director, Neuro-Oncology Center
University of Virginia
Charlottesville, Virginia

Setareh Shams'ili, MD *(Chapter 30)*
Laboratory Neuro-Oncology
Erasmus Medical Center
Rotterdam, The Netherlands

Edward G. Shaw, MD *(Chapter 24)*
Professor and Chairman
Department of Radiation Oncology
Wake Forest University School of Medicine
Winston-Salem, North Carolina

Tali Siegal, MD *(Chapter 27)*
Professor and Director
Leslie and Michael Center for Neuro-Oncology
Sharett Institute of Oncology
Hadassah Hebrew University Hospital
Jerusalem, Israel

Tzony Siegal, MD, DMD *(Chapter 27)*
Director, Chosen Specialties Clinics
Spinal Surgery Consultant
Assuta Hospital
Tel Aviv, Israel

Joao Siffert, MD *(Chapter 21)*
Medical Director
Neurology
Pfizer Global Pharmaceuticals
New York, New York

V. Siomin, MD *(Chapter 26)*
Cleveland Clinic
Cleveland, Ohio

Peter Sillevis Smitt, MD, PhD *(Chapter 30)*
Professor and Chairman
Department of Neurology
Erasmus Medical Center
Rotterdam, The Netherlands

Naganand Sripathi, MD *(Chapter 29)*
Director, Neuromuscular Clinic
Department of Neurology
Henry Ford Hospital
Detroit, Michigan

Volker W. Stieber, MD *(Chapter 24)*
Assistant Professor
Department of Radiation Oncology
Wake Forest University School of Medicine
Winston-Salem, North Carolina

Stephen B. Tatter, MD, PhD *(Chapter 24)*
Assistant Professor
Department of Neurosurgery
Wake Forest University School of Medicine
Winston-Salem, North Carolina

Michael D. Taylor, MD, PhD, FRCSC *(Chapter 6)*
Resident, Division of Neurosurgery
University of Toronto
Toronto, Ontario, Canada

Siew Koon Teoh, MD *(Chapter 3)*
Clinical Instructor in Radiology
Harvard Medical School
Department of Radiology
Mount Auburn Hospital
Boston, Massachusetts

L. Gerard Toussaint III, MD *(Chapter 22)*
Resident
Department of Neurosurgery
Mayo Clinic
Rochester, Minnesota

Joon H. Uhm, MD, FRCP *(Chapter 2)*
Assistant Professor of Neurology
Division of Neuro-Oncology
Mayo Clinic
Rochester, Minnesota

Mary Lee Vance, MD *(Chapter 19)*
Professor of Medicine
Department of Internal Medicine
University of Virginia Health System
Charlottesville, Virginia

Martin J. van den Bent *(Chapter 14)*
Neuro-Oncology Unit
Daniel den Hoed Cancer Clinic/Erasmus University Medical Center
Rotterdam, The Netherlands

Nicholas A. Vick, MD *(Foreword)*
Ruth Cain Ruggles Chairman
Evanston Northwestern Healthcare
Professor of Neurology
Feinberg School of Medicine
Northwestern University
Evanston, Illinois

M. A. Vogelbaum, MD *(Chapter 26)*
Cleveland Clinic Brain Tumor Center
Cleveland, Ohio

Patrick Y. Wen, MD *(Chapter 3)*
Associate Professor of Neurology
Harvard Medical School
Dana Farber Cancer Institute, Center for Neuro-Oncology
Boston, Massachusetts

Cynthia J. Wetmore, MD, PhD *(Chapter 12)*
Assistant Professor of Pediatrics and Neurology
Mayo Medical School
Rochester, Minnesota

Margaret Wrensch, MD *(Chapter 1)*
University of California, San Francisco
San Francisco, Califorinia

FOREWORD

It was not much more than 30 years ago that neurologists, or other physicians besides neurosurgeons or neuropathologists, had any interest in brain tumors. Douglas Buchanan's collaboration with Paul Bucy, leading to the classic *Intracranial Tumors of Infancy and Childhood* (1939), stood out as a unique contribution for decades. It was not until Jerome Posner began to explore the field, or better, began to create it, in the 1970s that neuro-oncology as a field of involvement by neurologists, oncologists, radiotherapists, and others began to emerge. Advances in anesthesia, neurosurgical techniques, radiotherapy, and imaging in the 1970s, added to the critical advent of the use of steroids in the 1960s, made it possible for the field to cohere and grow. In the last three decades, explosive advances in molecular biology, genetics, and brain imaging have carried the field to what now looks like a triumph, but nonetheless one that is still short of achieving major improvements in patient care and survival.

This book documents like no other available where we are today. It provides an encompassing look at neuro-oncology as it has just achieved its identity as a specialty. It is a hybrid specialty, not entirely sorted out, still awaiting official status, that includes physicians and basic scientists of differing orientations and interests. But the identity has emerged and the feeling of completeness that this book provides attests to it. It is hard to believe that the few who began meeting yearly in the early 1970s, with the leadership of Charles Wilson, would have been the predecessors of the Society for Neuro-Oncology, now a large and extraordinarily successful organization with its own journal and major connections to all of the important international organizations in the field. Wilson's willingness, as a neurosurgeon, to support the other specialties involved is still one possible model for success.

The grotesque disparity between current reimbursement for procedures, surgical or radiological, as contrasted to that for the neurology, oncology, nursing, and social work required for the total care of a patient with brain tumor demands creative financing. And this creativity must become institutional, not personal. The political and administrative factors involved in the organization and maintenance of comprehensive neuro-oncology programs at hospitals and universities are complex and vary greatly from place to place. These programs will have their best chance to prosper on behalf of the patients they serve when the field is organized around formal training programs. The obvious sense of multi-specialty collaboration among the diverse contributors to this book should be emblematic of the intellectual cohesion and generosity of spirit that will be needed to set up inclusive educational curricula.

The content of this book is exactly what needs to be mastered by trainees as well as referred to by those of us continuing our training as we work. It is all here, ready to be built on for the future. All we need to do is be smart enough to organize ourselves effectively. We have the wine; I have no illusion that it is perfect but it will surely improve with time. But when it is as good as it is now, however, as anyone can see by reading these 32 chapters, it is time for a good bottle to hold it in.

Nicholas A. Vick, MD
Ruth Cain Ruggles Chairman
Evanston Northwestern Healthcare
Professor of Neurology
Feinberg School of Medicine
Northwestern University
Evanston, Illinois

PREFACE

Brain tumors are a human disease with significant public health implications. Compared with other more common systemic tumors, brain tumors, particularly primary ones, are responsible for disproportionate morbidity and mortality because of their impact on cognition, memory, language, mobility, and adaptive skills. Within brain tumors is a melange of tumors with varying pathologies, epidemiologies, and prognoses. The most common primary brain tumor of adults, glioblastoma multiforme (GBM), is also disproportionally lethal. With standard treatment patients rarely live longer than twenty-four months and rarely longer than six months with surgery alone.

The neuro-oncology community has learned many of the underlying chromosomal, molecular genetic, and biologic alterations in human brain tumors. Nevertheless, there are still considerable gaps in our knowledge about the molecular etiology involved in these tumors. More importantly, little of what is known has been translated into clinical practice to relieve our patients and their families from the burden of disease.

Reliable figures predict an annual age-adjusted primary brain tumor incidence rate of 11.5 per 100,000 person years, more than half of who will develop malignant brain tumors. These latter tumors appear to be increasing in incidence, although this increase may be explained in part or entirely by improved detection capability and an increase in the size and life expectancy of the population. However, primary brain tumors are now the leading cause of cancer deaths for children and adolescents in the United States. Paradoxically, it is this group of patients for whom both the potential for cure or sustained remission and for long-term complications of therapy are the greatest.

Primary brain tumors are neurologic diseases due to cancer and cancers that are neurologic diseases. As such their study requires a unique knowledge base, one that is well-grounded in tumor biology and neuroscience. Similarly, clinicians have to be experienced and knowledgeable in clinical cancer medicine and the clinical neurosciences. The subspecialty of neuro-oncology crosses specialty and department boundaries and arguably, weaves basic, translational, population, and clinical science into a day-to-day management platform. As such, this textbook, *Principles of Neuro-Oncology*, is intended to provide the clinician with the necessary knowledge base for encountering both the tumor and the patient with the tumor. We have incorporated a section on the neurologic complications of metastatic disease, given the overall frequency of these problems and the commonality of many of the conceptual issues.

ACKNOWLEDGMENTS

I would like to thank the individual chapter authors who took the time from their busy academic schedules to prepare outstanding chapters in their area of expertise; I owe each of them a debt of gratitude. Brian O'Neill, a teacher, mentor, and friend, graciously accepted the task of co-editor, read every page of this volume, and made unfailingly insightful comments. He was more than an equal participant in this endeavor.

Many colleagues at University of Virginia helped make this effort possible. Fred Wooten, Mark Shaffrey, and Ed Laws brought me to the university and have helped to create an enviable environment for neuro-oncology; Bea Lopes and Isa Hussaini among others have contributed greatly as well. Bruce Leffler, an administrative assistant extraordinaire, provided indispensable organizational skills.

Most of all, I would like to thank my family, especially Harold Schiff and Tanya Nezzer, MD, for their encouragement to pursue this project and their love and support during its completion.

David Schiff, MD
Charlottesville, Virginia
June 2005

Very special thanks are in order for T. R. Johns who taught me how to think as a clinician, to William Blackwell who taught me how to think as a scientist, and my wife, Gayle Novelle O'Neill (a.k.a. Einstein) who taught me how to think as a human being.

Brian Patrick O'Neill, MD
Rochester, Minnesota
June 2005

PART I

Overview and Principles

CHAPTER 1

Epidemiology of Brain Cancer

Melissa L. Bondy / Randa El-Zein / Margaret Wrensch

The incidence rate of central nervous system tumors in 2000 reported from the Surveillance, Epidemiology, and End Results (SEER) registry was 6.7 per 100,000 persons (SEER Cancer Statistics Review 1975–2001), and gliomas account for approximately 51% of all central nervous system tumors.[1] *The American Cancer Society estimates that of 18,400 individuals diagnosed with malignant brain tumors in 2004, 12,690 will die from the disease.*[2] *The Central Brain Tumor Registry of the United States web site (http://www.cbtrus.org/) maintains comprehensive incidence and mortality data obtained from the state registries and updates the tables annually. These data are the most current available, and are updated annually.*

Although brain cancer accounts for only 1.4% of all cancers and 2.3% of cancer-related deaths, its high degree of lethality and inescapable traumatic impact on survivors and family members of patients make it an important subject of concern and investigation. Despite a recent increase in epidemiologic studies, research has achieved little consensus on the nature and magnitude of the risk factors for this disease. Contributing to disparate hypotheses are methodological differences in eligibility and the representativeness of the patients studied; variable use of proxies to report information about the case subjects; choice of control groups; substantial heterogeneity of primary brain tumors; inconsistencies in histologic diagnoses, definitions, and groupings; and the difficulties of retrospectively measuring exposure.

▶ HISTOLOGY AND MOLECULAR GENETICS OF BRAIN TUMORS

Although some brain tumors contain a mixture of cell types, primary brain tumors are currently classified by their predominant histologic appearance and location. Occurring in the support tissue or glial cells of the brain, gliomas, the most common primary brain tumors, account for more than 40% of all central nervous system neoplasms[3] and include as subtypes astrocytomas, oligodendrogliomas, and ependymomas. Gliomas display a broad spectrum of histologic features, and the variation in their behavior probably reflects the genes involved in their transformation.[3] Astrocytomas, the most frequently occurring gliomas, are classified into four major grades by the World Health Organization (WHO).[4] Figure 1-1 shows the distribution of brain tumors by histology and age, and the glioma subtypes are described below.

Astrocytomas

Astrocytomas, the most invasive as well as most commonly occurring brain tumors in all ages, develop in and take their name from the star-shaped astrocyte cells. Their WHO classification is based on increasing levels of malignancy, which rises with their invasiveness and loss of definition:

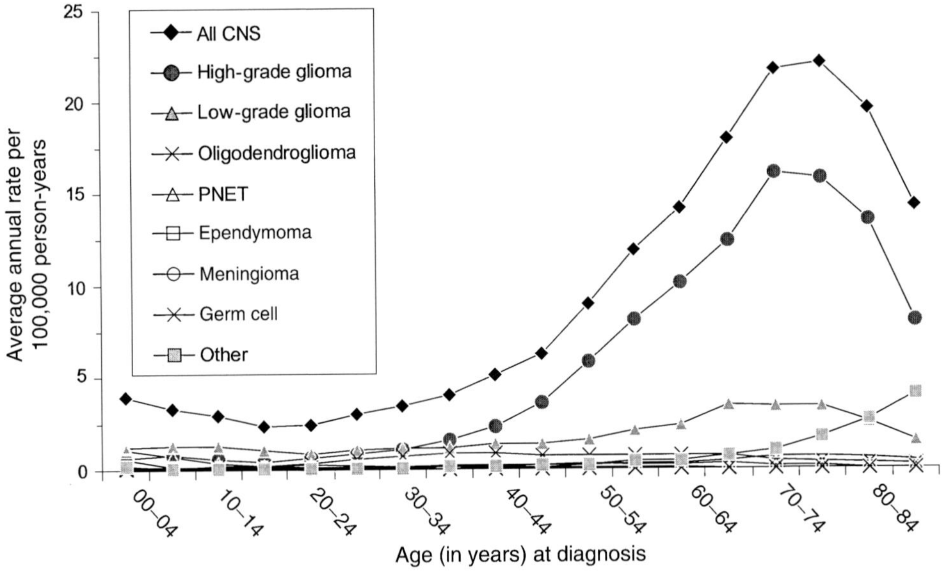

Figure 1-1. Incidence of malignant primary central nervous system (CNS) tumors by age and histology. (*Reproduced from SEER, 1986–2000.*)

1. WHO grade I or pilocytic astrocytomas are the most frequent brain tumors in children, but rarely undergo neoplastic transformation.
2. WHO grade II or low-grade astrocytomas account for 25% of all gliomas and are infiltrative in nature.
3. WHO grade III or anaplastic malignant astrocytomas are highly malignant gliomas and have an increased tendency to progress to glioblastoma.
4. WHO grade IV or glioblastoma multiforme is a highly malignant brain tumor, typically affecting adults. It has poor prognosis, largely because the tumor rapidly spreads to other regions of the brain.

The identification of the genetic alterations found in astrocytomas led to the recognition that a nonrandom series of genetic changes reflects increasing malignancy and clinical grade.[5] Several common chromosomal alterations that lead to changes in genetic expression have been observed. For example, in 40% of astrocytic tumors of all grades, mutations in the tumor suppressor *p53* gene (located on chromosome 17p) have been reported. They are primarily found in gliomas in young adults and not in supratentorial astrocytic tumors in children.[5] Another tumor suppressor gene frequently inactivated in astrocytic neoplasms is cyclin-dependent kinase N2 (*CDKN2*) or *p16*, located on chromosome 9p and inactivated by deletion of both copies of the gene. Its loss seldom occurs in low-grade astrocytomas but frequently in high-grade astrocytomas.[6] In astrocytomas, where considerable evidence supports the role of tumor suppressor genes, deletions of chromosome 10 commonly occur.[7] In approximately 70% of glioblastomas, loss of heterozygosity at 10q23 has been reported; in 40% of such cancers, mutated in multiple advanced cancers (*MMAC1*), or phosphatase tensin homologue (*PTEN*), a tumor suppressor gene located on 10q, is altered. Because *MMAC1* mutations are rarely found in low-grade gliomas, *MMAC1* is assumed to play an important role in progression from low-grade to high-grade tumors.[8]

In contrast to loss of tumor suppressor genes, another change reported is activation of oncogenes promoting cell proliferation. The epidermal growth factor receptor (*EGFR*) gene is most frequently amplified in malignant astrocytomas, having been found in mutated form in approximately one-third of glioblastomas but in no low-grade astrocytomas.[9,10]

Oligodendrogliomas

Accounting for less than 10% of intracranial tumors, oligodendrogliomas take their name and arise from the oligodendrocytes in the brain. Oligodendrogliomas are less aggressive than astrocytomas but, nevertheless, can invade and can even disseminate via the cerebral spinal fluid (CSF). Typically oligodendrogliomas are cortically based tumors and are potentially resectable. The ability of oligodendrogliomas to invade locally complicates their surgical removal, but because they are limited to the brain and CSF, they often permit a positive prognosis. Oligodendrogliomas characteristically exhibit loss of chromosomal regions on 1p and 19q13 and, less frequently, on 9q and 22.[11]

Ependymomas

Ependymomas arise from the ependymal cells lining the brain ventricles. Their growth may block the flow of CSF, causing notable swelling of the ventricle or hydrocephalus. Although ependymomas may move along the CSF, characteristically they do not infiltrate normal brain tissue and are sometimes amenable to surgical treatment, especially surgery of the spinal cord. The most commonly described genetic alterations in ependymomas are deletions of 17p and monosomy 22.[5]

Meningiomas

Meningiomas arise from the sheaths surrounding the brain. The growth of meningiomas and the pressure they produce lead to the symptoms of brain tumors. Meningiomas are common, accounting for approximately 50% of primary central nervous system tumors. Because they usually appear near the surface of the brain, they are often operable and benign. Malignant meningiomas are associated with deletions of loci on chromosome 1 and, to a lesser extent, with deletions on 6p, 9q, and 17p.[5] Mutations in the *p53* gene have also been reported in malignant meningioma.

Medulloblastomas

Medulloblastomas are primitive neuroectodermal tumors that arise in the cerebellum, replicate quickly, and frequently spread through the CSF. They occur most commonly in children. Chromosome 17p is a frequent site of deletions in medulloblastomas. Other less frequent sites of deletions are 2p, 6q 10q, 11p, 11q, and 16q.[5]

Ganglioglioma

Gangliogliomas are discrete low-grade tumors containing both neurons and glial cells. They have a high rate of cure by surgery alone or surgery combined with radiation therapy.

Schwannomas (Neurilemomas)

Schwannomas arise from Schwann cells, which surround cranial and other nerves. Schwannomas are usually benign tumors and often form near the cerebellum and in the cranial nerves responsible for hearing and balance.[5]

Chordomas

These tumors most frequently arise at the skull clivus and at the extremities of the spinal column and usually do not invade brain tissues and other organs. They are amenable to treatment but stubbornly recur over a span of 10 to 20 years.

▶ ETIOLOGY AND RISK FACTORS OF BRAIN TUMORS

Ionizing Radiation

Research consensus is that therapeutic ionizing radiation is a strong risk factor for intracranial tumors.[12–14] Even low doses (averaging 1.5 Gy) used to treat ringworm of the scalp (tinea capitis) have been associated with relative risks of 18, 10, and 3 for nerve sheath tumors, meningiomas, and gliomas, respectively.[12,13,15] Other studies showed a high (17%) prevalence of prior therapeutic radiation among patients with glioblastoma or glioma and an increased risk of brain tumors in children after radiation for acute lymphoblastic leukemia.

A study of 80,160 Nagasaki and Hiroshima atomic bomb survivors evaluated the role of radiation dose among survivors diagnosed with tumors of the nervous system and pituitary gland between 1958 and 1995.[16] Poisson regression analyses were computed to characterize radiation effects on tumor incidence, which are expressed as excess relative risk per sievert (ERR_{Sv}). They reported a statistically significant dose response for all nervous system tumors combined and for schwannomas considered separately, indicating that exposure to even moderate doses (i.e., <1 sievert [Sv]) of radiation is associated with an elevated incidence of nervous system tumors. Earlier studies of atomic bomb survivors from analyses of the Life Span Study cancer incidence data suggested an increased risk of extracranial neural tissue tumors, but there was little evidence of a radiation-associated increase in brain tumor risk.[17,18] Increased risks of meningioma associated with atomic bomb radiation exposure or distance from the bombs were reported in Hiroshima and in Nagasaki.[18]

The role of prenatal exposure to radiation in the etiology of childhood brain tumors is unclear. Japanese studies showed no increase of brain tumor incidence in individuals exposed in utero to atomic bomb radiation.[12] Other studies reporting increased relative risks of 1.2 to 1.6 for those exposed prenatally were statistically insignificant because of small sample size. Furthermore, relative risks of this low magnitude associated with a comparatively uncommon exposure would not account for many childhood brain tumors. Thus, parental exposure to ionizing radiation before conception of the affected child has not been shown to be a risk factor for childhood brain tumors.[13]

On the other hand, exposure to low doses from diagnostic radiation does not seem to play a role in glioma; three case-control studies reported relative risks of 0.4, 1.2, and 3.0 for exposure to dental x-rays. The evidence is slightly stronger for risk of meningioma, for which 3 of 4 studies have shown relative risks exceeding 2 for exposure to dental x-rays. Longstreth and associates[19] found elevated risk from full-mouth diagnostic x-rays only; however, they noted that full-mouth procedures are used far less frequently than formerly, so any increased incidence of meningioma associated with their use should decrease over time.[19]

Occupational studies of atomic energy and airline employees are equivocal. One reported a small, but statistically significant, elevated risk of 1.2 for brain tumors in nuclear facility employees and nuclear materials production workers, but was confounded by the possibility of the effect of chemical exposures.[20] More significantly, a cohort of U.S. nuclear workers was reexamined and, as in the first study, it was shown to have some 15% increased risk of brain tumors.[21] About the risk to airline pilots, no consensus exists, although some believe that exposure to cosmic radiation at high altitudes may contribute to brain tumors.[22,23] However, a study of British Airways flight deck workers showed no statistically significant mortality from brain tumors.[24]

Electromagnetic Fields

The debate on the impact of electromagnetic fields on brain cancer continues, despite largely negative findings. The debate has been prolonged by methodological difficulties with some studies. In 1979, Wertheimer and Leeper[24a] reported increased risks of brain tumors and leukemia in children living in homes in Denver near high-current versus low-current wiring. This triggered widespread public and scientific interest in the potential health effects of electromagnetic fields. One meta-analysis revealed a nonsignificant 50% increased risk of childhood brain tumors with residence in high- versus low-wire-coded homes.[25] In a meta-analysis of 29 studies of adult brain tumors in relation to occupational exposures to electric and magnetic fields, Kheifets and colleagues[26] found a significant 10% to 20% increased risk for brain cancer among electrical workers. However, they found no evidence for a consistent dose–response relationship with jobs considered to have higher rather than lower exposure. Three recent occupational studies reported an association among electromagnetic field (EMF)-exposed workers,[26–28] but others did not.[29,30] Studies have not found an association between maternal EMF exposures and brain tumors in their children.[31,32] A comprehensive assessment of childhood brain tumors in relation to residential EMF concluded that the evidence did not support an association.[33] Another epidemiologic study of adult brain tumors (reviewed in reference 34) and a recent large population-based study of adult glioma in the San Francisco Bay area did not provide strong support for the hypothesis that electromagnetic fields in homes may increase the risk of brain tumors.[35,36] In the San Francisco study, 492 adults with glioma and 463 controls were equally likely to have lived in homes with high-wire codes during the 7 years before diagnosis. Spot measurements taken in homes also showed no pattern of higher residential electromagnetic field exposures for cases when compared to controls.[36]

However, measurements of electromagnetic fields are not precise. Wire codes of electrical distribution to homes and spot measurements of electromagnetic fields in and around homes can lead to incorrect exposure estimates.[37] Wire codes also do not reflect exposures from internal wiring or sources such as appliances. Spot measurements change over time and do not always reflect the overall measurement in homes. The spot measurements can also be made at places where the subjects spend little or no time. Such assessments also neglect exposures outside the home, which may exceed those in the home. A positive Swedish study of adult leukemia and central nervous system tumors found increased risks in those exposed both residentially and occupationally but not in those with neither exposure or with only residential or only occupational exposure.[38] The Swedish study also was able to calculate residential magnetic field exposures over time because of detailed information available from Swedish power suppliers that is not available in the United States.[39]

EMF exposure has been suspected of influencing risk and progress of brain tumors, but no causal connection has been established. Methodological and conceptual issues of equivalency make it difficult (and perhaps impossible) to rule out EMF influence. Aside from the lack of information about total electromagnetic field exposure and its duration, a more basic limitation in assessing the relative risk is the failure, thus far, to show that electromagnetic fields induce mutations that in turn might promote tumorigenesis and brain tumors.[40] A recent brief communication even suggested that exposure to EMF might have a protective effect against brain tumors, because exposed subjects showed higher mean ages at diagnosis than did unexposed subjects.[40]

Cell Phones

Because of the intimate and often indeterminate exposures to radiation from cell phones—and their ubiquity—concerns have been voiced about their contribution to cancer risk. They produce non-ionizing radiation of the same type as microwave ovens, albeit in lower quantities. Studies of cell phone effects are inconclusive, especially because cell phone technology also continues to develop, so preliminary suggestions about risk or lack of it can only be tentative. The U.S. Food and Drug Administration study of cell phones concluded that no risk could be identified from cell phone use, but a Swedish study found a significant risk of acoustic neurinoma (odds ratio [OR] = 3.5) among analogue cellular telephone users. Elevated risk was also observed for tumors on the side of the brain used during phone calls.[41] A European study of cell phone use is ongoing and results will begin to be published over the next few years.

Diet

N-*Nitroso Compounds, Vitamins, Alcohol, Tobacco*

Several observations have led to studies of diet and brain tumors. First, in experimental animal studies, *N*-nitroso compounds have been clearly identified as neurocarcinogens.[42] Other investigators suggested several mechanisms involving DNA damage through which *N*-nitroso compounds might cause brain tumors.[43,44] These compounds can initiate neurocarcinogenesis through both prenatal and postnatal exposure, although in animals more tumors result from fetal than postnatal exposures.[43] Because there can be substantial lag between exposure and tumor formation, it is conceivable that early exposure could produce adult tumors. Animal studies show that a wide variety of primates and other mammals are susceptible to chemically induced brain tumors.

In humans, the ubiquity of *N*-nitroso compounds has complicated their epidemiologic evaluation as carcinogens. About half of all human exposures in the digestive system occurs when common amino compounds produced from fish, other foods, or drugs contact a nitrosating agent (such as nitrites from cured meats) in the right enzymatic milieu.[44] Equally common external exposures include agents such as tobacco smoke, cosmetics, auto interiors, and cured meats. To complicate matters further, some vegetables have nitrates that are convertible to nitrites but also contain a high level of vitamins that block formation of *N*-nitroso compounds. Comprehensive assessment of exposure to dietary and environmental compounds is thus difficult. Despite this, many studies have tried to examine major dietary sources of these chemicals and to assess the safeguards against formation of nitrosoureas presented by vitamins such as C and E, which are thought to inhibit *N*-nitroso formation.

No consensus has been achieved in human studies. Diet and vitamin supplementation investigations have provided only partial support for the hypothesis that dietary *N*-nitroso compounds increase the risk of both childhood and adult brain tumors.[43–46] However, increased consumption of foods cured with nitrosamines has been observed among brain tumor cases (or their mothers) compared with controls.[47,48] Additionally, lower rates after increased consumption of fruits and vegetables or vitamins that might block nitrosation or harmful effects of nitrosamines have been observed in some, but not all, studies.

Lee and associates[49] found that adults with glioma were more likely than controls to consume diets high in cured foods or nitrites and low in fruits and vegetables rich in vitamin C. The effect was more pronounced and only achieved statistical significance in men. Although the finding is compatible with the hypothesis that *N*-nitroso compounds might play a role in human neuro-oncogenesis, the observed patterns also support the hypothesis of oxidative burden and antioxidant protection. A recent meta-analysis found no association between cured meats and brain cancers and suggested uncontrolled confounding was the factor in previously found associations.[42]

After a comprehensive survey of nitrosamines in food and beverages, beer contamination with the nitrosamine derivative nitrosodimethylamine (NDMA) was considered a serious matter, especially in Germany. The source of the contamination was traced to oxidation of malt.[44] Beer in several countries was a major source of exposure to carcinogenic nitrosamines, because of the very large quantities consumed. NDMA was also present in whiskies of various kinds, but at lower concentrations than in beer, therefore posing a lower cancer risk, probably because of the smaller amounts consumed. In spite of much searching, particularly in connection with pediatric brain tumors, alcoholic products are not implicated in brain tumors.[50]

Because tobacco smoke contains polycyclic aromatic hydrocarbons and nitroso compounds, many studies have sought connections between brain tumors and cigarette smoke, but no significant effect has been established from smoke. Two studies report increased risk of adult glioma with smoking unfiltered, but not filtered cigarettes (reviewed in reference 51). However, a meta-analysis[52] found no clear association between a mother's smoking tobacco during pregnancy and risk for a brain tumor in the child. Another meta-analysis of 12 epidemiologic studies and 6566 subjects concurred but noted limits in study designs of size, lack of identification of tumor types, and lack of attention to dose–response relationships.[53]

The suspected role of secondary or passive smoking has more, but not universal, support. Several studies found slightly increased relative risks, generally smaller than 1.5; that is, the order of magnitude associated with some recognized hazards of exposure to passive smoking (1.2–1.3 for adult lung cancer and cardiovascular diseases).[52,54] Tumors most often found associated with maternal smoking in pregnancy or passive smoke exposures are childhood brain tumors and leukemia-lymphoma, with risks up to two or greater in selected studies.[55,56] A few studies have found elevated risk more closely associated with paternal smoking rather than maternal smoking; however, as one research team notes, study design issues limit definitive conclusions.[57] Even in the absence of definitive findings on the impact of the secondary smoke, the evidence from human studies coupled with demonstration of genotoxic effects on the fetus exposed to metabolites of tobacco smoke, and the demonstrable presence of adducts, should lead to strong recommendations aimed at eliminating tobacco smoke from the perinatal environment.[58–60]

A multifactorial managed care clinical cohort study of glioma with 21 years of follow-up produced ambiguous results, finding slightly elevated risk of glioma among cigarette smoking women but not men, an elevated risk—but no dose–response relationship—for marijuana smokers, an elevated risk for coffee drinkers who drink more than 7 cups per day, and no association between alcohol consumption and tumors.[61]

Industry and Occupation

Attempts to link specific chemicals to human brain tumors in occupationally or industrially exposed groups have proved inconclusive. In 1986, Thomas and Waxweiler[62] published a comprehensive review of occupational risk factors for brain tumors and established a group of suspect chemicals and occupations. Additional studies in the intervening 13 years have not established a conclusive link between any of these factors and brain tumor risk. Many occupational and industrial studies focused on individuals exposed to carcinogenic and/or neurotoxic substances such as organic solvents, lubricating oils, acrylonitrile, formaldehyde, polycyclic aromatic hydrocarbons, and phenols and phenolic compounds, which are part of workplace exposures and induce brain tumors in experimental animals. Animal neurocarcinogenicity studies, mainly in rats, have shown that susceptibility is significantly influenced by strain, gestational age, and fetal versus adult status, factors that cannot be accounted for in or generalized to human occupational cohort exposure studies.

Animal studies can also test exposures that cannot be tested in human studies. For instance, some compounds, such as polycyclic aromatic hydrocarbons, generally induce brain tumors only through direct placental implantation, not through inhalation or dermal exposure as in worker populations. Workers also are rarely exposed to a single chemical but rather are exposed to many chemicals that probably interact to affect risk. Followup studies of occupationally induced brain cancer usually consist of too few affected subjects to permit pinpointing the causal chemicals, physical agents, work processes, or interactions.

Consequently, no definitive link has been established between brain tumors and specific chemicals or strongly suspected carcinogens. For example, organochloride, alkyl urea, and copper sulfate compounds reliably induce cancer in laboratory animals. Yet studies of agricultural workers using these chemicals have about equally often produced negative and positive findings with regard to brain tumor risk. Additionally, studies do not show excess risk for workers involved in manufacturing these pesticides or fertilizers. In the meta-analysis of brain malignancies and farming by Khuder and associates,[63] the 33 studies yielded a relative risk of 1.3 (95% confidence interval [CI] 1.1–1.6). Although studies of workers in pesticide or fertilizer manufacturing have not shown an unusual risk of brain tumors, 4 of 5 studies of pesticide applicators have shown an increased risk of brain tumors with a nearly threefold median relative risk.[63] In an occupational study of women in the United States, insecticide or fungicide exposure was associated with a small but statistically significant increased risk for brain tumors (OR 1.3; 95% CI 1.1–1.5).[64] A recent study reported a positive association between wheat-producing acreage and brain tumor mortality in Minnesota, Montana, and the Dakotas, suggesting a possible role of chlorophenoxy herbicides employed in wheat agriculture.[65]

Because they involve production of many suspect carcinogens, synthetic rubber production and processing have received careful scrutiny by investigators who generally found a median increase in brain tumors of as much as 90%.[66] The by-products of synthetic rubber processing, such as coal tars, carbon tetrachloride, *N*-nitroso compounds, and carbon disulfide, might appear to account for this increased risk of brain tumors. However, several studies showed no increased risk or a decreased risk of brain tumors in this industry, and studies have usually failed to show a link with a single chemical.

The picture seems clearer with vinyl chloride. Vinyl chloride induces brain tumors in rats, and in 9 of 11 studies of polyvinyl chloride, production workers showed a median twofold increased relative risk of dying of brain tumors. Some argue, however, that the small number of brain tumor cases and statistical insignificance cast doubt on causality. A recent review of the association between vinyl chloride and cancers indicated that the role of vinyl chloride in the development of brain tumors is still inconclusive.[67] A large cohort study supports this notion, stating that mortality from brain cancer has attenuated, but the role of vinyl chloride is still unclear.[68] Another study also did not demonstrate a relationship of brain tumors to the extent of vinyl chloride exposure.[69] However, it has been difficult to determine whether the tumors were primary or metastatic in reviews of animal studies that indicated neurocarcinogenicity of vinyl chloride.[70] Future plans for trying to understand the role, if any, of vinyl chloride in causing human brain tumors need to reconsider the biologic plausibility of the association.

With formaldehyde, another long-suspected compound, the numbers are greater but the conclusions are just as elusive. Formaldehyde produces cancer in laboratory animals, and nearly 2 million workers in the United States are occupationally exposed to it. Thirty epidemiologic studies of segments of this large group were evaluated by Blair and associates.[71] The result was that the risk was elevated approximately 50% and existed for those exposed in professional roles such as embalmers, pathologists, and anatomists.[71] However, Blair and associates did not find a similar risk for industrial workers with formaldehyde exposure, and therefore rejected a causal role for formaldehyde in human brain tumorigenesis. Other unknown cofactors may obscure the true risk in industrially exposed workers and create a skewed estimate of risk in occupational groups. A National Cancer Institute (NCI) study by De Roos and associates[72] found no association between glioma and polymorphisms in genes involved in metabolism of suspect compounds contacted in occupational settings. A cluster of brain tumors were identified among long-term chemical researchers at the Amoco facility in Naperville, IL, which was closed in 1996. Six employees were diagnosed with glioma and another 13 were diagnosed with other benign intracranial tumors. After a thorough investigation, no specific cause was identified; however, two agents commonly used in experiments were ionizing radiation and *n*-hexane.[73]

Viruses

Certain viruses, like the suspect chemicals, induce brain tumors in animal studies, but, as in the chemical studies, small numbers and negative findings hinder epidemiologic evaluation.[74] Between 1955 and 1963, 92 million U.S. residents received Salk polio vaccines that may have been contaminated with simian virus 40 (SV40), varying among lots and manufacturers.[75,76] The vaccine was treated with formalin, but, being less susceptible to formalin inactivation than poliovirus, it may have contained infectious SV40. Early cohort studies of cancer in SV40-contaminated poliovirus vaccine recipients generally demonstrated no association between SV40 exposure and cancer mortality among children in the United States.[75–77] A cohort study specifically examined the risk of ependymoma, osteosarcoma, and mesothelioma among Americans who as children received SV40-contaminated poliovirus vaccine.[78,79] The study indicated such exposure was unassociated with significantly increased rates of brain cancers, osteosarcomas, mesotheliomas, or medulloblastomas.[78,79] As with other brain tumor investigations, studies of SV40 often resemble case reports, offering hints, clues, or coincidences that must be further tested. A study of SV40 concluded there is no apparent association between polio vaccination and brain tumors.[80]

Another subject of a few studies is the JC virus, commonly excreted in urine, particularly by immunosuppressed or immunodeficient patients or pregnant women. JC virus, a polyoma virus similar to SV40, induces brain tumors in experimental animals[81] and infects more than 70% of the human population worldwide.[82] Khalili and associates[83] recently detected JC virus in paraffin-embedded tissues from children with medulloblastoma. It was also found in a rare case of pleomorphic xanthoastrocytoma[84] and in oligodendrogliomas.[85] However, JC virus exists in cancer-free subjects and its connection, if any, to tumorigenesis is only a surmise.

Similarly, contradicting studies have found that more mothers of children with medulloblastoma than mothers of children without it were exposed to chicken pox, a herpes virus, during pregnancy. Wrensch and colleagues[86] found that adults in the San Francisco Bay area with glioma were significantly less likely than controls to report having had either chicken pox or shingles, an observation supported by serologic evidence.[87] The suggestion that viruses and infectious agents could be an explanation for a proportion of brain tumors, and therefore viral studies, still in their early stages, is intriguing and somewhat plausible.

Drugs and Medications

Few studies have examined the effects of medications and drugs on risk of adult brain tumors; the need for research is evident. An insignificant protective association was observed for headache, sleep, and pain medications. Ryan and colleagues[88] found that diuretics have insignificant protective association against meningioma but the opposite for adult glioma. They also found essentially no association between antihistamine use and adult glioma, but a 60% increased relative risk for meningioma. Insignificant findings resulted from three studies of childhood brain tumors and prenatal exposures to fertility drugs, oral contraceptives, sleeping pills, tranquilizers, pain medications, antihistamines, and diuretics, and prenatal exposure to barbiturates. Nonsteroidal antiinflammatory drugs may be protective against certain cancers, and their role in brain tumors should be investigated.

▶ GENETIC SUSCEPTIBILITY TO BRAIN TUMORS

The most generally accepted current model of carcinogenesis holds that cancers develop through accumulation of genetic alterations that allow the cells to grow out of control of normal regulatory mechanisms and/or escape destruction by the immune system. Some inherited alterations in crucial cell-cycle control genes, such as *p53*, as well as chemical, physical, and biologic agents that damage DNA, are therefore considered candidate carcinogens. Although rapid advances in molecular biology, genetics, and virology promise to help elucidate the molecular causes of brain tumors, continued epidemiologic work is necessary to clarify the relative roles of different mechanisms in the full scope of human brain tumors. Genetic and familial factors implicated in brain tumors are the subject of many studies and were previously reviewed.[89]

Familial Aggregation

Because heritable factors are the unique causes of only a minority of brain tumors, research is moving toward a consensus implicating gene–environment interaction. Findings of familial cancer aggregation may suggest a genetic etiology, but such aggregations may result from common familial exposure to environmental agents or an indirect heritability—heritable genetic mutability responding to exposures. This factor may explain why some case-control epidemiologic studies find significantly increased family histories of both brain tumors and of other cancers, whereas others find no increase for any cancer, with a relative risk ranging from 1 to 1.8 and from 1 to 9 for brain tumors.[90–92] Differences in study methodologies and locations, sample size, types of relatives included in the study, and how cancers were ascertained and validated might explain differences in the findings.

Apparently supporting genetic etiology were studies reporting a high frequency of siblings with brain tumors, but these were not validated by twin studies. A study of 250 childhood brain tumor patients showed by segregation analysis of the families of more than 600 adult glioma patients that familial aggregation, although small, supported multifactorial inheritance, and a polygenic environment-interactive model best explained the pattern of occurrence of brain tumors.[93] Segregation analyses of 2141 first-degree relatives of 297 glioma families did not find that an autosomal recessive model provided the best fit, but did not rule out a polyfactorial impact.[94] The study estimated that as few as 5% of all glioma cases were familial. Grossman and associates[95] showed brain tumors can occur in families without a known predisposing hereditary disease and that the pattern of occurrence in many families suggests environmental causes. Given the previously described complexities of environmental impact and multiplicity of possible heritable factors, more work is required to delineate how genetic susceptibility affects brain cancer risk.

Hereditary Syndromes

A few rare genes and chromosomal abnormalities can greatly increase the chances of developing brain tumors. Numerous case reports have associated central nervous system tumors with gross malformations, including medulloblastoma with gastrointestinal and genitourinary system abnormalities, ependymoma with multisystem abnormalities, astrocytoma with arteriovenous malformation of the overlying meninges, and glioblastoma multiforme with adjacent arteriovenous angiomatous malformation and pulmonary arteriovenous fistula. Central nervous system tumors may also be associated with Down syndrome, a disorder involving chromosome 21. Three epidemiologic studies found that brain tumor cases are two to five times more likely than controls to have a mentally retarded relative, although the result was statistically significant in only one study (reviewed in reference 89; see also Table 1-1). The heritability of brain tumors is also suggested by the many reports of these tumors in individuals with hereditary syndromes such as tuberous sclerosis, neurofibromatosis types 1 and 2, nevoid basal cell carcinoma syndrome, and syndromes involving adenomatous polyps (reviewed in reference 89).

Although there is convincing evidence that genetics plays a role in most cancers, including brain tumors, inherited predisposition to brain tumors probably account for only a very small percentage (5%–10%) of these tumors.[89] In a review of 16,564 cases of childhood cancers diagnosed from 1971 to 1983 and reported to the National Registry of Childhood Tumors in Great Britain, Narod and associates[96] estimated that the heritable fraction of childhood brain tumors was approximately 2%. In a population-based study of nearly 500 adults with glioma, only 4 individuals (less than 1%), all of whom were diagnosed in their thirties, reported having a known heritable syndrome (3 had neurofibromatosis and 1 had tuberous sclerosis).[89]

Another class of heritable conditions are the familial cancer syndromes (such as the Li-Fraumeni syndrome [LFS]), so-called because individuals in affected families have an increased risk of developing certain types of cancers. In

▶ TABLE 1-1. HEREDITARY SYNDROMES

Tumor	Syndrome	Chromosome
Medulloblastoma, GBM	Turcot syndrome	9q32-34, 11q
Glioma	Neurofibromatosis (NF-1)	17q12-22
Schwannoma, meningioma	Neurofibromatosis (NF-2)	22q
Medulloblastoma	Nevoid basal cell carcinoma syndrome	1q22 or 9q31
GBM, glioma	Turcot syndrome, familial polyposis, Gardner syndrome	5q

GBM = glioblastoma multiforme.

LFS, the cancers include brain tumors, sarcomas, breast cancer, and cancer of the adrenal gland. Individuals with LFS have inherited at least one copy of a defective gene, which can be passed from parent to child.[97]

In some families, LFS has been linked to a gene mutation in *p53* on chromosome 17p.[97] Li and associates[97] reported that *p53* mutation-positive patients were more likely to have a first-degree relative affected with cancer (58% vs. 42%) or a personal history of a previous cancer (17% vs. 8%). Further research needs to be done to determine the role of heredity, the frequency of *p53* mutations, and the interaction of *p53* mutations, whether spontaneous or germ line.

Metabolic Polymorphisms

Genetic traits involved in susceptibility refer to more common genetic alterations that influence oxidative metabolism, carcinogen detoxification, and DNA stability and repair. The role of genetic polymorphisms (alternative states of genes established in the population) in modulating susceptibility to carcinogenic exposures has been explored in some detail for tobacco-related neoplasms but much less so for other neoplasms, including gliomas. Because of rapid developments in genetic technology, an increasing number of potentially relevant polymorphisms are available for epidemiologic evaluation, including genes involved in carcinogen detoxification, oxidative metabolism, and DNA repair. The first study to report the role of metabolic polymorphisms in brain tumor risk found that the variants of cytochrome P450 2D6 (*CYP2D6*) and glutathione transferase (*GSTT1*) were significantly associated with increased risk of brain tumors.[98] Kelsey and associates[99] were unable to find an association of adult-onset glioma with either the *GSTT1* null genotype or homozygosity for the *CYP2D6* variant poor-metabolizer genotype. However, when they stratified the data by histologic subtype, there was a significant threefold increased risk for oligodendroglioma associated with the *GSTT1* null genotype. Trizna and associates[100] found no statistically significant associations between the null genotypes of glutathione transferase μ, *GSTT1*, and *CYP1A1* and the risk of adult gliomas. However, they observed an intriguing pattern with *N*-acetyltransferase acetylation status, with a nearly twofold increased risk for rapid acetylation and a 30% increased risk for intermediate acetylation. A study from the NCI reported that the *GSTP1* 105 Val/Val genotype was associated with a significantly increased glioma incidence (OR = 1.8), with the estimated effect following a trend of increasing magnitude by number of variant alleles (Ile/Ile: OR, 1.0; Ile/Val: OR, 1.3; Val/Val: OR, 2.1).[101] The *CYP2E1* RsaI variant was weakly associated with glioma (OR = 1.4) and acoustic neuroma (OR = 2.3), with some indication of stronger associations among younger subjects. Previously reported associations between the *GSTT1* null genotype and overall glioma incidence were not replicated, but an association with meningioma was found (OR = 1.5). It is unlikely that any single polymorphism will be sufficiently predictive of brain tumor risk. Therefore, a panel of relevant markers integrated with epidemiologic data should be assessed in a large number of study participants to clarify the role of genetic polymorphisms and brain tumor risk. Many more studies are forthcoming, and groups are beginning to combine their data to allow for larger samples that will provide stronger clues to the role of genetic polymorphisms and environmental determinants of brain tumors.

Mutagen Sensitivity

Cytogenetic assays of peripheral blood lymphocytes have been extensively used to determine response to genotoxic agents. The basis for these cytogenetic assays is that genetic damage reflects critical events in carcinogenesis in the affected tissue. To test this hypothesis Hsu and associates[102] developed a mutagen sensitivity assay in which the frequency of in vitro bleomycin-induced breaks in short-term lymphocyte cultures is used to measure genetic susceptibility. We[103] modified the assay by using gamma radiation to induce chromosome breaks because radiation is a risk factor for brain tumors and can produce double-stranded DNA breaks and mutations. It is believed that mutagen sensitivity indirectly assesses the effectiveness of one or more DNA repair mechanisms. The following observations support this hypothesis. First, the relationship between chromosome instability syndromes and cancer susceptibility is well-established.[104] Patients with these syndromes also have defective DNA repair systems.[105] Furthermore, patients with ataxia telangiectasia, who are extremely sensitive to the clastogenic effects of X-irradiation and bleomycin, differ from normal people in the speed with which aberrations induced by these agents are repaired, but not in the number of aberrations produced.[106]

Gamma radiation–induced mutagen sensitivity is one of the few significant independent risk factors for brain tumors.[103] DNA repair capability and predisposition to cancer are hallmarks of rare chromosome instability syndromes, and are related to differences in radiosensitivity. An in vitro study showed that individuals vary in lymphocyte radiosensitivity, which correlates with DNA repair capacity. Therefore, it is biologically plausible that increased sensitivity to gamma radiation results in increased risk of developing brain tumors because of individuals' inability to repair radiation damage. However, this finding needs to be tested in a larger study to determine the roles of mutagen sensitivity and radiation exposure in the risk of developing gliomas. The mutagen sensitivity assay has been shown to be an independent risk factor for other cancers, including head and neck and lung, suggesting the phenotype is constitutional.[107] The breaks are not affected by smoking status or dietary factors such as micronutrients.[108]

Chromosome Instability

A number of chromosomal loci have been reported to play a role in brain tumorigenesis because of the numerous gains and losses in those loci. For example, Bigner and associates[109] reported gain of chromosome 7 and loss of chromosome 10 in malignant gliomas and structural abnormalities involving chromosomes 1, 6p, 9p, and 19q; Bello and associates[110] reported involvement of chromosome 1 in oligodendrogliomas and meningiomas; and Magnani and associates[111] demonstrated involvement of chromosomes 1, 7, 10, and 19 in anaplastic gliomas and glioblastomas. Loss of heterozygosity for loci on chromosome 17p[112] and 11p15[113] have also been reported.

There are little data on chromosomal alterations in the peripheral blood lymphocytes of brain tumor patients. Information on such changes might shed light on premalignant changes that lead to tumor development. We demonstrated that compared with controls, glioma cases have less efficient DNA repair, measured by increased chromosome sensitivity to gamma radiation in stimulated peripheral blood lymphocytes. This inefficiency is an independent risk factor for glioma.[103] We[114] also investigated whether glioma patients have increased chromosomal instability that could account for their increased susceptibility to cancer. Using fluorescent in situ hybridization methods, background instability in these patients was measured at hyperbreakable regions in the genome. Reports indicate that the human heterochromatin regions are frequently involved in stable chromosome rearrangements.[115,116] Smith and Grosovsky[117] and Grosovsky and associates[118] reported that breakage affecting the centromeric and pericentromeric heterochromatin regions of human chromosomes can lead to mutations and chromosomal rearrangements and increase genomic instability. Our[114] study demonstrated that individuals with a significantly higher level of background chromosomal instability have a 15-fold increased risk of development of gliomas. A significantly higher level of hyperdiploidy was also detected. Chromosome instability leading to aneuploidy has been observed in many cancer types.[111] Although previous studies demonstrated the presence of chromosomal instability in brain tumor tissues,[119–123] our[114] study was the first to investigate the role of background chromosomal instability in the peripheral blood lymphocytes of patients with gliomas. This suggests that accumulated chromosomal damage in peripheral blood lymphocytes may be an important biomarker for identifying individuals at risk of developing gliomas.

▶ SUMMARY

In summary, the etiology of brain tumors remains largely unknown. Biologically intensive studies incorporating new molecular genetic techniques have the potential to increase our understanding of the etiology of gliomas. Use of more consistent applied histopathologic classification systems and greater understanding and use of molecular and genetic markers to classify tumors should help to create a more complete picture of the natural history and pathogenesis of brain tumors. We now know that primary brain tumors have many causes. Because not one cause thus far identified accounts for a very large proportion of cases, many possibilities remain that will enable us to discover important risk factors. Moreover, in the continuing search for explanations for this devastating disease, new concepts about neuro-oncogenesis might emerge, making the study of brain tumor epidemiology particularly exciting.

REFERENCES

1. Ries LAG, Eisner MP, Kosary CL, et al, eds. SEER cancer statistics review 1975–2001. Bethesda, MD: National Cancer Institute, 2004. Available at: http://seer.cancer.gov/csr/1975_2001/.
2. American Cancer Society. Cancer facts and figures–2004. American Cancer Society, 2005.
3. Kleihues P, Soylememzoglu F, Schauble B, et al. Histopathology, classification and grading of gliomas. Glia 1995;15:211–221.
4. Kleihues P, Cavenee WK, eds. Tumors of the central nervous system: pathology and genetics. Lyon, France: International Agency for Research on Cancer, 1997.
5. Hill JR, Kuriyama N, Kuriyama H, Israel MA. Molecular genetics of brain tumors. Arch Neurol 1999;56(4):439–441.
6. Ueki K, Ono Y, Henson JW, et al. CDKN2/p16 or RB alterations occur in the majority of glioblastomas and are inversely correlated. Cancer Res 1996;56:150–153.
7. Ichimura K, Schmidt EE, Miyakawa A, et al. Distinct patterns of deletion on 10p and 10q suggest involvement of multiple tumor suppressor genes in the development of astrocytic gliomas of different malignancy grades. Genes Chromosomes Cancer 1998;22:9–15.
8. Biernat W, Tohma Y, Yonekawa Y, et al. Alterations of cell cycle regulatory genes in primary (de novo) and secondary glioblastomas. Acta Neuropathol 1997;94:303–309.
9. Hunter SB, Abbot K, Varma VA, et al. Reliability of differential PCR for the detection of EGFR and MDM2 gene amplification in DNA extracted from FFPE glioma tissues. J Neuropathol Exp Neurol 1995;54:57–64.
10. Ritland SR, Ganju V, Jenkins RB. Region-specific loss of heterozygosity on chromosome 19 is related to the morphologic type of human glioma. Genes Chromosomes Cancer 1995;12:277–282.
11. Bondy M, Wiencke J, Wrensch M, et al. Genetics of primary brain tumors: a review. J Neurooncol 1994;18:69–81.

12. Hodges LC, Smith JL, Garrett A, Tate S. Prevalence of glioblastoma multiforme in subjects with prior therapeutic radiation. J Neurocsci Nurs 1992;24:79–83.
13. Socie G, Curtis RE, Deeg HJ, et al. New malignant diseases after allogeneic marrow transplantation for childhood acute leukemia. J Clin Oncol 2000;18:348–357.
14. Karlsson P, Holmberg E, Lundell M, et al. Intracranial tumors after exposure to ionizing radiation during infancy: a pooled analysis of two Swedish cohorts of 28,008 infants with skin hemangioma. Radiat Res 1998;150:357–364.
15. Wrensch M, Miike R, Lee M, Neuhaus J. Are prior head injuries or diagnostic x-rays associated with glioma in adults? The effects of control selection bias. Neuroepidemiology 2000;19:234–244.
16. Preston DL, Ron E, Yonehara S, et al. Tumors of the nervous system and pituitary gland associated with atomic bomb radiation exposure. J Natl Cancer Inst 2002; 94:1555–1563.
17. Thompson DE, Mabuchi K, Ron E, et al. Cancer incidence in atomic bomb survivors. Part II: solid tumors 1958–1987. Radiat Res 1994;137(2 Suppl):S17–S67.
18. Mabuchi K, Soda M, Ron E, et al. Cancer incidence in atomic bomb survivors. Part I: use of the tumor registries in Hiroshima and Nagasaki for incidence studies. Radiat Res 1994;137:S1–S16.
19. Longstreth WT, Phillips LE, Drangsholt M, et al. Dental x-rays and the risk of intracranial meningioma: a population-based case-control study. Cancer 2004;100:1026–1034.
20. Loomis DP, Wolf SH. Mortality of workers at a nuclear materials production plant at Oak Ridge, TN 1947–1990. Am J Ind Med 1996;29:131–141.
21. Alexander V, DiMarco JH. Reappraisal of brain tumor risk among U.S. nuclear workers: a 10-year review. Occup Med 2001;16:289–315.
22. Wrensch M, Bondy ML, Wiencke J, Yost M. Environmental risk factors for primary malignant brain tumors: a review. J Neurooncol 1993;17:47–64.
23. Gundestrup M, Storm HH. Radiation-induced acute myeloid leukaemia and other cancers in commercial jet cockpit crew: a population-based cohort study. Lancet 1999;354:2029–2031.
24. Irvine D, Davies DM. British Airways flight deck mortality study 1950–1992. Aviat Space Environ Med 1999;70:548–555.
24a. Wertheimer N, Leeper E. Electrical wiring configurations and childhood cancer. Am J Epidemiol 1979;109:273–284.
25. Minert R, Michaelis J. Meta-analysis of studies on the association between electromagnetic fields and childhood cancer. Radiat Environ Biophys 1996;35:11–18.
26. Kheifets LI, Afifi AA, Buffler PA, et al. Occupational electric and magnetic field exposure and brain cancer: a meta analysis. J Occup Environ Med 1995;37:1327–1341.
27. Savitz DA, Cai J, van Wijngaarden E, et al. Case-cohort analysis of brain cancer and leukemia in electric utility workers using a refined magnetic field job-exposure matrix. Am J Ind Med 2000;38:417–425.
28. Robinson CF, Petersen M, Palu S. Mortality patterns among electrical workers employed in the U.S. construction industry 1982–1987. Am J Ind Med 1999;36:630–637.
29. Minder CE, Pfluger DH. Leukemia, brain tumors, and exposure to extremely low frequency electromagnetic fields in Swiss railway employees. Am J Epidemiol 2001; 153:836–838.
30. Johansen C, Olsen JH. Risk of cancer among Danish electricity workers. A cohort study. Ugeskr Laeger 1999;161: 2079–2085.
31. Floderus B, Stenlund C, Persson T. Occupational magnetic field exposure and site-specific cancer incidence: a Swedish cohort study. Cancer Causes Control 1999;10:323–332.
32. Feychting M, Floderus B, Ahlbom A. Parental occupational exposure to magnetic fields and childhood cancer (Sweden). Cancer Causes Control 2000;11:151–156.
33. Sorahan T, Hamilton L, Gardiner K, et al. Maternal occupational exposure to electromagnetic fields before, during, and after pregnancy in relation to risks of childhood cancers: findings from the Oxford Survey of Childhood Cancers 1953–1981 deaths. Am J Ind Med 1999;35:348–357.
34. Kheifets LI, Sussman SS, Preston-Martin S. Childhood brain tumors and residential electromagnetic fields (EMF). Rev Environ Contam Toxicol 1999;159:111–129.
35. Wrensch M, Minn Y, Bondy ML. Epidemiology. In: Bernstein M, Berger M, eds. Neuro-oncology: the essentials. New York: Thieme, 1999:1–17.
36. Wrensch M, Yost M, Miike R, et al. Adult glioma in relation to residential power frequency electromagnetic field exposures in the San Francisco Bay Area. Epidemiology 1999;10:523–527.
37. EMF Science Review Symposium. Breakout group reports for epidemiological research findings. January 12–14, 1998, San Antonio, TX. Research Triangle, NC: National Institute of Environmental Health Sciences, National Institute of Health, 1998:121.
38. Floderus B, Tornqvist S, Stenlund C. Incidence of selected cancers in Swedish railway workers 1961–1979. Cancer Causes Control 1994;5:89–94.
39. Gurney JG, van Wijnagaarden E. Extremely low frequency electromagnetic fields (EMF) and brain cancer in adults and children: review and comment. Neurooncol 1999; 1:212–220.
40. Li CY, Lin RS, Sung FC. Elevated residential exposure to power frequency magnetic field associated with greater average age at diagnosis for patients with brain tumors. Bioelectromagnetics 2003;24:218–221.
41. Hardell L, Hallquist A, Mild KH, et al. Cellular and cordless telephones and the risk for brain tumours. Eur J Cancer Prev 2002;4:377–386.
42. Huncharek M, Kupelnick B, Wheeler L. Dietary cured meat and the risk of adult glioma: a meta-analysis of nine observational studies. J Environ Pathol Toxicol Oncol 2003;22:129–137.
43. Preston-Martin S. Epidemiological studies of perinatal carcinogenesis. In: Napalkov NP, Rice JM, Tomatis L, et al., eds. Perinatal and multigenerational carcinogenesis. Lyon, France: IARC, 1989:289–314.
44. Bondy M, Wiencke J, Wrensch M, et al. Genetics of primary brain tumors: a review. J Neurooncol 1994;18:69–81.
45. Wrensch M, Bondy ML, Wiencke J, et al. Environmental risk factors for primary malignant brain tumors: a review. J Neurooncol 1993;17:47–64.
46. Preston-Martin S, Mack WJ: Neoplasms of the nervous system. In: Schottenfeld D, Fraumeni JF, eds. Cancer

Epidemiology and Prevention, 2nd ed. New York: Oxford University Press, 1996:1231–1281.
47. Berleur MP, Cordier S. The role of chemical, physical, or viral exposures and health factors in neurocarcinogenesis: implications for epidemiologic studies of brain tumors. Cancer Causes Control 1995;6:240–256.
48. Preston-Martin S, Pogoda JM, Mueller BA, et al. Results from an international case-control study of childhood brain tumors: the role of prenatal vitamin supplementation. Environ Health Perspect 1998;106(Suppl 3):887–892.
49. Lee M, Wrensch M, Miike R. Dietary and tobacco risk factors for adult onset glioma in the San Francisco Bay Area. Cancer Causes Control 1997;8:13–24.
50. Mangino M, Scalan SR, O'Brien TJ. *N*-nitrosamines in beer. In: Scalan RA, Tannenbaum SR, eds. *N*-nitroso compounds. American Chemical Society Symposiuim Series, no. 174. 1981:229–245.
51. Norman MA, Holly EA, Preston-Martin S. Childhood brain tumors and exposure to tobacco smoke. Cancer Epidemiol Biomarkers Prev 1996;5:85–91.
52. Boffetta P, Tredaniel J, Greco A. Risk of childhood cancer and adult lung cancer after childhood exposure to passive smoke: a meta-analysis. Environ Health Perspect 2000;108:73–82.
53. Huncharek M, Kupelnick B, Klassen H. Maternal smoking during pregnancy and the risk of childhood brain tumors: a meta-analysis of 6566 subjects from twelve epidemiological studies. J Neurooncol 2002;57:51–57.
54. Scheidt S. Changing mortality from coronary heart disease among smokers and nonsmokers over a 20-year interval. Prev Med 1997;26:441–446.
55. Schwarz B, Schmeiser-Rieder A. Epidemiology of health problems caused by passive smoking. Wien Klin Wochenschr 1996;108:565–569.
56. Cordier S, Iglesias MJ, Le Goaster C, et al. Incidence and risk factors for childhood brain tumors in the Ile de France. Int J Cancer 1994;59:776–782.
57. Huncharek M, Kupelnick B, Klassen H. Paternal smoking during pregnancy and the risk of childhood brain tumors: results of a meta-analysis. In Vivo 2001;15:535–541.
58. Filippini G, Farinotti M, Lovicu G, et al. Mothers' active and passive smoking during pregnancy and risk of brain tumors in children. Int J Epidemiol 1994;57:769–774.
59. Magnani C, Pastore G, Luzzatto L, et al. Risk factors for soft tissue sarcomas in childhood cancer: a case-control study. Tumori 1989;75:396–400.
60. Sasco AJ, Vainio H. From in utero and childhood exposure to parental smoking to childhood cancer: a possible link and the need for action. Hum Exp Toxicol 1999;18:192–201.
61. Efird JT, Friedman GD, Sidney S, et al. The risk for malignant primary adult-onset glioma in a large, multiethnic, managed-care cohort: cigarette smoking and other lifestyle behaviors. J Neurooncol 2004;68:57–69.
62. Thomas TL, Waxweiler RJ. Brain tumors and occupational risk factors. Scand J Work Environ Health 1986;12:1–15.
63. Khuder SA, Mutgi AB, Schaub ES. Meta-analysis of brain cancer and farming. Am J Ind Med 1998;34:252–260.
64. Bohnen NL, Kurland LT. Brain tumor and exposure to pesticides in humans: a review of the epidemiologic data. J Neurol Sci 1995;132:110–121.
65. Schreinemachers DM. Cancer mortality in four northern wheat-producing states. Environ Health Perspect 2000; 108:873–881.
66. Straif K, Weiland SK, Bungers M, et al. Exposure to high concentrations of nitrosamines and cancer mortality among a cohort of rubber workers. Occup Environ Med 2000;57:180–187.
67. McLaughlin JK, Lipworth L. A critical review of the epidemiologic literature on health effects of occupational exposure to vinyl chloride. J Epidemiol Biostat 1999; 4:253–275.
68. Mundt KA, Dell LD, Austin RP, et al. Historical cohort study of 10,109 men in the North American vinyl chloride industry 1942–72: update of cancer mortality to 31 December 1995. Occup Environ Med 2000;57:774–781.
69. Simonato L, L'Abbé KA, Andersen A, et al. A collaborative study of cancer incidence and mortality among vinyl chloride workers. Scand J Work Environ Health 1991; 17:159–169.
70. Rice JM, Wilbourn JD. Tumors of the nervous system in carcinogenic hazard identification. Toxicol Pathol 2000; 28:202–214.
71. Blair A, Saracci R, Stewart PA, et al. Epidemiologic evidence on the relationship between formaldehyde exposure and cancer. Scand J Work Environ Health 1990;16:381–393.
72. De Roos AJ, Stewart PA, Linet MS, et al. Occupation and the risk of adult glioma in the United States. Cancer Causes Control 2003;14:139–150.
73. Buffler PA, Kelsh M, Chapman P, et al. Primary brain tumor mortality at a petroleum exploration and extraction research facility. J Occup Environ Med 2004;46:257–270.
74. Shah KV. SV40 infections in simians and humans. Dev Biol Stand 1998;94:9–12.
75. Fisher SG, Weber L, Carbone M. Cancer risk associated with simian virus 40 contaminated polio vaccine. Anticancer Res 1999;19:2173–2180.
76. Fraumeni JF Jr, Stark CR, Gold E, Lepow ML. Simian virus 40 in polio vaccine: follow-up of newborn recipients. Science 1970;167:59–60.
77. Heinonen OP, Shapiro S, Monson RR, et al. Immunization during pregnancy against poliomyelitis and influenza in relation to childhood malignancy. Int J Epidemiol 1973;2:229–235.
78. Mortimer EA Jr, Lepow ML, Gold E, et al. Long-term follow-up of persons inadvertently inoculated with SV40 as neonates. N Engl J Med 1981;305:1517–1518.
79. Geissler E. SV40 and human brain tumors. Prog Med Virol 1990;37:211–222.
80. Brenner AV, Linet MS, Selker RG, et al. Polio vaccination and risk of brain tumors in adults: no apparent association. Cancer Epidemiol Biomarkers Prev 2003;12:177–178.
81. Inskip PD, Linet MS, Heineman EF. Etiology of brain tumors in adults. Epidemiol Rev 1995;17:382–414.
82. Del Valle L, Gordon J, Assimakopoulou M, et al. Detection of JC virus DNA sequences and expression of the viral regulatory protein T-antigen in tumors of the central nervous system. Cancer Res 2001;61:4287–4293.
83. Khalili K, Krynska B, del Valle L, et al. Medulloblastomas and the human neurotropic polyomavirus JC virus. Lancet 1999;353:1152–1153.

84. Martin JD, King DM, Slauch JM, Frisque RJ. Differences in regulatory sequences of naturally occurring JC virus variants. J Virol 1985;53:306–311.
85. Rencic A, Gordon J, Otte J, et al. Detection of JC virus DNA sequence and expression of the viral oncoprotein, tumor antigen, in brain of immunocompetent patients with oligoastrocytoma. Proc Natl Acad Sci USA 1996;93:7352–7357.
86. Wrensch M, Weinberg A, Wiencke J, et al. Does prior infection with varicella zoster virus influence risk of adult glioma? Am J Epidemiol 1997;145:594–597.
87. Wrensch M, Weinberg A, Wiencke J, et al. Prevalence of antibodies to four herpesviruses among adults with glioma and controls. Am J Epidemiol 2001;154:161–165.
88. Ryan P, Lee MW, North JB, et al. Risk factors for tumors of the brain and meninges: results from the Adelaide adult brain tumor study. Int J Cancer 51:20–27, 1992.
89. Bondy M, Wiencke J, Wrensch M, et al. Genetics of primary brain tumors: a review. J Neurooncol 1994;18:69–81.
90. Wrensch M, Lee M, Miike R, et al. Family and personal medical history of cancer and nervous system conditions among adults with glioma and controls. Am J Epidemiol 1997;145:581–593.
91. Malmer B, Gronberg H, Bergenheim AT, et al. Familial aggregation of astrocytoma in northern Sweden: an epidemiological cohort study. Int J Cancer 1999;81:366–370.
92. Hemminki K, Li X, Vaittinen P, Dong C. Cancers in the first-degree relatives of children with brain tumours. Br J Cancer 2000;83:407–411.
93. de Andrade M, Barnholtz JS, Amos CI, et al. Segregation analysis of cancer in families of glioma patients. Genet Epidemiol 2001;20:258–270.
94. Malmer B, Iselius L, Holmberg E, et al. Genetic epidemiology of glioma. Br J Cancer 2001;84:429–434.
95. Grossman SA, Osman M, Hruban R, Piantadosi S. Central nervous system cancers in first-degree relatives and spouses. Cancer Invest 1999;17:299–308.
96. Narod SA, Stiller C, Lenoir GM. An estimate of the heritable fraction of childhood cancer. Br J Cancer 1991;63:993–999.
97. Li Y, Millikan RC, Carozza S, et al. p53 mutations in malignant gliomas. Cancer Epidemiol Biomarkers Prev 1998; 7:303–308.
98. Elexpuru-Camiruaga J, Buxton N, Kandula V, et al. Susceptibility to astrocytoma and meningioma: Influence of allelism at glutathione S-transferase (GSTT1 and GSTM1) and cytochrome P-450 (CYP2D6) loci. Cancer Res 1995;55:4237–4239.
99. Kelsey KT, Wrensch M, Zuo ZF, et al. A population-based case-control study of the CYP2D6 and GSTT1 polymorphisms and malignant brain tumors. Pharmacogenetics 1997;7:463–468.
100. Trizna Z, de Andrade M, Kryitsis AP, et al. Genetic polymorphisms in glutathione S-transferase μ and O N-acetyltransferase, and CYP1A1 and risk of gliomas. Cancer Epidemiol Biomarkers Prev 1998;7:553–555.
101. De Roos AJ, Rothman N, Inskip PD, et al. Genetic polymorphisms in GSTM1, -P1, -T1, and CYP2E1 and the risk of adult brain tumors. Cancer Epidemiol Biomarkers Prev 2003;12:14–22.
102. Hsu TC, Johnston DA, Cherry LM, et al. Sensitivity to genotoxic effect of bleomycin in humans: possible relationship to environmental carcinogenesis. Int J Cancer 1989;43:403–409.
103. Bondy ML, Kryitsis AP, Gu J, et al. Mutagen sensitivity and risk of gliomas: a case-control study. Cancer Res 1996; 56:1484–1486.
104. Busch D. Genetic susceptibility to radiation and chemotherapy injury: diagnosis and management. Int J Rad Oncol Biol Phys 1994;30:997–1002.
105. Wei Q, Spitz MR, Gu J, et al. DNA repair capacity correlates with mutagen sensitivity in lymphoblastoid cell lines. Cancer Epidemiol Biomarkers Prev 1996;5:199–204.
106. Hittelman WN, Sen P. Heterogeneity in chromosome damage and repair rates after bleomycin in ataxia telangiectasia cells. Cancer Res 1988;48:276–279.
107. Caporaso N. Genetics of smoking-related cancer and mutagen sensitivity. J Natl Cancer Inst 1999;91:1097.
108. Spitz MR, McPherson RS, Jiang H, et al. Correlates of mutagen sensitivity in patients with upper aerodigestive tract cancer. Cancer Epidemiol Biomarkers Prev 1997;6:687–692.
109. Bigner SH, Burger PC, Mahaley MS, et al. Specific chromosomal abnormalities in malignant gliomas. Cancer Res 1988;88:405–411.
110. Bello MJ, De Campos JM, Kusak ME, et al. Molecular analysis of chromosome 1 abnormalities in human gliomas reveals frequent loss of 1p in oligodendroglial tumors. Int J Cancer 1994;57:172–175.
111. Magnani I, Guerneri S, Pollo B, et al. Increasing complexity of the karyotype in 50 human gliomas: progressive evolution and de novo occurrence of cytogenetic alterations. Cancer Genet Cytogenet 1994;75:77–89.
112. Fults D, Tippets RH, Thomas GA, et al. Loss of heterozygosity for loci on chromosome 17p in human malignant astrocytoma. Cancer Res 1989;49:6572–6577.
113. Sonoda Y, Iizukam M, Yasuda J, et al. Loss of heterozygosity at 11p15 in malignant gliomas. Cancer Res 1995;55:2166–2168.
114. El-Zein R, Bondy ML, Wang LE, et al. Increased chromosomal instability in peripheral lymphocytes and risk of human gliomas. Carcinogenesis 1999;20:811–815.
115. Larizza L, Doneda L, Ginelli E, Fossati G. C-heterochromatin variation and transposition in tumor progression. In: Prodi G, Liotta LA, Lollini PL, et al, eds. Cancer metastasis: biological and biochemical mechanisms and clinical aspects. New York: Plenum Publishing, 1988:414–423.
116. Doneda L, Ginelli E, Agresti A, Larizza L. In situ hybridization analysis of interstitial C-heterochromatin in marker chromosomes of two human melanomas. Cancer Res 1989;49:433–438.
117. Smith LE, Grosovsky AJ. Genetic instability on chromosome 16 in a human B lymphoblastoid cell line. Somat Cell Mol Genet 1993;19:515–527.
118. Grosovsky AJ, Parks KK, Giver CR, Nelson SL. Clonal analysis of delayed karyotypic abnormalities and gene mutations in radiation-induced genetic instability. Mol Cell Biol 1996;16:6252–6262.
119. Lengauer C, Kinzler KW, Vogelstein B. Genetic instability in colorectal cancers. Nature 1997;386:623–627.
120. Arnoldus EPJ, Walters LBT, Voormolen JHC, et al. Interphase cytogenetics: a new tool for the study of genetic changes in brain tumors. J Neurosurg 1992;76:997–1003.

121. Mohapatra G, Kim DH, Feuerstein BG. Detection of multiple gains and losses of genetic material in ten glioma cell lines by comparative genomic hybridization. Genes Chromosomes Cancer 1995;13:86–93.
122. Wernicke C, Thiel G, Lozanova T, et al. Numerical aberrations of chromosomes 1, 2 and 7 in astrocytomas studied by interphase cytogenetics. Genes Chromosomes Cancer 1997;19:6–13.
123. Rosso SM, Van Dekken H, Krishnadath KK, et al. Detection of chromosomal changes by interphase cytogenetics in biopsies of recurrent astrocytomas and oligodendrogliomas. J Neuropathol Exp Neurol 1997;56:1125–1131.

CHAPTER 2

Translational Applications of Molecular Biology in Neuro-Oncology

JOON H. UHM

Patients diagnosed with glioblastoma know all too well the poor prognosis of their condition—that they perhaps have a 50/50 chance of being alive at the end of 1 year. Faced with this terrible condition, patients almost universally ask the same question: "How did this tumor grow in my head and do you have any new drugs to fight it?" A reply requires a working knowledge of molecular biology of gliomas, spanning the growth factor receptor at the cell surface that initiates the cascade of signaling events, to the gene induction events at the nucleus, and to the effector molecules that endow the tumor cell with its malignant characteristics. This chapter does not discuss each chemotherapy drug for all of the tumor types that affect the nervous system. Rather, it reviews both standard and novel chemotherapeutic agents in the context of recent advances in our understanding of the molecular genetics and signal transduction pathways that underlie the growth regulation of the malignant gliomas. Indeed, there has been intensive research into signal transduction pathways and effector molecules (i.e., molecules that mediate the malignant behavior of tumors, such as invasiveness, motility, and angiogenesis) in brain tumors. The importance of translating this body of research to the clinical arena is illustrated by the unfortunate fact that high-grade gliomas are synonymous with chemoresistance and, hence, the field of neuro-oncology, and our patients are in need of better therapeutics. Given the movement in all fields of oncology to identify and selectively target biochemical pathway components, the growth-regulatory pathways underlying high-grade gliomas (Fig. 2-1) provide an ideal template to illustrate both the standard and the emerging therapies in the context of the discoveries made in molecular biology.

▶ GROWTH-REGULATORY PATHWAYS IN TUMOR CELLS

Essentially all tumor types share the following sequential steps that collectively define the malignant phenotype (refer to Fig. 2-1) and therefore share the following common targets for therapeutics:

1. *Signal transduction*. This is a mechanism of amplifying and translating extracellular signals into ones that are understood at the level of the

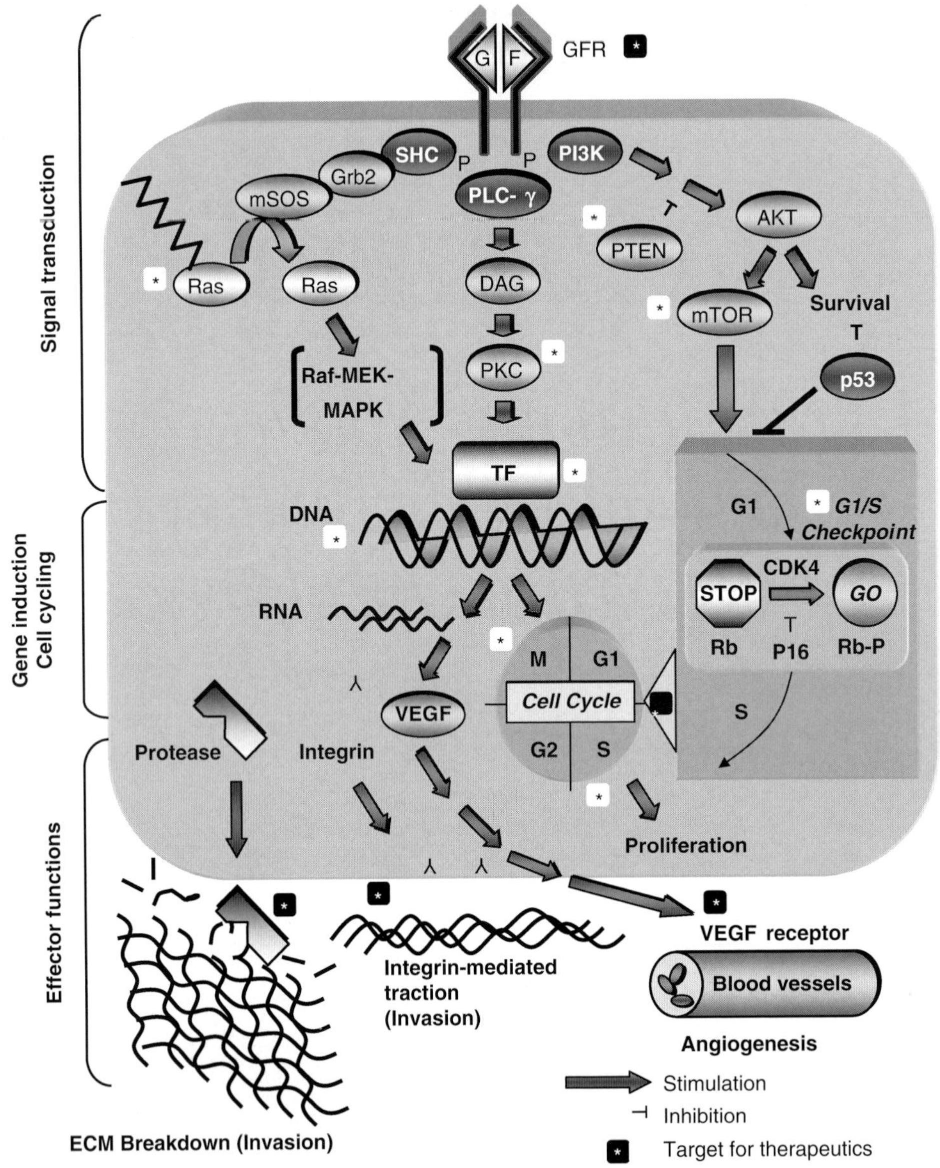

Figure 2-1. Signal transduction and effector molecules as therapeutic targets in glioma. Transduction of extracellular signals into the cell begins at the cell surface, leading to gene induction at the level of the DNA and, ultimately, in the synthesis of effector molecules that mediate the phenotypic changes (invasiveness, angiogenesis) that typify malignant tumors. The cascade occurs in the following sequence:

1. The interaction between the growth factor receptor (GFR) and its growth factor (GF) ligand leads to the phosphorylation (P) of specific tyrosine residues of the intracellular domain of the receptor.
2. The phosphorylated tyrosines bind specific signaling proteins, recruiting them to the inner leaflet of the plasma membrane (i.e., SHC, phospholipase C-γ [PLC-γ], phosphoinositide 3-kinase [PI3K]).
3. In turn, these adaptor proteins lead to activation of downstream signaling proteins: (a) SHC recruits Grb2 and mSOS, which, in turn, activates Ras; (b) PLC-γ generates diacylglycerol (DAG), which activates protein kinase C (PKC); (c) PI3K activates AKT downstream, which leads to enhanced cell survival and activation of mammalian target of rapamycin (mTOR).
4. These pathways converge upon the DNA, stimulating transcription factors (TFs) that lead to gene induction. As well, these pathways lead to events that "open" the checkpoint that regulates cell-cycle progression from G1 to the S (DNA synthesis) phase; this is the G1/S checkpoint. The retinoblastoma protein (Rb) in its native form blocks (*STOP* in inset) the G1/S checkpoint, but on phosphorylation by CDK4, Rb is inactivated, thereby permitting passage through to S phase (*GO* in inset).
5. The genes induced by the transcription factors encode proteins such as proteases, integrins, and soluble proteins such as vascular endothelial growth factor (VEGF). These proteins constitute the "effector" molecules that lead to the manifestation of the malignant phenotype, including invasiveness (proteases degrade proteins and cells that stand in the way of the advancing tumor), motility (integrins act as traction molecules to facilitate motility), and angiogenesis (VEGF acts in a paracrine fashion to stimulate endothelial proliferation).

Each intermediary in these complex pathways represent potential targets for therapeutic intervention (*), which are discussed further in the text.

nucleus to induce gene expression. The interaction between growth factors and their receptors at the cell surface leads to the intracellular recruitment and activation of second messenger components (i.e., Ras, protein kinase C [PKC]) that, in turn, provide a biochemical conduit linking components near the plasma membrane to the nucleus. At the nucleus, the transduced signals stimulate cell proliferation (cell cycling) and induce genes whose products endow the tumor cell with malignant characteristics, such as invasiveness. Drugs that target each of these signaling components represent the majority of the novel therapeutics emerging in brain tumor treatment.

2. *DNA replication and cell division.* Cell proliferation ensues in response to extracellular growth signals transduced to the nucleus. The act of cell division (mitosis) represents the final phase (termed *M phase* for mitosis) of a four-phase loop termed the *cell cycle*, which consists of the sequential passage through G1, S, G2, and M phases (see Fig. 2-1). One characteristic that distinguishes tumor cells from their nontransformed counterparts is that tumor cells possess the ability to repeat their cell-cycle loop in an uncontrolled fashion (and are therefore able to proliferate), while the entry of normal cells into the cell cycle is more tightly controlled. The point in the cell cycle at which this control is exerted is at the transition between G1 and S (S for synthesis of DNA) and is hence referred to as the *G1/S checkpoint* (see Fig. 2-1). Gliomas and other tumor cells are able to circumvent this checkpoint as they often possess a mutation in one or more of the protein components (p53, p16, Cdk4, Rb)[1] that collectively guard this checkpoint. Consequently, an area of research for therapeutics is to restore the function of this checkpoint by "fixing" the genetic defect in the checkpoint components (e.g., by gene transfer of the functionally normal *p16* gene into p16-deleted glioma tumors). For cells that still break through the G1/S checkpoint, pharmacologic agents that act distally at S phase (DNA synthesis inhibitors such as nucleoside analogues and topoisomerase poisons) or M phase (mitotic inhibitors such as vincristine that disrupt microtubules) are used. In addition to targeting DNA with cell-cycle–specific agents, DNA can also be targeted with agents whose mechanism of action is not dependent on the cell cycle. These agents constitute the classic "conventional" agents, the DNA alkylating drugs such as platinum and the nitrosoureas (e.g., 1,3-bis(2-chloroethyl)-1-nitrosourea [BCNU]).
3. *Effector molecules.* In addition to stimulating cell proliferation by way of enhancing cell-cycle progression, signal transduction from the membrane to the nucleus also leads to the expression of genes whose protein products endow the tumor cell with malignant characteristics, such as invasiveness and angiogenesis. Examples of such "effector molecules" consist of the proteases (i.e., matrix-degrading metalloproteinases [MMPs]) that mediate tumor invasion and soluble paracrine factors such as vascular endothelial growth factor (VEGF), which stimulates angiogenesis by inducing proliferation of endothelial cells. Given that invasiveness and angiogenesis are features shared by essentially all malignancies, therapeutics that target effector molecules are an exciting new focus in clinical trials.

Because every component along this cascade of events represents a potential target for antitumor therapeutics, Fig. 2-1 serves as a useful template to discuss these agents.

▶ COMPONENTS OF THE SIGNAL TRANSDUCTION PATHWAYS AS CHEMOTHERAPEUTIC TARGETS

Table 2-1 summarizes the potential targets and the drug or approach that has been proposed.

Cell Surface Growth Factor Receptors as Chemotherapeutic Targets

The initiation of signal transduction occurs at the plasma membrane upon the binding of a growth factor to its cognate receptor. Of the various types of growth factor receptors, the receptor protein tyrosine kinase (RPTK) receptor class is clearly linked to the pathogenesis of gliomas. These receptors are so-named because their activation (on binding their growth factor ligand) is associated with phosphorylation of specific tyrosine residues on the intracellular domain of the receptor.[2] Of the 14 subclasses of RPTKs identified to date, the 2 that have been implicated in the pathogenesis of gliomas include the epidermal growth factor receptor (EGFR) and the platelet-derived growth factor receptor (PDGFR).

Targeting Epidermal Growth Factor Receptor

Genetic alterations in the *EGFR* gene (*c-erbB* oncogene) that increase the activity of this RPTK represent one of the most frequently observed genetic aberrations in high-grade gliomas, occurring in approximately 40% to 50% of glioblastomas. Although point mutations have been observed, they are rare and the great majority of EGFR aberrations occur by the following two mechanisms[3]:

▶ TABLE 2-1. SIGNAL TRANSDUCTION COMPONENTS AS POTENTIAL THERAPEUTIC TARGETS

Signaling Component	Target	Mechanism Underlying Aberrant Expression	Drug/Approach
Growth factor receptor (receptor protein tyrosine kinase [RPTK])	EGFR	Amplification Truncated mutants	ZD1839 OSI-774 Neutralizing antibodies
	PDGFR	Amplification Increased activity	SU101
Intracellular signal transduction components	Ras	Increased activity secondary to activation by upstream RPTKs	Farnesyltransferase inhibitors (FTIs)
	PKC	Increased activity secondary to activation by upstream RPTKs	Tamoxifen (lipid)* UCN-01 (catalytic)* Hypericin (regulatory)* ISIS-3521 (PKC-α–selective antisense)
	PTEN	Deletion	Possible candidate for gene therapy
	mTOR	Increased activity secondary to (a) activation by upstream RPTKs and (b) PTEN deletion	CCI-779 (rapamycin analogue)

*Parentheses refer to PKC domain targeted by drug; e.g., hypericin binds to regulatory domain of PKC.

(a) increased copy number of the wild-type gene via gene amplification, and (b) gene rearrangements that delete regulatory domains of the protein, thereby giving rise to truncated EGFR proteins with increased biologic activity (Fig. 2-2 and Table 2-2). The most commonly observed truncation mutation is the deletion of the 5′ sequences giving rise to an EGFR molecule that lacks the N-terminal extracellular ligand-binding domain, rendering this mutant EGFR ligand-independent and hence constitutively activated. Because EGFR amplification/mutations increase glioma cell proliferation,[4] invasiveness,[5] and angiogenesis,[6] as well as chemoresistance,[7] inhibition of EGFR may have a widespread antitumor effect, with the potential to inhibit tumor growth at multiple levels.

Neutralizing Antibodies to EGFR

Given that EGFR is a cell surface protein, function-neutralizing antibodies have been developed for evaluation in a variety of EGFR-expressing tumors, including gliomas. Clinical testing has been performed with EGFR-specific

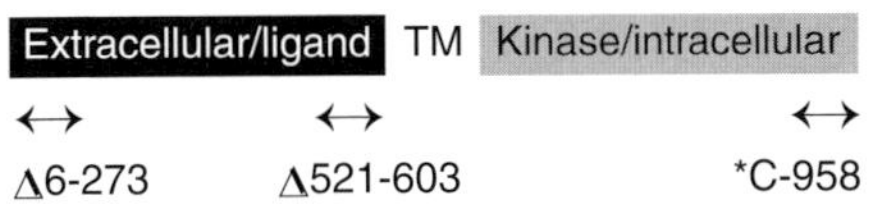

Figure 2-2. Structural and functional domains of EGFR and comparison with mutants identified in glioblastomas. This schematic of EGFR protein illustrates the three primary functional domains of this receptor protein tyrosine kinase: (a) the extracellular ligand (EGF) binding; (b) transmembrane (TM); and (c) the intracellular kinase domain. In addition to amplification of the wild-type gene, which increases EGFR activity via a gene dosage effect, various intragene deletion mutations (illustrated by *arrows* spanning the deleted codons) also augment the tyrosine kinase activity of EGFR. The functional consequences of these deletions are detailed in Table 2-2. *ATP-binding domain mutations in this domain are associated with sensitization of EGFR to EGFR-targeted therapy in lung carcinomas; thus far, this mutation has not been detected in gliomas (see Table 2-2 and chapter text).

▶ TABLE 2-2. MUTATIONS IN 48 GBMS WITH EGFR AMPLIFICATION

Mutation	
5′ Deletion (vIII mutant) (codons 6–273 deleted) Deletes ligand-binding domain Mutant is EGFR-independent	32 (67%)
3′ Deletion (C-958 mutant) Partial deletion of intracellular domain distal to tyr kinase domain	7 (15%)
Deletion of codons 521–603	7 (15%)
Other mutations (missense, insertions, etc.)	(3%–4%)
Multiple mutations in a given tumor	16 (33%)

EGFR = epidermal growth factor receptor; GBMS = glioblastoma multiformes.
Source: Reprinted with permission from Frederick L, Wang XY, Eley G, James CD. Diversity and frequency of epidermal growth factor receptor mutations in human glioblastomas. Cancer Res 2000; 60:1383–1387.

antibodies in patients with recurrent gliomas, demonstrating that this approach is feasible.[8]

Pharmacologic Inhibitors of EGFR

While the early generation tyrosine kinase inhibitors were disadvantaged by their relative lack of specificity for a given receptor type,[9–11] more recently developed inhibitors demonstrate superior specificity. The great majority of these agents act as competitive antagonists of the adenosine triphosphate (ATP)-binding intracellular domain of EGFR. Of these agents, ZD1839 is one that has generated considerable excitement with respect to evaluation in patients with EGFR-expressing tumors of central and peripheral histologies. Advantages boasted by this agent include (a) oral bioavailability; (b) selectivity for EGFR (concentration that inhibits 50% [IC_{50}] in micromolar range, with 100-fold less activity against other related Erb2 kinases and virtually no activity against other RPTKs); (c) lack of significant nausea/vomiting and bone marrow toxicity to patients in phase I studies. Phase II evaluation of ZD1839 (monotherapy) in newly diagnosed glioblastoma patients demonstrated that overall survival of ZD1839-treated patients was no better than historical controls and outcome did not appear to be influenced by EGFR status (amplification, mutation type). Despite these "negative" data, an encouraging observation was that patients who experienced adverse effects attributable to ZD1839 (loose stool/diarrhea) did have longer overall survival, underscoring the importance of adequate dosing for EGFR-targeted therapeutics.[12] A similar correlation between systemic adverse effects of ZD1839 and improved survival has also been reported in a study of recurrent glioblastoma patients.[13] Building on this experience, ZD1839 as well as other EGFR inhibitors, such as OSI-774, are currently in clinical studies in which these drugs are being evaluated in combinations with radiation as well as with other chemotherapeutic agents.

A specific mutation in the ATP-binding domain of EGFR sensitizes lung cancers that harbor that EGFR variant to ZD1839[14,15] (see Fig. 2-2 and Table 2-2 for further details), generating considerable excitement in the EGFR field for the potential of molecularly identifying those patient subgroups who may be most amenable to treatment with EGFR-directed small molecules such as ZD1839. The issue is less clear in gliomas, as reverse transcriptase polymerase chain reaction (RT-PCR) sequencing of the EGFR gene in 48 glioblastoma tumor samples did not detect this ATP-binding mutation in any of the 48 patient specimens.[3] Hence, if this mutation does occurs in glioblastoma multiforme (GBM) tumors, it would likely be a relatively rare occurrence. Nonetheless, for ongoing studies evaluating ZD1839 and similar drugs, EGFR will need to be sequenced to determine the presence of not only this mutation, but also any other point mutations that may be of prognostic/biologic importance.

Platelet-Derived Growth Factor Receptor Inhibitors

Platelet-derived growth factor receptor (PDGFR) is expressed as either PDGFR-α (chromosome 4) or PDGFR-β (chromosome 5). Ligands for PDGFR are also diverse, consisting of homo- or heterodimers of PDGF-A (chromosome 7) and PDGF-B (chromosome 22), thus giving rise to PDGF-AA, PDGF-AB, or PDGF-BB combinations. Of these various ligands, PDGF-BB is biologically the most potent, as it is capable of binding to either the α or β form of PDGFR.

PDGFR overexpression is a relatively common observation in gliomas, being present in approximately 25% of human astrocytomas.[16] However, unlike EGFR, the PDGFR gene is not frequently amplified or rearranged, with amplification being found in less than 10% of tumors in the case of the PDGFR-α gene, and in 0% of the PDGFR-β gene.[16] In addition to increased PDGFR, human gliomas also express high amounts of the ligand,[17] thus creating the setting for a paracrine (i.e., PDGF secreted by one glioma cell activating PDGFR on another glioma cell) or an autocrine (i.e., PDGF secreted by a glioma cell binds to and activates a receptor on the same cell) loop of growth stimulation. SU101, a parenteral agent with encouraging phase I/II results, is a PDGFR antagonist undergoing clinical evaluation in brain tumor patients. Thus far, SU101 has demonstrated encouraging results in gliomas, with evidence of tumor stabilization as well as, in a few cases, tumor shrinkage in phase I studies with recurrent glioma patients.[18] Future studies will likely combine this biologic agent with conventional brain tumor chemotherapy.

Intracellular Second Messenger Components

Conversion of the extracellular event of receptor-ligand interaction into an intracellular signal involves several key *adapter proteins* that are recruited to the vicinity of the receptor at the plasma membrane, as illustrated by the steps involved in the activation of Ras by EGFR (see Fig. 2-1): (a) On binding growth factor, the receptor (i.e., EGFR) dimerizes, with one member of the dimer phosphorylating specific tyrosine residues on the intracellular domain of its partner and vice versa. (b) As a result of the phosphorylation, these tyrosine residues are able to avidly bind the SHC adapter protein, which in turn binds Grb2 and mSOS. (c) This places mSOS at the plasma membrane, bringing it in close physical proximity to Ras, thereby permitting mSOS to activate Ras. (d) With the activation of Ras, signal transduction to the nucleus via sequential intermediaries (i.e., mitogen-activated protein kinase [MAPK]) ensues.

Targeting Ras with Farnesyltransferase Inhibitors

Ras is a signal transduction intermediary that becomes activated upon binding guanosine triphosphate (GTP). While oncogenic mutations in Ras (typically point mutations that give rise to a constitutively activated Ras) are found in approximately 25% of human cancers as a whole, Ras mutations in glioblastomas have not been identified; rather, the Ras overactivity frequently observed in glioblastomas is the consequence of mutant/aberrant upstream RPTKs that funnel their increased activity through Ras.[19]

The rationale for targeting Ras in gliomas is based on the following key observations: (a) The Ras mitogenic pathway (Ras-Raf-MEK-MAPK; see Fig. 2-1) lies downstream of many RPTKs, including ones that are frequently overactive in high-grade gliomas, such as EGFR and PDGFR (see "Cell Surface Growth Factor Receptors as Chemotherapeutic Targets" above). (b) Increased Ras activity is consistently observed in high-grade gliomas and is correlated with the rapid proliferation of these tumors.[19,20] (c) Inhibition of Ras leads to a dramatic reduction in glioma growth.[21]

To become activated, the Ras oncoprotein must be recruited to the plasma membrane where its activator (mSOS) resides (Fig. 2-1). As the anchoring of Ras to the plasma membrane requires "farnesylation," an enzymatic process by which a lipid moiety is covalently added to Ras, the development of farnesyltransferase inhibitors (FTIs) to target Ras-driven tumors gave rise to a novel class of antineoplastics.[22] Indeed, the antitumor effect of FTIs has been demonstrated in a wide variety of tumors,[22] including gliomas,[21,23] and has thus led to the proposal of clinical studies. However, many other cellular proteins other than Ras (approximately 1 in 200) also undergo farnesylation (e.g., nuclear lamins A and B, skeletal muscle phosphorylase kinase, three retinal proteins, as well as other members of the Ras superfamily).[24] While the potential for such a widespread effect on non-Ras proteins has raised serious concerns of adverse effects, these fears have not materialized in preclinical animal studies in which FTIs demonstrated dramatic antitumor effect without concomitant deleterious side effects. Interestingly, the ability of FTIs to inhibit farnesylation of proteins other than Ras has proven to be a potential benefit by having identified non-Ras targets such as Rho (involved in tumor motility/invasion) whose inhibition by FTIs is also associated with tumor growth inhibition. Evaluation of FTIs in brain tumor patients have recently commenced. As illustrated in Fig. 2-1, Ras represents both a point of convergence (i.e., *upstream* of Ras, many RPTKs funnel their signal transduction through Ras) as well as a point of *divergence* (i.e., *downstream* of Ras activation, multiple phenotypes/effector functions are stimulated, including proliferation, enhanced cell survival, and angiogenesis [Ras activation leads to expression of the potent angiogenic agent, VEGF]).[21] This central position of Ras in the pathways that determine the malignant phenotype of gliomas supports the premise that Ras represents not only a logical, but also a nearly ideal target in the treatment of patients afflicted with malignant gliomas.

Protein Kinase C Inhibitors

PKC represents a large family of phospholipid-dependent serine-threonine kinases, of which 12 isoforms have been identified to date.[25] The importance of this enzyme family in carcinogenesis was realized with the discovery that phorbol esters, which represent highly potent tumor promoters, were activating ligands for PKC. Like Ras, PKC also lies downstream of RPTKs such as EGFR and PDGFR and therefore transduces the extracellular growth factor signals to the nucleus (see Fig. 2-1). On binding its ligand (growth factor), specific intracellular tyrosine residues of the growth factor receptor become phosphorylated. These phosphorylated tyrosines bind phospholipase C-γ (PLC-γ), which, in turn, generates diacylglycerol (DAG), the endogenous activating ligand for PKC (phorbol esters, which induce tumors by way of PKC activation, represent a long-acting potent analogue of DAG).

Increased PKC activity in vitro is associated with the rapid growth rate of glioblastomas.[26–31] Similar to the situation with Ras, PKC overactivity in glioblastomas is not the result of mutations in the PKC gene but rather is a consequence of upstream RPTKs (that do bear function-enhancing mutations) signaling through PKC. Expectedly, PKC antagonists (see Table 2-1) inhibit glioma proliferation in vitro. PKC activity also is important in glioma invasiveness by way of increased production proteases (matrix-degrading metalloproteinases).[32] However, despite extensive encouraging in vitro data supporting PKC as a target for therapeutics, the experience in the clinical setting is less impressive.

Pending the evaluation of other agents, tamoxifen remains the PKC antagonist that is used most widely, largely because of its low toxicity profile. Currently, it is typically used for salvage therapy in patients with tumor recurrence.

▶ DRUGS THAT DIRECTLY DAMAGE DNA OR IMPAIR DNA REPLICATION

The majority of "standard chemotherapy" drugs act at this level, either by cell-cycle–independent mechanisms (covalent addition of adducts to the DNA chains, by alkylation of adduct formation), or by cell-cycle–dependent mechanisms (inhibition of DNA replication [S (synthesis) phase] or mitosis [M phase]). Given that DNA damage will hinder not only tumor but also all rapidly dividing cells, bone marrow suppression constitutes the most frequently encountered adverse effect.

Alkylating Agents

Drugs of this category that are commonly used in the treatment of gliomas include the nitrosoureas, procarbazine, platinum derivatives, and temozolomide (Table 2-3). Of these, all but platinum demonstrate significant penetration through the blood–brain barrier. Covalent modification of DNA strands by this class of drugs does not require that the cell be actively in cycle (i.e., passed through the G1/S checkpoint; see Fig. 2-1), which is therapeutically important, given that in a given glioma mass, only a minority of cells at any given time are cycling and therefore would predispose to relative resistance to pure cell-cycle–specific agents such as purine/pyrimidine analogues. In the setting of intermediate-grade gliomas, alkylating agents comprised of the nitrosoureas extend patient survival and thus represent the "standard of care" for these patients (Table 2-3). Previously, the three-drug combination of PCV—procarbazine, 1,3-*cis* (2-chloroethyl)-1-nitrosourea (CCNU) (orally bioavailable nitrosourea), and vincristine—had been shown to be superior to nitrosourea monotherapy (with the parenteral BCNU nitrosourea).[33] However, a more recent retrospective review of the data showed no difference between the two regimens.[34]

Recently, temozolomide, which is an orally bioavailable alkylating agent, has shown encouraging results in the setting of recurrent gliomas.[35] Furthermore, an important study published as this book was in press demonstrated improved survival in patients with newly diagnosed glioblastoma treated with temozolomide during and following radiotherapy (see Chap. 13).[35a] Compared to another orally administered alkylating agent procarbazine, temozolomide also had an added benefit of less toxicity (i.e., marrow suppression, nausea/vomiting) and faired better in quality-of-life scales. Temozolomide has been evaluated in numerous studies in which it is used in combination with either other cytotoxic (i.e., BCNU nitrosourea) or cytostatic agents (i.e., protease inhibitors, retinoids, interferon-α) in hopes of further augmenting the effectiveness of this drug.

Novel approaches directed toward enhancing drug delivery have been used as adjuncts in the setting of malignant gliomas. These approaches include drugs that enhance the permeability of the blood–brain barrier (e.g., RMP-7), interstitial delivery (direct implantation of a biodegradable polymer impregnated with BCNU chemotherapy into the surgical cavity; e.g., carmustine [Gliadel]), and convection methods (continuous infusion under pressure into brain parenchyma to enhance diffusion of drug into tissue). These are discussed in more detail in subsequent sections.

One of the most important discoveries in the last decade has been the identification of genetic "markers" that predict chemoresponsiveness among a subset of intermediate-grade glioma patients—those afflicted with tumors of oligodendroglial lineage. In these patients, deletions in the short arm of chromosome 1 (1p) alone

▶ **TABLE 2-3.** ALKYLATING AGENTS COMMONLY USED IN THE TREATMENT OF MALIGNANT GLIOMAS

Drugs	Dose	Route of Administration	Combinatorial Regimen
Nitrosoureas (BCNU, CCNU)	BCNU 200–240 mg/m^2 q 6–8 wk	IV	BCNU/6-TG
	BCNU wafers placed into surgical cavity	Implantation into surgical cavity	None
	CCNU 100–130 mg/m^2 q 6–8 wk	PO	PCV (procarbazine, CCNU, vincristine)
Procarbazine	50–150 mg/m^2 qd × 2 wk	PO	PCV (procarbazine, CCNU, vincristine)
Platinum derivatives (cisplatin, carboplatin)	Cisplatin 40–120 mg/m^2 q 6–8 wk	IV	Platinum derivative in combination with etoposide and nitrosourea
	Carboplatin 300–450 mg/m^2 q 6–8 wk	IV	
Temozolomide	150–200 mg/m^2 qd × 5 d each month	PO	In combination with other cytotoxic agents, biologic agents (i.e., interferon), protease inhibitors (i.e., marimastat)

or in combination with the long arm of chromosome 19 (19q) are highly (>90%) predictive of exquisite sensitivity to standard alkylating chemotherapeutic drugs such as the nitrosoureas and temozolomide.[36–38] Presumably, a gene at 1p or 19q encodes a product that renders the cell chemoresistant, and hence its deletion leads to the observed chemosensitivity. Current research is focused on the identification of these putative genes.

Unfortunately, despite its success in intermediate-grade oligodendrogliomas, alkylators—either in monotherapy or in combinatorial regimens—have shown little benefit in patients with glioblastoma. In regard to potential mechanism(s) of resistance to nitrosoureas, there has been considerable research focused on O^6-methyl-guanine-methyltransferase (MGMT). The cytotoxic effect of alkylators such as BCNU is dependent on alkylation of guanine residue at its O^6 position; MGMT repairs this DNA damage by removing the alkyl adduct. Both preclinical and clinical studies demonstrate a correlation between MGMT levels and resistance to nitrosoureas,[39–45] suggesting that inhibition of MGMT activity could sensitize glioma cells to alkylating agents. Indeed, in preclinical animal models, administration of MGMT inhibitors such as O^6-benzylguanine (O^6-BG) before treatment with BCNU has shown a benefit in tumors having high MGMT activity.[46] Despite these encouraging preclinical results and phase I studies,[47–49] O^6-BG did not restore sensitivity to BCNU in a more recent phase II study[50]; however, in that study, coadministration of O^6-BG with BCNU was associated with increased bone marrow suppression, mandating significant dose reductions of BCNU, which may, in part, explain the lack of activity of this regimen in the treatment of nitrosourea-resistant gliomas. Whether marrow suppression can be circumvented by way of locoregional administration of BCNU (e.g., use of BCNU-releasing polymer Gliadel) coupled with O^6-BG is being evaluated.[44]

Cell-Cycle Inhibitors

The process of cell division requires that the cell proceed in an orderly sequence through four phases that are collectively termed the *cell cycle*. Starting at G1, the cell contains its diploid DNA content. Prior to proceeding to the S phase, the phase of DNA replication, cells undergo a "screen" at the G1/S checkpoint (see Fig. 2-1). At its most basic level, this checkpoint functions as a border patrol to ensure that DNA does not possess oncogenic and other potentially deleterious mutations/rearrangements before it is replicated. At this checkpoint, numerous regulatory genes act coordinately to determine if a cell may pass or not. For cells that are stopped from proceeding, they are either sent back into G1 for repair of mutations or they are selected out for death by apoptosis. Table 2-4, as well as Fig. 2-1, summarizes the points at which the cell cycle is amenable to therapeutic intervention.

▶ TABLE 2-4. INHIBITORS OF THE CELL CYCLE

Phase of Cycle	Drug Class	Drugs	Mechanism of Action
G1/S checkpoint	Rapamycin analogues	CCI-779 Gene therapy approach	mTOR (mammalian target of rapamycin) is a protein that stimulates progression through the G1/S checkpoint specifically in glioma cells; rapamycin analogues inhibit mTOR (see Fig. 2-1)
	Gene therapy	Refer to Table 2-6	Aim is to replete genes (examples: p16, p53, Rb) that enforce the G1/S checkpoint (refer to Table 2-5 pertaining to gene therapy approaches for a more detailed discussion)
S (synthesis of DNA)	Nucleoside analogues	Fluorouracil Cytarabine Thioguanine	Incorporates into replicating DNA
	Topoisomerase inhibitors	Topotecan CPT-11 (irinotecan) Etoposide (VP16)	Inhibits unwinding of DNA at replication fork
M (mitosis)	Vinca alkaloids	Vincristine	Inhibits microtubule function during mitosis
	Taxanes	Paclitaxel (Taxol)	Inhibits microtubule function during mitosis
	Novel agents	CI-980	Binds to tubulin at the colchicine binding site; inhibits tubulin polymerization and blocks cell-cycle progression in mitosis

G1/S Checkpoint

Pharmacologic Therapy

As illustrated in Fig. 2-1, virtually all growth factor/RPTK signals—by way of pathways encoded by Ras/Raf/MEK/MAPK, PLC-γ/PKC, or phosphoinositide 3-kinase (PI3K)/AKT/mammalian target of rapamycin (mTOR)—ultimately stimulate cell-cycle progression. Of these pathways that lead to cell-cycle stimulation, mTOR activation (i.e., PI3K/AKT/mTOR pathway) has attracted attention for therapeutics. mTOR, as its acronym implies, is a target for analogues of rapamycin, a macrocyclic lactone originally isolated from *Streptomyces hygroscopicus*.[51,52] CCI-779, a potent analogue of rapamycin, is currently in phase I/II evaluation in patients with recurrent glioblastoma at several institutions. In addition to being a novel target for therapeutics in neuro-oncology, mTOR represents an example in which our knowledge of the molecular genetics of malignant gliomas may help identify patients whose tumors may be more sensitive to drugs that target mTOR. As shown in Fig. 2-1, mTOR activation can occur as a consequence of one of two molecular events: (1) EGFR overactivity (which stimulates PI3K/AKT pathway of mTOR activation) or by (2) inactivation of the tumor suppressor gene phosphatase tensin homologue (PTEN) (wild-type PTEN inhibits the PI3K/AKT pathway; therefore, mutations that inactivate PTEN lead to unopposed AKT activation of mTOR). As both mutations (i.e., EGFR overactivity and deletions in PTEN) are frequently observed in high-grade gliomas (either occurs in 40% of glioblastomas), tumors that harbor any one of these mutations would be expected to demonstrate elevated mTOR activity and hence be particularly sensitive to mTOR inhibition.

Gene Therapy Approaches Directed Toward Reinforcing the G1/S Blockade

Table 2-5 summarizes the rationale for targeting certain tumor suppressor genes for possible gene therapy approaches. As illustrated in Fig. 2-1, numerous gene products function coordinately to closely regulate this checkpoint. The retinoblastoma protein (Rb) represents the central component in the G1/S checkpoint. In its native unphosphorylated form, Rb blocks cell cycle progression into S phase ("Stop" in Fig. 2-1). On phosphorylation by cyclin-dependent kinase 4 (CDK4), Rb is no longer able to block cycle progression ("Go" in Fig. 2-1). The p16 gene product can inhibit CDK4-mediated inactivation of Rb.

The relative activities of the components that comprise the p16/CDK4/Rb axis determine whether a cell will pass or be blocked at the G1/S transition. In more than 90% of gliomas, the following mutations occur in any one of these three components leading to the common end result—inactivation of Rb and thus opening of

▶ TABLE 2-5. MUTATED TUMOR SUPPRESSOR GENES—POTENTIAL TARGETS FOR GENE THERAPY

Gene	Rationale for Candidate in Gene Therapy
PTEN	On binding ligand, growth factor receptors such as EGFR can activate PI3K (phosphotidylinositol-3-kinase), which leads to formation of intermediaries that activate AKT that in turn enhances cell cycle progression (via mTOR) and enhances survival (see Fig. 2-1). PTEN blocks the formation of AKT-stimulating intermediaries, hence the rationale for PTEN gene therapy. This is of particular relevance to glioblastomas, in which PTEN is frequently deleted.
P16/CDK4/Rb axis (regulation of G1/S checkpoint)	*Rb* (retinoblastoma protein), in its unphosphorylated form, blocks progression through the G1/S checkpoint. *CDK4* (cyclin-dependent kinase 4) phosphorylates Rb, thereby inactivating it, resulting in progression through the checkpoint. *P16* inhibits CDK4, enforcing arrest at G1/S checkpoint. Therefore, possible therapies would be aimed at stabilizing the G1/S checkpoint by: Replacement of p16 by gene therapy (p16 is often deleted in gliomas). Inhibition of CDK4. Replacement of Rb by gene therapy (which is also mutated frequently in gliomas).
P53	P53 functions as the "guardian of the genome," by way of preventing the replication of oncogenic mutations by two principal mechanisms: 1. *Arrest of cell cycle.* Cells that harbor mutations are arrested from progressing through the cell cycle, giving them the opportunity to repair DNA damage. 2. *Apoptosis.* In response to certain DNA damages, p53 induces programmed cell death. The inactivation of p53 function contributes to genetic instability (leading to further oncogenic mutations), as well as to resistance to apoptosis, which clinically is associated with resistance to chemo- and radiation therapy. Because p53-inactivating mutations are common in gliomas, p53 represents a viable candidate for repletion via gene therapy approaches.

the gate at the G1/S checkpoint: (a) direct inactivation of Rb by mutations/deletions of the Rb gene; (b) *CDK4* amplification, leading to a state in which Rb tends to exist in the phosphorylated inactive form; (c) deletion of *p16*, which leaves CDK4 unopposed to phosphorylate and thus inactivate Rb. Of these mutations, the deletions in *p16* or *Rb* represent ideal situations for possible gene therapy based approaches. In this regard, virally mediated gene transfer (adenovirus vectors containing the functional *p16* or *Rb* gene) has been used successfully to inhibit glioma growth in vitro, as well as in animal models.[53–57] However, although the rationale for gene therapy to replete cells that harbor inactivating mutations of tumor suppressor genes such as *Rb* and *p16* is exciting, clinical utility in the patient setting remains limited by the relative inability of the gene-carrying virus vectors to effectively disseminate into the tumor mass.[53,58] As such, an area of complementary research in the realm of gene therapy focuses on the generation of methods to enhance virus/gene delivery (see "Methods to Improve the Targeting of Therapeutic Agents to the Tumor" below).

Cell Cycle Phases Distal to the G1/S Checkpoint

As previously mentioned, more than 90% of malignant gliomas harbor mutations that permit the cells to pass through the G1/S checkpoint unimpeded as a result of mutations that affect the p16/CDK4/Rb axis. Therefore, for the great majority of cells that progress beyond the checkpoint, other therapies acting more distally in the cell cycle are of importance. S-phase–specific agents exert their mechanism of action by hindering the process of DNA synthesis. This is done by either targeting the DNA directly or by inhibiting the enzymes involved in replicating the DNA.

Inhibiting the DNA molecule directly is classically the mechanism of action used by nucleoside analogues, which mimic the pyrimidine and purine building blocks of DNA. These agents, such as fluorouracil and cytarabine (ara-C) (pyrimidine analogues) and thioguanine (purine analogue), disrupt DNA by their incorporation into the DNA molecule during replication. Unfortunately, with the exception of ara-C, which has demonstrated benefit in the setting of primary central nervous system (CNS) lymphoma, nucleoside analogues have faired poorly in the treatment of malignant gliomas or other tumors encountered in neuro-oncology.

Of the many enzymes involved in DNA replication, topoisomerases have been targeted by a variety of drugs, including ones that inhibit topoisomerase I (topotecan, irinotecan [CPT-11]) or topoisomerase II (etoposide [VP16]).[59–61] As the benefits demonstrated by these agents given as monotherapy have been modest at best, they (especially the topoisomerase I poisons) are the subject of combinatorial regimens under evaluation (e.g., CPT-11 in combination with nitrosourea, which has demonstrated synergy in both in vitro and animal models of malignant glioma).

For the M phase, numerous drugs exist that attempt to neutralize the cell in this final stage of the cell cycle. Typically, these drugs exert their antitumor effect by disrupting the function of microtubules, the protein filaments necessary for DNA partitioning and the actual process of cell division–cytokinesis. Vincristine, paclitaxel (Taxol), and CI-980 represent examples of this category of drugs. Similar to the topoisomerase inhibitors, the benefits of these drugs in the monotherapy setting has been disappointing and therefore are being used in combination with other drugs.

▶ EFFECTOR MOLECULES: TARGETING PROTEINASES, INTEGRINS, AND MEDIATORS OF ANGIOGENESIS

At the level of the DNA, cell surface signals are received in the form of activated transcription factors (TF in Fig. 2-1) that induce the expression of specific genes. Many of these induced genes encode proteins that participate in the cell-cycle progression—that is, proliferation. Other gene products induced by the signaling cascade constitute *effector molecules*, whose functions endow on the tumor cell additional phenotypes that render it malignant: invasiveness, motility, and angiogenesis. In addition to targeting the proliferation process, effective antitumor therapies must also encompass the effector functions (Table 2-6).

Of the various characteristics of a tumor cell, its capacity to invade underlies the poor prognosis associated with all malignant neoplasms.[62–64] While primary brain tumors—even the high-grade gliomas—do not metastasize (except very rarely) to distant organs, they are locally very invasive, disrupting and destroying adjacent brain tissue, thereby leading to further neurologic dysfunction that ultimately is the cause of the patient's demise. The process of invasion involves two processes: (a) proteolysis to degrade protein and cellular structures that constitute the barrier to invasion[64–67]; and (b) movement or motility of the tumor cell in the direction of the path that has been cleared. Powerful proteolytic enzymes mediate the first step, and the second by cell surface integrins that function as *traction* molecules (see Fig. 2-1).

Proteinases and Integrins as Mediators of Tumor Invasiveness

Proteinases

Numerous proteinases have been implicated in the invasiveness of gliomas. Of these, the MMPs have been the most studied and characterized. MMPs represent a large

► **TABLE 2-6.** EFFECTOR MOLECULES AS THERAPEUTIC TARGETS

Effector Molecules	Targets	Drugs
Proteases (invasion)	Matrix metalloproteinases (MMPs)	
	MMP-2 MMP-9 MT-MMP (MMP-14)	Marimastat AG3340 Chemically modified tetracyclines (CMTs—Metastat)
	Serine proteinases Urokinase (uPA) uPA receptor	Not yet targeted for therapeutics
	Cysteine proteinases Cathepsins	Not yet targeted for therapeutics
Integrins (invasion)	$\alpha_v\beta_3$	Neutralizing antibodies Small molecule inhibitors
Angiogenesis effectors	VEGFR (vascular endothelial growth factor receptor)	SU5416
	$\alpha_v\beta_3$	Neutralizing antibodies Small molecule inhibitors
	Inhibition of endothelial cell growth	Thalidomide

family of enzymes that share the common characteristic of requiring a Zn^{2+} cofactor at its active site, hence the "metallo" prefix.[66,68] Of the many MMPs, MMP-2,[32,69,70] MMP-9,[69–73] and MMP-14 (MT or membrane-type MMP)[74] are the ones most implicated in glioma invasiveness. Both in vitro and in vivo, the expression of these MMPs is correlated with increased invasive behavior and, conversely, their inhibition by endogenous or pharmacologic inhibitors leads to arrest of the invasive phenotype. The observation that virtually all malignant tumors use proteinases[65,66,75–78] to invade has led to the development of small molecule inhibitors that target these enzymes.

The first generation of MMP inhibitors was hydroxamate derivatives whose mechanism of action involved chelation of the Zn^{2+} cofactor from the active site of the enzyme.[79] In numerous tumor types, including gliomas, clinical trials evaluating MMP inhibitors have already been performed.[79,80] Marimastat, the orally bioavailable MMP inhibitor (inhibits all MMP isoforms),[80] was recently evaluated in a phase III randomized study (against placebo) in newly diagnosed glioblastoma patients (patients enrolled in study after completion of radiation treatment). As expected, the drug, lacking any nausea/vomiting or marrow-suppressive side effects, was well tolerated, apart from arthralgias; in this study, the proteinase inhibitor proved no better than placebo. While marimastat monotherapy showed no benefit, this drug, in combination with the alkylator temozolomide, did result in a modest increase in time to tumor progression.[81]

Other MMP inhibitors include AG3340, also a pan-MMP inhibitor that has demonstrated antiinvasive and antiangiogenic effects in several tumors,[82–84] including glioma.[85] Another exciting family of molecules is the tetracycline derivatives. Independent of its antimicrobial action, the tetracyclines exhibit potent anti-MMP activity.[86–90] In fact, a chemically modified tetracycline, Periostat, which lacks the antimicrobial activity but retains anti-MMP activity, was recently approved by the FDA for treatment of periodontal disease, a disease in which tissue damage is also MMP-mediated. A relative of this drug, Metastat, has been considered for phase I/II evaluation in malignant glioma patients. In addition to neutralizing tumor invasiveness, protease inhibitors also offer the potential added benefit of inhibiting angiogenesis, as neovascularizing blood vessels also use MMPs. Thus far, an important unresolved issue is whether MMP inhibitors should be used as monotherapy or in combination with other drugs. As MMP inhibitors are largely tumorostatic, rather than tumoricidal, their combination with a cytotoxic agent should offer a more effective treatment outcome. However, given that glioblastomas are resistant to essentially all cytotoxic therapies evaluated to date, an effective partner for combinatorial treatment is still wanting in the neuro-oncology field.

Integrins in Tumor Motility

As mentioned in the previous section, proteases function to degrade the barriers in the way of the tumor cell. Following proteolysis, the cell must then locomote to complete the invasion process.[91] This motility is enabled by cell surface integrins that grip the extracellular terrain to effectively pull the cell along. Of the many integrins expressed by glioma cells,[92] one heterodimer set that has received significant attention from a therapeutic standpoint is the $\alpha_V\beta_3$ complex. It is expressed abundantly in high-grade gliomas (being absent in low-grade tumors or normal brain)[91,93,94] and its expression does correlate with increased cell motility.[95] Moreover, ligation of this heterodimer is associated with enhanced chemoresistance by way of increased expression of antiapoptotic genes; consequently, treatments that target this integrin pair may impair both tumor motility/invasion and chemoresistance.[96] It is also important to note that the $\alpha_V\beta_3$ integrin is expressed by neovascularizing endothelial cells and that inhibition of this heterodimer leads to massive endothelial cell apoptosis[97–99]; thus, therapies directed toward this integrin pair may also impact on tumor growth by way of inhibiting angiogenesis. In this regard, pilot studies of a neutralizing monoclonal antibody against the $\alpha_V\beta_3$ integrin have been completed,[100] and further phase I evaluations are pending. As well, small molecule inhibitors of integrins are currently under development; thus far, a peptidomimetic inhibitor selective for the $\alpha_V\beta_3$ heterodimer has been tested in animal models of germ cell tumors with encouraging results[101] and is currently undergoing clinical evaluation in glioma patients.

Mediators of Angiogenesis

All tumors require neovascularization to sustain tumor growth; consequently, angiogenesis inhibitors represent an exciting area of potential therapeutics. Thalidomide, which inhibits endothelial cell growth, has undergone phase II evaluation in recurrent glioma patients. Under hypoxic conditions, the DNA promoter for the gene encoding VEGF, a potent mitogen for endothelial cells,[102,103] is induced in glioma cells.[23] The synthesized VEGF is secreted into the interstitium and interacts with the VEGFR expressed by endothelial cells. To interrupt this paracrine signaling, inhibitors of VEGFR were developed and are currently in clinical trials in a variety of tumors, including malignant gliomas. SU5416 is a selective inhibitor of VEGFR that has demonstrated potent antiangiogenic effect both in vitro and in animal models and is currently undergoing clinical trial evaluation. SU6668 is also a VEGFR inhibitor but is less selective than SU5416, inhibiting other tyrosine kinases such as PDGFR and fibroblast growth factor receptor (FGFR); it is also pending commencement of phase II evaluation in the setting of patients with recurrent gliomas.

Although VEGFR inhibitors target endothelial cell proliferation, other drug categories are directed at the effector molecules of endothelial cells that permit the neovascularizing cells to migrate and invade. Similar to tumor cells, endothelial cells that infiltrate tissue use proteinases (i.e., MMPs for proteolysis of barriers) in concert with cell surface integrins that mediate cell locomotion. In this setting, MMP inhibitors that are used to target tumor invasion may also have an added benefit of an antiangiogenic effect. With respect to integrins, the same integrin heterodimer pair—the $\alpha_V\beta_3$ pair—is expressed by neovascularizing endothelial cells. Importantly, the interaction between the $\alpha_V\beta_3$ integrin and the basement membrane constitutes an obligatory survival signal for endothelial cells, and disruption of this interaction leads to massive apoptosis of the endothelial cells. Thus, inhibitors of the $\alpha_V\beta_3$ heterodimer (i.e., neutralizing antibodies, small molecule inhibitors) used to target this integrin pair on glioma cell surfaces may also inhibit the $\alpha_V\beta_3$ present on endothelial cells, thereby inhibiting angiogenesis by way of inducing endothelial apoptosis.[97,99–101,104]

▶ METHODS TO IMPROVE THE TARGETING OF THERAPEUTIC AGENTS TO THE TUMOR

In addition to individual drugs designed to interfere at various points of signaling pathways, methods aimed at enhancing drug delivery also represent an important area of research. Improved delivery of therapy can be effected by at least two approaches: physical methods that simply increase the amount of drug penetrating the CNS (e.g., drugs that open the blood–brain barrier to enhance drug delivery into the brain interstitium), as well as biochemical methods that enhance the targeting of a given drug specifically to the tumor cell by taking advantage of molecular characteristics that distinguish tumor from adjacent nontumor cells.

Increasing the Amount of Drug Delivered to the Tumor: Agents That Increase the Permeability of the Blood–Brain Barrier

An important pharmacologic consideration in the choice of chemotherapy for tumors of the CNS is the drug's ability to penetrate the blood–brain barrier. For tumors that do not enhance significantly with contrast on imaging studies (i.e., low- to intermediate-grade gliomas), the intact blood–brain barrier is a significant impediment to drug delivery. Even with high-grade gliomas, in which the blood–brain barrier is breached at many sites, the blood–brain barrier is not universally impaired in all areas of a tumor mass and therefore drug delivery can be severely restricted.[105]

Platinum derivatives represent the archetypal example of a chemotherapeutic agent that demonstrates potent antitumor effects against glioma cells in vitro, but is limited in the clinical setting by the drug's hydrophilicity that severely impedes its entry into the central nervous system. For such reasons, considerable effort has been directed toward developing ways of permeabilizing the blood–brain barrier to improve the delivery of hydrophilic chemotherapeutic agents into brain tumors. Initial approaches involved physical disruption of the blood–brain barrier by the infusion of hyperosmotic agents such as mannitol and arabinose in high concentrations into the ipsilateral carotid artery.[106–108] Although this methodology was successful in achieving the primary goal of increased drug delivery, brain edema posed a significant risk, given that the blood–brain barrier perturbation induced by this approach was prolonged and also involved normal brain tissue as well.

Second-generation strategies focused on receptor-mediated, transient opening of the blood–brain barrier. One peptide that has received particular attention in this regard is bradykinin, which led to transient permeabilization of blood–brain barrier; moreover, this effect was more pronounced in tumor tissue than in nontumor tissue.[109,110] Building on this principle, RMP-7, a synthetic 9-amino-acid agonist of the bradykinin B_2 receptor, was developed; RMP-7 demonstrated more than 100 times the potency of endogenous bradykinin in blood–brain barrier permeabilization. These findings led to phase I[111] and subsequent phase II[112] studies in which intravenous dosing of RMP-7 preceded the administration of the platinum derivative carboplatin. While these studies confirmed the feasibility of administering the RMP-7/platinum combination, the response rate in patients treated with this regimen was less impressive than had been hoped. Whether the somewhat disappointing results were attributable to RMP-7 or its partner carboplatin is not clear. At present, it appears that RMP-7 may represent a viable mode to facilitate treatment, but it is in need of a more effective chemotherapeutic partner. Given the relative safety of RMP-7, the potential benefit of this approach may not be restricted to neuro-oncologic conditions, but may be generalizable to other neurologic conditions in which drug penetration into the nervous system is limited by blood–brain barrier.

Direct Administration of Chemotherapy into Brain Parenchyma: Interstitial Therapy

In contrast to the approach illustrated by bradykinin analogues such as RMP-7, in which the objective is to enhance drug penetration of the blood–brain barrier, interstitial approaches place the chemotherapeutic agent directly into the tumor site by way of surgical implantation. The approach involves impregnating a biodegradable polymer with a chemotherapeutic agent and intraoperatively implanting these polymer wafers into the surgical cavity of the tumor. Based on preclinical[113] and phase I data demonstrating the benefit of BCNU wafers (Gliadel),[114] this intracavitary approach was recently evaluated in a phase III randomized study in which recurrent glioma patients were stratified between the implantation of BCNU-containing wafer and placebo, in which the BCNU wafer implantation was associated with improved survival compared with placebo-treated patients.[115] However, the treatment did not appear to be superior to standard parenteral BCNU therapy; as a result, the use of interstitial therapy for malignant glioma has not been uniform. Nonetheless, the method offers several potential advantages: (a) it circumvents the blood–brain barrier altogether. Drugs are placed directly into the brain parenchyma with the objective of reaching higher local parenchymal drug concentrations than would be achievable with systemic drug administration; (b) there is less systemic toxicity (i.e., bone marrow suppression), given that the drug is administered locoregionally; and (c) the polymer approach is versatile. The polymer can be impregnated with a wide variety of chemotherapeutic agents.[113,116–118] As well, recently developed polymer microspheres,[119] which are much smaller than the wafers, can be implanted stereotactically in situations in which surgical resection is not feasible.

Increasing the Drug Distribution in the Brain: Convection Approaches

Although there are sophisticated means of delivering higher concentrations of chemotherapy to the brain, either by way of blood–brain barrier perturbation or by circumventing the blood–brain barrier altogether with intracavitary/interstitial approaches, the drug, once inside the brain, is still faced with the difficulty of slow diffusion within the brain parenchyma. Even following direct inoculation of drug into the brain (i.e., intratumoral injection or interstitially placed polymers), or into the cerebrospinal fluid (intrathecal therapy), diffusion of even small molecules into the parenchyma is typically inadequate, and for large molecules, is dismal. This is an important issue with respect to CNS tumors such as gliomas, because their ability to infiltrate deeply into the parenchyma away from the parent tumor mass renders locoregional therapies such as intratumoral injection approaches ineffective. As fluid convection, or bulk flow, in tissues occurs as a result of pressure gradients, several groups have attempted to augment tissue penetration by the application of a constant pressure gradient during interstitial infusion of drug (convection-enhanced delivery [CED]). In animal models, this approach has been very successful in achieving tissue penetration that was not only much higher (several orders of magnitude higher than intraparenchymal injection alone), but one that was more homogeneous throughout the white matter with distribution of the test agent even into the gray matter.[120,121] This approach may be of potential use not only in the delivery of small molecule drugs into the brain, but also in facilitating the volume distribution of larger molecules, such as the virus particles (i.e., adenovirus, herpes simplex) used as vectors in gene-therapy approaches.[122]

In regard to clinical trials, CED was used to intracranially deliver the *Pseudomonas* exotoxin conjugated recombinantly to interleukin (IL)-13 in a phase I study[123]; the rationale for this study is that IL-13 receptors are more abundantly expressed by glioblastoma cells, in contrast to minimal/no expression by normal brain glia/neurons.[124–126] Based on the initial phase I study results, there is a multiinstitutional phase III study (encompassing more than 60 institutions internationally) evaluating the IL-13/pseudomonal toxin conjugate delivered via CED. Given the obvious technological promises and advantages of CED in regards to drug penetration through the brain parenchyma, CED will no doubt be a focus of intense interest for future clinical studies.

Functional Targeting of the Therapeutic Agent to the Tumor Cell

Both of the methods described above—blood–brain barrier permeabilization and convection/diffusion—are directed toward increasing drug delivery to the tumor by way of physical means, either by opening up the tight junctions to facilitate drug entry into the brain or, once inside the brain, the drug is physically pushed to permeate the brain tissue. Of interest, there have also been methods recently to enhance treatment delivery by way of targeting a biochemical feature that distinguishes the tumor cell from its neighboring nonneoplastic cells. Although these methods are early in clinical development, they warrant mention, as they illustrate how molecular biology has led to the identification of not only physical targets (i.e., growth factor receptors, cell surface integrins, and other proteins that can be physically targeted by antibodies or inhibitors that will physically interact with them) but have also identified *functional* targets. Four examples of functional targets are discussed in the following sections: Ras activity (high in gliomas), MMP activity (high in gliomas), p53 function (low in gliomas), and Rb function (low in gliomas).

Overactive Ras

A Canadian group has exploited a unique biochemical feature of reovirus to selectively target tumors that express high Ras activity for viral infection. The life cycle of the reovirus requires that the host cell be high in Ras activity, as Ras leads to the derepression of viral RNA translation.[127] As a result, virus replication and, hence, host cell lysis occur preferentially in tumors such as high-grade gliomas that harbor high Ras activity in contrast to nontransformed glia and neurons. In animal models, intratumoral as well as systemic injection of reovirus led to dramatic regression of glioma tumors by an oncolytic effect.[128] Given that Ras overactivity is commonly observed in high grade gliomas, because of the position of Ras downstream of multiple RPTKs (i.e., EGFR, PDGFR) that activate it, functional targeting of Ras represents a novel approach to future therapeutics.

Overactive Proteolysis

Tumors capable of invading do so by using matrix-degrading enzymes, the principal category being that of the MMPs. High-grade gliomas express abundant amounts of MMPs, specifically MMP-2 and MMP-9 (see "Proteinases" above and Table 2-6). This high MMP activity can be exploited by developing viruses (for a gene-therapy approach) whose internalization by host cells is dependent on local MMP activity.[129] In this system, the internalization of the retrovirus requires a specific interaction between a protein on the viral membrane with a receptor on the host cell surface. The viral membrane protein is modified through recombinant DNA technology such that its ability to interact with the host cell receptor is hindered by a peptide moiety that has been added on. This peptide moiety is a cleavage substrate for MMP; consequently, when the virus is in the vicinity of high MMP activity, the blocking peptide is cleaved off, enabling the virus to interact with the host cell for internalization. The specificity of this virus construct for areas of high MMP activity permits this virus to potentially function as a gene-carrying vector to target not only tumors, but also other areas of increased MMP activity, such as neovascularizing blood vessels and inflammation.

Low Activity of Tumor Suppressors as Targets

Until recently, viruses in antitumor therapies had been used as gene therapy vectors to deliver the gene of interest. Typically, these viruses were engineered to be *replication-defective* such that the modified viruses were unable to complete their life cycle and hence unable to lyse the host cell. However, more recent approaches have focused on *replication-competent* viruses aimed at killing the tumor cell by way of direct viral oncolysis, rather than by gene transfer. An obvious pitfall of this approach is the potential danger of unleashing an active virus into the nervous system. Thus, through modification of the viral genome, viruses that can replicate selectively in tumor cells have been developed. In the design of tumor-selective viruses, the molecular genetic features that distinguish tumor from normal cells are exploited to ensure that the life cycle of the genetically engineered virus can be completed selectively in tumor cells, thereby leading to tumor lysis. The two examples discussed below exploit the protein–protein interaction that occurs between the E1 protein of adenovirus and p53 and Rb, two tumor suppressor gene products that are commonly inactivated by mutation in gliomas.

p53/E1 Interaction

Upon infection of a host cell, the wild-type E1 protein of the adenovirus sequesters cellular p53. The sequestered p53 is unable to block cell-cycle progression. As the virus life cycle is dependent upon cell cycling, sequestration of p53 permits the virus to complete its morphogenesis, leading to host cell lysis. Mutation of the viral E1 protein such that it cannot interact with cellular p53 protein renders the mutant virus to selectively replicate in tumor cells by the following mechanism[53]:

1. E1 mutant adenovirus infects a p53 wild-type cell (i.e., nontumor cell). Because the mutant E1 protein cannot bind p53, the wild-type p53 is left unopposed to block cell-cycle progression (see Fig. 2-1). The virus cannot complete its life cycle and the host cell survives.
2. E1 mutant adenovirus infects a tumor cell harboring a mutant (inactivated) p53. There is no functional p53 to block cell-cycle progression. Therefore, despite the mutated E1 protein, the adenovirus is able to replicate as the cell is permitted to cycle in the absence of p53. Viral replication ensues and the host cell is lysed. In this manner, mutating the E1 protein can genetically alter adenovirus, thereby generating a virus that selectively replicates in p53 mutant glioma (or other tumor types) cells. The potential pitfall of this approach is that in a given glioma tumor mass, the p53 status (i.e., mutant vs. wild-type) of the constituent cells is heterogeneous, thus the tumor cells containing wild-type p53 are resistant to the oncolytic effects of the mutant adenovirus.

E1/Rb Interaction

The wild-type E1 protein of the adenovirus is also capable of binding and sequestering the cellular Rb protein. The sequestered Rb is unable to block cell-cycle progression. As the virus life cycle is dependent on cell cycling, sequestration of Rb permits the virus to complete its morphogenesis, leading to host cell lysis. Mutation of the viral E1 protein such that it cannot interact with cellular Rb protein renders the mutant virus to selectively replicate in tumor cells by the following mechanism[53,54]:

1. Mutant E1 adenovirus infects the resting, nondividing cell (i.e., nontumor cell). In a resting, noncycling cell, Rb exists in its nonphosphorylated form, which is its active state. Rb thus blocks cell cycle ("Stop" sign in Fig. 2-1). The virus cannot replicate and the host cell lives.
2. Mutant E1 adenovirus infects dividing cell (i.e., tumor cell). As Rb is functionally inactivated in more than 90% of gliomas, these tumor cells are free to enter the cell cycle. The result is that the mutant E1 adenovirus can replicate, leading to tumor cell death.

▶ CONCLUSIONS AND PERSPECTIVES

The advances in our understanding of the molecular biology of brain tumors have led to the development of exciting new agents directed at newly identified targets. What does this mean for the future of "standard" or "conventional" chemotherapies such as procarbazine and CCNU in the treatment of brain tumor patients? Although there is no doubt that the field of oncology has been the most significant beneficiary of the molecular revolution, this revolution has actually brought certain conventional drugs *into*—rather than out of—the limelight. One of the best examples of this is the observation that the deletion of the chromosome 1p or of chromosomes 1p and 19q combined in intermediate-grade gliomas of oligodendroglial lineage (anaplastic oligodendrogliomas) is very reliably predictive of the tumor being exquisitely sensitive to standard alkylator chemotherapeutic drugs.[36–38] Presumably, a gene (or genes) on one or both of these chromosomes encodes a protein product(s) that renders the tumor cells chemoresistant, and hence its deletion leads to chemosensitivity. Therefore, progress in the molecular biology of brain tumors will play a pivotal role in not only the development of new drugs directed at novel targets, but will also help to more effectively use the armamentarium of conventional drugs by (a) better identifying those patients who are most likely to benefit from specific standard drugs and (b) determining the mechanisms underlying resistance to conventional chemotherapies. Thus, our understanding of the molecular biology and genetics of brain tumors offers not only the promise of novel drugs directed toward novel targets, but also of enhanced use of the standard therapies. Taken together, the future of neuro-oncology is a promising one.

REFERENCES

1. Fueyo J, Gomez-Manzano C, Yung WK, Kyritsis AP. Targeting in gene therapy for gliomas. Arch Neurol 1999; 56:445–448.
2. Feldkamp MM, Lau N, Guha A. Signal transduction pathways and their relevance in human astrocytomas. J Neurooncol 1997;35:223–248.
3. Frederick L, Wang XY, Eley G, James CD. Diversity and frequency of epidermal growth factor receptor mutations in human glioblastomas. Cancer Res 2000;60:1383–1387.

4. Sugawa N, Yamamoto K, Ueda S, et al. Function of aberrant EGFR in malignant gliomas. Brain Tumor Pathol 1998;15:53–57.
5. Berens ME, Rief MD, Shapiro JR, et al. Proliferation and motility responses of primary and recurrent gliomas related to changes in epidermal growth factor receptor expression. J Neurooncol 1996;27:11–22.
6. Goldman CK, Kim J, Wong WL, et al. Epidermal growth factor stimulates vascular endothelial growth factor production by human malignant glioma cells: a model of glioblastoma multiforme pathophysiology. Mol Biol Cell 1993;4:121–133.
7. Nagane M, Levitzki A, Gazit A, et al. Drug resistance of human glioblastoma cells conferred by a tumor-specific mutant epidermal growth factor receptor through modulation of Bcl-XL and caspase-3-like proteases. Proc Natl Acad Sci USA 1998;95:5724–5729.
8. Stragliotto G, Vega F, Stasiecki P, et al. Multiple infusions of anti-epidermal growth factor receptor (EGFR) monoclonal antibody (EMD 55,900) in patients with recurrent malignant gliomas. Eur J Cancer 1996;32A:636–640.
9. Graziani Y, Chayoth R, Karny N, et al. Regulation of protein kinases activity by quercetin in Ehrlich ascites tumor cells. Biochim Biophys Acta 1982;714:415–421.
10. Akiyama T, Ishida J, Nakagawa S, et al. Genistein, a specific inhibitor of tyrosine-specific protein kinases. J Biol Chem 1987;262:5592–5595.
11. Umezawa H, Imoto M, Sawa T, et al. Studies on a new epidermal growth factor-receptor kinase inhibitor, erbstatin, produced by MH435-hF3. J Antibiot 1986;39:170–173.
12. Uhm JH, Ballman KV, Giannini C, et al. Phase II study of ZD1839 in patients with newly diagnosed grade 4 astrocytoma. Proc Am Soc Clin Oncol 2004;22(145):1505.
13. Rich JN, Reardon DA, Peery T, et al. Phase II trial of gefitinib in recurrent glioblastoma. J Clin Oncol 2004;22: 133–142.
14. Paez JG, Janne PA, Lee JC, et al. GFR mutations in lung cancer: correlation with clinical response to gefitinib therapy [see comment]. Science 2004;304:1497–1500.
15. Lynch TJ, Bell DW, Sordella R, et al. Activating mutations in the epidermal growth factor receptor underlying responsiveness of non-small-cell lung cancer to gefitinib [see comment]. N Engl J Med 2004;350:2129–2139.
16. Fleming TP, Saint J, Oncolena A, et al. Amplification and/or overexpression of platelet-derived growth factor receptors and epidermal growth factor receptor in human glial tumors. Cancer Res 1992;52:4550–4553.
17. Nister M, Libermann TA, Betsholtz C, et al. Expression of messenger RNAs for platelet-derived growth factor and transforming growth factor-alpha and their receptors in human malignant glioma cell lines. Cancer Res 1988; 48:3910–3918.
18. Shapiro W, Ashby E, Obbens E, et al. A phase I/II study of SU101 in combination with carmustine (BCNU) in the treatment of patients newly diagnosed with malignant glioma. Proc Annu Meet Am Soc Clin Oncol 1999.
19. Guha A, Feldkamp MM, Lau N, et al. Proliferation of human malignant astrocytomas is dependent on Ras activation. Oncogene 1997;15:2755–2765.
20. Feldkamp MM, Lala P, Lau N, et al. Expression of activated epidermal growth factor receptors, Ras-guanosine triphosphate, and mitogen-activated protein kinase in human glioblastoma multiforme specimens. Neurosurgery 1999; 45:1442–1453.
21. Feldkamp MM, Lau N, Guha A. Growth inhibition of astrocytoma cells by farnesyl transferase inhibitors is mediated by a combination of anti-proliferative, pro-apoptotic and anti-angiogenic effects. Oncogene 1999;18:7514–7526.
22. Rowinsky EK, Windle JJ, Von Hoff DD. Ras protein farnesyltransferase: a strategic target for anticancer therapeutic development [review]. J Clin Oncol 1999;17:3631–3652.
23. Feldkamp MM, Lau N, Rak J, et al. Normoxic and hypoxic regulation of vascular endothelial growth factor (VEGF) by astrocytoma cells is mediated by Ras. Int J Cancer 1999;81:118–124.
24. Lebowitz PF, Prendergast GC. Non-Ras targets of farnesyltransferase inhibitors: focus on Rho [review]. Oncogene 1998;17:1439–1445.
25. Basu A. The potential of protein kinase C as a target for anticancer treatment. Pharmacol Ther 1993;59:257–280.
26. Baltuch GH, Couldwell WT, Villemure J-G, Yong VW. Protein kinase C inhibitors suppress cell growth in established and low passage glioma cell lines. A comparison between staurosporine and tamoxifen. Neurosurgery 1993;33:495–501.
27. Baltuch GH, Dooley NP, Couldwell WT, Yong VW. Staurosporine differentially inhibits glioma versus non-glioma cell lines. J Neurooncol 1993;16:141–147.
28. Couldwell WT, Antel JP, Apuzzo MLJ, Yong VW. Inhibition of growth of established human glioma lines by modulators of the protein kinase C system. J Neurosurg 1990; 73:594–600.
29. Couldwell WT, Uhm JH, Antel JP, Yong VW. Enhanced protein kinase C activity correlates with the growth rate of malignant gliomas in vitro. Neurosurgery 1991;29:880–887.
30. Couldwell WT, Antel JP, Yong VW. Protein kinase C (PKC) activity correlates with growth rate of gliomas. II: effects of glioma mitogens and modulators of PKC. Neurosurgery 1992;31:717–724.
31. Bredel M, Pollack IF. The role of protein kinase C (PKC) in the evolution and proliferation of malignant gliomas, and the application of PKC inhibition as a novel approach to anti-glioma therapy. Acta Neurochir 1997; 139:1000–1013.
32. Uhm JH, Dooley NP, Villemure J-G, Yong VW. Glioma invasion in vitro: regulation by matrix metalloprotease-2 and protein kinase C. Clin Exp Metastasis 1996;14:421–433.
33. Levin VA, Silver P, Hannigan J, et al. Superiority of post-radiotherapy adjuvant chemotherapy with CCNU, procarbazine, and vincristine (PCV) over BCNU for anaplastic gliomas: NCOG 6G61 final report. Int J Radiat Oncol Biol Phys 1990;18:321–324.
34. Prados MD, Scott C, Curran WJ Jr, et al. Procarbazine, lomustine, and vincristine (PCV) chemotherapy for anaplastic astrocytoma: a retrospective review of radiation therapy oncology group protocols comparing survival with carmustine or PCV adjuvant chemotherapy. J Clin Oncol 1999;17:3389–3395.
35. Yung WK, Prados MD, Yaya-Tur R, et al. Multicenter phase II trial of temozolomide in patients with anaplastic astrocytoma or anaplastic oligoastrocytoma at first

relapse. Temodal Brain Tumor Group. J Clin Oncol 1999;17:2762–2771.
35a. Stupp R, Mason WP, van den Bent MJ, et al. Radiotherapy plus concomitant and adjuvant temozolomide for glioblastoma. N Engl J Med 2005;352:987–996.
36. Cairncross JG, Ueki K, Zlatescu MC, et al. Specific genetic predictors of chemotherapeutic response and survival in patients with anaplastic oligodendrogliomas. J Natl Cancer Inst 1998;90:1473–1479.
37. Smith JS, Alderete B, Minn Y, et al. Localization of common deletion regions on 1p and 19q in human gliomas and their association with histological subtype. Oncogene 1999;18:4144–4152.
38. Smith JS, Perry A, Borell TJ, et al. Alterations of chromosome arms 1p and 19q as predictors of survival in oligodendrogliomas, astrocytomas, and mixed oligoastrocytomas. J Clin Oncol 2000;18:636–645.
39. Balana C, Ramirez JL, Taron M, et al. O^6-methyl-guanine-DNA methyltransferase methylation in serum and tumor DNA predicts response to 1,3-bis(2-chloroethyl)-1-nitrosourea but not to temozolomide plus cisplatin in glioblastoma multiforme. Clin Cancer Res 2003;9:1461–1468.
40. Chen ZP, Yarosh D, Garcia Y, et al. Relationship between O^6-methylguanine-DNA methyltransferase levels and clinical response induced by chloroethylnitrosourea therapy in glioma patients. Can J Neurol Sci 1999;26:104–109.
41. Silber JR, Blank A, Bobola MS, et al. O^6-methylguanine-DNA methyltransferase-deficient phenotype in human gliomas: frequency and time to tumor progression after alkylating agent-based chemotherapy. Clin Cancer Res 1999;5:807–814.
42. Jaeckle KA, Eyre HJ, Townsend JJ, et al. Correlation of tumor O^6-methylguanine-DNA methyltransferase levels with survival of malignant astrocytoma patients treated with bis-chloroethylnitrosourea: a Southwest Oncology Group study. J Clin Oncol 1998;16:3310–3315.
43. Silber JR, Bobola MS, Ghatan S, et al. O^6-methylguanine-DNA methyltransferase activity in adult gliomas: relation to patient and tumor characteristics. Cancer Res 1998; 58:1068–1073.
44. Rhines LD, Sampath P, Dolan ME, et al. O^6-benzylguanine potentiates the antitumor effect of locally delivered carmustine against an intracranial rat glioma. Cancer Res 2000;60:6307–6310.
45. Esteller M, Garcia-Foncillas J, Andion E, et al. Inactivation of the DNA-repair gene MGMT and the clinical response of gliomas to alkylating agents. N Engl J Med 2000; 343:1350–1354.
46. Kokkinakis DM, Bocangel DB, Schold SC, et al. Thresholds of O^6-alkylguanine-DNA alkyltransferase which confer significant resistance of human glial tumor xenografts to treatment with 1,3-bis(2-chloroethyl)-1-nitrosourea or temozolomide. Clin Cancer Res 2001;7:421–428.
47. Schold SC Jr, Kokkinakis DM, Chang SM, et al. O^6-benzylguanine suppression of O^6-alkylguanine-DNA alkyltransferase in anaplastic gliomas. Neuro-oncology 2004;6:28–32.
48. Friedman HS, Pluda J, Quinn JA, et al. Phase I trial of carmustine plus O^6-benzylguanine for patients with recurrent or progressive malignant glioma. J Clin Oncol 2000; 18:3522–3528.
49. Friedman HS, Kokkinakis DM, Pluda J, et al. Phase I trial of O^6-benzylguanine for patients undergoing surgery for malignant glioma. J Clin Oncol 1998;16:3570–3575.
50. Quinn JA, Pluda J, Dolan ME, et al. Phase II trial of carmustine plus O^6-benzylguanine for patients with nitrosourea-resistant recurrent or progressive malignant glioma. J Clin Oncol 2002;20:2277–2283.
51. Molnar-Kimber KL. Mechanism of action of rapamycin (Sirolimus, Rapamune). Transplant Proc 1996;28:964–969.
52. Hashemolhosseini S, Nagamine Y, Morley SJ, et al. Rapamycin inhibition of the G1 to S transition is mediated by effects on cyclin D1 mRNA and protein stability. J Biol Chem 1998;273:14424–14429.
53. Alemany R, Gomez-Manzano C, Balague C, et al. Gene therapy for gliomas: molecular targets, adenoviral vectors, and oncolytic adenoviruses [review] [71 refs]. Exp Cell Res 1999;252:1–12.
54. Fueyo J, Gomez-Manzano C, Alemany R, et al. A mutant oncolytic adenovirus targeting the Rb pathway produces anti-glioma effect in vivo. Oncogene 2000;19:2–12.
55. Fueyo J, Gomez-Manzano C, Yung WK, et al. Adenovirus-mediated p16/CDKN2 gene transfer induces growth arrest and modifies the transformed phenotype of glioma cells. Oncogene 1996;12:103–110.
56. Fueyo J, Gomez-Manzano C, Puduvalli VK, et al. Adenovirus-mediated p16 transfer to glioma cells induces G1 arrest and protects from paclitaxel and topotecan: implications for therapy. Int J Oncol 1998;12:665–669.
57. Fueyo J, Gomezmanzano C, Yung WKA, et al. Suppression of human glioma growth by adenovirus-mediated rb gene transfer. Neurology 1998;50:1307–1315.
58. Fueyo J, Gomez-Manzano C, Yung WKA, Kyritsis AP. Targeting in gene therapy for gliomas. Arch Neurol 1999; 56:445–448.
59. Lamond JP, Mehta MP, Boothman DA. The potential of topoisomerase I inhibitors in the treatment of CNS malignancies: report of a synergistic effect between topotecan and radiation. J Neurooncol 1996;30:1–6.
60. Weller M, Winter S, Schmidt C, et al. Topoisomerase-I inhibitors for human malignant glioma: differential modulation of p53, p21, bax and bcl-2 e expression and of CD95-mediated apoptosis by camptothecin and beta-lapachone. Int J Cancer 1997;73:707–714.
61. Macdonald D, Cairncross G, Stewart D, et al. Phase II study of topotecan in patients with recurrent malignant glioma. National Clinical Institute of Canada Clinical Trials Group. Ann Oncol 1996;7:205–207.
62. Dedhar S. Integrins and tumor invasion. Bioessays 1990; 12:583–590.
63. Ruoslahti E. Control of cell motility and tumor invasion by extracellular matrix interactions. Br J Cancer 1992; 66:239–242.
64. Furcht LT, Skubitz AP, Fields GB. Tumor cell invasion, matrix metalloproteinases, and the dogma [editorial; comment]. Lab Invest 1994;70:781–783.
65. Stetler-Stevenson WG, Liotta LA, Kleiner DE Jr. Extracellular matrix 6: role of matrix metalloproteinases in tumor invasion and metastasis. FASEB J 1993;7:1434–1441.
66. Mignatti P, Rifkin DB. Biology and biochemistry of proteinases in tumor invasion. Physiol Rev 1993;73:161–195.

67. MacDougall JR, Matrisian LM. Contributions of tumor and stromal matrix metalloproteases to tumor progression, invasion and metastasis. Cancer Metastasis Rev 1995;14: 351–362.
68. Matrisian LM. The matrix-degrading metalloproteinases. Bioessays 1992;14:455–463.
69. Chintala SK, Sawaya R, Gokaslan ZL, Rao JS. Modulation of matrix metalloprotease-2 and invasion in human glioma cells by alpha 3 beta 1 integrin. Cancer Lett 1996; 103:201–208.
70. Sawaya RE, Yamamoto M, Gokaslan ZL, et al. Expression and localization of 72 kDa type IV collagenase (MMP-2) in human malignant gliomas in vivo. Clin Exp Metastasis 1996;14:35–42.
71. Rao JS, Steck PA, Mohanam S, et al. Elevated levels of M(r) 92,000 type IV collagenase in human brain tumors. Cancer Res 1993;53:2208–2211.
72. Rao JS, Yamamoto M, Mohaman S, et al. Expression and localization of 92 kDa type IV collagenase/gelatinase B (MMP-9) in human gliomas. Clin Exp Metastasis 1996; 14:12–18.
73. Rao JS, Steck PA, Tofilon P, et al. Role of plasminogen activator and of 92-kDa type IV collagenase in glioblastoma invasion using an in vitro matrigel model. J Neurooncol 1994;18:129–138.
74. Yamamoto M, Mohanam S, Sawaya R, et al. Differential expression of membrane-type matrix metalloproteinase and its correlation with gelatinase A activation in human malignant brain tumors in vivo and in vitro. Cancer Res 1996;56:384–392.
75. Sato H, Takino T, Okada Y, Cao J, et al. Matrix metalloproteinase expressed on the surface of invasive tumor cells. Nature 1994;370:61–65.
76. Basset P, Wolf C, Chambon P. Expression of the stromelysin-3 gene in fibroblastic cells of invasive carcinomas of the breast and other human tissues: a review. Breast Cancer Res Treat 1993;24:185–193.
77. Moscatelli D, Rifkin DB. Membrane and matrix localization of proteinases: a common theme in tumor cell invasion and angiogenesis. Biochim Biophys Acta 1988;948:67–85.
78. Heino J. Biology of tumor cell invasion: interplay of cell adhesion and matrix degradation. Int J Cancer 1996; 65:717–722.
79. Brown PD. Matrix metalloproteinase inhibitors: a novel class of anticancer agents. Adv Enzyme Regul 1995; 35:293–301.
80. Brown PD. Synthetic matrix metalloproteinase inhibitors: from cancer models to cancer patients. Proc Am Assoc Cancer Res 1996;37:633–634.
81. Groves MD, Puduvalli VK, Hess KR, et al. Phase II trial of temozolomide plus the matrix metalloproteinase inhibitor, marimastat, in recurrent and progressive glioblastoma multiforme. J Clin Oncol 2002;20:1383–1388.
82. Shalinsky DR, Brekken J, Zou H, et al. Broad antitumor and antiangiogenic activities of AG3340, a potent and selective MMP inhibitor undergoing advanced oncology clinical trials. Ann NY Acad Sci 1999;878:236–270.
83. Shalinsky DR, Brekken J, Zou H, et al. Antitumor efficacy of AG3340 associated with maintenance of minimum effective plasma concentrations and not total daily dose, exposure or peak plasma concentrations. Invest New Drugs 1998;16:303–313.
84. Shalinsky DR, Brekken J, Zou H, et al. Marked antiangiogenic and antitumor efficacy of AG3340 in chemoresistant human non-small cell lung cancer tumors: single agent and combination chemotherapy studies. Clin Cancer Res 1999;5:1905–1917.
85. Price A, Shi Q, Morris D, et al. Marked inhibition of tumor growth in a malignant glioma tumor model by a novel synthetic matrix metalloproteinase inhibitor AG3340. Clin Cancer Res 1999;5:845–854.
86. Golub LM, Ramamurthy NS, Llavaneras A, et al. A chemically modified nonantimicrobial tetracycline (CMT-8) inhibits gingival matrix metalloproteinases, periodontal breakdown, and extra-oral bone loss in ovariectomized rats. Ann NY Acad Sci 1999;878:290–310.
87. Seftor RE, Seftor EA, De Larco JE, et al. Chemically modified tetracyclines inhibit human melanoma cell invasion and metastasis. Clin Exp Metastasis 1998;16:217–225.
88. Sipos EP, Tamargo RJ, Weingart JD, Brem H. Inhibition of tumor angiogenesis [review] [91 refs]. Ann NY Acad Sci 1994;732:263–272.
89. Tamargo RJ, Bok RA, Brem H. Angiogenesis inhibition by minocycline. Cancer Res 1991;51:672–675.
90. Weingart JD, Sipos EP, Brem H. The role of minocycline in the treatment of intracranial 9L glioma. J Neurosurg 1995;82:635–640.
91. Uhm JH, Gladson CL, Rao JS. The role of integrins in the malignant phenotype of gliomas. Front Biosci 1999; 4:188–199.
92. Paulus W, Tonn J. Basement membrane invasion of glioma cells mediated by integrin receptors. J Neurosurg 1994;80:515–519.
93. Gladson CL, Wilcox JN, Sanders L, et al. Cerebral microenvironment influences expression of the vitronectin gene in astrocytic tumors. J Cell Sci 1995;108:947–956.
94. Gladson CL, Cheresh DA. Glioblastoma expression of vitronectin and the α-vβ-3 integrin: adhesion mechanism for transformed glial cells. J Clin Invest 1991;88:1924–1932.
95. Gladson CL, Pijuan-Thompson VP. DGF stimulates vitronectin-directed migration and causes a localization of integrin alpha$_v$beta$_3$ and alpha$_v$beta$_5$ focal adhesions to the cell cortex in malignant astrocytoma cells. Proc Annu Meet Am Assoc Cancer Res 1997;38:A953.
96. Libermann TA, Nusbaum HR, Razon N, et al. Amplification, enhanced expression and possible rearrangement of EGF receptor gene in primary human brain tumors of glial origin. Nature 1985;313:144–147.
97. Brooks PC, Clark RAF, Cheresh DA. Requirement of vascular integrin $\alpha_v\beta_3$ for angiogenesis. Science 1994;264:569–571.
98. Stromblad S, Becker JC, Yebra M, et al. Suppression of p53 activity and p21$^{WAF/CIP1}$ expression by vascular cell integrin $\alpha_v\beta_3$ during angiogenesis. J Clin Invest 1996;98: 426–433.
99. Brooks PC, Montgomery AMP, Rosenfeld M, et al. Integrin $\alpha_v\beta_3$ antagonists promote further tumor regression by inducing apoptosis of angiogenic blood vessels. Cell 1994;79:1157–1164.
100. Gutheil JC, Campbell TN, Pierce PR, et al. Targeted antiangiogenic therapy for cancer using vitaxin: a humanized

monoclonal antibody to the integrin alpha(nu)beta(3). Clin Cancer Res 2000;6:3056–3061.
101. Carron CP, Meyer DM, Pegg JA, et al. A peptidomimetic antagonist of the integrin alpha(V)beta(3) inhibits Leydig cell tumor growth and the development of hypercalcemia of malignancy. Cancer Res 1998;58:1930–1935.
102. Lund EL, Spang-Thomsen M, Skovgaard-Poulsen H, Kristjansen PE. Tumor angiogenesis—a new therapeutic target in gliomas. Acta Neurol Scand 1998;97:52–62.
103. Plate KH. Mechanisms of angiogenesis in the brain. J Neuropathol Exp Neurol 1999;58:313–320.
104. Brooks PC, Montgomery AM, Rosenfeld M, et al. Integrin alpha v beta 3 antagonists promote tumor regression by inducing apoptosis of angiogenic blood vessels. Cell 1994;79:1157–1164.
105. Elliott PJ, Hayward NJ, Huff MR, et al. Unlocking the blood-brain barrier: a role for RMP-7 in brain tumor therapy. Exp Neurol 1996;141:214–224.
106. Neuwelt EA, Rapoport SI. Modification of the blood-brain barrier in the chemotherapy of malignant brain tumors. Fed Proc 1984;43:214–219.
107. Neuwelt EA, Hill SA, Frenkel EP. Osmotic blood-brain barrier modification and combination chemotherapy: concurrent tumor regression in areas of barrier opening and progression in brain regions distant to barrier opening. Neurosurgery 1984;15:362–366.
108. Neuwelt EA, Barnett PA, McCormick CI, et al. Osmotic blood-brain barrier modification: monoclonal antibody, albumin, and methotrexate delivery to cerebrospinal fluid and brain. Neurosurgery 1985;17:419–423.
109. Inamura T, Black KL. Bradykinin selectively opens blood-tumor barrier in experimental brain tumors. J Cereb Blood Flow Metab 1994;14:862–870.
110. Inamura T, Nomura T, Bartus RT, Black, KL. Intracarotid infusion of RMP-7, a bradykinin analog: a method for selective drug delivery to brain tumors. J Neurosurg 1994;81:752–758.
111. Ford J, Osborn C, Barton T, Bleehen NM. A phase I study of intravenous RMP-7 with carboplatin in patients with progression of malignant glioma. Eur J Cancer 1998; 34:1807–1811.
112. Gregor A, Lind M, Newman H, et al. Phase II studies of RMP-7 and carboplatin in the treatment of recurrent high grade glioma. RMP-7 European Study Group. J Neurooncol 1999;44:137–145.
113. Olivi A, Ewend MG, Utsuki T, et al. Interstitial delivery of carboplatin via biodegradable polymers is effective against experimental glioma in the rat. Cancer Chemother Pharmacol 1996;39:90–96.
114. McCawley LJ, Li S, Wattenberg EV, Hudson LG. Sustained activation of the mitogen-activated protein kinase pathway. A mechanism underlying receptor tyrosine kinase specificity for matrix metalloproteinase-9 induction and cell migration. J Biol Chem 1999;274:4347–4353.
115. Brem H, Piantadosi S, Burger PC, et al. Placebo-controlled trial of safety and efficacy of intraoperative controlled delivery by biodegradable polymers of chemotherapy for recurrent gliomas. The Polymer-Brain Tumor Treatment Group. Lancet 1995;345:1008–1012.
116. Williams JA, Dillehay LE, Tabassi K, et al. Implantable biodegradable polymers for IUdR radiosensitization of experimental human malignant glioma. J Neurooncol 1997;32:181–192.
117. Ramos-DeSimone N, French DL. Monoclonal antibodies to human MMP-9. Ann NY Acad Sci 1994;732:469–471.
118. French DL, Ramos-DeSimone N, Rozinski K, Nuovo GJ. Matrix metalloproteinase-9 in tumor cell invasion. Ann NY Acad Sci 1994;732:324–334.
119. Hudson LG, McCawley LJ. Contributions of the epidermal growth factor receptor to keratinocyte motility [review] [140 refs]. Microsc Res Tech 1998;43:444–455.
120. Bobo RH, Laske DW, Akbasak A, et al. Convection-enhanced delivery of macromolecules in the brain. Proc Nat Acad Sci USA 1994;91:2076–2080.
121. Kroll RA, Pagel MA, Muldoon LL, et al. Increasing volume of distribution to the brain with interstitial infusion: dose, rather than convection, might be the most important factor. Neurosurgery 1996;38:746–752.
122. Lieberman DM, Laske DW, Morrison PF, et al. Convection-enhanced distribution of large molecules in gray matter during interstitial drug infusion. J Neurosurg 1995; 82:1021–1029.
123. Kunwar S. Convection enhanced delivery of IL13-PE38QQR for treatment of recurrent malignant glioma: presentation of interim findings from ongoing phase 1 studies. Acta Neurochir (Suppl) 2003;88:105–111.
124. Debinski W, Gibo DM, Slagle B, et al. Receptor for interleukin 13 is abundantly and specifically over-expressed in patients with glioblastoma multiforme. Int J Oncol 15:481–486, 1999.
125. Debinski W, Obiri NI, Powers SK, et al. Human glioma cells overexpress receptors for interleukin 13 and are extremely sensitive to a novel chimeric protein composed of interleukin 13 and pseudomonas exotoxin. Clin Cancer Res 1995;1:1253–1258.
126. Debinski W, Gibo DM, Puri RK. Novel way to increase targeting specificity to a human glioblastoma-associated receptor for interleukin 13. Int J Cancer 1998;76:547–551.
127. Strong JE, Coffey MC, Tang D, et al. The molecular basis of viral oncolysis: usurpation of the Ras signaling pathway by reovirus. EMBO J 1998;17:3351–3362.
128. Coffey MC, Strong JE, Forsyth PA, Lee PW. Reovirus therapy of tumors with activated Ras pathway. Science 1998; 282:1332–1334.
129. Peng KW, Morling FJ, Cosset FL, et al. A gene delivery system activatable by disease-associated matrix metalloproteinases. Hum Gene Ther 1997;8:729–738.

CHAPTER 3

Presentation and Approach to Patient

PATRICK Y. WEN / SIEW KOON TEOH / DEBRA C. GIGAS / AND LISA MACDONALD

In recent years, the widespread availability of neuroimaging studies, such as computerized tomography (CT) scans and magnetic resonance imaging (MRI), has significantly changed the presentation and diagnosis of patients with brain tumors. The sensitivity of these neuroimaging modalities has resulted in patients presenting at an earlier stage of their illness. Although many patients still present with the classical symptoms of headaches, nausea, vomiting, and focal neurologic deficits, an increasing number of patients are diagnosed with brain tumors after developing relatively subtle symptoms such as simple partial seizures, loss of interest in activities, or reduced hearing for high frequencies. In addition, a growing number of asymptomatic brain tumors are being diagnosed in patients undergoing neuroimaging for unrelated symptoms. This chapter reviews the presentation and evaluation of patients suspected of having brain tumors.

▶ PRESENTATION

Patients with brain tumors typically present with headaches, seizures, nonspecific cognitive or personality changes, or focal neurologic deficits.[1–4] The precise combination of clinical features varies depending on the location, histology, and rate of growth of the tumor.

Headaches

Headaches are the presenting symptom in approximately 35% of patients with brain tumors and develop during the course of the disease in 40% to 70%.[1,3] The majority of these headaches are intermittent and nonspecific. They are usually dull, nonthrobbing, and often indistinguishable from tension headaches.[5] The headaches are usually located on the same side as the tumor. Supratentorial tumors tend to produce headaches with a frontal location because the majority of supratentorial pain-sensitive structures are supplied by the trigeminal nerve. The posterior fossa is innervated by cranial nerves IX and X and upper cervical nerves and usually produces pain in the occipital region and neck. Occasionally, posterior fossa tumors can produce headaches located in the vertex or retro-orbital region.[2]

Certain features of the headache increase the possibility of a tumor. These include headaches that wake the patient at night or are worse on awakening and improve over the course of the day; headaches exacerbated by postural change, coughing, or exercise; headaches of recent onset that are different from the patient's usual headaches or are greater in severity; as well as the presence of nausea or vomiting, papilledema, or focal neurologic signs.[2,5] Patients with these features require further evaluation with neuroimaging studies.

Papilledema

Papilledema is important evidence of increased intracranial pressure transmitted through the optic nerve sheath. The incidence of papilledema in an older series of patients with brain tumors has been reported to be greater than 50%.[1] However, advances in neuroimaging have resulted in patients being diagnosed at an increasingly earlier stage, and the incidence of papilledema in patients with brain tumor today is probably much lower. In a review of 100 consecutive patients with malignant gliomas who underwent surgery at Brigham and Women's Hospital, only 8% had papilledema at the time of diagnosis (El-Ouahabi and associates, unpublished data). Papilledema tends to be more common in children, in slowly growing tumors, and in posterior fossa tumors. It may be associated with symptoms of transient obscuration of vision, especially with postural change. Table 3-1 summarizes the differential diagnosis of papilledema.

Seizures

Seizures are the presenting symptom in approximately one-third of patients with brain tumors and are present at some stage of the illness in 40% to 60% of patients.[1–4] Approximately half the patients have focal seizures and the other half have generalized seizures. Slowly growing tumors are particularly likely to cause seizures, possibly because there is more time for an epileptogenic focus to develop. Seizures occur in 75% to 95% of patients with oligodendrogliomas, 65% to 70% of patients with astrocytomas, 39% to 57% of patients with meningiomas, 30% to 50% of patients with glioblastomas, and 10% to 30% of patients with brain metastases.

Tumor location is also important in determining the frequency of seizures. Supratentorial tumors, especially those located near the Rolandic fissure, are especially likely to cause seizures. Tumors in subcortical areas such as thalamus and the posterior fossa are much less epileptogenic. In patients with gliomas, seizures occur in 59% of frontal tumors, 42% of parietal tumors, 35% of temporal tumors, and 33% of occipital tumors.[6]

▶ **TABLE 3-1.** DIFFERENTIAL DIAGNOSIS OF PAPILLEDEMA

Causes of increased intracranial pressure
Brain tumor
Subdural hematoma
Benign intracranial hypertension (pseudotumor cerebri)
Venous sinus thrombosis
Hydrocephalus
Causes of abnormal optic disc
Optic neuritis
Drusen

Approximately 10% to 20% of adult patients with new-onset seizures have brain tumors,[7] and such patients should almost always have MR imaging as part of their evaluation, especially if they also have focal findings on examination or on electroencephalography (EEG). Patients with malignant gliomas who present with seizures tend to have a better prognosis, possibly because their tumors are diagnosed at an earlier stage than tumors presenting with mass effect and focal deficits.[8]

Altered Mental Status

Mental status changes are the initial symptom in 15% to 20% of patients with brain tumors and are frequently present in patients by the time of diagnosis.[1] These changes may range from subtle problems with concentration, memory, affect, personality, initiative, and abstract reasoning to severe cognitive problems and confusion. Changes in mentation are especially common in frontal lobe tumors, but will also occur in patients with increased intracranial pressure or gliomatosis cerebri. With increasing intracranial pressure there is also depression of the level of consciousness, resulting in drowsiness and eventually culminating in stupor and coma if appropriate therapy is not administered.

Focal Neurologic Symptoms and Signs

Whereas headaches, seizures, and altered mental status may be seen with tumors in many locations, certain clinical features have specific localizing value.

Cortical Tumors

Frontal lobe tumors are often clinically silent initially. As the tumor enlarges there may be personality changes such as disinhibition, irritability, impaired judgment, and lack of initiative (abulia). In addition, there may be hemiparesis, seizures, aphasia, urinary frequency and urgency, and gait difficulties. Gaze preference and primitive reflexes, such as forced grasping and snout, may be present. Meningiomas of the olfactory groove may produce anosmia.

Temporal lobe tumors frequently cause seizures. These include simple partial seizures characterized by olfactory and gustatory hallucinations, déjà vu, and feelings of fear and pleasure, and by complex partial seizures characterized by impairment of consciousness, repetitive psychomotor movements, and automatic behavior. Temporal lobe tumors may also cause memory disturbances, visual field defects (superior quadrantanopsia), and when the dominant temporal lobe is involved, aphasia.

Tumors of the parietal lobe can produce contralateral sensory loss, involving particularly joint position sense, two-point discrimination, stereognosis, and graphesthesia, although other modalities are also involved. Lesions in the dominant parietal lobe are associated with aphasia, whereas lesions in the nondominant parietal lobe may result in neglect of the contralateral side and the loss of ability to acknowledge deficits (anosognosia). There may also be hemiparesis, homonymous visual defects (or neglect), agnosias, apraxias, sensory seizures, and disturbance of visual spatial ability.

Occipital lobe astrocytomas may cause homonymous hemianopsia and, less commonly, visual seizures characterized by lights, colors, and formed geometric patterns. Tumors at the parietooccipital junction may produce visual agnosias such as prosopagnosia (inability to recognize faces) or Balint syndrome.

Brainstem Tumors

Thalamic tumors may produce contralateral sensory loss, hemiparesis, cognitive impairment, and occasionally visual defects and aphasia. Obstructive hydrocephalus occurs commonly and is associated with headache, nausea, vomiting, gait unsteadiness, and urinary incontinence.

Brainstem tumors produce cranial neuropathies, weakness, numbness, and ataxia, and occasionally vertigo, nausea, vomiting, and hiccups. As the tumor increases in size, compression of the aqueduct or the fourth ventricle may occur, producing hydrocephalus.

Pineal Region and Third Ventricular Tumors

Pineal tumors present either with symptoms of hydrocephalus as a result of compression of the third ventricle and aqueduct, or with symptoms produced by compression of the tectum of the midbrain. Midbrain compression may result in disturbance of extraocular function including Parinaud syndrome, characterized by impairment of upgaze and minimal pupillary reaction to light, with preservation of accommodation (pupillary light-near dissociation). Occasionally children may present with precocious puberty.

Tumors around the third ventricle may produce hydrocephalus. Valsalva maneuvers and positional changes may increase cerebral spinal fluid (CSF) obstruction and lead to severe headaches and occasionally leg weakness and syncope. Tumors in this region may also produce symptoms resulting from hypothalamic dysfunction, autonomic dysfunction, and impaired memory.

Cerebellar Tumors

Headaches and ataxia are the two most common symptoms in patients with cerebellar tumors. The headaches may be caused by the tumor or by hydrocephalus. They are often occipital and associated with nausea, vomiting, and occasionally neck stiffness. Some patients may experience vertigo. Midline cerebellar lesions may produce truncal ataxia, while lesions in the cerebellar hemispheres may cause appendicular ataxia, although frequently the findings are relatively subtle. Examination may also show nystagmus, hypotonia, and, frequently, cranial nerve and corticospinal tract signs from brainstem compression. Head tilt away from the lesion may occur with incipient tonsillar herniation.

Cranial Nerves

Skull base tumors frequently affect cranial nerves. The pattern of involvement and the presence of accompanying neurologic signs depend on the location of the tumor. Meningiomas of the olfactory groove may produce anosmia. Involvement of the optic nerve by optic nerve gliomas or meningiomas may produce unilateral visual loss and should be distinguished from optic neuritis or other primary optic nerve problems. Rarely, a large optic nerve meningioma may lead to optic atrophy in the ipsilateral eye as a result of compression of that nerve, and papilledema in the contralateral eye as a result of increased intracranial pressure from its mass effect (Foster-Kennedy syndrome). Visual field defects are common. Bitemporal hemianopia is caused by pituitary adenomas or suprasellar tumors; homonymous hemianopias are caused by intrinsic tumors involving the optic radiations. Ophthalmoplegia may occur with meningiomas of the cavernous sinus or brainstem gliomas. Unilateral sixth nerve palsy is frequently a false localizing sign reflecting increased intracranial pressure. Peripheral facial nerve weakness is uncommon as a tumor finding except with very large vestibular schwannomas. Hearing loss, on the other hand, is a common finding with large vestibular schwannomas, and sensorineural loss should be investigated by MR imaging. Lower cranial nerve deficits usually result from brainstem or posterior fossa tumors. Multiple cranial nerve palsies occur with leptomeningeal metastases, in which tumor nodules coat the cranial nerves.

False Localizing Signs

Occasionally, when tumors produce increased intracranial pressure, shifting of intracranial structures occurs and results in clinical features suggesting involvement of sites distant from the tumor, that is, false localizing signs. Examples of this include abducens (sixth) nerve palsy resulting from compression of the nerve as it passes forward over the petrous ligament, and compression of the cerebral peduncle by the free edge of the tentorium cerebelli contralateral to a herniating uncus, producing hemiparesis on the same side as the lesion.[2]

Differential Diagnosis

Clinically, many conditions producing increased intracranial pressure or progressive neurologic deficits mimic brain tumors (Table 3-2). These include subdural hematomas, brain abscesses, hydrocephalus, benign

▶ TABLE 3-2. DIFFERENTIAL DIAGNOSIS OF SINGLE BRAIN LESION

Tumors
- Primary brain tumor (including primary central nervous system lymphoma)
- Metastatic brain tumor

Hamartoma

Vascular
- Cerebral hemorrhage
- Cerebral infarction
- Aneurysm
- Arteriovenous malformation
- Cavernous angioma

Infection
- Abscess
- Progressive multifocal leukoencephalopathy (PML)
- Lyme disease
- Syphilis
- Viral encephalitis (e.g., herpes simplex encephalitis)

Inflammation
- Multiple sclerosis
- Postinfectious encephalomyelitis
- Systemic lupus erythematosus (SLE)
- Sarcoidosis
- Vasculitis

Degenerative disorders

Trauma

Benign cyst

intracranial hypertension, progressive multifocal leukoencephalopathy, multiple sclerosis, vascular malformations, cerebral infarctions, Alzheimer disease, and some congenital anomalies. Many of these conditions have characteristic radiologic appearances that enable them to be differentiated from brain tumors. However, some of these conditions cannot be distinguished from brain tumors on the basis of their radiologic appearances alone, and a definite diagnosis often requires biopsy. These include brain abscesses, certain inflammatory lesions, demyelinating disease, hamartomas, and congenital anomalies. Even when the imaging characteristics of a lesion are very suggestive of a tumor, a biopsy is usually indicated to obtain tissue for precise histologic diagnosis and grading of the tumor, because these factors will have an important influence on treatment.

▶ RADIOLOGIC DIAGNOSIS

The introduction of CT scanning and MR imaging has revolutionized the diagnosis and management of brain tumors.[9,10] Because radiologic studies play a central role in the evaluation of brain tumor patients, they are briefly discussed here. However, Chapter 4 provides a more comprehensive review of the topic.

Skull X-Rays

Plain skull films are rarely necessary today with the widespread availability of CT and MR imaging. Occasionally, they may be useful to demonstrate calcification, bony erosion, or hyperostosis. The presence of calcifications usually indicates a relatively slow-growing tumor. Calcification occurs in 70% to 80% of craniopharyngiomas, 50% to 60% of oligodendrogliomas, 50% of ependymomas, 35% of gangliogliomas, 20% of astrocytomas, and approximately 10% of meningiomas.[11] Persistent elevation of intracranial pressure can result in erosion of normally calcified structures. In children, erosion of the inner table of the skull may lead to a "hammered metal" appearance. Pituitary tumors may produce erosion of the clinoid processes and sella turcica. Slow-growing tumors such as meningiomas may produce hyperostosis of the adjacent skull.

Computed Tomography

Computed tomography remains the most widely used form of neuroimaging for the diagnosis of brain tumors because of its wider availability and lower cost, although magnetic resonance imaging (MRI) is used with increasing frequency. The use of contrast enhancement is indispensable in the evaluation of brain tumors and may help disclose an isodense lesion from the surrounding parenchyma or a hypodense lesion hidden within an area of edema. CT scans will detect more than 90% of brain tumors. Small tumors (<0.5 cm); tumors adjacent to bone such as pituitary adenomas, clival tumors, and vestibular schwannomas; brainstem tumors; and low-grade astrocytomas may be missed and are better detected by the more sensitive MRI. CT scans tends to be better tolerated than MRI because of shorter scanning time and are more sensitive for detecting acute hemorrhage, calcifications, and bony involvement. Although CT scans are generally less sensitive than MR scans, the CT appearances of certain tumors may be more specific. For example, small round cell tumors such as medulloblastomas are isodense or hyperdense compared to brain parenchyma before contrast administration, whereas astrocytomas are almost always hypodense. Thus medulloblastomas can frequently be differentiated from cerebellar astrocytomas with the use of CT scanning. MR appearances of tumors tend to be less specific and making a similar differentiation with MR imaging is often more difficult.

Magnetic Resonance Imaging

MRI has assumed an increasingly important role in the diagnosis of brain tumors. It is now the preferred modality for the definitive evaluation and followup of most brain tumors. MRI has the advantage of being more sensitive than CT scan, enabling the detection of small tumors that may be missed with CT scan. It provides much greater anatomic detail in multiple planes and is especially useful for visualizing skull base, brainstem, and posterior fossa tumors. MRI is also superior to CT scan in detecting hemorrhage and solid and cystic components within tumors, and in demonstrating the relationship of the tumors to intracranial vessels.[9] As with CT scans, the administration of contrast agents such as gadopentate dimeglumine (Magnevist), gadoteridol (ProHance), and gadodiamide (Omniscan) to T_1-weighted MR scans greatly increases the sensitivity of the test.[12]

MRI is evolving rapidly. Newer imaging sequences, such as echoplanar MRI, are continually being developed, reducing scan times and improving the information obtained from the images. Echoplanar MRI can scan images in less than 100 milliseconds and provide information on tumor diffusion and perfusion. Diffusion-weighted MR imaging allows the assessment of the mobility of water molecules and may be useful in helping to differentiate tumor from edema, cystic changes, and normal white matter.[13,14] However, the differences in diffusion constants between these entities are relatively small, potentially limiting the usefulness of this approach. With perfusion-weighted MR, multiple repeat images are taken during the first pass of a bolus of MR contrast agent. The resultant changes in signal intensity are used to determine the regional cerebral blood volume (rCBV) in tumors. The rCBV appears to be increased in higher grades of tumor.[15,16] rCBV images have been used to guide stereotactic brain biopsies to areas with potentially the highest grade of tumor and to differentiate recurrent tumor from radiation necrosis.[16]

Magnetic resonance spectroscopy (MRS) is a noninvasive method that allows direct investigation of tumor metabolism and provides information on the composition and spatial distribution of cellular metabolites.[17] Most MRS studies are done with proton (^1H) or phosphorus-31. With proton MRS, tumors tend to have increased lactate production, loss of *N*-acetylaspartate (NAA) (reflecting loss of neurons in the tumor area), and increased choline levels (reflecting active membrane biosynthesis).[17] There is currently great interest in evaluating the usefulness of MRS in noninvasively diagnosing tumors, determining tumor grade, and differentiating tumor from radiation effects.[17,18]

MR angiography provides a means of displaying blood vessels in the brain in a noninvasive manner. It is being used increasingly in place of conventional angiography, although angiography has better resolution and is still necessary in certain situations. MRI is also being integrated with advanced image-processing techniques to produce three-dimensional definition of brain tumors to aid in surgical planning.[19]

Angiography

The importance of angiography has diminished significantly with the availability of CT and MR imaging. It is no longer used for the routine diagnosis of brain tumors. Its role is limited to (a) the preoperative evaluation of the vascular anatomy in certain patients (e.g., sphenoid wing meningioma encircling the carotid artery), (b) assessment of the patency of venous sinuses in extracerebral tumors (e.g., falx meningioma), (c) as part of the procedure for embolizing large tumors such as meningiomas, and (d) ruling out the presence of arteriovenous malformations and aneurysms in patients who present with hemorrhage. However, MR angiography has increasingly taken the place of conventional angiography for most of these indications with the exception of embolization.

Positron Emission Tomography

Positron emission tomography (PET) is a versatile imaging modality that provides dynamic information regarding the blood flow, metabolism, and physiology of the brain and brain tumors.[20–22] Unfortunately, its use is limited by its high cost, restricted availability, and limited scanner resolution. PET is not used for the routine diagnosis of brain tumors, but it can provide important information complementing that obtained by CT and MR scanning.

Positron-emitting radioactive isotopes of oxygen (^{15}O), fluorine (^{18}F, a substitute for hydrogen), carbon (^{11}C), and nitrogen (^{13}N) are produced in a cyclotron, incorporated into a chosen metabolite, and injected intravenously. These isotopes decay spontaneously by emitting positrons. When these positrons encounter an electron there is annihilation of both the positron and electron with emission of two 511-kiloelectron volt (keV) photons traveling at 180 degrees to each other. The PET scanner contains a ring of collimators surrounding the subject's head to detect these photons. Computers are then used to measure the count density and reconstruct images. In this way an image of the brain can be produced reflecting the regional variation in positron emission.

The most commonly used PET brain imaging isotope is [^{18}F] fluorodeoxyglucose (FDG). This isotope is relatively easy to synthesize and has a relatively long half-life of 110 minutes.[20–22] PET with FDG has been used noninvasively to determine tumor grade and prognosis in patients with malignant gliomas and to differentiate radiation necrosis from recurrent tumor.[21,22] However, the usefulness of FDG-PET is limited by a relatively high false-positive and false-negative rate, and by poor spatial resolution; it is less sensitive than MR imaging–based techniques in detecting lesions less than 1 cm in diameter.[16] PET has also been used to study the metabolic effects of chemotherapy, radiation therapy, and steroids on tumor metabolism.[22] It is possible that newer technologies such as methionine, tyrosine, choline, and thymidine-labeled PET scanning, based on amino acid membrane transport, protein synthesis, phospholipid uptake, and DNA synthesis, respectively, may be potentially more useful.[16,21,22]

Single-Photon Emission Computed Tomography

Single-photon emission computed tomography (SPECT) involves the intravenous administration of radiopharmaceuticals, which are taken up by the brain and tumor cells. These radiopharmaceuticals emit photons detected by a rotating gamma camera. Standard tomography reconstruction algorithms are then used to generate cross-sectional images of the brain. Although SPECT is not used in the initial diagnosis of brain tumors, it is increasingly being used to complement information obtained by CT or MRI scanning. Thallium-201 chloride, a potassium analogue that is taken up by viable tumor cells, has been used to differentiate low-grade from high-grade gliomas and to identify residual astrocytoma after radiation therapy.[21] It has also been used in combination with technetium-99m hexamethylpropylene amine oxime (^{99}Tc-HMPAO), a blood flow tracer that crosses normal blood–brain barrier, to differentiate radiation necrosis from recurrent glioma.[23,24] The usefulness of thallium-201 SPECT for gliomas is reduced by its limited sensitivity and specificity and by its inferior spatial resolution compared with MRI, or even PET.

Thallium-201 SPECT scans have also been useful in differentiating primary central nervous system lymphoma (PCNSL) in patients with AIDS from other intracerebral mass lesions, such as toxoplasmosis. Areas of lymphoma usually show high thallium uptake, whereas toxoplasmosis and other lesions such as progressive multifocal leukoencephalopathy (PML) do not. In one study, the sensitivity and specificity of thallium-201 SPECT in depicting lymphoma were 100% and 93%, respectively.[25]

Other SPECT radioisotopes that have been evaluated for brain tumors include technetium-99m methoxyisobutylisonitrile, iodine-123 iodo-methyltyrosine, and indium-111 octreotide.[21] Indium-111 octreotide binds to somatostatin receptors and has been used to image meningiomas, which display high concentrations of these receptors.[26]

Ultrasonography

Ultrasonography is frequently the screening procedure of choice for fetal and infant tumors. It does not have a diagnostic role in adults, but may serve as a useful intraoperative guide for intracranial tumors.

▶ LABORATORY DIAGNOSIS

Perimetry

Visual fields can be quantitatively evaluated using a combination of Goldmann kinetic perimetry and static perimetry using Humphriss visual fields. Measurement of visual fields is especially important in the evaluation of tumors in the vicinity of the optic chiasm such as pituitary adenomas. Perimetry may be useful in confirming deficits found on examination, detecting subtle changes not found on confrontation, and monitoring the effects of treatment. However, the accuracy of this test is greatly dependent on patient cooperation. The results tend to be unreliable in patients who are confused or agitated, or who have difficulty with fixation.

Electroencephalography

As previously reviewed, seizures are the presenting symptom in approximately one-third of patients with brain tumors. The presence of focal slow waves and spikes or frank epileptiform activity on EEG may be the first indication of a focal lesion and the need for cerebral imaging. Large tumors producing mass effect and tumors involving the diencephalon may produce asynchronous generalized slowing. However, the EEG is often normal or shows nonspecific slowing in patients with brain tumors and thus has limited value as a screening test.[4]

Evoked Potentials

Evoked potentials have a role in the diagnosis of certain brain tumors. The brainstem auditory-evoked potentials (BSAEPs) are abnormal in 92% to 96% of patients with vestibular schwannomas and are a cost-effective screening test for patients with a low probability of these tumors.[27] The most useful indications of compression of the auditory nerve are prolongation of the wave I–III and wave I–V interwave latencies. When wave I cannot be visualized, the ear-to-ear difference and the absolute latency of wave V may be useful. Compression of the anterior visual pathway by tumors can reduce the amplitude of visual-evoked potentials (VEPs). However, these tumors are usually diagnosed by MRI, and VEPs are rarely necessary. Evoked potentials also have an important role in monitoring neurologic function during surgical resection of tumors.

Cerebrospinal Fluid Analysis

Examination of the CSF can be useful in the diagnosis of certain brain tumors and in evaluating the extent of leptomeningeal spread. However, it is important to recognize that lumbar puncture holds definite risks for patients with increased intracranial pressure and should be avoided in these patients.

Examination of the CSF is useful in patients with PCNSL. It helps eliminate infections, which are often an important differential diagnosis, and may establish the diagnosis if tumor cells are identified. In patients with AIDS-related PCNSL, the polymerase chain reaction (PCR) can be used to detect Epstein-Barr virus (EBV) DNA in the cerebrospinal fluid. The presence of EBV DNA in the CSF, together with increased uptake by the tumors of thallium on SPECT scans, is highly suggestive of PCNSL.[28] The detection of JC virus DNA by PCR is useful for diagnosing progressive multifocal leukoencephalopathy, which can mimic tumors.[29]

A positive cytology may also be helpful in the diagnosis of pineal region tumors, which are often difficult to biopsy. Examination of the CSF is important in postoperative staging of patients with medulloblastomas and primitive neuroectodermal tumors because the presence of leptomeningeal disease influences prognosis and treatment. Cytologic examination of the CSF may also be useful in the diagnosis of leptomeningeal metastases in patients with metastatic brain tumors and occasionally in patients with gliomas with leptomeningeal spread. CSF cytology is usually not helpful in the initial diagnosis of gliomas.

Germ cell tumors arising in the pineal region may produce biologic markers such as α-fetoprotein, β subunit of human chorionic gonadotrophin, and placental alkaline phosphatase. The presence of these markers helps in the diagnosis and subsequent followup of these germ cell tumors.

Audiometry

Audiometry can be a useful screening test for the diagnosis of cerebellopontine angle tumors. Of patients with vestibular schwannomas, 98% have sensorineural hearing loss on pure tone audiometry. The most common pattern is high-frequency hearing loss together with reduced speech discrimination. Vestibular testing, including electronystagmography, may be positive in patients with cerebellopontine angle tumors but is rarely needed.

Endocrine Evaluation

Tumors in the region of the pituitary gland and hypothalamus may be associated with a variety of endocrine abnormalities. Evaluation of the hypothalamic–pituitary axis involves measurement of hormonal levels in the blood and urine, dynamic testing, and, occasionally, hormonal sampling of venous sinuses to help localize the tumor.[30] Endocrine testing is becoming increasingly more important in the long-term management of brain tumor patients treated with radiotherapy. These patients frequently develop hypothyroidism, amenorrhea, and infertility, and in children, growth hormone deficiency.

▶ APPROACH TO PATIENT

The evaluation of patients suspected of having a brain tumor varies significantly, depending on the clinical setting and diagnostic suspicion. The general principles include:

1. Elimination of other potential nonneoplastic causes of the suspected lesion.
2. Determination of the extent of spread of the tumor throughout the nervous system and in the rest of the body, when appropriate.
3. Administration of supportive care (e.g., antiepileptic drugs, corticosteroids, emotional support).
4. Acquisition of tissue diagnosis by biopsy or surgical resection of the lesion.

Patients with a Single Brain Lesion

The evaluation of a patient who presents with new-onset neurologic symptoms and is found on neuroimaging studies to have a single, large, ring-enhancing mass is often fairly straightforward. Although there are many possibilities (see Tables 3-2 to 3-4), the most likely causes of intrinsic brain lesions are high-grade gliomas, metastasis, lymphoma, abscess, and demyelination, while the most likely cause of extraaxial lesions is a meningioma (Fig. 3-1). The differential diagnosis of single lesions in the pineal region, pituitary region, and cerebellopontine angle are summaried in Tables 3-5 to 3-7.

Diagnosis

Enhancing Lesions

GLIOMAS

The MR findings of patients with high-grade gliomas is usually fairly typical (Fig. 3-2). These patients should be placed on corticosteroids, if they are symptomatic, and referred for surgical resection or biopsy of the lesion.

▶ **TABLE 3-3.** DIFFERENTIAL DIAGNOSIS OF SUPRATENTORIAL TUMORS

Adults	Children	Infants
Metastases	Gliomas	Gliomas
Gliomas*	Ganglioglioma	PNET
Meningiomas	DNET	Germ cell tumors
Lymphomas	Neurocytoma	Choroid plexus tumors
Neurocytoma	PNET	Mesenchymal tumors (sarcoma, rhabdoid)
DNET		
Ependymomas		

*Includes variants such as ganglioglioma and pleomorphic xanthoastrocytoma.
DNET = dysembryoplastic neuroepithelial tumor; PNET = primitive neuroectodermal tumor.

▶ TABLE 3-4. DIFFERENTIAL DIAGNOSIS OF POSTERIOR FOSSA TUMORS

Adults	Children
Metastases	Cerebellar astrocytoma
Vestibular schwannoma	Medulloblastoma
Meningioma	Ependymoma
Hemangioblastoma	Brainstem glioma
Epidermoid	Dermoid
Brainstem glioma	Teratoma
Chordoma	Ganglioglioma
Ependymoma	Gangliocytoma (Lhermitte-Duclos)
Sarcoma	Choroid plexus papilloma and carcinoma
Paraganglioma	Neuroblastoma
Choroid plexus papilloma	

Increasingly, MR spectroscopy, PET scanning, and perfusion MRI are used to complement conventional MRI and allow the most active areas of the tumor to be targeted for biopsy or resection.[15,21,22]

▶ TABLE 3-5. DIFFERENTIAL DIAGNOSIS OF PINEAL REGION TUMORS

Germ cell tumors
Germinoma
Teratoma
Choriocarcinoma
Endodermal sinus (yolk sac tumor)
Embryonal carcinoma
Pineal parenchymal cell tumors
Pineocytoma
Pineoblastoma
Other tumors
Astrocytomas
Meningiomas
Metastases
Benign lesions
Pineal cyst
Lipomas
Epidermoid cyst
Arachnoid cyst
Vascular malformation

Brain Metastasis

In patients with a history of cancer or a history of smoking, a brain metastasis must be considered (Fig. 3-3). Patients without a history of cancer should have a complete general physical examination, complete blood count, sedimentation rate, urinalysis for hematuria, stool guaiac for occult blood, and chest radiograph. In selected patients, CT scans of the chest, abdomen, and pelvis and serum tumor markers (e.g., carcinoembryonic antigen [CEA], CA 15-3 and CA 27-29 for breast cancer, CA-125 for

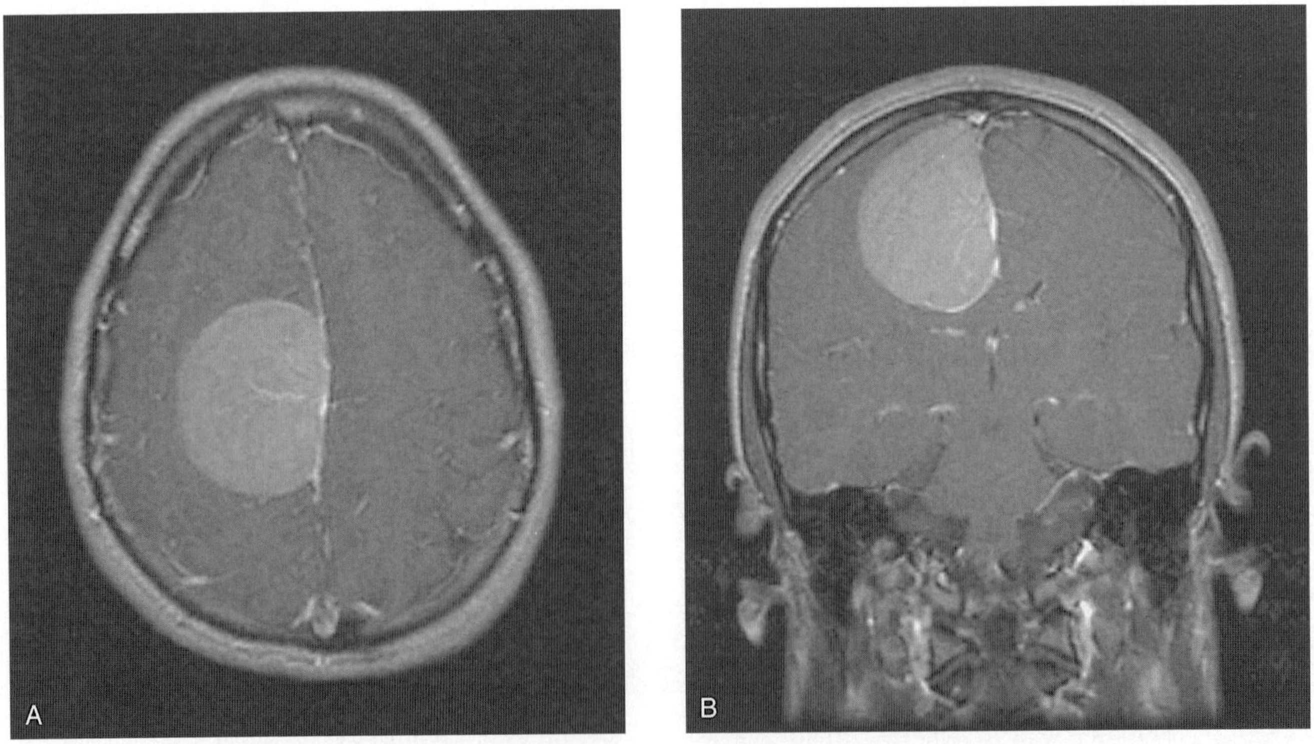

Figure 3-1. (A) Axial and (B) coronal T_1-weighted MRI of the brain with contrast showing large right parasagittal meningioma.

▶ TABLE 3-6. DIFFERENTIAL DIAGNOSIS OF PITUITARY REGION TUMORS

Tumors
Pituitary adenoma
Craniopharyngioma
Metastases
Meningioma
Glioma
Germinoma
Lymphoma
Dermoid/epidermoid
Lipoma
Nasopharyngeal carcinoma
Benign lesions
Hamartoma
Inflammatory lesions
Histiocytosis
Sarcoidosis
Hypophysitis
Cysts
Arachnoid
Rathke cleft
Colloid
Vascular lesions
Aneurysm

ovarian cancer) may be indicated to look for evidence of a primary tumor. If these tests are negative and there remains strong suspicion that the brain lesion is a metastasis, a PET scan may be helpful in detecting the primary tumor.[31] If a systemic primary tumor is found, it should be biopsied or resected to obtain a histologic diagnosis. The brain metastasis may be resected to obtain tissue if the systemic primary tumor is not easily accessible, or as part of the treatment of a single brain metastasis.[32]

▶ TABLE 3-7. DIFFERENTIAL DIAGNOSIS OF CEREBELLOPONTINE ANGLE TUMORS

Tumors
Vestibular schwannoma
Meningioma
Other schwannomas, e.g., trigeminal
Metastasis
Paraganglioma
Ependymoma
Choroid plexus papilloma
Lipoma
Exophytic glioma
Chordoma
Chondrosarcoma
Cystic lesions
Epidermoid cyst
Dermoid cyst
Arachnoid cyst
Vascular lesions
Aneurysm

For patients with a known underlying cancer, restaging studies (CT scan of the chest, abdomen, and pelvis, and possibly bone scans) and measurement of appropriate serum tumor markers should be performed. Patients with disseminated disease are more likely to have brain metastases, and the extent of the systemic disease is an important factor in determining the most appropriate therapy.

Primary Central Nervous System Lymphoma

A single enhancing mass may be caused by PCNSL, although this tumor frequently presents with multiple lesions. The diagnosis is usually made by biopsy, but examination of the cerebrospinal fluid is often useful, especially if biopsy is thought to be difficult. There may

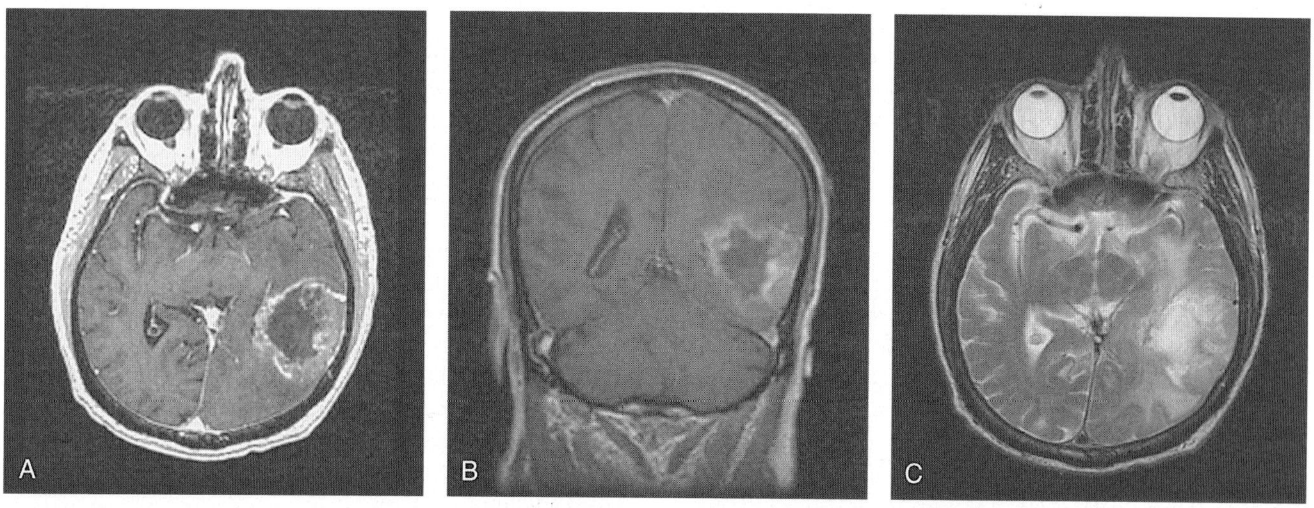

Figure 3-2. (A) Axial and (B) coronal T_1-weighted MRI of the brain with contrast showing left posterior temporal glioblastoma. (C) Axial T_2-weighted MRI showing extent of peritumoral edema.

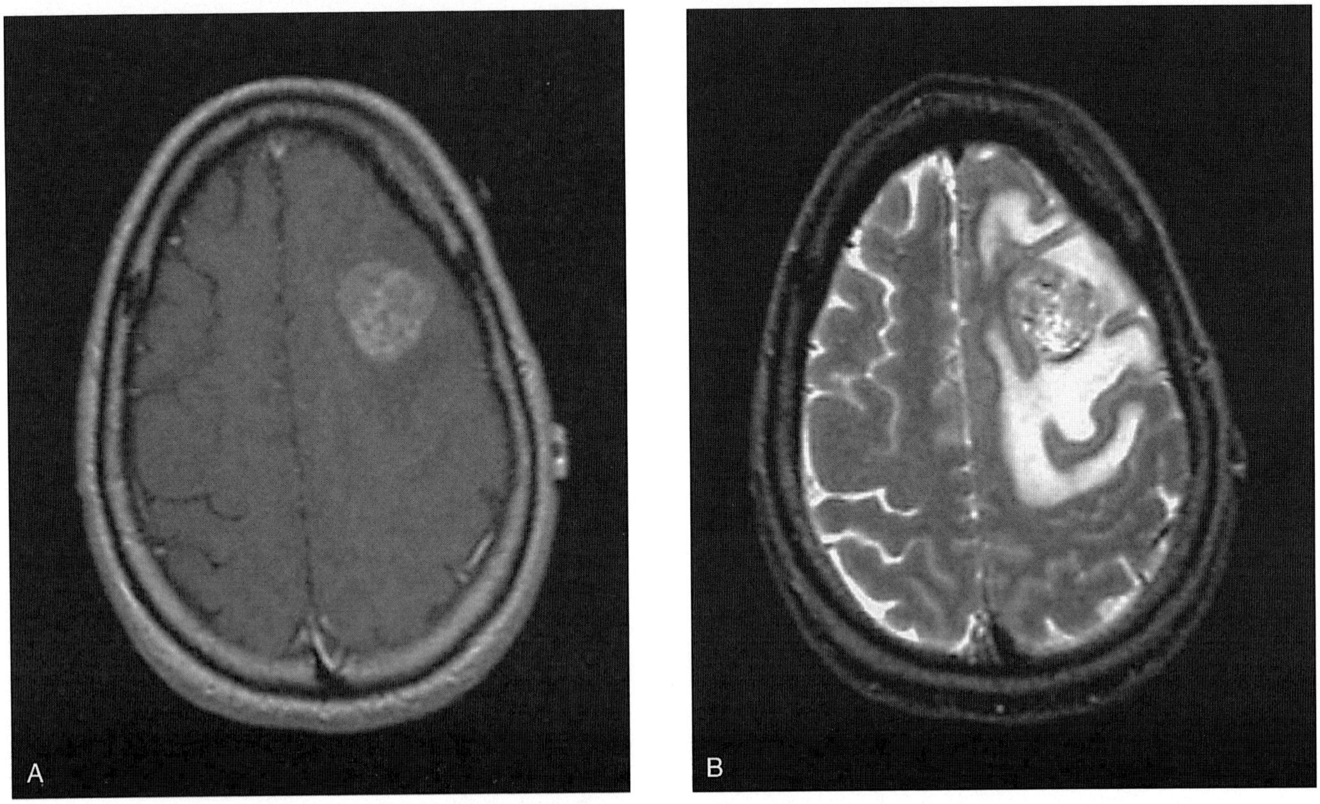

Figure 3-3. (A) Axial T_1-weighted MRI of the brain with contrast and (B) axial T_2-weighted MRI showing left frontal brain metastasis from a 58-year-old woman with breast cancer.

be lymphocytic pleocytosis (50%), elevated protein (85%) (rarely above 150 mg/dL), and in severe cases, low glucose. Cytologic examination may show neoplastic cells, although it may be difficult to differentiate these from reactive lymphocytes. When cytology is equivocal, the finding of a monoclonal B-cell population on immunoperoxidase or the demonstration of clonality of immunoglobulin gene rearrangement may help in establishing the diagnosis.[33] In patients infected with HIV, examination of the CSF for the EBV DNA by PCR may help with the diagnosis of lymphoma.[28]

In immunocompromised patients, the main differential diagnosis is toxoplasmosis. If the patient has toxoplasma antibodies, a therapeutic trial with antitoxoplasma therapy is often used to help make the diagnosis. Patients who do not respond to antitoxoplasma therapy have a high probability of having PCNSL and have traditionally undergone a stereotactic biopsy. There is increasing evidence that patients with both a positive thallium-201 SPECT scan and the presence of EBV DNA in the cerebrospinal fluid have a very high likelihood of having AIDS-related PCNSL (almost 100% sensitivity and negative predictive value).[28,34] Patients with these findings might reasonably undergo treatment without the need for a biopsy. In contrast, patients with hypoactive lesions on thallium-201 SPECT scans and negative EBV DNA should undergo empiric antitoxoplasma therapy, while patients with discordant SPECT/PCR results probably should undergo a biopsy.

Benign Conditions

Although there are many benign causes of a single enhancing lesion (see Table 3-2), the most common ones are abscesses and demyelination. The presence of fever and impaired immunity often help with the diagnosis of abscess. However, patients with impaired immunity may have both a tumor and infection (e.g., renal transplant recipients with lymphoma *and* infection).[35] Occasionally, CSF examination, blood cultures, serology, MRS, and PET imaging may be useful in differentiating abscesses from tumors. However, a stereotactic biopsy is usually needed.

Demyelinating disorders usually result in multiple lesions in the brain, but single enhancing demyelinating masses can occur, so-called tumefactive multiple sclerosis.[36] These patients tend to be young and there may be other evidence of demyelination in the nervous system on clinical examination or evoked potentials. Cerebrospinal fluid may show the presence of pleocytosis and oligoclonal bands; MRS and PET imaging may be helpful. If a demyelinating process is suspected, close observation is indicated. However, a biopsy is sometimes needed to make a definitive diagnosis.

Patients with Nonenhancing Lesions

The evaluation of a patient with a nonenhancing lesion with increased T_2 and fluid-attenuated inversion recovery (FLAIR) signal on MRI is often more complicated. The differential diagnosis includes low-grade gliomas (Fig. 3-4), nonenhancing high-grade gliomas, dysembryoplastic neuroepithelial tumors (DNT) (Fig. 3-5), hamartomas, encephalomalacia from prior trauma, cerebral infarctions, small vessel vascular disease, demyelination, infections, inflammation from a variety of causes such as systemic lupus erythematosus or Behçet disease, and vasculitis. MR spectroscopy is occasionally helpful in differentiating tumor from benign causes. Tumors may show an elevated choline and decreased NAA peaks. Conventional FDG-PET scans are often unhelpful as FDG uptake may be low both in low-grade neoplasms and in benign lesions. The number of lesions can be helpful because the presence of multiple lesions makes a primary brain neoplasm much less likely. The evaluation of these patients depends on the clinical suspicion. In young patients, especially women, the main differential diagnosis is between a low-grade tumor and demyelination. Careful examination of the patient for evidence of multiple lesions (e.g., optic atrophy or spinal cord lesion), a complete evoked potential battery, and in selected patients, CSF examination for oligoclonal bands and contrast-enhanced MRI of the spine, may be helpful in making the diagnosis of a demyelinating disorder. Other tests that may be helpful in selected patients include antinuclear antigen (systemic lupus erythematosus), Lyme antibody titer (Lyme disease), rapid plasma reagin (RPR) (syphilis), erythrocyte sedimentation rate (ESR), angiotensin-converting enzyme (sarcoidosis), CSF examination (infections, including PCR for JC virus in PML), and, in rare cases, angiography (vasculitis). Despite these tests, the diagnosis may still be in doubt. In this situation, patients should be followed closely with serial scans if the possibility of tumor is low, or undergo a stereotactic biopsy or resection if the likelihood of tumor is high.

STAGING

Most primary gliomas do not disseminate throughout the neuraxis, and staging studies are unnecessary. Medulloblastomas, pineoblastomas, and other primitive neuroectodermal tumors, pineal germ cells tumors, and

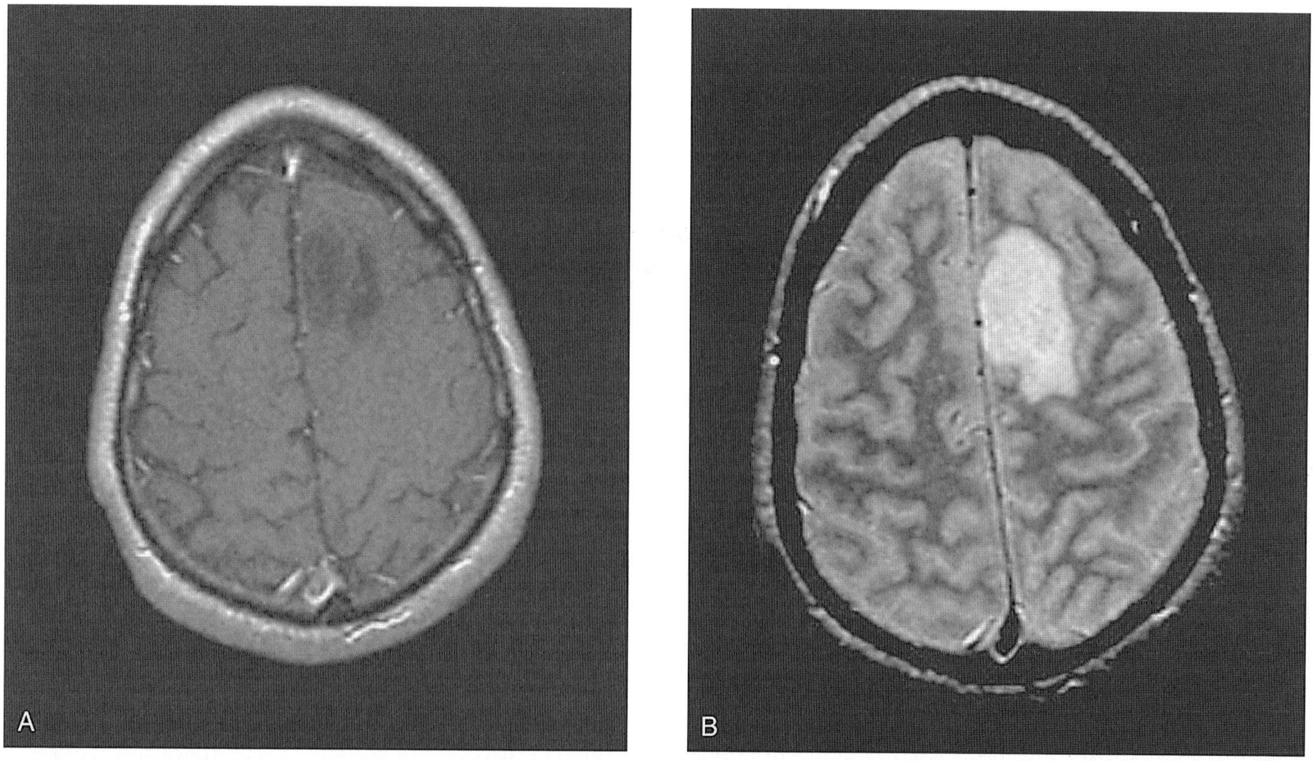

Figure 3-4. (A) Axial T_1-weighted MRI of the brain with contrast and (B) axial T_2-weighted MRI of the brain showing left frontal oligodendroglioma in a 32-year-old man who presented with new-onset seizures.

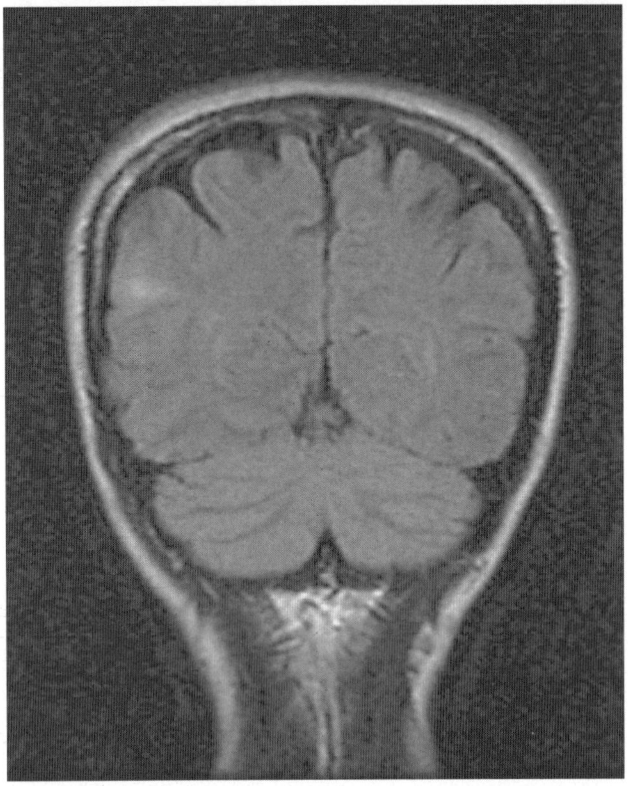

Figure 3-5. Coronal FLAIR MRI showing right parietal area of abnormal signal in a 36-year-old with a long history of seizures. Surgical resection showed a dysembryoplastic neuroepithelial tumor (DNT).

ependymomas may have drop metastases. Contrast-enhanced MRI of the spine and often examination of the CSF for tumor cells are indicated. These tests should ideally be performed prior to posterior fossa surgery, if it is safe to do so. For patients with primary CNS lymphoma, staging studies should include contrast-enhanced MRI of the spine and examination of the CSF (cytology is positive in 20%–40% of patients) and the eye (involved in 20% of patients) for evidence of tumor cells. CT scanning of the chest, abdomen, and pelvis and bone marrow examination in selected patients should also be performed but are rarely positive in immunocompetent patients. Patients with PCNSL should also have serologic testing for HIV.

▶ PATIENT WITH MULTIPLE BRAIN LESIONS

Table 3-8 details the differential diagnosis of a patient with multiple brain lesions. The most common cause is brain metastases (Fig. 3-6), and patients should undergo a full evaluation (as outlined above) to look for a systemic primary tumor. Other tests will vary depending on the diagnostic suspicion.

▶ TABLE 3-8. DIFFERENTIAL DIAGNOSIS OF MULTIPLE BRAIN LESIONS

Tumor
Brain metastases
Primary CNS lymphoma
Intravascular lymphoma
Lymphomatoid granulomatosis
Multifocal glioma
Leptomeningeal metastases
Vascular
Multiple cerebral infarction
Small vessel disease
Cavernous angiomas
Multiple hemorrhages (amyloid angiopathy, blood dyscrasias, anticoagulation)
Inflammatory
Systemic lupus erythematosus
Vasculitis
Demyelination
Multiple sclerosis
Acute disseminated encephalomyelitis
Behçet
Sarcoidosis
Infections
Abscesses
Bacterial
Tuberculosis
Syphilis
Fungal
Toxoplasma
Cysticercosis
Developmental
Heterotopia
Trauma

Supportive Care

These issues are discussed in greater depth in Chapter 9 and in a recent review.[37] They are outlined only briefly here.

Antiepileptic Drugs

Patients who present with seizures should be treated with standard antiepileptic drugs (AEDs). Although phenytoin remains the most commonly used medication, increasingly patients are treated with newer agents such as levetiracetam that are generally well-tolerated and do not require monitoring of serum drug levels and hematologic or liver function tests. Most of the newer AEDs also do not induce hepatic cytochrome P450 enzymes. This has become an increasingly important issue in brain tumor patients because many therapeutic agents are metabolized by the cytochrome P450 system. Patients receiving concomitant AEDs that induce hepatic P450 enzymes (e.g., phenytoin, phenobarbital, carbamazepine, and oxcarbazepine) frequently require much higher doses of the therapeutic agent than patients

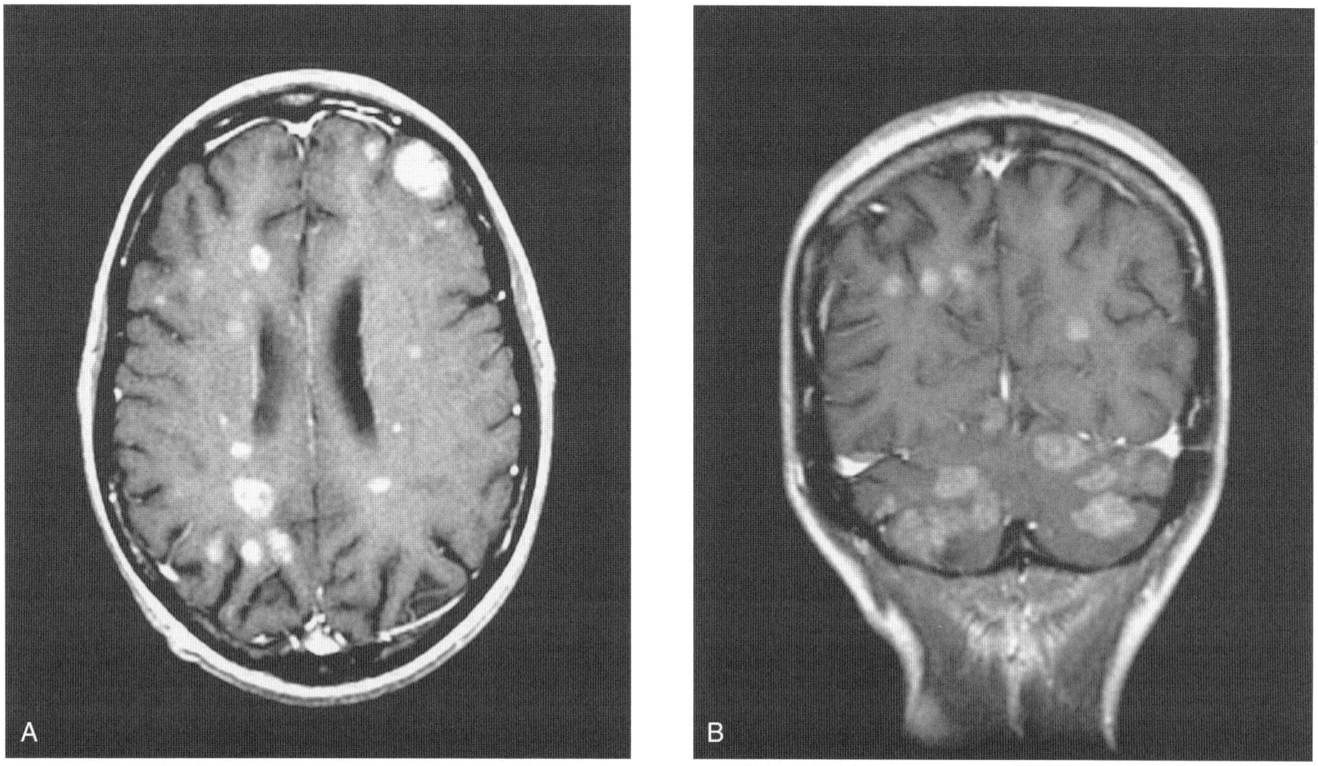

Figure 3-6. (A) Axial and (B) coronal T_1-weighted MRI of the brain with contrast showing multiple enhancing lesions in a 63-year-old man with non–small-cell lung cancer.

receiving non–enzyme-inducing AEDs.[38] Patients with posterior fossa tumors, pituitary tumors, or tumors involving the diencephalon or brainstem do not need AEDs. Patients with supratentorial tumors who have never had seizures probably do not need long-term AED,[39] but should be treated with an AED to prevent seizures during the perioperative period if surgery is planned.

Corticosteroids

Patients with suspected brain tumors who are symptomatic from peritumoral edema should begin treatment with corticosteroids (usually dexamethasone 16 mg a day in 2–4 divided doses). Corticosteroids are usually not required for patients with suspected low-grade gliomas or for asymptomatic patients. An exception may be asymptomatic patients with large tumors and mass effect who are scheduled to have surgery. The use of corticosteroids in these patients may help reduce the amount of peritumoral edema and facilitate surgical resection. For patients with suspected CNS lymphoma, every effort should be made to withhold corticosteroids until after tissue has been obtained for histologic diagnosis. Corticosteroids are cytotoxic to lymphoma cells, and their use prior to surgery may result in the biopsy specimen containing only nondiagnostic necrotic tissue (Fig. 3-7). The use of H_2 blockers and proton pump inhibitors should be restricted to patients receiving high doses of corticosteroids or for those who are at increased risk of gastritis and gastrointestinal bleeding, such as the elderly, those on anticoagulation, or those taking nonsteroidal anti-inflammatory medications.[37] Brain tumor patients on prolonged courses of corticosteroids are at increased risk of developing *Pneumocystis* pneumonitis[40] and benefit from prophylactic treatment. However, prophylactic treatment can be safely deferred until the postoperative period when it is usually apparent whether a patient will require prolonged corticosteroids therapy.

Prophylactic Therapy for Venous Thromboembolic Disease

Venous thromboembolic disease (VTED) is a common complication in patients with most malignant brain tumors and meningiomas, especially in the perioperative period.[37] Patients should receive prophylactic therapy for VTED, and there should be a low threshold for evaluating brain tumor patients for this complication.

Psychosocial Support

The diagnosis of a brain tumor is usually devastating, and most patients will benefit from support from social service, psychiatry, and patient support groups, and from information provided by societies such as the American

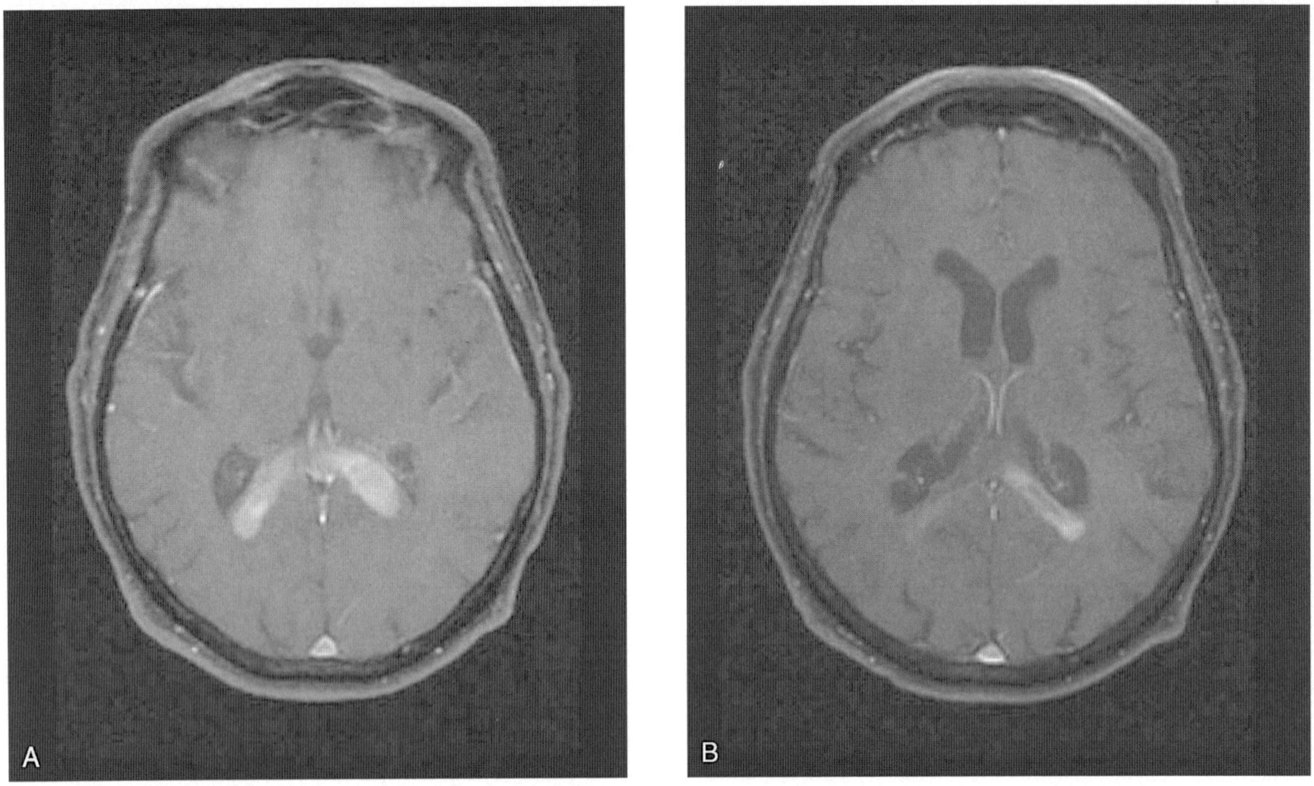

Figure 3-7. Axial T_1-weighted MRI of the brain with contrast before (A) and after 1 week on dexamethasone (B) in an 83-year-old woman with primary CNS lymphoma showing significant reduction in enhancement as a result of the corticosteroids therapy.

Brain Tumor Association [2720 River Road, Des Plaines, IL 60018; (847) 827-9910; Patient Line: (800) 886-2282; e-mail: info@abta.org], the Brain Tumor Society [124 Watertown Street, Suite 3-H, Watertown, MA 02472; (800) 770-TBTS (8287); e-mail: info@tbts.org], and the National Brain Tumor Foundation [414 Thirteenth Street, Suite 700, Oakland, CA 94612-2603; (510) 839-9777; Brain Tumor Information Line: (800) 934-CURE (2873), e-mail: nbtf@braintumor.org].

REFERENCES

1. Thomas DGT, McKeran RO. Clinical manifestations of brain tumors. In: Thomas DGT, ed. Neuro-oncology. Primary malignant brain tumors. Baltimore: Johns Hopkins University Press, 1990:94–121.
2. Jaeckle KA, Cohen ME, Duffner PK. Clinical presentation and therapy of nervous system tumors. In: Bradley WG, Daroff RB, Fenichel GM, Marsden CD, eds. Neurology in clinical practice, 2nd ed. Boston: Butterworth-Heinemann, 1996:1131–1149.
3. Wen PY. Diagnosis and management of brain tumors. In: Black P McL, Loeffler JS, eds. Cancer of the nervous system. Cambridge, UK: Blackwell Science, 1997:106–127.
4. Wen PY, Teoh SK, Black PM. Clinical, imaging and laboratory diagnosis of brain tumors. In: Laws E, Kaye A, eds. Brain tumors, 2nd ed. Edinburgh: Churchill Livingstone, 2001:217–248.
5. Forsyth P, Posner JB. Headaches in patients with brain tumors: a study of 111 patients. Neurology 1993;43:1678–1683.
6. Scott GM, Gibberd FB. Epilepsy and other factors in the prognosis of gliomas. Acta Neurol Scand 1980;61:227–239.
7. Dam AM, Fuglsang-Frederiksen A, Svarre-Olsen, et al. Late onset epilepsy: etiologies, type of seizure, and value of clinical investigation, EEG and computerized tomography scan. Epilepsia 1985;26:227–231.
8. Gehan EA, Walker MD. Prognostic factors for patients with brain tumors. Natl Cancer Inst Monogr 1977;46:189–195.
9. Ricci PE. Imaging of brain tumors. Neuroimaging Clin N Am 1999;9:651–669.
10. Stark AA, Bradley WG. Magnetic resonance imaging, 3rd ed. St. Louis: Mosby, 1999.
11. Segall HD, Destian S, Nelson S, et al. CT and MR imaging in malignant gliomas. In: Apuzzo MLJ, ed. Malignant cerebral glioma. Park Ridge, IL: American Association of Neurologic Surgeons, 1990:63–78.
12. Abdullah ND, Mathews VP. Contrast issues in brain tumor imaging. Neuroimaging Clin N Am 1999;9:733–749.
13. Nelson SJ. Imaging of brain tumors after therapy. Neuroimaging Clin N Am 1999;9:801–819.

14. Rowley HA, Grant PE, Roberts TPL. Diffusion MR imaging. Neuroimaging Clin N Am 1999;9:343–361.
15. Aronen HJ, Perkio J. Dynamic susceptibility contrast MRI of gliomas. Neuroimaging Clin N Am 2002;12(4):501–523.
16. Lev MH, Rosen BR. Clinical applications of intracranial perfusion MR imaging. Neuroimaging Clin N Am 1999; 9(2):309–331.
17. Nelson SJ, McNight TR, Henry RG. Characterization of untreated gliomas by magnetic resonance spectroscopy. Neuroimaging Clin N Am 2002;12:599–614.
18. Rand SD, Prost R, Li S-J. Proton MR spectroscopy of the brain. Neuroimaging Clin N Am 1999;9:379–395.
19. Grimson WEL, Kikinis R, Jolesz FA, Black PMcL. Image guided surgery. Sci Am 1999;280:63–69.
20. Di Chiro G. Positron emission tomography using (18F) fluorodeoxyglucose in brain tumors. A powerful diagnostic and prognostic tool. Invest Radiol 1987;22:360–371.
21. Hustinx R, Alavi A. SPECT and PET imaging of brain tumors. Neuroimaging Clin N Am 1999;9:751–766.
22. Spence AM, Mankoff DA, Muzi M. Positron emission tomography of brain tumors. Neuroimaging Clin N Am 2003;13:715–739.
23. Carvalho PA, Schwartz, RB, Alexander E, et al. Detection of recurrent gliomas with quantitative thallium-201/technetium-99m HMPAO single-photon emission computerized tomography. J Neurosurg 1992;77:565–570.
24. Schwartz RB, Holman BL, Polak JF, et al. Dual-isotope single-photon emission computerized tomography scanning in patients with glioblastoma multiforme: association with patient survival and histopathological characteristics of tumor after high dose radiotherapy. J Neurosurg 1998;89:60–68.
25. Kessler LS, Ruiz A, Donovan Post MJ, et al. Thallium-201 brain SPECT of lymphoma in AIDS patients: pitfalls and technique optimization. Am J Neuroradiol 1998;19:1105–1109.
26. Klutmann S, Bohuslavizki KH, Brenner W, et al. Somatostatin receptor scintigraphy in post-surgical follow-up examinations of meningiomas. J Nucl Med 1998;39:1913–1917.
27. Welling DB, Glasscock ME, Woods CI, Jackson CG. Acoustic neuroma: a cost effective approach. Otolaryngol Head Neck Surg 1990;103:364–370.
28. Antinori A, De Rossi G, Ammassari A, et al. Value of combined approach with thallium-201 single-photon emission computed tomography and Epstein-Barr virus DNA polymerase chain reaction in CSF for the diagnosis of AIDS-related primary CNS lymphoma. J Clin Oncol 1999;17:554–560.
29. Koralnik IJ, Boden D, Mai VX, et al. JC virus DNA load in patients with and without progressive multifocal leukoencephalopathy. Neurology 1999;52:253–260.
30. Simard MF. Pituitary tumor endocrinopathies and their endocrine evaluation. Neurosurg Clin N Am 2003;14(1): 41–54.
31. Rees JH, Hain SF, Johnson MR, et al. The role of [18F]fluoro-2-deoxyglucose-PET scanning in the diagnosis of paraneoplastic neurological disorders. Brain 2001;124:2223–2231.
32. Wen PY, Loeffler JS. Management of brain metastases. Oncology 1999;13:941–961.
33. Ferreri AJ, Abrey LE, Blay JY, et al. Summary statement on primary central nervous system lymphomas from the Eighth International Conference on Malignant Lymphoma, Lugano, Switzerland, June 12 to 15, 2002. J Clin Oncol 2003;21(12):2407–2414.
34. Lorberboym M, Wallach F, Estok L, et al. Thallium-201 retention in focal intracranial lesions for differential diagnosis of primary lymphoma and nonmalignant lesions in AIDS patients. J Nucl Med 1998;39:1366–1369.
35. Phan TG, O'Neill BP, Kurtin PJ. Posttransplant primary CNS lymphoma. Neuro-oncology 2000;2:229–238.
36. Kepes JJ. Large focal tumor-like demyelinating lesions of the brain: intermediate entity between multiple sclerosis and acute disseminated encephalomyelitis? A study of 31 patients. Ann Neurol 1993;33:18–27.
37. Wen PY, Marks PW: Medical management of patients with brain tumors. Curr Opin Oncol 2002;14(3):299–307.
38. Prados MD, Yung WYK, Jaeckle KA, et al. Phase I trial of irinotecan (CPT-11) in patients with recurrent malignant glioma: a North American Brain Tumor Consortium study. Neuro-oncology 2004;6:44–54.
39. Glantz MJ, Cole BF, Forsyth PA, et al. Practice parameter: anticonvulsant prophylaxis in patients with newly diagnosed brain tumors. Report of the Quality Standards Subcommittee of the American Academy of Neurology. Neurology 2000;54(10):1886–1893.
40. Slivka A, Wen PY, Shea WM, et al. *Pneumocystis carinii* pneumonia during steroid taper in patients with primary brain tumors. Am J Med 1993;94(2):216–219.

CHAPTER 4

Neuroimaging

L. BURT NABORS

The evaluation of patients with intracranial tumors is highly dependent on neuroimaging. The importance of the neuroimaging procedure and the role of different procedures vary and are dependent on the clinical setting. Patients who are newly diagnosed with brain tumors may require radiographic studies more suited to anatomic definition and detection of structural abnormalities. The utility of imaging studies may evolve during the course of a patient's treatment, with radiographic studies used more for the evaluation of tumor response to therapy or the differentiation of effects of treatment from tumor progression. The parameters of importance to both the neuroradiologist and clinician include signal contrast of the tumor, structural features, tumor extent or margins, the presence of contrast enhancement, and associated tumor phenomena such as necrosis and vasogenic edema. Until recently, imaging techniques have primarily relied on the discrimination of intracranial anatomy. Current advancements, however, are making it possible to measure noninvasively both physiologic and biochemical properties of intracranial tumors with perfusion, diffusion, or spectral acquisitions.

▶ MEDICAL IMAGE STORAGE AND RETRIEVAL

The advent of several medical imaging modalities including ultrasonography, computerized tomography (CT), magnetic resonance imaging (MRI), positron emission tomography (PET), and single-photon emission computed tomography (SPECT) has brought about the need for hardware and software alike that can save, retrieve, and interpret these images on a common platform. It is not unusual to acquire multiple modality acquisitions for a single patient. Consequently, unification of medical image databases and technology services has led to an increase in operational efficiency and reduction in medical error. This is evidenced by many hospitals integrating radiology information systems (RIS) and picture archiving and communication systems (PACS) to deliver the best radiology services. Indeed, neuroimaging stands to benefit significantly from such developments.

With the increasing use of computers in clinical and radiological applications, the American College of Radiology (ACR) and the National Electrical Manufacturers Association (NEMA) recognized the emerging need for a standard method for transferring images and associated information between devices manufactured by various vendors. These devices produce a variety of digital image formats. The ACR and the NEMA formed a joint committee in 1983 to develop a standard to

- Promote communication of digital image information, regardless of device manufacturer.
- Facilitate the development and expansion of PACS that can also interface with other systems of hospital information.

- Allow the creation of diagnostic information databases that can be interrogated by a wide variety of devices distributed geographically.

ACR-NEMA *Standards Publication No. 300-1985*, published in 1985 was designated version 1.0. This standard has since evolved and is currently designated *Digital Imaging and Communications in Medicine* (DICOM). It embodies a number of major enhancements to previous versions of the ACR-NEMA standard. In addition to universal standards such as DICOM, most medical imaging equipment manufacturers have their own image formats.

The basic PACS organizational units are the image acquisition unit(s), the standardization protocols, the image management control, the telemedicine interface, and the display/evaluation. Important issues in PACS management include connectivity, reliability, security, and ease of operation. A large fraction of developments in radiology and imaging technology are specific to neuroimaging.

▶ BASIC CONCEPTS

The need for less invasive diagnostic tests and followup examinations has promoted the widespread use of neuroimaging in neuro-oncology. Depending on the patient's diagnosis, some of the different possible evaluations are MRI, CT, PET, and SPECT. Table 4-1 compares these techniques.

Computerized Tomography

Computerized tomography is created by a rotating x-ray beam, whose altered attenuation is registered by detectors situated around the patient as the ray goes through the body. Dense objects, such as bone, attenuate the ray more and appear brighter in the image, whereas less dense objects, such as brain tissue, have a lower attenuating effect and appear darker. Flowing blood has a higher density than brain tissue and appears lighter in the image; therefore it is possible to recognize the vascular system and any of its abnormalities possibly caused by trauma or tumor masses. The application of a contrast medium will enhance the image as a result of the breakdown at the blood–brain barrier, creating a lighter boundary in diseased tissue with a leaky blood–brain barrier compared with normal brain tissue. However, some of these agents can cause unwanted reactions in the patients.

Magnetic Resonance Imaging

MRI is the gold standard for diagnosis of brain tumors. In addition to high-resolution anatomic visualization, variants of MRI, such as functional MRI (fMRI), magnetic resonance (MR) spectroscopy (MRS) or MR spectroscopic imaging (MRSI), MR angiography (MRA), and perfusion and diffusion MRI, have been successfully used to study brain tumors in a clinical setting, including radiologic diagnosis, description of tumor characteristics, evaluation of size and volume, blood flow and volume computation, and determination of biochemical information. The chief advantage of using MRI over other imaging modalities is the excellent tissue contrast it affords coupled with very good resolution and sensitivity. MRI is also advantageous because it can image directly in several planes.

Protons (^{1}H) in water usually present low signal intensity on T_1-weighted images and high signal intensity on T_2-weighted images. Pathologic processes such as brain tumors and associated physiology produce an increase in extracellular water. MRI tissue contrast is hence most apparent in T_2 images. Nonetheless, most intracranial lesions possess great MR signal heterogeneity, especially higher grade neoplasms.

Magnetic resonance imaging allows rapid image acquisition and excellent analysis of the tissue architecture of the central nervous system. The retrieval of the images is possible because of the magnetization of dipoles containing ^{1}H, later altered by a radiofrequency (RF).

▶ TABLE 4-1. COMPARISON OF NEUROIMAGING TECHNIQUES

Technique	Special Requirements	Limitations	Advantages
CT	None	Resolution Bone artifact	Low cost Fast Easy to visualize blood
MRI	Implanted devices may be contraindicated	Time Expense	Resolution Signal-to-noise ratio Flexible
PET	Cyclotron	Expense Reimbursement Resolution	Metabolic profile
SPECT		Resolution	Inexpensive

CT = computerized tomography; MRI = magnetic resonance imaging; PET = positron emission tomography; SPECT = single-photon emission computed tomography.

This frequency flips the molecules and as these regain their equilibrium magnetization, the molecules create a response frequency, which is gathered by a coil. These frequencies are weighted against the rate at which the proton recuperates 63.2% of its longitudinal alignment (T_1) and also by its spin–spin relaxation time (T_2) in which it loses 63.2% of its maximum transverse magnetization. The intensity of the volume element, or image pixel, depends on the concentration of ^{1}H atoms, which varies between tissue types. This intensity variation between tissues allows an easy detection of any irregularity, such as tumors, irregular vascularity, tissue necrosis, and other injury. Bone is not perceived by this imaging process, making it difficult to diagnose skull trauma through this examination, yet it facilitates a better image in soft tissue–bone interfaces, areas in which CT is prone to create artifact.

MRI does have the following limitations in the context of brain tumor imaging:

- Lack of specificity, caused most often by infarctions and abscesses
- Enhancement does not always equate with histologic grade or define tumor borders
- Choice of treatment (e.g., corticosteroids) may influence enhancement
- Decreased sensitivity for cases involving calcification
- Prior treatment, particularly with radiation therapy and surgery may influence both T_2 signal and extent of postcontrast enhancement
- Patient limitations such as pacemakers, foreign metallic objects, claustrophobia

Positron Emission Tomography

In comparison to CT and MRI, where enhancement agents are optional, the injection of a radiopharmaceutical is necessary for PET imaging. These labeled compounds are injected into the venous circulation and the isotope's positrons combine with electrons. During this combination two photons are released and a signal is detected by the positron detectors. Different radiopharmaceuticals serve different purposes, like measuring the permeability of the blood–brain barrier, cerebral perfusion, and cerebral metabolism, as well as detecting certain neurotransmitters and binding with specific cerebral receptors. This allows detection of tumors as a result of their neurochemical and physiologic processes, such as increase of blood flow to the tumor, protein production, or glucose consumption.

PET limitations in the context of brain tumor imaging include

- Production of the isotope requires proximity to a cyclotron
- Rapid decay time of isotopes
- Poor anatomic resolution
- Few useful surrogates
- Expense and reimbursement

Single-Photon Emission Computed Tomography

In SPECT, the labeled compound injected into the patient creates a flux of photons that is detected by a gamma camera. This camera detects potentials created by the photons within a certain interval later used to reconstruct the images through computer software. This type of tomography serves the same purposes of PET, but at a lower cost and higher accessibility (see Table 4-1).

▶ APPROACH TO THE PATIENT

Neuroimaging is an essential component to the care of patients with brain cancer. In the newly diagnosed patient, the utility of neuroimaging as a tool to determine tumor location and volume is well-established. The interpretation is relatively straightforward and not influenced by outside influences. In the followup of patients under active treatment, neuroimaging is combined with clinical parameters to determine patient response to treatment. In this setting, imaging changes may not only be influenced by tumor changes but also current or prior treatments. The incorporation of treatment effects into the imaging interpretation is often not straightforward. Although emerging imaging methodologies may be able to offer ancillary assistance, it is important to understand the current state of imaging and the role of additional imaging studies, or sequences, and functional studies.

The care of patients with brain malignancies is best performed in a multidisciplinary fashion. The team members include those directly involved in treatment, such as neurosurgeons, radiation oncologists, and medical or neuro-oncologists, as well as experts in neuropathology and neuroradiology. The incorporation of imaging studies and the selection of the study types and techniques is best preformed in coordination with neuroradiology. The primary imaging technique used is MRI and the selection of the sequence choice should include the following considerations: patient time and comfort, delineation of central nervous system anatomy, characterization of tumor volume, and functional considerations. There are multiple sequence choices from which to build a brain tumor MRI protocol. The inclusion of appropriate sequences should be based on the clinical task to be addressed. For example, the sequence choice at initial diagnosis and used for surgical planning may differ from that used for patients at routine follow-up. In addition, studies that address specific functional or biochemical processes such as diffusion, perfusion, or spectral sequences may be included. The basic building block sequences should include a sequence that is weighted toward T_2. Pathologic processes affecting the central nervous system (CNS) and that are related to neoplasms commonly involve changes in the distribution and density of water. Therefore, when weighted toward T_2, these lesions appear bright. Brain tumor sequences should include a T_2-weighted and fluid-attenuated inversion recovery (FLAIR) sequence. The FLAIR sequences provide a cerebral spinal fluid (CSF) nulling effect that allows for visualization of pathologic processes affecting the cortical and periventricular structures. The T_2-weighted sequence and FLAIR sequence are important for delineation of the extent of pathologic processes related to brain tumors. This includes extent of tumor infiltration, amount of vasogenic edema, and composition of cystic fluids. T_1-weighted sequences should be included for high-definition anatomic images and to evaluate for the presence of substances that may cause T_1 shortening, such as fat and proteinaceous cystic fluids. A T_1 sequence should also be dedicated to the administration of contrast in order to detect disruption of the blood–brain barrier and to characterize tumors by their enhancement patterns.

Neuroimaging plays a critical role in the delineation of response to treatment in brain cancer. The most commonly used criteria for response assessment in clinical investigation are the Macdonald criteria.[1] Four response categories are defined: complete response (CR), partial response (PR), stable disease (SD), and progressive disease (PD). The criteria include measurements of the maximum cross-sectional tumor area, corticosteroid use, and clinical status. The imaging criteria for a CR require a complete resolution of contrast-enhancing volume on CT or MRI; for PR there should be a 50% decrease in enhancing volume that is maintained for two sequential imaging studies separated by 4 weeks; and for PD there is a 25% increase in the enhancing volume on postcontrast studies.

▶ NEUROIMAGING OF ASTROCYTIC TUMORS

Tumors derived from astrocytes comprise the most common primary brain tumor and account for the majority of the 18,000 new cases of primary brain cancer a year in the United States (Table 4-2). The World Health Organization (WHO) histopathologic classification of CNS tumors is as follows: (a) pilocytic astrocytoma (grade I), (b) subependymal giant cell astrocytoma (grade I), (c) pleomorphic xanthoastrocytoma (PXA) (grade I), (d) astrocytoma (grade II), (e) anaplastic (malignant) astrocytoma (grade III), and (f) glioblastoma multiforme (GBM) (grade IV). The malignant gliomas include the anaplastic astrocytoma and glioblastoma multiforme. The majority of newly diagnosed astrocytomas are malignant. The predominant location of astrocytomas in adults is supratentorial in contrast to a predominant infratentorial location in children. The general imaging features of malignant astrocytomas at times overlap with features of uncommon CNS tumors that are amenable to complete surgical resection and thus potential cure. These include pilocytic astrocytomas, PXA, subependymal giant cell astrocytoma, dysembryoplastic neuroepithelial tumor (DNET), and ganglioglioma. As a result, it is critical not to overestimate the potential behavior or diagnosis of a CNS tumor from the imaging study alone.

Computerized Tomography

MRI has largely replaced CT as the modality of choice for the assessment of astrocytomas; however, CT is a more commonly used modality, particularly for patients presenting with new neurologic symptoms. The CT appearance of astrocytomas is characterized by variable degrees of mass effect and contrast enhancement. The low-grade astrocytomas, with the exception of the pilocytic, typically have limited mass effect and do not enhance. Pilocytic astrocytomas will often have a cystic component with a tumor nodule that homogeneously enhances after contrast. Mass effect may exist in pilocytics from the cytic component. Anaplastic astrocytomas and GBM will demonstrate increasing degrees of mass effect and moderate to significant enhancement patterns. CT is useful for the demonstration of calcification in primary brain tumors. Low-grade astrocytomas will often demonstrate calcifications.

Magnetic Resonance Imaging

The appearance of astrocytomas on MRI varies, depending on the histologic grade. Low-grade astrocytomas include pilocytic astrocytomas, subependymal giant cell astrocytomas, PXA, and infiltrative astrocytoma WHO grade II. Pilocytic astrocytomas, subependymal giant cell astrocytomas, and PXA are localized, usually well circumscribed lesions, whereas the infiltrative low-grade astrocytoma, anaplastic and its malignant relatives (anaplastic astrocytoma and glioblastoma) are poorly localized and highly disseminated into the surrounding brain. Pilocytic astrocytomas are the most common primary brain tumor of children, typically found in the cerebellum. In adults, pilocytic astrocytomas (PAs) may occur in the thalamus or walls of the third ventricle. These tumors may have associated cystic components but almost always demonstrate a high degree of contrast enhancement. The pilocytic astrocytoma is unique in the intense degree of enhancement for a low-grade tumor. Subependymal giant cell astrocytomas are present in the periventricular area, usually near the foramen of Monro. These tumors are primarily seen in patients with tuberous sclerosis. They are

▶ **TABLE 4-2.** SUMMARY OF PRIMARY BRAIN TUMOR IMAGING FEATURES

Tumor Type	Imaging Features
Pilocytic astrocytoma (WHO grade I)	• Cerebellar, thalamic, or third ventricle location • Tumor nodules show intense enhancement • Cysts are hypointense on T_1WI and hyperintense on T_2WI
Subependymal giant cell astrocytoma (WHO grade I)	• Lateral ventricle in proximity to foramen of Monro location • Heterogenous T_2 signal with areas of hypointensity • Enhance with contrast administration
Pleomorphic xanthoastrocytoma (WHO grade I)	• Temporal or parietooccipital location • Hypo- to isointense on T_1 • Hyperintense on T_2 • Solid portion enhances with contrast
Astrocytoma (WHO grade II)	• Calcification present in 50% of the case, although seldom appreciated in MRI • Well-defined homogenous masses • Hypointense on T_1WI and hyperintense on T_2WI • Enhancement usually absent
Anaplastic astrocytoma (WHO grade III)	• Heterogeneous on MRIs • Less well defined borders and greater mass effect, vasogenic edema and enhancement • In noncontrast T_1 and T_2 images heterogeneous signal intensity is present • Necrosis and heterogeneous ring enhancement are *not* common features
Glioblastoma multiforme (WHO grade IV)	• MRI reflects heterogeneous pathology—heterogeneous signal intensity on both T_1WI and T_2WI • Poorly defined with mass effect and vasogenic edema • Hemorrhage is common and useful in distinguishing from lower grade astrocytomas • Signature—large region of high signal on T_2WI (edema + microscopic tumor infiltration) • T_2 FLAIR provides good visualization
Oligodendroglioma	• High frequency of calcification • Heterogeneous in signal intensity • Predominantly isointense with gray matter on T_1WI and hyperintense on T_2WI • GE imaging is more sensitive to calcification and hemorrhaging than SE, and is useful in imaging these tumors • 50% demonstrate faint enhancement
Medulloblastoma	• Location: midline in young, more lateral in adults • T_2 may be isointense to gray matter • Homogeneous enhancement • Cyst, necrosis, and hemorrhage are atypical features
Ependymoma	• Posterior fossa in children; spinal cord in adults • Hyperintense on T_2 • Hypo- to isointense on T_1 • Majority enhance with contrast regardless of histologic grade
Ganglioglioma	• Temporal or parietooccipital location • Cystic component common • Hyperintense on T_2 • Solid component enhances with contrast
Meningioma	• Extraaxial and dural based • Isointense on T_2 • Hypo- to isointense on T_1 • Homogeneous enhancement • Presence of vasogenic edema with more malignant histology

(*Continued*)

▶ TABLE 4-2. SUMMARY OF PRIMARY BRAIN TUMOR IMAGING FEATURES (*CONTINUED*)

Tumor Type	Imaging Features
Craniopharyngioma	• Sellar to suprasellar location • Calcifications present on CT • Cystic components may contain cholesterol: hypointense to isointense on T_1 • Hyperintense on T_2 • Solid portions enhance with contrast
Brainstem glioma	• Location: pons > midbrain > medulla • May be diffuse or focal • Hypointense on T_1 • Hyperintense on T_2 • Often do not enhance with contrast
Hemangioblastoma	• Posterior fossa location • May be solid or cystic • Solid portion is isointense on T_1 • Hyperintense on T_2 • Solid portion enhances with contrast
Primary central nervous system lymphoma	• Immunocompetent: single lesion more peripheral location • Immunosuppressed: multiple lesions with deeper location (basal ganglia) • Hypo- to isointense on T_1 • Hyperintense on T_2 • Intense enhancement with contrast

CT = computerized tomography; FLAIR = fluid-attenuated inversion recovery; GE = gradient echo; MRI = magnetic resonance imaging; SE = spin echo; T_1WI = T_1-weighted image; T_2WI = T_2-weighted image.

usually well-defined, homogenous masses with variable enhancement. The PXA is distinctive in terms of location and imaging features when compared to the other low-grade astrocytomas. Typically affecting patients in their teens or twenties, these tumors are often located in the temporal or parietooccipital regions. MR appearance varies with hypo- and isointense lesions described on T_1 weighting and hyper- and isointense on T_2 weighting. The solid portion usually enhances with contrast administration and the surrounding brain may demonstrate hypointense signal consistent with vasogenic edema.[2] Malignant astrocytomas are more heterogeneous on MRI and have a greater degree of mass effect, vasogenic edema, and enhancement. Anaplastic astrocytomas (WHO grade III) present the least consistent findings on MRI. Anaplastic astrocytomas have poorly defined borders secondary to their infiltrative nature. There is usually a moderate degree of mass effect and these tumors typically enhance with the administration of gadolinium. Fourteen percent to 45% of anaplastic astrocytomas will not enhance with contrast.[3] The risk of a nonenhancing, supratentorial cerebral tumor being anaplastic increases with a patient's age.[4] The lack of enhancement on routine imaging studies in a subset of anaplastic astrocytomas is important because it may lead to undertreatment of a malignant tumor. Glioblastoma multiformes, which represent 50% of all astrocytic tumors, are poorly defined lesions that may be multifocal. The most common locations are the frontal and temporal lobes but may occur anywhere throughout the neuraxis, including the brainstem and spinal cord. These tumors have significant mass effect and surrounding edema due in large part to the robust development of new, leaky blood vessels. Hemorrhage is common and T_2-weighted images are hyperintense to normal brain. Accurate tumor characterization often goes hand in hand with identifying and isolating necrosis, edema, hemorrhage, calcification, mass effect, signal and flow voids, and motion-related artifacts. The high-grade astrocytoma enhances intensely after the administration of contrast. The pattern is often one of a ring enhancement with a central area of hypointensity reflective of tumor necrosis[5] (Figs. 4-1 to 4-4).

▶ NEUROIMAGING OF OLIGODENDROGLIOMA

Oligodendroglioma is a glioma subtype that originates from the oligodendrocyte, the cell that produces and maintains myelin. It may be pure or mixed, and may be located as a parenchymal or intraventricular tumor. As with other brain tumors, CT and MRI can readily determine the spatial configuration of the oligodendrogliomas, and the radiographic findings are often characteristic. The importance of an early diagnosis of oligodendrogliomas may lead to consideration of a surgical option for treatment.

Pilocytic astrocytoma

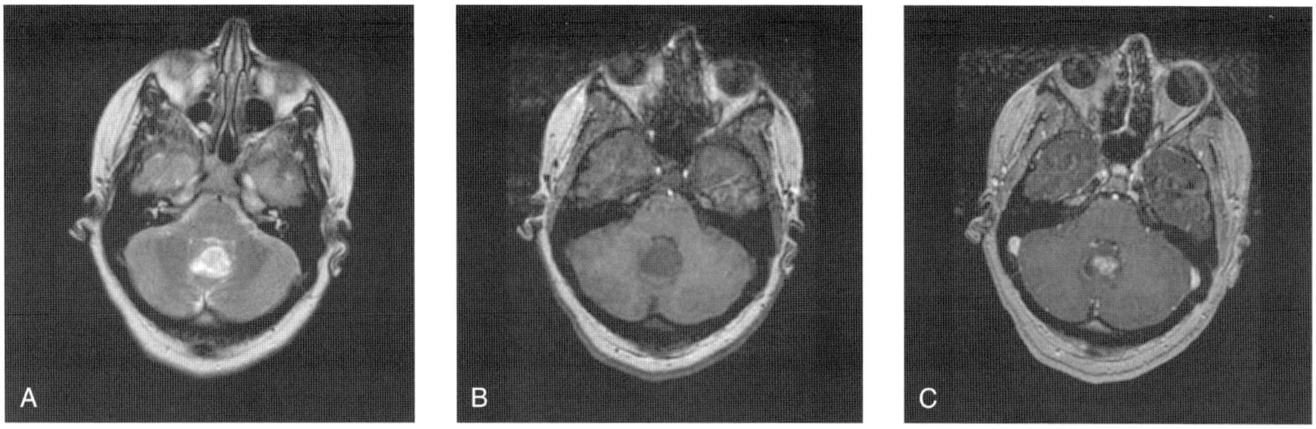

Subependymal giant cell astrocytoma

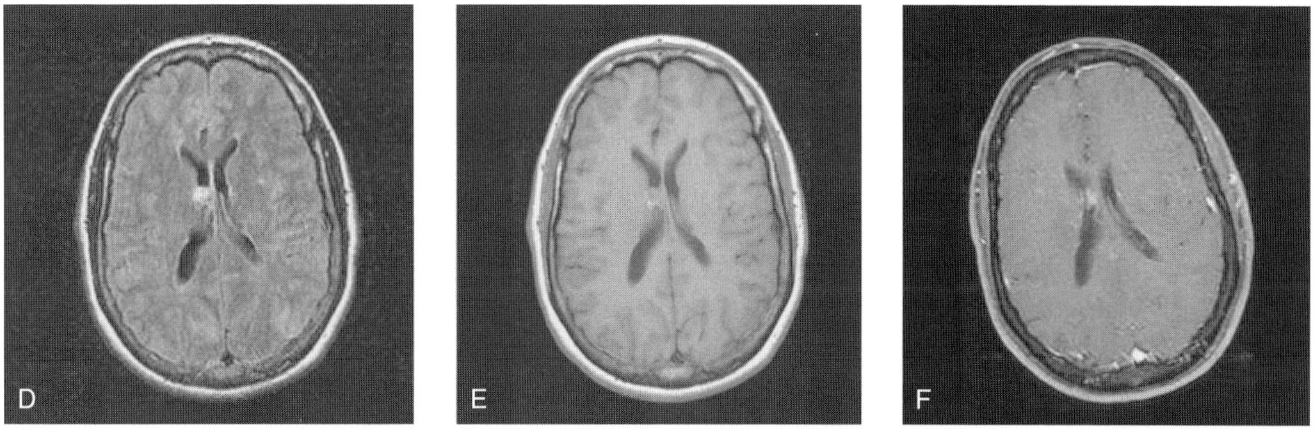

Pleomorphic xanthoastrocytoma

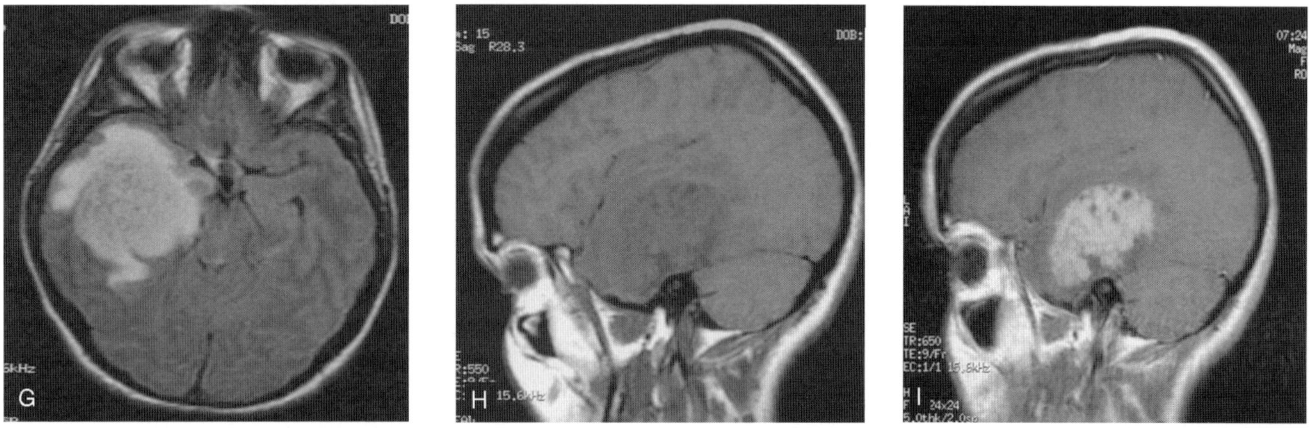

Figure 4-1. Astrocytoma grade I includes (upper panel) the pilocytic astrocytoma, (middle panel) subependymal giant cell astrocytoma, and (lower panel) pleomorphic xanthoastrocytoma. The studies include FLAIR (A, D, G), precontrast T_1 (B, E, H), and postcontrast T_1 (C, F, I) imaging.

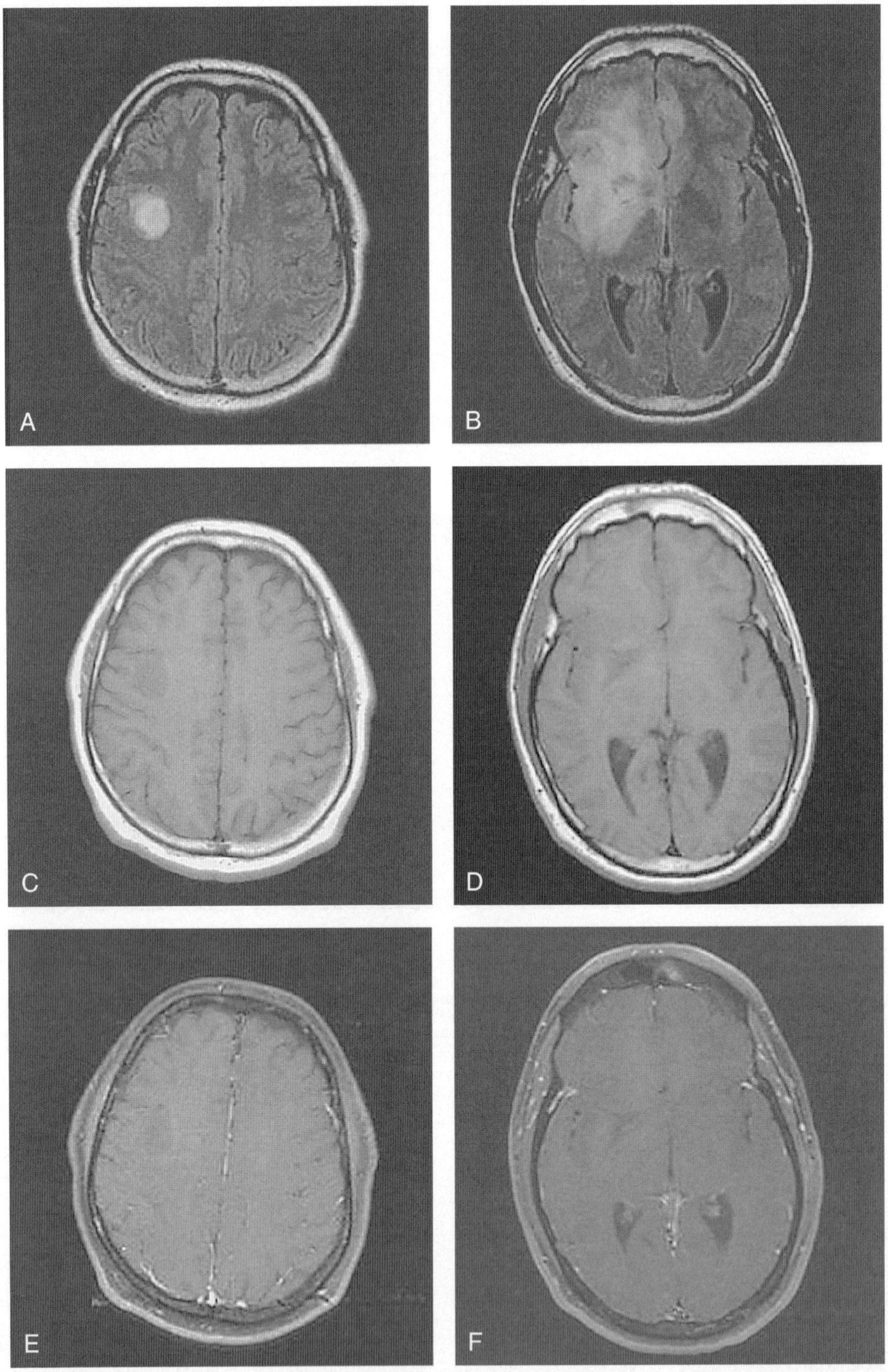

Figure 4-2. The astrocytoma grade II is a low-grade but infiltrative tumor. The imaging features include tumors that are well delineated and compact (A, C, E) versus the diffuse and widespread (B, D, F). FLAIR (A and B), precontrast T_1 (C and D), and postcontrast T_1 (E and F) imaging.

General Imaging Findings

Oligodendrogliomas occur most often in frontal lobe, and then temporal lobe. They often tend to extend to cortical surface, and may even erode the overlying calvaria in some cases. Oligodendrogliomas are divided histologically into low-grade and high-grade tumors. The low-grade tumors represent WHO grades I and II and the high-grade tumors represent WHO grades III and IV. The mixed oligoastrocytic tumors are generally large at the time of

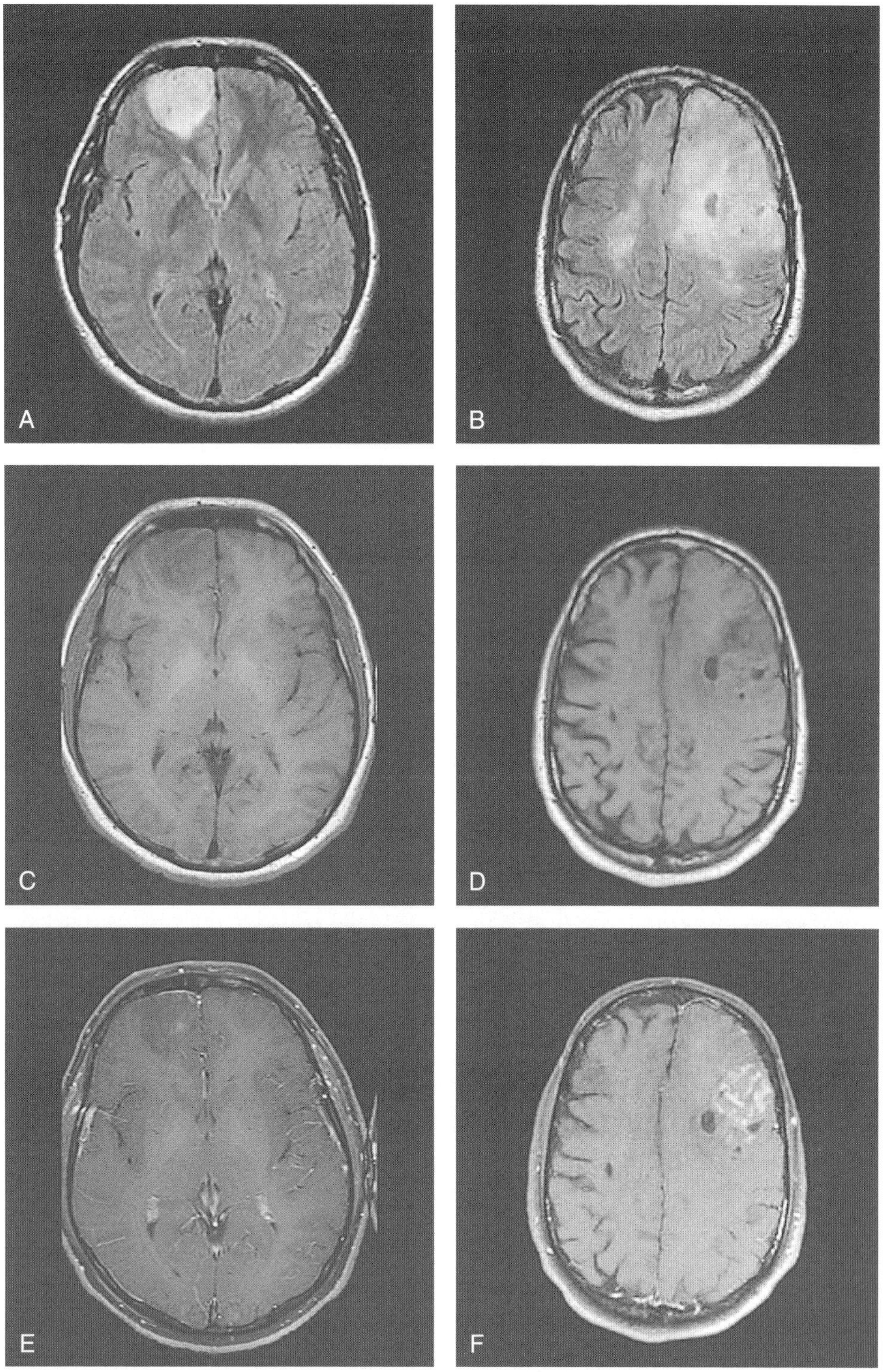

Figure 4-3. The astrocytoma grade III (anaplastic astrocytoma) may have both the features of a lower-grade infiltrative tumor (left panel) or of the more malignant glioblastoma multiforme (right panel).

diagnosis, whereas the pure oligodendrogliomas are somewhat smaller. Peritumoral edema is usually mild or absent in either the mixed or pure low-grade oligodendroglioma but may be significant in high-grade tumors mimicking malignant astrocytomas.[6]

Computerized Tomography

Oligodendrogliomas are typified by their calcific hyperdensity on CT scans. Calcifications often present a coarse appearance; punctate or linear calcifications also may

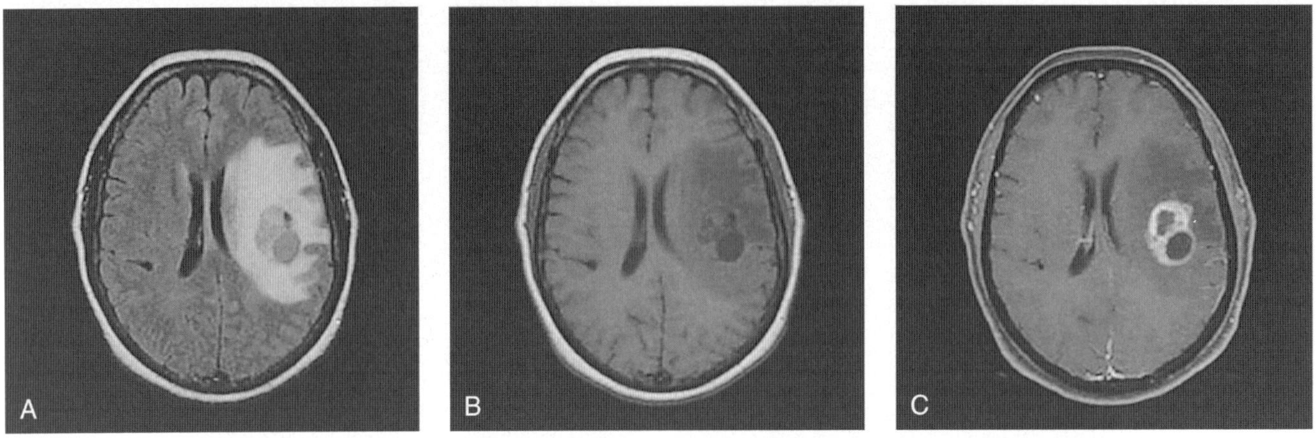

Figure 4-4. The glioblastoma multiforme is characterized by a mass lesion that enhances intensely with contrast (C). The neoplasm may be cystic and surrounded by areas of hyperintense FLAIR signal (A) or hypointense signal on precontrast T_1 imaging (B).

occur. As a consequence of their typically peripheral location and slow-growing nature, oligodendrogliomas may cause calvarial erosion.[7] Although calcification is common, it is not diagnostic for oligodendroglioma, because astrocytomas may also calcify and are more common. In general, contrast enhancement is minimal on CT. But when it becomes moderate or marked (either patchy or homogeneous), it may indicate more aggressive tumor.[8]

Magnetic Resonance Imaging

Although CT shows the calcium deposits better than MRI, the tumor margins are still poorly delineated by CT scans. MRI is more sensitive than CT for tumor delineation and margination. The best delineation is obtained on T_2-weighted MRI. The lower-grade oligodendroglioma will often be a hyperintense lesion exhibiting regular shape and sharp margination. Higher-grade tumors may appear more infiltrative and resemble the MRI findings of high-grade astrocytomas. A unique feature of oligodendrogliomas is the involvement of the cortex with infiltration and thickening of the gyri from the surface to its deeper part.[9] This contrasts with astrocytic tumors, which arise in the deeper white matter.[10]

Tumors are hypointense on T_1-weighted images, but the T_1 low signal volume is often less than the T_2 high signal volume. Intense spongiosis and/or microcystic changes seen on histologic examination can be identified in T_1-weighted images.[11] Compared with CT scans, contrast enhancement is better seen on MRI. In the presence of calcifications, contrast enhancement not seen on CT scans may be demonstrated by MRI. It has been reported that the presence or absence of contrast enhancement on MRI is strongly correlated with the tumor growth patterns.[11,12] Therefore performance of postcontrast MRI appears to be necessary if tumors show calcifications on CT scans.

Positron Emission Tomography

Although the radiographic findings are often characteristic, they are not sufficiently specific for differential diagnostic purpose. For example, calcifications and contrast enhancements, when present on CT and MRI scans, are not consistent features of oligodendrogliomas. Preliminary studies indicate that functional and metabolic PET imaging may represent an important source of support. PET image can give quantitative information about glucose metabolism, blood flow, and amino acid metabolism. Carbon-11-methionine (^{11}C-MET) PET is reported to be a noninvasive means of differentiating between low-grade astrocytoma and oligodendroglioma, and as a means for grading oligodendrogliomas, that is, distinguishing between low- and high-grade tumors.[13] [^{18}F]fluorodeoxyglucose (FDG) PET has been used as a tool in estimating the proliferating activity of oligodendrogliomas and assisting in assessing residual tumors and in the early detection of tumor recurrence.[14]

PET scans can be coregistered with MR images to combine the metabolic data provided by PET with the superior anatomic resolution achievable using MRI. Therefore, although studies with large numbers of patients still need to be conducted, PET seems to hold promise for future use in the management of patients with oligodendroglioma (Fig. 4-5).

▸ NEUROIMAGING OF MEDULLOBLASTOMA

Medulloblastomas comprise approximately 15% to 20% of pediatric brain tumors. Medulloblastomas occur in adults but are extremely rare with an annual incidence of 0.05 per 100,000 adults. The adult age group is typically the third decade of life. The location of medulloblastomas is the

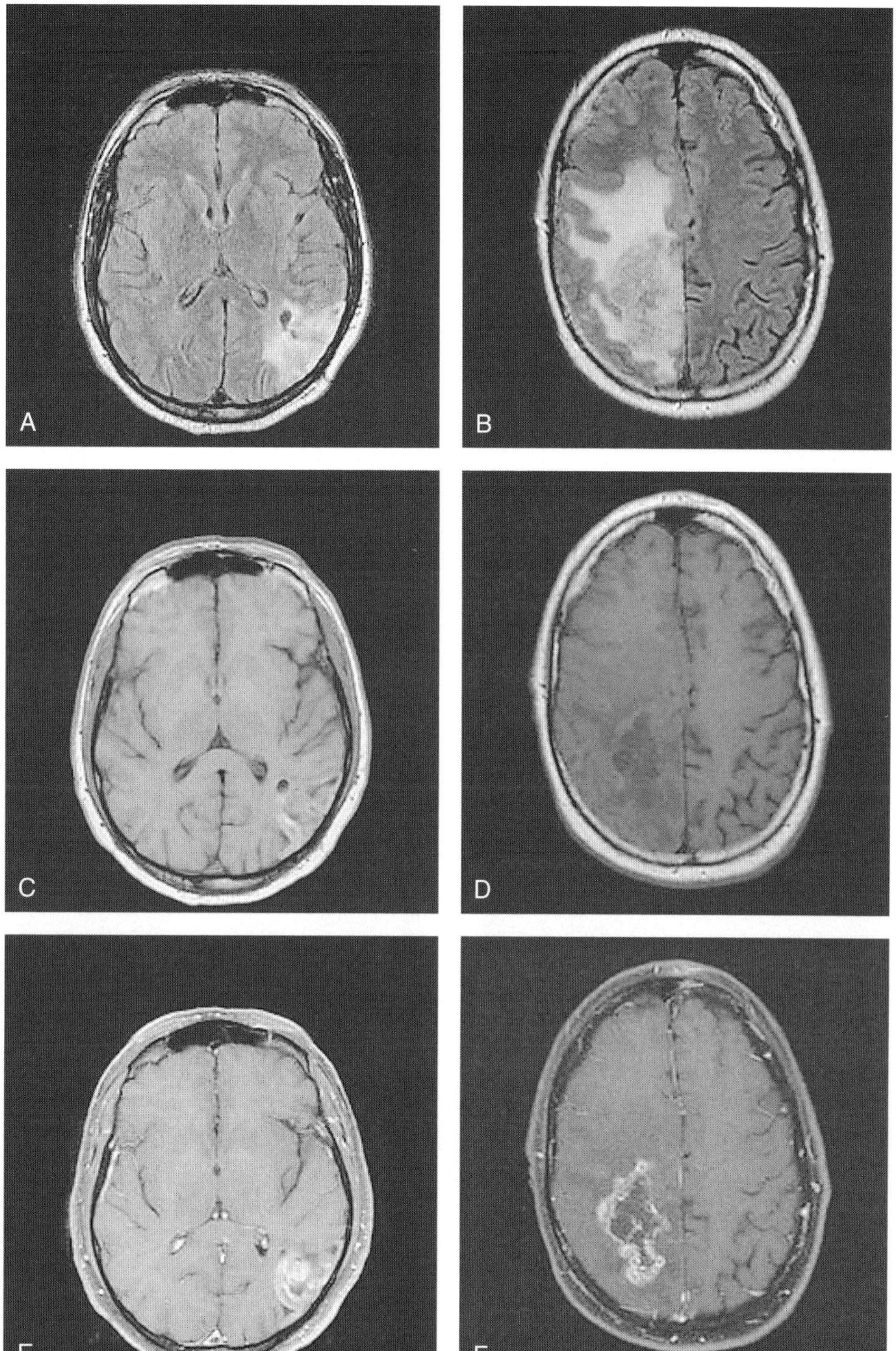

Figure 4-5. The left panel (A, C, E) illustrates an oligodendroglioma grade II. The FLAIR sequence (A) demonstrates a cortical location with a regular shape and sharp borders. Cystic areas are noted on the precontrast T_1 imaging (C) and the tumor demonstrates a mild degree of enhancement with contrast (E). The anaplastic oligodendroglioma is in the right panel (B, D, F). The FLAIR sequence (B) demonstrates a deeper mass in the white matter with poor margins. Following the administration of contrast (F), there is a ring-enhancing lesion.

posterior fossa arising often from the floor of the fourth ventricle and presenting clinically as a consequence of obstruction of CSF flow and the development of hydrocephalus. Survival for both children and adults has improved with the use of craniospinal irradiation and adjuvant chemotherapy.[15]

Computerized Tomography

The CT findings of medulloblastoma in children are of a midline cerebellar mass with extension into the fourth ventricle. Depending on the degree of CSF obstruction, hydrocephalus may be present. The tumor is characteristically hyperintense on precontrast studies, attributed to the high cellularity and high nuclear-to-cytoplasm ratio. The mass enhances homogeneously with contrast administration and usually has well-delineated margins.[16,17] In adults, CT findings vary, with tumors being more lateral in the cerebellar hemispheres, often in contact with the tentorium or cerebellopontine angle. The precontrast signal may not be hyperintense. Atypical findings such as cyst or necrosis are more common in adults.[16]

Magnetic Resonance Imaging

The T_2 signal of medulloblastomas is either iso- or hyperintense to gray matter, in contrast to other CNS tumors that are routinely hyperintense.[18] Following the administration of contrast, tumors typically enhance homogenously, particularly in children. Enhancement in adults with more laterally located tumors is variable.[16] Cyst, necrosis, and hemorrhage may be atypical features noted on MRI. In children, tumor location is typically in the midline; however, in adolescents and young adults, a more lateral location into the cerebellar hemisphere is not uncommon.

Neuroimaging is an important component to the staging of medulloblastoma and should include postoperative cranial as well as total spine studies.[19] The timing of the spinal studies is of some debate. Preoperative studies with contrast-enhanced MRI would be ideal, although often not feasible. When performed postoperatively, an interval of at least 2 weeks helps to minimize the chance of false-positives in the assessment of disseminated leptomeningeal disease[20] (Fig. 4-6).

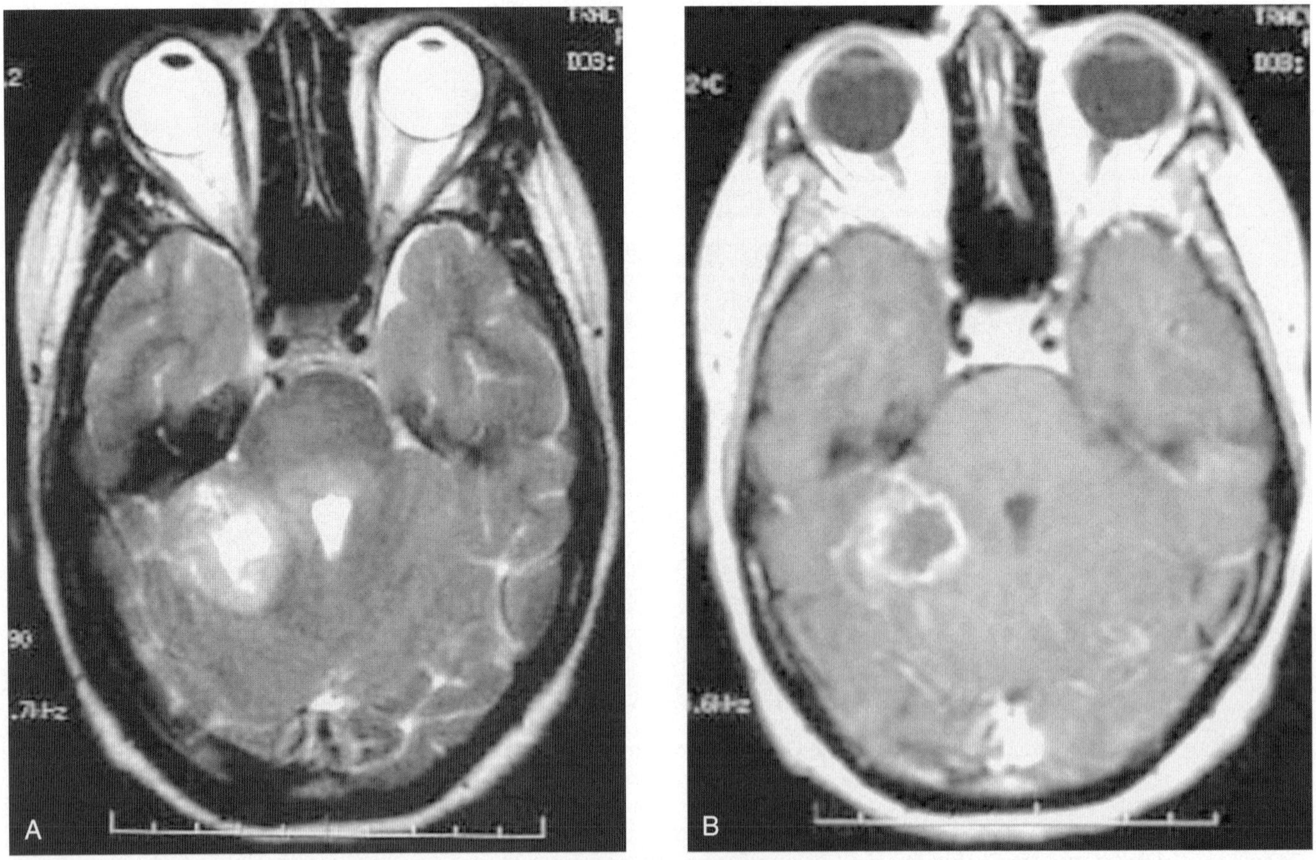

Figure 4-6. The panel demonstrates a medulloblastoma in a young adult. Unlike in children, the location in adults is more lateral, as in this case, within the right cerebellar peduncle. The tumor is isointense to brain on T_2 imaging (A), but there is a central cystic component that is an atypical feature of medulloblastoma. Following the administration of contrast (B), there is mild enhancement.

▶ NEUROIMAGING OF EPENDYMOMA

Ependymomas are glial tumors derived from differentiated ependymal cells lining the ventricles of the brain and the central canal of the spinal cord. They are usually found in children and young adults. The majority of ependymomas occur infratentorially, arising from the floor of the fourth ventricle, whereas most others arise from the outer wall of the lateral ventricles or within the spinal canal.[21]

Most infratentorial ependymomas are intraventricular, frequently arising within the fourth ventricle and extending through the outlet foramina of the fourth ventricle into the subarachnoid space of the posterior cranial fossa. Supratentorial ependymomas, on the other hand, are more commonly extraventricular, primarily occurring within either the frontal or parietal lobes.[22] Spinal cord ependymomas can be cervical, thoracic, or filar, usually located centrally in an expanded spinal cord. Supratentorial ependymomas are usually large lesions, typically between 4 and 8 cm, with an average size of 4 to 5 cm.[23,24] Their large size at the time of presentation is, at least in part, likely a function of their usual extraventricular location. In contrast, most infratentorial ependymomas are significantly smaller, because of ventricular obstruction at an early stage of growth. The extent of spinal cord ependymomas often ranges from 1 to 10 vertebral segments, with a mean length around 4 segments.

Computerized Tomography

On CT scan, the signal intensity of the soft-tissue components of ependymomas is generally isointense or hypointense to white matter.[24] Dense, punctate calcification occurs in approximately 50% of both infratentorial and supratentorial ependymomas. The enhancement characteristics of infratentorial and supratentorial ependymomas are similar, and both enhance moderately or markedly. The enhancement patterns, however, are quite variable, varying from heterogeneous to homogeneous or ring-enhancing.[22]

Supratentorial ependymomas often contain a cystic component, while the incidence of a cystic component in infratentorial ependymomas is significantly lower. Hydrocephalus nearly always occurs when infratentorial ependymomas are present because of their frequent intraventricular location with concomitant obstruction of the fourth ventricle or cerebral aqueduct. This is not the case with supratentorial ependymomas, because they are more frequently intraparenchymal. Intratumoral hemorrhage is not a typical CT feature of supratentorial or infratentorial ependymomas. Peritumoral edema is a frequent accompaniment of supratentorial ependymoma.[22]

For spinal cord ependymomas, CT scan is rarely useful, because the resolution within the spinal canal is limited and only indirect signs of thinning of the pedicles and enlargement of the spinal canal, when present, may be seen.

Magnetic Resonance Imaging

The signal intensity of ependymomas on MRI is nonspecific. Regardless of their location within the neuraxis, they are hypo- to isointense to gray matter on nonenhanced T_1-weighted imaging, and hyperintense on T_2-weighted imaging, findings that are similar to those of other CNS tumors. In some tumors, the nonenhanced T_1-weighted images are heterogeneous as a result of combined presence of calcification, hemorrhage, and cyst.[24] Signal decay on T_2-weighted images is also observed in some cases, probably as a result of high cellular density and high nuclear-to-cytoplasm ratio.[25] Intratumoral hemorrhage occurs infrequently in ependymomas. On T_2 imaging, however, the presence of a low-signal rim along the rostral or caudal margin of a spinal cord tumor is a fairly specific indicator of ependymoma. Peritumoral edema is mild or absent in infratentorial and spinal tumors because of space limitation imposed by their intraventricular or intraspinal location. Most ependymomas show contrast enhancement; however, the pattern of this varies, ranging from heterogeneous to homogeneous. The most characteristic feature of enhancement is that the margins of the enhanced areas are almost always sharply defined, though isolated tumor cell infiltration may exist outside the margin of contrast enhancement[21] (Fig. 4-7).

▶ NEUROIMAGING OF GANGLIOGLIOMA AND GANGLIOCYTOMA

Gangliogliomas and gangliocytomas compromise a group of rare neoplasms of the central nervous system characterized histologically as composed of neuronal elements.[26] The two are often referred to as ganglion cell tumors and are distinct from hamartomatous processes. Ganglion cell tumors are seen in the young age group, typically adolescent or young adult. Their locations are often in the temporal lobe followed by the parietal or occipital but are also seen in the thalamus, cerebellum, and optic nerve. Gangliogliomas that occur in the cervical cord, optic nerve, and craniocervical junction seem to behave differently.

Computerized Tomography

The CT appearance of ganglion cell tumors is of a mass lesion with a cystic component. The tumor on CT may be hypointense in signal with contrast enhancement in nodular components. Calcifications are frequent and apparent on CT. The lesions appear well circumscribed.[27]

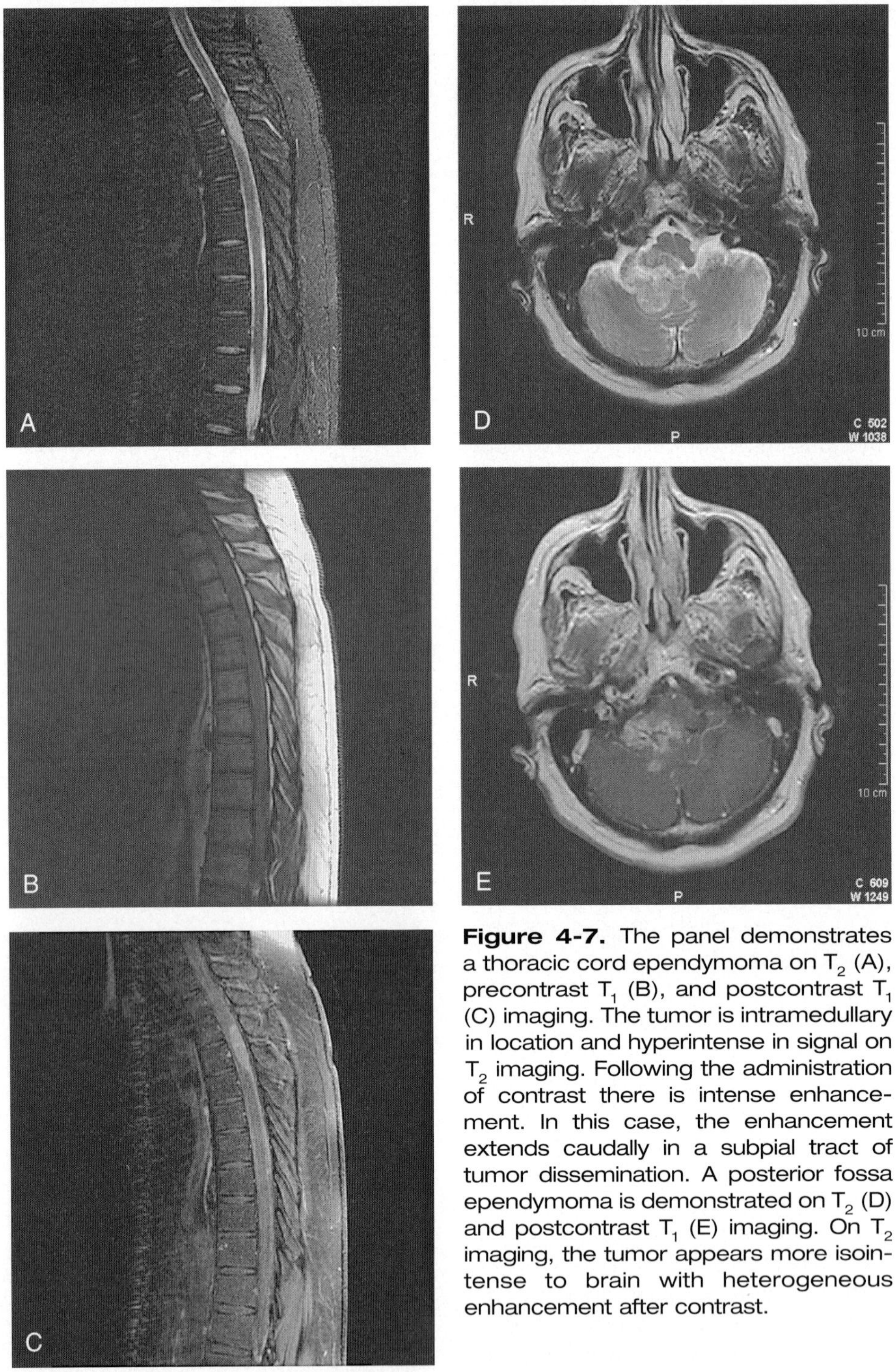

Figure 4-7. The panel demonstrates a thoracic cord ependymoma on T_2 (A), precontrast T_1 (B), and postcontrast T_1 (C) imaging. The tumor is intramedullary in location and hyperintense in signal on T_2 imaging. Following the administration of contrast there is intense enhancement. In this case, the enhancement extends caudally in a subpial tract of tumor dissemination. A posterior fossa ependymoma is demonstrated on T_2 (D) and postcontrast T_1 (E) imaging. On T_2 imaging, the tumor appears more isointense to brain with heterogeneous enhancement after contrast.

Magnetic Resonance Imaging

MRI offers improved delineation of the tumor extent. Ganglion cell tumors typically do not have an infiltrative appearance. The tumor is again often seen with a cystic component. The tumor mass is hyperintense on T_2 imaging. Following the administration of contrast, the solid component of the tumor may enhance (Fig. 4-8).

▶ NEUROIMAGING OF MENINGIOMA

Meningiomas are the most common type of primary nonglial intracranial tumors and account for approximately 15% to 20% of all primary brain tumors.[26] Symptoms are variable and depend on the size and location of the tumor. Meningiomas are neoplasms that arise mainly from meningothelial cells, which are located in the arachnoid

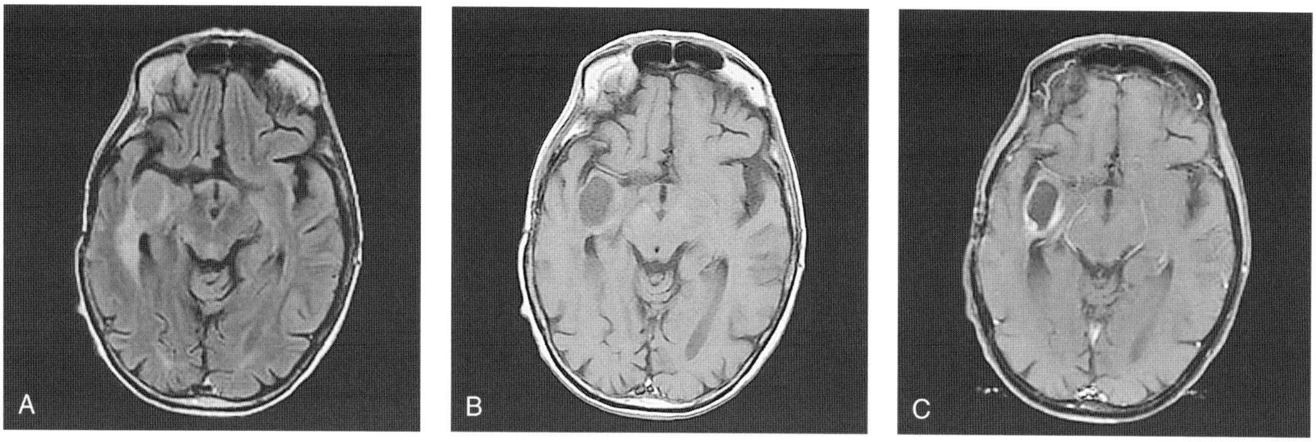

Figure 4-8. The panel demonstrates a ganglioglioma on FLAIR (A), precontrast T_1 (B), and postcontrast T_1 (C) imaging. The tumor has a cystic component that is hyperintense on T_2 imaging but isointense because of CSF nulling on FLAIR. The location is typically temporal and the solid portion of the tumor does enhance after contrast administration.

granulations. None of the three meningeal layers can be singled out as the source of these tumors. Genetic influences, such as loss of chromosome 22 and sex hormones, are implicated in meningioma formation. Occasionally, meningiomas will occur in unusual locations, such as in the ventricle.

Histologic classifications of meningioma usually include the meningotheliomatous (syncytial), fibrous, transitional, and angioblastic types. The more recent WHO classifications are typical benign, atypical, and anaplastic. Most meningiomas occur in adults with a stronger predilection for females (annual incidence 2 to 7 per 100,000 women and 1 to 5 per 100,000 men). Most meningiomas are extraaxial dural-based lesions and approximately 90% are supratentorial. Optic nerve sheath, intraspinal, ventricular system, epidural, and ectopic variants of meningiomas have been reported in the literature. About half of meningiomas cause edema.

Computerized Tomography

In radiographic terms, intracranial meningiomas are usually globular, highly vascular, contrast enhancing, and dural based.[26] Early in their development, vascular supply is usually from the dural branches of the external carotid artery. As the tumor grows, pial arteries become involved in supplying the peripheral regions of the tumor. CT shows a well-marginated oval or lobulated mass attached to the dura at an obtuse angle. The classic "dural tail" of enhancement is a noted radiologic feature. About a quarter of meningiomas are calcified, although the calcification can vary from diffuse to focal. Variable peripheral edema is often seen. Meningiomas also produce marked enhancement following contrast administration. The degree of contrast enhancement does not correlate with specific features of the tumor such as size, location, and growth rate. Attempts have been made to correlate CT features with histologic findings.[28] Also, the utility of computed tomography and angiography in distinguishing malignant meningiomas from benign ones has been questioned.[29] Ten percent to 15% of meningiomas follow atypical patterns, exhibiting features such as rim-like enhancement, prominent cyst formation, intratumoral hemorrhage, and metaplasia.[30]

Hyperostosis and, rarely, bone erosion are findings on plain films of meningiomas that may also be noted on CT. CT with contrast detects 85% to 95% of meningiomas. On noncontrast CT, meningiomas appear as sharply circumscribed masses that displace brain and often are associated with significant edema. A wide range of densities may be present and are discernible from normal brain tissue. Hypodense lesions are present in less than 5% of cases.

Magnetic Resonance Imaging

MRI appearances of meningiomas are very diverse. On unenhanced T_1-weighted images, they are usually only slightly hypointense or isointense to gray matter. On T_2-weighted images, most meningiomas are isointense or slightly hyperintense compared to gray matter. On T_2-weighted images, a correlation has been reported between histologic subtype of the tumor and signal characteristics.[31] The T_2-weighted images are generally more variable and inhomogeneous because of the intrinsic tumor vascularity, calcification, and cystic foci. Intratumoral calcifications are less well defined with MRI than with CT. MR venous angiography has also been used to image conditions such as a thrombosed sinus resulting from compression or invasion by tumor.

Several researchers have examined the correlations between MRI and histology in the context of intracranial

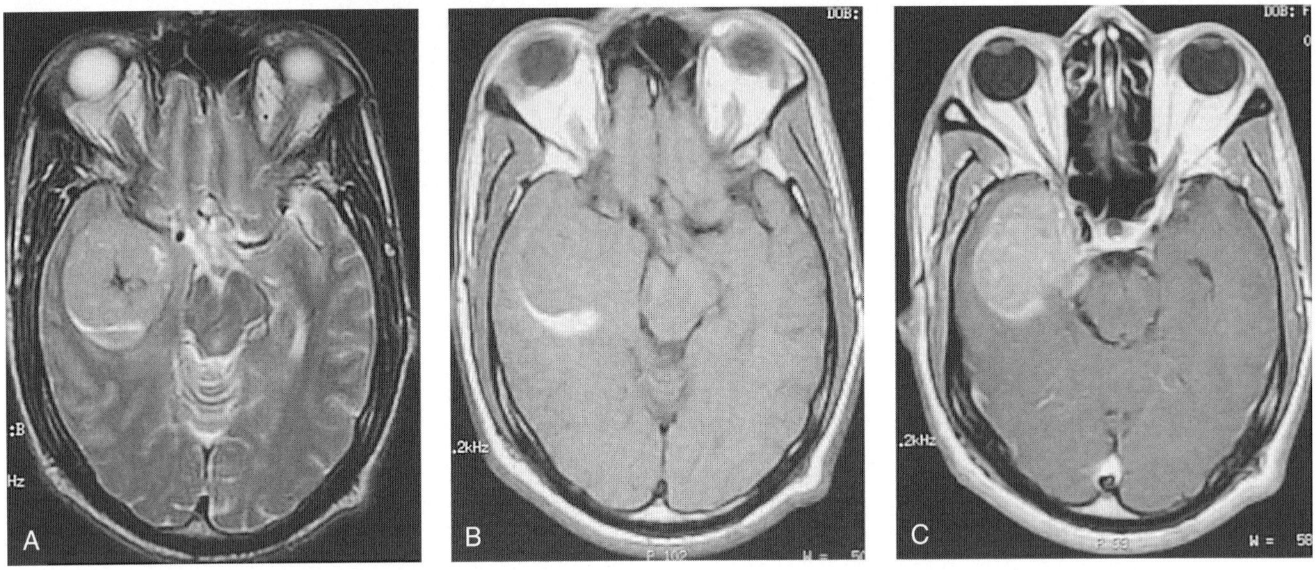

Figure 4-9. The panel demonstrates a meningioma on T_2 (A), precontrast T_1 (B), and postcontrast T_1 (C) imaging. The tumor is extraaxial, arising from the dural lining of the petrous ridge. It is isointense to brain on T_2 and precontrast T_1 imaging. Following the administration of contrast, the tumor has homogeneous and intense enhancement.

meningiomas. It has been suggested that signal intensity of MRI may be useful in the preoperative characterization of such tumors.[32] T_1-weighted images may predict the presence of cysts and intratumoral blood vessels, whereas T_2-weighted images can reveal information about histologic subtype, vascularity, and consistency. The accuracy of MR-based meningioma diagnosis is estimated to be 95%. The presence of vasogenic edema extending into brain parenchyma surrounding a meningioma has been reported to be associated with a more aggressive histology.[33] More recently, diffusion-weighted MRI has been used[34] in the radiologic evaluation and assessment of meningiomas in tandem with attempts to correlate such findings with histopathologic features. Contrast-enhanced T_1-weighted MR sequences are useful in distinguishing benign from nonbenign intracranial meningiomas.[35] Advances in MRI have permitted usage of multiple modalities such as diffusion, perfusion, and spectroscopy[36] for better understanding of meningiomas and hold the promise of improving their understanding, clinical diagnosis, and surgical intervention. Addition of such techniques affords physicians more structural and metabolic hints, which were not available through either standard CT or MRI (Fig. 4-9).

▶ NEUROIMAGING OF CRANIOPHARYNGIOMA

The craniopharyngioma is a tumor of the sellar region and is often classified into two types: adamantinomatous and papillary. The adamantinomatous type tends to have solid and cystic areas that are histologically composed of epithelial islands with central regions that degenerate into dark viscous fluid and are usually compared with motor oil because of the consistency and color. The papillary type is composed of sheets and pseudopapillary tissue of mature squamous epithelium. Calcification is frequently seen in craniopharyngioma; however, in adult cases, the tumor tends to have a more homogeneous cystic composition. Because the usual treatment involves surgery that is often followed by radiotherapy, imaging to delineate the tumor margins and extent is important.[26]

Even though craniopharyngioma is thought to be a childhood tumor, 60% of these cases are seen in patients older than age 16 years. Craniopharyngioma represents 1.2% to 4% of all intracranial brain tumors, having a peak incidence in 5- to 10-year-old patients, and later in adults between the ages of 50 and 60 years, with an overall slim predominance in males (55%) compared to females (45%).[37,38]

The tumor tends to have a slow growth rate and a benign histology, but a malignant behavior as it compresses the hypothalamus and the visual apparatus, causing visual, endocrinologic, and hypothalamic dysfunctions. It typically situates itself in the infundibular–hypophysial axis, frequently growing into the infrasellar and suprasellar regions.

Common symptoms are headache, nausea, vomiting, visual degeneration, and endocrinologic or hypothalamic dysfunctions. Plain radiographs may demonstrate an enlarged sella turcica and suprasellar region, as well as the calcification of the tumor. Definitive diagnosis usually requires MR scanning.

Computerized Tomography

CT imaging allows detection of the craniopharyngioma by presence of a calcified mass in the appropriate area. The calcification tends to present itself as chunks within the solid or as a border around it, and is better demonstrated by using thin slices and bone algorithm. A better image of the tissue is obtained by using contrast. The mass tends to be hypotense or isointense, the latter occurring more frequently in noncalcified masses.[39,40] CT with bone windows is particularly useful in the surgical planning and assessment.

Magnetic Resonance Imaging

In the case of MRI, the anatomic separation between structures and tumor is more noticeable, but the calcification is almost imperceptible. Conversely, the advantage of a better-defined topography allows a superior detection of the location of the tumor, the soft-tissue involvement, and the displacement of structures, facilitating a better planning of the surgical approach, but it tends to fail in detecting if the mass is inside or outside of the chiasm. Depending on the cholesterol content of a cystic homogenous mass, the signal will be high and uniform on T_1-weighted images; for inhomogeneous tumors containing solid parts, the T_1-weighted image will range from hypointense to isointense, and it will be hyperintense on T_2-weighted images. Contrast, such as gadolinium-diethylenetriamine pentaacetic acid (Gd-DTPA) intensifies the signal on T_1-weighted images of homogeneous parts of the tumor[41,42] (Fig. 4-10).

▶ NEUROIMAGING OF BRAINSTEM GLIOMA

Brainstem gliomas account for 10% to 15% of pediatric brain tumors.[43] Tumors of the brainstem are also seen in adults. Tumors of the brainstem are a heterogeneous group with differences in clinical outcomes based on location and growth patterns.

Computerized Tomography

CT has been used to describe brainstem tumors and the characteristics that may assist in operative planning and determining prognosis. The four categories of CT criteria are described based on location within the brainstem and growth patterns: group I tumors are contrast-enhancing with dorsally exophytic components; group IIa are hypodense intrinsic brainstem masses without contrast enhancement; group IIb tumors are both intrinsic with an exophytic component into the cerebellopontine and prepontine cisterns; group III are intrinsic but with a cystic, enhancing capsule; and group IV are focal intrinsic lesions that enhance homogeneously.[44] Patients in groups II, III, and IV have a poor prognosis and patients in group I have a good prognosis. The only advantage CT offers in brainstem tumors is the improved ability to detect calcification. This, however, is an uncommon finding in brainstem glioma. MRI has largely replaced CT for the evaluation of posterior fossa tumors in all patient populations.

Magnetic Resonance Imaging

MRI reveals the majority of brainstem tumors to be located in the pons, followed by the midbrain and medulla. Tumors are typically hypointense on T_1-weighted studies

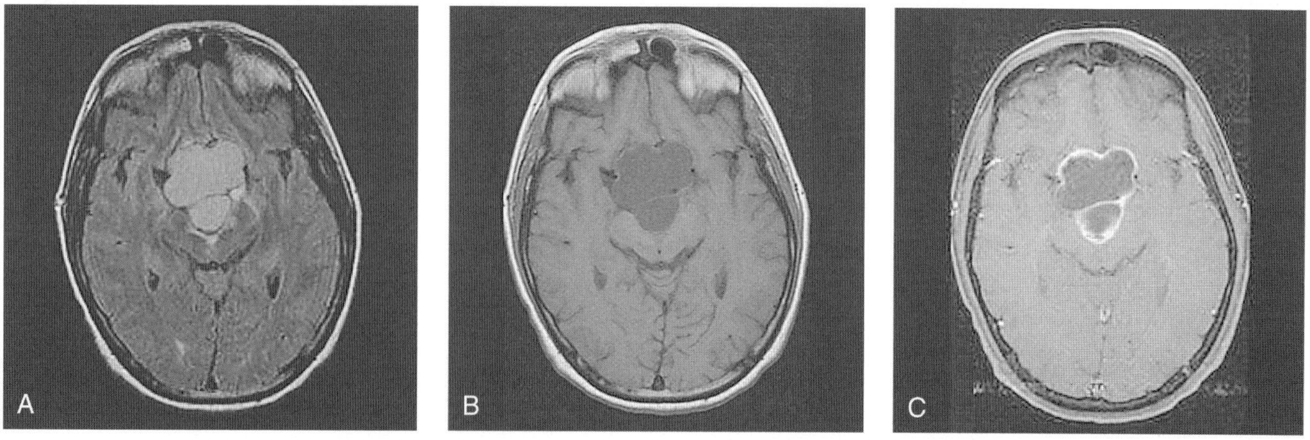

Figure 4-10. The panel demonstrates a craniopharyngioma on FLAIR (A), precontrast T_1 (B), and postcontrast T_1 (C) imaging. The tumor is suprasellar in location with a notable cystic component. The signal intensity of the cystic fluid in this example is low on precontrast T_1 imaging, indicating a low cholesterol content. Following the administration of contrast, the rim and solid portions of tumor do enhance.

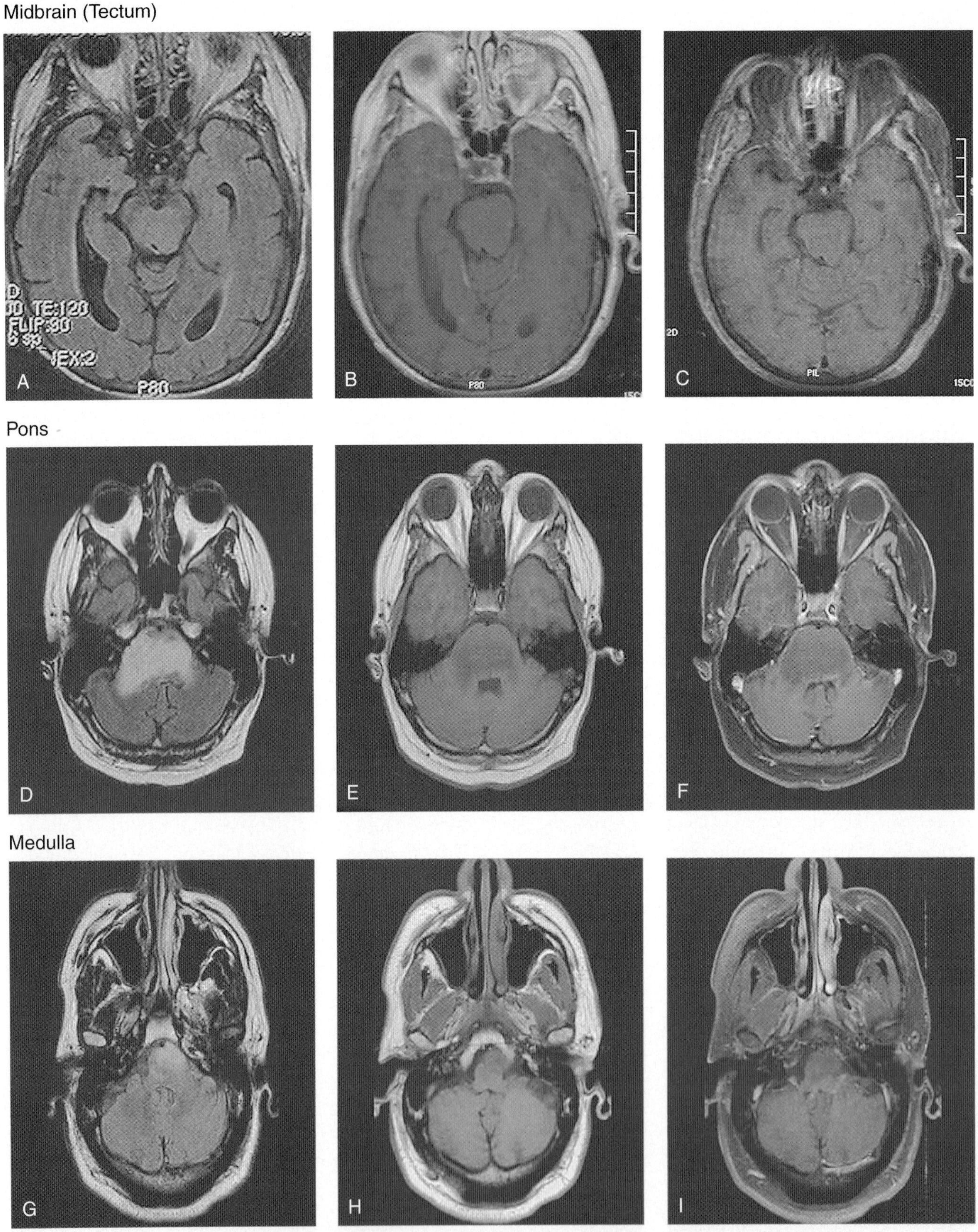

Figure 4-11. The series of panels depict brainstem gliomas based on location. The upper panel shows a tectal tumor located in the dorsal aspect of the midbrain. The middle panel illustrates a pontine glioma. This example is primarily intrinsic with an infiltrative component extending into the cerebellar peduncles bilaterally. This is best seen on the FLAIR sequence (D). The lower panel is an exophytic tumor located in the medulla. The imaging sequences are FLAIR (A, D, G), precontrast T_1 (B, E, H), and postcontrast T_1 (C, F, I).

and hyperintense on T_2-weighted studies. Contrast enhancement is present in less than 50% of cases.[45–47] Pontine and midbrain lesions may be further classified as focal or diffuse, with the majority being diffuse. Hydrocephalus is rare in both locations, with the exception of tectal midbrain lesion. Tectal lesions are viewed as a separate entity and typically have associated hydrocephalus but a much improved survival compared to the more diffuse pontine or midbrain lesions. The lesions in the medulla may also be classified as focal or diffuse. Both groupings in the medulla may have a dorsally exophytic component (Fig. 4-11).

▶ NEUROIMAGING OF HEMANGIOBLASTOMA

Hemangioblastomas are slow growing and are histologically unusual, uncommon, and of uncertain origin. Despite their unknown origin, there are some patients who develop these neoplasms as part of a genetic syndrome called von Hippel-Lindau disease (VHL).[26]

Hemangioblastomas account for 1% to 2.5% of all intracranial neoplasms, but are the most common primary cerebellar tumor with approximately 85% of these tumors being found in the cerebellum. The remainder can be found in the spinal cord, medulla, and, rarely, in the supratentorial compartment and optic nerve. Hemangioblastomas can be found in all age groups; however, they are most frequent in the 35- to 45-year-old age group. These neoplasms are more common in men than in women with a male-to-female ratio of approximately 2:1 in clinical series.

There are two basic forms in which hemangioblastomas occur: solid and cystic. Solid tumors consist entirely of tumor cells; cystic tumors are composed of a generally small solid component, adjacent to an oftentimes much larger cystic portion of tumor. Both the solid portion and wall of the cyst are neoplastic. With either form of hemangioblastoma, contrast and noncontrast CT or MRI scans can be used as a key diagnostic tool because plain radiographs do not usually aid diagnosis. Hemangioblastomas can occasionally mimic other tumors, such as meningioma, brain metastases, or, in some cases, an arteriovenous malformation, but typically they are easily differentiated.

Computerized Tomography

In approximately 60% of cases, the tumor is primarily cystic with a mural nodule of variable size. On noncontrast CT, the cystic portions of hemangioblastomas are isodense and the nodule is often inapparent because it is so isodense or slightly hyperdense relative to white matter. Solid hemangioblastomas are often isodense to brain tissue, with little surrounding edema. CT scans with intravenous contrast show uniform enhancement of the tumor nodule.[48,49]

Magnetic Resonance Imaging

Radiographically, hemangioblastomas are best diagnosed with MRI, which permits visualization of the margins and inner structures of the tumors. In addition, magnetic resonance imaging usually shows the enhancing mass clearly delineated from the surrounding brain or spinal cord tissue. Because of its ability to delineate the degree of cerebellar involvement, MRI is important not only in surgical treatment but also in the long-term management of the patient. On noncontrast T_1-weighted MR images, the solid portion of the tumor is typically isointense with brain tissue, and this intensity increases with contrast. On T_2-weighted images, the solid portion of the tumor is usually hyperintense to white matter but is occasionally isointense[50,51] (Fig. 4-12).

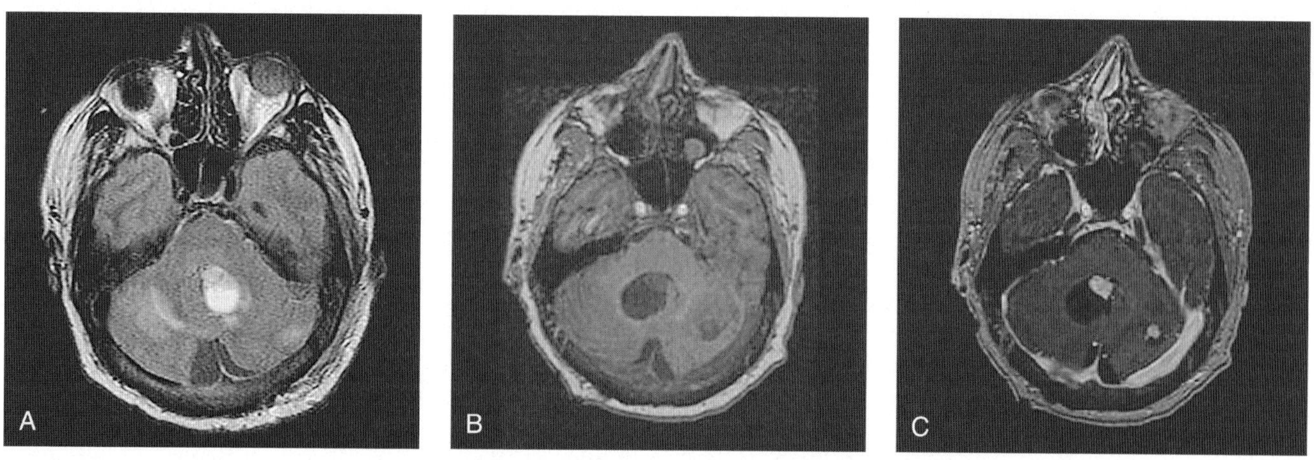

Figure 4-12. The panel demonstrates multiple hemangioblastomas in the cerebellum of a patient with von Hippel-Lindau disease on FLAIR (A), precontrast T_1 (B), and postcontrast T_1 (C) imaging. The tumors have a cystic component with a solid nodule. The nodules enhance after contrast administration.

▶ NEUROIMAGING OF PRIMARY CENTRAL NERVOUS SYSTEM LYMPHOMA

Primary central nervous system lymphoma (PCNSL) is a malignant non-Hodgkin B-cell lymphoma confined to the central nervous system. PCNSLs comprise 1% to 6% of primary brain cancers.[52] This malignancy is thought to be more common in the immunocompromised population but is reported to have an increasing frequency in the immunocompetent. The age of the population is younger in the immunocompromised and older in the immunocompetent. PCNSL usually presents as a solitary lesion in the immunocompetent and is more likely to be multiple in the immunocompromised.[53,54] The location is supratentorial with a slight frontal and is parietal predominance. The majority of lesions are reported as peripheral but deep lesions involving the basal ganglia or corpus callosum occur in a significant proportion.[53]

Computerized Tomography

PCNSL is iso- to hyperintense on cranial CT imaging. The lesions are associated with surrounding signal attenuation consistent with vasogenic edema but proportionally little mass effect. Cyst or calcification is rarely seen on CT. With the administration of contrast, there is moderate to marked homogeneous enhancement.[55] Calcification and cyst are rarely seen with PCNSL.[53]

Magnetic Resonance Imaging

MRI of PCNSL shows hypo- to isointense lesion on T_1-weighted sequences. The lesions are predominantly hyperintense on T_2-weighted sequences. The administration of contrast results in intense homogeneous enhancement in the majority of PCNSL. Large mass lesions often demonstrate surrounding hypointense signal on T_1 images, and hyperintense signal on T_2 images, consistent with vasogenic edema.[56] PCNSL is, however, far more infiltrative than imaging studies reveal. Autopsy studies of patients with PCNSL reveal extensive infiltration outside of areas that demonstrate imaging abnormalities even on T_2 images.[57] Clinical response to therapy and improved overall survival correspond to imaging decrease and resolution of mass lesions.[58] Thus, from a clinical standpoint, the utility of imaging studies in established cases remains relevant for following the course of the disease and response to treatment. The MR features of PCNSL are more variable in immunosuppressed patients. Multifocal presentation is more common and a basal ganglia location is far more common.[54] Tumor hemorrhage and lack of contrast enhancement, which are uncommon in the immunocompetent, are seen in a significant percentage in the immunosuppressed (Fig. 4-13).

▶ SPECIAL IMAGING STUDIES

Magnetic Resonance Spectroscopy

While conventional, perfusion, and diffusion MRI sequences acquire anatomic and flow-related information, these methods do not provide biochemical information. Such information clearly has the potential to aid in tumor diagnosis and characterization. This is achieved using MRS or MRSI.

MRS can be performed on commercial scanners using special acquisition sequences. At present most clinical scanners come with prepackaged spectroscopic modules that enable not only acquisition but also spectral reconstruction and analysis. Improvements in hardware and measurement techniques have made in vivo spectroscopic studies practical. In many cases, spectra with an acceptable signal-to-noise ratio (SNR) and spatial resolution can be obtained with only a minimal increase in the total patient examination time. Based on the pathology under investigation, spectroscopy may be performed using one of several nuclei, for example, hydrogen, nitrogen, fluorine, phosphorus, or carbon. Hydrogen nuclei-based spectroscopy (^{1}H MRS or proton MRS) is the most used technique for brain tumor assessment. State-of-the-art procedures for acquiring and analyzing multivoxel MRS data are well reviewed and documented.[59,60]

Most available evidence suggests that MRS provides additional diagnostic information that improves the management and outcomes of patients who are being evaluated for brain tumors. ^{1}H MRS is the major clinically applied method in neurospectroscopy[61] as it provides information on markers of neuronal function, myelin, cell membranes, and metabolic compounds. Generally speaking, the use of MRS information for patient management depends on the clinical condition and may typically influence the decisions on biopsies. MRS is based on the fact that nuclei in different chemicals and metabolites have varying characteristic resonance patterns that depend not only on their chemical structure but also on the neighboring chemical structures and the interactions between these various chemical structures. Typical waveforms produced by an MRS examination show different peaks corresponding to nuclei in different chemical environments. Hence the spectra provide information not only about the chemical components of a tissue but also about their concentrations. Single voxel spectroscopy (SVS) techniques are extremely popular because of their ease of use. SVS techniques use selective excitation pulses to localize the signal to a relatively small volume of tissue. Two popular techniques are stimulated echo acquisition mode (STEAM)[62] and point-resolved spectroscopy (PRESS).[63]

Metabolic parameters found most useful in distinguishing tumor from normal and necrotic tissue are levels

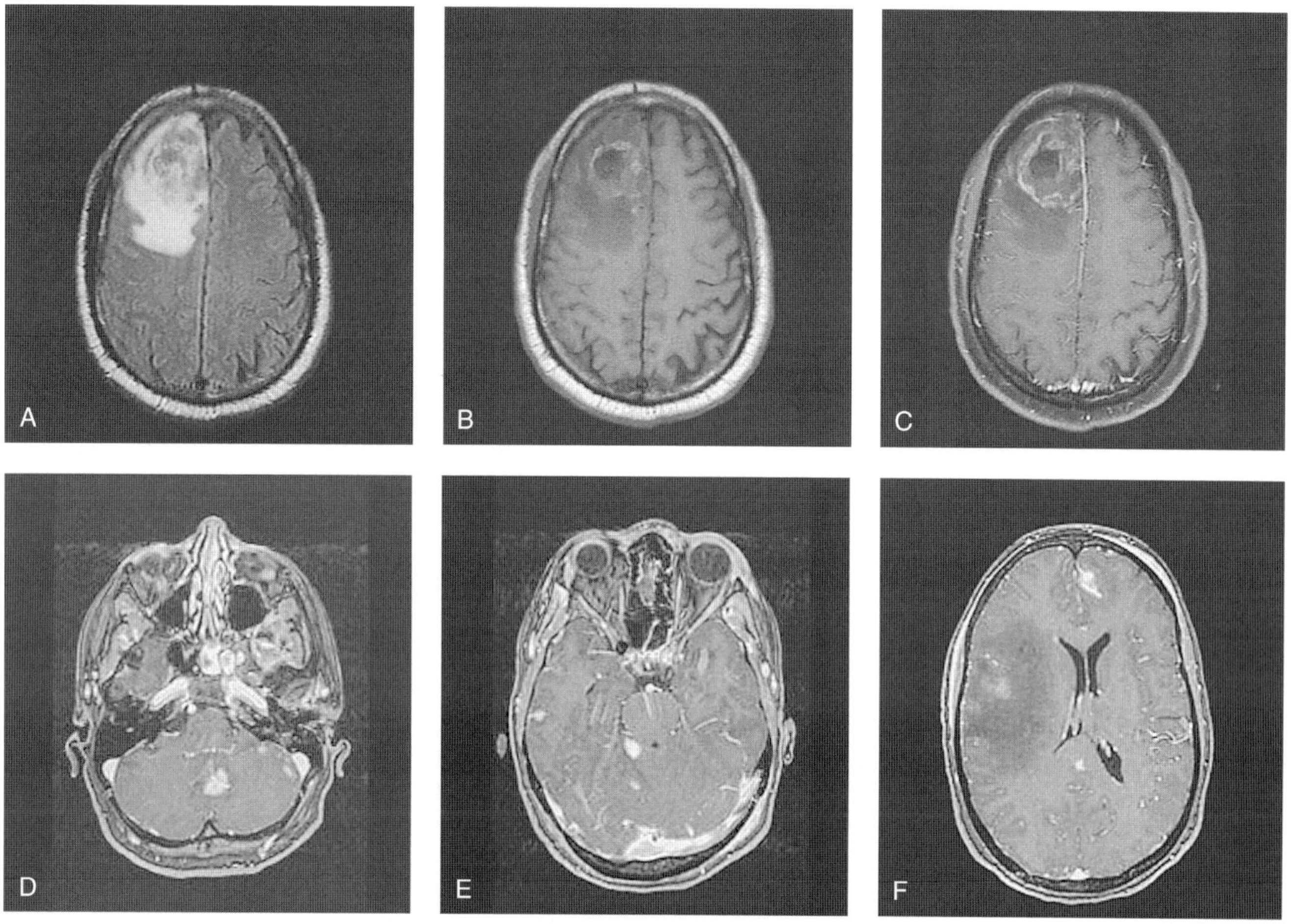

Figure 4-13. The upper panel represents a PCNSL in an immunocompromised patient. The tumor is a mass with signal intensity of brain on FLAIR (A) with surrounding hyperintense signal from vasogenic edema or infiltrative tumor. Following the administration of contrast, there is significant contrast enhancement, although the pattern is heterogeneous because of the presence of tumor necrosis. The precontrast T_1 image (B) is compared to the postcontrast T_1 image; (C) illustrates the presence of blood products. The lower panel represents an immunocompetent patient with multifocal disease. There are areas of abnormal enhancement seen on this series of postcontrast slices in multiple areas of the CNS.

of choline and *N*-acetyl aspartate (NAA).[64] It has been also shown that combination of conventional volumetric MRI and multivoxel localized MRSI data provides the potential for quantifying variations in tissue morphology and function. Other combined approaches for evaluation of cerebral gliomas, such as using a combination of MRS, perfusion, diffusion, and other techniques, have been published.[65–71] Attempts have been made to correlate kinetic parameters such as cerebral blood volume, the apparent diffusion coefficient, and metabolite information obtained from proton MRS. These techniques are complementary to each other, while aiding in the diagnosis and differentiation of tumors. Several significant metabolite correlations have been proposed which suggest that critical aspects of tumor proliferation such as neuronal damage, energy metabolism, necrotic transformation, and metastases may be better understood by using techniques that provide spectral information. Tumor heterogeneity has also been analyzed using spectroscopic techniques.[72] Tumor burden measured using the extent of metabolic abnormalities or the metabolic levels in the most abnormal voxels was correlated with the degree of malignancy of the tumor. Such information about metabolites could potentially provide valuable information about the biochemistry of tumor-specific processes such as survival, proliferation, invasion, and angiogenesis (Fig. 4-14).

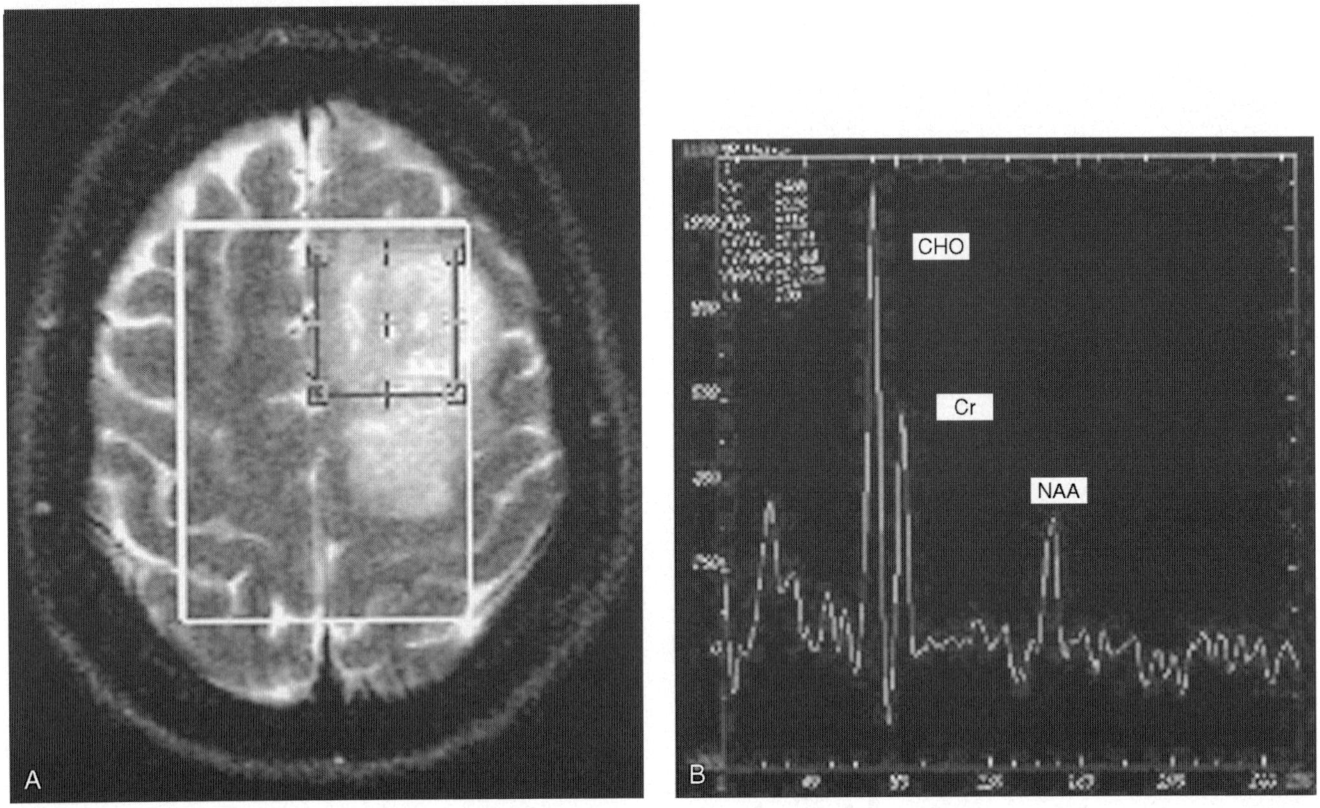

Figure 4-14. A single voxel proton MRS study of a patient with an anaplastic glioma. Panel A localizes placement of the VOI (voxel of interest) over the hyperintense T_2 signal. The spectra in this area are illustrated in panel B with NAA (*N*-acetylaspartate), CHO (choline), and CR (creatine compounds).

Perfusion Magnetic Resonance

Perfusion refers to the physiologic state of the delivery of blood to the microcirculation. The quantification of tissue perfusion may be obtained with MR by combining fast image acquisition with timed contrast administration. The resultant maps may be useful in characterizing alterations in perfusion that occur in pathologic states. Malignant gliomas are noted for their intense neovascularization or angiogenesis. The presence of endothelial cell proliferation is one of the histologic hallmarks of glioblastoma multiforme and is a clear property that separates the low-grade from the high-grade glial tumors. As a result, this property is useful in tumor grading and may be used as a marker of tumor transformation or progression.

The utility of MR to quantitate tissue perfusion was initially noted as an early indicator of tissue at risk in the clinical setting of stroke. Perfusion MR has also been used to characterize glial neoplasms. The technical aspects of perfusion MR rely on the acquisition of serial images before, during, and after contrast administration. This tracking of a contrast bolus is referred to as dynamic contrast-enhanced (DCE) or bolus-tracking MRI. The resultant images may be used to generate a signal-change-versus-time curve from which properties related to the tumor vascular state may be extracted.

DCE-MRI may be acquired with a T_1-weighting or T_2^* bolus tracking. In both instances, serial images are acquired during contrast administration in order to generate a signal-change-to-time curve. The analysis of these curves may differ but have been shown to provide useful information related to the tumor-associated features of permeability, blood volume, and blood flow. In the clinical setting of glial neoplasms, these parameters have been shown to be altered; depending upon the grade of astrocytic tumors,[73,74] they may be useful for directing surgical interventions[75] and in the assessment of tumor response to antiangiogenic or chemotherapeutic agents (Fig. 4-15).[76,77]

Diffusion Magnetic Resonance

The basic principle of diffusion-weighted imaging (DWI) comes from a very common physical phenomenon: brownian motion of water molecules. The energy carried

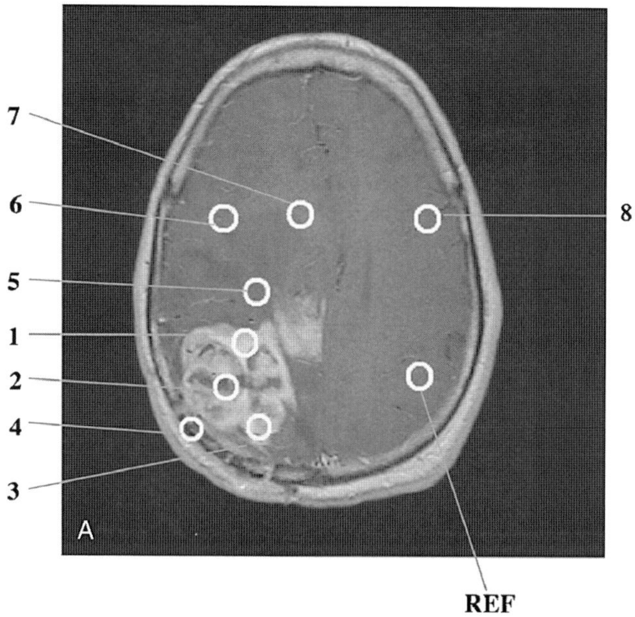

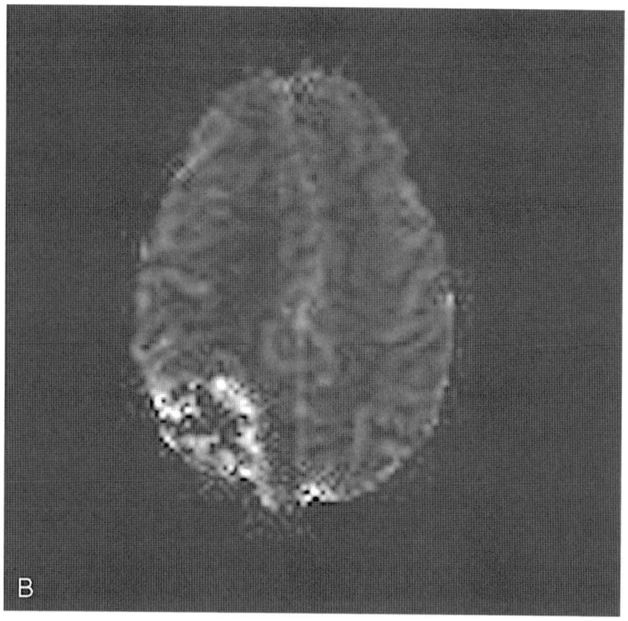

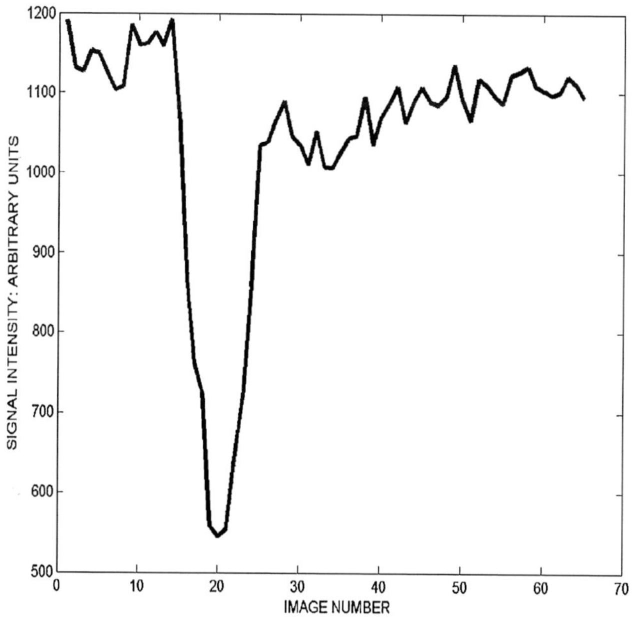

C

ROI Number	Normalized CBV Ratio	Normalized CBF Ratio
1	11.72	3.62
2	0.76	0.86
3	8.89	6.38
4	0.00	0.00
5	0.36	0.37
6	0.35	0.35
7	1.69	1.71
8	1.91	1.69

D

Figure 4-15. Perfusion MR using a T_2* dynamic contrast susceptibility study allows demonstration of relative cerebral blood volume (CBV) and flow (CBF). Panel A provides the postcontrast T_1 study that illustrates a right parietal mass of heterogeneous enhancement consistent with a glioblastoma multiforme. ROIs (regions of interest) have been placed in multiple areas corresponding to the extraaxial space, enhancing rim, central area of necrosis, peritumoral region, and a reference in the contralateral uninvolved hemisphere. The CBV parametric map is generated from the signal-loss-versus-time curve illustrated in (C) and displayed in (B). Table D provides the ratios of CBV and CBF from the different ROIs following normalization with the REF ROI. There are significant increases in these values in the ROIs that correspond to the enhancing border of the tumor. Also of note is a decrease in CBV and CBF in the peritumoral area consistent with loss of cerebral autoregulation and peritumoral ischemia.

by water molecules leads to a random motion of these molecules. The pattern of this random, diffusion-driven motion is correlated with the tissue structure. Through the detection of the movement of water molecules within tissues, DWI provides an additional MRI modality to study tissue structures and diagnose diseases.

During DWI, a pair of dephasing and rephasing magnetic field gradients is applied in a specified direction to probe water molecule motion in that direction.[78] The rephasing gradient is able to refocus the signal dephased by the prior dephasing gradient. If there were no random motion of molecules, we could expect that the signal would be refocused perfectly; that is, no signal attenuation could be observed. During this interval protons diffuse to new positions in the gradient direction in the time between the applications of dephasing and rephasing gradients, causing signal loss or attenuation. The information of the diffusivity in a particular direction can be obtained through the measurement of the amount of signal attenuation. The signal intensity S following application of the diffusion gradients is $S = S_0 \exp(-bD)$, where S_0 is the signal intensity with no diffusion gradients applied, b is a function of the diffusion gradient strength and duration, and D is diffusion value or *apparent diffusion coefficient* (ADC).

Diffusion is a three-dimensional process. If the water molecule motion was independent of direction (i.e., isotropic diffusion), ADC would be sufficient to describe tissue diffusivity. However, directionally dependent motion (i.e., anisotropic diffusion) is observed in muscle, spinal cord, and white matter, in which diffusion along a certain direction is favored while restricted in other directions. For example, in white matter, diffusion in the direction of the fibers is much faster than in the perpendicular direction. To fully characterize the diffusion anisotropy in this situation, a more complex technique of diffusion tensor imaging (DTI) must be used.[79] A diffusion tensor is a 3×3 matrix derived by applying diffusion gradients along at least 6 noncollinear directions.[80] Diagonalizing diffusion tensor matrix gives eigenvalues and eigenvectors, the effective principal diffusivities along the orthotropic axis of the tissue, which can be used to measure the mean diffusivity and diffusion anisotropy. Assuming that water tends to diffuse along white matter fibers, white matter tracts can be mapped by identifying the direction of the longest axis of principal diffusivities (Fig. 4-16).

Application in Brain Tumor Diagnosis

Although conventional contrast-enhanced T_1- and T_2-weighted images can provide information about the location and extent of a brain tumor, these modalities are limited in their ability to reliably define tumor boundaries and grade. DWI and DTI have been increasingly used for tumor delineation, grading, and invasion assessment. Although their usefulness in brain tumor diagnosis and treatment is still controversial, their potential applications in this area have been well recognized.

Tumor Delineation

In several studies, ADC values were used to differentiate tumor, edema, and normal brain tissue.[81–83] The results suggested that ADC values might be helpful for identifying different tissues and depicting tumor border, because cystic or necrotic areas have the highest ADC values and contrast-enhancing tumors have lower ADC values than both cystic or necrotic areas and edema. On the contrary, some studies demonstrated that DWI has no significant advantage in characterizing brain tumor and peritumoral tissue[84–86] because the ADC values from tumor, edema, and normal tissue overlapped. The contradictory results are probably caused by different image acquisition and postimage processing techniques among the studies. Currently, no firm conclusion can be drawn as to whether ADC values are useful in tumor demarcation and further studies are still required.

Mean diffusivity (D) and fractional anisotropy (FA) obtained from DTI were also used to delineate brain tumors.[82,83] The results show that D is highest in the necrotic tumor core followed by edematous brain, enhancing tumor core, enhancing tumor margin, and normal brain. Therefore D values can be used to differentiate brain tissues. Diffusion anisotropic data FA, however, demonstrated no significant difference among tissues.

Tumor Grading

ADC values have also been used in grading tumor types. Because cellularity is one of the most important factors for determining grade, these studies tried to correlate the cellularity with ADC value.[86,87] The results show that ADC value is inversely proportional to tumor cellularity, that is, the higher the grade of tumor, the lower the ADC value it has. This observation may be explained by the fact that more highly cellular tumor has a smaller interstitial space, restricting the motion of water in the interstitium and reduces the ADC value.

Tumor Invasion Assessment

Assessing tumor invasion is probably one of the most exciting and potential applications of DTI and is expected to be intensely used in clinical medicine in the future. Usually, brain tumor tends to spread out from its core, especially along white matter. Unfortunately, this is rarely observable in conventional MRI. After tumor invasion, the diffusivity, anisotropy, and structure of white matter may change, reflecting the displacement, invasion, and disruption of white matter.[88,89] These changes can be detected by using information from eigenvalues and

Figure 4-16 (PLATE 1). Diffusion-weighted MR of a normal volunteer (left panel) and a patient with a right frontal GBM (right panel). ADC map (A, B), FA map (C, D), DTI with color overlay (E, F), and fiber tracking on color map (G, H).

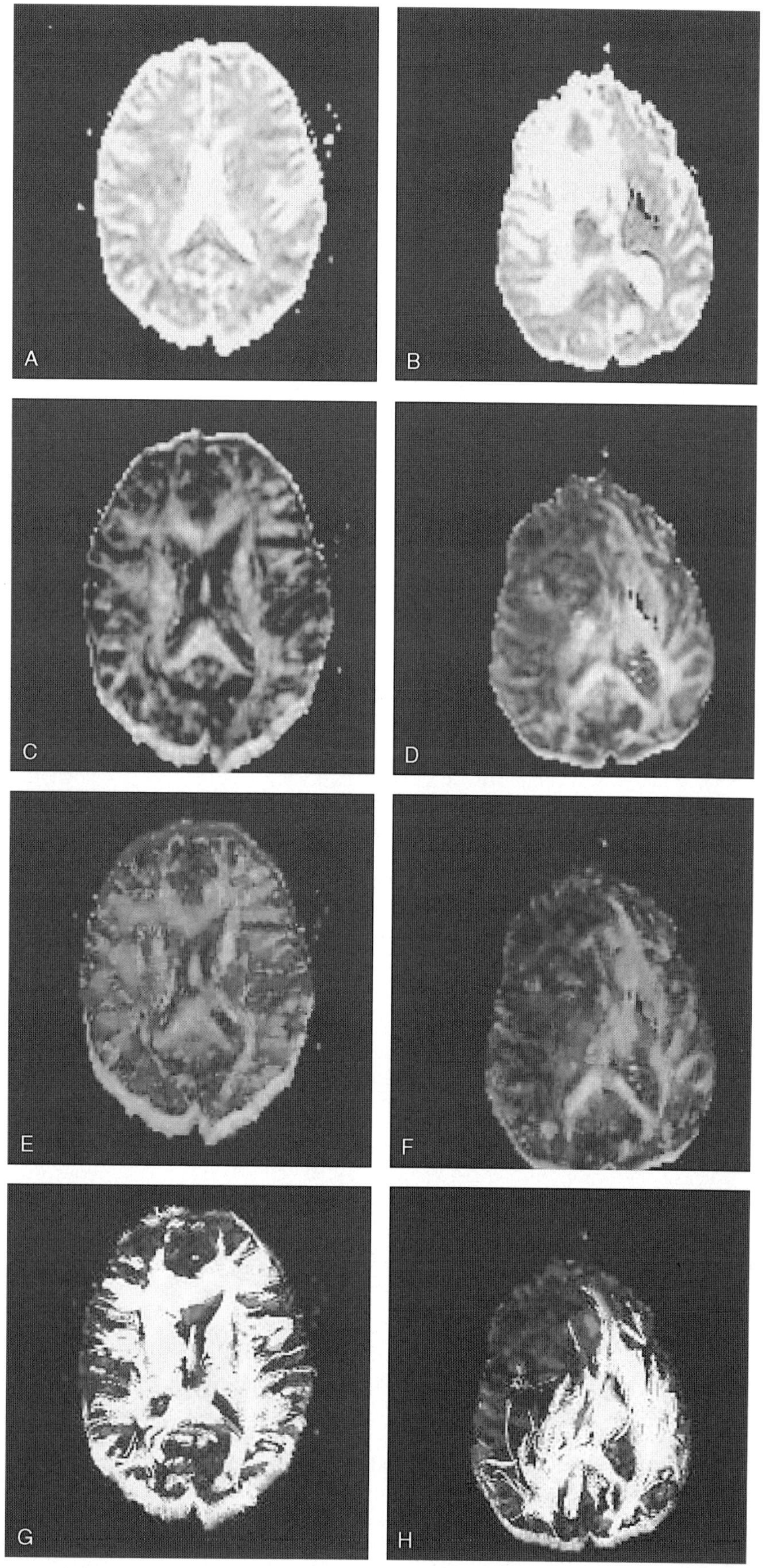

eigenvectors derived from diffusion tensor matrix as mentioned above. Thus patterns of tumor infiltration can be mapped, making treatment procedures (surgical resection, radiotherapy, and chemotherapy) more targeted.

REFERENCES

1. Macdonald DR, Cascino TL, Schold SC Jr, et al. Response criteria for phase II studies of supratentorial malignant glioma. J Clin Oncol 1990;8(7):1277–1280.
2. Lipper MH, Eberhard DA, Phillips CD, et al. Pleomorphic xanthoastrocytoma, a distinctive astroglial tumor: neuroradiologic and pathologic features. Am J Neuroradiol 1993; 14:1397–1404.
3. Scott JN, Brasher PM, Sevick RJ, et al. How often are nonenhancing supratentorial gliomas malignant? A population study. Neurology 2002;59:947–949.
4. Barker FG II, Chang SM, Huhn SL, et al. Age and the risk of anaplasia in magnetic resonance-nonenhancing supratentorial cerebral tumors. Cancer 1997;80:936–941.
5. Graif M, Bydder GM, Steiner RE, et al. Contrast-enhanced MR imaging of malignant brain tumors. Am J Neuroradiol 1985;6:855–862.
6. Lee C, Duncan VW, Young B. Magnetic resonance features of the enigmatic oligodendroglioma. Invest Radiol 1998;33(4): 222–231.
7. Vonofakos D, Marcu H, Hacker H. Oligodendrogliomas: CT patterns with emphasis on features indicating malignancy. J Comput Assist Tomogr 1979;3(6):783–788.
8. Engelhard HH, Stelea A, Mundt A. Oligodendroglioma and anaplastic oligodendroglioma: clinical features, treatment, and prognosis. Surg Neurol 2003;60:443–456.
9. Lee Y-Y, Van Tassel P. Intracranial oligodendrogliomas: imaging findings in 35 untreated cases. Am J Neuroradiol 1989;10:119–127.
10. Daumas-Duport C, Varlet P, Tucker M-L, et al. Oligodendrogliomas. Part I: Patterns of growth, histological diagnosis, clinical and imaging correlations: A study of 153 cases. J Neurooncol 1997;34:37–59.
11. Daumas-Duport C, Tucker M-L, Kolles H, et al. Oligodendrogliomas. Part II: a new grading system based on morphological and imaging criteria. J Neurooncol 1997;34:61–78.
12. Reiche W, Grunwald I, Hermann K, et al. Oligodendrogliomas. Acta Radiol 2002;43(5):474–482.
13. Derlon JM, Chapon F, Noel MH, et al. Non-invasive grading of oligodendrogliomas: correlations between in vivo metabolic pattern and histopathology. Eur J Nucl Med 2000;27(7): 778–787.
14. Mineura K, Shioya H, Kowada M, et al. Blood flow and metabolism of oligodendrogliomas: a positron emission tomography study with kinetic analysis of F-fluorodeoxyglucose. J Neurooncol 1999;43:49–57.
15. Brandes AA, Palmisano V, Monfardini S. Modulloblastoma in adults: clinical characteristics and treatment. Cancer Treatment Reviews 1999;25:3–12.
16. Blaser SI, Harwood-Nash DCF. Neuroradiology of pediatric posterior fossa medulloblastoma. J Neurooncol 1996;29: 23–34.
17. Hubbard JL, Scheithauer BW, Kispert DB, et al. Adult cerebellar medulloblastomas: the pathological, radiographic, and clinical disease spectrum. J Neurosurg 1989;70:526–544.
18. Packer RJ, Cogen P, Vezina G, et al. Medulloblastoma: clinical and biologic aspects. Neuro-oncol 1999;1(3):232–250.
19. Minn AY, Pollock BH, Garzarella L, et al. Surveillance neuroimaging to detect relapse in childhood brain tumors: a Pediatric Oncology Group study. J Clin Oncol 2001;19(21): 4135–4140.
20. Meyers SP, Wildenhain SL, Chang J-K, et al. Postoperative evaluation for disseminated medulloblastoma involving the spine: contrast-enhanced MR findings, CSF cytologic analysis, timing of disease occurrence, and patient outcomes. Am J Neuroradiol 2000;21:1757–1765.
21. Choi J-Y, Chang K-H, Yu IK, et al. Intracranial and spinal ependymomas: review of MR images in 61 patients. Korean J Radiol 2002;3(4):219–228.
22. Armington WG, Osborn AG, Cubberley DA, et al. Supratentorial ependymoma: CT appearance. Radiology 1985; 157:367–372.
23. Fine MJ, Kricheff IK, Freed D, et al. Spinal cord ependymomas: MR imaging features. Radiology 1995;197:655–658.
24. Furie DM, Provenzale JM. Supratentorial ependymomas and subependymomas: CT and MR appearance. J Comput Assist Tomogr 1995;19(4):518–526.
25. Tortori-Donati PM, Fondelli P, Cama A, et al. Ependymomas of the posterior cranial fossa: CT and MRI findings. Neuroradiology 1995;37:238–243.
26. Luyken C, Blumoke I, Fimmers R, et al. Supratentorial gangliogliomas: histopathologic grading and tumor recurrence in 184 patients with a median follow-up of 8 years. Cancer 2004;1:146–155.
27. Demierre B, Stichnoth FA, Hori A, et al. Intracerebral ganglioglioma. J Neurosurg 1986;65:177–182.
28. Dufresne MC, Bedard F. X-ray computed tomographic aspects of malignant meningioma and meningeal hemangiopericytoma. Can Assoc Radiol J 1996;47(4):279–287.
29. Servo A, Porras M, Jaaskelainen J, et al. Computed tomography and angiography do not reliably discriminate malignant meningiomas from benign ones. Neuroradiology 1990;32(2): 94–97.
30. Buetow MP, Buetow PC, Smirniotopoulos JG. Typical, atypical, and misleading features in meningioma. Radiographics 1991;11(6):1087–1106.
31. Elster AD, Challa VR, Gilbert TH, et al. Meningiomas: MR and histopathologic features [see comment]. Radiology 1989; 170(3 Pt 1):857–862.
32. Maiuri F, Iaconetta G, de Divitiis O, et al. Intracranial meningiomas: correlations between MR imaging and histology. Eur J Radiol 1999;31(1):69–75.
33. Goldman CK, Bharara S, Palmer CA, et al. Brain edema in meningiomas is associated with increased vascular endothelial growth factor expression. Neurosurgery 1997;40(6):1269–1277.
34. Filippi CG, Edgar MA, Ulug AM, et al. Appearance of meningiomas on diffusion-weighted images: correlating diffusion constants with histopathologic findings. Am J Neuroradiol 2001;22(1):65–72.
35. Tanaka Y, Matsuo M. Role of MR imaging in the differentiation of benign and nonbenign intracranial meningiomas:

the utility of contrast-enhanced T_1-weighted images. Nippon Igaku Hoshasen Gakkai Zasshi 1996;56(1):1–8.
36. Harting I, Hartmann M, Bonsanto MM, et al. Characterization of necrotic meningioma using diffusion MRI, perfusion MRI, and MR spectroscopy: case report and review of the literature. Neuroradiology 2004;46(3):189–193.
37. Nishi T, Kuratsu J, Takeshima H, et al. Prognostic significance of the MIB-1 labeling index for patient with craniopharyngioma. Int J Mol Med 1999;3(2):157–161.
38. Brummitt ML, Kline LB, Wilson ER. Craniopharyngioma: pitfalls in diagnosis. J Clin Neuroophthalmol 1992;12(2): 77–81.
39. Linden CN, Martinez CR, Gonzalvo AA, et al. Intrinsic third ventricle craniopharyngioma: CT and MR findings. J Comput Assist Tomogr 1989;13(2):362–363.
40. Mark RJ, Lutge WR, Shimizu KT, et al. Craniopharyngioma: treatment in the CT and MR imaging era. Radiology 1995;197(1):195–198.
41. Ahmadi J, Destian S, Apuzzo ML, et al. Cystic fluid in craniopharyngiomas: MR imaging and quantitative analysis. Radiology 1992;182(3):783–785.
42. Ikezaki K, Fujii K, Kishikawa T. Magnetic resonance imaging of an intraventricular craniopharyngioma. Neuroradiology 1990;32(3):247–249.
43. Packer RJ, Nicholson HS, Vezina LG, et al. Brainstem gliomas. Neurosurg Clin N Am 1992;3(4):863–879.
44. Stroink AR, Hoffman HJ, Hendrick EB, et al. Diagnosis and management of pediatric brain-stem gliomas. J Neurosurg 1986;65(6):745–750.
45. Zimmerman RA. Neuroimaging of primary brainstem gliomas: diagnosis and course. Pediatr Neurosurg 1996;25: 45–53.
46. Fishbein NJ, Prados MD, Wara W, et al. Radiologic classification of brain stem tumors: correlation of magnetic resonance imaging appearance with clinical outcome. Pediatr Neurosurg 1996;24:9–23.
47. Kaplan AM, Albright AL, Zimmerman RA, et al. Brainstem gliomas in children. A Children's Cancer Group review of 119 cases. Pediatr Neurosurg 1996;24(4):185–192.
48. Hasuo K, Uchino A, Matsumoto S, et al. MR imaging compared with CT, angiography, and myelography supplemented with CT in the diagnosis of spinal tumors. Radiat Med 1993;11(5):177–186.
49. Wierzba-Bobrowicz T, Schmidt-Sidor B, Szpak GM, et al. Haemangioblastoma of the posterior cranial fossa: clinico-neuropathological study. Folia Neuropathol 2003;41(4): 245–249.
50. Wolansky LJ, Malantic GP, Heary R, et al. Preoperative MRI diagnosis of Lhermitte-Duclos disease: case report with associated enlarged vessel and syrinx. Surg Neurol 1996;45(5): 470–475.
51. Escott EJ, Kleinschmidt-DeMasters BK, Brega K, et al. Proximal nerve root spinal hemangioblastomas: presentation of three cases, MR appearance, and literature review. Surg Neurol 2004;61(3):262–273.
52. Ling SM, Roach M 3rd, Larson DA, et al. Radiotherapy of primary central nervous system lymphoma in patients with and without human immunodeficiency virus. Ten years of treatment experience at the University of California San Francisco. Cancer 1994;73(10):2570–2582.
53. Coulon A, Lafitte F, Hoang-Xuan K, et al. Radiographic findings in 37 cases of primary CNS lymphoma in immunocompetent patients. Eur Radiol 2002;12:329–340.
54. Thurnher MM, Rieger A, Kleibl-Popov C, et al. Primary central nervous system lymphoma in AIDS: a wider spectrum of CT and MRI findings. Neuroradiology 2001;43:29–35.
55. Gliemroth J, Kehler U, Gaebel C, et al. Neuroradiological findings in primary cerebral lymphomas of non-AIDS patients. Clin Neuroradiol Neurosurg 2003;105:78–86.
56. Buhring U, Herrlinger U, Krings T, et al. MRI features of primary central nervous system lymphomas at presentation. Neurology 2001;57:393–396.
57. Lai R, Rosenblum MK, DeAngelis LM. Primary CNS lymphoma: a whole-brain disease? Neurology 2002;59:1557–1562.
58. Batchelor T, Carson K, O'Neill A, et al. Treatment of primary CNS lymphoma with methotrexate and deferred radiotherapy: a report of NABTT 96–07. J Clin Oncol 2003;24(6): 1044–1049.
59. Nelson SJ. Multivoxel magnetic resonance spectroscopy of brain tumors. Mol Cancer Ther 2003;2(5):497–507.
60. Rudkin TM, Arnold DL. Proton magnetic resonance spectroscopy for the diagnosis and management of cerebral disorders. Arch Neurol 1999;56(8):919–926.
61. Burtscher IM, Holtas S. Proton MR spectroscopy in clinical routine. J Magn Reson Imaging 2001;13(4):560–567.
62. Frahm J, Bruhn H, Gyngell ML, et al. Localized high-resolution proton NMR spectroscopy using stimulated echoes: initial applications to human brain in vivo. Magn Reson Med 1989; 9(1):79–93.
63. Bottomley PA. Spatial localization in NMR spectroscopy in vivo. Ann NY Acad Sci 1987;508:333–348.
64. Nelson SJ. Analysis of volume MRI and MR spectroscopic imaging data for the evaluation of patients with brain tumors. Magn Reson Med 2001;46(2):228–239.
65. Law M, Cha S, Knopp EA, et al. High-grade gliomas and solitary metastases: differentiation by using perfusion and proton spectroscopic MR imaging. Radiology 2002;222(3): 715–721.
66. Law M, Yang S, Wang H, et al. Glioma grading: sensitivity, specificity, and predictive values of perfusion MR imaging and proton MR spectroscopic imaging compared with conventional MR imaging. Am J Neuroradiol 1989;24(10): 1989–1998.
67. Howe FA, Barton SJ, Cudlip SA, et al. Metabolic profiles of human brain tumors using quantitative in vivo 1H magnetic resonance spectroscopy. Magn Reson Med 2003;49(2): 223–232.
68. Moller-Hartmann W, Herminghaus S, Krings T, et al. Clinical application of proton magnetic resonance spectroscopy in the diagnosis of intracranial mass lesions. Neuroradiology 2002;44(5):371–381.
69. Gupta RK, Sinha U, Cloughesy TF, et al. Inverse correlation between choline magnetic resonance spectroscopy signal intensity and the apparent diffusion coefficient in human glioma. Magn Reson Med 1999;41(1):2–7.
70. Yang D, Korogi Y, Sugahara T, et al. Cerebral gliomas: prospective comparison of multivoxel 2D chemical-shift imaging proton MR spectroscopy, echoplanar perfusion and diffusion-weighted MRI. Neuroradiology 2002;44(8):656–666.

71. Tzika AA, Astrakas LG, Zarifi MK, et al. Multiparametric MR assessment of pediatric brain tumors. Neuroradiology 2003;45(1):1–10.
72. Li X, Lu Y, Pirzkall A, et al. Analysis of the spatial characteristics of metabolic abnormalities in newly diagnosed glioma patients. J Magn Reson Imaging 2002;16(3):229–237.
73. Roberts HC, Roberts TP, Bollen AW, et al. Correlation of microvascular permeability derived from dynamic contrast-enhanced MR imaging with histologic grade and tumor labeling index: a study in human brain tumors [see comment]. Acad Radiol 2001;8(5):384–391.
74. Shin JH, Lee HK, Kwun BD, et al. Using relative cerebral blood flow and volume to evaluate the histopathologic grade of cerebral gliomas: preliminary results. Am J Roentgenol 2002;179(3):783–789.
75. Knopp EA, Cha S, Johnson G, et al. Glial neoplasms: dynamic contrast-enhanced T_2*-weighted MR imaging. Radiology 1999;211(3):791–798.
76. Gossmann AT, Helbich H, Kuriyama N, et al. Dynamic contrast-enhanced magnetic resonance imaging as a surrogate marker of tumor response to anti-angiogenic therapy in a xenograft model of glioblastoma multiforme. J Magn Reson Imaging 2002;15(3):233–240.
77. Aronen HJ, Glass J, Pardo FS, et al. Echo-planar MR cerebral blood volume mapping of gliomas. Clinical utility. Acta Radiol 1995;36(5):520–528.
78. Thomsen C, Henriksen O, Ring P. In vivo measurement of water self-diffusion in the human brain by magnetic resonance imaging. Acta Radiol 1987;28:353–361.
79. Basser PJ, Mattiello J, LeBihan D. MR diffusion tensor spectroscopy and imaging. Biophys J 1994;66(1):259–267.
80. Basser PJ, Mattiello J, LeBihan D. Estimation of the effective self-diffusion tensor from the NMR spin echo. J Magn Reson B 1994;103(3):247–254.
81. Krabbe K, Gideon P, Wagn P, et al. MR diffusion imaging of human intracranial tumours. Neuroradiology 1997;39(7):483–489.
82. Sinha SM, Bastin E, Whittle IR, et al. Diffusion tensor MR imaging of high-grade cerebral gliomas. Am J Neuroradiol 2002;23(4):520–527.
83. Lu S, Ahn D, Johnson G, et al. Peritumoral diffusion tensor imaging of high-grade gliomas and metastatic brain tumors. Am J Neuroradiol 2003;24(5):937–941.
84. Castillo MJ, Smith K, Kwock L, et al. Apparent diffusion coefficients in the evaluation of high-grade cerebral gliomas. Am J Neuroradiol 2001;22(1):60–64.
85. Stadnik TW, Chaskis C, Michotte A, et al. Diffusion-weighted MR imaging of intracerebral masses: comparison with conventional MR imaging and histologic findings. Am J Neuroradiol 2001;22(5):969–976.
86. Kono K, Inoue Y, Nakayama K, et al. The role of diffusion-weighted imaging in patients with brain tumors [see comment]. Am J Neuroradiol 1981;22(6):1081–8.
87. Sugahara T, Korogi Y, Kochi M, et al. Usefulness of diffusion-weighted MRI with echo-planar technique in the evaluation of cellularity in gliomas. J Magn Reson Imaging 1999;9(1):53–60.
88. Price SJ, Burnet NG, Donovan T, et al. Diffusion tensor imaging of brain tumours at 3T: a potential tool for assessing white matter tract invasion? Clin Radiol 2003;58(6):455–462.
89. Witwer BP, Moftakhar R, Hasan KM, et al. Diffusion-tensor imaging of white matter tracts in patients with cerebral neoplasm. J Neurosurg 2002;97(3):568–575.

CHAPTER 5

Neuropathology

M. Beatriz S. Lopes

Diagnosis in neuropathology is based on the integration of several steps, including a traditional morphologic examination of the tissues, a topographic/radiologic analysis of the lesion, an evaluation of these findings in view of the clinical data, and, at times, the analysis of the molecular and cytogenetic profile of the tumor. In the analysis of a brain biopsy for a tumor, the integration of pathologic findings and clinical data is essential.

This chapter presents the reader with a brief description of the most common tumors occurring within the nervous system, combined with suggestions regarding practical issues from handling of the surgical specimens to adequate communication between clinicians and pathologists to obtain the most appropriate diagnoses. Comprehensive and detailed reviews of pathologic features of all tumors of the nervous system are available in many neuropathology textbooks.

▶ GENERAL CONSIDERATIONS

Brain tumors account for approximately 3% of all malignant primary tumors. However, in children, the central nervous system (CNS) is the second most common site of primary tumors, leukemias being the most common. The distribution and categories of neoplasms that arise in the CNS of children and adults reflect the unique histogenesis of the CNS. Although the pathogenesis of brain tumors remains largely unknown, the diverse cell populations present in the immature nervous system, in contrast with the adult brain, present vulnerable targets for neoplastic transformation.[1] These distinctive histogenetic targets are reflected in the incidence of the most frequent tumors in children and adults and their distinct locations. The majority of the tumors of the adult brain are localized in the cerebral hemispheres, whereas approximately two-thirds of the tumors in children are infratentorial. Although the most common malignant tumor arising in children is an embryonal neoplasm, the cerebellar medulloblastoma, in adults glioblastomas multiforme (astrocytoma grade IV), are the most frequent malignant tumors. Molecular genetic studies also show that gliomas with similar histologic features follow different genetic pathways in pediatric and adult population. For example, oligodendrogliomas in the pediatric population have infrequent 1p and 19q chromosome alterations, whereas deletions of 1p and 19q are considered a genetic "signature" of oligodendrogliomas in adults.[2] These age- , location- , and histogenetic-related specificities serve as important reminders that the diagnosis of tumors of the CNS cannot be accurately assessed in the absence of clinical data.

Classification and Grading

The classification of nervous system tumors employed in this chapter follows the now widely adopted classification of the World Health Organization (WHO).[3] This scheme is based on the principle of a hypothesized cell of origin of the tumor and modified by associated classical histologic features of cellular and tissue arrangements and indicators of anaplastic transformation.

Grading of CNS tumors has been a controversial issue since the initial classifications of tumors, primarily as a result of somewhat imperfect qualifiers and subjective evaluation of histologic parameters of tumors. Nevertheless, the need for a systematic approach for treatment of the patients and their inclusion in many neuro-oncology protocols, necessitates a more universal and systematic designation of the different grade of tumors. The WHO classification designates gliomas and nonglial CNS tumors as grades I to IV tumors. Grade I is reserved for pilocytic astrocytoma and a few other gliomas and neuronal/dysplastic lesions. It is generally accepted that significant mitotic activity is a feature of grade III and grade IV tumors, necrosis and/or endothelial proliferation are features of grade IV tumors, and the absence of necrosis and significant mitotic activity is a feature of grade II tumors.

Prognostic Features

In addition to the histologic features discussed above, there are now several additional techniques for establishing prognostic indicators in CNS tumors. The evaluation of tumor cell proliferation, commonly by immunohistochemistry for the antigen Ki-67 (monoclonal MIB-1), has shown increasingly importance for diagnostic and therapeutic accuracy in CNS tumors. The Ki-67 antigen is a nuclear, nonhistone protein that is required for maintaining the cell cycle and is expressed during G1, S, G2, and M phases of the cell cycle, but is absent in the G0 phase. The measurement of the Ki-67 labeling index is therefore a reflection of cells within the proliferative phases of the cell cycle, including the mitotic phase. Cytogenetic and molecular profiles of CNS tumors are now emerging not just as factors of significance in the complete evaluation of CNS tumors, but as required information for clinical trial eligibility. For example, many neuro-oncology centers routinely require that gliomas with an oligodendroglial component be analyzed for alterations of chromosomes 1p and 19q before determination of specific treatments.

▶ INTRAOPERATIVE DIAGNOSIS AND HANDLING OF THE SPECIMEN

The role of the neuropathologist during intraoperative consultations of neurosurgical cases is to guide the neurosurgeon on making clinically relevant intraoperative decisions. In the great majority of cases, the intraoperative consultation consists of confirming that a neoplasm is present and determining whether it is primary or secondary, benign or malignant, and of a morphologic type that may lend itself to total excision and surgical cure. In some ways, the increased use of stereotactic biopsies has altered the significance of the role of intraoperative consultations. Pathologists are often called on to render "conclusive" diagnoses on diminutive tissue fragments. This limited tumor sampling emphasizes the importance of combining cytologic and histopathologic findings with neuroimaging data for accurate assessment of tumor diagnosis, especially considering the morphologic heterogeneity of the more anaplastic gliomas. However, both the pathologist and neurosurgeon must recognize that the intraoperative diagnosis is no more than the first step in establishing a diagnosis, and that it has its limitations. Definitive and refined diagnosis is based upon permanent sections in every case.

An intraoperative diagnosis is significantly jeopardized when performed without the benefit of clinical data and without consideration of neuroimaging data. Accurate identification of the process is based on such factors as well as patient age, clinical presentation, symptom duration, and gross operative features. Patient age and location of the mass lesion are extremely critical data in the differential diagnosis of CNS tumors. The importance of personal communication between pathologist and neurosurgeon cannot be overstated.

Although the frozen section method provides a reliable tissue diagnosis for intraoperative consultation, several centers, including ours, have demonstrated that the tissue smear technique (Fig. 5-1) represents an accurate and effective method for the intraoperative evaluation of CNS biopsies with diagnostic accuracy similar to frozen sections of neurosurgical biopsies. The great advantage of smears resides in the fact that multiple areas from small biopsy specimens may be carefully examined while conserving most tissue for optimal preservation and processing methods. In addition, smear preparations eliminate the need to perform frozen sections on small specimens and minimize the risk of distorting or losing valuable diagnostic material.

Handling of the Surgical Specimen

Because the intraoperative consultation is not the final step in the evaluation of a tumor specimen, but a diagnostic guide for the neurosurgeon, care must be taken to warrant that sufficient tissue remains for routine histology and special procedures. In any tumor case, material should be reserved for routine histology and special stains including immunohistochemistry and electron microscopy if possible. In cases with suspicion of hematopoietic disorders and lymphomas, fresh material should be submitted to flow cytometric studies for better characterization of tumor clonality. Tumor material should also be separated for immediate freezing in liquid nitrogen so that molecular biology assays can be carried out if available.

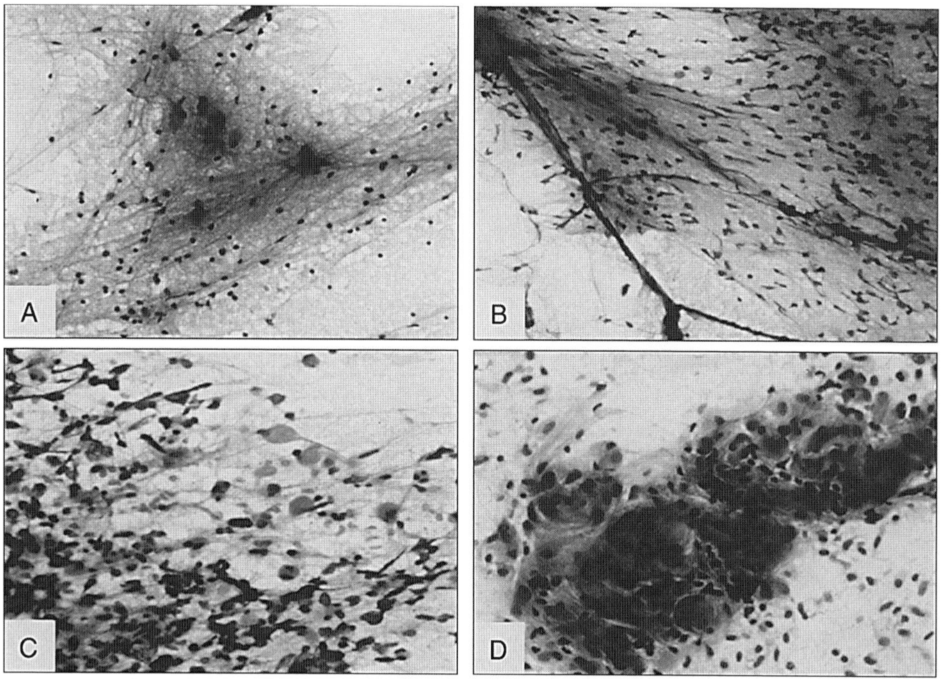

Figure 5-1 (PLATE 2). Smear preparations. (A) Smear preparation of an inflammatory process showing stellate, reactive astrocytes, edema, and mild inflammatory lymphocytic infiltration. (B) Smear preparation of a low-grade astrocytoma with cells showing fibrillary processes and mild atypia. Note the thin, delicate vessel intermixed with the cells. (C) Smear preparation of a high-grade astrocytoma composed of pleomorphic cells with variable size nuclei. Note the gemistocytic forms and the granular, necrotic background. (D) Smear preparation of a meningioma readily demonstrate typical meningothelial cells with ill-defined cytoplasmic borders. The nuclei are homogeneous. Whorl formation is prominent in this case. (A to D: Morris stain.)

▶ GENERAL APPROACH TO TISSUE EVALUATION

The analysis of histologic tissue sections is based on a systematic evaluation of several steps. As in every pathologic analysis of a tissue sample, the pathologist must first decide whether this is normal or abnormal tissue. Apparently an obvious step, in neuropathology this becomes a crucial point mainly in the setting of stereotactic biopsies that, unfortunately, may sometimes fail to yield diagnostic tissue. Once the adequacy of a specimen has been established, the identification of either an inflammatory/infectious or a neoplastic process is performed. Infectious and inflammatory diseases may mimic CNS tumors in both clinical presentation and neuroimaging findings, and these differential diagnoses may be a challenge for the pathologist. Acute demyelinating disease such as multiple sclerosis may present as hypercellular lesions composed of bizarre, pleomorphic astrocytes intermixed with variable degree of infiltration of macrophages and lymphocytes. Careful analysis of the cytologic features and the application of special histochemical and immunohistochemical stains yield a more precise diagnosis. Stains for myelin (e.g., Luxol-fast blue) and axons (e.g., Bielschowsky) facilitate the confirmatory features of demyelination with relative preservation of axonal processes. Immunohistochemistry for macrophages and leukocyte antigens confirm the presence of these cell types within the astrocytic proliferation. Most of the time, it is simple to identify basic lesions, such as abscesses, metastatic carcinomas, lymphomas, and, obviously, malignant gliomas. More problematic, however, is the distinction between gliosis and a low-grade glioma.

Conventional steps in the analysis of primary brain tumors include examination of

1. The general tumor architecture and the degree of cellularity.
2. The presence or absence of histologic cellular arrangements; for instance, rosette or pseudorosette formation in ependymomas, and specialized arrangements like meningothelial whorls in meningiomas.
3. The cytologic features of the tumor cells including the characteristics of cytoplasm, presence or absence of cellular processes, quality of the

chromatin, and presence or absence of prominent nucleoli. The presence of cellular fibrillary processes is particularly useful in identifying gliomas, especially astrocytomas of any grade, while scarce cytoplasm or the presence of perinuclear halos is more consistent with an oligodendroglial tumor.

4. The degree of cytologic atypia and other features suggestive of malignancy. The several grading systems that the WHO recommends should be applied to the individual groups of tumors. For example, in diffusely infiltrating astrocytomas, four histologic criteria should be examined in a given tumor, including cellular atypia, mitotic activity, presence or absence of microvascular endothelial proliferation, and presence or absence of tumoral necrosis.

The use of ancillary techniques to further characterize a pathologic process is applied in many situations in neuropathology. In cases of inflammatory/infectious process, special histochemical stains for microorganisms (bacteria, fungi, and mycobacteria) are always employed. However, these tissue stains do not always produce sufficient information about a specific microorganism. Consequently, the pathologist should advise the neurosurgeon to send material for microbiologic studies directly from the operating room in cases of suspected infectious process. In tumors, several immunohistochemical markers may help to define a specific glioma, assess a proliferative index, and other specific oncogenes and tumor suppressor genes. As is discussed in several sections of this chapter, immunohistochemical stains for glial (glial fibrillary acidic protein [GFAP], S100, vimentin) and neuronal (neurofilaments, synaptophysin, neuron-specific nuclear protein [NeuN]) markers are routinely used in any pathology laboratory. In addition, a battery of antibodies against specific cellular markers may be applied in cases of metastatic tumors.

Finally, the pathologist must always be prepared to admit that pathologic findings are negative or mention that they are inconsistent with the clinical-radiologic data. Comparison of the radiographic and pathologic findings is an essential step in arriving at the correct diagnosis.

▶ PRIMARY CENTRAL NERVOUS SYSTEM TUMORS

This chapter reviews the tumors of the central nervous system as classified by the WHO.[3] Especially mentioned are the most common tumors in the category of neuroepithelial tumors and those of the meninges. Other more uncommon categories of tumors, including pineal parenchymal tumors and germ cell tumors, are reviewed in other chapters. This review emphasizes the distinctive cytologic and histopathologic properties of these tumors, their salient clinical features, and their molecular genetic profile.

Neuroepithelial Tumors

Gliomas

Gliomas are the most common tumors of the CNS in all age groups, representing approximately 45% of all CNS tumors.[4] They are classified according to the predominant cell type that presumably gives origin to the tumors, and are thus classified as astrocytomas, oligodendrogliomas, and ependymomas (Table 5-1).

Astrocytic Tumors

Astrocytomas are tumors composed of proliferating neoplastic astrocytes and comprise a group of neoplasms that vary greatly in morphologic features and biologic behavior. Astrocytomas constitute approximately 70% of all gliomas and are classically divided into two groups according to their capacity to infiltrate the surrounding brain: (a) diffuse infiltrating astrocytomas and (b) circumscribed astrocytomas.

Diffuse Infiltrating Astrocytomas The diffuse infiltrating astrocytomas constitute nearly 60% of all brain tumors.[5] They comprise a continuous spectrum of differentiation and malignancy degree, and represent prognostically unfavorable diffuse tumors. In this group are included the *astrocytoma* (astrocytoma WHO Grade II), the *anaplastic astrocytoma* (astrocytoma WHO Grade III), and the *glioblastoma multiforme* (astrocytoma WHO Grade IV).

Diffuse infiltrating astrocytomas show a capacity for infiltration of the adjacent brain regardless of histologic grade. In addition, these tumors have an intrinsic tendency to progress to more malignant phenotypes with remarkable intratumoral heterogeneity, both morphologic and genetic, which increases with progressive anaplastic transformation. The intrinsic tendency towards anaplastic transformation of diffuse astrocytomas contributes to the general poor prognosis of these tumors.

Astrocytoma Astrocytomas (WHO grade II) are low-grade, diffusely infiltrative neoplasms composed of astrocytes. These tumors may occur in patients of all ages and may arise at any location of the neuraxis. However, site predilection varies according to the patient's age; in adults, they are more common in the cerebral hemispheres, whereas in children these tumors usually arise in the brainstem. Both grossly and microscopically, astrocytomas are ill-defined masses that diffusely infiltrate the surrounding brain. Astrocytomas have been traditionally subdivided into three major variants—*fibrillary, protoplasmic,*

▶ TABLE 5-1. HISTOLOGICAL CLASSIFICATION OF NEUROEPITHELIAL TUMORS

1. Tumors of the Glial Tissue—Gliomas
   - A. Astrocytic tumors
     - Diffuse astrocytomas
       - Astrocytoma
       - Anaplastic astrocytoma
       - Glioblastoma multiforme and variants
     - Special subtypes of astrocytomas
       - Pilocytic astrocytoma
       - Pleomorphic xanthoastrocytoma
       - Subependymal giant cell astrocytoma
       - Desmoplastic infantile astrocytoma
       - Gliofibroma
   - B. Oligodendroglial tumors
     - Oligodendroglioma
     - Anaplastic oligodendroglioma
     - Oligoastrocytoma
     - Anaplastic oligoastrocytoma
   - C. Ependymal tumors
     - Ependymoma
     - Anaplastic ependymoma
     - Myxopapillary ependymoma
     - Subependymoma
   - D. Choroid plexus tumors
     - Choroid plexus papilloma
     - Choroid plexus carcinoma
2. Neuronal and mixed neuronal-glial tumors
   - A. Neuronal tumors
     - Gangliocytoma
     - Dysplastic gangliocytoma of the cerebellum
     - Central neurocytoma and variants
   - B. Mixed neuronal-glial tumors
     - Ganglioglioma
     - Anaplastic ganglioglioma
     - Desmoplastic infantile ganglioglioma
     - Dysembryoplastic neuroepithelial tumor
3. Embryonal tumors
   - Medulloblastoma
     - Classical medulloblastoma
     - Desmoplastic/nodular medulloblastoma
     - Medullomyoblastoma
     - Melanotic medulloblastoma
   - Supratentorial primitive neuroectodermal tumor
   - Medulloepithelioma
   - Ependymoblastoma
   - Central neuroblastoma
   - Atypical teratoid/rhabdoid tumor

and *gemistocytic astrocytomas*—according to their resemblance to typical morphologic subtypes of astrocytes in normal and reactive brain. This subclassification of astrocytomas has significant limitations, and in reality, the majority of tumors have a mixed population of the different subtypes. However, particular consideration should be given to astrocytomas with a significant gemistocytic component (see below).

Histologically, low cellularity and minimal cellular/nuclear atypia characterize low-grade astrocytomas (Fig. 5-2). Histologic features suggestive of anaplasia, including increased mitotic activity, endothelial microvascular proliferation, and necrosis, are absent in these tumors. Tumors with more fibrillary cellular components have prominent cytoplasmic processes that form a rich fibrillary stroma. In other examples, the tumors may be composed of large numbers of protoplasmic astrocytes with stellate-shaped cells intermixed within an abundant eosinophilic matrix. Microcystic formation and a loose matrix may be present.

Astrocytomas with a major component of gemistocytic cells are classified as *gemistocytic astrocytomas*. Gemistocytic astrocytomas are characterized by cells with abundant eosinophilic, round to slightly angulated cytoplasm, and eccentric nuclei. The fibrillary matrix, commonly seen in the more fibrillary tumors, is less conspicuous. Tumor comprised solely of gemistocytic astrocytes are rare,[6] but the presence of significant numbers of gemistocytes is a sign of poor prognosis in low-grade astrocytomas.[6,7] In a large series of cases, low-grade astrocytomas containing more than 5% gemistocytes had a significantly shorter time to progression than those tumors with less than 5% gemistocytes.[7]

Special stains are helpful for the characterization of the astrocytic nature of low-grade astrocytomas. Astrocytomas are conspicuously immunoreactive for GFAP and vimentin in both cytoplasm and cellular processes. Tumor cells also show immunoreactivity to S100 protein in the nucleus and in cellular processes.

Mitotic activity is absent or low in low-grade astrocytomas, and assessment of proliferative activity by immunohistochemistry against the antigen Ki-67 shows low labeling index (LI) with mean values ranging from 2% to 4%.[8–10]

Although considered "low-grade" tumors, astrocytomas actually behave in a rather aggressive fashion, and the prognosis is guarded. The incidence of progression within astrocytomas is variable but may be as high as 80%,[11] and the median survival is about 7 years.[5] The time interval for astrocytomas to progress to glioblastoma appears to be shorter in those astrocytomas carrying a *TP53* mutation.[7]

Anaplastic Astrocytoma Anaplastic astrocytomas (WHO grade III) constitute a group of astrocytic neoplasms that, although exhibiting more prominent histologic features of anaplasia than low-grade astrocytomas, do not exhibit the degree of anaplasia seen in glioblastomas multiforme. Similar to astrocytomas, anaplastic astrocytomas arise most frequently in the cerebral hemispheres; however, they tend to occur in patients a decade older than those with astrocytomas (median age 41 years).[5] Although anaplastic astrocytomas may arise from progression of an astrocytoma, these tumors also apparently arise *de novo* without undergoing malignant transformation from a low-grade astrocytoma.

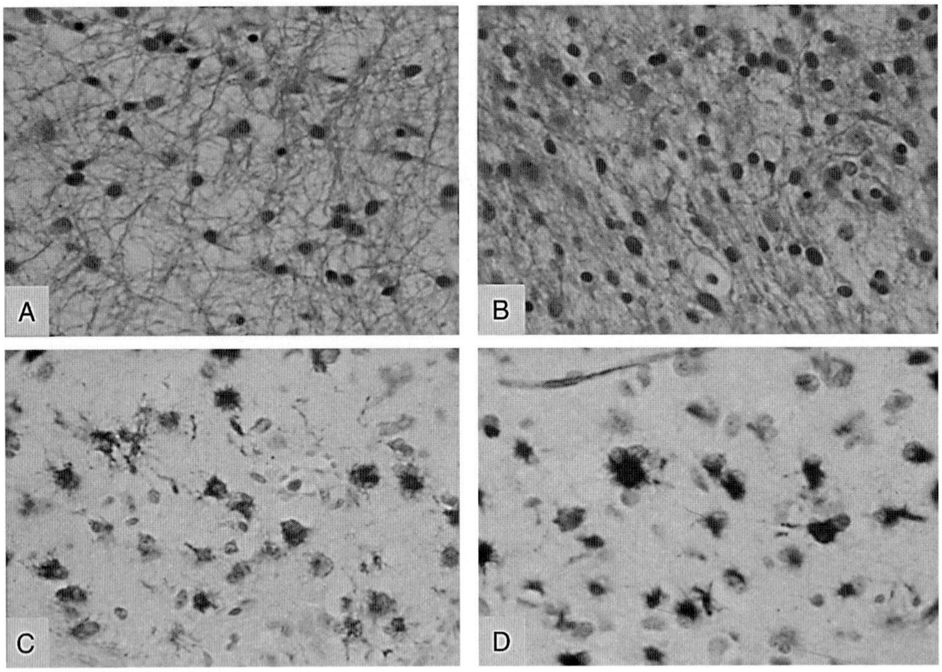

Figure 5-2 (PLATE 3). Astrocytoma grade II. (A) Astrocytoma grade II infiltrating cortex, with focal increased cellularity (B). Immunohistochemistry for GFAP (C) and vimentin (D) highlights the cellular processes of the tumor cells.

Microscopically, anaplastic astrocytomas are hypercellular compared to astrocytomas, and exhibit a variable degree of cytoplasmic and nuclear pleomorphism (Fig. 5-3). Gemistocytic elements are more commonly seen. Anaplastic astrocytomas typically display increased mitotic activity and higher levels of Ki-67 LI than do low-grade astrocytomas, with mean values around 12% to 14%.[9,12] Endothelial microvascular proliferation and necrosis should be absent in accordance with the WHO classification.

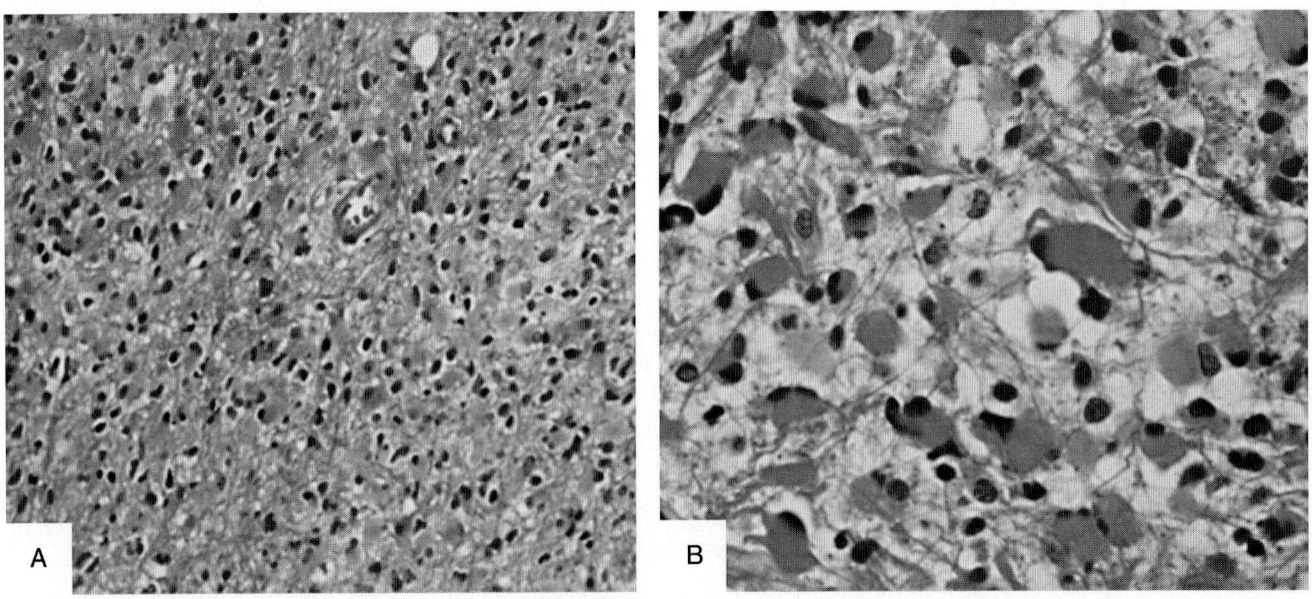

Figure 5-3 (PLATE 4). Anaplastic astrocytoma grade III. (A) Anaplastic astrocytoma with moderate cellular atypia and increased cellularity. (B) Note the large numbers of gemistocytic cells.

Glioblastoma Multiforme Glioblastomas (WHO grade IV) are the most malignant form of astrocytoma and represent approximately 25% of all intracranial tumors and approximately 50% of gliomas in adults.[4] These tumors tend to arise in older patients than astrocytomas and anaplastic astrocytomas, with a peak incidence in the fifth and sixth decades of life.[13] Glioblastomas may arise *de novo*, or develop from low-grade astrocytomas, or, more often, develop from anaplastic astrocytomas. These two types of glioblastomas are designated respectively as *primary glioblastoma* and *secondary glioblastoma*.[14] *Primary glioblastomas* occur more commonly in older patients (median age 55 years) and have a short clinical history. *Secondary glioblastomas* often develop from lower grade astrocytomas over months or years, and typically occur in younger patients (median age 39 years). Glioblastomas are much less common in children and adolescents.[13]

As in the lower grades of diffuse astrocytomas, glioblastomas most often arise in the cerebral hemispheres in adults and in the brainstem in pediatric patients. Glioblastomas are diffusely infiltrative lesions; however, most tumors show a central necrotic area surrounded by infiltrating tumor, giving the appearance of a circumscribed ring-enhancing lesion on neuroimaging. Glioblastomas frequently infiltrate the adjacent brain in an aggressive manner. Common routes of spread include the white matter tracts, particularly the corpus callosum with invasion of the contralateral cerebral hemisphere ("butterfly" pattern), ventricular ependymal areas, and cerebral spinal fluid (CSF) pathways. The great tendency of glioblastomas to spread accounts in part for these tumors' poor prognosis.

Microscopically, glioblastomas manifest a variety of histologic aspects, which give the denomination of "multiforme" to the tumors (Figs. 5-4 through 5-6). The tumors are hypercellular and exhibit a high degree of cytoplasmic and nuclear pleomorphism. Nonetheless, the fibrillary character of the neoplasms with obvious elongated, delicate GFAP-immunoreactive processes is always present. Tumors may range from closely packed small cells with scant cytoplasm to larger cells with a gemistocytic appearance of ample cytoplasm. Multinucleated giant cells are common. Mitotic figures are numerous, and Ki-67 immunohistochemical studies show high labeling indices (mean values range from 14% to 20%), although these may significantly vary within an individual tumor (Fig. 5-7).[8–10] Microvascular endothelial proliferation is seen throughout the tumor, but is especially prominent in areas surrounding necrosis and at the tumor–brain interface. Geographic necrosis with pseudopalisading of the adjacent tumor cells is present in varying degrees. In addition, large areas of ischemic necrosis accompanied by thrombosed vessels are also observed.

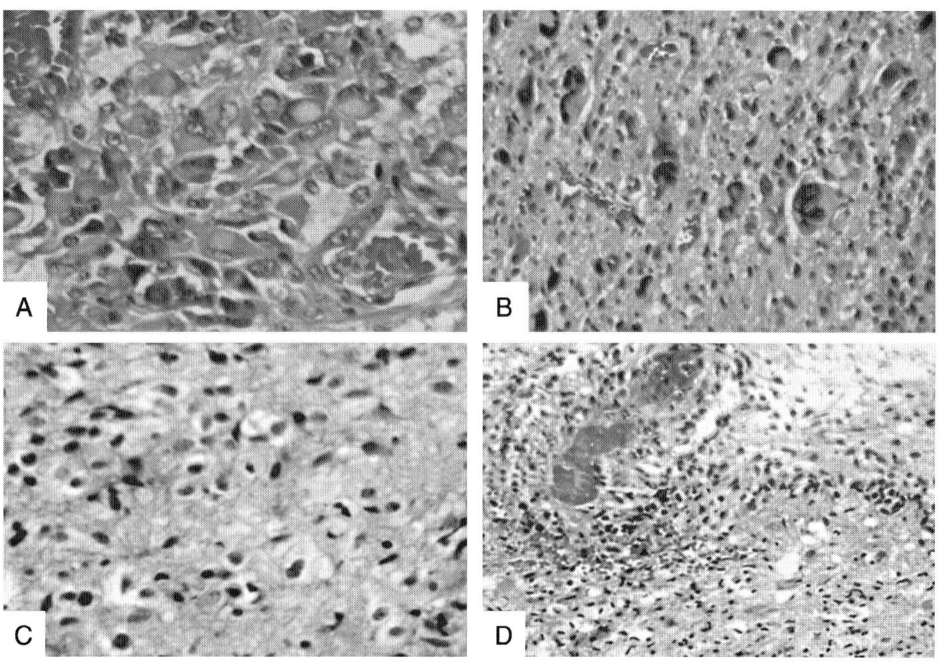

Figure 5-4 (PLATE 5). Astrocytoma grade IV (glioblastoma). Glioblastomas have an abundance of cellular types and arrangements ranging from gemistocytic forms (A) to multinucleated giant cells (B) and small cells (C). Mitotic activity (C) and areas of necrosis (D) are characteristic of glioblastomas.

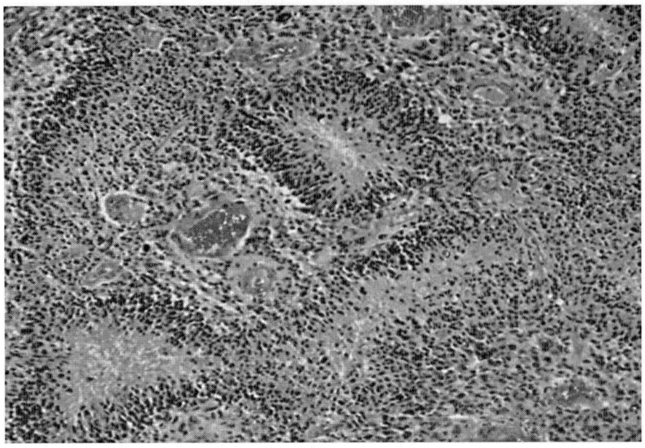

Figure 5-5 (PLATE 6). Astrocytoma grade IV (glioblastoma). Areas of necrosis, particularly with pseudopalisading arrangement of tumor cells, are common in glioblastomas.

Giant Cell Glioblastoma

The giant cell glioblastoma is a glioblastoma variant worthy of mention because of its distinctive clinical presentation, histology, and molecular genetics profile. Giant cell glioblastomas account for approximately 5% of all glioblastomas.[15] The majority of giant cell glioblastomas are *de novo* tumors with a short preoperative history.[16] In contrast to ordinary glioblastomas, giant cell glioblastomas tend to arise in younger patients and to be more circumscribed lesions with less infiltrative growth. These particular features of giant cell glioblastomas may account for their better prognosis as reported by some authors.[15] However, only a few patients with survival times of more than 5 years have been reported, including a long-term survival of 17 years after surgical resection.[17,18]

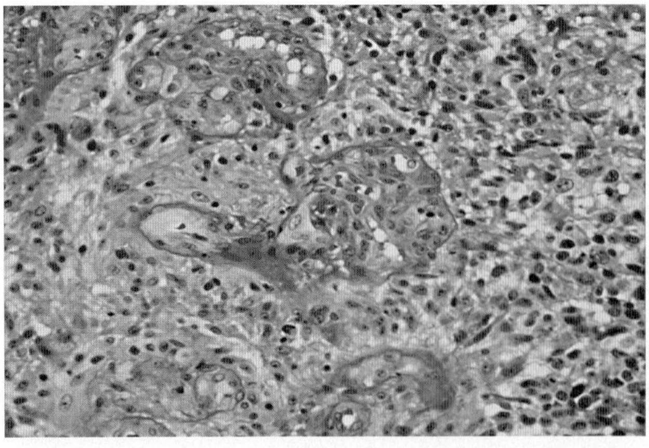

Figure 5-6 (PLATE 7). Astrocytoma grade IV (glioblastoma). Vascular endothelial proliferation is another typical feature of glioblastomas.

A predominance of bizarre, multinucleated giant cells and extensive areas of necrosis and hemorrhage characterize giant cell glioblastomas (Figs. 5-8 and 5-9). An increase of the stromal reticulin network is also seen, particularly related to blood vessels.

Studies demonstrate that the molecular genetics of giant cell glioblastomas resemble *secondary glioblastomas* with *TP53* gene mutations and rare epidermal growth factor receptor (*EGFR*) gene or *MDM2* gene amplification[16,19] (see below), a feature in contrast to their clinical presentation as *de novo* neoplasms in the majority of the cases.

Gliosarcoma

The *gliosarcoma* is a glioblastoma variant that demonstrates a biphasic tissue pattern with intermixed areas of glial and mesenchymal proliferation. Gliosarcomas account for approximately 2% of all glioblastomas.[20] The glial component shows the typical features of glioblastoma as previously described. The sarcomatous component often shows a diverse histologic appearance, most often resembling fibrosarcoma, malignant fibrous histiocytoma, or angiosarcoma. The proportions of glial and sarcomatous components are variable. GFAP immunohistochemistry confirms the glial elements, whereas vimentin, other mesenchymal-related markers, and reticulin stains highlight the sarcomatous portions.

Immunohistochemical and ultrastructural studies had suggested that the sarcomatous components were probably derived from an undifferentiated mesenchymal cell associated with the adventitia of tumor vessels.[21] However, more recent molecular genetic analyses show that both glial and mesenchymal elements of gliosarcomas share similar genetic alterations.[22–24] Identical *TP53* gene mutations in both gliomatous and sarcomatous elements have been identified,[23,24] suggesting that the sarcomatous areas may represent a phenotypic change of the glial cells.

Molecular Genetics of Diffuse Astrocytomas

Molecular genetic studies have provided much insight in the tumorigenesis of diffuse infiltrating astrocytomas with the recognition of specific alterations that correlate with the different grades of tumor, from astrocytomas to glioblastomas (reviewed in reference 25). These genetic mechanisms are complex and are discussed in detail in other chapters. Similar to many other tumors, astrocytomas accumulate a number of genetic events during their formation and progression. Studies of glioblastoma provide the largest source of data in astrocytoma tumorigenesis. It appears that at least three main pathways may be involved in the tumorigenesis of glioblastomas: (a) inactivation of the *TP53* gene; (b) amplification of *EGFR* gene; and (c) alternative pathways.

Briefly, inactivation of *TP53* gene occurs in approximately one-third of glioblastomas. However, loss of alleles

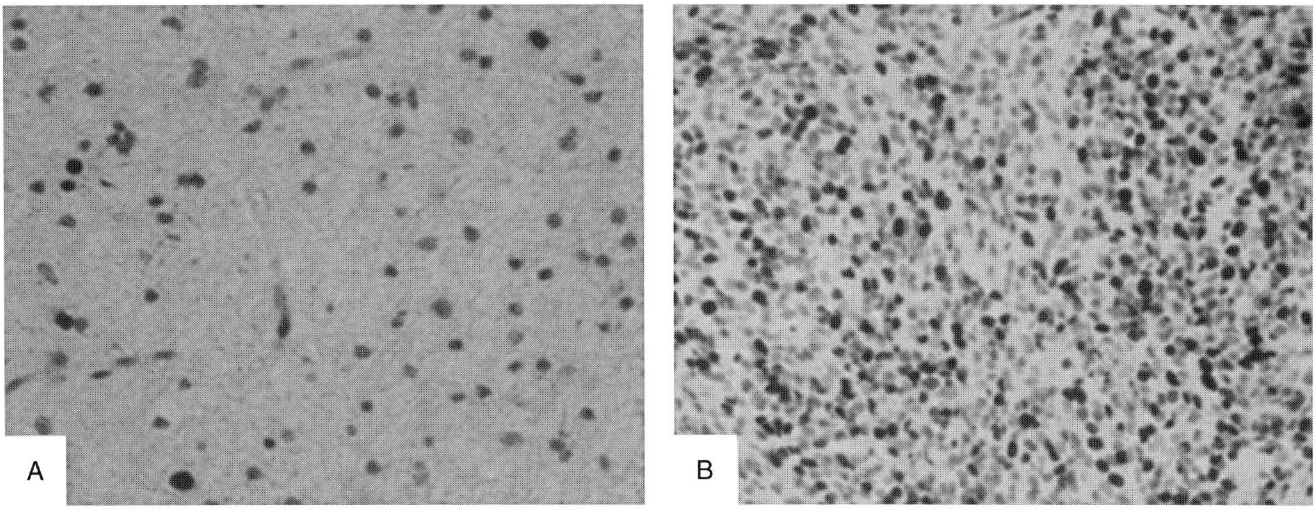

Figure 5-7 (PLATE 8). Ki-67 immunostain. Note the contrast between the Ki-67 labeling index in a grade II (A) and a grade IV astrocytoma (B).

on chromosome 17p, including the *TP53* locus, is present in more than 60% of astrocytomas (grade II) and anaplastic astrocytomas (grade III), indicating that the p53 pathway is altered as an early event in astrocytoma tumorigenesis. There are, however, several additional mechanisms by which the p53 pathway may be inactivated in astrocytomas, including amplification or overexpression of *MDM2* gene and alterations and/or deletion of $p14^{ARF}$ gene (reviewed in reference 26). The second main genetic alteration in glioblastomas is *EGFR* gene amplification, which is present in another one-third of tumors.[26] Overexpression of EGFR may be present in glioblastomas even when amplification of *EGFR* gene is not present. *EGFR* gene amplification almost never occurs in glioblastomas with *TP53* mutation or loss of chromosome 17p. These two genetic pathways denote not only different genetic trails of tumor formation, but also seem to reflect different courses of glioblastomas. Primary or *de novo glioblastomas* arise as high-grade from the onset (i.e., without progression from a lower grade astrocytoma), exhibit *EGFR* gene amplification, and arise in elderly patients. *Secondary glioblastomas* are associated with *TP53* gene inactivation, evolve from lower grade astrocytomas, either astrocytoma (grade II) or anaplastic astrocytoma (grade III), and arise in younger patients. The clinical and epidemiologic data concerning these two sets of glioblastomas are well characterized.[14] From the histologic viewpoint, these two types of glioblastomas are indistinguishable.

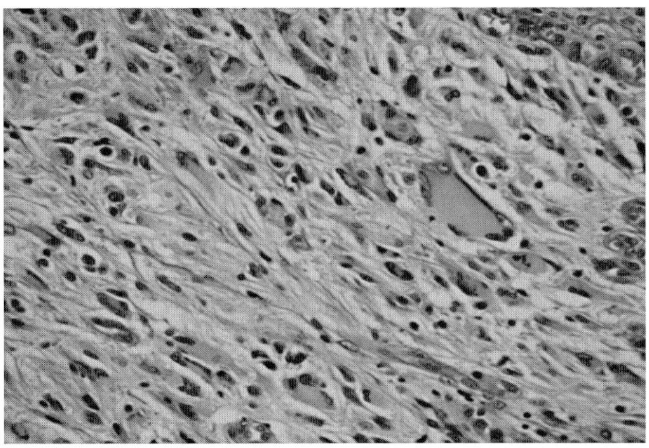

Figure 5-8 (PLATE 9). Giant cell glioblastoma (grade IV). Giant cell glioblastoma with typical multinucleated giant cell intermixed with smaller astrocytic cells.

Alternative pathways to those previously discussed have been described in the progression of diffuse astrocytomas. One mentioned above is the giant cell glioblastoma, despite clinically presenting as a *primary glioblastoma*, showing *TP53* gene mutation, a trait seen most commonly in *secondary glioblastomas*.[18,25] Glioblastomas in the pediatric population also show patterns of genetic alterations different from those previously described in glioblastomas arising in adults. For example, *TP53* gene mutations in pediatric cerebral glioblastomas have been detected at variable frequency varying from 0 to 35% of cases,[27–31] whereas in glioblastomas arising in the brainstem, the frequency of *TP53* mutations can be as high as 70%.[32]

Special Categories of Astrocytomas

The second group of astrocytomas includes tumors that are relatively circumscribed neoplasms by radiographic and gross appearances when compared to diffusely infiltrating astrocytomas. This category includes the *pilocytic*

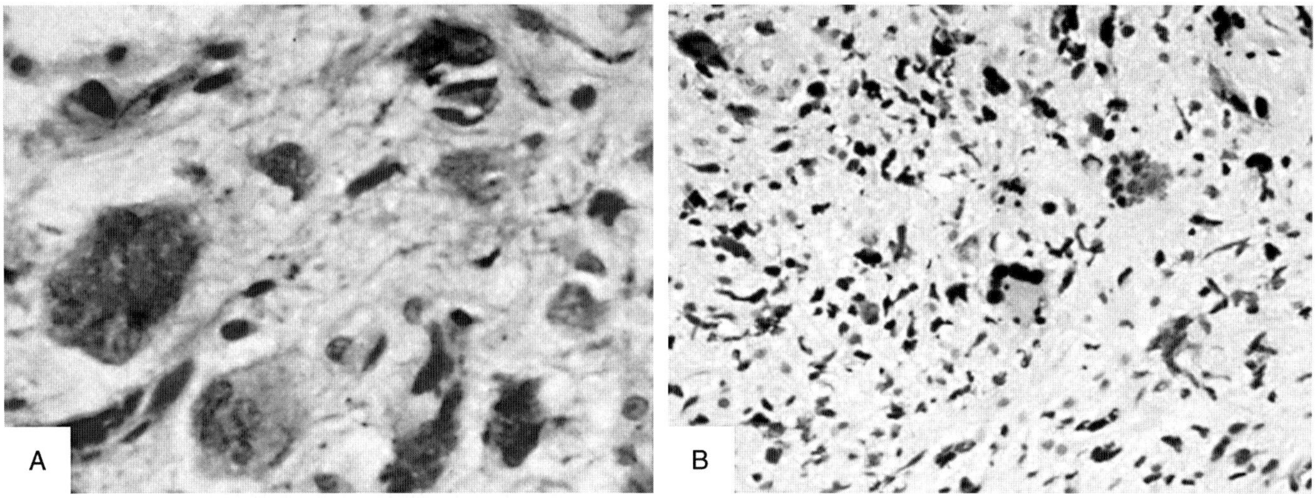

Figure 5-9 (PLATE 10). Giant cell glioblastoma (grade IV). (A) Multinucleated giant cells immunoreactive for GFAP in a giant cell glioblastoma. (B) Characteristically, this variant of glioblastoma is highly immunoreactive for p53 immunostain as a consequence of common p53 mutation seen in these tumors.

astrocytoma, the *pleomorphic xanthoastrocytoma,* and the *subependymal giant cell astrocytoma*. These astrocytic tumors exhibit distinctive clinicopathologic features and prognostically tend to be more favorable tumors with slow growth, relatively indolent biologic behavior, and rare anaplastic progression.

Pilocytic Astrocytoma Pilocytic astrocytomas (WHO grade I) are relatively well-circumscribed tumors that occur most frequently in children and young adults, with a peak incidence in the second decade of life.[33] Pilocytic astrocytomas are typically located in midline structures, including the cerebellum, optic pathways, hypothalamus and third ventricular regions, and brainstem. Less frequently, these tumors arise in the cerebral hemispheres and spinal cord. The latter location is most commonly seen in adults. They occur both sporadically and in association with neurofibromatosis type 1 (NF1). Fifteen percent of patients with NF1 develop pilocytic astrocytoma of the optic nerve (also called optic glioma),[33] and approximately 70% of optic gliomas are associated with NF1.[34]

Most tumors are cystic lesions with a solid component or mural nodule. The nodule is usually soft and gray with variably sized cysts containing yellow fluid. Pilocytic astrocytomas arising in the optic pathways are remarkable for infiltrating diffusely the optic nerve, producing a fusiform, expanded mass.

A biphasic pattern of growth with bipolar, piloid cells arranged in dense fascicles, alternating with a loose, microcystic tissue formed by stellate astrocytic cells, characterizes the histology of pilocytic astrocytomas (Figs. 5-10 and 5-11). Characteristically, these tumors also contain Rosenthal fibers and eosinophilic granular bodies. Although these structures are not pathognomonic or a precondition for the diagnosis of pilocytic astrocytomas, they are helpful for establishing the diagnosis.

Both compact and loose cellular elements of the pilocytic astrocytoma are GFAP-immunoreactive, but the piloid cells are more strongly positive than the stellate cells of the loose areas. Vimentin immunoreactivity is equally conspicuous in both cellular patterns. Some degree of cellular atypia, including multinucleated cells, may be present in pilocytic astrocytomas. These are considered degenerative features rather than anaplastic attributes of the tumors. In fact, anaplastic progression of pilocytic astrocytoma is a rare event, occurring in only 0.9% of cases.[35] Mitotic activity is relatively low in pilocytic astrocytomas. Studies using proliferative markers, including Ki-67, have also shown low proliferative potential, although with some intratumoral variation.[10,36]

Pilocytic astrocytomas are highly vascular lesions. Hyalinized vessels are often seen and may be accompanied by perivascular lymphocytic infiltrates. Microvascular proliferation may be present, sometimes simulating the glomeruloid type of vascular hyperplasia in glioblastomas, but this does not connote malignant transformation. Although the tumors are macroscopically circumscribed, some degree of parenchymal infiltration may occur. More importantly, they show a significant propensity to invade the leptomeninges,[35] and when arising in the optic nerve, they commonly diffusely infiltrate the entire optic pathway. Despite the rather indolent behavior

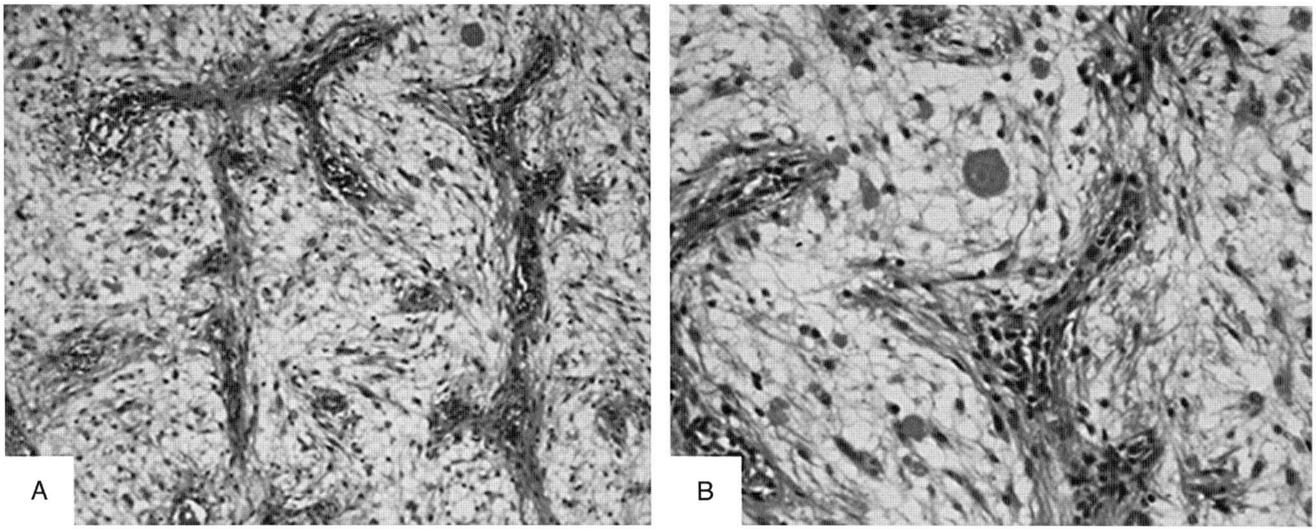

Figure 5-10 (PLATE 11). Pilocytic astrocytoma: (A) Pilocytic astrocytoma with alternating areas of dense, fibrillary cells and areas of looser stroma forming a biphasic pattern. (B) Degenerative structures, including hyaline droplets, are commonly seen in these tumors.

of pilocytic astrocytomas, recurrence is possible, particularly after incomplete resection.[37]

Allelic loss on chromosome 17 has been described in sporadic pilocytic astrocytomas, including the region encoding the *NF1* gene.[38] Nevertheless, the role for *NF1* as a tumor suppressor gene in the genesis of pilocytic astrocytomas is not confirmed.[33] In contrast to diffuse astrocytomas, the *TP53* gene mutation does not seem to play a role in the tumorigenesis of the pilocytic astrocytoma.

Pleomorphic Xanthoastrocytoma Pleomorphic xanthoastrocytomas (WHO grades II to III) are superficially located tumors in the cerebral hemispheres that arise most frequently in children and young adults with

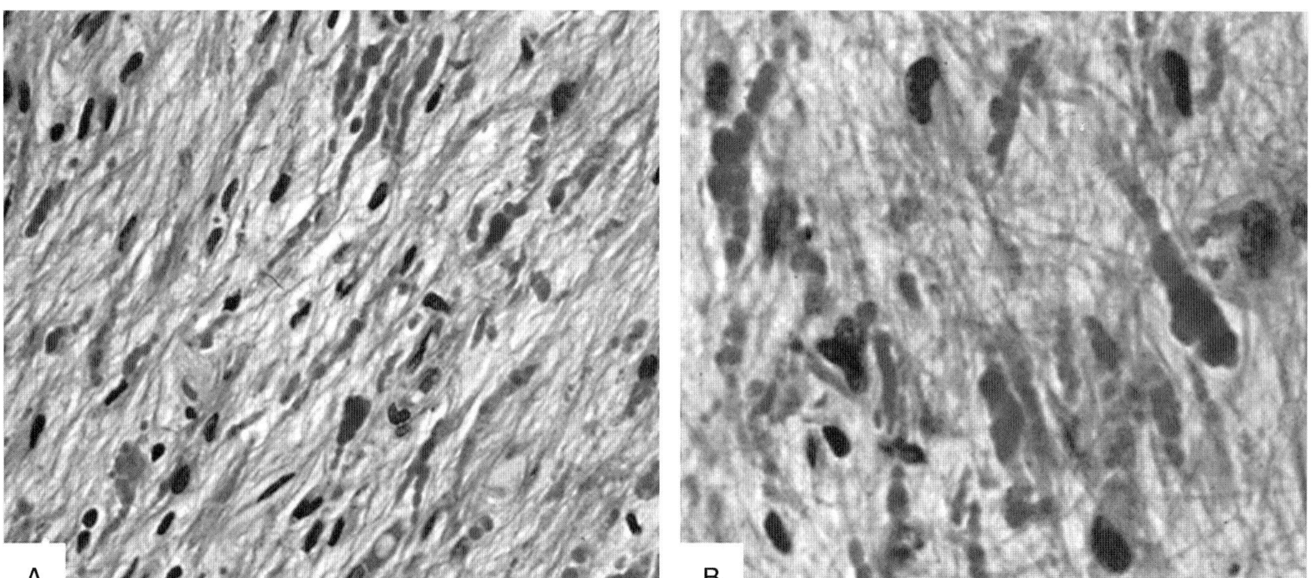

Figure 5-11 (PLATE 12). Pilocytic astrocytoma. (A and B) Dense areas of fibrillary cells with the formation of Rosenthal fibers in a pilocytic astrocytoma of the third ventricular region.

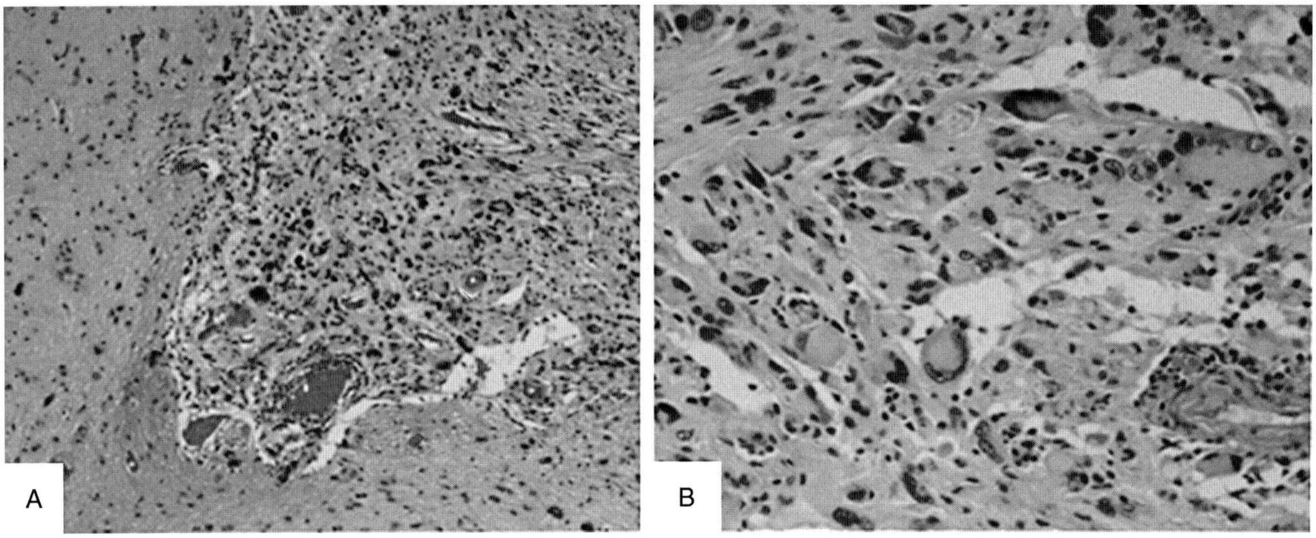

Figure 5-12 (PLATE 13). Pleomorphic xanthoastrocytoma. (A) Pleomorphic astrocytoma are superficial tumors involving the cortical ribbon with infiltration of the subpial area. (B) The tumor has a variety of cell types with large pleomorphic and xanthomatous cells.

long histories of seizures.[39] These tumors are frequently located in the temporal region and exhibit leptomeningeal involvement. In many cases, they have a cystic component.

The histologic hallmark of pleomorphic xanthoastrocytoma is their remarkable cellular heterogeneity with a combination of spindle and polygonal astrocytes and pleomorphic, lipid-vacuolated cells arranged in interlacing bundles (Figs. 5-12 and 5-13). Bizarre hyperchromatic nuclei, as well as multinucleated giant cells, are invariably present. Tumor cells are usually arranged in fascicular patterns. A notable feature of these tumors is the presence of a dense intercellular reticulin network delineating either individual cells or fascicles of cells. This latter feature reflects the presence of a pericellular basement membrane-like deposition seen at the ultrastructural level.[40,41] Although this distinct stroma may be present in any portion of the tumor, it is most conspicuous in areas

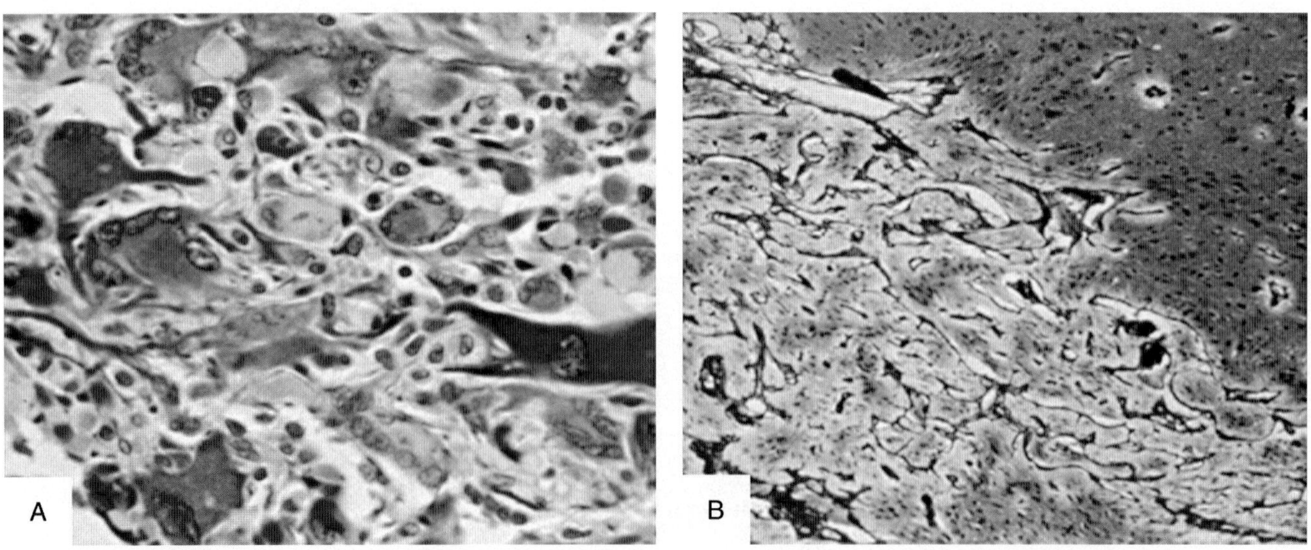

Figure 5-13 (PLATE 14). Pleomorphic xanthoastrocytoma. (A) GFAP immunoreactivity in both spindle and xanthomatous glial cells. (B) Characteristically, pleomorphic xanthoastrocytoma has a dense reticulin network mainly when infiltrating the subpial area.

of leptomeningeal involvement.[42] Mitotic activity is generally low. Microvascular endothelial proliferation and areas of necrosis are absent. The presence of increased mitotic activity, vascular endothelial proliferation, or necrosis is considered evidence of histological malignant transformation and a poor prognosis in pleomorphic xanthoastrocytomas.[40,41,43]

In general, pleomorphic xanthoastrocytomas are associated with a relatively favorable prognosis. Many patients have long-term survival after tumor resection. Nevertheless, tumor recurrence and malignant progression may occur in a subset of cases. There are no histopathologic criteria for the prospective identification of malignant biologic potential in these tumors. Tumors with low mitotic activity are designated as WHO Grade II, whereas tumors that show focal histologic indicators of anaplasia are designated as "anaplastic pleomorphic xanthoastrocytoma," WHO Grade III. Astrocytomas with features that resemble the pleomorphic xanthoastrocytoma but with frank anaplastic features, that is, a high mitotic index, necrosis, and/or microvascular proliferation, should be designated as glioblastomas rather than pleomorphic xanthoastrocytomas.[39]

Thus far no definitive molecular genetic profile has been distinguished in the pleomorphic xanthoastrocytoma. The genetic mutations seen in diffuse astrocytomas, mainly *TP53* gene mutation and *EGFR* gene amplification, are probably not implicated in the pathogenesis of these tumors.[39] However, *TP53* mutations have been described in a few pleomorphic xanthoastrocytomas, including recurrent tumors and tumors that later underwent malignant transformation.[44–46] Amplification of the *EGFR* gene was observed in the recurrence of an ordinary pleomorphic xanthoastrocytoma that presented with anaplastic progression.[45]

Subependymal Giant Cell Astrocytoma Subependymal giant cell astrocytomas (WHO grade I) are tumors that typically arise in the first two decades of life, and are the most common CNS neoplasm in association with the tuberous sclerosis complex (TSC).[47] However, these tumors may also occur without other apparent signs of the phakomatosis.

Subependymal giant cell astrocytomas are circumscribed, nodular tumors arising in the wall of the lateral ventricles at the level of the basal ganglia. Less frequently, they arise in the third ventricle. Microscopically, the tumors are composed by a variety of astroglial cellular types with spindle cells, polygonal cells, and distinctive ganglion-like cells merged in a variably fibrillated matrix (Fig. 5-14). Some cellular pleomorphism and occasional multinucleate cells may be present. A conspicuous microvasculature with dilated vessels with hyalinized walls is present, which may hemorrhage, either spontaneously or after surgical manipulation. Calcifications are common.

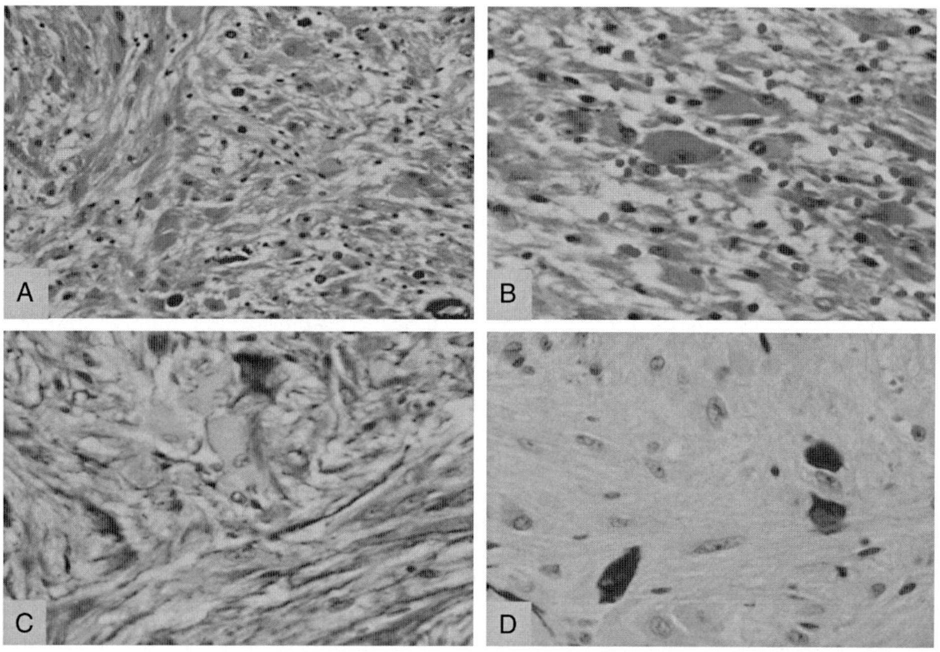

Figure 5-14 (PLATE 15). Subependymal giant cell astrocytoma (SEGA). (A and B) The SEGAs are composed of a variety of cellular elements, ranging from spindle to polygonal to ganglion-like cells (B). Giant cells in SEGAs may show glial (GFAP) (C) and/or neuronal (neurofilament) (D) markers by immunohistochemistry.

Subependymal giant cell astrocytomas have a uniformly favorable prognosis despite the occasional finding of atypia, mitoses, and even necrosis. Despite a few examples of recurrent tumor, no cases with malignant transformation have been described.[47]

Although subependymal giant cell astrocytomas are designated as a special variant of astrocytoma, these tumors have the capacity for divergent phenotypic expression with mixed glioneuronal differentiation. Their primary astrocytic nature is confirmed by GFAP and S100 protein immunoreactivities. Most tumors, however, also express focal neuronal-associated proteins, including neurofilament proteins and neuronal-associated class III β-tubulin.[48] Ultrastructural profiles suggestive of neuronal differentiation, including microtubules, rare dense-core granules, and occasional synapse formation have confirmed these observations.[49] Similar findings are seen in the cortical tubers of the TSC. As a result, some authors have proposed that these tumors be designated subependymal giant cell tumors.[5]

Loss of heterozygosity in *TSC2* gene region (16p13) has been described in a few cases of subependymal giant cell astrocytoma.[47,50] Studies by immunohistochemistry for tuberin, the *TSC2* gene product, show loss of tuberin immunostaining in a number of subependymal giant cell astrocytomas, confirming the presumed tumor suppressor function of this gene.[51,52]

Oligodendroglial Tumors

Oligodendroglioma

Oligodendrogliomas (WHO grade II) constitute approximately 5% to 15% of intracranial gliomas.[53] Although the majority of tumors occur in adults, with a peak incidence in the fourth and fifth decades of life, tumors arising in children and adolescents comprise approximately 6% of oligodendrogliomas.[54] The great majority of oligodendrogliomas manifest slow clinical evolution and are associated with a long history of seizures.[54]

Oligodendrogliomas can arise at any region in the neuraxis. However, they most frequently involve the cerebral hemispheres, particularly the frontotemporal region. Involvement of multiple lobes is not rare; nor are bilateral tumors.[54] The cerebellum, brainstem, and spinal cord are very rarely affected.

Oligodendrogliomas are grossly soft, gelatinous masses that extend from the white to gray matter obliterating the gray–white junction. Areas of cystic degeneration are common as well as calcifications visible on neuroimaging studies. Areas of hemorrhage are occasionally seen.

Microscopically, oligodendrogliomas are highly distinctive (Figs. 5-15 and 5-16). In optimally fixed specimens, the tumor cells have scant, indistinct cytoplasm and the nuclei are typically round with a delicate particulate chromatin pattern. The cells are dispersed in a poorly fibrillated matrix, commonly within a pseudolobulated pattern resulting from subdivision of the cells into variably sized groups by delicate, geometric branching vessels. This distinctive vascular pattern is often referred as a "chicken wire" pattern. On paraffin sections, a common artifact seen in oligodendrogliomas is the clearing of the cytoplasm that gives the cell a characteristic "fried egg" appearance. The lack of a conspicuous fibrillary matrix of cell processes helps to distinguish oligodendrogliomas from astrocytomas. Oligodendrogliomas frequently diffusely infiltrate the cerebral cortex, exhibiting characteristic secondary structures such as perineuronal satellitosis, perivascular accumulations, and subpial infiltration. Frequently, neoplastic oligodendrocytes display a small rim of eosinophilic cytoplasm and eccentric nuclei. These cells are referred to as "gliofibrillary oligodendrocytes" or "mini-gemistocytes."[55–57] Although the presence of these cellular elements does not have any prognostic value,[57] their distinction from reactive and/or neoplastic astrocytes within an oligodendroglioma may be problematic. Reactive astrocytes are often found scattered throughout the tumor, but particularly around blood vessels and in the areas of cortical infiltration.

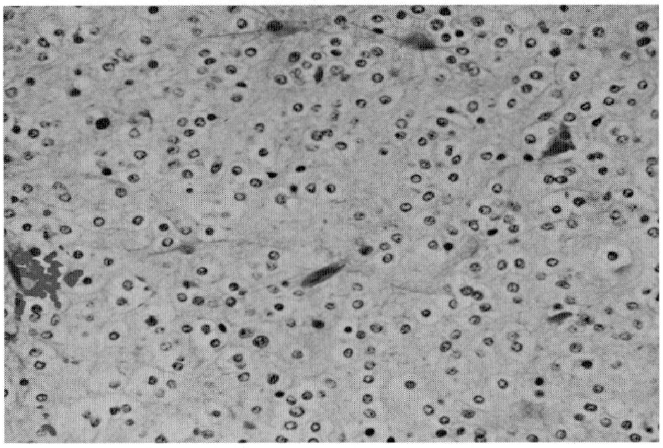

Figure 5-15 (PLATE 16). Oligodendroglioma grade II. Typical "fried egg" appearance of a low-grade oligodendroglioma.

Histopathologic features of anaplasia are not present in grade II oligodendrogliomas. Mitotic figures can be observed in low numbers without other evidence for malignant transformation. Ki-67 labeling indices are generally low, with mean values around 2%.[58] Grade II oligodendrogliomas with Ki-67 LI greater than 5% are associated with shorter survival.[58]

Establishing a diagnosis of oligodendrogliomas may be problematic when the typical histologic features are not readily appreciated or when an "astrocyte-like" component is present in the tumor. Currently there are no reliable immunocytochemical markers for neoplastic oligodendrocytes for the purpose of diagnosis and tumor

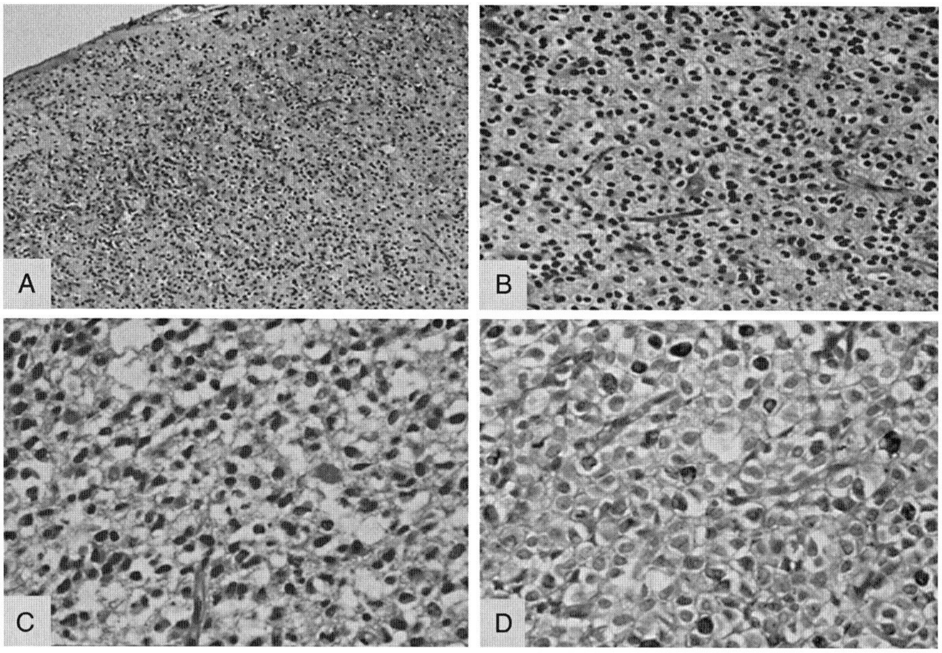

Figure 5-16 (PLATE 17). Oligodendroglioma grade II. Typical features of oligodendrogliomas include diffuse infiltration of the cortex and subpial areas (A) and perineuronal satellitosis (B). The presence of cells with a small rim of cytoplasm, the so-called mini-gemistocytes (C), can be easily appreciated with GFAP immunohistochemistry (D).

classification. The diagnosis of oligodendrogliomas is mainly based on observations of hematoxylin and eosin (H&E)-stained sections and the analysis of lack of reactivity for markers associated with astroglial differentiation. To date, most markers expressed by developing and mature oligodendrocytes are inconstantly expressed by neoplastic oligodendrocytes and are unsatisfactory for characterizing oligodendrogliomas.[59–61]

In recent years, several studies have tried to correlate the expression of the transcription factors OLIG-1 and OLIG-2 in oligodendrogliomas. This newly identified class of oligodendrocyte-specific genes, named *OLIG-1/2*, encodes basic helix–loop–helix transcription factors, which are thought to have a major role in the specification of oligodendrocyte precursors, but are also expressed by oligodendrocytes in the mature CNS.[62,63] Initial studies confirmed that oligodendroglial tumor cells overexpress OLIG-1/2 RNA by in situ hybridization, and this expression appeared to be specific to oligodendrogliomas and the oligodendroglial component of oligoastrocytomas and glioblastomas.[64–66] Nevertheless, more recent studies using larger numbers of gliomas and new specific antibodies to OLIG-1/2 have demonstrated that these markers are not exclusively expressed by gliomas with oligodendroglial elements. OLIG-1/2 has been detected in high levels in all astrocytomas (low and high grade), including pilocytic astrocytomas,[67,68] and in low levels in ependymomas.[67] Preliminary data demonstrate, however, that the OLIG family is not expressed in nonglial tumors, which includes both neuronal and nonneural tumors.[68] This may be of practical advantage when differentiation between oligodendroglial and neuronal tumors is necessary, as between central neurocytoma and dysembryoplastic neuroepithelial tumor.

The majority of oligodendrogliomas do not express the intermediate filaments GFAP and vimentin. Minigemistocytic oligodendrocytes, however, commonly show intense GFAP immunoreactivity[56,69] and anaplastic oligodendrogliomas are more likely to show vimentin expression.[70] Consequently, these markers are not completely reliable. In our experience, the combination of GFAP and vimentin may be helpful in a few situations. One situation is to distinguish a reactive or neoplastic astrocytic population from mini-gemistocytic oligodendrocytes, because the latter are most commonly negative for vimentin and astrocytes are positive. Another situation is to help differentiate low-grade oligodendrogliomas from astrocytomas and ependymomas. Because vimentin is expressed in neoplastic astrocytic and ependymal cells, the lack of vimentin in a low-grade glioma may be more diagnostic of an oligodendrogliomas than an astrocytoma or an ependymoma in a particular case.

Anaplastic Oligodendroglioma

Anaplastic oligodendrogliomas (WHO grade III) represent a minority of oligodendroglial tumors and account for fewer than 5% of new malignant gliomas.[71] Anaplastic oligodendrogliomas either evolve from low-grade oligodendroglioma by a process of anaplastic transformation or appear de novo. The recognition of anaplastic oligodendrogliomas and their differentiation from other anaplastic gliomas has both clinical and prognostic implications as a result of their distinct chemosensitivity.[71,72]

Anaplastic oligodendrogliomas demonstrate histologic features of low-grade oligodendrogliomas in addition to evidence of anaplastic transformation similar to that accompanying anaplasia in diffusely infiltrating astrocytomas (Fig. 5-17). These include increased nuclear/cytoplasm pleomorphism, increased mitotic activity, prominent endothelial proliferation, and areas of necrosis including palisading necrosis. Although there is no systematic grading system for oligodendrogliomas, the same criteria as those for diffuse astrocytomas are used in daily practice.

Conflicting results have been reported regarding whether any histopathologic feature seen in anaplastic oligodendrogliomas has prognostic value in predicting tumor behavior. Some authors found that conventional parameters, such as mitotic activity and necrosis, are the most important prognostic indicators.[73] Other investigators identified proliferative activity assessed by Ki-67 as more strongly associated with patient survival.[74,75] However, it appears that the molecular genetic profile of oligodendrogliomas has greater prognostic value (see "Molecular Genetics of Oligodendroglial Tumors").

Mixed Oligoastrocytoma

Mixed oligoastrocytomas (WHO grade II) are tumors composed of oligodendrocytes and a significant proportion of neoplastic astrocytes. Mixed oligoastrocytomas arise primarily in the cerebral hemispheres, with the frontal lobes most frequently affected, followed by the temporal lobes.[76] Similar to low-grade oligodendrogliomas, patients often present with a long-standing history of seizures.

Currently, there are no definitive histologic criteria to make the diagnosis of a mixed oligoastrocytoma. The distinction between oligodendrogliomas and oligoastrocytomas is problematic because of the great variability in the composition of the two cell populations within the tumor and the lack of clearly discriminating parameters. The two glial neoplastic cell populations may be focally or diffusely distributed. Frequently, the predominant cell component is oligodendroglial. Some investigators have defined a mixed glioma as a tumor in which a second minor glial component may be present in at least one ×100 field.[77]

As in low-grade oligodendrogliomas, mixed oligoastrocytomas show a mild degree of pleomorphism

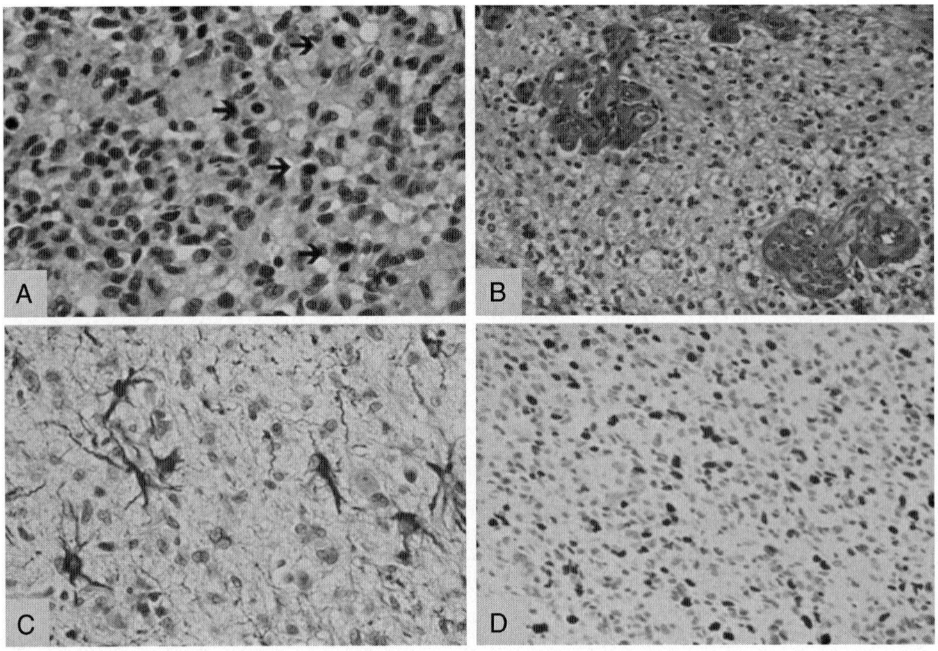

Figure 5-17 (PLATE 18). Anaplastic oligodendroglioma grade III. (A) Anaplastic oligodendrogliomas are characterized by increased cellularity and atypia in combination with areas of necrosis (not shown) and (B) microvascular endothelial proliferation. (C) GFAP immunoreaction highlights increased reactive astrocytes in malignant oligodendrogliomas with absence of immunoreaction in the tumor cells. Increased mitotic activity (A, arrows) and high Ki-67 labeling index (D) are present in anaplastic oligodendrogliomas.

and few mitotic figures (Fig. 5-18). Endothelial proliferation and necrosis are absent.

Anaplastic Oligoastrocytoma

Anaplastic oligoastrocytomas (WHO grade III) (also known as mixed anaplastic gliomas [MAGs]) are mixed gliomas with histologic evidence of anaplasia, including increased cellularity, nuclear atypia, and high mitotic activity. Vascular endothelial proliferation and focal areas of necrosis are commonly seen. In the majority of tumors, the anaplastic changes are evident in both oligodendroglial and astrocytic components (see Fig. 5-18). However, the astrocytic component appears more prone to undergo anaplastic progression.

The distinction between anaplastic oligoastrocytoma and anaplastic astrocytoma or glioblastoma multiforme is of clinical relevance because of the potential chemosensitivity of these mixed gliomas. Although the prognosis of these anaplastic oligoastrocytomas is guarded, the median survival is considerably better than that of patients with glioblastoma.[78]

Molecular Genetics of Oligodendroglial Tumors

Oligodendroglial tumors have a more distinct molecular genetic profile than do astrocytomas.[76] Somatic deletions of chromosomes 1p and 19q are the most significant events in tumorigenesis of oligodendrogliomas, and occur in 40% to 70% of tumors. Point mutations of *TP53* in oligodendrogliomas are much less common than in astrocytic tumors[79] and mutations are limited to less than 10% of cases; but mutations may be more common with progression to anaplastic oligodendrogliomas. During transformation to anaplastic forms, in addition to losses on chromosomes 1p and 19q, oligodendrogliomas accumulate losses of chromosome 9p (including the CDKN2A region), losses of chromosome 10q, and mutations of *TP53*.[80] Data show that molecular profiling of anaplastic oligodendrogliomas is the most powerful predictor for both the response of the tumors to chemotherapy treatment and longer recurrence-free survival.[72]

Mixed oligoastrocytomas are, however, a genetically more heterogeneous group of tumors. From 30% to 70% of oligoastrocytomas have allelic losses on chromosomes 1p and 19q, thus resembling oligodendrogliomas,[81–83] whereas another 30% of tumors have genetic aberrations frequently found in diffuse astrocytomas including mutations of the *TP53* gene and/or loss of heterozygosity on chromosome 17p.[81,82] In both groups, identical genetic alterations have been identified in astrocytic and oligodendroglial elements, indication a clonal origin of these mixed gliomas.[83] The presence of *TP53* mutations and/or 17p loss and 1p and 19q deletion appears to be mutually exclusive in the individual groups.[81,82]

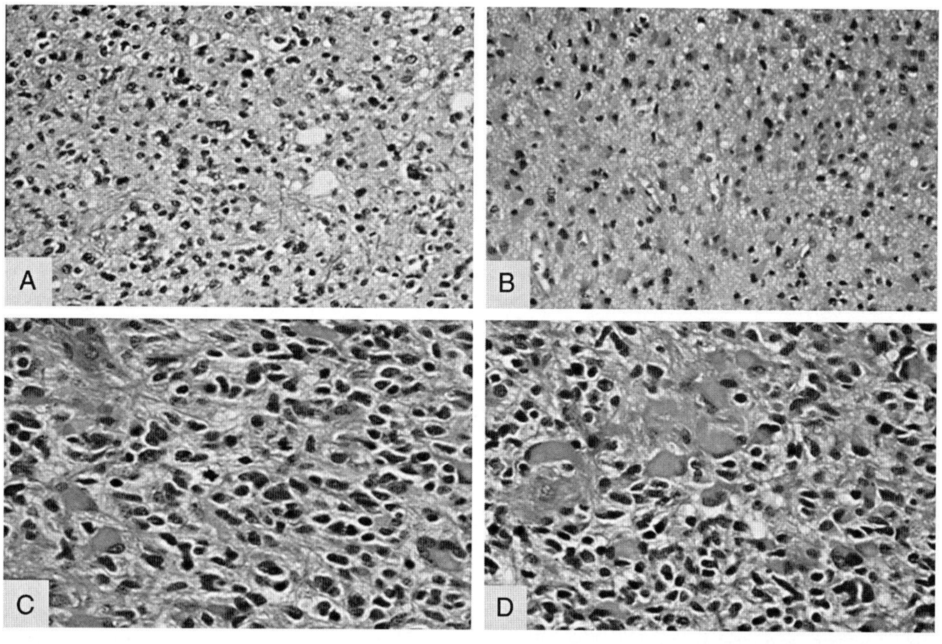

Figure 5-18 (PLATE 19). Mixed oligoastrocytoma. (A and B) Low-grade oligoastrocytoma (grade II) with a mixed population of oligodendroglial- and astrocytic-like cells. (C and D) In high-grade tumors (anaplastic oligoastrocytoma grade III), increased cellular atypia and gemistocytic forms may be seen.

Ependymal Tumors

Ependymoma

Ependymomas (WHO grade II) represent approximately 10% of brain tumors in children and 3% to 9% of all neuroepithelial tumors.[84] They are more common in children and adolescents than in adults, and have an equal gender distribution. Ependymomas typically arise near the ventricular system; the fourth ventricle is the most frequent site, followed by the lateral ventricles, the aqueduct, and the spinal cord. In children, ependymomas commonly arise in the fourth ventricle, whereas in adults ependymomas are more commonly seen in the spinal cord. Multiple spinal cord ependymomas are typically associated with neurofibromatosis type 2 (NF2).[85]

Ependymomas are well-demarcated tumors that produce less infiltration and more compression of surrounding brain than other gliomas. They are usually soft masses with numerous cystic areas. Areas of hemorrhage are commonly seen at gross examination because of the highly vascular network of these tumors. Despite the circumscribed nature of ependymomas, intraventricular tumors not uncommonly extend beyond the ventricular system to involve the subarachnoid space, sometimes encasing extraventricular structures like the cerebellopontine angle, the cisterns, the brainstem, and cervical cord. Spinal cord tumors tend to be well circumscribed as well, and syrinx cavities may accompany these lesions. Ependymomas may also develop outside the CNS in the sacrococcygeal or subcutaneous regions.[86]

Ependymomas are composed of a monotonous population of compactly arranged cells within a variably fibrillated matrix (Figs. 5-19 and 5-20). The cells typically contain an oval nucleus with an open, salt-and-pepper-like chromatin, and have long, tapering, fibrillated processes. A characteristic histologic feature of ependymomas is the polarized orientation of the tumor cells around blood vessels to form the so-called pseudorosettes. True ependymal rosettes and epithelial-lined tubules, although pathognomonic of these gliomas, are less common. Ependymomas may contain areas of myxoid degeneration, hemorrhage, and calcification. Hyalinization of the tumor vessels is commonly seen. Mitotic figures, nuclear atypia, and even small foci of necrosis may be present without indicating anaplastic change.

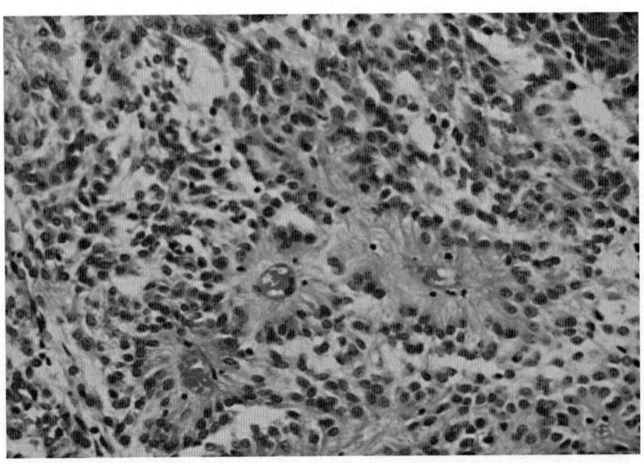

Figure 5-19 (PLATE 20). Ependymoma. Typical pseudorosetting formation in a spinal cord ependymoma.

Ependymomas are immunoreactive for GFAP and vimentin, particularly the cellular processes forming pseudorosettes around blood vessels. Ependymal rosettes are also immunoreactive for GFAP but in a more variable pattern.

Four histologic variants of ependymomas are recognized in the WHO classification: *cellular, papillary, tanycytic*, and *clear cell*.[84] These tumors have essentially the same clinical behavior, but the histopathologic features differ from ordinary ependymomas. *Cellular ependymomas* are characterized by prominent cellularity and only a few perivascular pseudorosettes and ependymal rosettes. As a result of the lack of these specialized structures, the differentiation of ependymoma from other gliomas can be problematic. Besides location, other indicators that help in the correct diagnosis are the chromatin pattern of the tumor cells and the very fibrillary nature of the intercellular matrix of all types of ependymoma. The *papillary ependymomas* are remarkable by conspicuous formation of papillary and tubular structures, somewhat similar to choroid plexus papillomas. The *tanycytic ependymoma* is characterized by its highly fibrillated and elongated cells with less pseudorosette formations that resemble astrocytomas. *Clear cell ependymomas* are a rare subtype; they show a distinctive appearance of perinuclear halo formation resembling that seen in oligodendroglial cells.[87] This may present a problem in differential diagnosis with other neuroepithelial tumors, including oligodendrogliomas and central neurocytomas. The correct diagnosis is suggested by other clinicopathologic features, such as tumor location and distinct tumor demarcation, as well as adequate immunohistochemistry, including prominent GFAP and vimentin-immunoreactive fibrils, and the presence of a 9 + 2 cilia arrangement, microvilli, and junctional complexes at the ultrastructural level.[87]

Anaplastic Ependymoma

Anaplastic features of ependymomas (WHO grade III) may be present in tumors at most sites, but are very rare in spinal cord ependymomas.[88] Features of anaplasias include hypercellularity, cellular and/or nuclear atypia, increased mitotic activity, endothelial microvascular proliferation, and large areas of necrosis.[89] Although these tumors are morphologically recognizable, the correlation

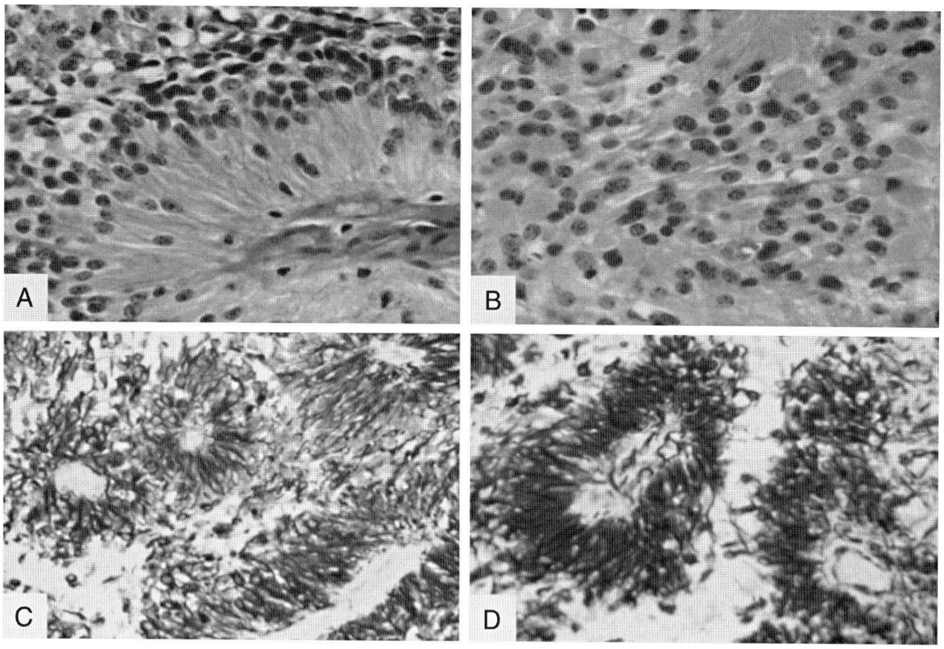

Figure 5-20 (PLATE 21). Ependymoma. (A) Fibrillary cellular processes in a high-power view of a pseudorosette. The ependymoma cells are typically characterized by a homogeneous distribution of the nuclear chromatin (B). Immunohistochemical stains for GFAP (C) and vimentin (D) emphasize the dense fibrillary processes of ependymoma cells.

between histopathology and clinical outcome of patients with anaplastic ependymomas is not as clearcut as that seen in other gliomas.[90] Anaplastic ependymomas have a high tendency to disseminate along the neuraxis.[91]

Tumor cell proliferation as reflected in mitotic index and/or proliferative labeling index appears to be the most important prognostic factor in ependymomas, particularly in the supratentorial tumors. Immunohistochemistry for Ki-67 shows that high labeling indices have a positive correlation with histologic grade and early tumor recurrence.[91–93] The presence of microvascular endothelial proliferation appears to be less relevant to the prognosis of these patients.[94]

Special Variants of Ependymomas

Myxopapillary Ependymoma

Myxopapillary ependymomas (WHO grade I) are a distinct variant of ependymoma that most commonly develop in the cauda equina and filum terminale of adult patients.[95] Less frequently, tumors may arise in the upper levels of the spinal cord and lateral ventricles. Ectopic tumors located in the extradural and presacral or retrosacral areas have also been reported.[86] The tumors are slow-growing and usually have a favorable prognosis.

Myxopapillary ependymomas are macroscopically well-circumscribed, encapsulated, sausage-shaped masses arising from the filum terminale and involving the spinal nerve roots of the cauda equina. Histologically, these tumors are characterized by extensive papillary formation with blood vessels showing hyaline and mucinous degeneration. Mucin accumulation in the form of small "mucin lakes" may also be seen intermixed with the tumor cells. Although the papillary arrangements dominate the histologic picture, focal formation of ependymal tubules can also be seen.

The majority of myxopapillary ependymomas are slow-growing tumors with a benign clinical course. However, local recurrence and dissemination along the neuraxis are not uncommon.[91] The prognosis of myxopapillary ependymoma appears to be directly related to successful total resection.[91]

Subependymoma

Subependymomas (WHO grade I) are well-circumscribed, generally asymptomatic masses of variable size located in the walls of the fourth and lateral ventricles.[96,97] Other tumor sites are the septum pellucidum, the foramen of Monro, and, less commonly, the spinal cord. Most tumors are found incidentally at autopsy. Symptomatic subependymomas may present with signs of increased intracranial pressure because of obstruction of CSF flow or spontaneous tumor hemorrhage. Tumors are found in both genders and in all age groups, but most frequently the symptomatic ones affect middle-aged patients (mean age 48 years).[97]

Subependymomas exhibit histologic features of both ependymal and astrocytic cellular differentiation, reflecting the hypothesized lineage of these tumors.[98] The tumors are mostly hypocellular with a dense fibrillary matrix. Ependymal features include perivascular pseudorosettes and, less frequently, true ependymal rosettes, whereas astroglial features are characterized by elongate, fibrillary to somewhat gemistocytic cells intermixed in a dense fibrillary matrix. The association of astrocytic and ependymal features has also been confirmed with electron microscopic and tissue culture studies. Microcalcifications and microcystic degeneration are common. Hyalinized blood vessels and signs of prior subclinical hemorrhage including hemosiderin deposition are often present.

Tumor location and surgical resection, particularly related to tumors situated on the floor of the fourth ventricle, are the most important prognostic factors.[96]

Molecular Genetics of Ependymal Tumors

The molecular genetic alterations in ependymomas are complex and still not completely understood.[84] Unlike astrocytomas, mutations of the *TP53* gene have only occasionally been demonstrated.[99] About a third of ependymomas show abnormalities involving chromosome 22, and a tumor suppressor gene on 22q may be present. Although some investigators have demonstrated evidence of mutations of the *NF2* suppressor gene at 22q12,[100] others have been unable to identify such mutations in a large number of ependymomas.[101–103]

Neuronal and Mixed Neuronal-Glial Tumors

Neuronal Tumor

This category of neuroepithelial tumors includes tumors in which the cellular elements show either ganglionic or neurocytic-like features without a true neoplastic glial component. The majority of neuronal tumors arises in childhood and early adulthood and are associated with a history of seizures. Although some authors consider some of these tumors as dysplastic (hamartomatous) lesions, they are considered true neoplasms in the WHO classification. Nevertheless, all neuronal tumors have a benign clinical behavior and are classified as grade I or II tumors.

Gangliocytoma and Dysplastic Gangliocytoma of the Cerebellum

Gangliocytomas (WHO grade I) are rare tumors composed of mature ganglionic neurons. The tumors are generally well circumscribed and most commonly arise in the temporal lobe and cervicothoracic spinal cord.[104,105] Other locations include the hypothalamus and pituitary region, and, rarely, the pineal gland.[104,106,107] Most lesions become symptomatic within the first three decades. Although temporal lobe tumors may be associated with seizure disorders, in other locations, gangliocytomas may present with specific symptomatology. For example, tumors arising in the pituitary region are associated with endocrine disorders,[107] and hypothalamic gangliocytomas may present with precocious puberty.[108]

Gangliocytomas are characterized by a proliferation of neoplastic ganglion cells in a scanty cellular glial–mesenchymal stroma (Fig. 5-21). The ganglionic population is irregularly distributed and exhibits great cytologic pleomorphism, including bizarre and binucleate forms. Abnormal ganglionic cells and neuritic processes can be highlighted with silver stains such as modified Bielschowsky and immunohistochemical stains for neuronal-associated markers. Because the glial elements of the lesion are not neoplastic in nature, these tumors have no potential for anaplastic progression.[104]

The *dysplastic gangliocytoma of the cerebellum*, also known as Lhermitte-Duclos disease, is a rare form of gangliocytoma restricted to the cerebellum. The lesion usually becomes clinically apparent during the fourth decade of life, although patients with symptoms earlier in life have been reported, mainly as a result of megacephaly and intracranial hypertension.[109] Lhermitte-Duclos disease is associated with Cowden syndrome and phosphatase tensin homologue (*PTEN*) mutation in approximately 50% of cases,[110] suggesting that this entity may have features of both a hamartoma and neoplasm.

Hypertrophic cerebellar folia as a result of the proliferation of abnormal ganglion and neuronal cells that occupy both the normal granular and Purkinje cell layers characterize this lesion (Fig. 5-22). The histogenesis of these ganglionic and neuronal cells is still not well understood. Although they resemble small Purkinje cells histologically, immunohistochemical studies suggest a histogenetic relationship to both Purkinje cell and granular cell neuronal lineages.[111] Hypermyelinated fibers and enlarged neurites replace the normal molecular layer and the adjacent white matter.

Central Neurocytoma

Central neurocytomas (WHO grade II) are rare, benign neuronal tumors most commonly found in the region of the lateral ventricles and/or the third ventricle.[112] These tumors usually occur in young patients, with a mean age of 24 years in one large series.[113] Most tumors present as well-delineated, partially calcified masses in or adjacent to the lateral ventricles, typically in the region of the foramen of Monro. Massive tumors involving both the lateral and third ventricles have also been described.

Central neurocytomas are histologically distinguished by a homogeneous population of cells with round lobulated nuclei and scant cytoplasm in a conspicuously

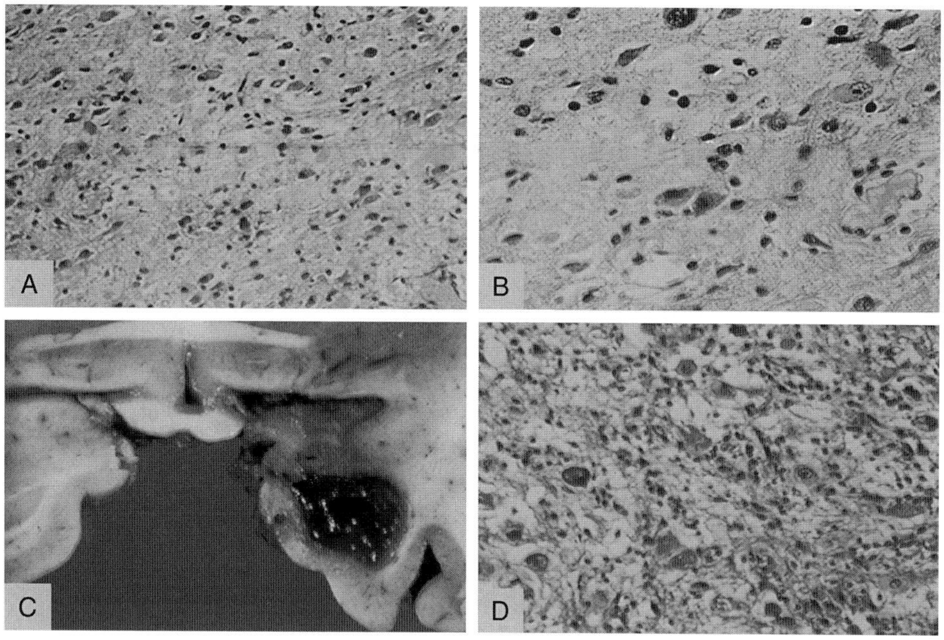

Figure 5-21 (PLATE 22). Neuronal and mixed neuronal-glial tumors. (A and B) Gangliocytomas are characteristically hypocellular and composed of ganglion-like cells. In contrast, gangliogliomas have a mixture of glial and neuronal cells (D). The formation of cysts is a common feature of gangliogliomas (C).

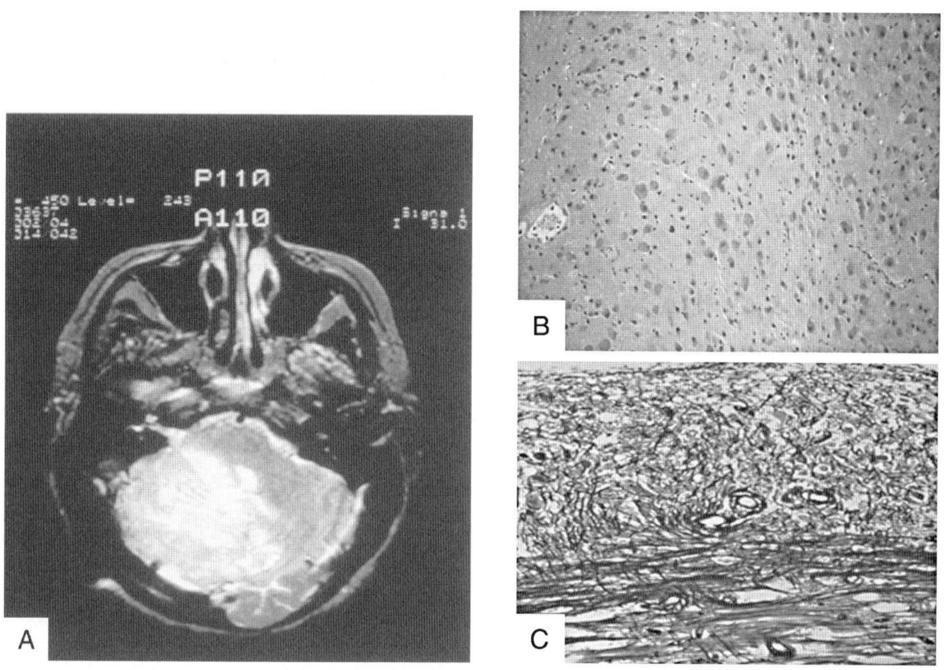

Figure 5-22 (PLATE 23). Dysplastic gangliocytoma of the cerebellum: (A) A magnetic resonance imaging (MRI) scan of a case of dysplastic gangliocytoma of the cerebellum showing the enlarged cerebellar folia and hemispheric hypertrophy. Large ganglionic cells resembling Purkinje cells (B) and abnormally shaped and thick neuritic process (Bielschowsky silver) (C) histologically characterize the tumor.

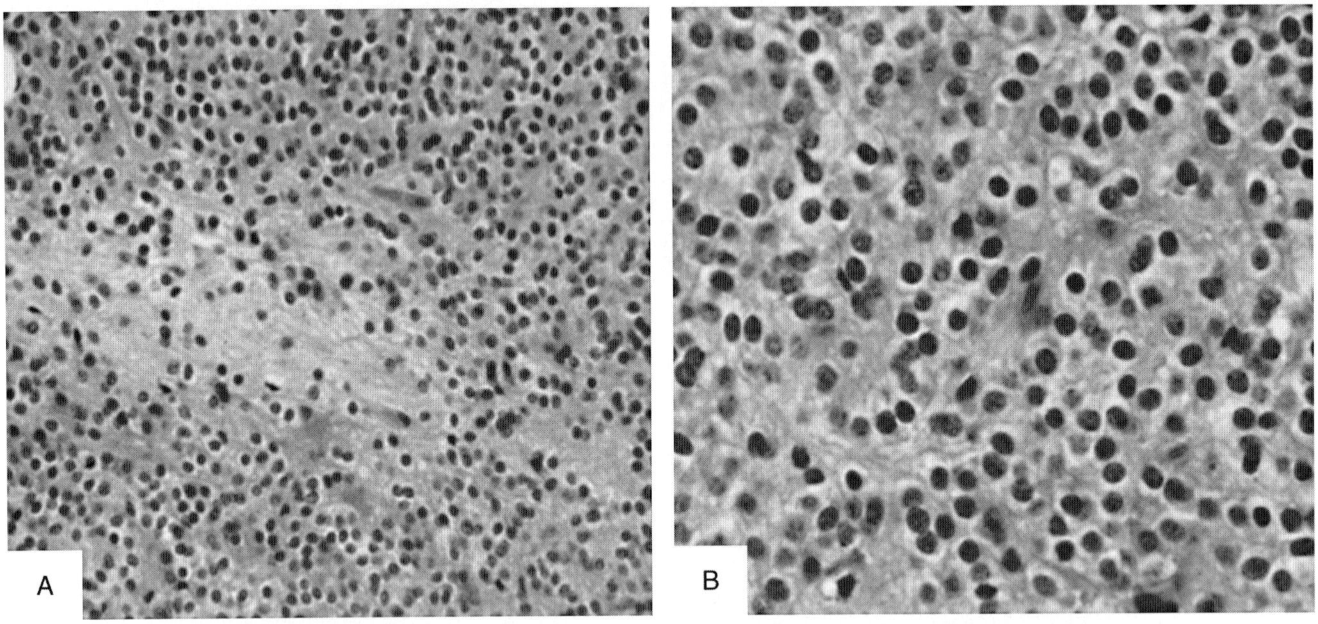

Figure 5-23 (PLATE 24). Central neurocytoma. (A and B) The appearance of central neurocytomas typically consists of a homogeneous population of cells with oval to round nuclei that resemble oligodendrogliomas.

fibrillated matrix (Figs. 5-23 and 5-24). A distinctive feature of these tumors is the presence of anuclear islands composed of a delicate fibrillary matrix resembling neuropil. Perinuclear halos may be prominent, and a delicate branching microvasculature is typically seen—two features that resemble oligodendrogliomas. Focal calcification and small areas of necrosis may be rarely observed. Mitotic activity is low and Ki-67 LI is generally low.[114]

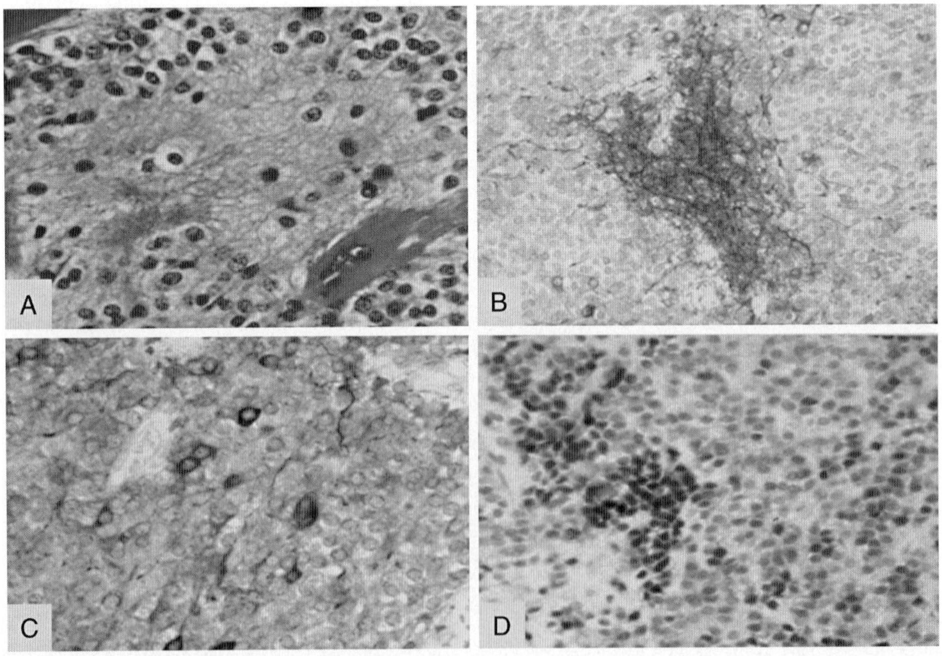

Figure 5-24 (PLATE 25). Central neurocytoma. Close examination of central neurocytoma demonstrates anuclear, neuropil-like areas (A) that are strongly immunoreactive for neuronal markers (B) (synaptophysin). Individual or group of tumor cells show immunoreactivity for neuronal-associated markers MAP2 (C) and NeuN (D).

Endothelial proliferation is not present (see below). Mature ganglion cells are rarely reported in central neurocytomas.[115]

The neuronal differentiation of central neurocytomas is readily confirmed with immunohistochemistry for synaptophysin and other neuronal-associated proteins including neurofilament proteins and NeuN.[113,115,116] GFAP immunoreactivity has been described in a few reported cases.[115] but in the majority of cases it is restricted to reactive stromal astrocytes.[113]

Central neurocytomas are benign lesions, with most tumors behaving as a grade II neoplasm. However, tumor recurrence has been reported in several cases,[114,117,118] generally after incomplete resection. Some tumors have exhibited ventricular and subarachnoid dissemination at the time of recurrence.[118] Several reports have described tumors with moderate mitotic activity, vascular proliferation, and focal necrosis.[116] Some authors contend that the proliferative potential of central neurocytomas correlates with their clinical behavior,[119] and that central neurocytomas with Ki-67 LI greater than 2% have a higher chance of recurrence. In addition, their study demonstrates a highly significant correlation between the presence of vascular endothelial proliferation and the Ki-67 LI. These authors suggest that such tumors should be termed "atypical central neurocytoma."

Other tumors with histologic features similar to those of central neurocytomas have been described in extraventricular locations. These tumors are designated as "neurocytomas" by the WHO classification, including the cerebellar liponeurocytoma.[120] The relationship between these tumors and the typical central neurocytoma remains unclear.

Mixed Neuronal-Glial Tumors

Ganglioglioma and Malignant Ganglioglioma

Gangliogliomas (WHO grade I-III) represent approximately 1% of all brain tumors[121] and approximately 1% to 4% of all pediatric CNS tumors.[122] They are the most common mixed neuronal-glial tumors, and the majority arise within the first three decades of life.[123] Gangliogliomas present with seizure disorders, most frequently with complex partial seizures.[122]

Gangliogliomas are most frequently located in the temporal lobes followed by parietal and frontal lobes.[121–124] The tumors are relatively well demarcated on computerized tomography (CT) and magnetic resonance imaging (MRI) scans, commonly showing cystic and calcified components. Some cases are associated with cortical dysplasia in the vicinity of the tumor.[121,124] Leptomeningeal involvement may be present.

Gangliogliomas are composed of a mixture of neoplastic, abnormal ganglion cells and glial cells (most commonly fibrillary and pilocytic astrocytes) (see Fig. 5-21). Oligodendroglial elements are considerably less common.[124] The ganglion cells may show substantial variation in size and density. Bizarre and binucleate forms are present, but the latter may be rare in some tumors. Another prominent feature of gangliogliomas is the presence of a rich fibrous stroma often accompanied by perivascular lymphocytic infiltrates.

Silver stains and immunohistochemistry for neuronal-associated proteins including neurofilament proteins, synaptophysin, and NeuN greatly facilitate the identification of the ganglionic elements in gangliogliomas.[121,123] Immunostains for GFAP, vimentin, and S100 protein highlight the usually astrocytic glial elements.

Gangliogliomas are graded as grade I or II according to their glial elements. The glial component contributes to the potential for recurrence and anaplastic progression. Although Ki-67 LI is low in the great majority of gangliogliomas, labeling appears to be confined to the glial component.[121,123] High labeling values are associated with a more aggressive behavior of these tumors.[123]

Malignant transformation in gangliogliomas is reported to occur in approximately 10% of cases.[125] These tumors are designated *anaplastic gangliogliomas* (WHO grade III), and represent anaplastic progression invariably occurring in the glial component. The histopathology may resemble an anaplastic astrocytoma or even a glioblastoma. The ganglionic elements are less readily detected in these anaplastic tumors. Immunohistochemical stains for neuronal-associated markers are frequently helpful in this context.

Dysembryoplastic Neuroepithelial Tumor

Dysembryoplastic neuroepithelial tumor (DNT) (WHO grade I) is a particular type of mixed neuronal–glial neoplasm that arises in children and young adults with long-standing complex partial seizures.[126] DNTs are rare tumors and may represent less than 1% of all brain tumors.[127] However, in specialized centers for epilepsy surgery, the frequency may be higher.

The tumors most frequently involve the temporal lobes.[126] A few cases involving other sites, including the caudate nucleus and cerebellum, have also been reported.[128] The lesions are predominantly intracortical and multinodular, but subcortical white matter involvement also occurs. A multicystic appearance is frequently appreciated on MRI.[129] A common radiographic sign is an overlying skull defect, suggesting a long-standing lesion.

The distinct histopathologic presentation of DNT is the multinodular architecture of the tumor, best appreciated at low-power magnification (Fig. 5-25). The tumor nodules are composed of a mixture of small cells resembling oligodendroglia (the so-called oligodendroglial-like cell [OLC]), astrocytes, and neuronal cells embedded

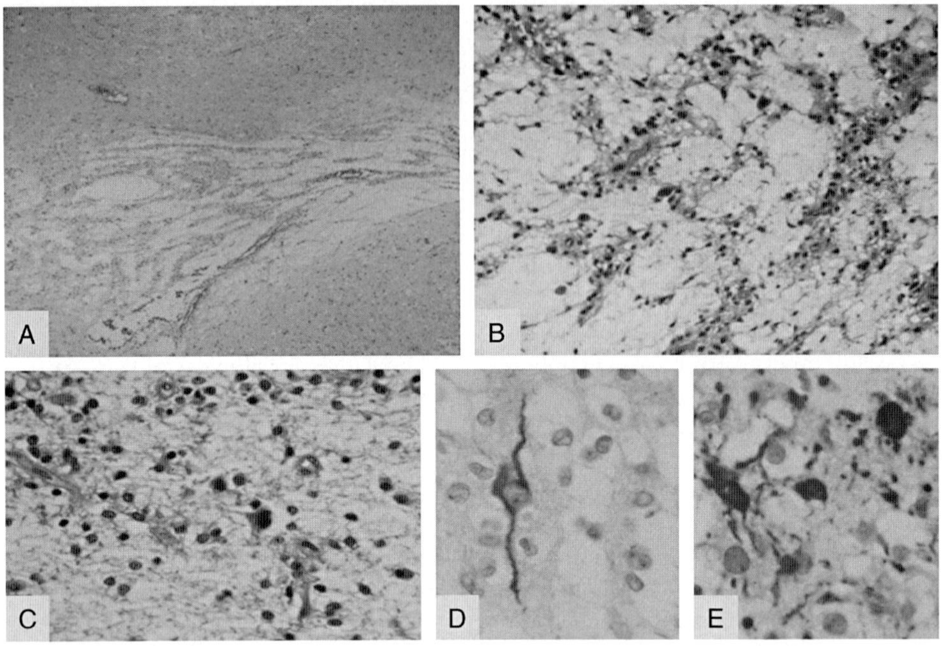

Figure 5-25 (PLATE 26). Dysembryoplastic neuroepithelial tumor (DNT). An example of DNT at low magnification shows a mildly cellular neoplasm with microcystic changes (A). The mixed cellular elements of DNT are composed of oligodendroglial-like cells, astrocytes, and neurons in variable proportions (B to C). Floating neurons are typically seen in these areas (D) (neurofilament), intermixed with other glial cells (E) (GFAP).

within a mucinous and microcystic matrix. The neuronal component is mostly composed of large cells floating within the mucinous matrix. The small OLCs appear to be a mixture of cells with early glial and neuronal differentiation.[130] Mitotic activity may be observed, but proliferative indexes are generally low with Ki-67 LI generally around 1%.[131] Neuronal-associated markers (synaptophysin, neurofilament proteins, class III β-tubulin, NeuN) confirm the distinct neuronal component, whereas GFAP, vimentin, and S100 stains verify the glial elements.[130,132] Typically, the brain surrounding a DNT has a variable degree of cortical dysplasia.[126]

Considering the heterogeneity of these tumors, adequate sampling is very important for the correct diagnosis of DNTs. The major differential diagnoses to be considered include oligodendroglioma and mixed oligoastrocytoma. The recognition of DNT is significant because surgical resection results in an extremely favorable prognosis. DNTs are benign, grade I tumors, but recurrence has been observed in cases with incomplete initial surgical resection.[131]

Embryonal Tumors

The embryonal tumors are a group of clinically aggressive neuroepithelial tumors that typically occur in childhood. The histogenesis of the tumors is hypothesized as the result of transformation of immature or primitive neuroepithelial progenitor cells that are believed to be present throughout the neuraxis.[133] All embryonal tumors have a number of common histologic features, including high cellularity, primitive-appearing small cells, and high mitotic activity. Additionally, these tumors exhibit a high tendency for cerebrospinal fluid seeding. All these features reflect the clinically aggressive behavior of embryonal tumors and their designation as grade IV neoplasms by the WHO classification.

Despite the common properties shared by these neoplasms, a number of embryonal tumors are individualized on the basis of their distinctive histopathologic and molecular features and presumed histogenesis. The current WHO classification recognizes the central neuroblastoma and the ependymoblastoma as embryonal tumors demonstrating differentiation toward neuronal and ependymal lineages, respectively. The medulloepithelioma, a very rare embryonal neoplasm that has a characteristic histomorphology, is also a separate entity in the WHO classification. Atypical teratoid/rhabdoid tumors are also distinguished in this category because of their specific clinical, pathologic, and genetic characteristics. The most common of these tumors is the medulloblastoma that arises in the cerebellum. Embryonal tumors indistinguishable from medulloblastomas but located at other sites of the neuraxis are designated supratentorial primitive neuroectodermal tumor (sPNET).

Medulloblastomas

Medulloblastomas (WHO grade IV) are the most common malignant CNS tumor arising in childhood[134] and are the prototype of primitive neuroepithelial neoplasms. Medulloblastomas comprise approximately 25% of all intracranial tumors in children, occurring primarily during the first decade of life with a peak occurrence in children age 7 years.[134] However, medulloblastomas may also arise in early adulthood, and rarely in the fifth and sixth decades of life.[134]

The tumors are situated in the cerebellum, the majority in the cerebellar midline, although they may also arise in the cerebellar hemispheres. Grossly, they are soft and relatively demarcated from the adjacent brain. Necrosis may be focal or confluent, but massive necrosis is infrequent.

Medulloblastomas are hypercellular neoplasms composed of relatively small cells with scant cytoplasm and hyperchromatic nuclei (Fig. 5-26). The cells are usually arranged in sheets, although focal formation of rhythmic nuclear palisades can be seen. The tumor cells diffusely infiltrate the cerebellar cortex with obliteration of the granular and molecular layers. Although the tumors are poorly differentiated by routine microscopy, approximately one-third of medulloblastomas reveal neuroblastic differentiation manifested by the presence of neuroblastic (Homer Wright) rosettes, prominent intercellular fibrillated matrix, and the proliferation of cells with large and vesicular nuclei, similar to neurocytic cells. Mitoses are frequently seen. Apoptotic figures and necrosis are frequently encountered, but endothelial vascular proliferation is rare.

Immunohistochemistry demonstrates that more than half of medulloblastomas show neuronal differentiation. Neuronal-associated markers, including synaptophysin and neurofilament proteins, are seen. Astrocytic differentiation, highlighted by GFAP reactivity, has been convincingly shown in several cases, but in the majority of the cases is restricted to a small percentage of tumor cells.[5,134]

Variants of medulloblastomas (see Table 5-1) include the *desmoplastic medulloblastoma,* which comprises approximately 10–12% of tumors.[5] These tumors are remarkable both for their firm consistency and striking amount of connective tissue and their biphasic architecture with a follicular or nodular arrangement of tumor cells (Fig. 5-27). The nodules are characterized by hypocellularity alternating with hypercellular internodular areas. In addition, the cells forming the nodules have a neurocytic-like appearance, that is, larger cells with larger nuclei within a neuropil-like background; immunoreactivity for neuronal-associated markers also demonstrate these neuronal-like differentiation features.[134–136] In contrast, the hypercellular areas are composed of small, primitive-appearing cells with increased mitotic activity and proliferative labeling indexes. This unique biphasic arrangement of desmoplastic medulloblastoma is most apparent on reticulin stain wherein, in contrast to the reticulin-rich hypercellular areas, the hypocellular nodules are markedly free of staining. More significantly, this variant of medulloblastoma appears to have a distinct clinical behavior from the classic medulloblastoma, making its recognition important in the treatment of medulloblastomas (see below).

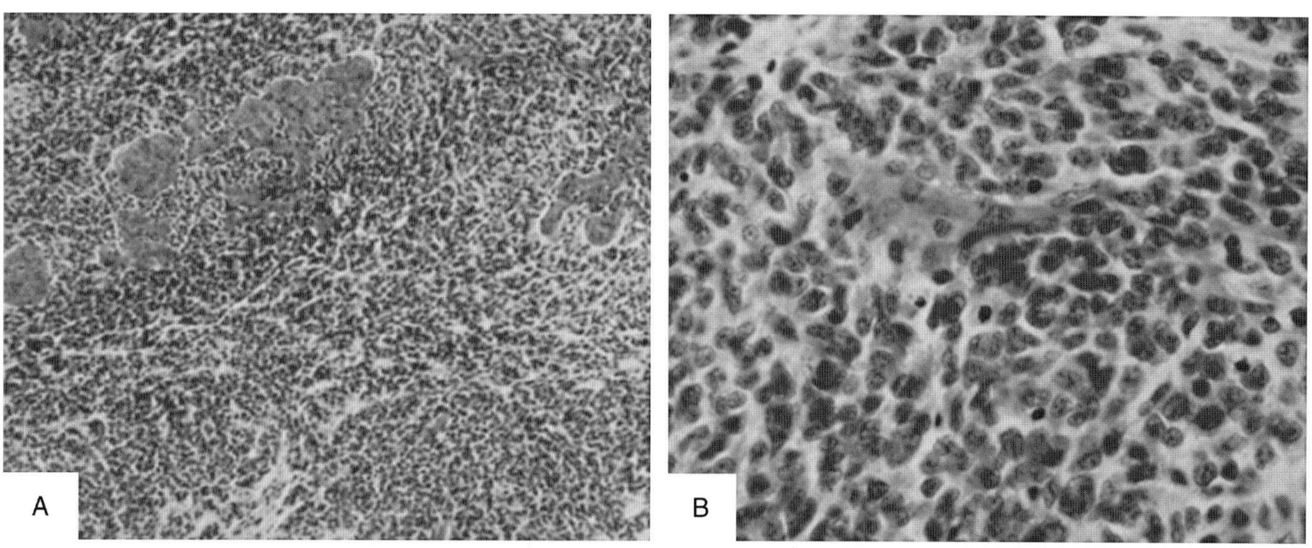

Figure 5-26 (PLATE 27). Medulloblastoma (classical variant). (A and B) Medulloblastomas are densely cellular tumors composed of closely packed primitive cells. (B) High mitotic activity and apoptotic figures are commonly seen.

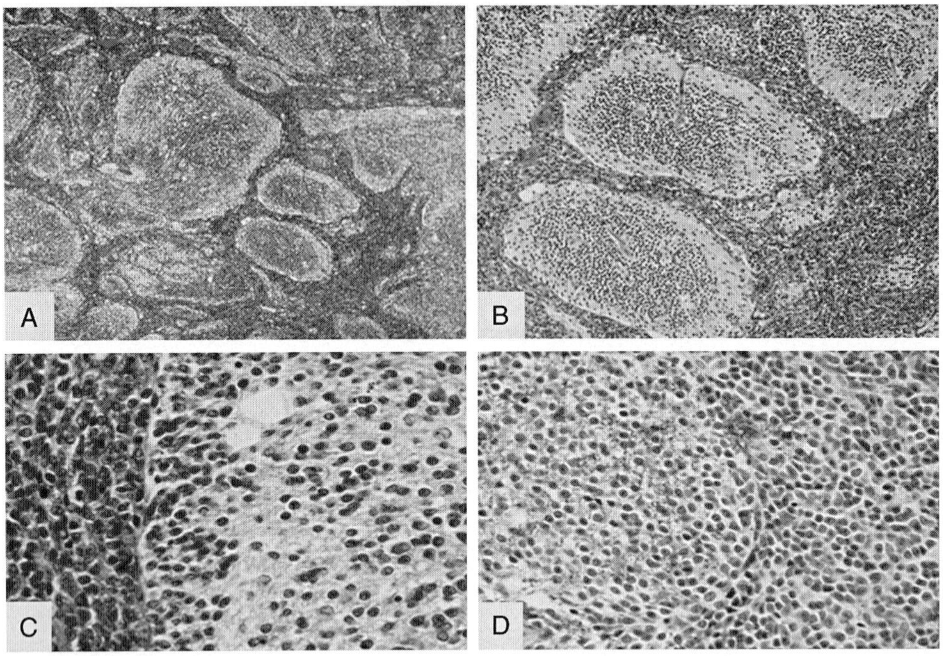

Figure 5-27 (PLATE 28). Medulloblastoma (desmoplastic variant). (A and B) The desmoplastic or nodular variant of medulloblastoma is characterized by a lobular appearance with hypercellular areas alternating with less cellular nodules. The nodules are reticulin free (not shown), and show more differentiated cells (C) and neuronal differentiation by immunohistochemistry (D) (neurofilament).

Another recognized variant that has significant prognostic value is the *large cell/anaplastic medulloblastoma*.[134,137] These tumors represent approximately 4% of medulloblastomas and have a very poor prognosis. Tumor cells have large and pleomorphic nuclei and ample cytoplasm. The tumor shows large areas of necrosis, high mitotic activity, and apoptosis.

Some other rare variants of medulloblastoma are also described (see Table 5-1). The *medullomyoblastoma*, which show striated muscle cell differentiation, and the *melanotic medulloblastoma*. The relationship of these variants to the more common classic medulloblastoma is not understood.

It has been noted in large clinical cohorts that patients with medulloblastomas receiving similar therapies may have completely different clinical outcomes.[134] Attempts to understand prognostic predictors from the clinical, pathologic, molecular, and therapeutic standpoints have been actively undertaken in recent years (reviewed in reference 138). Medulloblastomas appear to present a spectrum of histologic features associated with best or worst clinical outcome. The two extremes of the histologic spectrum are the desmoplastic/nodular medulloblastoma and the large cell/anaplastic medulloblastoma as previously discussed. Although an official grading system is not widely accepted for medulloblastomas, some authorities advocate stratification of tumors according to their degree of differentiation/anaplasia.[138,139] Medulloblastomas displaying features of anaplasia, including increased nuclear size, marked cytologic anaplasia, and increased mitotic and apoptotic rates, are associated with aggressive clinical behavior.[139,140] Tumors that show some features of neuronal differentiation, including nodularity, however, have a statistically longer survival than do classic (non-nodular) medulloblastomas.[138–140]

Molecular Genetics of Medulloblastomas and sPNETs

Cytogenetic studies show that isochromosome 17q [i(17q)] is the most frequent abnormality in medulloblastomas, occurring in about a third of tumors.[134] Molecular studies have confirmed this finding with the frequent loss of heterozygosity (LOH) for chromosome 17p.[141] Although this region contains the *TP53* gene locus, *TP53* mutations are rarely seen in medulloblastomas.[27,31,141]

In contrast to medulloblastomas, relatively little is known about the genetic abnormalities of sPNETs. At present, data indicate that the chromosomal and genetic aberrations in sPNETs differ from those usually seen in medulloblastomas. For example, isochromosome 17q is exceptional in sPNETs.[142] Similarly, the commonly seen LOH at 17p in medulloblastomas is not present in sPNETs.[31,143]

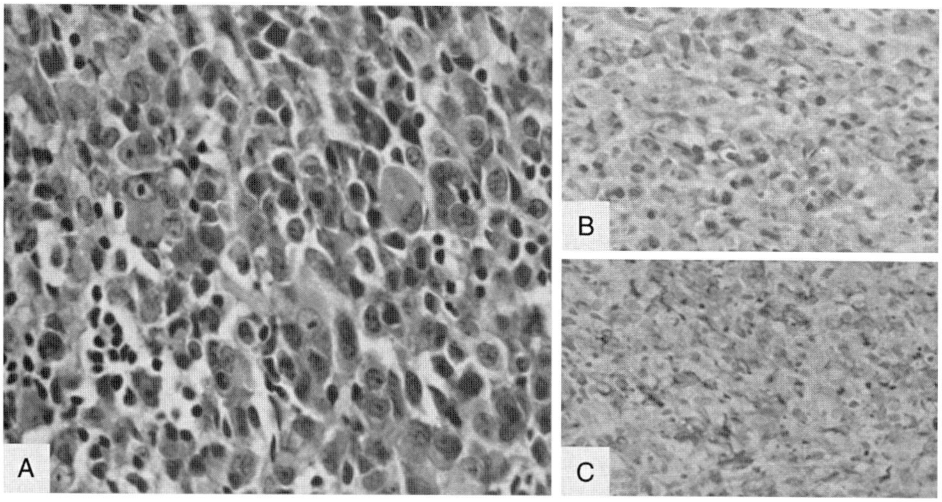

Figure 5-28 (PLATE 29). Atypical teratoid/rhabdoid tumor. (A) The abundant eosinophilic cytoplasm of the tumor cells gives the rhabdoid appearance to the tumor. Immunohistochemistry for vimentin (B) highlights the cytoplasmic inclusions, while focal reactivity may also be seen for neuronal markers (C) (neurofilament).

Atypical Teratoid/Rhabdoid Tumor

This childhood brain tumor (a WHO grade IV tumor) shows histologic features of rhabdoid cells similar to those seen in tumors of the kidneys. These rare tumors arise most often in the posterior fossa, although supratentorial tumors and tumors involving multiple sites are not uncommon.[144] Seventy-five percent of the patients are 3 years of age or younger, with males more commonly affected than females. The tumors grossly are often large, soft, focally necrotic, and hemorrhagic, with occasional regions of firm white tissue. One-third of the tumors are disseminated at the time of diagnosis with involvement of cranial nerves and vessels.

The tumors are characteristically composed of rhabdoid cells, that is, large and polygonal cells with eccentric nuclei and prominent single nucleoli, and an eosinophilic cytoplasm containing spherical fibrillary intracytoplasmic inclusions (Fig. 5-28). These cells may be abundant or may be incorporated into a complex mix of primitive neuroepithelial tumor resembling medulloblastoma, glial, epithelial, and mesenchymal elements. Immunohistochemically, the rhabdoid cells are strongly immunoreactive for vimentin, and variably reactive for epithelial membrane antigen (EMA) and smooth muscle actin (SMA); on occasion, they may react with GFAP, cytokeratin, and neurofilament proteins. The cells are mostly unreactive for desmin and germ cell markers (placental alkaline phosphatase [PLAP], α-fetoprotein [AFP], beta human chorionic gonadotropin [bhCG]).

Genetic analyses of these tumors were essential in the characterization of such separate entity among the group of embryonal tumors. Cytogenetic analysis revealed chromosome 22 abnormalities, either monosomy of chromosome 22 or partial deletion on 22q11.2.[145] This region contains the *INI1/hSNF5* gene, which encodes a component of the SWI/SNF chromatin remodeling complex.[146,147] Alterations of the *INI1* tumor suppressor gene have been documented in the majority of these tumors by either deletion of one or both copies and/or mutation of *INI1/hSNF5* gene.[146]

Atypical teratoid/rhabdoid tumors are extremely aggressive tumors. Median survival is 6 months, with overall 2-year survival being less than 20%.[148] The very poor prognosis of the tumor is probably partly a result of its proclivity for craniospinal tumor seeding.[149]

▶ MENINGEAL TUMORS

Meningiomas

Meningiomas are tumors arising from the meningothelial/arachnoidal cells. They account for approximately 28% of all primary CNS tumors,[4] 15% of intracranial tumors, and approximately 25% of intraspinal tumors.[150] Meningiomas typically manifest in middle age (peak incidence between 45 and 55 years)[5] and are rarely seen in childhood. A marked female predominance (3:1) is seen in adults,[150] and some series in children report a significant male predilection.[151] Meningiomas may occur sporadically or associated with NF2. This association is particularly high in childhood, where approximately 40% of children with meningiomas have NF2.[151] Rare familial non–NF2-associated meningiomas may also occur.[150]

Multiple meningiomas occur in nearly 8% of the cases, particularly in association with NF2.[150]

Meningiomas may potentially arise at any place in the neuraxis where meningothelial cells are present. However, certain sites are favored. In the supratentorium, meningiomas are most frequently seen in the falx, cerebral convexities, tuberculum sellae and parasellar region, olfactory grooves, sphenoidal ridge, and pineal region. Intraventricular meningiomas are not rare, and they presumably arise from arachnoidal cells within the tela choroidea or stroma of the choroid plexus. In the posterior fossa, the cerebellopontine angle proximate to the petrous bone is a common site. In the spinal canal, meningiomas occur in the thoracic, cervical, and lumbar regions, in order of decreasing frequency. In comparison with adults, meningiomas in children tend to present in unusual locations, including the ventricles, posterior fossa, and spinal dural regions.[151]

Most meningiomas are well-demarcated, dural-based globular masses that push the brain and erode into adjacent structures. The exception to this pattern is the so-called meningioma "en plaque"—carpet-like tumors that typically occur at the base of the skull and over the sphenoid ridge. Invasion of dura and bone are commonly seen.

Several histologic variants of meningiomas are listed in the WHO classification, reflecting both epithelial and mesenchymal phenotypic aspects of meningothelial cells (Fig. 5-29). Meningiomas are also graded on the basis of histologic anaplasia and potential for aggressive behavior (Table 5-2). Three major groups—*meningioma* (WHO grade I), *atypical meningioma* (WHO grade II), and *anaplastic (malignant) meningioma* (WHO grade III)—are listed according to histologic features of anaplasia. In addition, special variants of meningiomas are highlighted because of their particular potential for aggressive behavior. These are the *clear cell* and *chordoid* meningiomas (WHO grade II) and *papillary* and *rhabdoid* meningiomas (WHO grade III).

Meningioma

Although meningiomas (WHO grade I) are notable for the extraordinary diversity of their histologic patterns, the histologic hallmark remains the cellular meningothelial whorl. The *meningotheliomatous* and *transitional* meningiomas display the most typical meningothelial appearance. These are characterized by group of cells with poorly defined cell borders forming the typical whorls around individual cells, blood vessels, and stromal elements. Psammoma bodies, lamellated, calcified structures normally seen intermixed with meningothelial cells in the arachnoid membrane, are commonly seen in these tumors; but when psammoma bodies are a predominant feature, the tumor is designated *psammomatous* meningioma. *Fibroblastic* meningiomas are composed of spindled cells arranged in fascicles and variable degree of reticulin-positive stroma and presence of extracellular matrix proteins, including laminin.

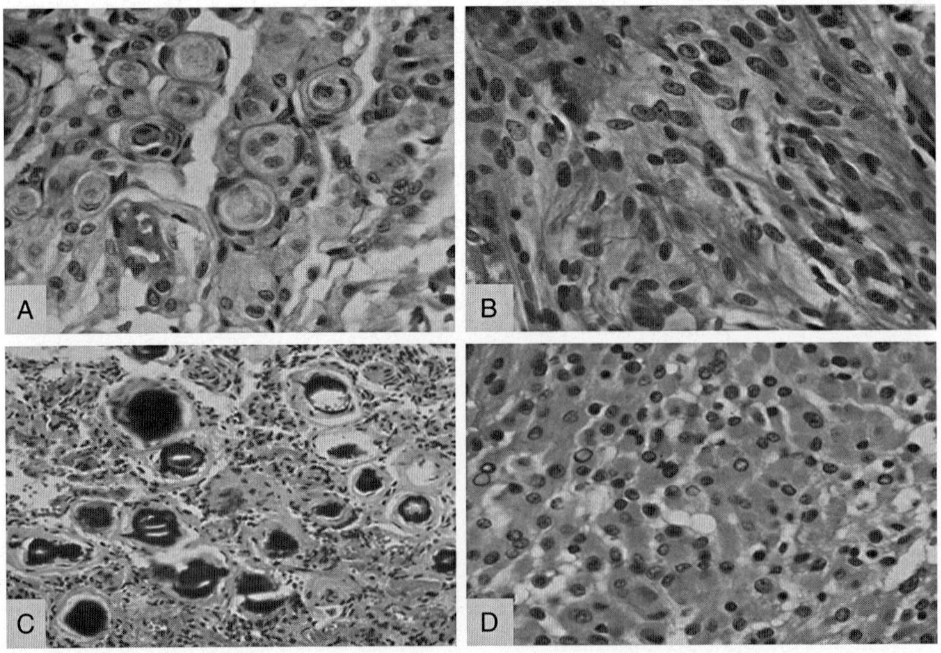

Figure 5-29 (PLATE 30). Meningioma. Meningiomas may present a variety of tissue arrangements, including meningothelial (A), fibroblastic (B), psammomatous (C), and rhabdoid (D).

▶ **TABLE 5-2.** TUMORS OF THE MENINGOTHELIAL TISSUE

Meningioma Variant	WHO Grading
Meningothelial	WHO grade I
Fibrous (fibroblastic)	
Transitional (mixed)	
Psammomatous	
Angiomatous	
Microcystic	
Secretory	
Lymphoplasmacyte-rich	
Metaplastic	
Clear cell	WHO grade II
Chordoid	
Atypical*	
Rhabdoid	WHO grade III
Papillary	
Anaplastic (malignant)*	

*Meningiomas of any subtype may be classified as atypical or anaplastic.

The *microcystic, secretory, clear cell,* and *papillary* meningiomas are the "epithelial" variants of meningiomas. As previously mentioned, the *clear cell* and the *papillary* tumors are special category of meningiomas prone to malignant transformation.

Meningiomas are strongly immunoreactive for vimentin, confirming their mesenchymal nature. However, the epithelial marker EMA is also immunoreactive in the majority of the meningiomas (Fig. 5-30). Meningiomas are also variably immunoreactive for S100 protein, cytokeratin, and carcinoembryonic antigen (CEA); the last two markers are mostly found in the secretory variants.

Grade I meningiomas are benign tumors with low proliferative indices, with reported mean Ki-67 LI around 4%.[152]

Atypical Meningiomas

Atypical meningiomas (WHO grade II) are tumors that exhibit histologic features associated with potential for recurrence.[150] The WHO classification recognizes atypical meningiomas as those tumors with high mitotic index (≥ 4/10 high-powered fields [HPFs]) or at least 3 of 5 histologic features (sheet-like architecture, macronucleoli, small cell formation, hypercellularity, necrosis). These features may be identified in any histologic variant without specific predilections. Frequently these features are not uniformly distributed throughout the tumor, emphasizing the necessity for very careful examination of multiple tissue sections for evaluating meningiomas.

Ki-67 labeling indices tend to correlate with increase of tumor grade. Atypical meningiomas usually present a mean value of around 7%.[152]

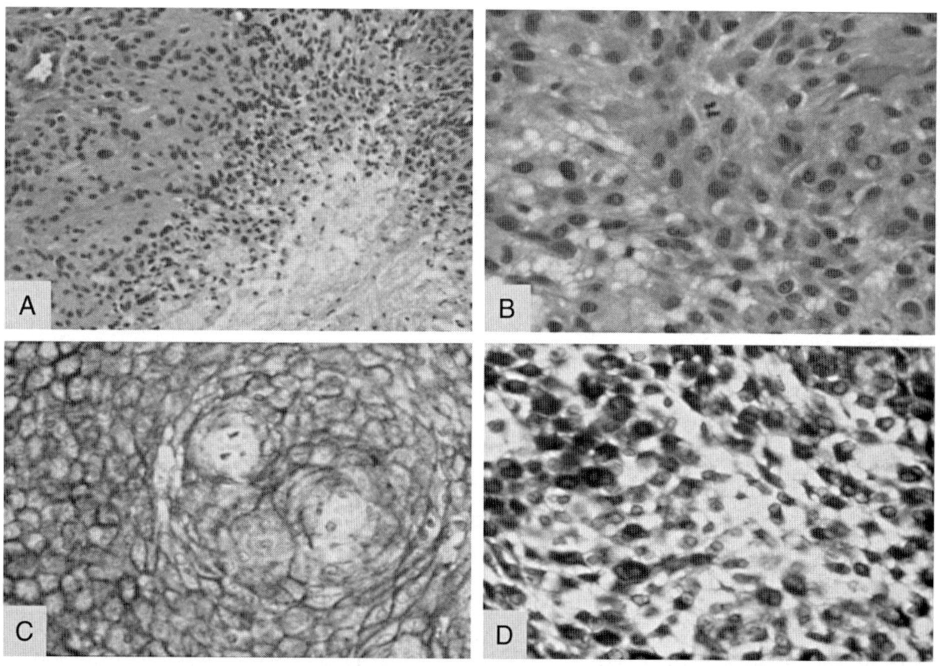

Figure 5-30 (PLATE 31). Anaplastic meningioma. Areas of necrosis (A) and high mitotic activity (B) are some of the features of anaplastic meningiomas. The characteristic immunohistochemical profile of all malignancy grades of meningiomas includes strong EMA (C) and vimentin (D) positivity.

The clinical importance in recognized atypical meningioma resides in the increased propensity of these tumors to recur compared to the usual meningioma.[153]

Anaplastic (Malignant) Meningiomas

Anaplastic meningiomas (WHO grade III) are tumors that display frank anaplasia (carcinoma-, sarcoma-, or melanoma-like appearance) or a very high mitotic index (at least 20/10 HPF)[150] (see Fig. 5-30). Nonetheless, the histologic features of meningioma as described above are retained and are distinct from sarcomas that may arise in the meninges. Anaplastic meningiomas are rare, and the prognosis for patients with anaplastic meningiomas is very poor, with a median survival of less than 2 years.[154]

Clinically, anaplastic meningiomas arise in the elderly (6th decade) with a virtual equal male-to-female ratio.[155] Recurrence following surgery is 100% at 15 years versus 2% for ordinary meningiomas.[155]

Meningiomas with brain invasion and incorporation of cerebral parenchyma into tumor have previously been considered anaplastic meningiomas. Although direct invasion of the brain is considered a strong indicator of aggressive clinical behavior of meningioma, regardless of histologic degree of anaplasia, the morbidity and mortality are equivalent to that encountered in atypical meningiomas. Therefore, such tumors are classified as grade II rather than grade III meningiomas.[150]

Molecular Genetics of Meningiomas

The most common cytogenetic abnormality in meningiomas is allelic loss of 22q (reviewed in reference 150). This chromosome is also the site for the neurofibromatosis gene *NF2*, a finding in agreement with the high incidence of meningiomas in this familial disorder. However, mutations of the *NF2* gene are not restricted to tumors arising in patients with NF2. The frequency of *NF2* mutation in sporadic meningiomas is as high as 60%.[150] Several other genes appear to be implicated in the tumorigenesis of meningiomas. A detailed discussion of these findings is found in Chapter 18 and in Louis and associates.[150]

Hemangiopericytoma

Hemangiopericytoma (WHO grades II to III) is a highly cellular and richly vascularized mesenchymal tumor of the meninges, indistinguishable from hemangiopericytoma of the soft tissue. Once considered a particular vascular (angioblastic) variant of meningiomas, hemangiopericytomas are now classified as a separate entity and are linked to one of the most controversial entities in soft-tissue pathology.[156]

Hemangiopericytomas arise from dura, often in or about the tentorium, and may compress or even invade underlying brain tissue. They may produce lytic lesions of the overlying skull, and unlike meningiomas do not elicit osteoblastic/hyperostotic lesions. These tumors comprise less than 1% of all primary CNS tumors and affect males slightly more often than females, with a slightly younger age range (30–50 years) than meningiomas.[157]

Grossly, hemangiopericytomas are usually spherical, firm, and highly vascular, making surgical resection difficult. The tumors are histologically hypercellular and composed of sheets of oval to spindle-shaped tumor cells, interspersed with slit-like (staghorn) blood vessels (Fig. 5-31). Mitotic figures are present, but highly variable in number, even within the same tumor. Immunohistochemical immunoreactivity of the tumor cells is seen with vimentin and CD34. Unlike meningiomas, EMA and other epithelial markers are negative. The Ki-67 LI is variable but averages 10%.[157] High mitotic rate (≥ 5–6/10 HPF), together with evidence of nuclear pleomorphism and tumor necrosis, is associated with decreased survival.[158]

The histogenesis of hemangiopericytomas is uncertain, and pathologists debate the relationship of these tumors to other soft-tissue tumors including solitary fibrous tumor.[156] Hemangiopericytoma of the meninges is considered a low-grade sarcoma because of its high recurrence rate despite apparently complete surgical excision and tendency to metastasize outside the CNS. Risk of recurrence is as high as 90% at 15 years.[159]

Solitary Fibrous Tumor

The solitary fibrous tumor (SFT), once thought unique to the pleura, has been identified throughout the body, including in meninges.[160] The tumor may arise in cranial or spinal compartments and encroach upon brain, spinal cord, or nerves.

Grossly, these tumors are firm, tan-to-white, and usually well-circumscribed. Microscopically, they are a spindle cell tumor of variable cellularity with distinctive interspersed islands of eosinophilic collagen. The main differential diagnoses are fibroblastic meningioma and hemangiopericytoma. Immunohistochemical studies offer diagnostic help for differentiating it from meningiomas because the SFT is strongly reactive with CD34 but negative with EMA. However, as previously discussed, the differentiation between SFT and hemangiopericytoma is more problematic.[156] CD99 and Bcl-2 immunostains may be of help in this regard.

▶ TUMORS OF THE CRANIAL AND PERIPHERAL NERVES

This category includes tumors derived from supportive or stromal cells of the peripheral nerves. The tumors comprising the great majority of nerve sheath neoplasms are the *schwannoma* and the *neurofibroma*. In both cases,

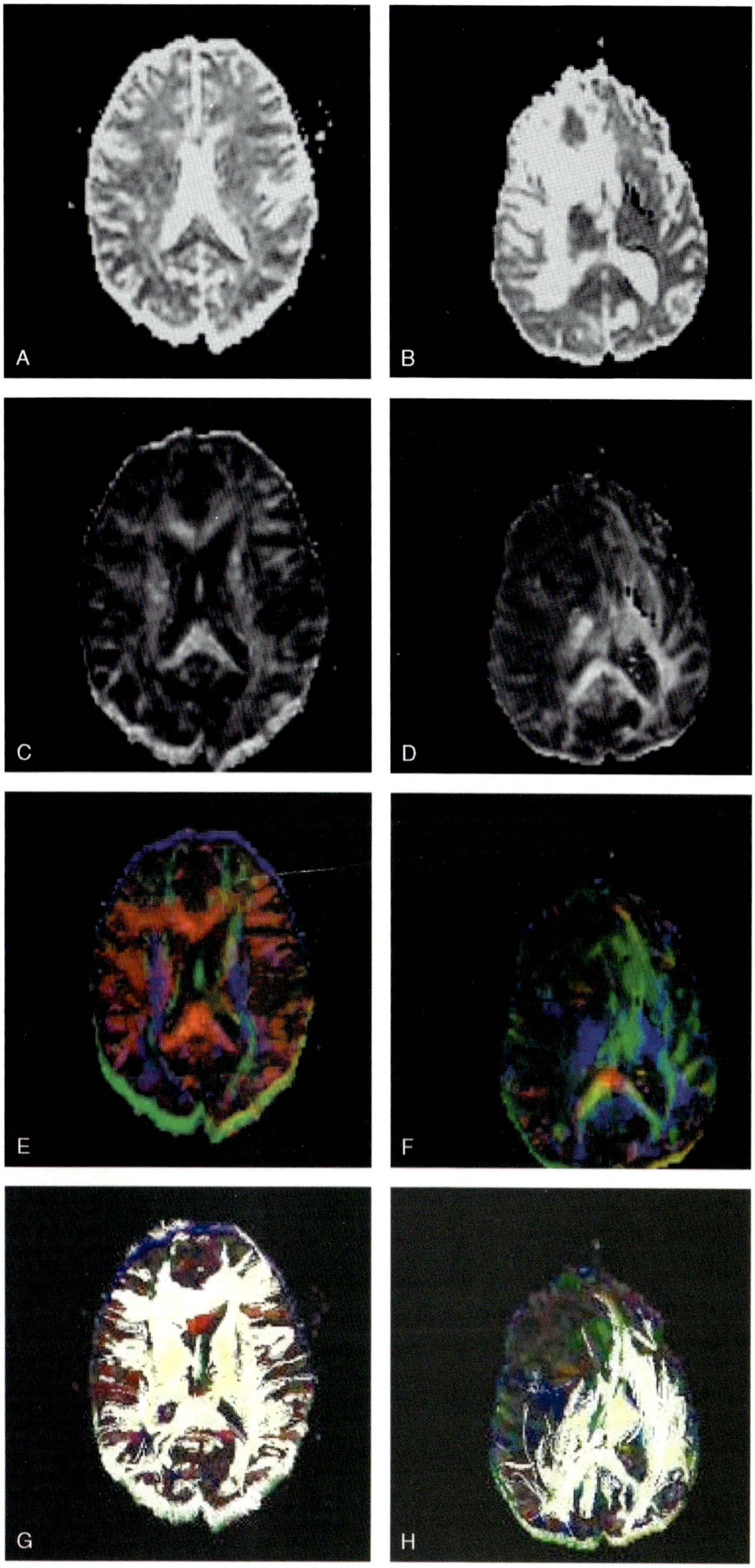

PLATE 1 (Figure 4-16). Diffusion-weighted MR of a normal volunteer (left panel) and a patient with a right frontal GBM (right panel). ADC map (A, B), FA map (C, D), DTI with color overlay (E, F), and fiber tracking on color map (G, H).

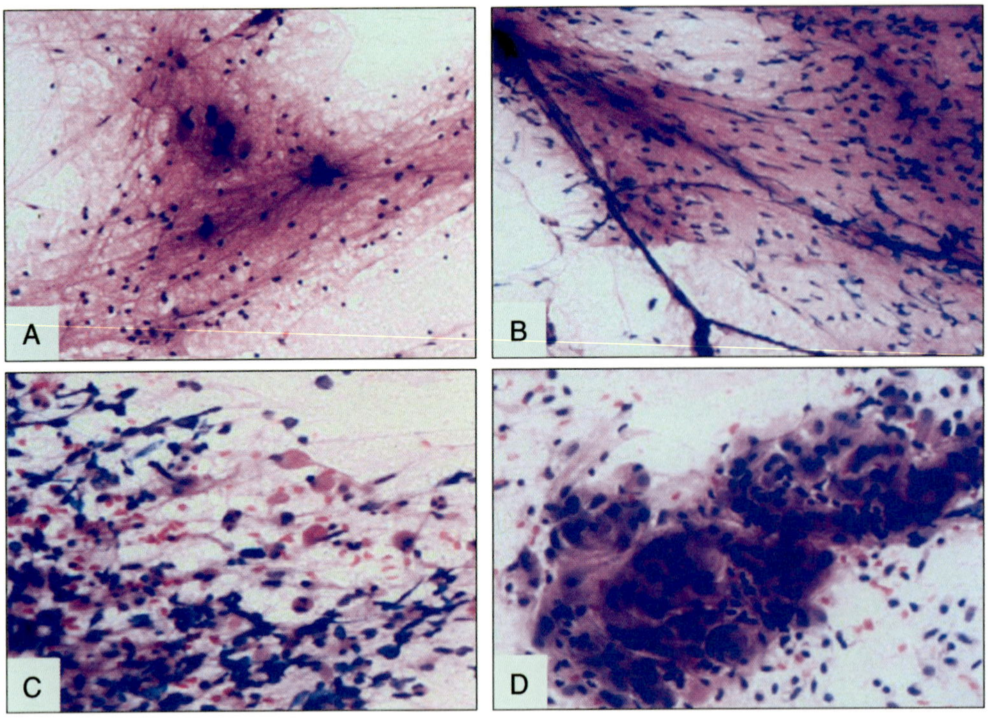

PLATE 2 (Figure 5-1). Smear preparations. (A) Smear preparation of an inflammatory process showing stellate, reactive astrocytes, edema, and mild inflammatory lymphocytic infiltration. (B) Smear preparation of a low-grade astrocytoma with cells showing fibrillary processes and mild atypia. Note the thin, delicate vessel intermixed with the cells. (C) Smear preparation of a high-grade astrocytoma composed of pleomorphic cells with variable size nuclei. Note the gemistocytic forms and the granular, necrotic background. (D) Smear preparation of a meningioma readily demonstrate typical meningothelial cells with ill-defined cytoplasmic borders. The nuclei are homogeneous. Whorl formation is prominent in this case. (A to D: Morris stain.)

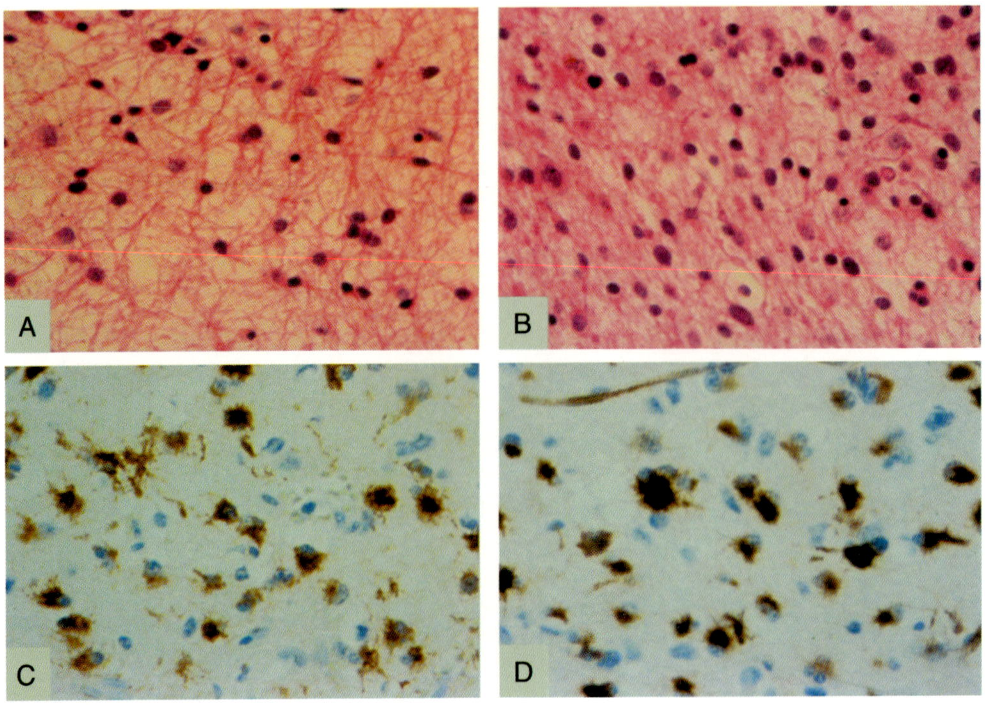

PLATE 3 (Figure 5-2). Astrocytoma grade II. (A) Astrocytoma grade II infiltrating cortex, with focal increased cellularity (B). Immunohistochemistry for GFAP (C) and vimentin (D) highlights the cellular processes of the tumor cells.

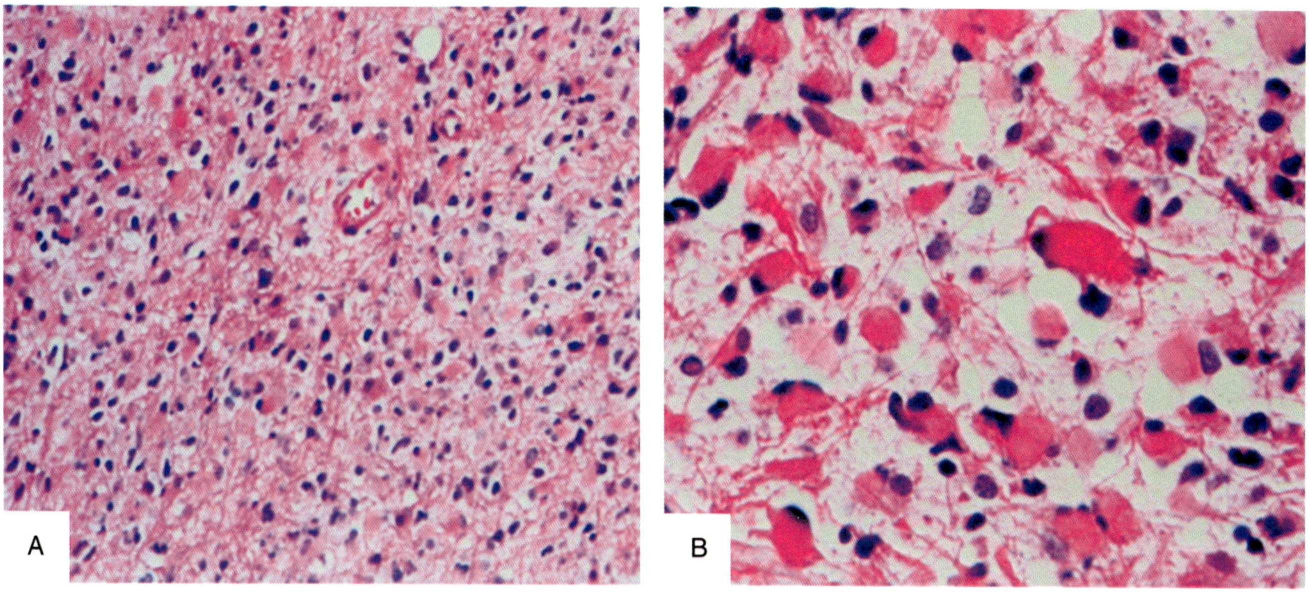

PLATE 4 (Figure 5-3). Anaplastic astrocytoma grade III. (A) Anaplastic astrocytoma with moderate cellular atypia and increased cellularity. (B) Note the large numbers of gemistocytic cells.

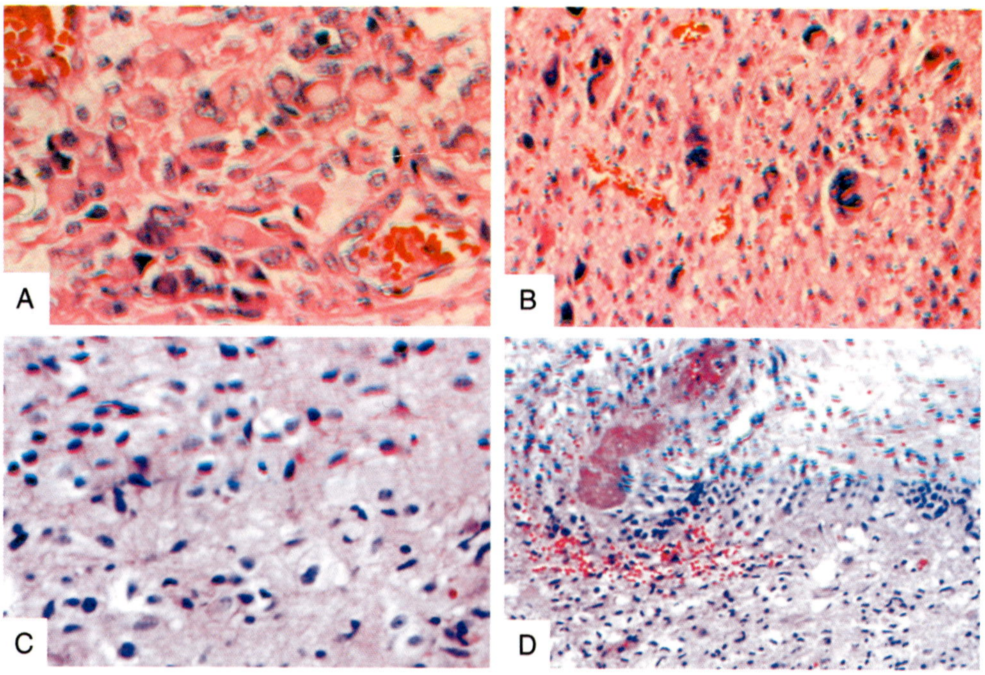

PLATE 5 Figure 5-4. Astrocytoma grade IV (glioblastoma). Glioblastomas have an abundance of cellular types and arrangements ranging from gemistocytic forms (A) to multinucleated giant cells (B) and small cells (C). Mitotic activity (C) and areas of necrosis (D) are characteristic of glioblastomas.

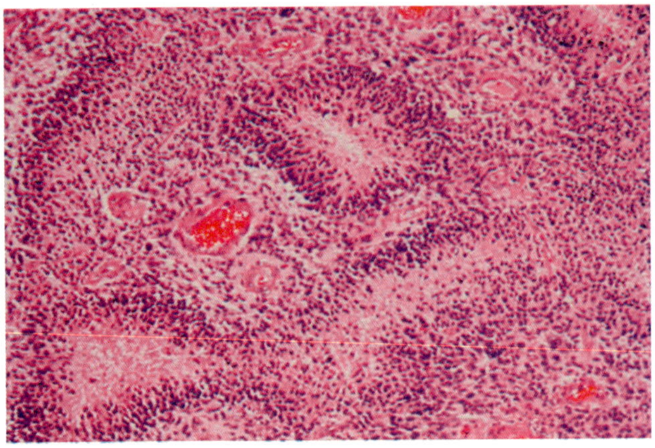

PLATE 6 (Figure 5-5). Astrocytoma grade IV (glioblastoma). Areas of necrosis, particularly with pseudopalisading arrangement of tumor cells, are common in glioblastomas.

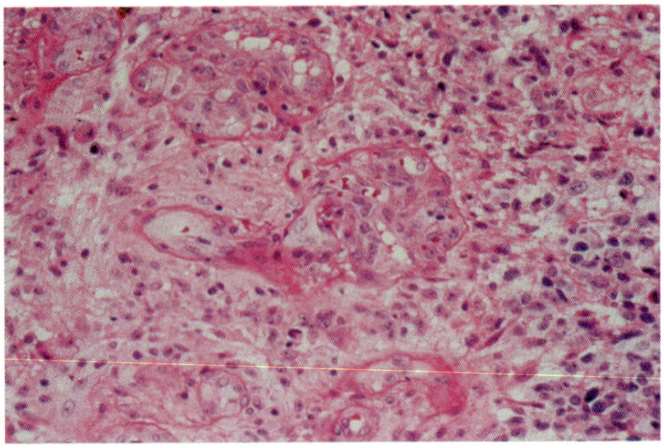

PLATE 7 (Figure 5-6). Astrocytoma grade IV (glioblastoma). Vascular endothelial proliferation is another typical feature of glioblastomas.

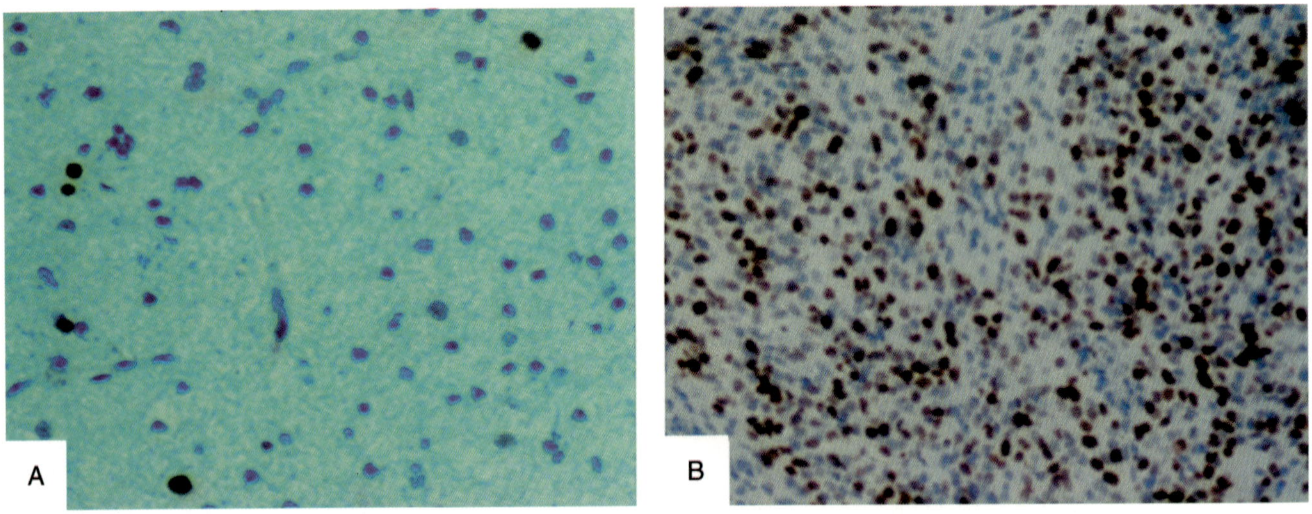

PLATE 8 (Figure 5-7). Ki-67 immunostain. Note the contrast between the Ki-67 labeling index in a grade II (A) and a grade IV astrocytoma (B).

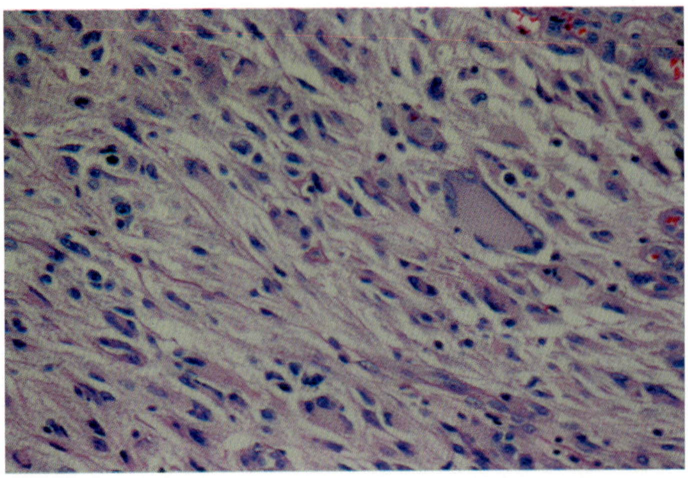

PLATE 9 (Figure 5-8). Giant cell glioblastoma (grade IV). Giant cell glioblastoma with typical multi-nucleated giant cell intermixed with smaller astrocytic cells.

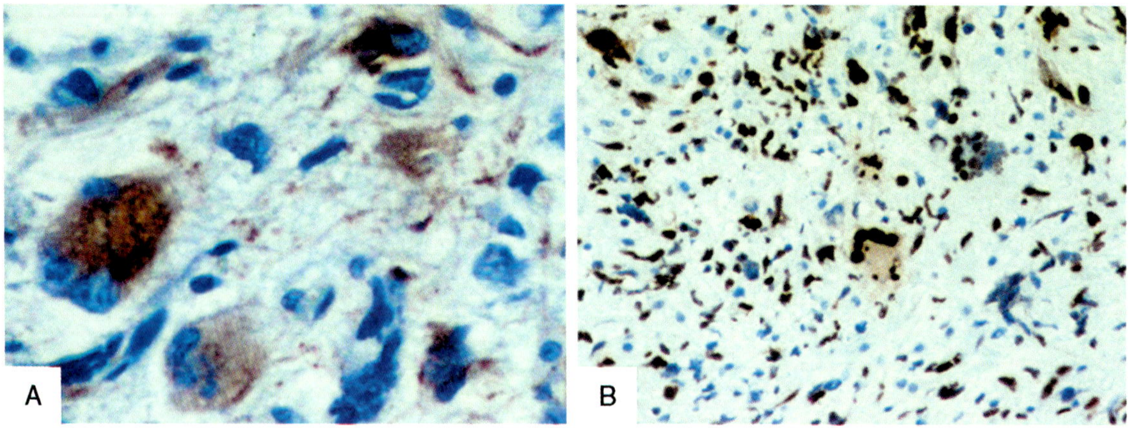

PLATE 10 (Figure 5-9). Giant cell glioblastoma (grade IV). (A) Multinucleated giant cells immunoreactive for GFAP in a giant cell glioblastoma. (B) Characteristically, this variant of glioblastoma is highly immunoreactive for p53 immunostain as a consequence of common p53 mutation seen in these tumors.

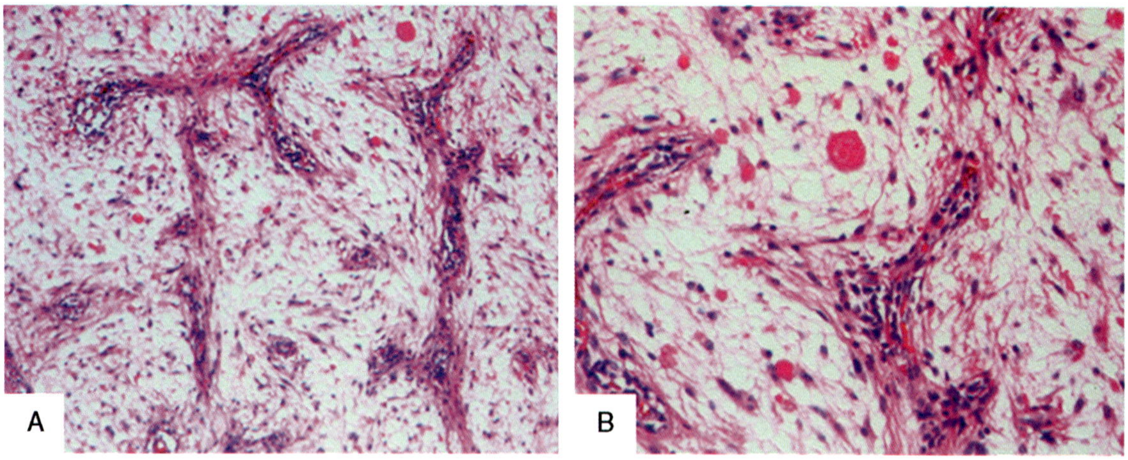

PLATE 11 (Figure 5-10). Pilocytic astrocytoma: (A) Pilocytic astrocytoma with alternating areas of dense, fibrillary cells and areas of looser stroma forming a biphasic pattern. (B) Degenerative structures, including hyaline droplets, are commonly seen in these tumors.

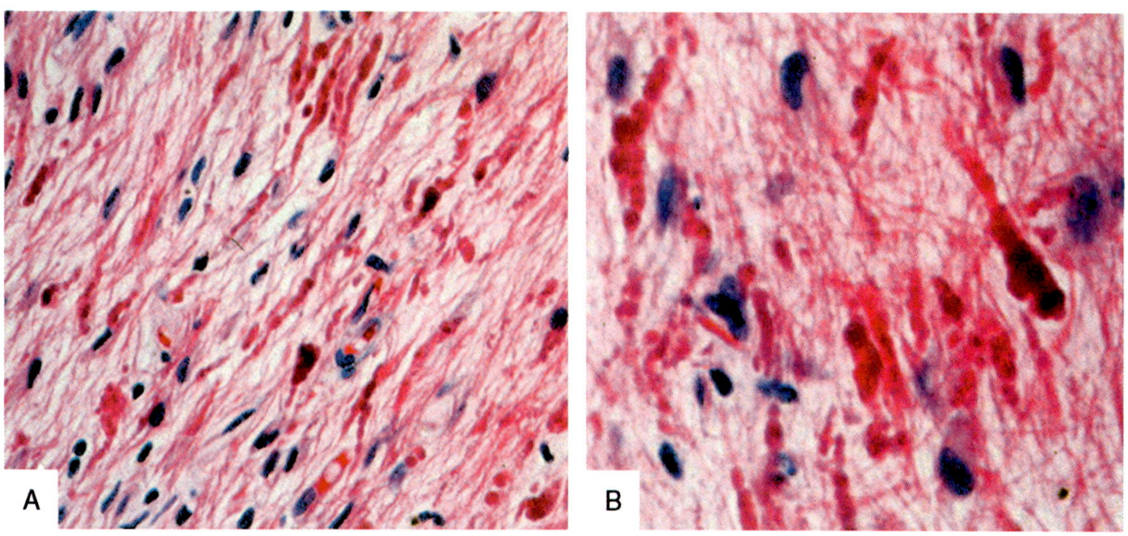

PLATE 12 (Figure 5-11). Pilocytic astrocytoma. (A and B) Dense areas of fibrillary cells with the formation of Rosenthal fibers in a pilocytic astrocytoma of the third ventricular region.

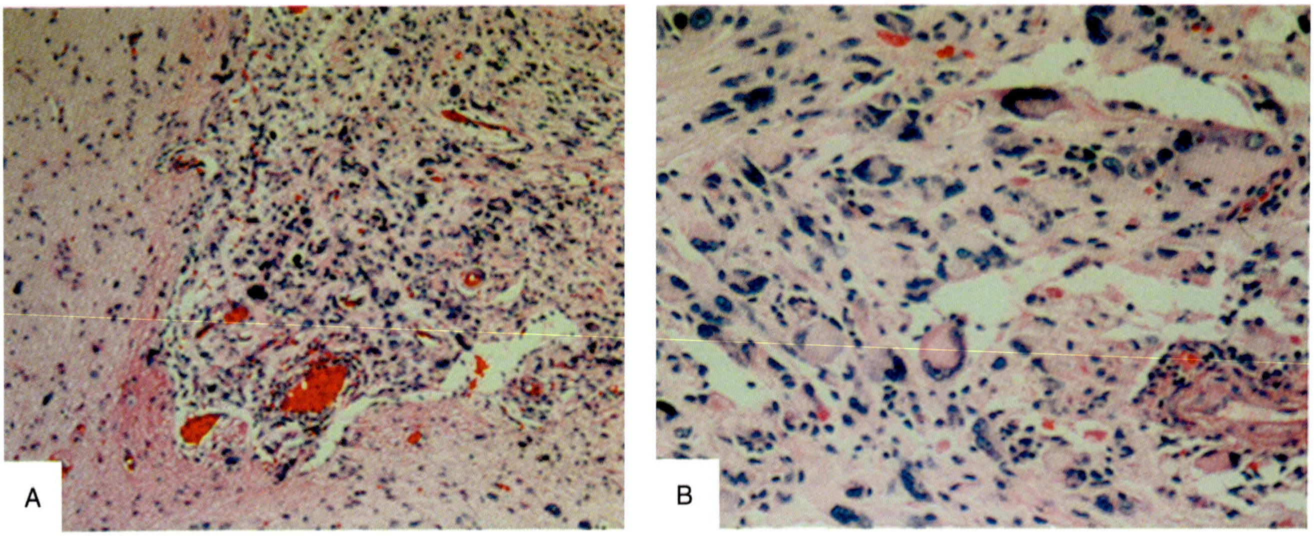

PLATE 13 (Figure 5-12). Pleomorphic xanthoastrocytoma. (A) Pleomorphic astrocytoma are superficial tumors involving the cortical ribbon with infiltration of the subpial area. (B) The tumor has a variety of cell types with large pleomorphic and xanthomatous cells.

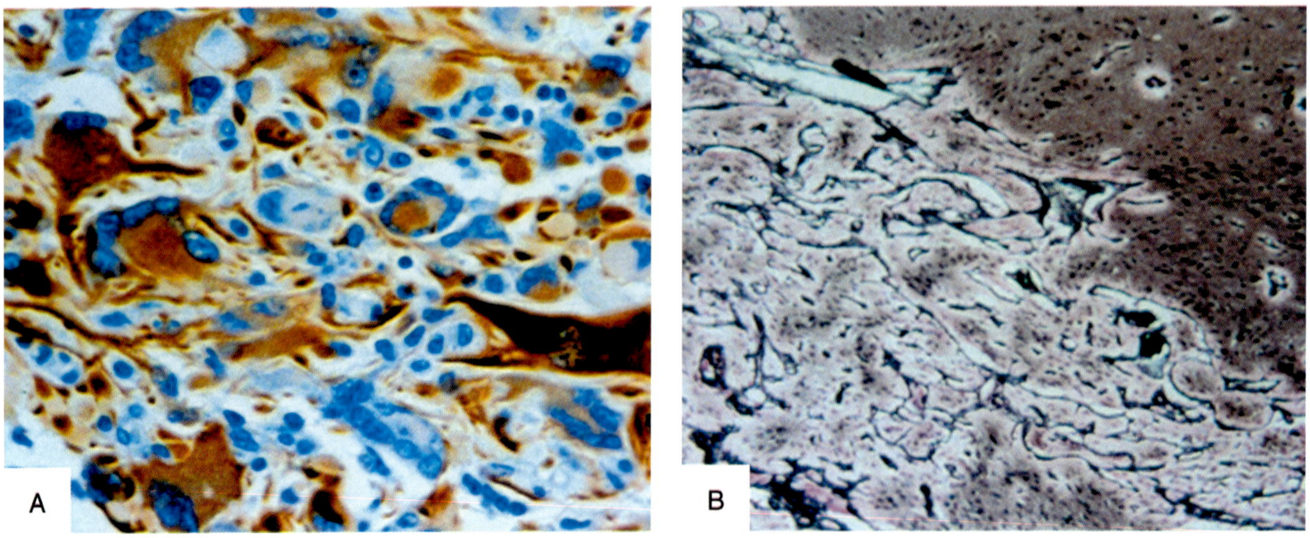

PLATE 14 (Figure 5-13). Pleomorphic xanthoastrocytoma. (A) GFAP immunoreactivity in both spindle and xanthomatous glial cells. (B) Characteristically, pleomorphic xanthoastrocytoma has a dense reticulin network mainly when infiltrating the subpial area.

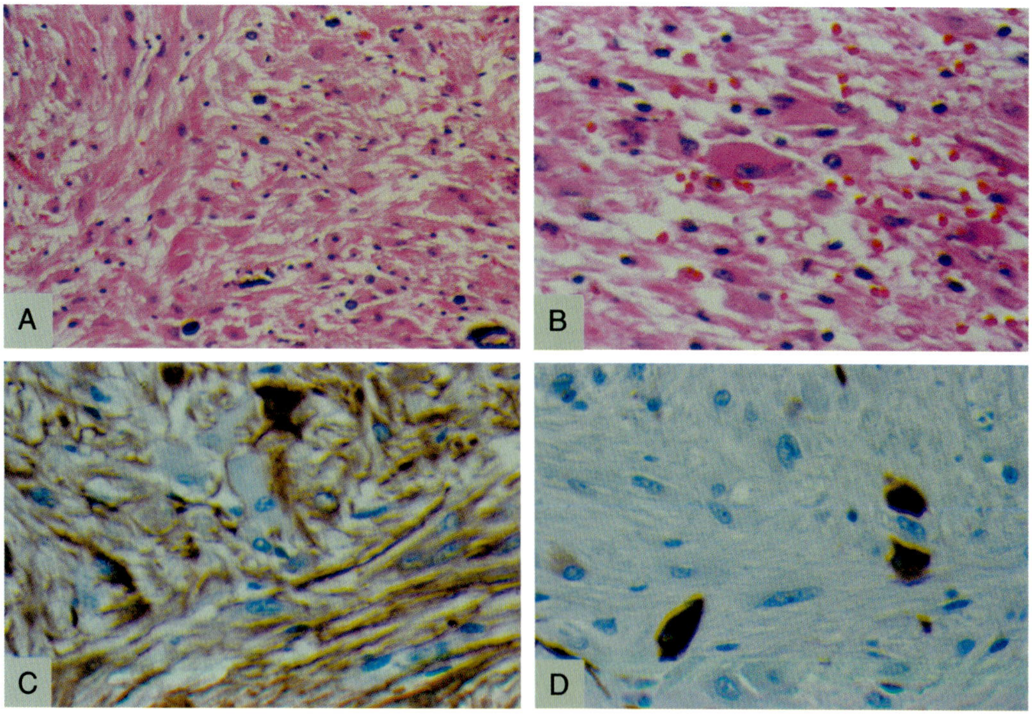

PLATE 15 (Figure 5-14). Subependymal giant cell astrocytoma (SEGA). (A and B) The SEGAs are composed of a variety of cellular elements, ranging from spindle to polygonal to ganglion-like cells (B). Giant cells in SEGAs may show glial (GFAP) (C) and/or neuronal (neurofilament) (D) markers by immunohistochemistry.

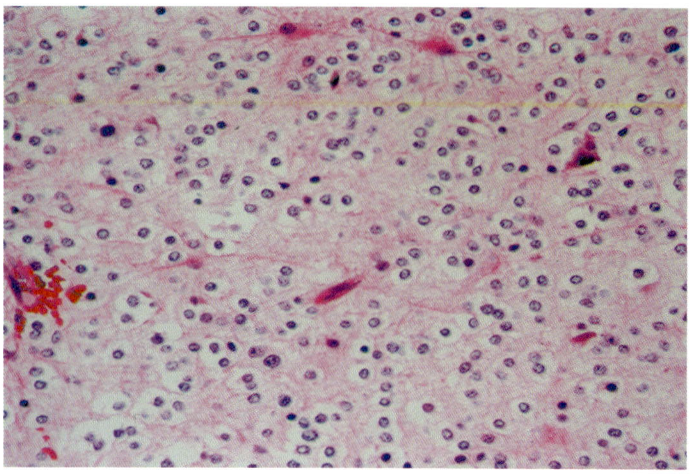

PLATE 16 (Figure 5-15). Oligodendroglioma grade II. Typical "fried egg" appearance of a low-grade oligodendroglioma.

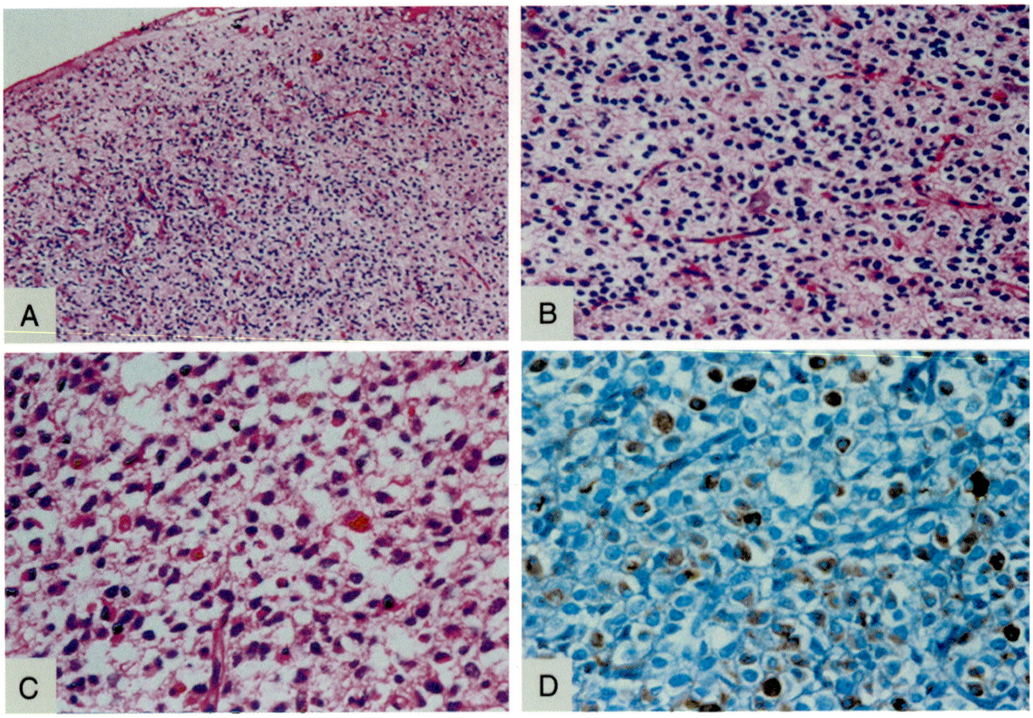

PLATE 17 (Figure 5-16). Oligodendroglioma grade II. Typical features of oligodendrogliomas include diffuse infiltration of the cortex and subpial areas (A) and perineuronal satellitosis (B). The presence of cells with a small rim of cytoplasm, the so-called minigemistocytes (C), can be easily appreciated with GFAP immunohistochemistry (D).

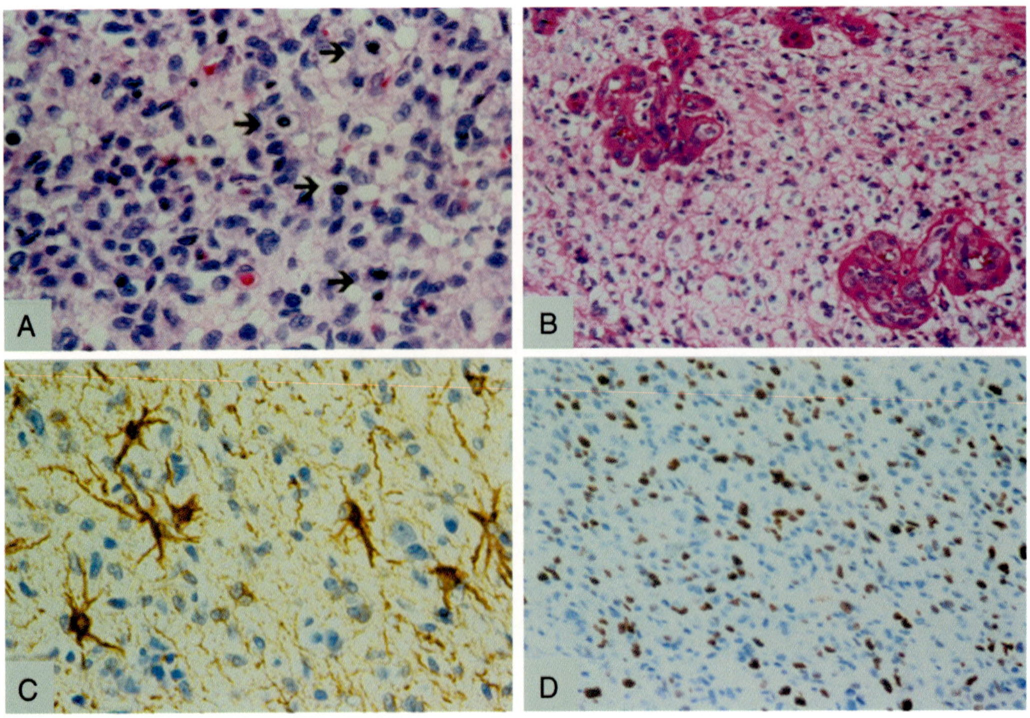

PLATE 18 (Figure 5-17). Anaplastic oligodendroglioma grade III. (A) Anaplastic oligodendrogliomas are characterized by increased cellularity and atypia in combination with areas of necrosis (not shown) and (B) microvascular endothelial proliferation. (C) G FAP immunoreaction highlights increased reactive astrocytes in malignant oligodendrogliomas with absence of immunoreaction in the tumor cells. Increased mitotic activity (A, arrows) and high Ki-67 labeling index (D) are present in anaplastic oligodendrogliomas.

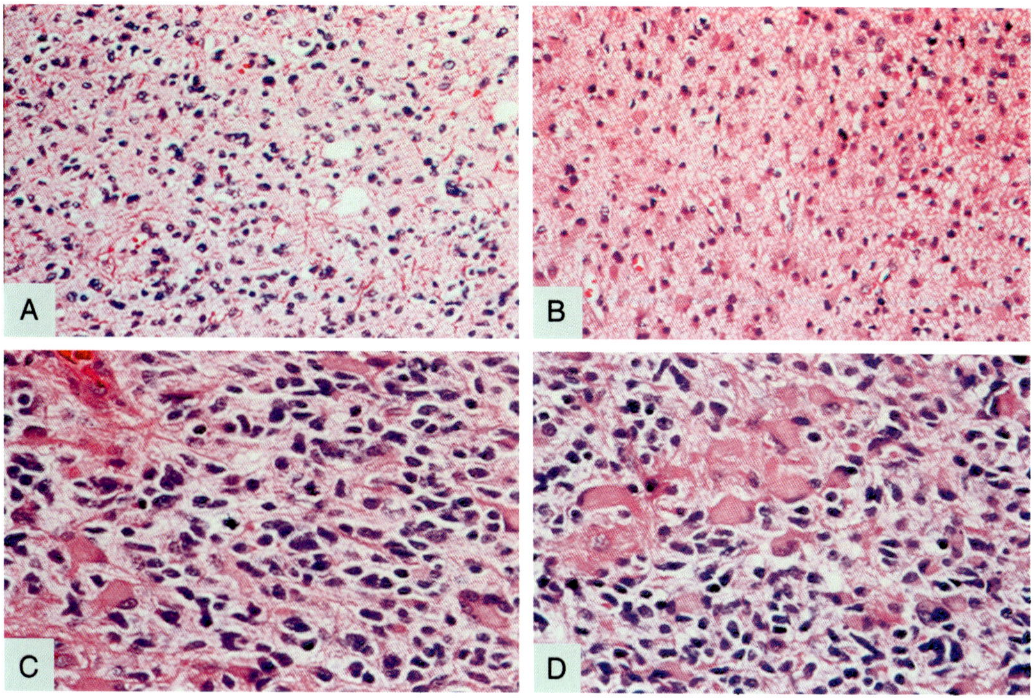

PLATE 19 (Figure 5-18). Mixed oligoastrocytoma. (A and B) Low-grade oligoastrocytoma (grade II) with a mixed population of oligodendroglial- and astrocytic-like cells. (C and D) In high-grade tumors (anaplastic oligoastrocytoma grade III), increased cellular atypia and gemistocytic forms may be seen.

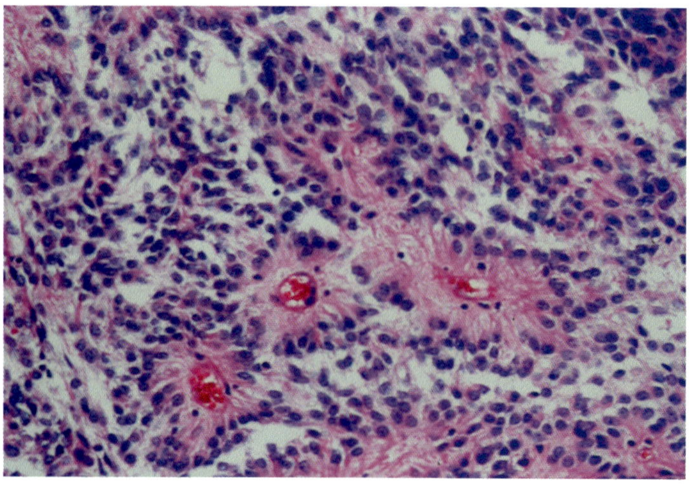

PLATE 20 (Figure 5-19). Ependymoma. Typical pseudo-rosetting formation in a spinal cord ependymoma.

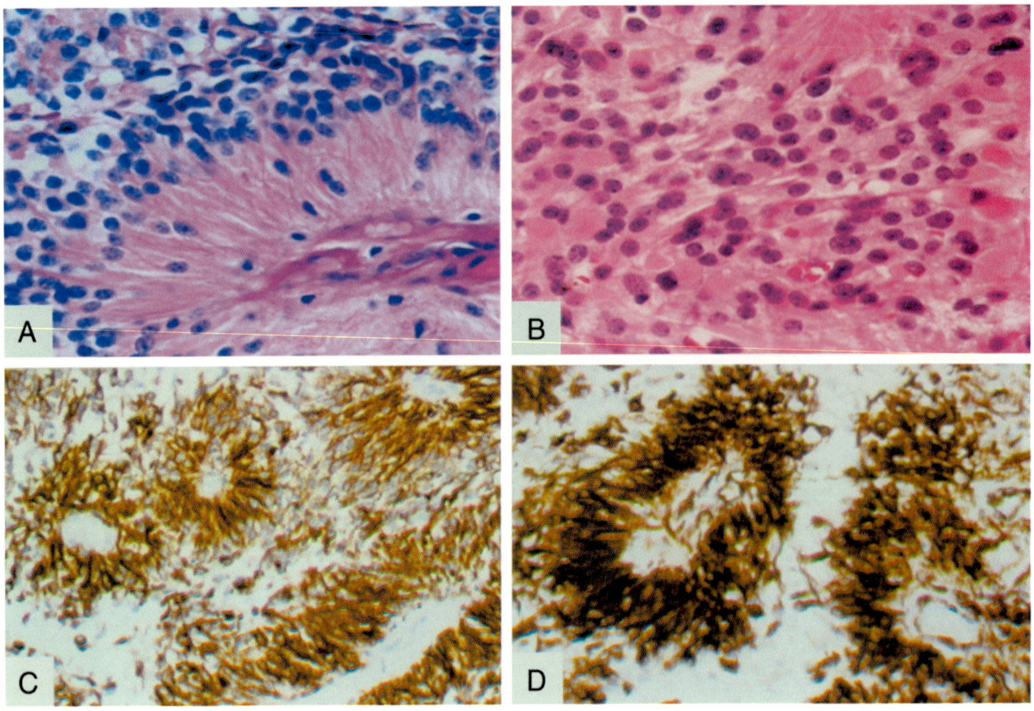

PLATE 21 (Figure 5-20). Ependymoma. (A) Fibrillary cellular processes in a high-power view of a pseudorosette. The ependymoma cells are typically characterized by a homogeneous distribution of the nuclear chromatin (B). Immunohistochemical stains for GFAP (C) and vimentin (D) emphasize the dense fibrillary processes of ependymoma cells.

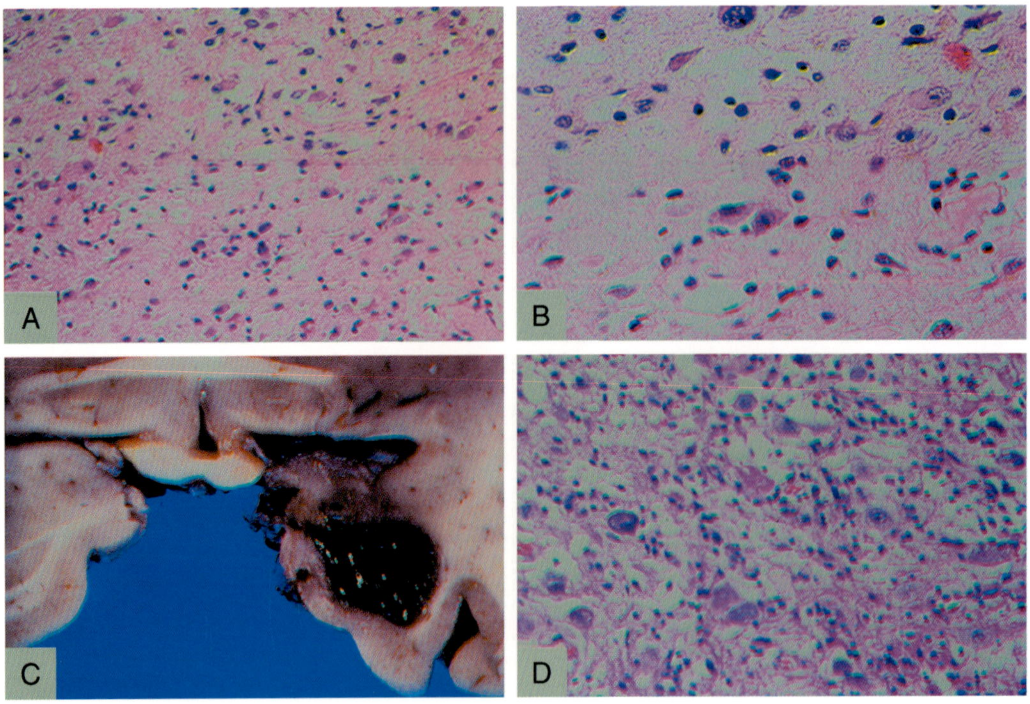

PLATE 22 (Figure 5-21). Neuronal and mixed neuronal-glial tumors. (A and B) Gangliocytomas are characteristically hypocellular and composed of ganglion-like cells. In contrast, gangliogliomas have a mixture of glial and neuronal cells (D). The formation of cysts is a common feature of gangliogliomas (C).

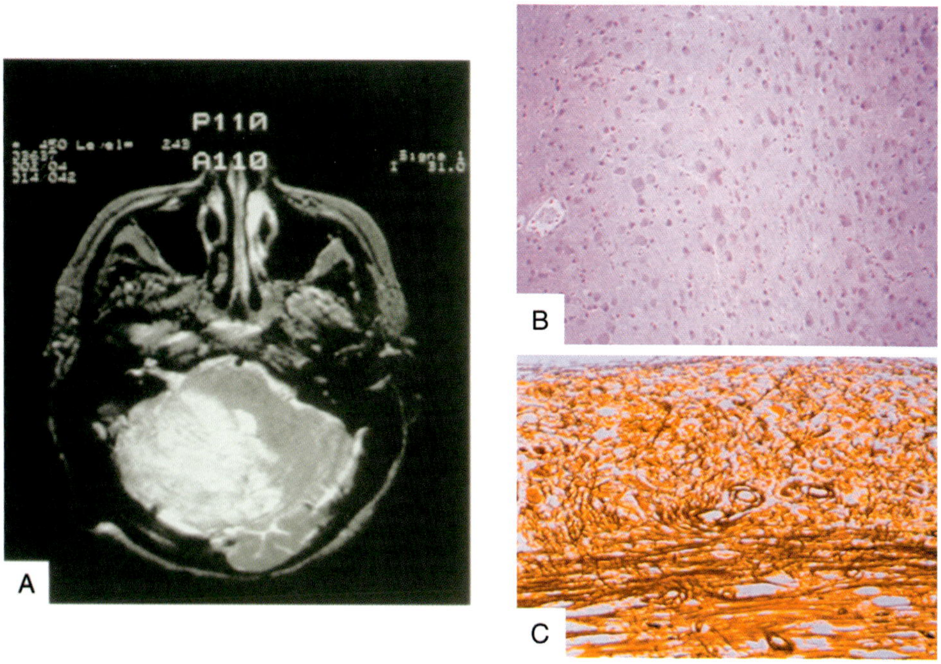

PLATE 23 (Figure 5-22). Dysplastic gangliocytoma of the cerebellum: (A) A magnetic resonance imaging (MRI) scan of a case of dysplastic gangliocytoma of the cerebellum showing the enlarged cerebellar folia and hemispheric hypertrophy. Large ganglionic cells resembling Purkinje cells (B) and abnormally shaped and thick neuritic process (Bielschowsky silver) (C) histologically characterize the tumor.

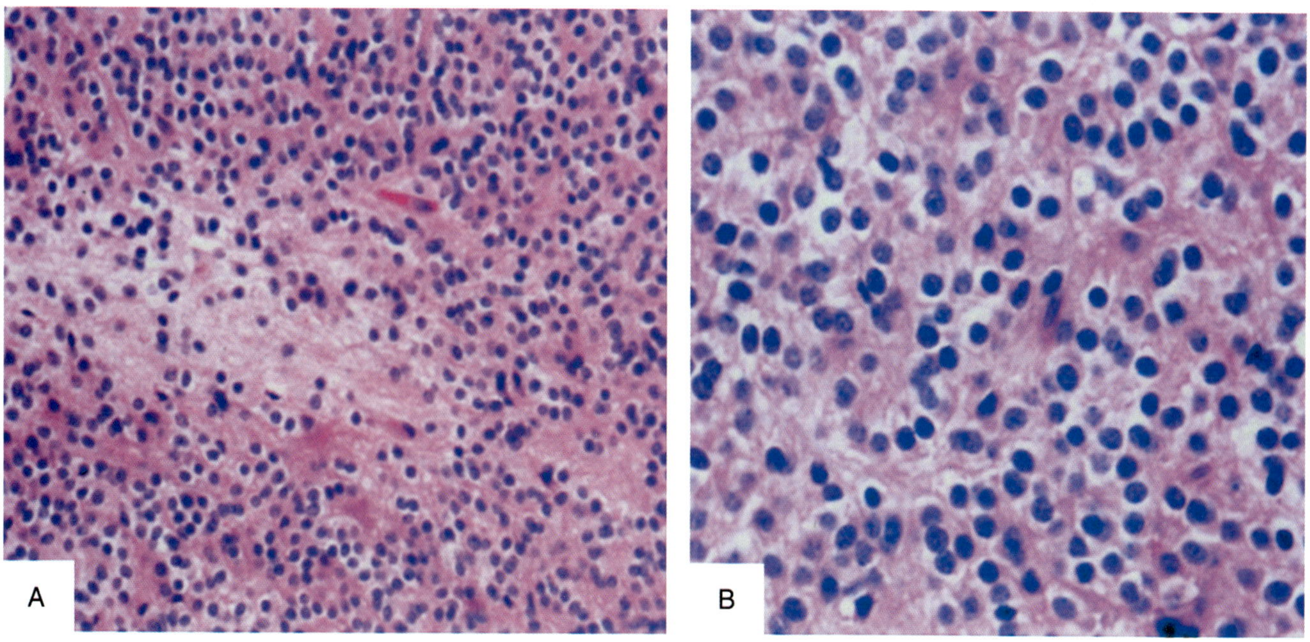

PLATE 24 (Figure 5-23). Central neurocytoma. (A and B) The appearance of central neurocytomas typically consists of a homogeneous population of cells with oval to round nuclei that resemble oligodendrogliomas.

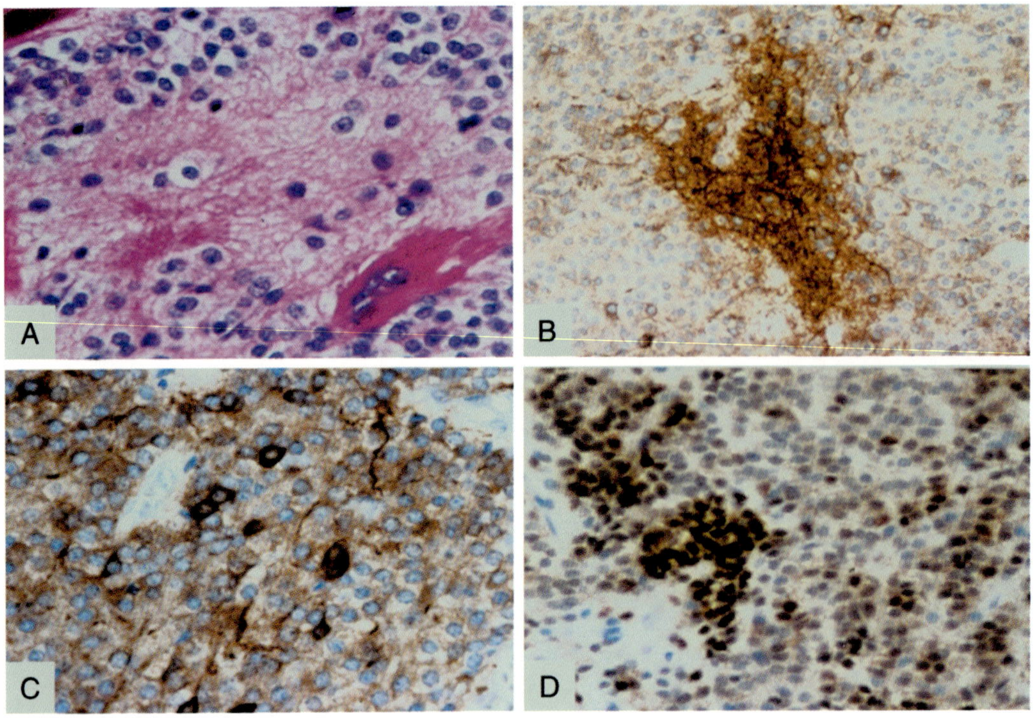

PLATE 25 (Figure 5-24). Central neurocytoma. Close examination of central neurocytoma demonstrates anuclear, neuropil-like areas (A) that are strongly immunoreactive for neuronal markers (B) (synaptophysin). Individual or group of tumor cells show immunoreactivity for neuronal-associated markers MAP2 (C) and NeuN (D).

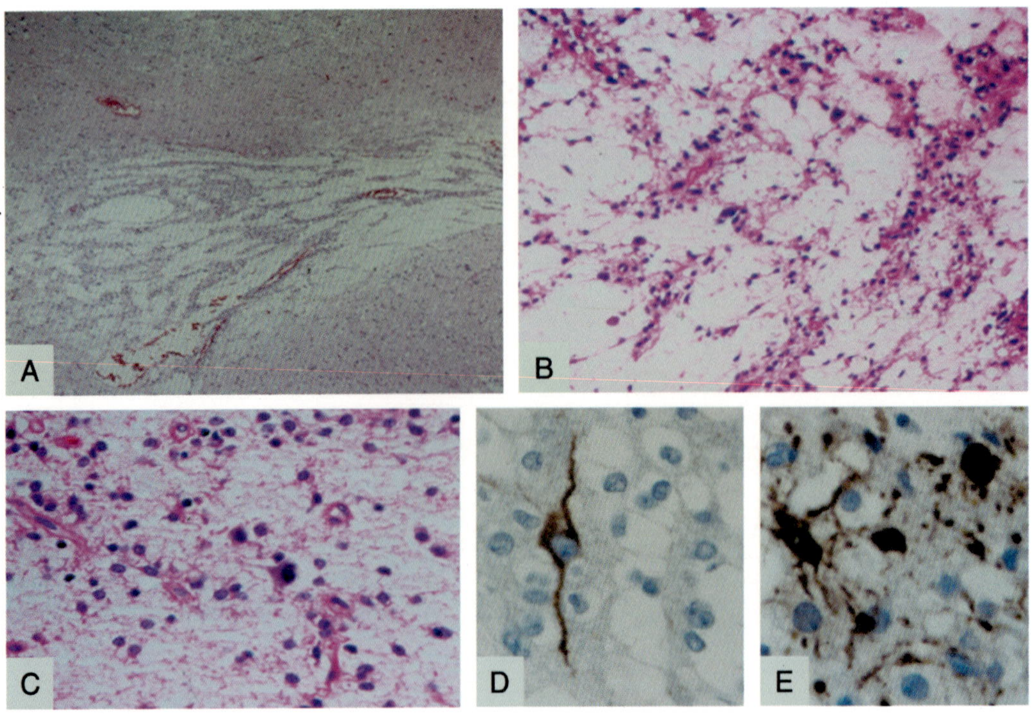

PLATE 26 (Figure 5-25). Dysembryoplastic neuroepithelial tumor (DNT). An example of DNT at low magnification shows a mildly cellular neoplasm with microcystic changes (A). The mixed cellular elements of DNT are composed of oligodendroglial-like cells, astrocytes, and neurons in variable proportions (B to C). Floating neurons are typically seen in these areas (D) (neurofilament), intermixed with other glial cells (E) (GFAP).

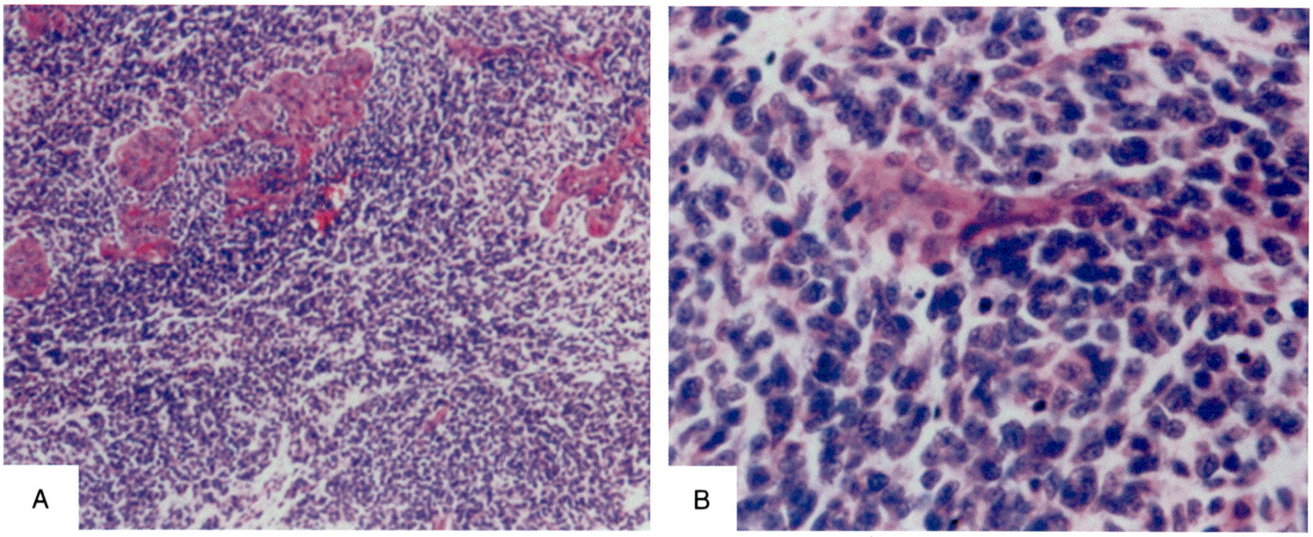

PLATE 27 (Figure 5-26). Medulloblastoma (classical variant). (A and B) Medulloblastomas are densely cellular tumors composed of closely packed primitive cells. (B) High mitotic activity and apoptotic figures are commonly seen.

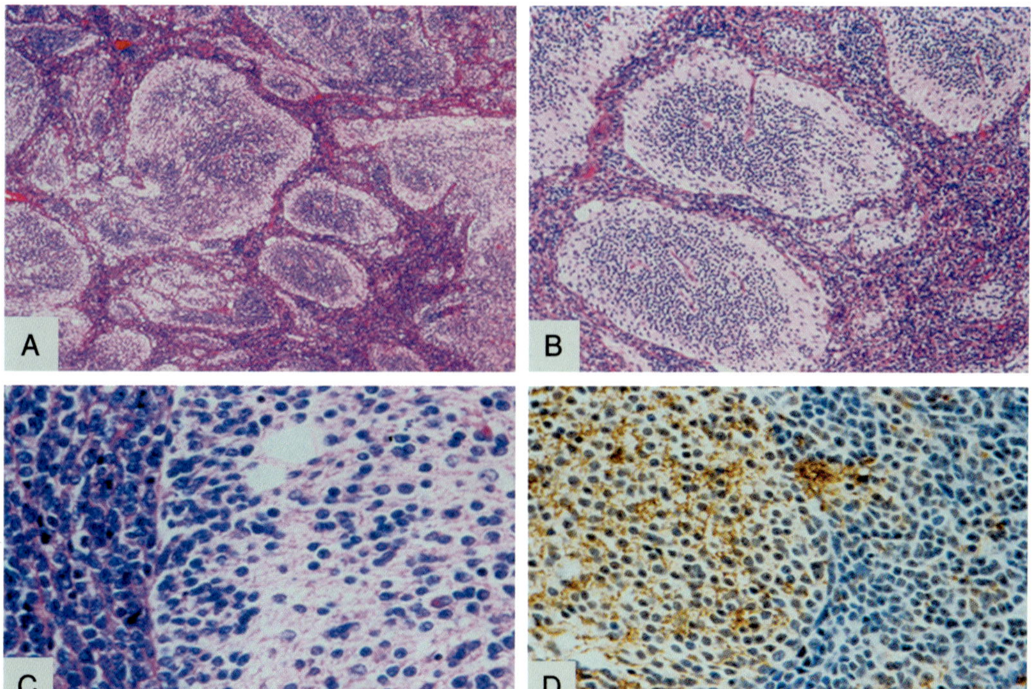

PLATE 28 (Figure 5-27). Medulloblastoma (desmoplastic variant). (A and B) The desmoplastic or nodular variant of medulloblastoma is characterized by a lobular appearance with hypercellular areas alternating with less cellular nodules. The nodules are reticulin free (not shown), and show more differentiated cells (C) and neuronal differentiation by immunohistochemistry (D) (neurofilament).

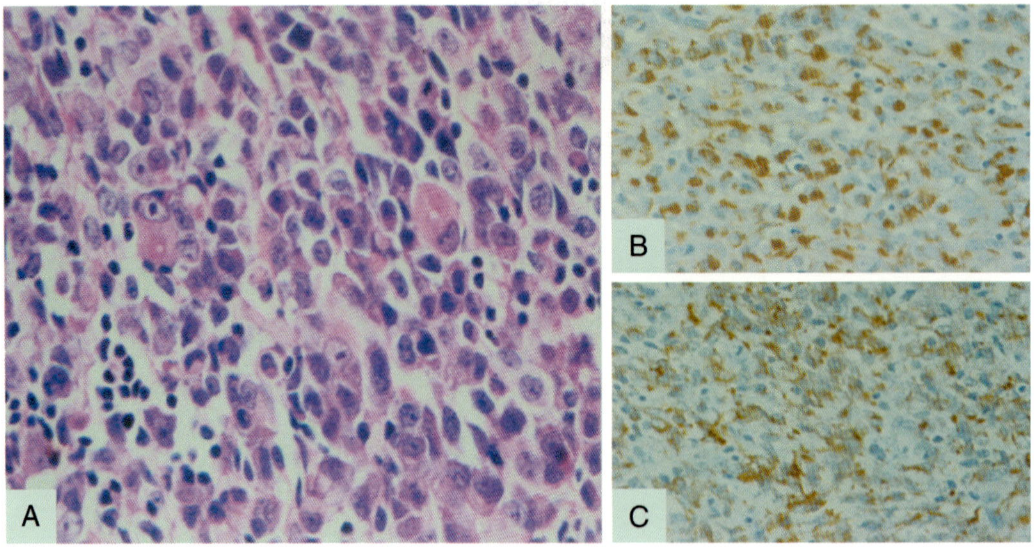

PLATE 29 (Figure 5-28). Atypical teratoid/rhabdoid tumor. (A) The abundant eosinophilic cytoplasm of the tumor cells gives the rhabdoid appearance to the tumor. Immunohistochemistry for vimentin (B) highlights the cytoplasmic inclusions, while focal reactivity may also be seen for neuronal markers (C) (neurofilament).

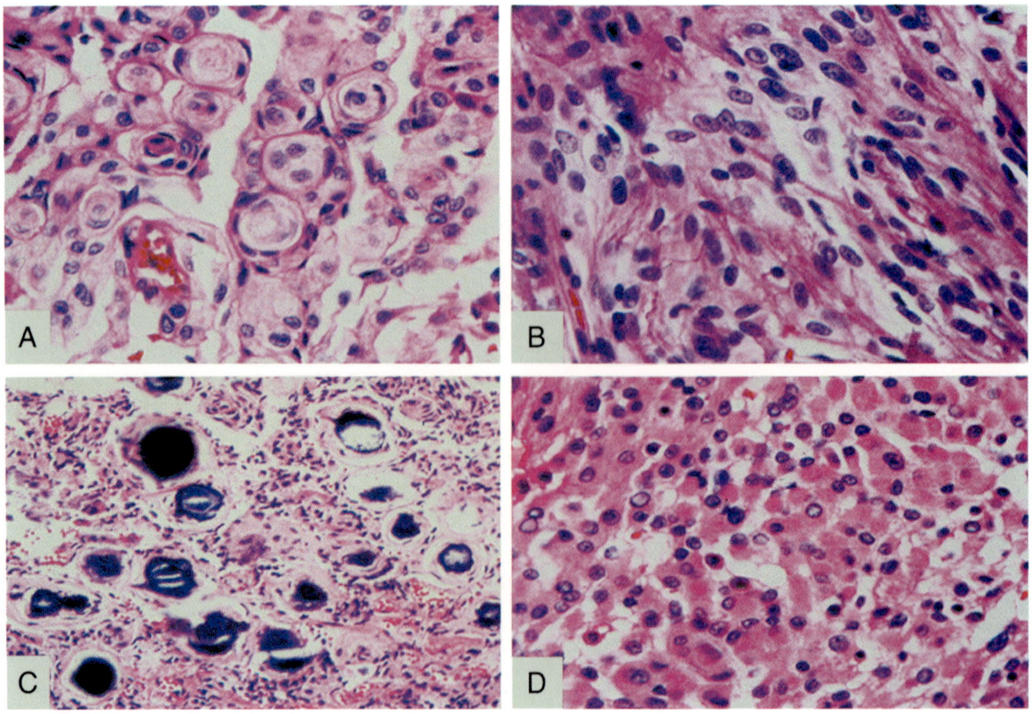

PLATE 30 (Figure 5-29). Meningioma. Meningiomas may present a variety of tissue arrangements, including meningothelial (A), fibroblastic (B), psammomatous (C), and rhabdoid (D).

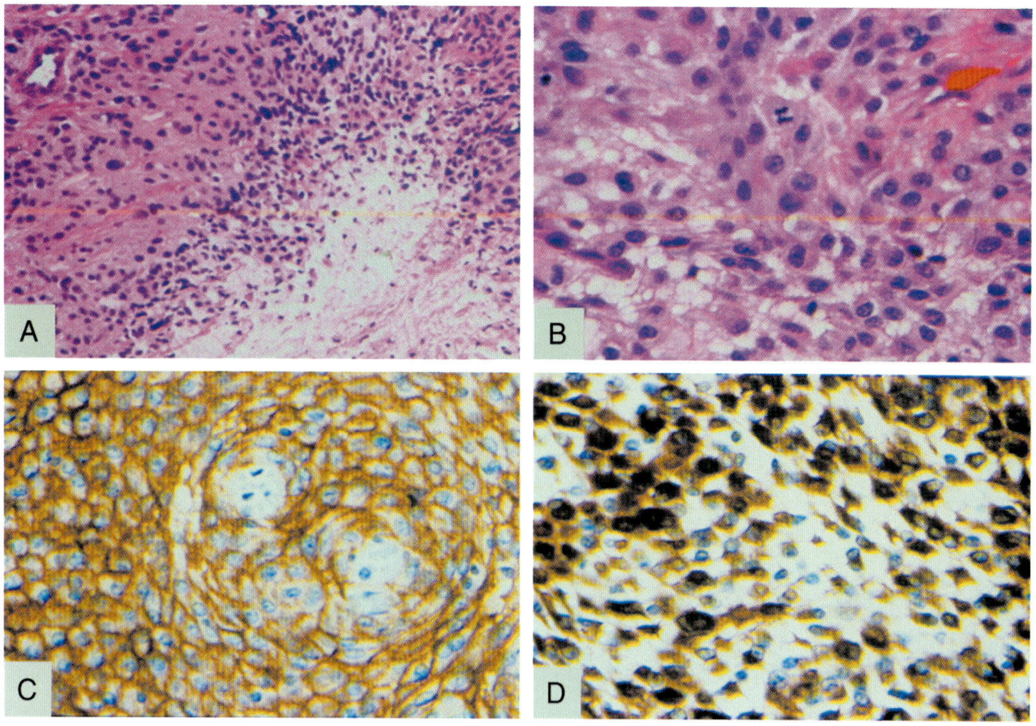

PLATE 31 (Figure 5-30). Anaplastic meningioma. Areas of necrosis (A) and high mitotic activity (B) are some of the features of anaplastic meningiomas. The characteristic immunohistochemical profile of all malignancy grades of meningiomas includes strong EMA (C) and vimentin (D) positivity.

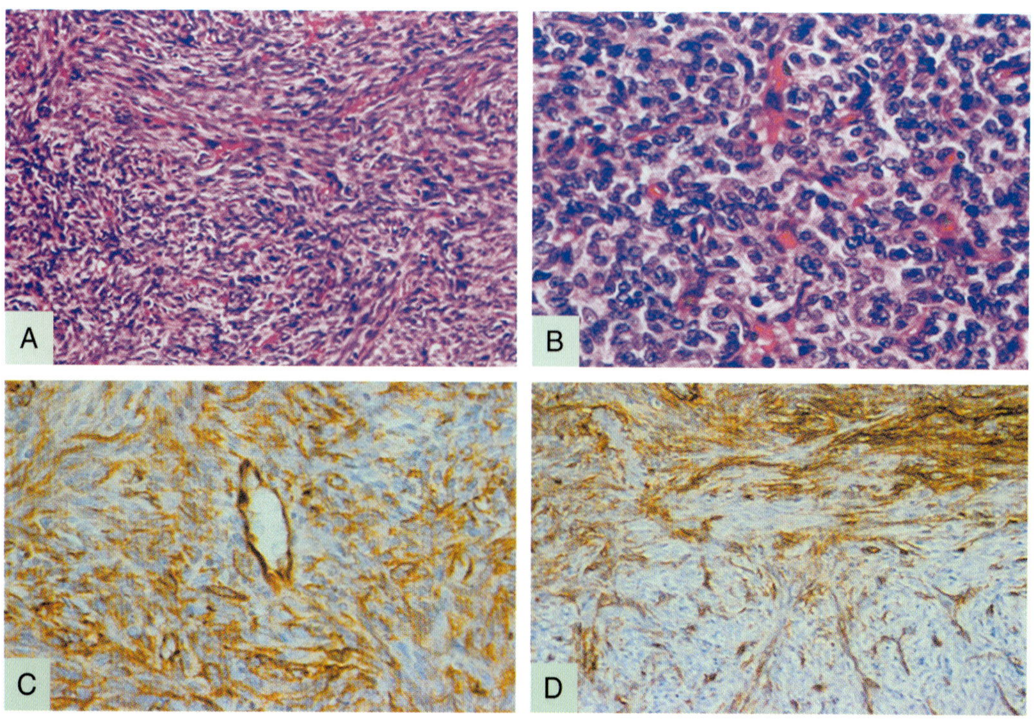

PLATE 32 (Figure 5-31). Hemangiopericytoma. Histologic appearance of hemangiopericytomas includes high cellularity, spindle to plump cells, and a rich vascular network (A and B). The vascular channels of the tumor may be highlighted by immunohistochemistry for mesenchymal markers including CD34 (C) and CD99 (D).

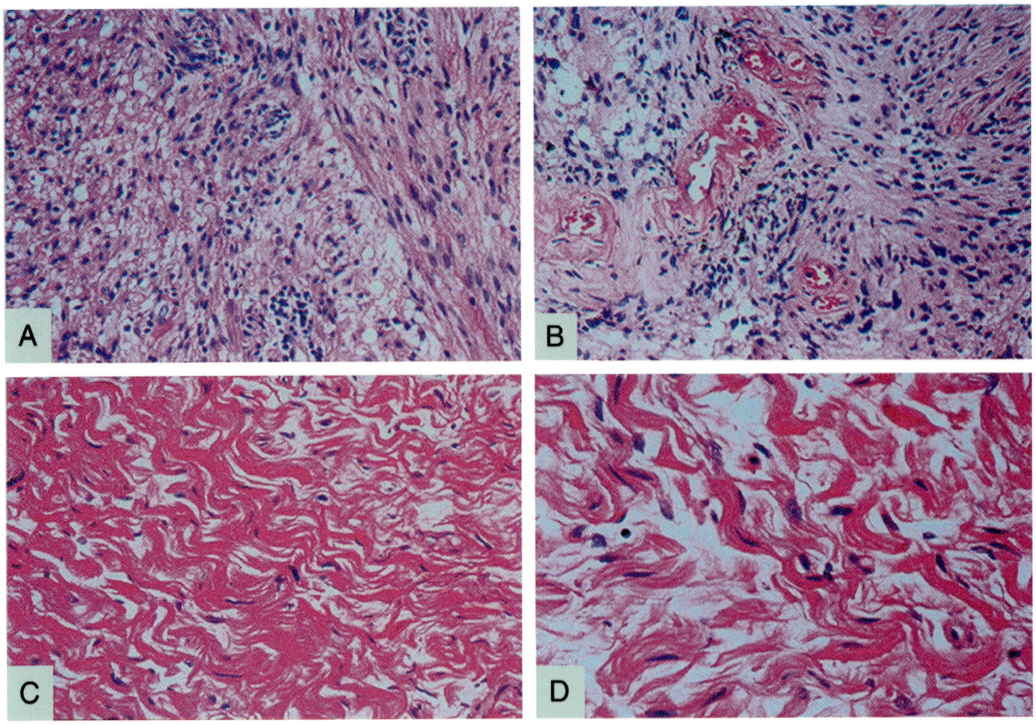

PLATE 33 (Figure 5-32). Peripheral nerve sheath tumors: (A) Schwannomas are typically characterized by alternating hypercellular areas (Antoni A) and looser areas (Antoni B) of spindle-shaped cells. (B) Focal areas of old hemorrhage and blood vessels with hyalinized walls are commonly seen. (C) Neurofibromas are composed of a mix of cellular types including Schwann cells. (D) A myxoid stroma is also a typical feature of these tumors.

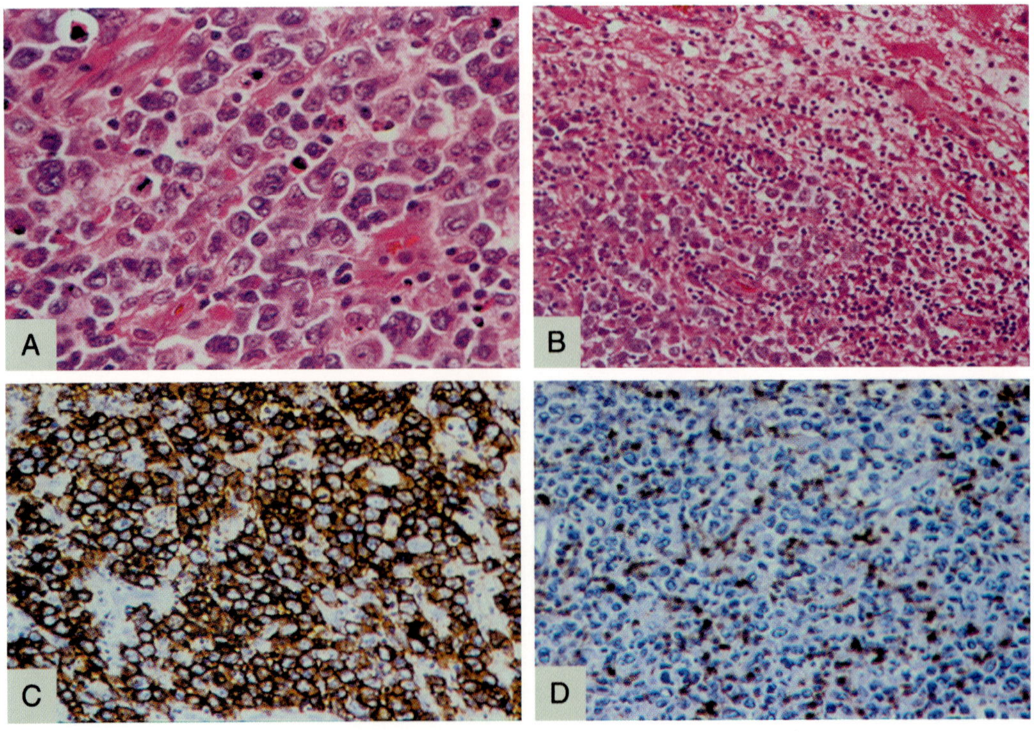

PLATE 34 (Figure 5-33). Primary CNS lymphoma. (A) High-grade large cell lymphomas are most commonly seen in the brain. (B) Diffusely infiltrating pattern is seen along with a more angiocentric infiltration of the tumor cells. B-cell markers (CD79a) (C) highlight the malignant large cell component, whereas small reactive T cells (CD3) (D) commonly infiltrate the neoplasm.

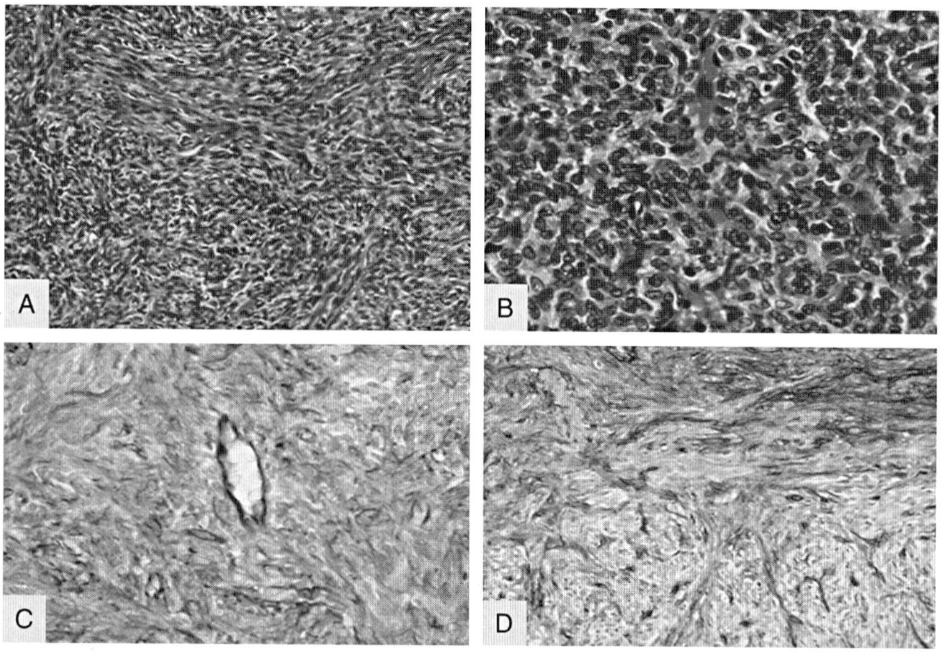

Figure 5-31 (PLATE 32). Hemangiopericytoma. Histologic appearance of hemangiopericytomas includes high cellularity, spindle to plump cells, and a rich vascular network (A and B). The vascular channels of the tumor may be highlighted by immunohistochemistry for mesenchymal markers including CD34 (C) and CD99 (D).

Schwann cells constitute their primary cell component. In schwannomas, Schwann cells are the exclusive cellular constituent, whereas in neurofibromas, perineurial cells and fibroblasts are also part of the tumoral proliferation. Both tumors exhibit distinct growth patterns and histologic features.

Schwannomas and neurofibromas occur either sporadically or as part of both NF1 and NF2. Bilateral acoustic schwannomas are characteristic of NF2. In NF1, neurofibromas are the principal lesions. These affect peripheral nerves and are far more common than schwannomas. Nerve sheath tumors account for almost 8% of all primary brain and nervous tissue tumor.[4]

Schwannoma

Schwannomas (WHO grade I) tend to be solitary masses arising more frequently from cranial and spinal nerve roots than from peripheral nerves. The intracranial schwannoma comprises approximately 8% of all primary intracranial tumors,[161] and approximately 80% of them arise from the vestibular division of the acoustic nerve.[162] Spinal schwannomas arise most frequently from sensory nerve roots, but motor and autonomic nerves may also be involved. Schwannomas rarely are intraparenchymal within the cerebrum, brainstem, cerebellum, or spinal cord.[163,164] Tumors most commonly are found in females in the age 40 to 50 years range and are solitary in 95% of cases.[162]

Schwannomas are lobular, often spherical tumors with a golden yellow hue, the result of frequent hemorrhage. Histologically, the tumors are composed of spindle-shaped cells alternating in two characteristic histologic arrangements: the cellular or compact Antoni A and the loosely cohesive Antoni B patterns (Fig. 5-32). Other diagnostic features include elongated tumor cells arranged in parallel nuclear arrays (the so-called Verocay bodies) and frequent foci of degeneration including large atypical nuclei, hemorrhage, hemosiderin-laden macrophages, hyalinized blood vessels, and foamy histiocytes.

Immunohistochemical features include strong reactivity for S100 with both cytoplasmic and nuclear expression. Leu-7, CD34, and vimentin are also consistently reactive. GFAP, especially the polyclonal antibodies, may react and create diagnostic confusion.

An important variant, the cellular schwannoma, consists exclusively of the Antoni A cellular pattern accompanied by nuclear pleomorphism and increased mitotic activity (as high as 2–4/10 HPF). Despite these histologic features suggestive of anaplasia and the increased mitotic rate, this tumor behaves in a benign fashion.[161]

Neurofibroma

The neurofibroma (WHO grade I) is a complex mixture of Schwann cells, fibroblasts, and perineurial cells that expands a diffuse segment of nerve; in contrast, the circumscribed schwannoma arises from, but displaces,

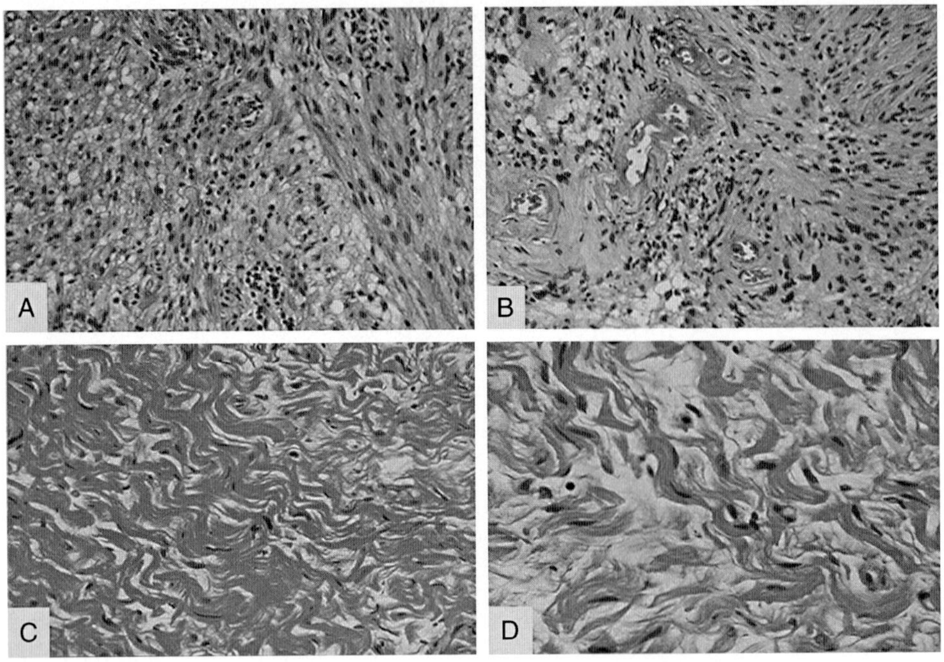

Figure 5-32 (PLATE 33). Peripheral nerve sheath tumors: (A) Schwannomas are typically characterized by alternating hypercellular areas (Antoni A) and looser areas (Antoni B) of spindle-shaped cells. (B) Focal areas of old hemorrhage and blood vessels with hyalinized walls are commonly seen. (C) Neurofibromas are composed of a mix of cellular types including Schwann cells. (D) A myxoid stroma is also a typical feature of these tumors.

nerve. Neurofibromas chiefly arise in the spine and peripheral nerves, whereas intracranial neurofibromas are very uncommon. Neurofibromas are classically multiple and usually involve major peripheral nerves or their branches (plexiform neurofibromas). Neurofibromas are also largely cutaneous tumors. Intraspinal neurofibromas arise from dorsal sensory nerve roots and are most frequently associated with NF1.[165]

Neurofibromas display a uniform array of delicately waving Schwann cells with comma-shaped nuclei intermixed with perineurial-like cells and fibroblasts within a frequently myxoid background matrix (see Fig. 5-32). Immunohistochemical reactivity with S100 is present, but less pronounced than in schwannoma. EMA reactivity may be focally present as a consequence of the presence of perineurial cells within the tumor. CD34 is also present, especially in more myxoid sites. Although mitotic activity of mild-to-moderate degree is of only minor prognostic concern in schwannomas, even mild mitotic activity in a neurofibroma (1–2/10 HPF) is cause for concern and when coupled with hypercellularity and nuclear atypia is grounds for a diagnosis of malignancy.

Malignant Peripheral Nerve Sheath Tumor

Malignant peripheral nerve sheath tumors (MPNSTs) (WHO grade III or IV) are, in almost all cases, malignant counterparts of neurofibromas. Anaplastic transformation of schwannomas is an extremely rare event.[166] Although MPNST may occur *de novo*, in the majority of tumors a coexisting neurofibroma can be demonstrated.[167] The overall incidence of MPNST in the general population is very low (approximately 0.001%); however, it is higher among patients with NF1 (4.6%). MPNSTs occur mainly in adults and are slightly more frequent in females. Radiation-induced tumors have been reported in both patients with and without NF1.[168] Intracranial examples of such malignant tumors are rare with the trigeminal (fifth) and the eighth cranial nerves most commonly involved.[167]

Histologically, MPNSTs show features of a spindle cell sarcoma, resembling fibrosarcoma, with fascicles of hyperchromatic spindle cells with elongate nuclei. Most tumors have a diffuse growth pattern, but arrangements resembling hemangiopericytoma or malignant fibrous histiocytomas may be seen. Increased mitotic activity (≥ 4/10 HPF) and areas of geographic necrosis are commonly present. MPNST cases may show unusual histologic features such as epithelioid morphology and divergent differentiation.[169]

Molecular Genetics of Schwannomas and Neurofibromas

Deletion or mutation of selected loci on chromosome 22q, coinciding with the *NF2* gene, is characteristic of schwannoma. The *NF2* gene codes for merlin, a protein that may participate in cellular remodeling and growth regulation. The gene mutation is germ line in *NF2* and the deletion is somatic in sporadic schwannoma (reviewed in reference 170).

The *NF1* gene on chromosome 17q12 is associated with neurofibromas occurring in the setting of neurofibromatosis. This gene is probably associated with sporadic neurofibromas as well (reviewed in reference 171).

▶ TUMORS OF THE HEMATOPOIETIC SYSTEM

Primary Central Nervous System Lymphoma

Primary CNS lymphomas are extranodal non-Hodgkin lymphomas arising in the CNS in the absence of obvious lymphoma outside the nervous system. The historic rarity of this tumor (formerly ≈1% to 5% of primary CNS tumors) has increased steadily in recent decades with an incidence approaching almost 7% of all primary CNS tumors in some series.[172] Although much of this increase may be attributed to increase in the immunocompromised population (transplantation and AIDS related), there is also clear evidence that CNS lymphomas are increasing in all age groups and in both genders, regardless of the immunologic status of the population.[173–175] Primary CNS lymphomas arise most commonly in males in their sixth and seventh decades of life. However, in the immunocompromised population, the age of manifestation is lower, with a median in the thirties.[176]

CNS lymphomas usually arise in the supratentorial compartment, with deep white matter of the frontal lobe being the most common location. Other locations include the posterior fossa and basal ganglia with common involvement of the periventricular regions. Unlike most primary CNS tumors, the tumors are often multiple and multifocal, simulating metastatic tumor. Multiple lesions are particularly prevalent in the AIDS and post-transplantation population.

On gross examination, CNS lymphoma is often pale white and soft with ill-defined margins. Following therapy, tumors are often necrotic, hemorrhagic, and deceptively well-defined. Histologically, CNS lymphomas are characteristically angiocentric neoplasms with tumor cells arranged in vascular concentric cuffings with invasion of the vascular walls and increase reticulin deposition. The tumor cells also diffusely infiltrate brain parenchyma (Fig. 5-33). An intense reactive astrocytosis is seen in the areas of infiltration.

The great majority of primary CNS lymphomas are of the diffuse, large cell or immunoblastic variety.[176] Immunohistochemical evaluation reveals a B-cell histogenesis in more than 90% of cases, usually with immunoglobulin (Ig) M kappa production. T-cell CNS lymphoma, typically of peripheral T-cell type, is exceptionally rare and

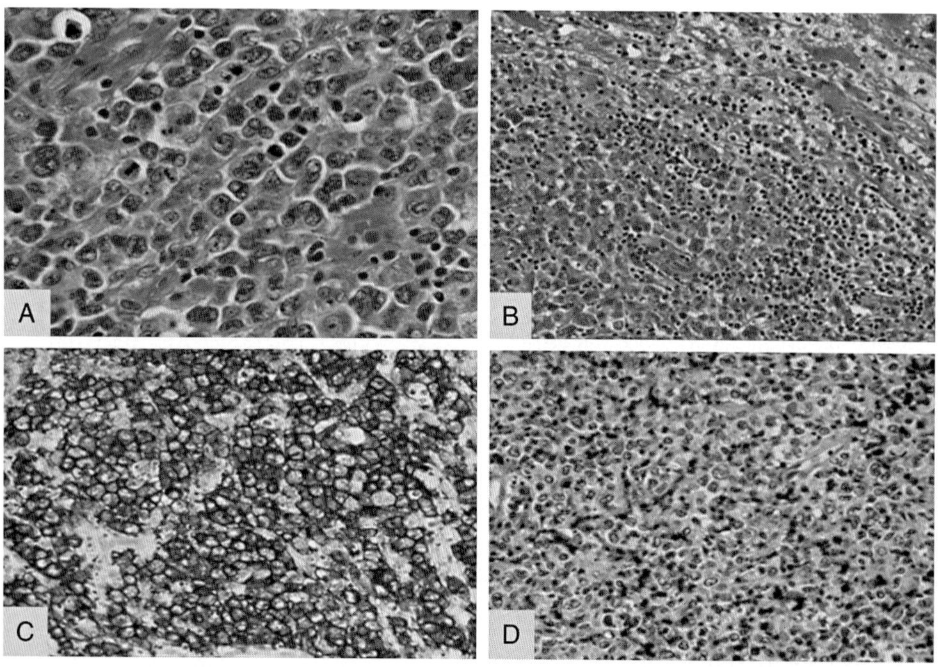

Figure 5-33 (PLATE 34). Primary CNS lymphoma. (A) High-grade large cell lymphomas are most commonly seen in the brain. (B) Diffusely infiltrating pattern is seen along with a more angiocentric infiltration of the tumor cells. B-cell markers (CD79a) (C) highlight the malignant large cell component, whereas small reactive T cells (CD3) (D) commonly infiltrate the neoplasm.

accounts for only 2% of these tumors.[176] T-cell lymphomas often involve the leptomeninges and are mostly seen in immunocompetent individuals.[177] Much more rare are anaplastic lymphomas (Ki-1, often T-cell subtype),[178] and Hodgkin disease.[176] The CNS may, however, be involved in the setting of disseminated Hodgkin's disease.[176]

Molecular studies of CNS lymphomas have confirmed the typical gene rearrangements of B-cell lymphomas.[176] The Epstein-Barr virus has been identified as the great majority of CNS lymphomas arising in immunocompromised patients, but it is uncommon in CNS lymphomas arising in the immunocompetent.[179]

REFERENCES

1. Lopes MBS, Scheithauer BW, VandenBerg SR. Ontogeny and classification of brain tumors. In: Vincken PJ, Bruyn GW, Vecht CJ, eds. Neuro-oncology, vol 1. Amsterdam: Elsevier Science, 1998:1–16.
2. Raghavan R, Balani J, Pery A, et al. Pediatric oligodendrogliomas: a study of molecular alterations on 1p and 19q using fluorescence in situ hybridization. J Neuropathol Exp Neurol 2003;62:530–537.
3. Kleihues P, Cavenee WK: Pathology and genetics of tumours of the nervous system. Lyon, France: IARC, 2000.
4. CBTRUS. (2002). Statistical report: primary brain tumors in the United States, 1995–1999. Central Brain Tumor Registry of the United States.
5. Lantos PL, Louis DN, Rosenblum MK, et al. Tumours of the nervous system, vol II. In: Graham DI, Lantos PL, eds. Greenfield's neuropathology, 7th ed. London: Arnold, 2002: 767–1052.
6. Krouwer HG, Davis RL, Silver P, et al. Gemistocytic astrocytomas. a reappraisal. J Neurosurg 1991;74:399–406.
7. Watanabe K, Osamu T, Yonekawa Y. Role of gemistocytes in astrocytoma progression. Lab Invest 1997;76:277–284.
8. Karamitopoulu E, Perentes E, Diamantis I, et al. Ki-67 immunoreactivity in human central nervous system tumors. A study with MIB 1 monoclonal antibody on archival material. Acta Neuropathol 1994;87:47–54.
9. Montine TJ, Vandersteenhoven JJ, Aguzzi A, et al: Prognostic significance of Ki-67 proliferation index in supratentorial fibrillary astrocytic neoplasms. Neurosurgery 1994;34: 674–679.
10. Giannini C, Scheithauer BW, Burger PC, et al. Cellular proliferation in pilocytic and diffuse astrocytomas. J Neuropathol Exp Neurol 1999;58:46–53.
11. Lopes MBS, Laws ER. Low-grade central nervous system tumors. Neurosurg Focus 2002;12:1–4.
12. Raghavan R, Steart PV, Weller RO. Cell proliferation patterns in the diagnosis of astrocytomas, anaplastic astrocytomas and glioblastoma multiforme. A Ki-67 study. Neuropathol Appl Neurobiol 1990;16:123–133.
13. Kleihues P, Burger PC, Collins VP, et al. Glioblastoma. In: Kleihues P, Cavenee WK, eds. Pathology and genetics of tumours of the nervous system. Lyon, France: IARC, 2000: 29–39.
14. Watanabe K, Tachibana O, Sato K, et al: Overexpression of the EGF receptor and p53 mutations are mutually exclusive in the evolution of primary and secondary glioblastomas. Brain Pathol 1996;6:217–224.
15. Ohgaki H, Peraud A, Nakazato Y, et al. Giant cell glioblastoma. In: Kleihues P, Cavenee WK, eds. Pathology and genetics of tumours of the nervous system. Lyon, IARC, 2000:40–41.
16. Peraud A, Watanabe K, Plate KH, et al. p53 mutations versus EGF receptor expression in giant cell glioblastomas. J Neuropathol Exp Neurol 1997;56:1236–1241.
17. Scott JN, Rewcastle NB, Brasher PMA, et al. Which glioblastoma multiforme patient will become a long-term survivor? A population-based study. Ann Neurol 1999; 46:183–188.
18. Sabel M, Reifenberger J, Weber RG, et al. Long-term survival of a patient with giant cell glioblastoma. J Neurosurg 2001;94:605–611.
19. Meyer-Puttlitz B, Hayashi Y, Waha A, et al. Molecular genetic analysis of giant cell glioblastomas. Am J Pathol 1997;151:853–857.
20. Ohagaki H, Biernat W, Reis R, et al. Gliosarcoma. In: Kleihues P, Cavenee WK, eds. Pathology and genetics of tumours of the nervous system. Lyon, France: IARC, 2000:42–44.
21. Haddad SF, Moore SA, Schelper RL, et al. Smooth muscle cells can comprise the sarcomatous component of gliosarcomas. J Neuropathol Exp Neurol 1992;51:493–498.
22. Paulus W, Bayas A, Ott G, et al. Interphase cytogenetics of glioblastoma and gliosarcoma. Acta Neuropathol 1994;88:420–423.
23. Biernat W, Aguzzi A, Sure U, et al. Identical mutations of the p53 tumor suppressor gene in the glial and sarcomatous part of gliosarcomas suggest a common origin from glial cells. J Neuropathol Exp Neurol 1995;54:651–656.
24. Boerman RH, Anderl K, Herath J, et al. The glial and mesenchymal elements of gliosarcoma share similar genetic alterations. J Neuropathol Exp Neurol 1996;55:973–981.
25. Cavenee WK, Furnari FB, Nagane M, et al. Diffusely infiltrating astrocytomas. In: Kleihues P, Cavenee WK, eds. Pathology and genetics of tumours of the nervous system. Lyon, IARC, 2000:10–21.
26. Collins VP. Cellular mechanisms targeted during astrocytoma progression. Cancer Lett 2002;188:1–7.
27. Raffel C, Thomas GA, Tishler DM, et al. Absence of p53 mutations in childhood central nervous system primitive neuroectodermal tumors. Neurosurgery 1993;33:103–106.
28. Litofsky NS, Hinton D, Raffel C: The lack of a role for p53 in astrocytomas in pediatric patients. Neurosurgery 1994;34:967–973.
29. Schiffer D, Cavalla P, Di Sapio A, et al. Mutations and immunohistochemistry of p53 and proliferation markers in astrocytic tumors of childhood. Childs Nerv Syst 1995;11:517–522.
30. Sure U, Ruedi D, Tachibana O, et al. Determination of p53 mutations, EGFR overexpression, and loss of p16 expression in pediatric glioblastomas. J Neuropathol Exp Neurol 1997;56:782–789.
31. Kraus JA, Felsberg J, Tonn JC, et al. Molecular genetic analysis of the TP53, PTEN, CDKN2A, EGFR, CDK4 and

MDM2 tumour-associated genes in supratentorial primitive neuroectodermal tumours and glioblastomas of childhood. Neuropathol Appl Neurobiol 2002;28:325–333.
32. Louis DN, Rubio M-P, Correa KM, et al. Molecular genetics of pediatric brain stem gliomas. Application of PCR techniques to small and archival brain tumor specimens. J Neuropathol Exp Neurol 1993;52:507–515.
33. Burger PC, Scheithauer BW, Paulus W, et al. Pilocytic astrocytoma. In: Kleihues P, Cavenee WK, eds. Pathology and genetics of tumours of the nervous system. Lyon, France: IARC, 2000:45–51.
34. Listernick R, Louis DN, Packer RJ, et al. Optic pathway gliomas in children with neurofibromatosis 1. Consensus from the NF1 optic pathway glioma task force. Ann Neurol 1997;41:143–149.
35. Tomlinson FH, Scheithauer BW, Hayostek CJ, et al. The significance of atypia and histologic malignancy in pilocytic astrocytoma of the cerebellum. A clinicopathologic and flow cytometric study. J Neurooncol 1994;9:301–310.
36. Dirven CM, Koudstaal J, Mooji JJ, et al. The proliferative potential of the pilocytic astrocytoma. The relation between MIB-1 labeling and clinical and neuro-radiological follow-up. J Neurooncol 1998;37:9–16.
37. Brown MT, Friedman HS, Oakes J, et al. Chemotherapy for pilocytic astrocytoma. Cancer 1993;71:3165–3172.
38. von Deimling A, Louis DN, Menon AG, et al. Deletions on the long arm of chromosome 17 in pilocytic astrocytoma. Acta Neuropathol 1993;86:81–85.
39. Kepes JJ, Louis DN, Giannini C, et al. Pleomorphic xanthoastrocytoma. In: Kleihues P, Cavenee WK, eds. Pathology and genetics of tumours of the nervous system. Lyon, France: IARC, 2000:52–54.
40. Weldon-Linne CM, Victor TA, Groothuis DR, et al. Pleomorphic xanthoastrocytoma. Ultrastructural and immunohistochemical study of a case with a rapidly fatal outcome following surgery. Cancer 1983;52:2055–2063.
41. Kepes JJ, Rubinstein LJ, Ansbacher L, et al. Histopathological features of recurrent pleomorphic xanthoastrocytomas. Further corroboration of the glial nature of this neoplasm. A study of three cases. Acta Neuropathol 1989;78:585–593.
42. Kawano N. Pleomorphic xanthoastrocytoma (PXA) in Japan. Its clinico-pathologic features and diagnostic clues. Brain Tumor Pathol 1991;8:5–10.
43. Daita G, Yonemasu Y, Muraoka S, et al. A case of anaplastic astrocytoma transformed from pleomorphic xanthoastrocytoma. Brain Tumor Pathol 1991;8:63–66.
44. Muñoz, EL, Eberhard DA, Lopes MBS, et al. Proliferative activity and p53 mutation as prognostic indicators in pleomorphic xanthoastrocytoma. J Neuropathol Exp Neurol 1996;55:606.
45. Paulus W, Lisle DK, Tonn JC, et al. Molecular genetic alterations in pleomorphic xanthoastrocytoma. Acta Neuropathol 1996;91:293–297.
46. Nasuha NA, Daud AH, Ghazali MM, et al. Molecular genetic analysis of anaplastic pleomorphic xanthoastrocytoma. Asian J Surg 2003;26:120–125.
47. Wiestler OD, Lopes BS, Green AJ, et al. Tuberous sclerosis complex and subependymal giant cell astrocytoma. In: Kleihues P, Cavenee WK, eds. Pathology and genetics of tumours of the nervous system. Lyon, France: IARC, 2000:227–230.
48. Lopes MBS, Altermatt HJ, Scheithauer BW, et al. Immunohistochemical characterization of subependymal giant cell astrocytoma. Acta Neuropathol 1996;91:368–375.
49. Hirose T, Scheithauer BW, Lopes MB, et al. Tuber and subependymal giant cell astrocytoma associated with tuberous sclerosis. An immunohistochemical, ultrastructural, and immunoelectron microscopic study. Acta Neuropathol 1995;90:387–399.
50. Henske EP, Scheithauer BW, Short MP, et al. Allelic loss is frequent in tuberous sclerosis kidney lesions but rare in brain lesions. Am J Hum Genet 1996;59:400–406.
51. Henske EP, Wessner LL, Golden J, et al. Loss of tuberin in both subependymal giant cell astrocytomas and angiomyolipomas supports a two-hit model for the pathogenesis of tuberous sclerosis tumors. Am J Pathol 1997;151:1639–1647.
52. Mizuguchi M, Kato M, Yamanouchi H, et al. Tuberin immunohistochemistry in brain, kidneys and heart with or without tuberous sclerosis. Acta Neuropathol 1997;94: 525–531.
53. Reifenberger G, Kros JM, Burger PC, et al. Oligodendroglioma. In: Kleihues P, Cavenee WK, eds. Pathology and genetics of tumours of the nervous system. Lyon, France: IARC, 2000:56–61.
54. Shaw EG, Scheithauer BW, O'Fallon JR, et al. Oligodendrogliomas. The Mayo Clinic experience. J Neurosurg 1992;76:428–434.
55. Wondrusch E, Huemer M, Budka H. Production of glial fibrillary acidic protein (GFAP) by neoplastic oligodendrocytes. Gliofibrillary oligodendroglioma and transitional oligoastrocytoma revisited. Brain Tumor Pathol 1991;8: 11–15.
56. Kros JM, de Jong AA, van der Kwast ThH. Ultrastructural characterization of transitional cells in oligodendrogliomas. J Neuropathol Exp Neurol 1992;51:186–193.
57. Schiffer D, Dutto A, Cavalla P, et al. Prognostic factors in oligodendrogliomas. Can J Neurol Sci 1997;24:313–319.
58. Coons SW, Johnson PC, Pearl DK. The prognostic significance of Ki-67 labeling indices for oligodendrogliomas. Neurosurgery 1997;41:878–884.
59. Noble M, Ataliotis P, Barnett SC, et al. Development, regeneration and neoplasia of glial cells in the central nervous system. Ann N Y Acad Sci 1991;633:35–47.
60. Landry CF, Verity MA, Cherman L, et al. Expression of oligodendrocytic mRNAs in glial tumors: changes associated with tumor grade and extent of neoplastic infiltration. Cancer Res 1997;57:4098–4104.
61. Shoshan Y, Nishiyama A, Chang A, et al. Expression of oligodendrocyte progenitor cell antigens by gliomas. Implications for the histogenesis of brain tumors. Proc Natl Acad Sci U S A 1999;96:10361–10366.
62. Lu QR, Yuk D, Alberta JA, et al. Sonic hedgehog-regulated oligodendrocyte lineage genes encoding bHLH proteins in the mammalian central nervous system. Neuron 2000; 25:317–329.
63. Zhou Q, Wang S, Anderson DJ. Identification of a novel family of oligodendrocyte lineage-specific basic helix-loop-helix transcription factors. Neuron 2000;25:331–343.

64. Lu QR, Park JK, Noll E, et al. Oligodendrocyte lineage genes (OLIG) as molecular markers for human glial brain tumors. Proc Natl Acad Sci U S A 2001;98:10851–10856.
65. Marie Y, Sanson M, Mokhtari K, et al. OLIG2 as a specific marker of oligodendroglial tumour cells. Lancet 2001;358: 298–300.
66. Hoang-Xuan K, Aguirre-Cruz L, Mokhtari K, et al. OLIG-1 and 2 gene expression in oligodendroglial tumours. Neuropathol Appl Neurobiol 2002;28:89–94.
67. Bouvier C, Bartoli C, Aguirre-Cruz L, et al. Shared oligodendrocyte lineage gene expression in gliomas and oligodendrocyte progenitor cells. J Neurosurg 2003;99:344–350.
68. Ligon KL, Alberta JA, Kho AT, et al. The oligodendroglial lineage marker OLIG2 is universally expressed in gliomas. J Neuropathol Exp Neurol 2004;63:499–509.
69. Kros JM, Van Eden CG, Stefanko SZ, et al. Prognostic implications of glial fibrillary acidic protein containing cell types in oligodendrogliomas. Cancer 1990;66:1204–1212.
70. Cruz-Sanchez FF, Rossi ML, Buller JR, et al: Oligodendrogliomas. A clinical, histological, immunocytochemical and lectin-binding study. Histopathology 1991;19: 361–367.
71. Cairncross JG, Macdonald DR, Ramsay DA. Aggressive oligodendroglioma. A chemosensitive tumor. Neurosurgery 1992;31:78–82.
72. Cairncross JG, Ueki K, Zlatescu MC, et al. Specific genetic predictors of chemotherapeutic response and survival in patients with anaplastic oligodendrogliomas. J Natl Cancer Inst 1998;90:1473–1479.
73. Burger PC. The grading of astrocytomas and oligodendrogliomas. In: Fields WS, ed. Primary brain tumors. A review of histologic classification. New York: Springer Verlag, 1989:171–180.
74. Schiffer D, Dutto A, Cavalla P, et al. Prognostic factors in oligodendrogliomas. Can J Neurol Sci 1997;24:313–319.
75. Coons SW, Johnson PC, Pearl DK. The prognostic significance of Ki-67 labeling indices for oligodendrogliomas. Neurosurgery 1987;41:878–884.
76. Reifenberger G, Kros JM, Burger PC, et al. Oligoastrocytoma. In: Kleihues P, Cavenee WK, eds. Pathology and genetics of tumours of the nervous system. Lyon, France: IARC, 2000:65–67.
77. Coons SW, Johnson PC, Scheithauer BW, et al. Improving diagnostic accuracy and interobserver concordance in the classification and grading of primary diagnosis. Cancer 1997;79:1381–1393.
78. Reifenberger G, Kros JM, Burger PC, et al. Anaplastic oligoastrocytoma, in Kleihues P, Cavenee WK, eds. Pathology and genetics of tumours of the nervous system. Lyon, France: IARC, 2000:68–69.
79. Ohgaki H, Eibl RH, Wiestler OD, et al. p53 mutations in nonastrocytic human brain tumors. Cancer Res 1991;51: 6202–6205.
80. Reifenberger G, Louis DN. Oligodendroglioma: toward molecular definitions in diagnostic neuro-oncology. J Neuropathol Exp Neurol 2003;62:111–126.
81. Maintz D, Fielder K, Koopmann J, et al. Molecular genetic evidence for subtypes of oligoastrocytomas. J Neuropathol Exp Neurol 1997;56:1098–1104.
82. Reifenberger J, Reifenberger G, Liu L, et al. Molecular genetics analysis of oligodendroglial tumors shows preferential allelic deletions on 19q and 1p. Am J Pathol 1994;145:1175–1190.
83. Kraus JA, Koopmann J, Kaskel P, et al. Shared allelic losses on chromosomes 1p and 19q suggest a common origin of oligodendroglioma and oligo-astrocytoma. J Neuropathol Exp Neurol 1995;54:91–95.
84. Wiestler OD, Schiffer D, Coons SW, et al. Ependymoma. In: Kleihues P, Cavenee WK, eds. Pathology and genetics of tumours of the nervous system. Lyon, France: IARC, 2000:72–76.
85. Louis DN, Ramesh V, Gusella JF. Neuropathology and molecular genetics of neurofibromatosis 2 and related tumors. Brain Pathol 1995;5:163–172.
86. Kline MJ, Kays DW, Rojiani AM. Extradural myxopapillary ependymoma. Report of two cases and review of the literature. Pediatr Pathol Lab Med 1996;16:813–822.
87. Min KW, Scheithauer BW. Clear cell ependymoma. A mimic of oligodendroglioma. Clinicopathologic and ultrastructural considerations. Am J Surg Pathol 1997;21:820–826.
88. Russell DS, Rubinstein LJ. Pathology of tumours of the nervous system, 5th ed. London: Edward Arnold, 1989: 187–219.
89. Wiestler OD, Schiffer D, Coons SW, et al. Anaplastic ependymoma. In: Kleihues P, Cavenee WK, eds. Pathology and genetics of tumours of the nervous system. Lyon, France: IARC, 2000:76–77.
90. Figarella-Branger D, Gambarelli D, Dollo C, et al. Infratentorial ependymomas of childhood. Correlation between histological features, immunohistochemical phenotype, silver nucleolar organizer region staining values and post-operative survival in 16 cases. Acta Neuropathol 1991;82:208–216.
91. Rezai AR, Woo HH, Lee M, et al. Disseminated ependymomas of the central nervous system. J Neurosurg 1996;85:618–624.
92. Rushing EJ, Brown DF, Hladik CL, et al. Correlation of bcl-2, p53, and MIB-1 expression with ependymoma grade and subtype. Mod Pathol 1998;11:464–470.
93. Prayson RA. Clinicopathologic study of 61 patients with ependymoma including MIB-1 immunohistochemistry. Ann Diagn Pathol 1999;3:11–18.
94. Schiffer D, Chio A, Cravioto H, et al. Ependymoma. Internal correlations among pathological signs. The anaplastic variant. Neurosurgery 1991;29:206–210.
95. Wiestler OD, Schiffer D, Coons SW, et al. Myxopapillary ependymoma. In: Kleihues P, Cavenee WK, eds. Pathology and genetics of tumours of the nervous system. Lyon, France: IARC, 2000:78–79.
96. Ernestus RI, Schroder R. Clinical aspects and pathology of intracranial subependymoma—18 personal cases and review of the literature. Neurochirurgica 1993;36:194–202.
97. Chiechi MV, Smirniotopoulus JG, Jones RV. Intracranial subependymomas. CT and MR imaging features in 24 cases. AJR Am J Roentgenol 1995;165:1245–1250.
98. Wiestler OD, Schiffer D. Subependymoma. In: Kleihues P, Cavenee WK, eds. Pathology and genetics of tumours of the nervous system. Lyon, France: IARC, 2000:80–81.

99. Fink KL, Rushing EJ, Schold SC Jr, et al. Infrequency of p53 gene mutations in ependymomas. J Neurooncol 1996;27:111–115.
100. Birch BD, Johnson JP, Parsa A, et al. Frequent type 2 neurofibromatosis gene transcript mutations in sporadic intramedullary spinal cord ependymomas. Neurosurgery 1996;39:135–140.
101. Rubio MP, Correa KM, Ramesh V, et al. Analysis of the neurofibromatosis 2 gene in human ependymomas and astrocytomas. Cancer Res 1994;54:45–57.
102. Slavc I, MacCollin MM, Dunn M, et al. Exon scanning for mutations of the NF2 gene in pediatric ependymomas, rhabdoid tumors and meningiomas. Int J Cancer 1995; 64:243–247.
103. von Haken MS, White EC, Daneshvar Shyesther L, et al. Molecular genetic analysis of chromosome arm 17p and chromosome arm 22q DNA sequences in sporadic pediatric ependymomas. Genes Chromosomes Cancer 1996; 17:37–44.
104. Russell DC, Rubinstein LJ. Pathology of tumours of the nervous system, 5th ed. London: Edward Arnold, 1989:289–306.
105. Russo CP, Katz DS, Corona RJ, et al. Gangliocytoma of the cervicothoracic spinal cord. AJNR Am J Neuroradiol 1995; 16:889–891.
106. Beal MF, Kleinman GM, Ojemann RG, et al. Gangliocytoma of third ventricle. Hyperphagia, somnolence, and dementia. Neurology 1981;31:1224–1228.
107. Towfighi J, Salam MM, McLendon RE, et al. Ganglion cell-containing tumors of the pituitary gland. Arch Pathol Lab Med 1996;120:369–377.
108. Boyko OB, Curnes JT, Oakes WJ, et al. Hamartomas of the tuber cinereum. CT, MR, and pathologic findings. AJNR Am J Neuroradiol 1991;12:309–314.
109. Tuli S, Provias JP, Bernstein M. Lhermitte-Duclos disease. Literature review and novel treatment strategy. Can J Neurol Sci 1997;24:155–160.
110. Vinchon M, Blond S, Lejeune JP, et al. Association of Lhermitte-Duclos and Cowden disease. Report of a new case and review of the literature. J Neurol Neurosurg Psychiatry 1994;57:699–704.
111. Yachnis AT, Trojanowski JQ, Memmo M, et al. Expression of neurofilament proteins in the hypertrophic granule cells of Lhermitte-Duclos disease. An explanation for the mass effect and the myelination of parallel fibers in the disease state. J Neuropathol Exp Neurol 1988;47:206–216.
112. Hassoun J, Gambarelli D, Grisoli F, et al. Central neurocytoma. An electron-microscopic study of two cases. Acta Neuropathol 1982;56:151–156.
113. Hessler RB, Lopes MBS, Frankfurter A, et al. Cytoskeletal immunohistochemistry of central neurocytomas. Am J Surg Pathol 1991;16:1031–1038.
114. Robbins P, Segal A, Narula S, et al. Central neurocytoma. A clinicopathological, immunohistochemical and ultrastructural study of 7 cases. Pathol Res Pract 1995;191:100–111.
115. von Deimling A, Janzer R, Kleihues P, Wiestler OD. Patterns of differentiation potential in central neurocytoma. Acta Neuropathol 1990;79:473–479.
116. Figarella-Branger D, Söylemezogly F, Kleihues P, et al. Central neurocytoma. In: Kleihues P, Cavenee WK, eds. Pathology and genetics of tumours of the nervous system. Lyon, France: IARC, 2000:107–109.
117. Kim DG, Kim JS, Chi JG, et al. Central neurocytoma: proliferative potential and biological behavior. J Neurosurg 1996;84:742–747.
118. Eng DY, DeMonte F, Ginsberg L, et al. Craniospinal dissemination of central neurocytoma. J Neurosurg 1997;86: 547–552.
119. Söylemezoglu F, Scheithauer BW, Esteve J, et al. Atypical central neurocytoma. J Neuropathol Exp Neurol 1997;56: 551–556.
120. Kleihues P, Chimelli L, Giangaspero F. Cerebellar liponeurocytoma. In: Kleihues P, Cavenee WK, eds. Pathology and genetics of tumours of the nervous system. Lyon, France: IARC, 2000:110–111.
121. Wolf HK, Muller MB, Spanle M, et al. Ganglioglioma. A detailed histopathological and immunohistochemical analysis of 61 cases. Acta Neuropathol 1994;88:166–173.
122. Johnson JH Jr, Hariharan S, Berman J, et al. Clinical outcome of pediatric gangliogliomas. Ninety-nine cases over 20 years. Pediatr Neurosurg 1997;27:203–207.
123. Hirose T, Scheithauer BW, Lopes MB, et al. Ganglioglioma. An ultrastructural and immunohistochemical study. Cancer 1997;79:989–1003.
124. Prayson RA, Khajavi K, Comair YG. Cortical architectural abnormalities and MIB1 immunoreactivity in gangliogliomas. A study of 60 patients with intracranial tumors. J Neuropathol Exp Neurol 1995;54:513–520.
125. Russell DS, Rubinstein LJ. Pathology of tumours of the nervous system, 5th ed. London: Edward Arnold, 1989; 289–302.
126. Daumas-Duport C. Dysembryoplastic neuroepithelial tumours. Brain Pathol 1993;3:283–295.
127. Rosemberg S, Vieira GS. Dysembryoplastic neuroepithelial tumor. An epidemiological study from a single institution. Arq Neuropsiquiatr 1998;56:232–236.
128. Kuchelmeister K, Demirel T, Schlorer E, et al. Dysembryoplastic neuroepithelial tumour of the cerebellum. Acta Neuropathol 1995;89:385–390.
129. Ostertun B, Wolf HK, Campos MG, et al. Dysembryoplastic neuroepithelial tumors. MR and CT evaluation. AJNR Am J Neuroradiol 1996;17:419–430.
130. Hirose T, Scheithauer BW, Lopes MBS, et al. Dysembryoplastic neuroepithelial tumor (DNT). An immunohistochemical and ultrastructural study. J Neuropathol Exp Neurol 1994;53:184–195.
131. Prayson RA, Morris HH, Estes ML, et al. Dysembryoplastic neuroepithelial tumor. A clinicopathologic and immunohistochemical study of 11 tumors including MIB1 immunoreactivity. Clin Neuropathol 1996;15:47–53.
132. Wolf HK, Buslei R, Schmidt-Kastner R, et al. NeuN: a useful neuronal marker for diagnostic histopathology. J Histochem Cytochem 1996;44:1167–1171.
133. VandenBerg SR. The developing brain and cellular targets for neoplastic transformation. In: Kaye AH, Laws ER Jr, eds. Brain tumors, an encyclopedic approach, 2nd ed. London: Churchill Livingstone, 2001:9–28.
134. Giangaspero F, Bigner SH, Kleihues P, et al. Medulloblastoma. In: Kleihues P, Cavenee WK, eds. Pathology

and genetics of tumours of the nervous system. Lyon, France: IARC, 2000:129–137.
135. Katsetos CD, Herman MM, Frankfurter A, et al. Cerebellar desmoplastic medulloblastomas. A further immunohistochemical characterization of the reticulin-free pale islands. Arch Pathol Lab Med 1989;113: 1019–1029.
136. Eberhart CG, Kaufman WE, Tihan T, et al. Apoptosis, neuronal maturation, and neurotrophin expression within medulloblastoma nodules. J Neuropathol Exp Neurol 2001;60:462–469.
137. Giangaspero F, Rigobello L, Badiali M, et al. Large cell medulloblastomas. A distinct variant with highly aggressive behavior. Am J Surg Pathol 1992;16:687–693.
138. Eberhart CG, Burger PC. Anaplasia and grading in medulloblastomas. Brain Pathol 2003;13:376–385.
139. Eberhart CG, Kepner JL, Goldthwaite PT, et al. Histopathologic grading of medulloblastomas: a Pediatric Oncology Group Study. Cancer 2002;94:552–560.
140. McManamy CS, Lamont JM, Taylor RE, et al. Morphophenotypic variation predicts clinical behavior in childhood non-desmoplastic medulloblastomas. J Neuropathol Exp Neurol 2003;62:627–632.
141. Steichen-Gersdorf E, Baumgartner M, Kreczy A, et al. Deletion mapping on chromosome 17p in medulloblastoma. Br J of Cancer 1997;76:1284–1287.
142. Russo C, Pellarin M, Tingby O, et al. Comparative genomic hybridization in patients with supratentorial and infratentorial primitive neuroectodermal tumors. Cancer 1999;86:331–339.
143. Thomas GA, Raffel C. Loss of heterozygosity on 6q, 16q, and 17p in human central nervous system primitive neuroectodermal tumors. Cancer Res 1991;51:639–643.
144. Rorke LB, Biegel JA. Atypical teratoid/rhabdoid tumour. In: Kleihues P, Cavenee WK, eds. Pathology and genetics of tumours of the nervous system. Lyon, France: IARC, 2000:145–148.
145. Biegel JA, Zhou JY, Rorke LB, et al. Germ-line and acquired mutations of INI1 in atypical teratoid rhabdoid tumors. Cancer Res 1999;59:74–79.
146. Biegel JA, Kalpana G, Knudsen ES, et al. The role of INI1 and the SWI/SNF complex in the development of rhabdoid tumors: meeting summary from the workshop on childhood atypical teratoid/rhabdoid tumors. Cancer Res 2002;62:323–328.
147. Gessi M, Giangaspero F, Pietsch T. Atypical teratoid/rhabdoid tumors and choroid plexus tumors: when genetics "surprise" pathology. Brain Pathol 2003;13:409–414.
148. Rorke LB, Packer RJ, Biegel JA. Central nervous system atypical teratoid/rhabdoid tumors of infancy and childhood. J Neurosurg 1996;85:56–65.
149. Burger PC, Yu IT, Tihan T, et al. Atypical teratoid/rhabdoid tumor of the central nervous system: a highly malignant tumor of infancy and childhood frequently mistaken for medulloblastoma: a Pediatric Oncology Group study. Am J Surg Pathol 1998;22:1083–1092.
150. Louis DN, Scheithauer BW, Budka H, et al. Meningiomas. In: Kleihues P, Cavenee WK, eds. Pathology and genetics of tumours of the nervous system. Lyon, France: IARC, 2000:176–184.
151. Perry A, Dehner LP. Meningeal tumors of childhood and infancy. An update and literature review. Brain Pathol 2003;13:386–408.
152. Perry A, Stafford SL, Scheithauer BW, et al. The prognostic role of MIB-1, p53 and DNA flow cytometry in completely resected primary meningiomas. Cancer 1998;82: 2262–2269.
153. Chen WYK, Liu HC. Atypical (anaplastic) meningioma. Relationship between histological features and recurrence—a clinicopathologic study. Clin Neuropathol 1990;9:74–81.
154. Perry A, Scheithauer BW, Stafford SL, et al. "Malignancy" in meningiomas: a clinicopathologic study of 116 patients. Cancer 1999;85:2046–2056.
155. Mahmood A, Caccamo DV, Tomecak FJ, et al. Atypical and malignant meningiomas. A clinicopathological review. Neurosurgery 1993;33:955–963.
156. Guillov L, Fletcher JA, Fletcher CDM, et al. Extrapleural solitary fibrous tumor and haemangiopericytoma. In: Fletcher CDM, Unni KK, Merters F, eds. World Health Organization classification of tumours. Pathology and genetics of tumours of soft tissue and bone. Lyon, France: IARC, 2002.
157. Jääskeläinen J, Louis DN, Paulus W, et al. Haemangiopericytoma. In: Kleihues P, Cavenee WK, eds. Pathology and genetics of tumours of the nervous system. Lyon, France: IARC, 2000:190–192.
158. Mena H, Ribas JL, Pezeshkour GH, et al. Hemangiopericytoma of the central nervous system. A review of 94 cases. Hum Pathol 1991;22:84–91.
159. Vuorinen V, Salinen P, Haapasalo H, et al. Outcome of 31 intracranial hemangiopericytomas. Poor predictive value of cell proliferation indices. Acta Neurochir 1996;138: 1399–1408.
160. Carneiro SS, Scheithauer BW, Nascimento AG, et al. Solitary fibrous tumor of the meninges. A lesion distinct from fibrous meningioma. A clinicopathologic and immunohistochemical study. Am J Clin Pathol 1996; 106:217–224.
161. Woodruff JM, Kourea HP, Louis DN, et al. Schwannoma. In: Kleihues P, Cavenee WK, eds. Pathology and genetics of tumours of the nervous system. Lyon, France: IARC, 2000:164–166.
162. Consensus Development Panel: NIH health consensus development conference statement on acoustic neuroma. Arch Neurol 1991;51:201–207.
163. Beskonakli E, Cayli S, Turgut M, et al. Intraparenchymal schwannomas of the central nervous system. An additional case report and review. Neurosurg Rev 1997;20: 139–144.
164. Sharma MC, Karak AK, Gaikwad SB, et al. Intracranial intraparenchymal schwannomas. A series of eight cases. J Neurol Neurosurg Psychiatry 1996;60:200–203.
165. Woodruff JM, Kourea HP, Louis DN, Scheithauer BW. Neurofibroma. In: Kleihues P, Cavenee WK, eds. Pathology and genetics of tumours of the nervous system. Lyon, France: IARC, 2000:167–168.
166. Woodruff JM, Selig AM, Crowley K, et al. Schwannoma (neurilemoma) with malignant transformation. Am J Surg Pathol 1994;18:882–895.

167. Woodruff JM, Kourea HP, Louis DN, et al. Malignant peripheral nerve sheath tumour (MPNST). In: Kleihues P, Cavenee WK, eds. Pathology and genetics of tumours of the nervous system. Lyon, France: IARC, 2000: 172–174.
168. Wanebo JE, Malik JM, VandenBerg SR, et al. Malignant peripheral nerve sheath tumors. A clinicopathologic study of 28 cases. Cancer 1993;71:1247–1253.
169. Scheithauer BW, Woodruff JM, Erlandson RA. Tumors of the peripheral nervous system. Washington, DC: Armed Forces Institute of Pathology, 1999.
170. Baser ME, Evans DGR, Gutmann DH. Neurofibromatosis 2. Curr Opin Neurol 2003;16:27–33.
171. Lynch TM, Gutmann DH. Neurofibromatosis 1. Neurol Clin 2002;20:841–865.
172. Miller DC, Hochberg FH, Harris NL, et al. Pathology with clinical correlations of primary central nervous system non-Hodgkin's lymphoma. Cancer 1994;74: 1383–1397.
173. Eby NL, Grufferman S, Flannelly CM, et al. Increasing incidence of primary brain lymphomas in the U.S. Cancer 1988;62:2461–2465.
174. Hao D, DiFrancesco LM, Brasher PM, et al. Is primary CNS lymphoma really becoming more common? A population-based study of incidence, clinicopathological features and outcome in Alberta from 1975 to 1996. Ann Oncol 1999;10:65–70.
175. Olson JE, Janney CA, Rao RD, et al. The continuing increase in the incidence of primary central nervous system non-Hodgkin lymphoma. Cancer 2002;95: 1504–1510.
176. Paulus W, Jellinger K, Morgello S, et al. Malignant lymphomas. In: Kleihues P, Cavenee WK, eds. Pathology and genetics of tumours of the nervous system. Lyon, France: IARC, 2000:198–203.
177. Nitta T, Uda K, Ebato M, et al. Primary peripheral-postthymic T-cell lymphoma in the central nervous system: immunological and molecular approaches to diagnosis. J Neurosurg 1995;82:77–82.
178. Paulus W, Ott MM, Strik H, et al. Large cell anaplastic (Ki-1) brain lymphoma of T-cell genotype. Hum Pathol 1994;25: 1253–1256.
179. Morgello S. Pathogenesis and classification of primary central nervous system lymphoma: an update. Brain Pathol 1995;5:383–393.

CHAPTER 6

Surgical Management

MICHAEL D. TAYLOR / MARK BERNSTEIN

At first glance, gliomas appear to be a disease ideally suited to surgical treatment and cure. They very infrequently metastasize; making their treatment a problem of local tumor control. However, their eloquent location within the central nervous system, as well as their consistent propensity to local invasion, belies this hypothesis, as even radical surgery for adult gliomas is not curative. Indeed, almost 100 years ago Ballance remarked, "infiltrating growths, such as glioma and sarcoma of the brain, can but seldom be completely removed, chiefly because in the living brain there is often no visible and obvious line of demarcation between the brain and the tumor tissue."[1]

Even so, surgery remains one of the core, integral treatment modalities for patients with brain tumors. The neurosurgeon is often the brain tumor patient's gateway to the neuro-oncology team, as surgery is often the initial modality of treatment. In spite of this, not all patients with brain tumors need surgery, and the type or extent of surgery for a given brain tumor is often controversial. Surgery for intraaxial brain tumors has a set of possible goals, as outlined in Table 6-1.

▶ INDICATIONS FOR SURGERY

Diagnosis

When a patient presents with an intraaxial central nervous system (CNS) mass lesion, the histology of the lesion is one of the most important predictors of both natural history and response to therapy. Currently, a definitive diagnosis is made by histopathology and immunohistochemistry performed on tissue removed from the lesion. Although preoperative imaging in combination with a patient's history can be highly suggestive of a specific pathologic entity, the final diagnosis is never certain until the pathologist's report is available. Many, if not most, experienced brain tumor surgeons have operated on a "glioblastoma" only to find an abscess at surgery, or to have the pathology report come back as "demyelination" or "chronic hematoma." Some experts recommend taking multiple biopsies from different areas of the tumor in order to avoid a so-called sampling error. This occurs when the lesion is heterogeneous; for example, when a glioblastoma arises from a low-grade glioma (LGG). If the LGG portion of the tumor alone is unwittingly biopsied in such a case, the pathology report will not reflect the true biology of the lesion. A tissue diagnosis can be obtained by stereotactic biopsy, or by open craniotomy. Avoidance of a sampling error is one of the benefits of open resection of gliomas caused by the larger volume of tumor available for pathologic analysis. If a tumor histology that would benefit from cytoreductive surgery is found at the time of stereotactic biopsy, the patient can then undergo a craniotomy in the future.

▶ **TABLE 6-1.** GOALS OF BRAIN TUMOR SURGERY

Obtain a diagnosis
Cytoreduction (bulk tumor removal)
Improvement in symptoms and signs
Increase duration of life/quality of life

Cytoreduction

One of the most contentious issues in neuro-oncology is the value of cytoreduction in the treatment of gliomas. There are brain tumors where we know that cytoreduction is of no value (i.e., primary CNS lymphoma), and tumors where good evidence exists that cytoreduction alters the natural history (i.e., medulloblastoma). No high-quality evidence exists to support or refute the value of cytoreduction in adult gliomas. Although there are many papers written on this topic, most contain several biases, predominantly selection bias, in which patients with a poor prognosis underwent biopsies, whereas patients with a better prognosis underwent resections. Many papers dealing with the value of cytoreduction in adult glioma surgery rely on the operating surgeon's estimate of the extent of resection, which is now well known to be a poor reflection of the actual extent of resection. It has been suggested that it is not the extent of tumor that is removed that is most prognostically relevant, but rather the volume of tumor that is left at the end of the operation.[2–4] For example, if a 100-cm^3 tumor had 95 cm^3 removed, this would be a 95% resection, but there would be 5 cm^3 of tumor left. Conversely if a 10-cm^3 tumor had 8 cm^3 removed, this would only be an 80% resection, but there would only be 2 cm^3 of residual tumor. Whether the extent of resection, or the volume of residual tumor, or both or neither are prognostic for adults with malignant glioma is not known. Indeed, a Cochrane library review of biopsy versus resection for malignant glioma concluded that randomized trials are needed before any recommendations can be established. As a result, a 50-year-old man presenting with headaches secondary to a nondominant frontopolar glioblastoma will receive a stereotactic biopsy prior to adjuvant therapy at some centers, and a craniotomy for gross total resection in other centers.

Numerous papers in the literature support cytoreductive surgery for malignant gliomas; however, many of these papers are written by neurosurgeons.[2–16] A smaller number of papers claim that it has little or no effect on survival.[17,18] Most of these papers are retrospective, and even among the prospective studies, in no case was the extent of surgery randomized. Indeed, the better evidence in support of cytoreduction comes from prospective trials examining the role of other therapeutics (e.g., chemotherapy) in the treatment of glioma, where extent of resection was looked at as a side issue. Critics of cytoreduction claim that this results in two groups of patients: younger patients with higher Karnofsky performance status (KPS) scores and superficial tumors that are most likely to receive a gross total resection, and older patients with low KPS scores and deep tumors who receive a biopsy. These two groups of patients will have widely disparate outcomes regardless of the extent of surgery, but casual analysis could credit the better outcome in the former group to their more extensive resection. Some authors suggest that more extensive cytoreduction is associated with fewer complications during subsequent radiotherapy, and may result in a better response to adjuvant treatments (radiotherapy and chemotherapy).[19,20]

The study to answer whether cytoreduction is of value in the treatment of malignant gliomas has been debated and discussed in the neurosurgical community but has not yet been carried out. This is because neurosurgeons on both sides of the argument believe that it would be "unethical" to randomize their patients to the other treatment arm (biopsy for the supporters of cytoreduction, craniotomy for the proponents of biopsy) in spite of the lack of definitive evidence to support either protocol. As a result, many neurosurgeons attempt cytoreductive surgery for adult malignant gliomas as long as it is deemed safe for the patient (will not lead to additional deficits or death) (Fig. 6-1). This middle road is probably a good compromise in the absence of good evidence.

Similar low-quality evidence exists to support or refute the value of cytoreductive surgery for LGGs, specifically for low-grade astrocytoma. Supporters hope to decrease the numbers of cells in the tumor, thereby statistically delaying the chance that any one cell in the tumor will sustain additional genetic hits and progress on to a malignant tumor. Opponents of cytoreduction will point out the diffuse nature of most LGGs, making complete resection difficult if not impossible, as well as the fact that most of these patients have many years of productive life left and to burden them with the possibility of an additional postoperative neurologic deficit will have profound results. A wide spectrum of practice is currently seen in various centers where large numbers of patients with LGG are seen and treated. At one end of the spectrum patients are biopsied and observed (or perhaps even just followed by serial imaging); and at the other end of the spectrum, patients receive large, aggressive resections that are successful in removing all, or most of the abnormality seen on T_2-weighted magnetic resonance imaging (MRI) scan. The clinical trial to determine the value of cytoreductive surgery in LGG would be even more difficult than for malignant gliomas and is unlikely to be carried out in the near future. This controversy has been discussed by many authors, both in primary data papers and in a number of reviews, but no consensus is apparent.[21–39]

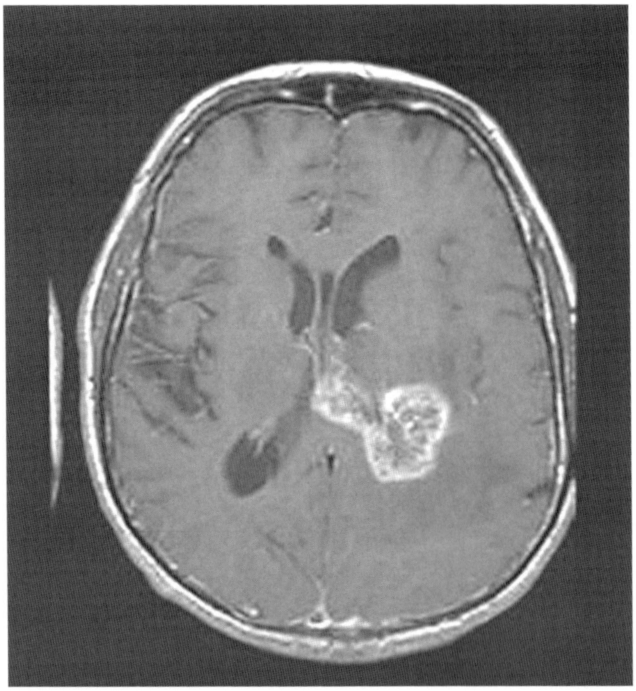

Figure 6-1. Axial T_1 gadolinium-enhanced magnetic resonance imaging (MRI) of a 58-year-old healthy man with a 1-month history of mild weakness and sensory inattention on the right side. Stereotactic biopsy was recommended over craniotomy because of the deep, eloquent location of the tumor, its involvement of the corpus callosum, and the belief that there was essentially no chance of making him better with debulking, but a great chance of making him worse. The diagnosis was glioblastoma.

Improvement in Symptoms and Signs

Surgery for adult gliomas is largely palliative and can offer some patients great relief from their symptoms. Cytoreductive surgery in patients with headaches secondary to increased intracranial pressure can provide excellent symptom relief. The rare patient with a supratentorial glioma and concomitant hydrocephalus will benefit from opening up of the cerebral spinal fluid (CSF) pathways either by tumor removal or placement of a ventriculoperitoneal shunt. Patients presenting with chronic epilepsy who have a mass lesion on imaging are excellent candidates for epilepsy surgery, part of which includes removal of the mass lesion. These patients should be assessed by a multidisciplinary epilepsy surgery team to determine the origin of the seizures and whether more extensive surgery than just removal of the tumor (lesionectomy) is required for good epileptic control (i.e., should intraoperative electrocorticography [ECOG] be performed).[27,40–44] Seizure disorders are much more common in patients with slow-growing, more benign lesions such as pilocytic astrocytoma or dysembryoplastic neuroepithelial tumor (DNT), and less common with malignant tumors like glioblastoma multiforme.

Gliomas usually cause a focal neurologic deficit in one of two ways: they either invade an eloquent area of brain (cortex or white matter), or they compress an eloquent area of brain. Rarely Todd's postictal paralysis may be seen, but this should be evident on the basis of history and serial exams. If the area of eloquent brain has been invaded, the patient's neurologic deficit will be the same or worse postoperatively. If the area in question was only compressed, there is likely to be some recovery of function postoperatively, sometimes after a temporary decline in function. When operating on a patient with a focal neurologic deficit, especially a language deficit, the surgeon should consider the use of an awake craniotomy (see "Awake Craniotomy" below) to minimize the chances of exacerbating the neurologic deficit postoperatively.

Improvement in the Duration and/or Quality of Life

As previously mentioned, surgery for adult gliomas, with the possible exception of pilocytic astrocytoma is not curative. The value/lack of value of cytoreduction to improve survival in patients with malignant gliomas is discussed above (see "Cytoreduction"). There exists a subgroup of patients for whom no trial or study is necessary to show the benefit of surgery in extending life. For those patients presenting in extremis with a large necrotic or hemorrhagic tumor and very high intracranial pressure, surgery can be lifesaving in the short-term. A patient dying from uncal herniation secondary to a large necrotic temporal lobe glioblastoma needs immediate surgical intervention, and this group of patients could never be randomized in a prospective trial. This type of patient is only a small subgroup among patients with malignant glioma.

The role of cytoreductive surgery in improving quality of life and/or functional independence in glioma patients has not been the subject of any randomized prospective, controlled trials. There is some soft evidence that more complete resections of adult supratentorial gliomas leads to a better postoperative quality of life than do less extensive resections.[2,3,6,15,19,21] Ammirati and associates[15] reported that among patients who are functionally independent preoperatively, those who underwent gross total resection were independent longer than were the patients who underwent subtotal resection (185 weeks vs. 12.5 weeks). These investigators observed similar benefit of gross total resection among patients who were "semi-independent" (KPS score >60).[15] Keles and associates[2] reported that most patients undergoing cytoreductive surgery for glioma had a drop in their KPS score postoperatively, except for patients who had a gross total resection. Another group reported that patients who underwent gross total resection had a slight improvement in their KPS score, as compared to biopsy patients who had a slight drop.[3] In none of these studies was the extent of surgery randomized; consequently, a selection bias is highly likely, and the true value of cytoreductive surgery in maintaining/improving quality of life and/or functional independence is not clear.

▶ CRANIOTOMY FOR BRAIN TUMOR: THE PROCEDURE

Craniotomy for brain tumor can be performed under general anesthetic, or local anesthetic (see "Awake Craniotomy" below). Although craniotomy is a well-tolerated procedure, patients with significant medical comorbidities, especially cardiorespiratory problems, should have a preoperative anesthetic consultation. Preoperative workup includes blood work to rule out a coagulopathy or anemia. The patient's blood group should be determined in case an intra- or postoperative blood transfusion is necessary. The most important part of the preoperative workup is for the operating surgeon to obtain an informed consent. An informed consent consists of telling the patient what the operation will entail, why it needs to be done, what the possible alternatives are, and what the material risks of the procedure are. It includes the components of disclosure, voluntariness, and capacity. If the patient is deemed incapable to fully comprehend (usually because of dysphasia and/or cognitive effects of the tumor), the patient's substitute decision maker must give consent.

After the induction of general anesthesia, the patient is positioned on the operating table such that the operative site is most superior, and all points on the body (especially those over peripheral nerves) are padded. The site of the tumor is mapped out on the surface of the scalp using the surgeon's best judgment as compared to the preoperative imaging, or, more recently, using a surgical navigation device or frameless stereotaxy (see "Surgical Navigation" below). After having marked the incision, the area is shaved. Some neurosurgeons shave widely because this facilitates surgery and may decrease infection rates. Other neurosurgeons prefer to shave little or no hair. Patients highly desirous of keeping their hair should discuss this with their surgeon preoperatively. A scalp flap, similar to a trap door, is elevated to expose the skull, although linear or curvilinear incisions are also very satisfactory. Holes in the skull (*burr holes*) are now made at the periphery of the exposed skull. Typically these holes are made blindly by a drill (burr) that cuts through solid bone, but which comes to a stop automatically when soft dura is found. Once the burr holes are made, a high-speed air-powered saw is used to connect the holes, and the "bone flap" is removed, to be replaced later. The exposed dura is now incised, and tented out of the way to expose the underlying brain.

Now that the brain is exposed, superficial tumors are easily localized (Fig. 6-2). Deeper tumors can be found by observing an expanded gyrus or abnormal vessels coursing over the surface of the brain. The light touch of a gloved finger can occasionally palpate a tumor underlying the cortex. Frameless stereotaxy (a surgical navigation device) is the ideal method for localizing a subcortical tumor. By placing the pointer from the frameless stereotaxy system on the surface of the brain, the surgeon can determine where the surgeon is, where the tumor is, and the location of important adjacent structures. If frameless stereotaxy is unavailable, intraoperative ultrasonography is another valuable technique for localizing a deep tumor.

After the tumor has been localized, the first order of business is to obtain a quick section diagnosis. Most experienced brain tumor surgeons have operated on a lesion that appeared on the preoperative imaging to be a neoplasm, only to have the neuropathologist tell them it was an infarct or a demyelinating pseudotumor. Patients with primary CNS lymphoma are not helped by cytoreductive surgery, and the craniotomy should probably be terminated if that diagnosis comes back from the pathologist with a degree of certainty. If the pathology is a glioma, the tumor is removed piecemeal using a combination of ultrasonic aspirator, suction, and bipolar cautery. As there is no definite tissue plane between most glial tumors and the surrounding brain, most neurosurgeons will start the resection within the tumor, working outward until they reach an area that resembles normal brain. The extent of tumor removal will vary from surgeon to surgeon (see the discussion of the benefits of cytoreduction in glioma surgery under "Cytoreduction" above), but most surgeons will resect until they perceive a danger to the patient. Once the decision has been made to stop the operation, hemostasis is obtained and the dura is reapproximated. The bone flap is replaced and held in place by small plates and screws. The layers of the scalp are sewn together and a bandage is placed over the wound. Typically, surgery for a supratentorial glioma takes 2 to 4 hours. Neuroanesthesia is different from other types of anesthesia in that it is desirous for the patient to wake up as soon as possible after the operation in order that CNS function can be examined and followed to rule out intraoperative and postoperative complications.

Postoperative Care After Craniotomy

Patients are watched very closely in the immediate postoperative period to assure that they regain consciousness and that they have not acquired new neurologic deficits. They are then observed for a period of time in some sort of intensive monitoring unit, either a recovery room (postanesthetic care unit) or the intensive care unit. Depending on the patient and the location of the

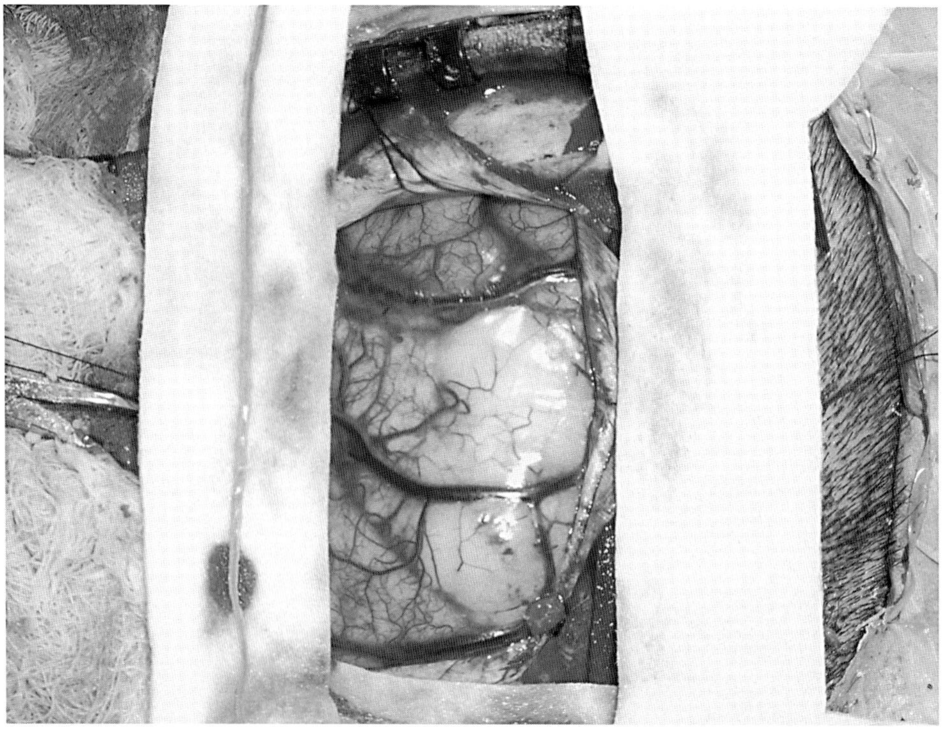

Figure 6-2. Intraoperative photograph of the surface of the brain. A typical low-grade glioma appears as a pale area in an expanded gyrus that comes up to, but does not penetrate, the pia mater.

tumor, the patient's CNS is monitored by checking the level of consciousness (usually the Glasgow Coma Scale), pupillary size and reactivity, and motor function in the extremities. A diminished level of consciousness is unusual in preoperative/postoperative glioma patients. In those rare cases when a patient presents acutely in coma because of an intratumoral bleed, hydrocephalus, or a rapid increase in cerebral edema, the coma may persist postoperatively. In those patients it may be beneficial to leave an intracranial pressure monitor at the time of surgery, as the postoperative neurologic exam is less sensitive in comatose patients. The pressure monitor is used to measure intracranial pressure (ICP), and thereby measure cerebral perfusion pressure (mean arterial blood pressure minus the ICP). A rise in ICP or a fall in cranial perfusion pressure (CPP) postoperatively can signal an accumulating postoperative blood clot, hydrocephalus, or an increase in cerebral edema. Early intervention during these complications can improve outcome.

All patients should be placed on maintenance isotonic intravenous fluids (normal saline or Ringer lactate) postoperatively until they are able take adequate fluids orally. There is no place for the use of hypotonic intravenous fluids (e.g., dextrose 5% in water [D_5W]) in the treatment of postoperative brain tumor patients, as these solutions will cause increased cerebral edema with possible grave consequences. Patients should also be maintained on corticosteroids. Patients with low-grade tumors who are neurologically stable can have their steroids weaned over the next week or so if they were not on chronic therapy preoperatively. Patients with malignant tumors should be maintained on a moderate dose of steroids in anticipation of future radiotherapy.

In comparison to surgery on the torso or the extremities, craniotomy is well tolerated from a pain perspective. Both IV/IM and PO opiates and PR/PO acetaminophen are used for postoperative pain control. Some neurosurgeons prefer to use codeine rather than other opiates in the belief that it causes less miosis (diminishing the value of the pupillary exam in the postoperative period), although there is scant support for this in the literature. Once they are taking fluids orally, most patients have their pain controlled with oral formulations of combined codeine and acetaminophen. Skin stitches or staples are removed between 1 and 2 weeks postoperatively, and most centers delay radiotherapy at least until the stitches are removed. In many centers, postoperative imaging with and without intravenous contrast is obtained within 5 days of surgery to determine the amount of residual tumor (Fig. 6-3). Imaging in the period from 5 days to 2 to 3 weeks can show areas of spurious enhancement secondary to postoperative changes.[45,46] Once patients are neurologically stable, and are eating and drinking well, they can be discharged home. A typical hospital stay after craniotomy for supratentorial glioma is 1 to 4 days.

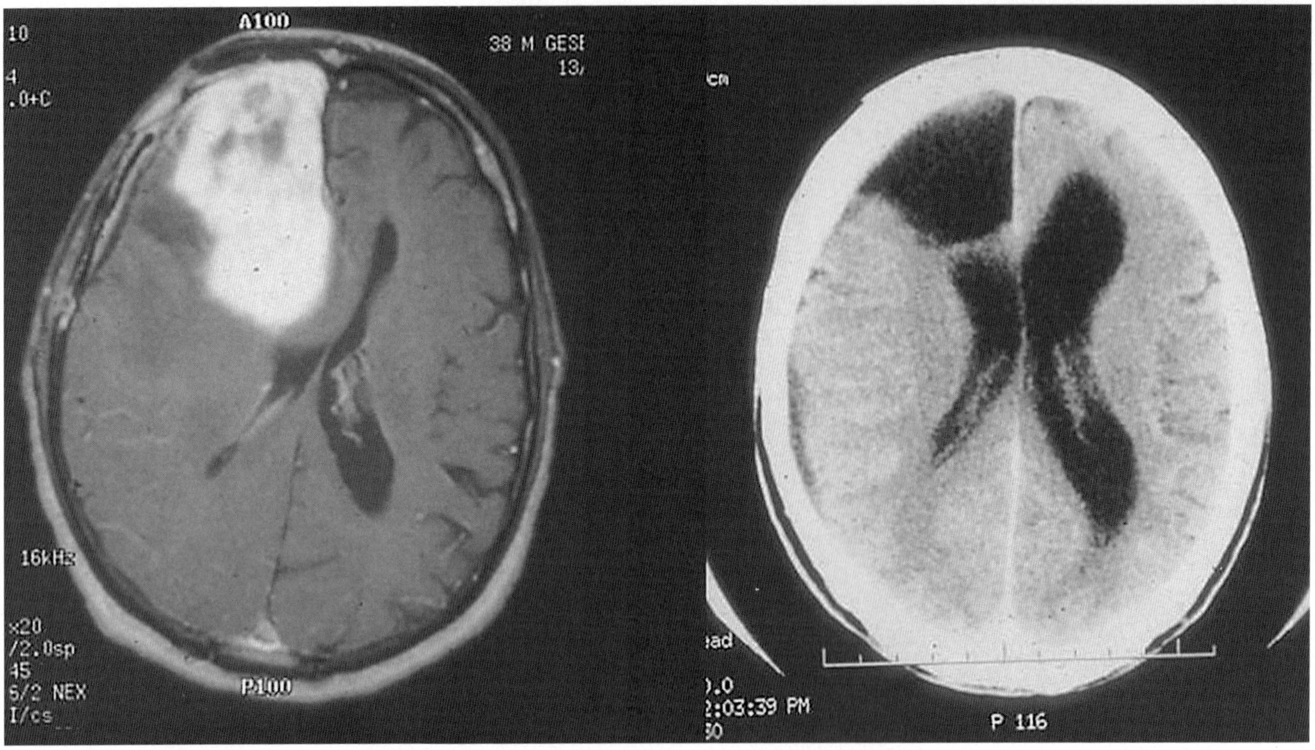

Figure 6-3. The left-hand panel shows a preoperative magnetic resonance imaging (MRI) scan of a large, right frontal, peripherally enhancing lesion that turned out to be glioblastoma multiforme. This lesion underwent gross total resection. The right-hand panel shows a postoperative computerized tomography (CT) scan with contrast, demonstrating that the entire lesion, indeed, has been resected.

At the time of presentation, 20% to 40% of brain tumor patients have experienced a seizure, and another 20% to 45% will ultimately develop seizures.[47] Among brain tumor patients who present with a seizure disorder, the need for anticonvulsant therapy is clear. Anticonvulsants have also been used in the attempt to prevent a first seizure in brain tumor patients. Anticonvulsants are not without risks, including allergic reaction, toxicity, discomfort, expense, inconvenience of serum level monitoring, cognitive impairment, myelosuppression, liver dysfunction, and dermatologic reactions.[47] Side effects of anticonvulsants are much more common in patients with brain tumors, probably as a result of the concomitant administration of other drugs including corticosteroids and antineoplastics. Anticonvulsant drugs (ACDs) also reduce the efficacy of corticosteroids and some antineoplastics. In addition, despite a large body of literature, there is no evidence that prophylactic administration of ACDs can lower the incidence of first seizure in brain tumor patients. This has led the American Academy of Neurology to publish the following guideline: "Prophylactic anticonvulsants should not be used routinely in patients with newly diagnosed brain tumors."[47] Many neurosurgeons administer ACDs to their patients around the time of craniotomy in an attempt to decrease the incidence of perioperative seizures. Randomized trials have either found no efficacy of prophylactic anticonvulsants in the postcraniotomy setting, or have shown a limited duration of benefit (less than 3 days).[47] This has led the American Academy of Neurology to recommend as a guideline that, in patients with a brain tumor and no prior history of seizures, tapering followed by discontinuing ACDs should be done 1 week after surgery.[47]

Complications After Craniotomy

Complications can be broken up into those seen in any patient undergoing general anesthesia, patient-specific complications, and complications seen as a consequence of the specific operation. General complications caused by general anesthesia are rare, but include benign transient events such as postoperative nausea and vomiting, as well as more serious events such as an anaphylactic reaction. Complications specific to the patient are caused by underlying medical disorders, especially of the cardiovascular and respiratory systems. Those patients with significant medical comorbidities should have a preoperative anesthesia consultation in an attempt to minimize their risk of complications and to plan for adequate postoperative monitoring.

Complications have been seen in up to 28% of patients undergoing craniotomy for supratentorial glioma, with mortality rates of 1% to 2% in modern series.[48,49] New postoperative neurologic deficits are seen in 10% to 15% of patients, but are permanent in only approximately 5%.[49] Postoperative neurologic deficits are much more common in patients with preoperative deficits, probably as a result of the location of the tumor. Infections, including wound infections, osteomyelitis, meningitis, and cerebral abscess, can be seen postoperatively, and it is probably possible to decrease their incidence with the administration of perioperative antibiotics that cover skin flora (gram-positives).[50] Infections remote from the surgical site such as bladder infection and pneumonia are also commonly seen. The incidence of deep venous thrombosis (DVT) during the 6 weeks after glioma surgery has been reported to be as high as 60%.[51] Risk factors predisposing to DVT include leg paresis, glioblastoma pathology, large tumor size, use of chemotherapy, age greater than or equal to 60 years, and surgical time greater than 4 hours.[51] Patients at high risk for DVT who do not mobilize quickly after surgery should probably be placed on low-molecular-weight heparin subcutaneously to prevent DVT and pulmonary embolism.

One of the most feared complications of intracranial surgery is the formation of a postoperative intracranial hematoma that compresses the brain, which if left untreated can raise intracranial pressure, leading to the death of the patient. Indeed, intensive postoperative neurologic monitoring is done to allow early diagnosis of this potentially treatable problem. The classic clinical portrait of a postoperative hematoma is that of a patient who initially awakens after surgery with no additional neurologic deficit, but who over a period of hours, or at most days, develops a new neurologic deficit or has a progressive loss of consciousness. These patients need to be treated emergently by resuscitating their CNS (oxygen, mannitol, urgent imaging, intubation, and possibly hyperventilation if there is a severely decreased level of consciousness) followed by emergent craniotomy to remove the clot. Taylor and associates[52] published a report of more than 2000 intracranial procedures and found a postoperative hematoma rate of 2.2%. Importantly, 44 of 50 postoperative clots occurred within the first 6 hours of surgery, and the other 6 occurred more than 24 hours postoperatively. This highly suggests that most patients having glioma surgery only need 6 hours of intensive-care-type postoperative monitoring, after which they can be transferred to a less intense environment such as the neurosurgical ward.

Complication Avoidance

Complication avoidance starts with patient and tumor selection. Extensive operations on elderly, sick patients with severe medical comorbidities are doomed to produce an unsatisfactory outcome. Similarly, attempting a gross total resection of a thalamic LGG in a young, healthy, intact patient is probably inadvisable because of a poor risk-to-benefit ratio. Although opinions differ from center to center, most neurosurgeons know which patients and what tumors they can operate on safely.

Surgical Navigation

There are a number of adjuncts that can be used during glioma surgery to minimize the incidence of complications. Most of these adjuncts assist the surgeon by identifying normal anatomic structures (including the tumor itself), or by determining the neurophysiologic function of a given area of brain. Some authors recommend the use of the operative microscope to better appreciate the difference between the surrounding brain and the tumor.[53] While superficial gliomas are readily identified once the brain is exposed, deeper tumors are not found so easily. Deep lesions can be located through the use of a traditional stereotactic frame or through the use of frameless stereotactic technologies (Fig. 6-4). The use of a "pointer" device allows the surgeon to match the exposed brain in real time to imaging (either MRI or computerized tomography [CT]) obtained preoperatively to determine if they are taking the most direct and/or the safest route through brain to approach the tumor. These devices can also be used to gauge the extent of resection, but they tend to fail over the course of the operation as the brain shifts with the resection, and therefore the real-time brain no longer corresponds with the preoperative imaging. In times past, when these technologies were unavailable, "digging through the brain" looking for a tumor was responsible for considerable morbidity. A small minority of centers now have available the technology to do intraoperative MRI. These centers have special surgical suites that contain an MRI unit, enabling the surgeon to periodically image the patient during the procedure to guide the resection (Fig. 6-5).[54–57] Besides their obvious expense, these systems are troubled by the inability of the surgeon to use ferromagnetic instruments within the magnetic field.

A more economical alternative to intraoperative MRI/CT is the use of intraoperative ultrasonography for tumor localization.[58] Intraoperative ultrasonography is available in most operating rooms and is technically straightforward. The advantage of ultrasonography over frameless stereotaxy is that the latter is based on preoperative imaging, and if the brain shifts during surgery, the navigation information can be incorrect. Ultrasonography, in contrast, offers real-time information in spite of brain shift. Ultrasonography remains a useful

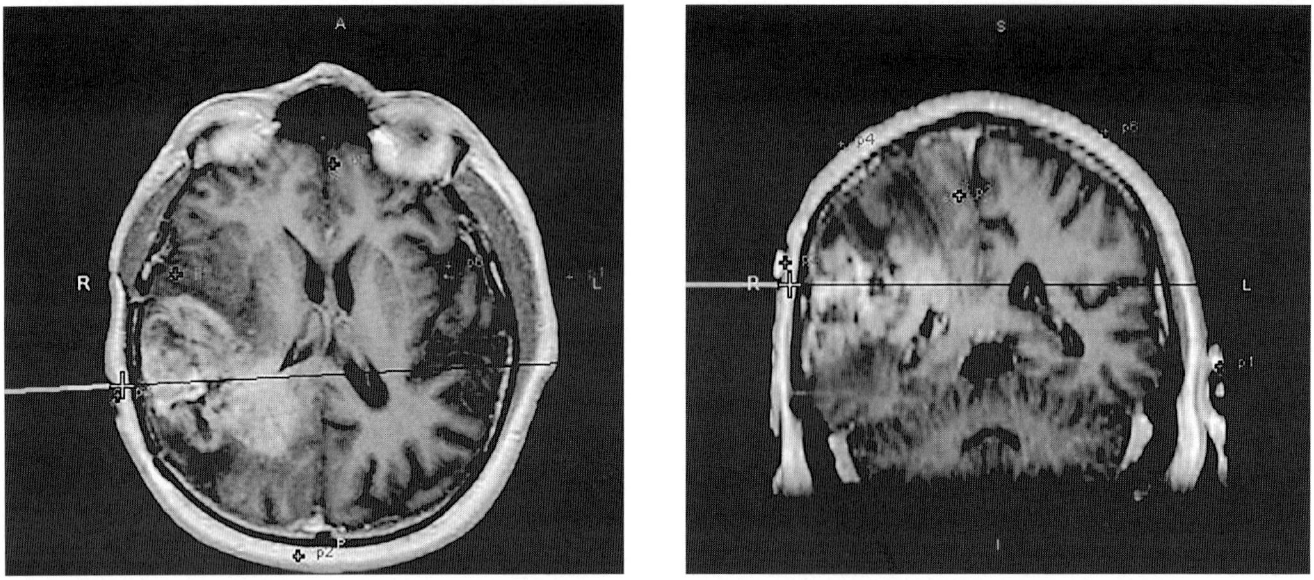

Figure 6-4 (PLATE 35). In-house (i.e., not commercially available) surgical navigation system (frameless stereotaxy) used to localize a recurrent tumor prior to the scalp incision. This was done to see if the previous scalp and/or bone flap would require revision to access the tumor. The navigation system was also used during the tumor resection. The end of the pointer tool in the surgeon's hand is demonstrated on the screen as the tip of the line.

tool for localizing subcortical tumors in those cases where frameless stereotaxy is not used.

Functional Magnetic Resonance Imaging

In addition to anatomic adjuncts, there are also neurophysiologic adjuncts that attempt to identify the function of peritumoral brain, or, alternatively, to identify the location of specific, important brain functions (e.g., language or hand function). A noninvasive technique for the identification of functional cortical areas and their relation to the tumor is the use of functional MRI. This robust and now more commonly used technique is

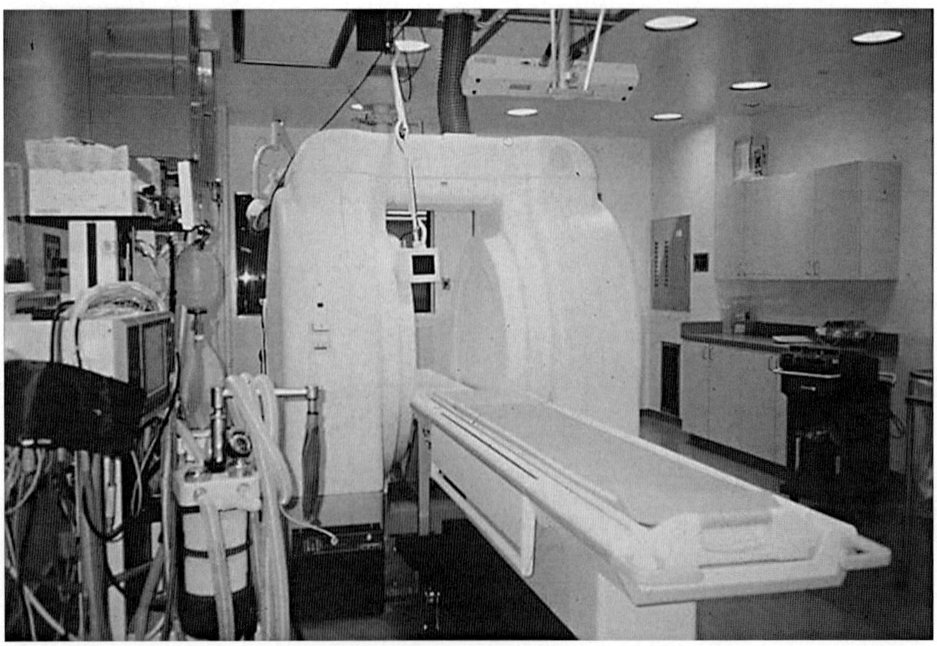

Figure 6-5. Example of an intraoperative MRI unit. This is the first iteration of the intraoperative MRI used at the Toronto Western Hospital from 1996 to 2003.

excellent at identifying language and motor areas, and can show their relationships in terms of both direction and distance from the tumor (Fig. 6-6).[53] Preoperative identification of cortex important for language function through the use of functional MRI can be particularly valuable in patients who might not be left-hemisphere dominant (i.e., who are left-handed patients). Functional MRI can be particularly powerful when married to intraoperative frameless stereotactic neuronavigation devices as outlined above (see "Surgical Navigation"). With the brain exposed and the patient under general anesthesia, cortical areas important for movement (primary motor

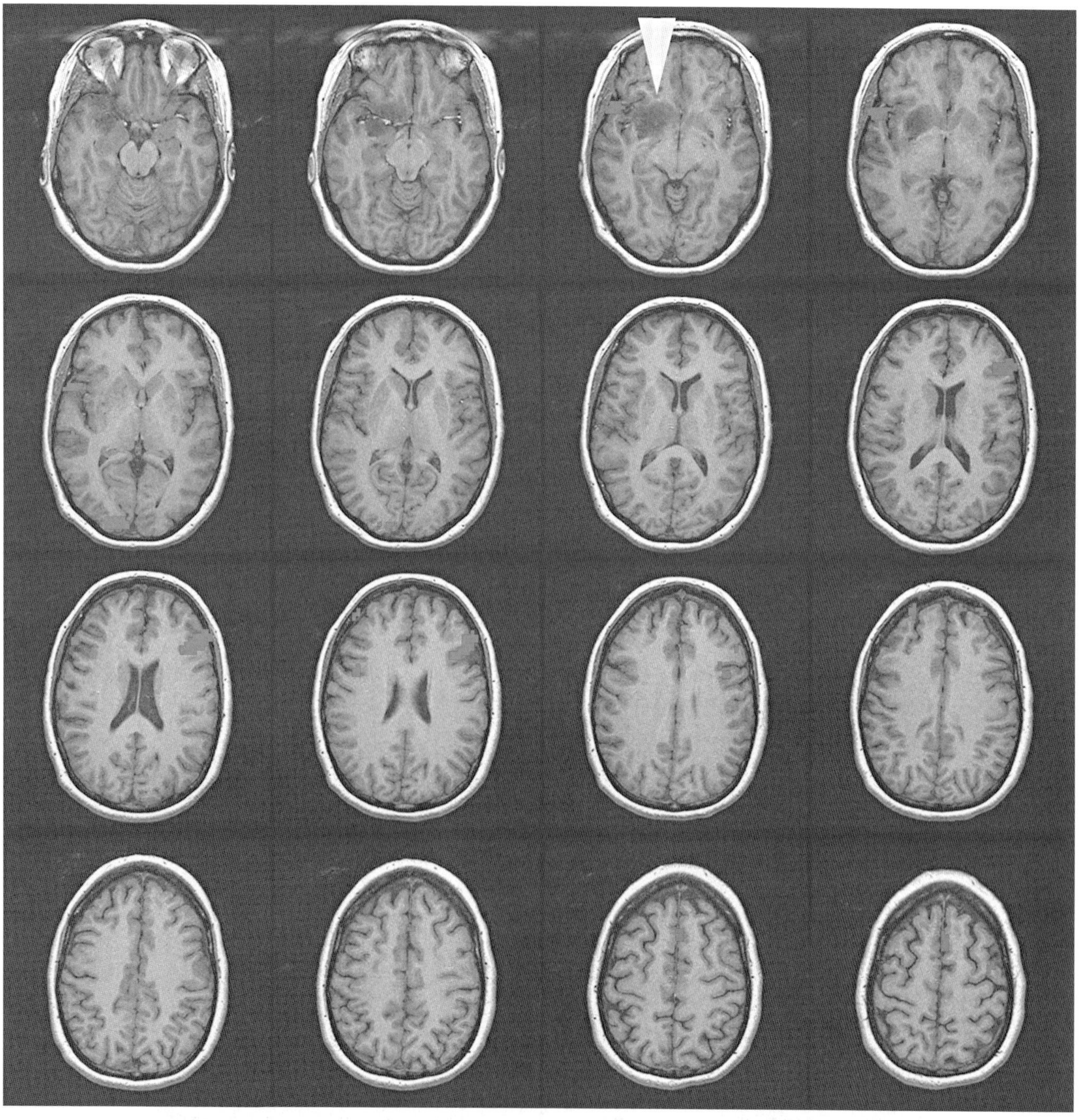

Figure 6-6 (PLATE 36). A 51-year-old left-handed lady presented with seizures and a right-sided perisylvian low-grade glioma (see arrowhead). Functional MRI in this left-handed patient revealed that her speech center was located in her left frontal lobe, thereby increasing the surgeon's confidence that this lesion could be safely resected without causing aphasia.

cortex) can be identified using somatosensory-evoked potentials (SSEPs) and motor-evoked potentials (MEPs). These electrical tests allow for the identification of sensory and motor areas through direct excitation of neural elements, followed by monitoring the effects of the stimulation (i.e., discharge of the primary sensory cortex for the arm after electrical stimulation of the median nerve at the wrist). An effective test for the intraoperative identification of speech cortex in a patient under general anesthesia has not yet been developed.

Awake Craniotomy

The gold standard for neurophysiologic monitoring during glioma surgery is use of the so-called awake craniotomy technique.[49,59–64] In this technique, the patient has a craniotomy under local anesthetic, with the preservation of consciousness. The technique is well tolerated by almost all brain tumor patients and may have a better postoperative side-effect profile with regards to pain, nausea, and vomiting as compared to traditional craniotomy under general anesthesia.[65,66] After the scalp, skull, and dura are opened, the exposed brain is stimulated with an electric current (Fig. 6-7). The awake patient describes phenomena that they feel, and the contralateral limbs are observed for movement. Those areas identified as causing movement during stimulation (usually the primary motor area) are avoided during the tumor resection. Mapping of the language cortex is done by testing the patient's language (i.e., asking them to name various objects) while simultaneously moving a stimulator over the exposed cortex. When the areas of cortex vital for language are stimulated, the speech is

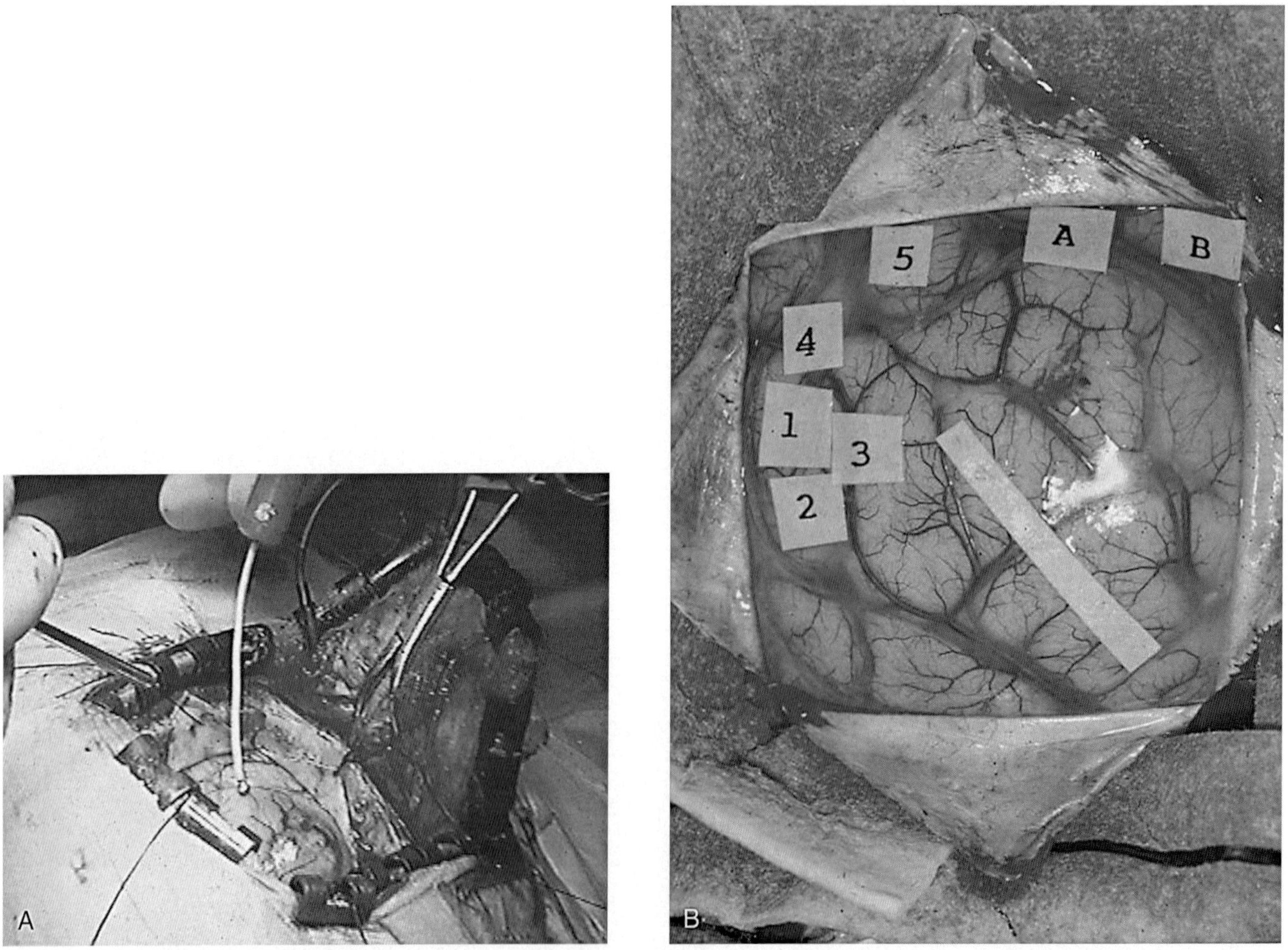

Figure 6-7. (A) During an awake craniotomy, the surface of the exposed brain is stimulated with an electrical stimulator. During this time, the patient undergoes neurophysiologic testing to detect abnormalities of speech, motor function, and sensory function. For example, if the patient experiences speech arrest during stimulation, that cortical site is likely important for speech function. (B) Cortical sites identified as subserving important neurologic functions are labeled with small, sterile paper tickets so that they can be avoided during the tumor resection.

affected, most commonly by speech arrest. In experienced hands, neurologically intact brain tumor patients uncommonly have a new, permanent postoperative neurologic deficit after tumor resection during an awake craniotomy.[49]

In many centers, anatomic and neurophysiologic techniques are used in combination to further increase the safety of surgery, minimize the size of the operative site, and, in some cases, safely maximize the extent of resection. Common examples would be an awake craniotomy using a frameless stereotaxy neuronavigational device or, more recently, awake craniotomy in the intraoperative MR unit. The latter example is a very powerful technique that gives the surgeon real-time, accurate information on both anatomy and physiology.

▶ STEREOTACTIC BRAIN TUMOR BIOPSY

Stereotactic brain biopsy (SBB) differs from craniotomy in that only a very small piece of the tumor is removed in order to make a diagnosis. In most brain tumor cases, stereotactic brain biopsy has no therapeutic effect. SBB is chosen over craniotomy when the patient is too old, or too infirm for a craniotomy, or the lesion is too deep, diffuse, multiple, or of uncertain histology. Patients who likely harbor a histology that will not benefit from cytoreduction (e.g., primary CNS lymphoma) are also excellent candidates for SBB. While imaging alone can highly suggest a histologic diagnosis, it lacks specificity. In one series of 100 consecutive stereotactic biopsies, the initial preoperative diagnosis was wrong in 26 cases. Tumors with the imaging characteristics of a glioblastoma were instead due to other conditions, including brain abscess, lymphoma, metastatic tumor, and an infarct.[67] This study was performed in the CT scanning era, however, and modern MRI would undoubtedly decrease these numbers, but not reduce them to zero.

Some surgeons are reluctant to offer SBB to a patient with very high intracranial pressure, as even a small intraoperative or postoperative hemorrhage could tip the patient's intracranial pressure volume curve into the critical zone, with resultant brain herniation and death. Tumors that are very superficial (cortical or subpial) may also be dangerous for stereotactic biopsy because of the proximity of the leptomeningeal vessels.

SBB is usually done under local anesthetic, but rarely can be done under general anesthesia because of patient delirium or extreme patient anxiety. A stereotactic frame is placed over and around the patient's head. After the injection of local anesthetic, the frame is then screwed to the patient's skull using sharp pins (Fig. 6-8). This is done to fix the frame in relation to the patient's head and, therefore, in relation to the brain tumor. Placement of the frame is the most uncomfortable portion of the procedure, and patients can be reassured once it is in place that the rest of the procedure is much less uncomfortable. Frame in place, the patient is subject to some cross-sectional imaging (CT or MRI) to visualize the tumor and surrounding important intracranial contents in relation to the frame. Various measurements are made using frame-specific software after the location for the biopsy within the tumor is chosen. The patient is then taken from the radiology department to the operating room.

In the operating room, the adjustable parts of the stereotactic frame are set to the measurements provided by the software. The scalp is frozen with local anesthetic and then incised, followed by a small twist burr hole in the skull. The stereotactic biopsy needle is then passed through the burr hole into the brain along the trajectory dictated by the stereotactic frame to the depth indicated by the computer. The biopsy needle, held by the frame and passed to the calculated depth will be within the tumor. One or more biopsies are taken and sent for quick section diagnosis. If the pathologist returns a diagnosis of "lesional tissue," regardless of the actual diagnosis, the procedure is over. If the quick section diagnosis comes back "normal or reactive brain," the settings on the stereotactic brain are triple checked, and the biopsy is repeated. The diagnostic success rate of SBB in cases of brain tumor is very high (> 90%), but it falls sharply in immunocompromised patients and in patients with nonenhancing lesions or inflammatory pathologies. Complications of SBB include a death or major complication rate of up to 2%, with other complications occurring in another 4% of patients.[68] Complications include exacerbation of a neurologic deficit, a new neurologic deficit, infection (meningitis, brain abscess), seizures, cerebrospinal fluid leak, pin-site infection, tumor seeding, and a postoperative intracerebral hematoma.[69] Postoperatively patients are monitored through serial neurologic exams. Most patients are able to go home the next day. In some centers, SBB is a day surgery procedure.[70] Final pathology results are discussed with the patient at a followup appointment 1 to 2 weeks after the operation and appropriate adjunctive therapy, radiation or chemotherapy, is arranged. In some centers, neurosurgeons are performing stereotactic biopsy of brain tumors using frameless neuronavigation systems rather than using a traditional frame that is bolted to the skull. This is a more recently developed technique, and time will tell if the success rate and complications are comparable to or better than biopsy using a standard frame.

Noninvasive Tissue Diagnosis

Magnetic resonance spectroscopy is being developed as a noninvasive alternative to stereotactic biopsy for determining the histology of brain tumors. For example, MR

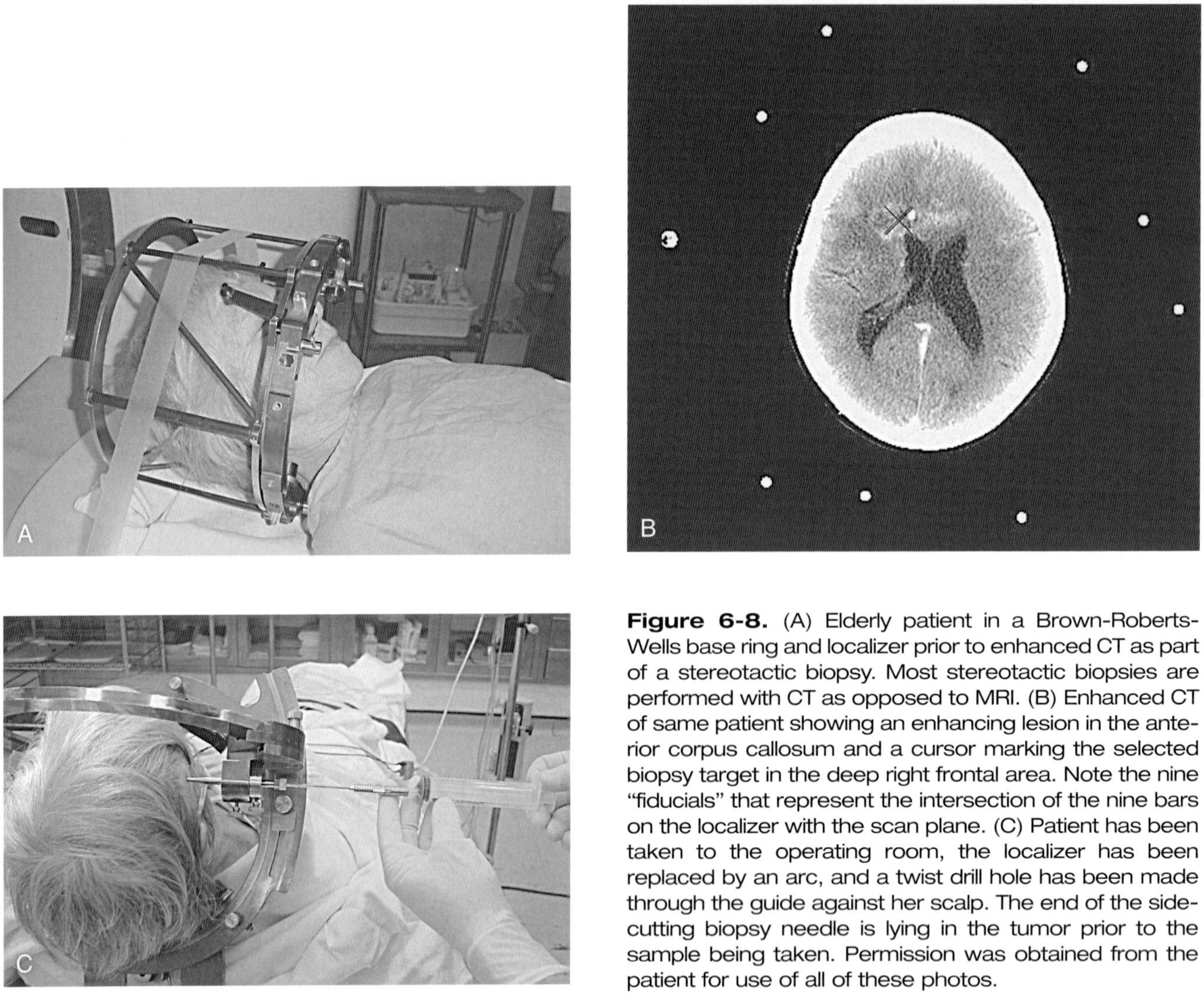

Figure 6-8. (A) Elderly patient in a Brown-Roberts-Wells base ring and localizer prior to enhanced CT as part of a stereotactic biopsy. Most stereotactic biopsies are performed with CT as opposed to MRI. (B) Enhanced CT of same patient showing an enhancing lesion in the anterior corpus callosum and a cursor marking the selected biopsy target in the deep right frontal area. Note the nine "fiducials" that represent the intersection of the nine bars on the localizer with the scan plane. (C) Patient has been taken to the operating room, the localizer has been replaced by an arc, and a twist drill hole has been made through the guide against her scalp. The end of the side-cutting biopsy needle is lying in the tumor prior to the sample being taken. Permission was obtained from the patient for use of all of these photos.

spectroscopy has been used as a preliminary tool to differentiate primary CNS lymphoma from glioma.[71] In some centers, MR spectroscopy has become part of the routine imaging assessment of intracranial mass lesions, and has been shown to be of value in addition to regular MRI.[72] Currently, there are few cases where MR spectroscopy has replaced stereotactic biopsy because of MR spectroscopy's lack of specificity. MR spectroscopy is, however, an evolving technology, and we believe that it, or a similar noninvasive technology, will be developed in the not too distant future to allow noninvasive preoperative accurate prediction of brain tumor histology. In spite of this, stereotactic biopsy will likely remain in use. Although histology was all that was necessary for planning adjuvant treatments in the past, in the future adjuvant therapies for glioma patients will be chosen based on molecular markers such as gene expression profiles or genetic changes (i.e., loss of heterozygosity [LOH] on chromosomes 1p and 19q in oligodendrogliomas), which means that tissue is likely to be required for the foreseeable future.[73,74]

▶ MISCELLANEOUS SURGICAL INTERVENTIONS IN GLIOMA PATIENTS

Cerebrospinal Fluid Diversion

Although hydrocephalus is rarely seen at the time of presentation in adult patients with supratentorial gliomas, it is commonly seen in brainstem tumors, and is occasionally observed in thalamic or cerebellar gliomas. These latter groups are, of course, more commonly seen in children. Stenosis or occlusion of the aqueduct is particularly common with so-called periaqueductal midbrain tumors. In many cases where hydrocephalus is present, it will resolve with resection of the tumor. Should resection of the tumor fail to resolve the hydrocephalus, or should the tumor be in a location difficult or impossible to resect (i.e., the dorsum of the midbrain), and if the patient has a reasonable KPS and a reasonable prognosis, the hydrocephalus should be treated. Treatment options include third ventriculostomy in cases of noncommunicating hydrocephalus, and ventriculoperitoneal shunt in almost all cases of hydrocephalus. There is a very small risk of disseminating a CNS malignancy with a ventriculoperitoneal shunt. A small percentage of glioma patients will also develop hydrocephalus after craniotomy, particularly if the ventricular system has been entered during surgery.[75] Postsurgical hydrocephalus is an uncommon but treatable entity to consider in a glioma patient who undergoes deterioration late after surgery. A final group of patients present with communicating hydrocephalus because of diffuse leptomeningeal dissemination of their glioma. These patients are usually preterminal, and treatment of their hydrocephalus is rarely advisable.

Cerebrospinal Fluid Access

As well as diverting CSF flow in the treatment of hydrocephalus, it is necessary, on occasion, to have repeated access to the CSF for the administration of intrathecal chemotherapy. This is done to treat tumors that have disseminated through the CSF axis, so-called leptomeningeal gliomatosis. Clinically, this manifests as increased intracranial pressure, seizures, and multiple cranial neuropathies. This clinical picture is only rarely seen in glioma patients, but is not uncommon in patients with systemic malignancies metastatic to the CNS (so-called neoplastic meningitis). As repeated lumbar puncture for intrathecal chemotherapy is painful and inconvenient, neurosurgeons can implant a device called an Ommaya reservoir in which a reservoir placed subcutaneously in the scalp is connected to a catheter whose tip lies in the lateral ventricle. Successful implantation of an Ommaya reservoir makes repeated CSF access almost trivial, while minimizing patient suffering. Current treatment of gliomas with intrathecal therapy is mostly palliative—to alleviate or arrest cranial neuropathies—or investigational in nature.

Brachytherapy

Brachytherapy has been used in some centers as a treatment for gliomas, both at the time of the initial presentation, as well as at tumor recurrence. This technique involves the temporary (high-activity implant) or, in some cases, permanent (low-activity implant) surgical implantation of a radiation source into the tumor bed, either at the time of open resection or by stereotactic methods. Brachytherapy is commonly combined with standard external beam radiotherapy, allowing extremely large doses of more than 100 Gy to be delivered to the tumor. In spite of these massive radiation doses, two randomized, prospective, controlled trials of brachytherapy in adult patients with supratentorial malignant gliomas treated at the time of the initial presentation showed no survival benefit to the brachytherapy arm.[76,77] The role of brachytherapy in the treatment of gliomas at the time of recurrence is less well defined, and is still used in some centers. As a consequence of the recent popularity of the noninvasive alternative, stereotactic radiosurgery, for which results are similar to brachytherapy, brachytherapy is used less commonly these days.

Intratumoral Chemotherapy

After removing all of the grossly visible disease that can be safely resected, the neurosurgeon is faced with a cavity in the brain, the walls of which presumably contain normal brain cells as well as infiltrating glioma cells. Those infiltrating cells are the target of postoperative radiotherapy and chemotherapy. Recently, strategies have been developed to apply local therapies at the time of surgery targeted at these infiltrating cells. The most well-known of these strategies is a chemotherapy impregnated polymer, which comes in the form of wafers (carmustine [Gliadel]). These wafers are used to line the resection cavity and are designed to slowly leak out chemotherapy over time. There have been three randomized trials of Gliadel in the treatment of gliomas, two at the time of initial surgery and one in patients with recurrent tumors. Westphal and associates[78] conducted a placebo-controlled, multicenter, double-blind, randomized trial of Gliadel for the initial treatment of malignant gliomas. They found that the median survival in the Gliadel arm was 13.9 months compared with 11.6 months in the placebo arm ($p = 0.03$).[78] There were some methodological problems with the trial as there was a slight excess of glioblastomas in the placebo arm (88% vs. 84%), and some patients who were enrolled in the study were not within the age range specified for inclusion in the trial. Valtonen and associates[79] published a small trial of 32 patients who were randomized at the time of initial surgery for adult supratentorial malignant glioma to either Gliadel or a placebo. This trial was designed to enroll 100 patients, but the authors could not obtain enough Gliadel, causing the trial to be terminated. They found a median survival of 58.1 weeks in the Gliadel arm, versus 39.9 weeks in the placebo arm ($p = 0.012$). However, there was an imbalance in the trial in that 16 of 16 patients in the placebo arm had glioblastoma multiforme, while only 11 of 16 in the Gliadel arm had glioblastoma multiforme. Brem and associates[80] conducted a randomized trial of 222 patients with recurrent malignant gliomas who were randomized to either Gliadel or placebo. The median survival in the Gliadel arm was 31 weeks, versus 23 weeks in the placebo arm ($p = 0.006$). Although these three trials are not perfect, the fact that all three show benefit to patients receiving Gliadel as opposed to placebo certainly suggests that in some cases Gliadel may be beneficial. Detractors of Gliadel point out the not inconsiderable cost of the treatment, as well as the modest increase in median survival (around 2 months). This type of technology is potentially very exciting and perhaps, when combined with more effective chemotherapeutics, will form part of the standard treatment of malignant gliomas.

▶ LOW-GRADE GLIOMA

Prognostic factors including age, histology, and presentation are much more important than surgical resection in predicting outcome for patients with LGG. However, these variables are fixed. As discussed above for malignant gliomas, the roles of surgery in the treatment of LGG—to provide a tissue diagnosis and to relieve neurologic deficits secondary to mass effect—are well accepted by the neuro-oncology community.[81] Although many neurosurgeons continue to advise craniotomy and resection of LGGs, there are no prospective, randomized trials to support this. There are numerous papers on the topic, both refuting and supporting the role that resection of adult LGG plays in increasing overall survival. As a result of the inadequacy of the available evidence, the truth remains unknown.[82–89] Consequently, there is a broad spectrum of practice, with some surgeons removing most LGGs, whereas others only obtain a biopsy in most cases of adult LGG. A third set of surgeons takes each case on its own merit, resecting some, biopsying others,[81] and following some with imaging without establishing a tissue diagnosis (Fig. 6-9).

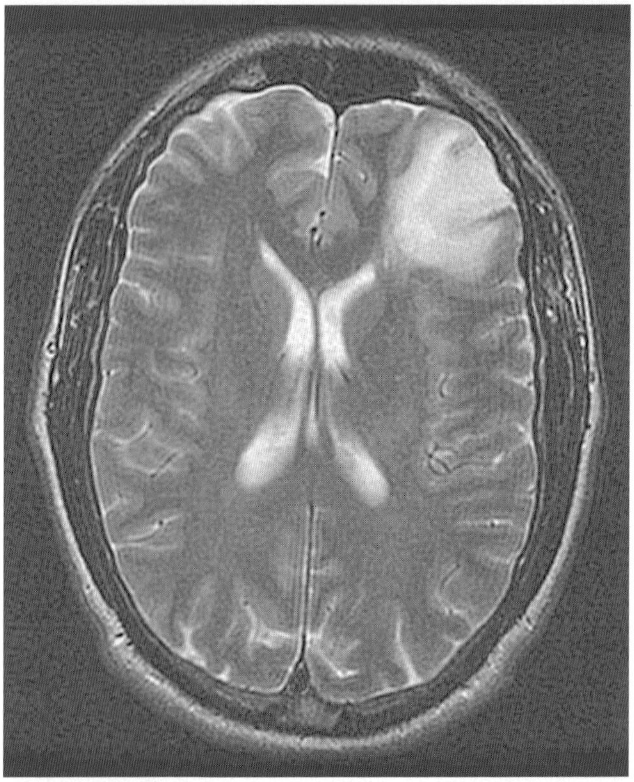

Figure 6-9. T_2-weighted MRI of a man in his thirties presenting with a single seizure. Imaging shows a typical left frontal low-grade glioma. There was no enhancement on T_1-weighted MRI. The tumor is very accessible surgically, but in this situation one could use the "wait and see" approach with periodic MRI. Intervention would be reserved for when the tumor grows and/or shows enhancement.

A randomized European Organization of Research and Treatment of Cancer (EORTC) trial, which had some study design limitations, showed that both the location and the size of a LGG are predictive of both overall and progression-free survival, with the best prognosis seen in young patients with unifocal tumors less than 3 cm in diameter that are situated away from the midline.[90] Other investigators have reported that larger tumors behave differently, have a poorer prognosis, and/or have a greater tendency toward malignant evolution.[91]

A recent randomized trial of adults with supratentorial LGG compared radiation at the time of diagnosis to radiation at the time of clinical progression; radiation at the time of diagnosis showed some benefit in terms of progression-free survival, but no benefit in terms of overall survival.[92] Some neurosurgeons cite this article as additional proof that deferred treatment is an acceptable initial approach to young patients with a LGG. Because of earlier diagnoses, some studies are now quoting median survivals greater than 10 years for patients with LGG, making it hard to justify doing a biopsy or surgery early on and subjecting the patient to the risk, albeit small, of a neurologic deficit that will be with them for a decade (Fig. 6-10). With median survivals over a decade being reported, some clinicians are reluctant to offer upfront biopsy and treatment because of the side effects of radiation therapy, which can worsen and accumulate with time. Long-term survivors of CNS radiotherapy are at risk for neurocognitive impairment, hypothalamic–pituitary dysfunction, radiation necrosis, and secondary neoplasms.[93] It has been argued that deferring treatment minimizes these risks. If a tumor chosen for deferred treatment should show rapid clinical or radiological progression, it is still feasible to proceed with biopsy or craniotomy followed by radiotherapy. On the converse side, a young patient rendered aphasic after surgery for a LGG is in an irreversible situation.

The sort of patient typically chosen for deferred treatment is an individual younger than age 40 years who presents with a seizure, has no deficits or minimal

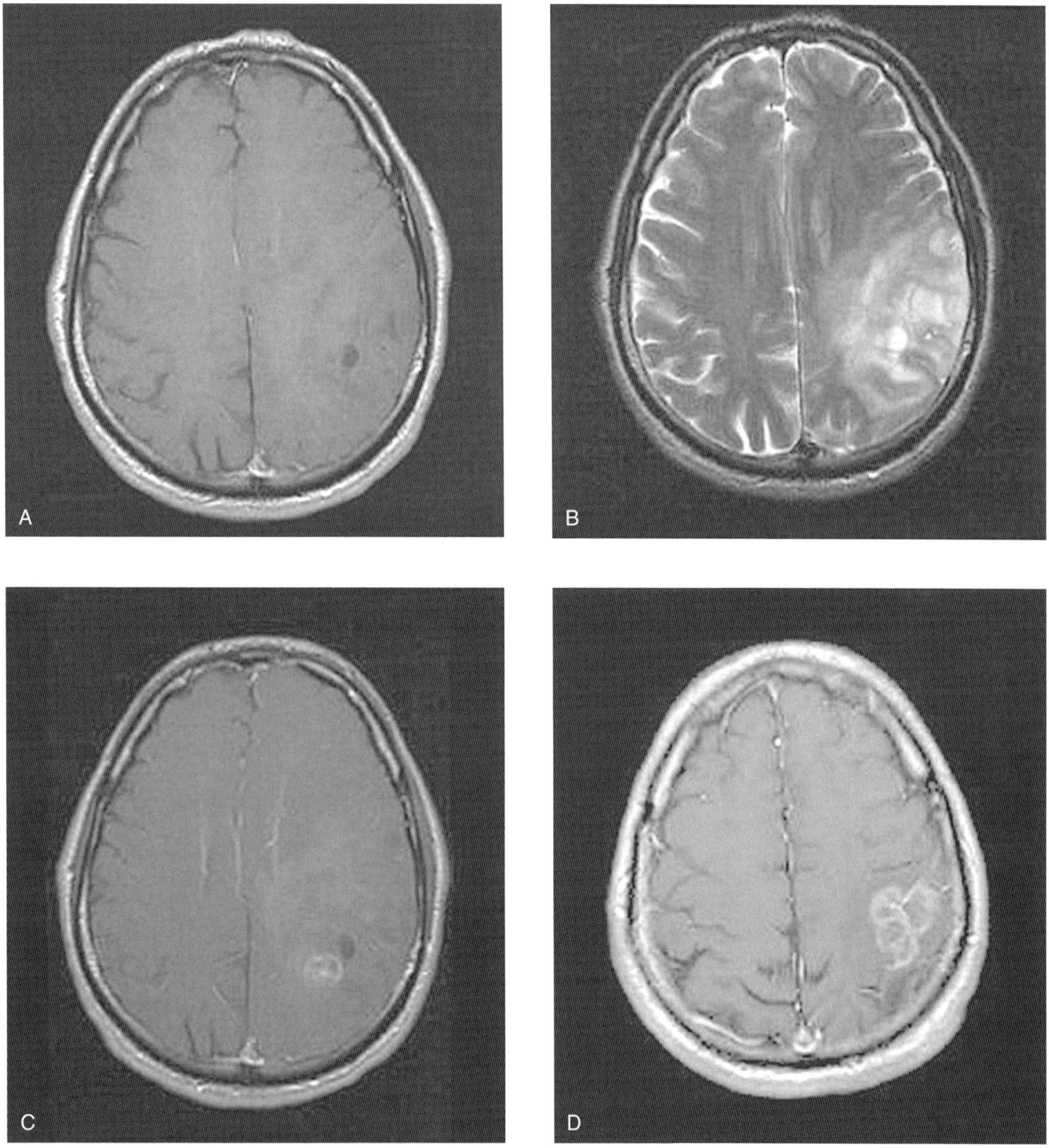

Figure 6-10. (A) T_1 axial postgadolinium MRI of a 40-year-old man who has been followed with yearly MRI after presenting with a seizure 6 years prior. MRIs have remained stable as has the patient. (B) T_2 axial image. (C) Axial T_1 postgadolinium MRI of same patient 6 years later showing asymptomatic progression 12 years after initial seizure. Stereotactic biopsy revealed an anaplastic oligodendroglioma. Treatment consisted of fractionated radiation and chemotherapy with temozolomide. (D) Axial T_1 postgadolinium MRI 2 years later showing progression. The patient was asymptomatic, so reoperation was not recommended; instead, treatment with a novel chemotherapeutic regimen was initiated.

neurologic deficits, no enhancement on imaging, and minimal or no mass effect from the lesion.[81] One risk of deferred treatment is making the diagnosis of LGG based on imaging when the pathology is actually something else (e.g., a higher-grade glial tumor, a nonglial neoplasm, or even a nonneoplastic pathology such as an infarct or demyelination). The incidence of wrong diagnosis in modern series probably ranges from 5% to 10% of cases, but only a small proportion of those suffer any harm as a result of deferring their diagnosis and treatment. Although enhancement is good evidence of malignancy in a supratentorial glioma, in one publication, nonenhancing adult supratentorial gliomas were malignant in up to 30% of cases, especially in older adults.[94] Conversely, a small percentage (10%–15%) of true adult LGGs will enhance on imaging, and these must be biopsied at a minimum to rule out a more aggressive tumor requiring upfront treatment.[85] These uncertainties with an imaging diagnosis of LGG have led some authors to conclude that all tumors with an imaging diagnosis of LGG should be biopsied up front. Authors on the other side of the argument suggest that those tumors that are not LGG will quickly show a different biologic behavior and declare themselves and that a short delay in diagnosis is not harmful to the patient. As a result of this controversy, deferring treatment is a standard of practice in some centers, but has been described as "unjustifiable" by other groups.[69]

Even if deferred treatment is the initial choice of the treating clinicians, surgery will eventually become necessary when the patient's clinical status deteriorates, or when the lesion is shown to grow or acquire enhancement on imaging (Table 6-2). These three events are characteristic of malignant progression of the tumor, a switch in its biology from LGG to either an anaplastic tumor or glioblastoma multiforme. Almost all LGGs will eventually progress to a more malignant biology if observed over time.

Cytoreductive surgery in patients with mass effect and either increased intracranial pressure or a focal neurologic deficit often results in some recovery, if the tumor is not located very deep or in eloquent cortex. Removal of tumor may also decrease the amount of vasogenic edema, thereby decreasing the patient's reliance on steroids and minimizing their well-known side effects. Lesionectomy (taking out the tumor) with or without electrocorticography decreases the number of seizures and/or the dosage of anticonvulsant medications in patients with a LGG and chronic epilepsy.

The controversial issue in the surgery of LGG is whether or not cytoreductive surgery increases time to progression, overall survival, and/or quality of life. A number of articles support and refute the value of cytoreductive surgery, but there are no randomized, prospective trials, so the truth remains unknown.[81,83,86,87,95–101] There is an appealing, logical argument that extent of resection (cytoreductive surgery) should delay the time to progression in cases of LGG. A LGG progresses to a more malignant glioma by the random acquisition of additional genetic abnormalities ("hits") in one cell of the tumor. That cell subsequently undergoes clonal expansion, followed by additional genetic hits until it eventually becomes a glioblastoma. By reducing the number of cells in the tumor (e.g., from 9×10^9 cells to 1×10^9 cells), it could be argued that one decreases the chance of one cell accumulating the additional genetic abnormalities needed to become a malignant neoplasm. There is further support for this argument in that recent randomized trials showed a worse prognosis for larger LGG as compared to smaller ones.[90,92] What is not apparent from this trial data is whether the tumors that were larger preoperatively had a more malignant biology *ab initio*, and whether one can improve the patient's prognosis by leaving a small postoperative residual. As there is some support in the literature for cytoreduction, many surgeons exercise the practice option of removing as much LGG as can be done safely at the time of surgery. Safety and extent of resection can be increased through the use of anatomic and physiologic adjuncts as described above, including modern frameless neuronavigational devices and awake craniotomy with neurophysiologic monitoring.[49,59] Surgery for low-grade fibrillary astrocytomas is not a curative operation, and there is no reason to subject a patient to a planned neurologic deficit in the pursuit of a complete resection.

▶ TABLE 6-2. REASONS TO TREAT LOW-GRADE GLIOMA AGGRESSIVELY AB INITIO

Any enhancement on imaging
Significant mass effect on imaging
Increased intracranial pressure/papilledema
Focal neurologic deficit
Age older than 40 years
Lesion crossing the midline
Large lesion (> 3–5 cm in maximal diameter)

▶ PEDIATRIC GLIOMAS

Although the value of extent of resection in the treatment of adult gliomas has been highly debated, it is well accepted for most pediatric low- and high-grade gliomas.[102] In particular, resection of pediatric pilocytic astrocytomas, which have a completely distinct biology, is definitely of benefit to the child in most cases.[81] Indeed 20-year survivals of greater than 90% are not uncommon in pediatric pilocytic astrocytoma, and these tumors should only very rarely be irradiated as this predisposes them to malignant degeneration.[103]

Postoperative imaging within 48 hours of surgery in order to minimize postsurgical enhancement should be undertaken in most cases. In some children, a postoperative residual may be an indication for a return to the operating room to complete the resection. In other cases (e.g., pilocytic astrocytoma) residual tumor may not need to be treated at all, just observed with serial imaging. The importance of surgical resection in the treatment of pediatric gliomas is supported by the toxicity of radiation to the developing nervous system. Furthermore, many pediatric gliomas (especially pilocytic astrocytomas) almost never undergo malignant progression in the absence of radiotherapy, further increasing the value of reoperation for residual tumor.[103] Techniques for stereotactic biopsy and craniotomy for childhood gliomas are similar to the treatment of adult lesions, with modifications for the fragility of the child, especially younger children.[102]

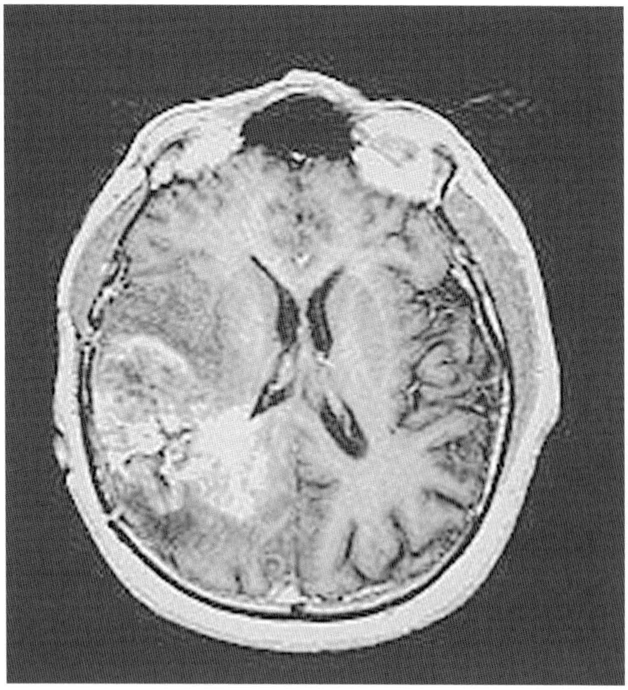

Figure 6-11. T_1 axial gadolinium-enhanced MRI of a 54-year-old man with progressive left hemiparesis 1 year after initial surgery and radiation and two chemotherapy regimens for right parietal glioblastoma. Reoperation was offered (a) because the recurrence is focal; (b) because the interval from initial surgery is favorable; (c) to decrease mass effect; (d) to improve symptoms; and (e) to prolong life for further chemotherapy.

▶ RECURRENT GLIOMAS

In almost every case, a malignant glioma will recur and will eventually lead to the death of the patient. There may be a role for reoperation in some patients at the time of recurrence. Older patients with a diffuse recurrence and a low KPS are unlikely to benefit from repeat surgery. Young patients with a focal recurrence, high KPS, and a long interval since their last surgery are more likely to receive a meaningful benefit from a second craniotomy.[104] Reoperation may be indicated when the volume of recurrent tumor is significant enough to cause increased intracranial pressure and/or focal neurologic deficit (Fig. 6-11).[104] Most surgeons would be unwilling to offer reoperation unless it is to be followed by some sort of adjuvant therapy, or experimental protocol, because reoperation in isolation is not very effective. Reirradiation using stereotactic methods (radiosurgery) or brachytherapy may be appropriate in some patients after reoperation. Similar to the surgical approach to the initial treatment of gliomas, the indications can be broken down into diagnostic, neurologic, and oncologic.

When a patient with a treated LGG returns with a recurrent mass lesion on imaging, it is not always clear whether the new imaging abnormality represents regrowth of the LGG or progression of the LGG to a more malignant histology, such as anaplastic astrocytoma or glioblastoma multiforme. In cases such as this, a histologic diagnosis, either at the time of resection or by stereotactic biopsy, may be helpful in planning future treatment.

Similarly, when a patient with a glioma (either low-grade or malignant) returns with a recurrent ring-enhancing mass after having received radiotherapy, it is not clear whether the new lesion is recurrent tumor, radiation necrosis, a mixture of both, or a radiation-induced tumor (rare because of the short survival of glioblastoma patients). Radiation necrosis is much more common following focused radiation such as brachytherapy or stereotactic radiation.[105] When it occurs, it has most commonly been a combination of radiation necrosis and recurrent tumor; that is, pure radiation necrosis is uncommon. Various imaging techniques have attempted to distinguish between radiation necrosis and recurrent tumor, but in most studies they lack specificity. The nature of the mass lesion can be reliably determined by stereotactic biopsy, and the histology is predictive of future survival (better survival with radiation necrosis).[106] The specific histology may also guide treatment, as additional radiation (e.g., radiosurgery) is probably not a good treatment for radiation necrosis, although it may help in cases of recurrent tumor.

Patients likely to benefit from reoperation have large, focal tumors that are causing generalized or focal neurologic deficits. Surgery is an excellent method to

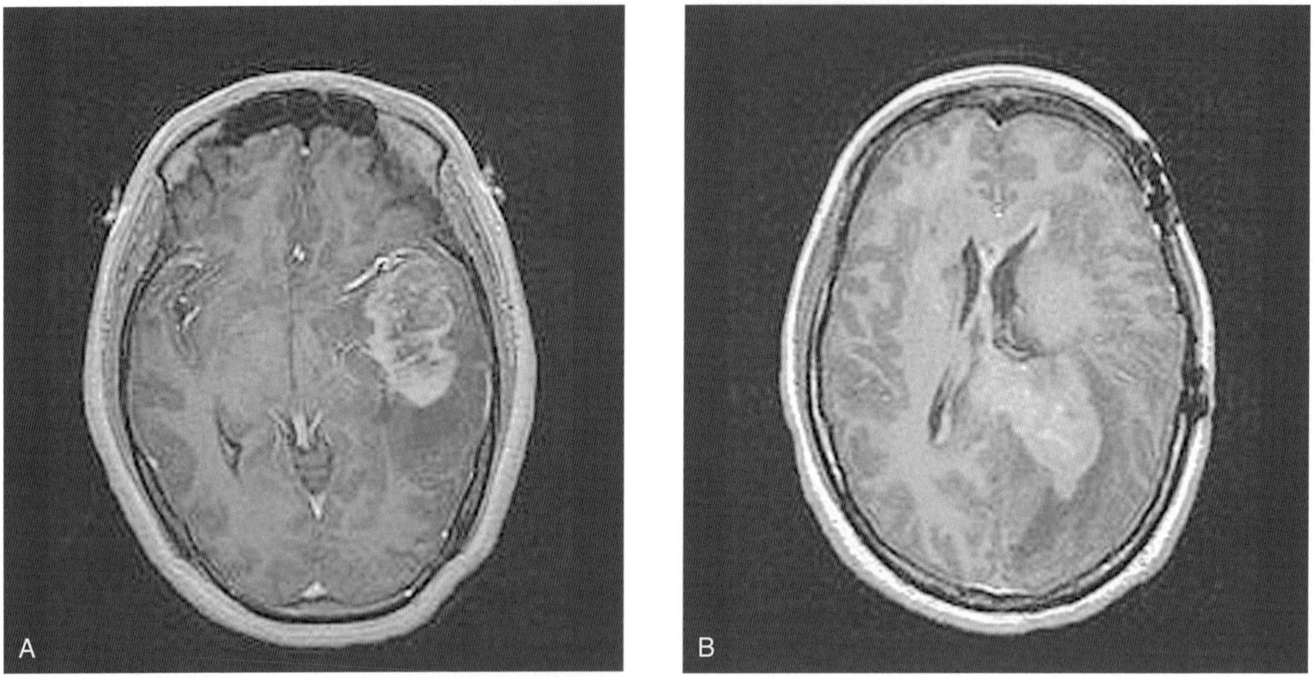

Figure 6-12. (A) Preoperative enhanced T_1 axial MRI of 27-year-old woman. She was treated with aggressive resection, fractionated radiation, and chemotherapy for glioblastoma. (B) She recurred a year later and was treated with a new chemotherapy regimen but further progressed at 22 months as shown by this MRI. In spite of her young age, reoperation was not offered because the recurrence is in a different location, and the tumor is deep in the dominant hemisphere and involves corpus callosum and ventricular walls.

rapidly decrease intracranial pressure or decompress a vital functional area of the brain in order to relieve neurologic deficit. After reoperation for recurrent glioblastoma, 25% of patients have an improvement in their KPS, 50% remain stable, and 25% deteriorate.[107]

The role of cytoreduction at the time of reoperation for malignant gliomas is even less clear than at the time of initial surgery. Some authors suggest that repeat resection may improve the efficacy of adjuvant treatments by removing treatment-resistant hypoxic cells.[104] Bulk tumor removal may also allow a patient's corticosteroid dose to be decreased, thereby avoiding their well-known side effects. Patients with glioblastoma multiforme who do have a reoperation are reported to have a longer survival time than those who do not, but there is a huge selection bias that obscures the meaning of these data.[107]

Median survival after reoperation for glioblastoma in a number of retrospective clinical trials has ranged up to 36 weeks.[107–111] Some of the older literature suggested that the morbidity and mortality from reoperation for glioma was much higher than the initial operation. Recent prospective data from the Glioma Outcomes Project do not support this.[112] The Project found that systemic infections (but not local infections) and depression were more common after reoperation, but that most other complications were not statistically different from patients undergoing a first craniotomy. It is unlikely that a prospective, randomized trial of reoperation for glioblastoma will be undertaken any time soon, and patients such as this should continue to be evaluated on a case-by-case basis by experienced neurosurgeons with an interest in neuro-oncology (Fig. 6-12).

▶ FUTURE DIRECTIONS

The cure for gliomas is not likely to be mechanical in nature. An especially dexterous surgeon, with a wonderful new microscope and an intraoperative MRI is not going to be able to cure this infiltrative disease. The future of glioma treatment lies in biologic modifiers. Surgery, however, will likely continue to play a role in the management of patients with gliomas.

As the treatment and assessment of gliomas becomes increasingly complex, it will be necessary to obtain tissue samples to assess the biology of the tumor through genetic and functional genomic assays (e.g., LOH of 1p for the assessment of oligodendrogliomas). Therapeutically, neurosurgeons will provide direct access to the CNS and the tumor for a growing number of locally delivered technologies such as biodegradable wafer placement, gene therapy, immunotherapy, and conjugated toxin therapy. Finally, in addition to these high-technology examples, there is a subset of patients who present in extremis, with necrotic and/or hemorrhagic tumors, who need the immediate decompression currently offered only by craniotomy.

REFERENCES

1. Salcman M. Historical development of surgery for glial tumors. J Neurooncol 1999;42(3):195–204.
2. Keles GE, Anderson B, Berger MS. The effect of extent of resection on time to tumor progression and survival in patients with glioblastoma multiforme of the cerebral hemisphere. Surg Neurol 1999;52(4):371–379.
3. Kiwit JC, Floeth FW, Bock WJ. Survival in malignant glioma: analysis of prognostic factors with special regard to cytoreductive surgery. Zentralbl Neurochir 1996;57(2):76–88.
4. Rostomily RC, Spence AM, Duong D, et al. Multimodality management of recurrent adult malignant gliomas: results of a phase II multiagent chemotherapy study and analysis of cytoreductive surgery. Neurosurgery 1994;35(3):376–388; discussion 388.
5. Vuorinen V, Hinkka S, Farkkila M, et al. Debulking or biopsy of malignant glioma in elderly people—a randomised study. Acta Neurochir (Wien) 2003;145(1):5–10.
6. Lacroix M, Abi-Said D, Fourney DR, et al. A multivariate analysis of 416 patients with glioblastoma multiforme: prognosis, extent of resection, and survival. J Neurosurg 2001;95(2):190–198.
7. Shinoda J, Sakai N, Murase S, et al. Selection of eligible patients with supratentorial glioblastoma multiforme for gross total resection. J Neurooncol 2001;52(2):161–171.
8. Mohan DS, Suh JH, Phan JL, et al. Outcome in elderly patients undergoing definitive surgery and radiation therapy for supratentorial glioblastoma multiforme at a tertiary care institution. Int J Radiat Oncol Biol Phys 1998;42(5):981–987.
9. Kowalczuk A, Macdonald RL, Amidei C, et al. Quantitative imaging study of extent of surgical resection and prognosis of malignant astrocytomas. Neurosurgery 1997;41(5): 1026–1036; discussion 1036–1038.
10. Slotman BJ, Kralendonk JH, van Alphen HA, et al. Hypofractionated radiation therapy in patients with glioblastoma multiforme: results of treatment and impact of prognostic factors. Int J Radiat Oncol Biol Phys 1996;34(4):895–898.
11. Nitta T, Sato K. Prognostic implications of the extent of surgical resection in patients with intracranial malignant gliomas. Cancer 1995;75(11):2727–2731.
12. Quigley MR, Flores N, Maroon JC, et al. Value of surgical intervention in the treatment of glioma. Stereotact Funct Neurosurg 1995;65(1–4):171–175.
13. Albert FK, Forsting M, Sartor K, et al. Early postoperative magnetic resonance imaging after resection of malignant glioma: objective evaluation of residual tumor and its influence on regrowth and prognosis. Neurosurgery 1994;34(1):45–60; discussion 60–61.
14. Kelly PJ, Hunt C. The limited value of cytoreductive surgery in elderly patients with malignant gliomas. Neurosurgery 1994;34(1):62–66; discussion 66–67.
15. Ammirati M, Vick N, Liao YL, et al. Effect of the extent of surgical resection on survival and quality of life in patients with supratentorial glioblastomas and anaplastic astrocytomas. Neurosurgery 1987;21(2):201–206.
16. Andreou J, George AE, Wise A, et al. CT prognostic criteria of survival after malignant glioma surgery. Am J Neuroradiol 1983;4(3):486–490.
17. Kreth FW, Berlis A, Spiropoulou V, et al. The role of tumor resection in the treatment of glioblastoma multiforme in adults. Cancer 1999;86(10):2117–23.
18. Bricolo A, Turazzi S, Cristofori L, et al. Experience in "radical" surgery of supratentorial gliomas in adults. J Neurosurg Sci 1990;34(3–4):297–298.
19. Sawaya R. Extent of resection in malignant gliomas: a critical summary. J Neurooncol 1999;42(3):303–305.
20. Hess KR. Extent of resection as a prognostic variable in the treatment of gliomas. J Neurooncol 1999;42(3):227–231.
21. Keles GE, Lamborn KR, Berger MS. Low-grade hemispheric gliomas in adults: a critical review of extent of resection as a factor influencing outcome. J Neurosurg 2001;95(5):735–745.
22. Schmidt MH, Berger MS, Lamborn KR, et al. Repeated operations for infiltrative low-grade gliomas without intervening therapy. J Neurosurg 2003;98(6):1165–1169.
23. Berger MS. Surgery of low-grade gliomas—technical aspects. Clin Neurosurg 1997;44:161–180.
24. Berger MS, Rostomily RC. Low grade gliomas: functional mapping resection strategies, extent of resection, and outcome. J Neurooncol 1997;34(1):85–101.
25. Rostomily RC, Keles GE, Berger MS. Radical surgery in the management of low-grade and high-grade gliomas. Baillieres Clin Neurol 1996;5(2):345–369.
26. Berger MS, Deliganis AV, Dobbins J, et al. The effect of extent of resection on recurrence in patients with low grade cerebral hemisphere gliomas. Cancer 1994; 74(6):1784–1791.
27. Berger MS, Ghatan S, Haglund MM, et al. Low-grade gliomas associated with intractable epilepsy: seizure outcome utilizing electrocorticography during tumor resection. J Neurosurg 1993;79(1):62–69.
28. Rees JH. Low-grade gliomas in adults. Curr Opin Neurol 2002;15(6):657–661.
29. Yeh SA, Lee TC, Chen HJ, et al. Treatment outcomes and prognostic factors of patients with supratentorial low-grade oligodendroglioma. Int J Radiat Oncol Biol Phys 2002;54(5):1405–1409.
30. Lo SS, Cho KH, Hall WA, et al. Does the extent of surgery have an impact on the survival of patients who receive postoperative radiation therapy for supratentorial low-grade gliomas? Int J Cancer 2001;96(Suppl):71–78.
31. Arienti VM, Botturi A, Boiardi A, et al. Adult brain low-grade astrocytomas: survival after surgery and radiotherapy. Neurol Sci 2001;22(3):233–238.

32. Nakamura M, Konishi N, Tsunoda S, et al. Analysis of prognostic and survival factors related to treatment of low-grade astrocytomas in adults. Oncology 2000;58(2):106–116.
33. Bauman G, Lote K, Larson D, et al. Pretreatment factors predict overall survival for patients with low-grade glioma: a recursive partitioning analysis. Int J Radiat Oncol Biol Phys 1999;45(4):923–929.
34. Rudoler S, Corn BW, Werner-Wasik M, et al. Patterns of tumor progression after radiotherapy for low-grade gliomas: analysis from the computed tomography/magnetic resonance imaging era. Am J Clin Oncol 1998;21(1): 23–27.
35. Lote K, Egeland T, Hager B, et al. Survival, prognostic factors, and therapeutic efficacy in low-grade glioma: a retrospective study in 379 patients. J Clin Oncol 1997; 15(9):3129–3140.
36. Eyre HJ, Crowley JJ, Townsend JJ, et al. A randomized trial of radiotherapy versus radiotherapy plus CCNU for incompletely resected low-grade gliomas: a Southwest Oncology Group study. J Neurosurg 1993;78(6):909–914.
37. Miralbell R, Balart J, Matias-Guiu X, et al. Radiotherapy for supratentorial low-grade gliomas: results and prognostic factors with special focus on tumour volume parameters. Radiother Oncol 1993;27(2):112–116.
38. Shibamoto Y, Kitakabu Y, Takahashi M, et al. Supratentorial low-grade astrocytoma. Correlation of computed tomography findings with effect of radiation therapy and prognostic variables. Cancer 1993;72(1):190–195.
39. Singer JM. Supratentorial low grade gliomas in adults. A retrospective analysis of 43 cases treated with surgery and radiotherapy. Eur J Surg Oncol 1995;21(2):196–200.
40. Lombardi D, Marsh R, de Tribolet N. Low grade glioma in intractable epilepsy: lesionectomy versus epilepsy surgery. Acta Neurochir Suppl (Wien) 1997;68:70–74.
41. Britton JW, Cascino GD, Sharbrough FW, et al. Low-grade glial neoplasms and intractable partial epilepsy: efficacy of surgical treatment. Epilepsia 1994;35(6):1130–1135.
42. Haglund MM, Berger MS, Kunkel DD, et al. Changes in gamma-aminobutyric acid and somatostatin in epileptic cortex associated with low-grade gliomas. J Neurosurg 1992;77(2):209–216.
43. Luyken C, Blumcke I, Fimmers R, et al. The spectrum of long-term epilepsy-associated tumors: long-term seizure and tumor outcome and neurosurgical aspects. Epilepsia 2003;44(6):822–830.
44. Duffau H, Capelle L, Lopes M, et al. Medically intractable epilepsy from insular low-grade gliomas: improvement after an extended lesionectomy. Acta Neurochir (Wien) 2002;144(6):563–572; discussion 572–573.
45. Cairncross JG, Pexman JH, Rathbone MP, et al. Postoperative contrast enhancement in patients with brain tumor. Ann Neurol 1985;17(6):570–572.
46. Forsyth PA, Petrov E, Mahallati H, et al. Prospective study of postoperative magnetic resonance imaging in patients with malignant gliomas. J Clin Oncol 1997;15(5):2076–2081.
47. Glantz MJ, Cole BF, Forsyth PA, et al. Practice parameter: anticonvulsant prophylaxis in patients with newly diagnosed brain tumors. Report of the Quality Standards Subcommittee of the American Academy of Neurology. Neurology 2000;54(10):1886–1893.
48. Ciric I, Ammirati M, Vick N, et al. Supratentorial gliomas: surgical considerations and immediate postoperative results. Gross total resection versus partial resection. Neurosurgery 1987;21(1):21–26.
49. Taylor MD, Bernstein M. Awake craniotomy with brain mapping as the routine surgical approach to treating patients with supratentorial intraaxial tumors: a prospective trial of 200 cases. J Neurosurg 1999;90(1):35–41.
50. Barker FG 2d. Efficacy of prophylactic antibiotics for craniotomy: a meta-analysis. Neurosurgery 1994;35(3): 484–490; discussion 491–492.
51. Marras LC, Geerts WH, Perry JR. The risk of venous thromboembolism is increased throughout the course of malignant glioma: an evidence-based review. Cancer 2000; 89(3):640–646.
52. Taylor WA, Thomas NW, Wellings JA, Bell BA. Timing of postoperative intracranial hematoma development and implications for the best use of neurosurgical intensive care. J Neurosurg 1995;82(1):46–50.
53. Vives KP, Piepmeier JM. Complications and expected outcome of glioma surgery. J Neurooncol 1999;42(3): 289–302.
54. Bernstein M, Al-Anazi AR, Kucharczyk W, et al. Brain tumor surgery with the Toronto open magnetic resonance imaging system: preliminary results for 36 patients and analysis of advantages, disadvantages, and future prospects. Neurosurgery 2000;46(4):900–907; discussion 907–909.
55. Moriarty TM, Quinones-Hinojosa A, Larson PS, et al. Frameless stereotactic neurosurgery using intraoperative magnetic resonance imaging: stereotactic brain biopsy. Neurosurgery 2000;47(5):1136–1145; discussion 1145–1146.
56. Alexander E 3d, Moriarty TM, Kikinis R, et al. The present and future role of intraoperative MRI in neurosurgical procedures. Stereotact Funct Neurosurg 1997;68(1–4 Pt 1): 10–17.
57. Moriarty TM, Kikinis R, Jolesz FA, et al. Magnetic resonance imaging therapy. Intraoperative MR imaging. Neurosurg Clin N Am 1996;7(2):323–331.
58. Hammoud MA, Ligon BL, el Souki R, et al. Use of intraoperative ultrasound for localizing tumors and determining the extent of resection: a comparative study with magnetic resonance imaging. J Neurosurg 1996;84(5):737–741.
59. Blanshard HJ, Chung F, Manninen PH, et al. Awake craniotomy for removal of intracranial tumor: considerations for early discharge. Anesth Analg 2001;92(1):89–94.
60. Signorelli F, Guyotat J, Isnard J, et al. The value of cortical stimulation applied to the surgery of malignant gliomas in language areas. Neurol Sci 2001;22(1):3–10.
61. Meyer FB, Bates LM, Goerss SJ, et al. Awake craniotomy for aggressive resection of primary gliomas located in eloquent brain. Mayo Clin Proc 2001;76(7):677–687.
62. Yamamoto F, Kato R, Sato J, et al. Anaesthesia for awake craniotomy with non-invasive positive pressure ventilation. Br J Anaesth 2003;90(3):382–385.
63. Sarang A, Dinsmore J. Anaesthesia for awake craniotomy—evolution of a technique that facilitates awake neurological testing. Br J Anaesth 2003;90(2):161–165.
64. Brock-Utne JG. Awake craniotomy. Anaesth Intensive Care 2001;29(6):669.

65. Manninen PH, Tan TK. Postoperative nausea and vomiting after craniotomy for tumor surgery: a comparison between awake craniotomy and general anesthesia. J Clin Anesth 2002;14(4):279–283.
66. Danks RA, Rogers M, Aglio LS, et al. Patient tolerance of craniotomy performed with the patient under local anesthesia and monitored conscious sedation. Neurosurgery 1998;42(1):26–34; discussion 34–36.
67. Lunsford LD, Martinez AJ. Stereotactic exploration of the brain in the era of computed tomography. Surg Neurol 1984;22(3):222–230.
68. Bernstein M, Parrent AG. Complications of CT-guided stereotactic biopsy of intra-axial brain lesions. J Neurosurg 1994;81(2):165–168.
69. Kondziolka D, Lunsford LD. The role of stereotactic biopsy in the management of gliomas. J Neurooncol 1999;42(3):205–213.
70. Bhardwaj RD, Bernstein M. Prospective feasibility study of outpatient stereotactic brain lesion biopsy. Neurosurgery 2002;51(2):356–361; discussion 361–364.
71. Harting I, Hartmann M, Jost G, et al. Differentiating primary central nervous system lymphoma from glioma in humans using localised proton magnetic resonance spectroscopy. Neurosci Lett 2003;342(3):163–166.
72. Bulakbasi N, Kocaoglu M, Ors F, et al. Combination of single-voxel proton MR spectroscopy and apparent diffusion coefficient calculation in the evaluation of common brain tumors. Am J Neuroradiol 2003;24(2):225–233.
73. Nutt CL, Mani DR, Betensky RA, et al. Gene expression-based classification of malignant gliomas correlates better with survival than histological classification. Cancer Res 2003;63(7):1602–1607.
74. Cairncross JG, Ueki K, Zlatescu MC, et al. Specific genetic predictors of chemotherapeutic response and survival in patients with anaplastic oligodendrogliomas. J Natl Cancer Inst 1998;90(19):1473–1479.
75. Marquardt G, Setzer M, Lang J, et al. Delayed hydrocephalus after resection of supratentorial malignant gliomas. Acta Neurochir (Wien) 2002;144(3):227–231.
76. Laperriere NJ, Leung PM, McKenzie S, et al. Randomized study of brachytherapy in the initial management of patients with malignant astrocytoma. Int J Radiat Oncol Biol Phys 1998;41(5):1005–1011.
77. Selker RG, Shapiro WR, Burger P, et al. The Brain Tumor Cooperative Group NIH Trial 87–01: a randomized comparison of surgery, external radiotherapy, and carmustine versus surgery, interstitial radiotherapy boost, external radiation therapy, and carmustine. Neurosurgery 2002; 51(2):343–355; discussion 355–357.
78. Westphal M, Hilt DC, Bortey E, et al. A phase 3 trial of local chemotherapy with biodegradable carmustine (BCNU) wafers (Gliadel wafers) in patients with primary malignant glioma. Neuro-oncol 2003;5(2):79–88.
79. Valtonen S, Timonen U, Toivanen P, et al. Interstitial chemotherapy with carmustine-loaded polymers for high-grade gliomas: a randomized double-blind study. Neurosurgery 1997;41(1):44–48; discussion 46–49.
80. Brem H, Piantadosi S, Burger PC, et al. Placebo-controlled trial of safety and efficacy of intraoperative controlled delivery by biodegradable polymers of chemotherapy for recurrent gliomas. The Polymer-Brain Tumor Treatment Group. Lancet 1995;345(8956):1006–1012.
81. Bampoe J, Bernstein M. The role of surgery in low grade gliomas. J Neurooncol 1999;42(3):259–269.
82. Daumas-Duport C, Varlet P, Tucker ML, et al. Oligodendrogliomas. Part I: Patterns of growth, histological diagnosis, clinical and imaging correlations: a study of 153 cases. J Neurooncol 1997;34(1):37–59.
83. Berger MS. Functional mapping-guided resection of low-grade gliomas. Clin Neurosurg 1995;42:437–452.
84. Leighton C, Fisher B, Bauman G, et al. Supratentorial low-grade glioma in adults: an analysis of prognostic factors and timing of radiation. J Clin Oncol 1997;15(4):1294–1301.
85. Piepmeier J, Christopher S, Spencer D, et al. Variations in the natural history and survival of patients with supratentorial low-grade astrocytomas. Neurosurgery 1996;38(5):872–878; discussion 876–879.
86. Lunsford LD, Somaza S, Kondziolka D, et al. Survival after stereotactic biopsy and irradiation of cerebral nonanaplastic, nonpilocytic astrocytoma. J Neurosurg 1995;82(4):523–529.
87. Philippon JH, Clemenceau SH, Fauchon FH, et al. Supratentorial low-grade astrocytomas in adults. Neurosurgery 1993;32(4):554–559.
88. Vertosick FT Jr, Selker RG, Arena VC. Survival of patients with well-differentiated astrocytomas diagnosed in the era of computed tomography. Neurosurgery 1991;28(4): 496–501.
89. McCormack BM, Miller DC, Budzilovich GN, et al. Treatment and survival of low-grade astrocytoma in adults—1977–1988. Neurosurgery 1992;31(4):636–642.
90. Karim AB, Maat B, Hatlevoll R, et al. A randomized trial on dose-response in radiation therapy of low-grade cerebral glioma: European Organization for Research and Treatment of Cancer (EORTC) Study 22844. Int J Radiat Oncol Biol Phys 1996;36(3):549–556.
91. Bahary JP, Villemure JG, Choi S, et al. Low-grade pure and mixed cerebral astrocytomas treated in the CT scan era. J Neurooncol 1996;27(2):173–177.
92. Karim AB, Afra D, Cornu P, et al. Randomized trial on the efficacy of radiotherapy for cerebral low-grade glioma in the adult: European Organization for Research and Treatment of Cancer Study 22845 with the Medical Research Council study BR04: an interim analysis. Int J Radiat Oncol Biol Phys 2002;52(2):316–324.
93. Lunsford LD, Kondziolka D. Adverse long-term effects of brain radiotherapy in adult low-grade glioma patients. Neurology 2001;57(11):2150–2151.
94. Scott JN, Brasher PM, Sevick RJ, et al. How often are nonenhancing supratentorial gliomas malignant? A population study. Neurology 2002;59(6):947–949.
95. Piepmeier JM. Observations on the current treatment of low-grade astrocytic tumors of the cerebral hemispheres. J Neurosurg 1987;67(2):177–181.
96. Rajan B, Pickuth D, Ashley S, et al. The management of histologically unverified presumed cerebral gliomas with radiotherapy. Int J Radiat Oncol Biol Phys 1994; 28(2):405–413.
97. Recht LD, Lew R, Smith TW. Suspected low-grade glioma: is deferring treatment safe? Ann Neurol 1992;31(4):431–436.

98. Smith DF, Hutton JL, Sandemann D, et al. The prognosis of primary intracerebral tumours presenting with epilepsy: the outcome of medical and surgical management. J Neurol Neurosurg Psychiatry 1991;54(10):915–920.
99. Laws ER Jr, Taylor WF, Bergstralh EJ, et al. The neurosurgical management of low-grade astrocytoma. Clin Neurosurg 1986;33:575–588.
100. Laws ER Jr, Taylor WF, Clifton MB, et al. Neurosurgical management of low-grade astrocytoma of the cerebral hemispheres. J Neurosurg 1984;61(4):665–673.
101. Morantz RA. Radiation therapy in the treatment of cerebral astrocytoma. Neurosurgery 1987;20(6):975–982.
102. Pollack IF. The role of surgery in pediatric gliomas. J Neurooncol 1999;42(3):271–288.
103. Dirks PB, Jay V, Becker LE, et al. Development of anaplastic changes in low-grade astrocytomas of childhood. Neurosurgery 1994;34(1):66–78.
104. Tatter SB. Recurrent malignant glioma in adults. Curr Treat Options Oncol 2002;3(6):509–524.
105. Siddiqi SN, Provias J, Laperriere N, et al. Effects of iodine-125 brachytherapy on the proliferative capacity and histopathological features of glioblastoma recurring after initial therapy. Neurosurgery 1997;40(5):910–917; discussion 917–918.
106. Forsyth PA, Kelly PJ, Cascino TL, et al. Radiation necrosis or glioma recurrence: is computer-assisted stereotactic biopsy useful? J Neurosurg 1995;82(3):436–444.
107. Barker FG 2d, Chang SM, Gutin PH, et al. Survival and functional status after resection of recurrent glioblastoma multiforme. Neurosurgery 1998;42(4):709–720; discussion 720–723.
108. Harsh GRT, Levin VA, Gutin PH, et al. Reoperation for recurrent glioblastoma and anaplastic astrocytoma. Neurosurgery 1987;21(5):615–621.
109. Salcman M, Kaplan RS, Ducker TB, et al. Effect of age and reoperation on survival in the combined modality treatment of malignant astrocytoma. Neurosurgery 1982; 10(4):454–463.
110. Ammirati M, Galicich JH, Arbit E, et al. Reoperation in the treatment of recurrent intracranial malignant gliomas. Neurosurgery 1987;21(5):607–614.
111. Dirks P, Bernstein M, Muller PJ, et al. The value of reoperation for recurrent glioblastoma. Can J Surg 1993; 36(3): 271–275.
112. Chang SM, Parney IF, McDermott M, et al. Perioperative complications and neurological outcomes of first and second craniotomies among patients enrolled in the Glioma Outcome Project. J Neurosurg 2003;98(6):1175–1181.

CHAPTER 7

Principles of Radiotherapy and Radiosurgery

PAUL D. BROWN / BRUCE E. POLLOCK

The use of radiation for scientific and medical purposes dates back more than 100 years to the discovery of the X-ray by Conrad Roentgen in 1895.[1] This was followed by the isolation of radium by Marie and Pierre Curie in 1897.[2] Almost immediately after this discovery, radium was used in the treatment of cancer, often with great success in patients with otherwise incurable disease.[3–5] External beam techniques took much longer to develop. The first clinical uses of radiation delivered with roentgen-type machines were unsatisfactory. These early machines produced very low-energy rays resulting in poor tissue penetration and severe skin damage. In the 1920s, Coutard and Regaud followed up on biologic experiments and showed that by dividing the total dose into many smaller treatments delivered over several weeks, tumors could be cured without severe normal-tissue damage.[6] This method was quickly adopted by others and ushered in the concept of fractionation *of treatment into a sequence of daily doses usually given over a few to several weeks. Later, higher energy machines capable of depositing their maximum dosage below the surface of the skin began to appear. However, the first high-energy machines were expensive and complex units.*

The start of the modern era of external-beam therapy began with the appearance of the cobalt-60 (^{60}Co) machines in the mid-1950s. Cobalt machines were less complex and delivered high-energy rays in the megavoltage (MV) range. In the 1960s, and more significantly in the 1970s, cobalt machines gave way to the multiple advantages of the linear accelerator. In addition to photons, linear accelerators are able to produce electrons, which have a finite range in tissue that allows one to tailor the depth of penetration to the exact clinical situation. The edge of the treatment field is much more sharply defined with linear accelerators compared to cobalt units. This allows greater precision in the delivery of radiation with linear accelerators. The dose rate (amount of radiation dose produced per minute) is variable with linear accelerators but with cobalt units is fixed and determined by the cobalt in the machine. Therefore, linear accelerators are now the predominant machines operating, albeit with much greater sophistication than their predecessors (Fig. 7-1). The technology of radiation therapy continues to undergo rapid development and change. To better understand these modern, sophisticated linear accelerators and radiation in general, a review of the physical and biologic properties of radiation is necessary.

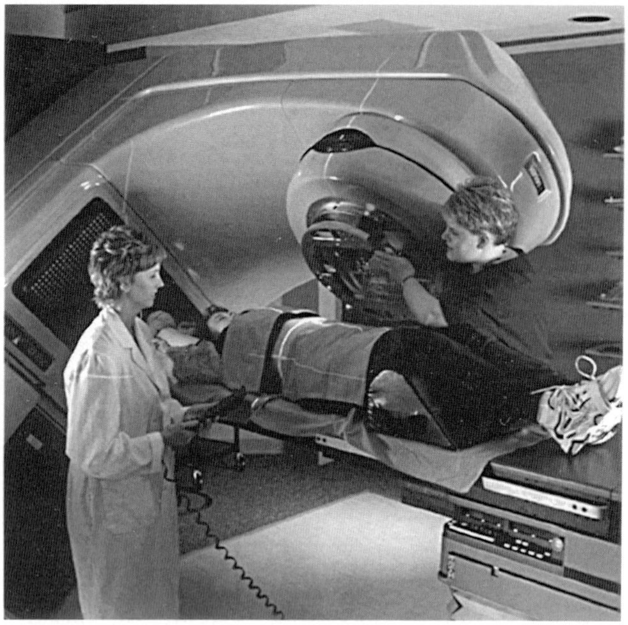

Figure 7-1. A modern high-energy linear accelerator. Note the room lasers used for setup and positioning of the patient.

▶ PHYSICAL PROPERTIES OF RADIATION

Photons

Radiation oncologists use ionizing radiation to eradicate malignancies. Ionizing radiation is composed of particulate radiation and electromagnetic radiation. Radiation oncologists use electrons (particulate) frequently and a few radiation centers use neutrons or protons (particulate), but the vast majority of radiation treatments are delivered via photons (electromagnetic radiation). Electromagnetic radiation is part of a continuum of waveform energy known as the *electromagnetic spectrum*. All waves from the electromagnetic spectrum behave in part like continuous waves but also behave in part like particles of energy. The particles of energy are often referred to as photons. The electromagnetic spectrum has a wide spectrum of different energies, from low-energy, long-wavelength, low-frequency radio waves to high-energy, short-wavelength, high-frequency cosmic waves. Only a small portion of the electromagnetic spectrum constitutes visible light. Near the high-energy (short wavelength), deeply penetrating end of this spectrum lie X-rays and gamma rays, the electromagnetic waves used therapeutically to treat cancer. Gamma rays and X-rays are essentially identical, with the only difference being their origin. X-rays are obtained from an extranuclear process when an accelerated electron strikes a target (e.g., tungsten) with a high atomic number (Z). This results in deceleration of the electron, producing polyenergetic X-rays through the process of *bremsstrahlung* (braking radiation). Linear accelerators produce high-energy X-rays by this process. In contrast, gamma rays are emitted from the nucleus during nuclear decay. Cobalt machines and gamma knife radiosurgical units produce high-energy radiation by this method.

Electromagnetic radiation on the higher end of the spectrum (X-rays, gamma rays, cosmic rays) interacts with matter, removing electrons from their orbits, resulting in *ionization* and the release of energy. These electrons may then produce secondary electrons, releasing more energy, as they pass through matter. However, photons interact differently with matter depending on the energy of the radiation.[7] At lower photon energies (<100,000 electron volts or 100 keV), characteristic of diagnostic radiology, the *photoelectric effect* predominates. An inner orbital electron absorbs the radiation resulting in the electron's ejection from the atom. This interaction is highly dependent on the atomic number of the substance irradiated. Thus bone, which has a high atomic number (high Z), absorbs more radiation than do soft tissues. This difference in absorption is the basis for imaging in diagnostic radiology. Thus older radiation machines with lower-energy X-rays (Grenz rays and even orthovoltage units) had the disadvantage of increased absorption of radiation in bone, which often led to severe radiation damage.

At higher energies, characteristic of cobalt units or linear accelerators, the *Compton effect* dominates. In this process, the photon interacts with an outer shell electron, resulting in the release of the electron and a photon of lower energy deflected from its original course. These interactions are not dependent on the atomic number of the substance with which the X-ray is interacting, but only dependent on the density of the absorbing material. The amount of radiation absorbed is roughly equal gram for gram, whether the material is soft tissue or bone. Therefore, films exposed on the high-energy linear accelerator (port films used to verify patient and radiation field setup accuracy) are difficult to interpret because the bone with these high-energy X-rays does not absorb vastly different amounts of energy compared with the soft tissues. This also explains why body lead is protective in the energies typically used for diagnostic radiology, but entirely impractical with the higher energies typically used in radiation oncology.

Particulate Radiation

Electrons are the most commonly used particulate radiation in general radiotherapy practice (e.g., skin cancers). However, because of the lack of penetration of electrons, they are rarely used in the treatment of brain tumors. In contrast, other forms of particulate radiation, such as protons and neutrons, are used in the treatment of brain tumors. X-ray photons interact with orbital electrons and release electrons.[7] Electrons are very light, negatively charged particles. In contrast, neutrons interact with the nuclei of atoms and produce much heavier particles such as protons, alpha particles (nuclei of helium atoms), and even heavier nuclear fragments. As can be imagined, the density of ionizations along the pathway of these particles is much greater than the density of X-rays.

An intriguing approach when treating brain tumors with neutrons is boron neutron capture therapy (BNCT). Boron neutron capture therapy is based on the nuclear reaction that occurs when boron is irradiated with neutrons to produce high-energy alpha particles and nuclear fragments. In principle, a drug containing boron would localize only in tumors, thereby producing alpha particles when bombarded with neutrons. Because these alpha particles have a very short range (about the length of a cell), ionization and damage occurs only at the site of the tumor. One difficulty with this approach is the heterogeneity of uptake of boron in brain tumors. Another concern is deposition of boron in normal adjacent structures causing severe toxicity. Therefore, although boron neutron capture therapy is promising in theory, the results to date have not been substantially better for patients with high-grade gliomas compared with standard radiotherapy,[8] although ongoing studies continue.[9]

In contrast with neutrons, the advantage of protons is in their dose distribution.[10] Protons deposit most of their energy at the end of their track range in tissue, called the *Bragg peak*. The energy delivered to tissue proximal to the peak is minimal; the energy delivered at the peak is high; and essentially no energy passes beyond the peak. This allows energy to be deposited in large amounts in a region, while sparing, in a fairly dramatic fashion, an adjacent area. Consequently, protons are often used to treat tumors near critical structures such as the brainstem (e.g., chordomas), lesions next to the optic chiasm, choroid melanomas, and paraspinal neoplasms.[11] However, because of the complexity of particle beam treatment planning, the need for a cyclotron to generate the protons, and the expense of these units, there is a limited number of facilities around the world.

Radiation Measurements

One of the first units of radiation measurement defined was the roentgen (R).[12] The roentgen is a unit of exposure and is related to the ability of radiation to ionize air. The rad is a unit of absorbed dose and is defined as 100 ergs absorbed per gram of tissue. The rad was later replaced with the gray (Gy), which corresponds to one joule absorbed per kilogram (1 Gy = 100 rads). Often the unit centigray (cGy) is used with 1 cGy equal to 1 rad.

▶ BIOLOGIC PROPERTIES OF RADIATION

When photon radiation hits a cell it will most likely interact with water because cells are primarily composed of water.[13] This creates unstable molecules, called *free radicals*, that may interact with DNA. The free radicals damage the DNA, possibly resulting in permanent cell injury or death. This is called the *indirect effect* of radiation. Less commonly, photon radiation may interact directly with DNA or other cellular molecules, leading to damage and possibly cell death. This *direct effect* is the predominant process in heavy particle radiation (e.g., alpha particles, neutrons).

The majority of evidence supports DNA as the primary target for radiation-induced death. An elegant experiment by Munro confirmed this concept.[14] Individual cells attached to a glass coverslip were radiated with a polonium microneedle. The alpha particles from the polonium have a well-defined range making it possible to radiate only the cytoplasm and not the nucleus of the cell. Doses in excess of 250 Gy delivered to the cytoplasm had no effect on cell proliferation, whereas a few alpha particles into the nucleus were lethal.

Radiation of the cell leads to damage of the DNA, but not all of the damage is equally capable of producing biologic damage. DNA–protein cross-links, direct base damage, and single-strand breaks seem to play a relatively minor role in the lethality of ionizing radiation compared with double-strand breaks.[15] As long as the opposite strand is intact, the cell remains capable of repairing single-strand breaks with great efficiency. Therefore, the critical lesions caused by radiation are double-strand breaks.

Cell Death Caused by Radiation

The most common types of cell death after radiotherapy are mitotic cell death and apoptosis. If a cell accumulates sufficient radiation damage, its later progeny may be unable to go through mitosis successfully, and will die. Several cell divisions may occur before the lethal effects of radiation are expressed.[16] As a consequence of this phenomenon, rapidly dividing normal tissues (e.g., oral cavity mucosa) or tumors (e.g., small cell lung cancer) will express radiation damage sooner than either slower-dividing tissues (e.g., brain) or tumors (e.g., meningioma). This raises the concept that acute responses and toxicity do not necessarily predict long-term local control or late toxicity, respectively. For example, not all tumors that rapidly regress with radiotherapy enjoy long-term control, and many tumors that seem to change little with radiotherapy will have slow regression or stability that leads to a local cure.

Some cells do not have to go through mitosis to succumb to radiation, but instead die as a consequence of programmed cell death or apoptosis.[17] Lymphocytes, spermatogonia (germ cells), small intestinal crypt cells, and parotid acinar cells are known to die very quickly after radiation exposure (an intermitotic death).[18] An apoptotic event is irreversible, and there is no capability for repair of radiation damage that characterizes cells dying from mitotically expressed DNA damage. This extraordinary sensitivity to radiation extends to many tumors such as low-grade non-Hodgkin lymphoma and seminoma, such that doses as low as 400 cGy (4 Gy) can yield long-term control of a lesion.[19]

Therapeutic Ratio

Radiation can cause damage to tumor, as well as normal, cells. To have a therapeutic effect, radiation must cause less damage to the normal tissues while causing more damage to the tumor. This is accomplished physically by designing radiation treatments that deliver higher doses of radiation to tumor while sparing normal structures these higher doses. Simple opposed fields will provide adequate dose coverage of the planning target volume (PTV) but will also treat a large amount of normal brain and other tissues to the same dose as the prescription dose (Fig. 7-2A). By treating the PTV with multiple fields, adequate dose coverage of the target is still achieved; however, a significantly less amount of brain receives the full prescribed dose of radiation compared to the simple opposed lateral plan (Fig. 7-2B). Instead, with the more complex plan, a larger amount of normal brain receives a lower dose of radiation. It is expected the normal structures will have a much lower risk of toxicity with lower doses of radiation than higher doses of radiation.

The therapeutic ratio can also be improved biologically by using the advantages of differential radiosensitivity of normal tissues and tumors with fractionated (i.e., a sequence of daily doses usually given over a period of a few to several weeks) radiotherapy. In general, normal tissues are better able to repair DNA damage than tumors because of aberrant cell-cycle control mechanisms in tumors. In general, tumors are more acutely sensitive to the effects of radiotherapy (much like oral mucosa) than are most other normal tissues that are slowly dividing (e.g., muscle, neural tissue).[20] These slowly dividing tissues are able to repair low doses of radiation. However,

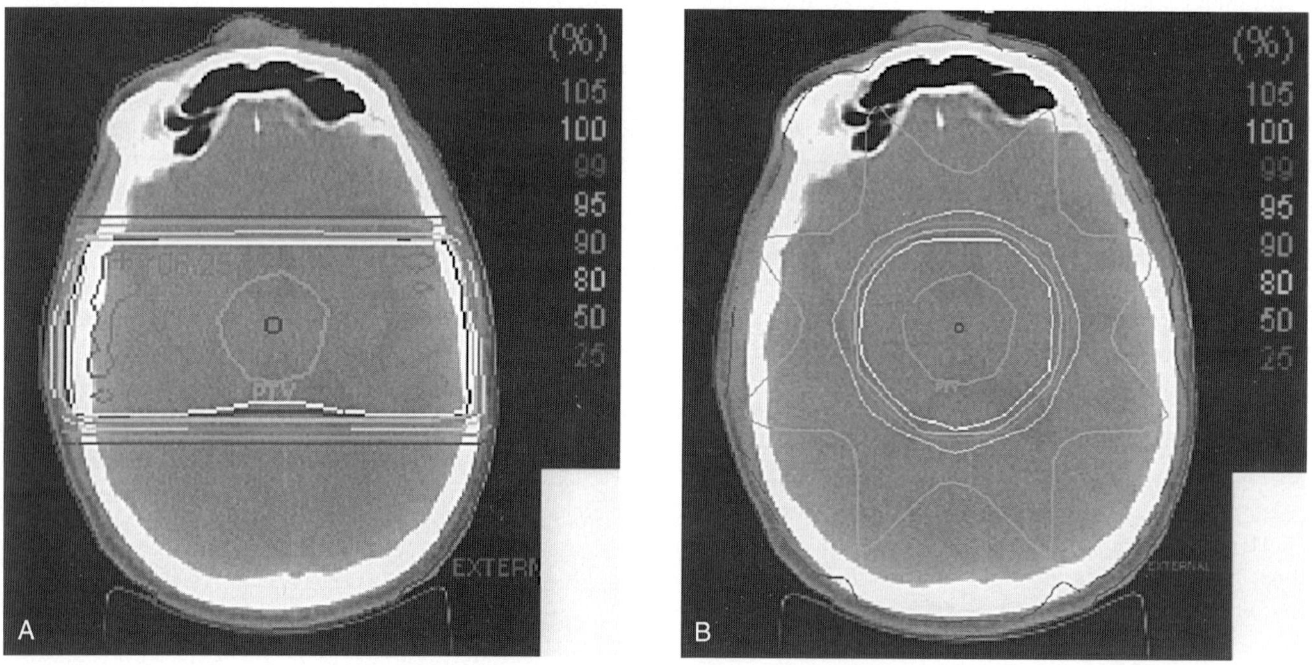

Figure 7-2 (PLATES 37 AND 38). These two radiation plans illustrate one of the basic principles of three-dimensional conformal radiotherapy. For plan (A), a pair of equally weighted parallel opposed fields treat a centrally positioned lesion. In plan (B), four pairs of opposed fields treat the lesion. Both radiation plans encompass the target lesion with the 100% isodose curve. For plan (B) there is an approximately fourfold reduction in dose per field while maintaining the full dose at the intersection of all fields. This results in a significant reduction in the amount of brain receiving the full dose of radiation while increasing the amount of brain receiving lower doses of radiation.

a single, large dose of radiation is able to overcome these repair mechanisms and damage normal tissues along with tumor.[21] Thus it is advantageous to deliver multiple small doses of radiation with the normal cells inherent superiority in repairing sublethal damage compared to tumor cells.

Radiation Tolerance of Normal Tissues in the Central Nervous System

For a more detailed review of the tolerance of normal CNS tissues to radiotherapy, see Chapter 32. Cranial radiotherapy is usually well tolerated acutely. Some patients do develop headache, nausea, and somnolence. These symptoms are related to cerebral edema and can be treated with corticosteroids, although it is important to be cognizant of the possibility of tumor progression during treatment as the cause of increased intracranial pressure. Alopecia is common and can be permanent if the scalp receives 50 Gy or more or in regions of tangential radiation.

The subacute side effects of radiation are believed to be caused by transient demyelination mediated by damage to oligodendrocytes. The clinical manifestations are numbness, tingling, or even "electric" sensations with head flexion (Lhermitte sign) following spinal cord irradiation, or somnolence, anorexia, and irritability (somnolence syndrome) after cranial irradiation. The sleep somnolence syndrome is usually seen in pediatric patients (although it does occur in adults) approximately 10 weeks after cranial radiotherapy has been completed.[22,23] Both Lhermitte sign and sleep somnolence syndrome are self-limiting and are not associated with subsequent neurologic difficulties when standard radiation doses have been delivered.

Late effects following cranial or spinal radiotherapy tend to occur several months to many years after treatment. Clinical and radiographic changes vary from asymptomatic white matter changes[24] (Fig. 7-3) to neurocognitive difficulties,[25] hypothalamic–pituitary dysfunction,[26] optic neuropathy,[27] myelopathy,[28] brain necrosis,[29,30] or second malignancies. With the exception of second malignancies, each of these late effects is function of total dose and dose per fraction.

Myelopathy can occur several months to years after spinal cord irradiation, but fortunately is quite rare with conventional fractionation and sufficient time between treatments.[31] A review of 1112 patients treated with multiple different fractionation schedules to a range of doses (30 Gy to more than 60 Gy) to the cervical spine found 2 (0.18%) cases of radiation myelitis. Because of the rarity of myelopathy after standard doses of conventionally fractionated radiotherapy, spinal cord myelopathy caused by radiation is a diagnosis of exclusion, with recurrence of tumor being the most common cause of neurologic complications. Brain necrosis also occurs

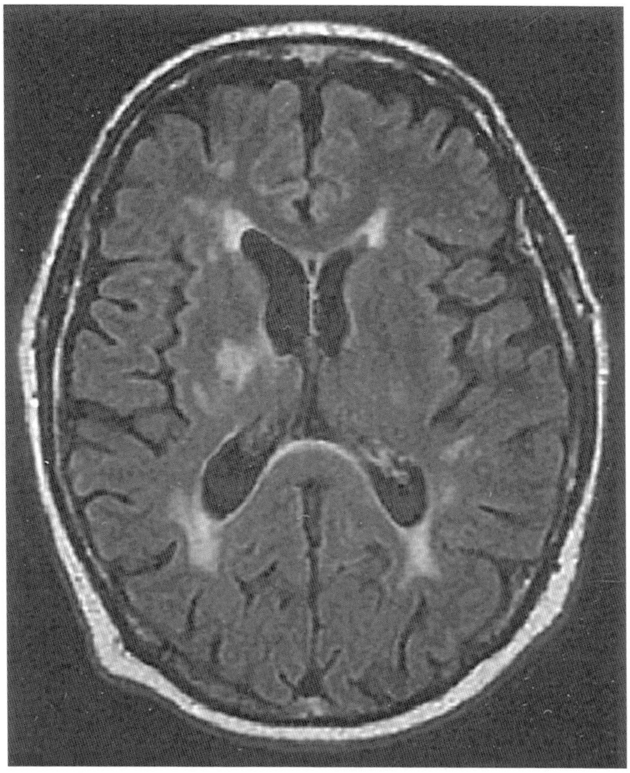

Figure 7-3. Axial fluid-attenuated inversion recovery (FLAIR) image of an asymptomatic patient who had received whole-brain radiotherapy (3000 cGy in 10 fractions) for multiple brain metastases 9 months prior to this magnetic resonance imaging (MRI). Increased signal in the right internal capsule consistent with a recurrent brain metastasis. There is also increased periventricular signal. Note the symmetry of the increased periventricular signal consistent with prior radiotherapy delivered via opposed lateral fields.

several months to years[29] after cranial irradiation. It can be very difficult to differentiate from recurrence (Fig. 7-4) even with imaging studies such as magnetic resonance spectroscopy (MRS) and positron emission tomography (PET). A randomized trial of 50.4 Gy/28 fractions versus 64.8 Gy/36 fractions localized radiation therapy for 203 patients with low-grade gliomas found a 5-year actuarial incidence of severe, late radiation toxicity (e.g., necrosis) of 2% in the 50.4-Gy arm and 10% in the 64.8-Gy arm.[30] This study and a large body of retrospective and prospective data provide the radiation oncologist the ability to estimate the risk of necrosis for a patient based on the planned total dose, fractionation schedule, and irradiated volume.

Neurocognitive difficulties may develop many years after radiotherapy and are not uncommon after cranial radiation for pediatric patients (especially children younger than age 4 years).[32,33] However, radiation-induced neurocognitive deterioration in adults is quite

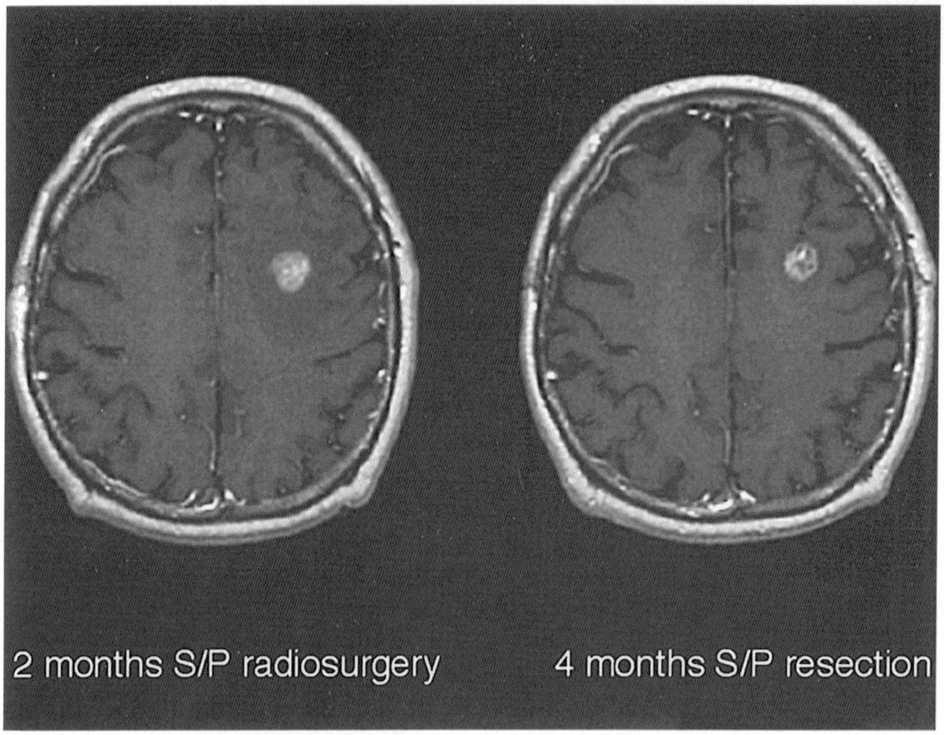

Figure 7-4. Magnetic resonance imaging (MRI) of the head demonstrates a gadolinium-enhancing mass in the left frontal lobe 2 months after gamma knife radiosurgery (20 Gy to the margin at the 50% isodose) for a renal cell carcinoma metastasis. The lesion was resected, proving (in-field) recurrence of the renal cell metastasis. Four months after resection of the left frontal lesion, MRI of the head again demonstrates recurrence of a contrast-enhancing lesion in the left frontal lobe. Resection of this lesion revealed lymphohistiocytic infiltrate and fibrosis consistent with radionecrosis. There was no evidence of cancer.

rare if high total dose,[30] whole-brain fields[34] (Fig. 7-5), and larger fraction sizes (3 Gy or greater) are avoided.[25] Prospective studies following high-grade[35] and low-grade glioma patients[36] after radiotherapy have found the predominant cause of neurocognitive difficulties to be tumor progression and not prior treatment with radiotherapy. Several retrospective studies have found increased neurocognitive difficulties after cranial radiotherapy. However, these studies have suffered from many deficiencies, besides the weaknesses inherent in retrospective studies, including outdated radiotherapy techniques (using whole-brain radiotherapy for low-grade glioma patients),[34,37] unknown number of patients treated but not studied (unidentified denominator),[38] extremely heterogenous groups,[39] and, most importantly, the lack of baseline neurocognitive testing to evaluate the effects of both the tumor and individual patient comorbidity.[34,37,40]

In sharp contrast, a number of studies have prospectively performed extensive neuropsychological testing on adult patients with low-grade neoplasms before (baseline) and after radiotherapy (up to 6 years after radiotherapy) and have not found significant neurocognitive deficits when compared to either baseline[24,41–44] or to a cohort of patients with low-grade gliomas not treated with radiotherapy (Table 7.1).[36,45]

Therefore, the weight of evidence indicates a low incidence of neurocognitive difficulties after focal, conventionally fractionated radiotherapy using modern techniques to deliver moderate doses in adults (Fig. 7-6).[49]

▶ CLINICAL APPLICATIONS OF RADIATION THERAPY

The vast majority of radiotherapy treatments are delivered by a linear accelerator using photons, although other modalities are occasionally used (particulate radiation, brachytherapy). The interface of computer verification systems, coupled with computerized tomography (CT)- or magnetic resonance imaging (MRI)-based treatment planning and the delivery of precise treatments through multiple complex beams allows the reliable distribution of therapeutic doses to the tumor volume while excluding the normal tissues from the high-dose region. These advances have significantly increased the

▶ TABLE 7-1. PROSPECTIVE NEUROCOGNITIVE TRIALS (WITH BASELINE TESTING) OF LOW-GRADE NEOPLASMS

Author	Histology (Number Receiving RT)	Radiation Total Dose/Fraction Size (Gray)	Mean Follow-Up (year)	Extensive Neurocognitive Assessment at Each Evaluation	Neurotoxicity After RT
Glosser[46]	Chordoma, chondrosarcoma (17)	Proton RT median 67.4 CGE/1.8 CGE	4	Yes	No; mild decline in psychomotor speed with high doses
Vigliani[45]	LGG, AA (17)	Focal RT 54/1.8	4	Yes	No; transient decline in reaction time
Armstrong[24]	LGG, pituitary, pineal, meningioma (26)	Focal RT Mean 54.6/1.8–2.0	3	Yes	No; mild decline in visual memory after 5 years
Brown[47]	LGG (203)	Focal RT 50.4/1.8 or 64.8/1.8	7.4 (median)	No (MMSE and NFS)	5.3% with MMSE decline at 5 years
Torres[36]	Meningioma, LGG, GBM, ependymoma, adenoma (15)	Focal RT Mean 54/1.8	2	Yes	No; decline in memory and attention only if tumor progression
Laack[48]	LGG (20)	Focal RT 50.4/1.8 or 64.8/1.8	3	Yes	No

AA = anaplastic astrocytoma; CGE = centigray equivalent; GBM = glioblastoma multiforme; LGG = low-grade glioma; MMSE = Folstein Mini Mental State Examination; NFS = neurologic function scores; RT = radiotherapy.

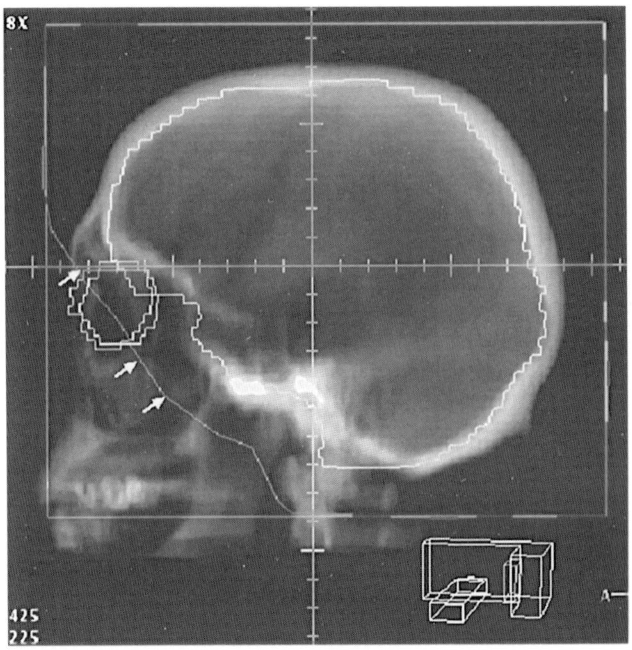

Figure 7-5. A typical whole-brain (lateral) radiotherapy field. Cerrobend blocks or multileaf collimators (arrows) are used to shape the beam, thereby "blocking" the eyes and oral cavity from radiation. When the blocks are designed, adequate margin is maintained between the target (the intracranial contents in this situation) and the edge of the block to allow the delivery of adequate doses of radiation.

therapeutic ratio and advanced the field of radiotherapy significantly when compared with where the field was even just 20 years ago. It is important to emphasize this point because basing treatment decisions on toxicities experienced with antiquated radiation techniques is akin to basing treatment decisions on neurosurgery or chemotherapy performed 20 to 30 years ago when morbidity was still quite high and fatalities occasionally occurred.

Patient Assessment

A complete assessment by the radiation oncologist is essential before initiating radiation therapy. This assessment includes a thorough history and physical, with special attention to specific neurologic signs and symptoms and the overall health and performance status of the patient. A review of the surgical procedures, pathology, and imaging is conducted ideally in a multidisciplinary setting with neuroradiologic, neuropathologic, neurosurgical, and neuro-oncologic input.

Immobilization and Simulation

Once the decision has been made to proceed with radiation therapy, the next step is immobilization. Patient positioning is a critical part of radiation therapy, especially for focal localized radiotherapy, but also for whole-brain radiotherapy. Proper immobilization and consistent

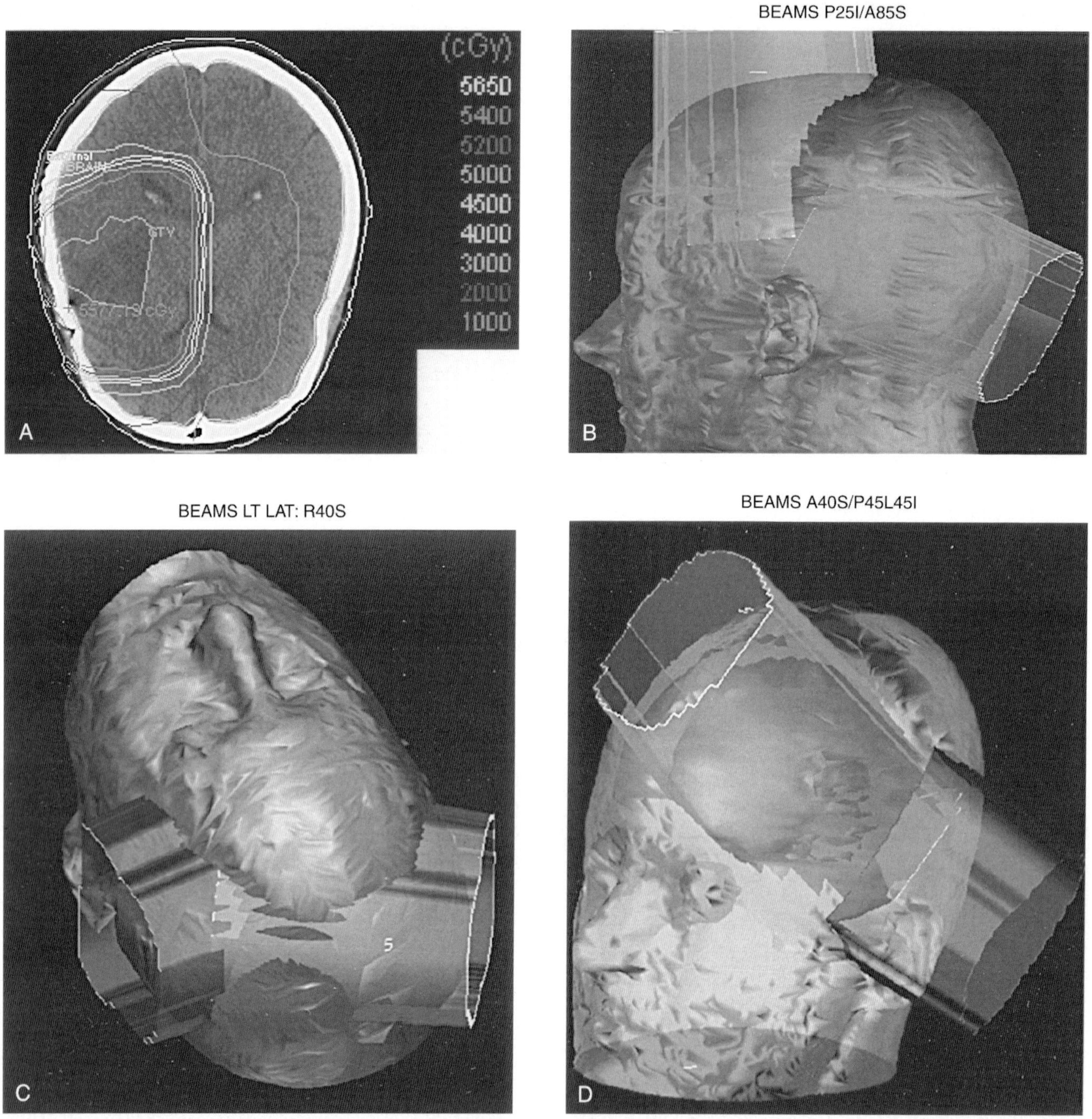

Figure 7-6 (PLATE 39). (A) Axial isodose distribution through the geometric center of a recurrent oligodendroglioma. The patient was placed in the prone position to obviate mechanical constraints of the linear accelerator, allowing a wider selection of beam angles. A thermoplastic mask was fabricated to immobilize the patient's head. Axial T_2-weighted MRI images were fused with a planning CT scan to define the gross tumor volume (GTV). Two-centimeter margins were added to the tumor volume to account for patient setup variability and subclinical tumor infiltration. The margin was decreased medially because the tumor did not involve the corpus callosum and therefore contralateral hemispheric involvement was not a concern. This step was taken to decrease the dose to the contralateral hemisphere. The three-dimensional treatment plan called for six beams (B, posterior 25 degrees inferior and anterior 85 degrees superior; C, left lateral and right 40 degrees superior; D, anterior 40 degrees superior and posterior 45 degrees left 45 degrees inferior) employing various wedging (to improve dose homogeneity) to deliver a total dose of 5400 cGy in 30 fractions.

reproducibility of the treatment position is essential. Consequently, a device is needed to accurately reposition the patient on a day-to-day basis. This is accomplished through many measures, but most radiation therapy centers custom fabricate a thermoplastic mask for each individual patient (Fig. 7-7). These masks prevent the head from moving during treatment (immobilization). To provide consistent reference points, fiducial markers are placed on the mask. Each day during treatment setup these markers are aligned with lasers in the linear accelerator treatment room, allowing precise alignment of patients on a daily basis (see Fig. 7-1). Current plastic masks can achieve a setup accuracy of 2 to 3 mm.[50]

Once an immobilization device has been constructed, the patient will undergo a treatment simulation and planning session in the treatment position. In the past, most simulators were conventional fluoroscopic units and decisions were based on bony anatomic landmarks using fluoroscopy and plain radiographs. Now most radiation centers use CT simulators to acquire a set of axial images through the volume of interest to plan the treatments. The planning CT scanners are similar to diagnostic scanners, except planning scans are conducted under the same conditions (on a flat table with custom immobilization devices) used for treatment of the patient on the linear accelerator. The CT simulators incorporate powerful imaging workstations allowing efficient target contouring, image manipulation, and "virtual" simulation of beam arrangements (Fig. 7-8). Image fusion between CT and other imaging modalities, such as MRI, can also be performed on these workstations, and this additional imaging information can significantly facilitate tumor volume definition.[51]

Once the planning CT images are in the treatment planning computer, the radiation oncologist defines the gross tumor volume (GTV), volumes at risk for tumor spread (clinical target volume [CTV]) without obvious gross disease on imaging, and critical normal structures (e.g., optic nerves, brainstem, middle ear, pituitary). A planning target volume (PTV) is then generated by enlarging the CTV with a margin of approximately 5 mm to account for patient setup error and inaccuracies in imaging. The radiation dosimetrist then designs a treatment plan to deliver a homogenous radiation dose (as prescribed by the radiation oncologists) to cover the PTV while minimizing dose to critical structures outside the PTV. By achieving a homogenous dose distribution, areas of excessive dose ("hot spots") are avoided, decreasing the risk of toxicities (e.g., necrosis). The radiation oncologist reviews the computerized dose distributions (isodoses) displayed (most commonly) on axial CT slices through the volume of interest and determines if the plan is acceptable or needs to be modified.

In the recent past, as a result of the constraints of limited planning abilities and advanced imaging, avoiding critical structures such as normal surrounding brain was not possible and large portions of normal structures were treated to the same dose as prescribed to the tumor volume. With the advent of sophisticated computerized planning systems and detailed imaging, it is now possible to deliver high doses of radiation to a tumor while significantly sparing surrounding normal structures from these high doses of radiation. This is accomplished by the use of multiple, nonoverlapping, conformal radiation beams shaped by custom-made blocks to the configuration of the tumor volume in the "beam's eye view" (Fig. 7-9) or,

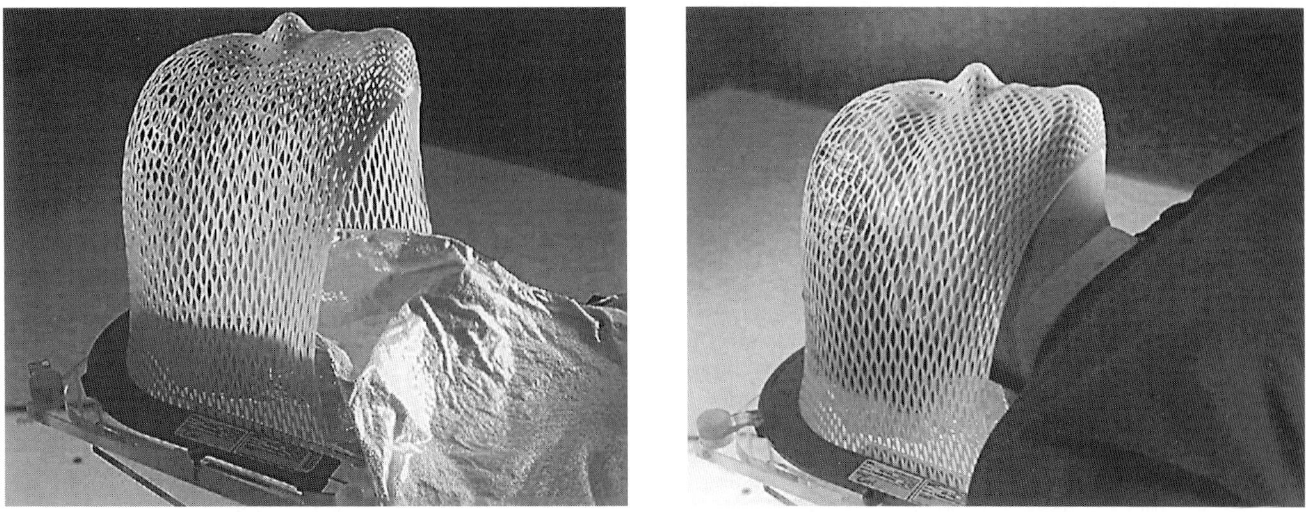

Figure 7-7. Thermoplastic head immobilization device. Note also the custom molding neck rest to better immobilize the back of the head.

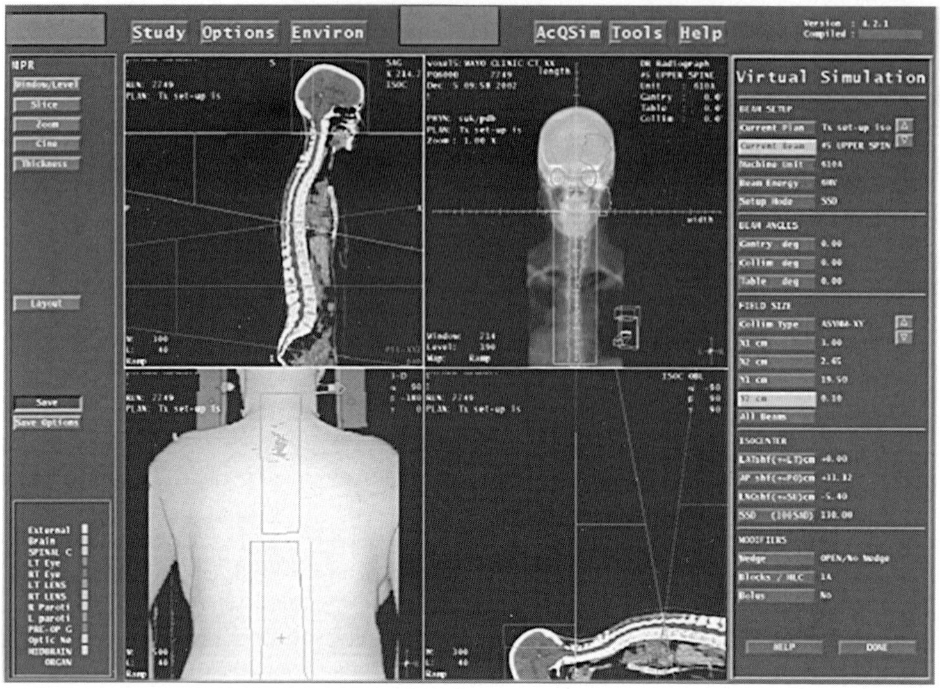

Figure 7-8. A sagittal isocentric, reformatted image (top left and lower right box) of a 33-year-old female with a primitive neuroectodermal tumor (PNET) undergoing cranial spinal axis radiation therapy. The virtual simulation of all fields demonstrates the precise matching of the cranial and spine fields achieved by interactive collimator rotation of the spine fields and the creation of a "beam-split" cranial field and upper spine field on the workstation.

R10I Beam

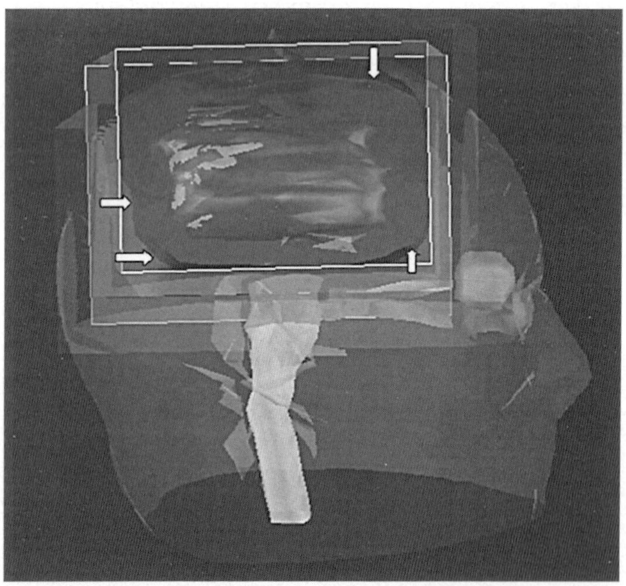

Figure 7-9. A 57-year-old male with a glioblastoma multiforme treated with three-dimensional conformal radiotherapy. Five non-coplanar beams and one compensating beam (to increase dose homogeneity) were used to treat the initial volume of abnormal contrast enhancement and edema with margin. Only the right 10 degrees inferior (R10I) beam is shown to illustrate the shaping of blocks (arrows) to *conform* the beam of radiation to the shape of the target while avoiding critical structures by manipulating the beam angle.

as it is often named, three-dimensional (3D) conformal radiotherapy. In the past these custom-made blocks were lead-alloy and quite heavy (Fig. 7-10A). These lead-alloy blocks were placed, between the linear accelerator and the patient, in a tray (Fig. 7-10B). Each separate field required a therapist reentering the treatment room and changing the block. This process was taxing on the therapist as well as time-consuming, especially for complex treatments requiring multiple fields. Therefore, computer-controlled tungsten leaves, or multileaf collimators (MLCs), were created. (Fig. 7-11). These individual leaves shift to form specific patterns, conforming the radiation beam to the target just as the lead-alloy blocks do.[52] This advance in technology relieves the physical strain on the therapist and significantly decreases treatment time for the patient. In addition to blocks, wedges are often added to alter the radiation beam dose distribution to allow more uniform dose distribution within the treatment volume. The planning and designing of beams in this process is done manually and guided by experience and comparison of a few different sets of beam arrangements to achieve the "best" treatment plan.

A recent innovation, intensity-modulated radiation therapy (IMRT), provides a completely different approach to treatment planning. Instead of clinicians defining beam directions, beam weights, wedges, blocks, and margins, and then computing and displaying dose distributions to assess whether the treatment plan will lead to an acceptable outcome, they do the opposite, or "inverse" treatment

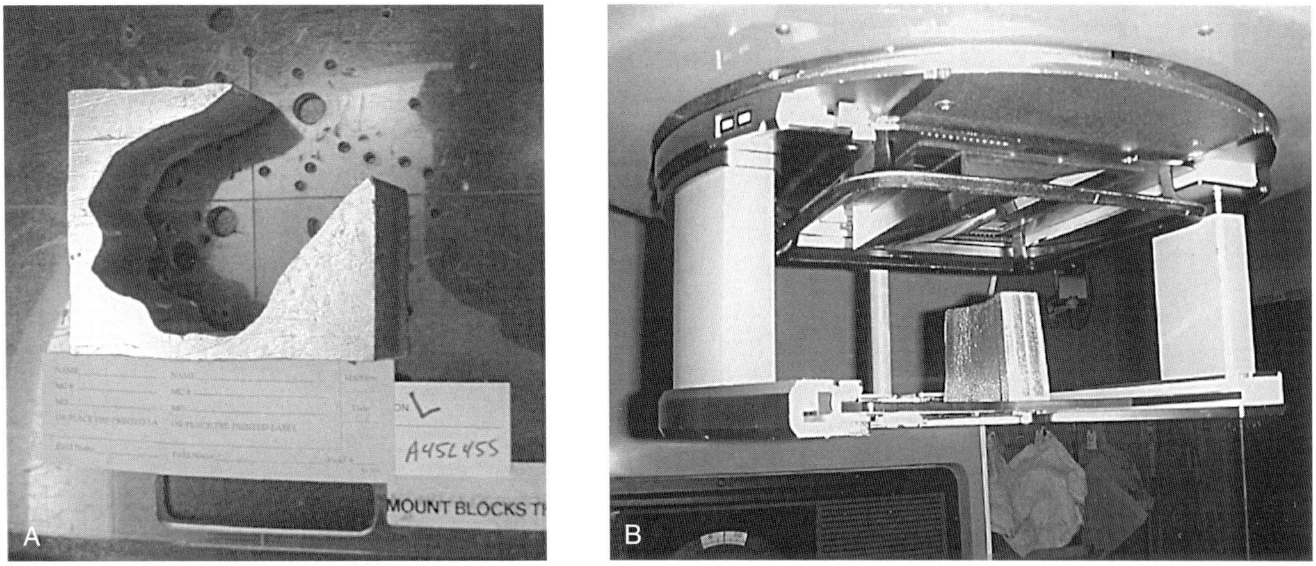

Figure 7-10. (A) A lead-alloy custom-made block used to shape and conform the radiation beam to the target. (B) A view of the head of the linear accelerator with the block placed in position on the tray between the linear accelerator and the patient.

planning. The radiation oncologist specifies the prescribed target dose and the dose constraints for normal structures. The radiation oncologist then prioritizes these dose specifications. The sophisticated algorithms of the inverse treatment planning system allows the evaluation of millions of possible beam arrangements and determines the clinically optimized treatment plan, maximizing the dose to the tumor while minimizing exposure to surrounding healthy tissue. MLCs and computer-controlled tungsten leaves can shift during treatment to form specific patterns, selectively blocking the radiation to create beams of varying intensities. Hundreds to thousands of small, modulated radiation beams strike a tumor site with varying intensities and from many angles to attack the target in a

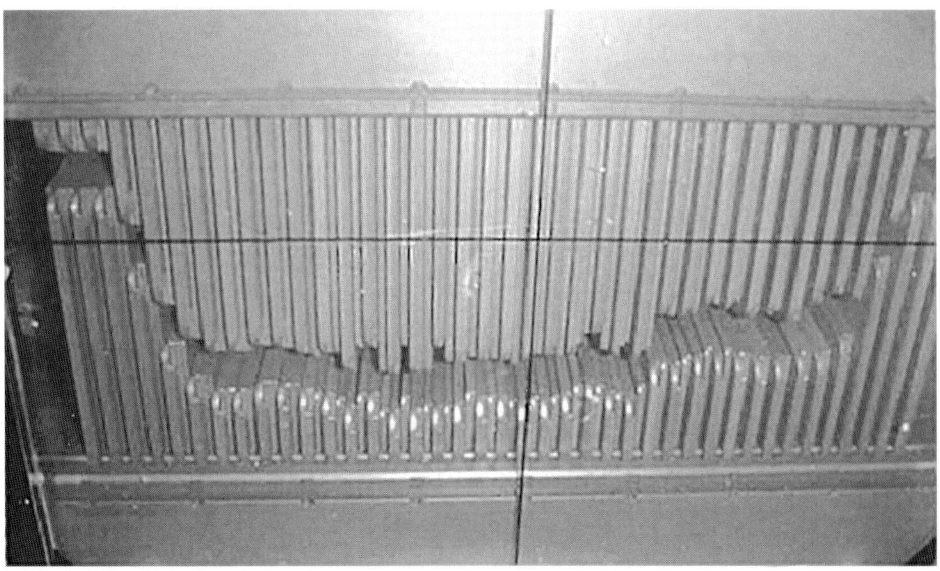

Figure 7-11. A close-up view of the head of a linear accelerator showing the multileaf collimator (MLC) leaves in position to treat a radiotherapy field.

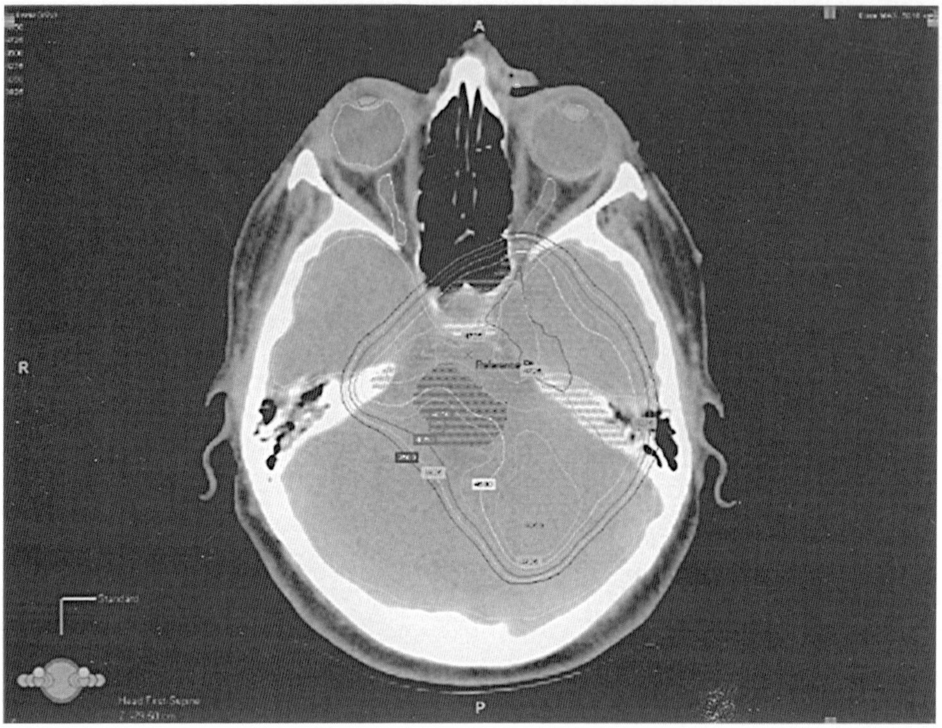

Figure 7-12 (PLATE 40). Dose distribution of an intensity-modulated radiation therapy plan for a 51-year-old female with an extensive skull-based meningioma (shaded) with involvement of clivus, left petrous apex, and left tentorium. The plan conforms the dose to the irregular tumor volume, allowing greater sparing of the brainstem and other critical structures.

complete three-dimensional manner. The combination of these beams produces the final dose distribution that conforms to the targets and avoids organs at risk (Fig. 7.12). IMRT is usually delivered using a "step-and-shoot" technique. There are two versions of step-and-shoot treatments: static and sliding window. In both instances, while the radiation beam is on, the gantry remains stationary. The gantry then moves (or steps) to the next position. With static step and shoot, MLC leaves change shape only when radiation is not being produced. With sliding window, MLC leaves change shape while radiation is being delivered. A comparison of linear accelerator–based radiosurgery (five non-coplanar arcs), fixed non-coplanar 3D custom-blocked (six) fields, and IMRT (six non-coplanar intensity-modulated beams) did find improved dose conformity and decreased dose to nontarget brain in high and low isodose (i.e., a line of constant dose akin to the contours on a topography map) regions for the IMRT plans for the irregular tumor targets.[53]

Another innovation, stereotactic radiotherapy, combines the advantages of high precision radiosurgery with the biologic benefit of fractionation. Stereotactic radiotherapy is able to achieve this by using the physical advantages of stereotactic radiosurgery of accurately depositing the radiation in the target with sparing of normal tissues along with the differential radiosensitivity of normal tissues and the neoplasms with fractionated radiotherapy. These advantages are helpful when treating lesions near dose-limiting structures such as the optic nerves (Fig. 7-13).

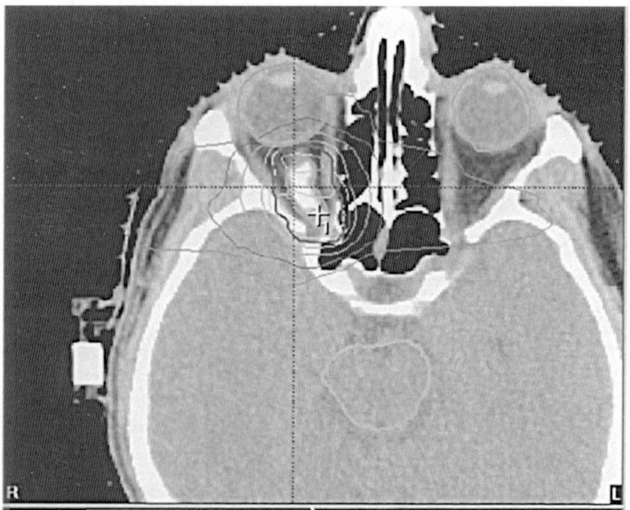

Figure 7-13 (PLATE 41). A patient with a right optic nerve sheath meningioma treated to 50.4 Gy with fractionated stereotactic radiotherapy system using a relocatable head frame stabilized by a mouth-guard bite block.

Image-guided target localization and image-integrated dose planning are essential. Additionally, because the treatment may last several weeks, a repeatable head fixation device is an absolute requirement for any facility performing stereotactic radiation therapy.[54] These devices often include a relocatable head frame stabilized by a mouthguard-type bite block. Although these "pinless" stereotactic systems are less accurate than the standard, fixed-head frames often used in radiosurgery, they can achieve an accuracy of better than 2 mm.[55,56]

Treatment Delivery

Each treatment day the patient is repositioned into the exact position in which the planning scan was performed. During a typical 20-minute treatment session, most of the time is spent positioning the patient. To aid in this procedure, lasers in the horizontal and vertical directions are used to align the patient with fiducial markers. Computer systems verify and record multiple parameters of each treatment including wedging, blocks, patient position, dose, and beam energy.[57] If any of these parameters are not set properly, the software will not allow the radiation treatment to proceed. These computer systems along with the manual quality checklists significantly increase the level of accuracy and patient safety. Portal films (or port films) are periodically obtained using the treatment machine with the patient setup for treatment. These port films, although of poorer quality as a consequence of the Compton effect, verify patient position, blocking, and beam arrangement throughout treatment. In the past, these were "hard" films that required much of the therapist's time for processing and developing. With the introduction of electronic portal imaging devices (EPIDs), these port films are now obtained during the treatment procedure and are digitally stored enabling intra- and intertreatment assessment of patient position and blocking.[58] The EPID films are equivalent or superior to traditional port films[59] and significantly decrease the amount of labor required.

Typically the patient will receive five treatments a week, once a day, Monday through Friday, although there can be variations on this schedule. In addition to the treatment schedule, the patient will visit with the radiation oncologists once a week (or more) to assess his or her status and manage any potential toxicities or other difficulties. Most conventional fractionation schedules are delivered with 1.8 to 2 Gy fractions daily. Hyperfractionation involves delivering multiple (two to three), smaller (1–1.2 Gy) fractions per day, with the goal of delivering a higher total dose. The smaller doses per fraction allow more healing of sublethal damage between treatments and therefore permit modest dose escalations of 15% to 20%. This approach has been tested in prospective randomized studies in high-grade gliomas[60] and brainstem gliomas[61,62] and, unfortunately, has resulted in little success. Accelerated hypofractionation uses fewer fractions but larger doses per fraction (typically 3–5 Gy) to achieve a lower total dose (20–40 Gy) over 1 to 3 weeks. These schedules are often used for palliation of brain metastases and spinal cord compression. The goal is to minimize the number of treatments for patient convenience while providing palliation for patients with a poor prognosis.

Brachytherapy

As reviewed earlier, the use of brachytherapy, the placement of radioactive sources into or next to tumors, dates back approximately 100 years. Brachytherapy is advantageous because it can deliver a large dose of radiation to the target with significant fall-off of dose within the normal surrounding structures. Brachytherapy can be achieved by direct implantation of radioactive "seeds" or, more often, by placing hollow closed-end catheters into the target volume and afterloading these catheters with "ribbons" of radioactive seeds. Brachytherapy is highly technical and if the radiation is not properly distributed, it can result in significant overdosing in regions of the brain; therefore, a limited number of institutions have sufficient experience to perform this task. There was an initial enthusiasm for brachytherapy in the high-grade gliomas, but with two prospective randomized trials showing no significant benefit for brachytherapy[63,64] and the complex, labor-intensive nature of the process, this procedure has now been relegated to research protocols at a handful of institutions.

▶ STEREOTACTIC RADIOSURGERY

Stereotactic radiosurgery is a surgical procedure that combines the principles of stereotactic localization with the precise delivery of radiation to an imaging-defined target. Lars Leksell, a Swedish neurosurgeon, conceived the concept of stereotactic radiosurgery in 1951.[65] His goal was to provide a method for the noninvasive destruction of intracranial lesions that were high risk for surgical resection. To accomplish this goal, Leksell coupled stereotactic localization with the delivery of a large, single-fraction dose of ionizing radiation.[66,67] The early devices used low-energy X-rays (280 kV) to treat primarily functional disorders including obsessive-compulsive states and trigeminal neuralgia. Leksell later explored the utility of linear accelerators (LINACs) and proton beams for radiosurgery. In 1967, Leksell, in collaboration with Börje Larsson, developed the first cobalt-60 gamma unit (the Gamma Knife, Elekta Instruments, Norcross, GA). However, it has only been in the past two decades that radiosurgery has gained acceptance and has become an integral part of both neurosurgery and radiation oncology. Recent years have seen an exponential growth in the number of radiosurgical sites across the world. Advances in neuroimaging and improved computer software have made radiosurgery safer and more effective in the management of a wide range of disorders affecting the nervous system. Today, radiosurgery is available to patients at the majority of large medical centers.

The goal of radiosurgery is to deliver a high radiation dose in a single fraction to an imaging-defined target while minimizing the radiation exposure to the adjacent tissues. In contrast to conventional fractionated radiation therapy, radiosurgery does not rely on the increased radiation sensitivity of the target compared with the normal brain. Rather, radiosurgical treatment spares normal structures using conformal dose plans that deposit large radiation doses into the target with a rapid fall-off of radiation at the edges of the dose plan (Fig. 7-14). Stereotactic imaging and target localization using CT, MRI, and/or angiography must be fully integrated with the radiation delivery device to achieve pinpoint localization of the target. The irradiation isocenter must accurately coincide with the desired target. Different radiosurgical systems satisfy these essential criteria by using various technical solutions. Similarly, a variety of computer-based approaches to radiosurgical dose planning provide a three-dimensional representation of isodose contours superimposed on the stereotactic images of the target and surrounding intracranial structures.

A key element in stereotactic radiosurgery is the use of multiple radiation fields (isocenters) distributed over space to create a conformal dose plan to cover the desired target. A single field (or a pair of opposed fields) will deliver full dose to the target but will also treat a large portion of the normal tissues to full dose. By increasing the number of isocenters, the high-dose region tends to conform to the target (Fig. 7-15).

▶ RADIOSURGICAL INSTRUMENTS

The Gamma Knife

The first gamma unit was installed at the Sofiahemmet Hospital in Stockholm in 1968. Leksell and Larsson designed the first 179-source ^{60}Co gamma unit as a "practical, precise and simple tool which could be handled by the surgeon himself."[66] Despite improvements in the device and clinical usage in Sweden, Sheffield, and Buenos Aires, the clinical usefulness of the Gamma Knife became widely appreciated only after the initial experience from the University of Pittsburgh was published by Lunsford and his colleagues.[68] The current version of this device contains 201 individual ^{60}Co sources that naturally decay to nickel (^{60}Ni) (Figs. 7-16 and 7-17). During this process gamma photons are released with energies of 1.17 MeV and 1.33 MeV. The emitted photons are precisely directed through circular channels drilled into a high-density metal helmet. Each of these channels houses an individual collimator. The collimators are removable

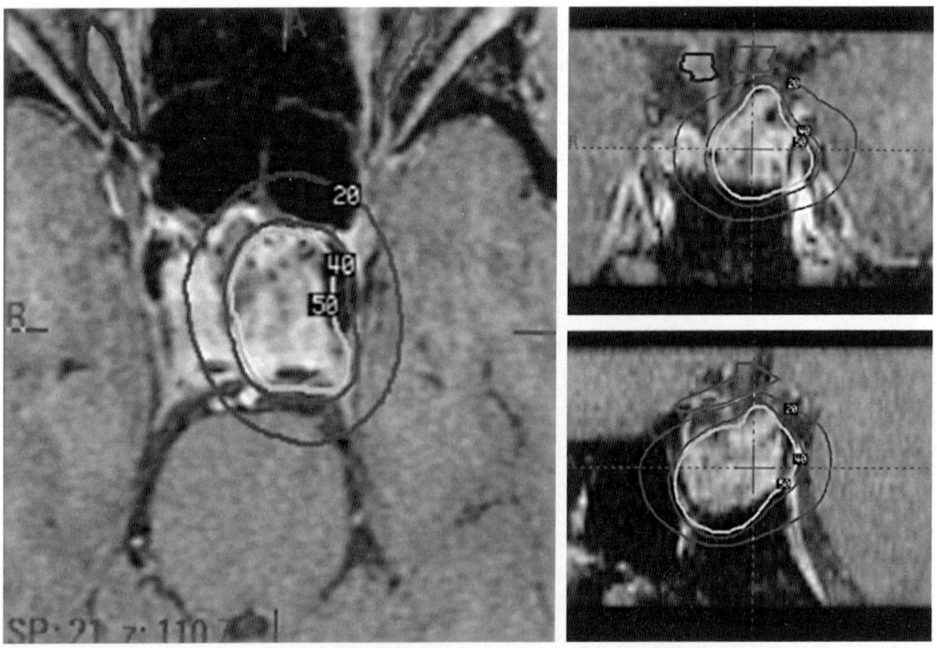

Figure 7-14 (PLATE 42). Dose plan of a patient with an enlarging nonfunctional pituitary adenoma after prior transsphenoidal resection. Six isocenters of radiation were used to cover a volume of 3.2 cm^3. The tumor margin dose was 16 Gy; the maximum radiation dose to the adjacent left optic nerve was 6.1 Gy.

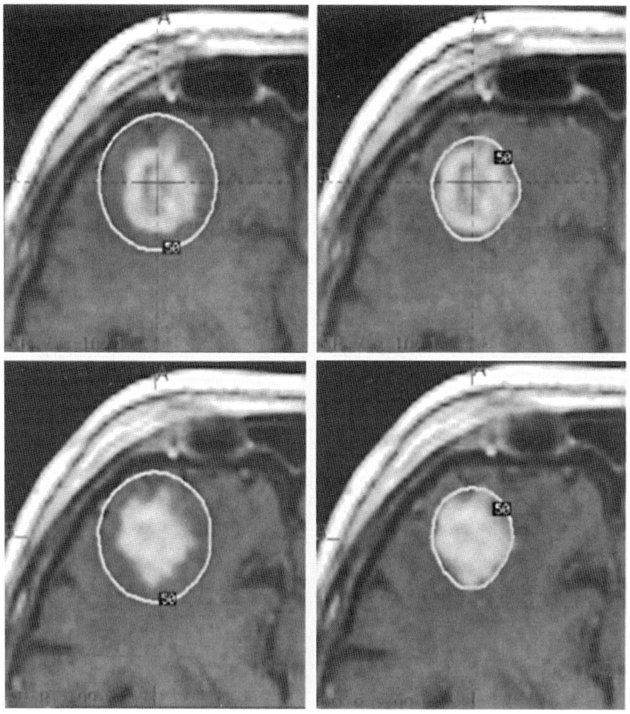

Figure 7-15. Two possible dose plans for a patient with a right frontal metastasis. (Left) Dose plan consisting of a single 18-mm isocenter of radiation. The volume inside the 50% isodose line is 5.9 cm^3. (Right) Dose plan consisting of two 14-mm and four 8-mm isocenters of radiation. The volume inside the 50% isodose line is 3.2 cm^3. Although both dose plans provide good tumor coverage, the more conformal plan is 46% smaller in volume.

with diameters of 4, 8, 14, or 18 mm. One or more of these collimators can be removed and replaced with a plug with no aperture to block radiation from that particular source. Plugging of individual sources is typically performed to limit radiation to radiosensitive structures such as the optic nerves or chiasm. The target coordinates, collimator size, and relative weighting of each isocenter are entered into the treatment-planning computer. Commercially available dose-planning systems provide an interactive video display of multiplanar isodose contours superimposed on the stereotactic images, plus a three-dimensional analysis of isodose volumes in relation to adjacent intracranial structures. Because the Gamma Knife employs fixed sources with a constant relation to the collimator helmet and stereotactic frame, isocenter verification films or port films are unnecessary. The majority of targets are treated at the 50% isodose (see Fig. 7-15) line or higher. Dose prescription at such isodose lines contributes to dose inhomogeneity, which correlates to a higher risk of radiation-related complications if the dose plans are not conformal (i.e., doses shaped—conformed—to the contour of the treatment

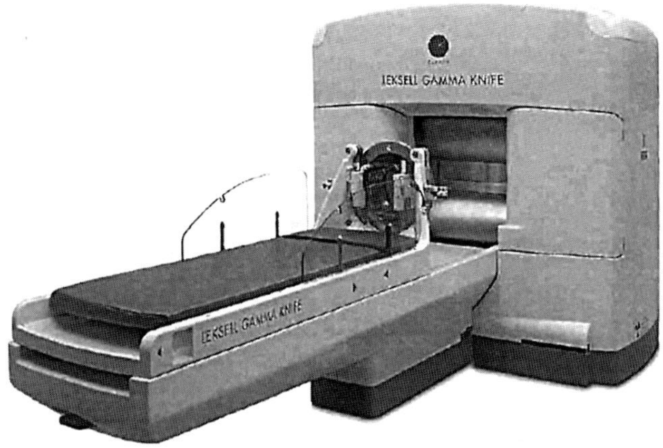

Figure 7-16. Photograph of the Model C Leksell Gamma Knife. (*Courtesy of Elekta Instruments, Norcross, GA.*)

area) and significant portions of normal tissue fall within the prescription isodose line. The dose distribution can be modified by several variables including the number of isocenters, the placement of isocenters, the choice of different collimator helmets, plugging individual beam channels, and weighting of isocenters. The latest version of the Gamma Knife (Model C) features an automatic positioning system (APS) (Fig. 7-18). The APS is a fully motorized system that automatically sets the head frame coordinates, repositioning the patient at each isocenter by digitally transferred information from the operator's console.[69] Advantages of the APS system include a reduction in the time needed to treat individual patients and a decreased chance of radiation misadministration because of human error. In addition, this system encourages the creation of dose plans consisting of a large number of small isocenters of radiation, thereby allowing for even more conformal radiosurgical plans.

Linear Accelerator–Based Radiosurgery

The development of LINAC-based radiosurgical systems began in the 1980s.[70] Betti,[71] Colombo,[72,73] Hartmann,[74] and their respective associates, Winston and Lutz[75]; and others contributed to the innovation and growth of this technology. These systems generally consist of a stereotactic head frame, floorstand, and a 6-MV linear accelerator. Multiple (often four or more) sagittally oriented irradiation arcs are delivered using a wide range of circular collimators. Detection of mechanical inaccuracy is performed by a phantom-target film technique for every treatment arc. Friedman and Bova further refined LINAC-based radiosurgery by adding a high-precision attachment to control movements of the patient's head and the tertiary collimators (5–35 mm diameter) independent of potential variations in gantry or treatment couch alignment.[76]

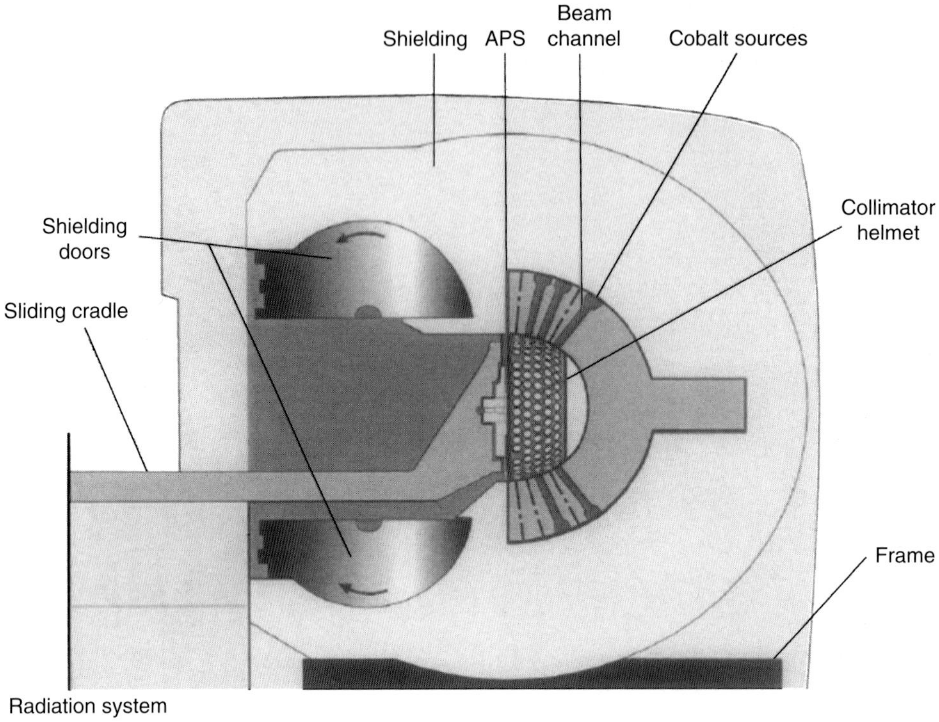

Figure 7-17. Cross-sectional schematic of the Gamma Knife (*Courtesy of Elekta Instruments, Norcross, GA*) showing the orientation of the cobalt-60, the secondary collimators, and the patient couch.

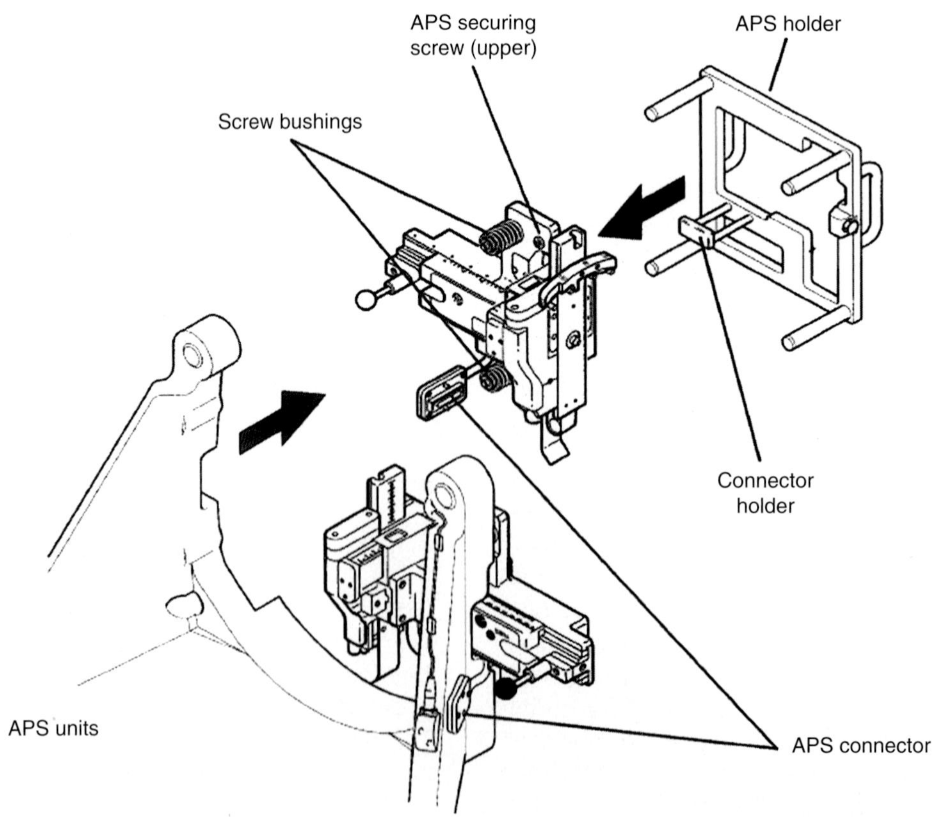

Figure 7-18. Schematic of the Leksell Gamma Knife Automatic Positioning System (APS). (*Courtesy of Elekta Instruments, Norcross, GA.*)

The CyberKnife

John Adler and colleagues at Stanford University developed a radiosurgical device called the CyberKnife (Accuray, Sunnyvale, CA) that incorporates recent advances in robotics and computerized image recognition.[77] The CyberKnife has a compact, lightweight linear accelerator mounted on a robotic arm (Fig. 7.19). For intracranial targets, patients are fitted with a noninvasive flexible mesh mask to limit large movements. Because skeletal landmarks are used to define stereotactic space, fixation with a conventional "fixed" stereotactic head frame is not required. For extracranial targets, small, radiopaque fiducial markers are placed near the target and are tracked as reference points during treatments. Radiographs of the treatment site are taken and image registration performed to determine the target's coordinates with respect to the LINAC. The target coordinates are transferred to the robot, which directs the beam to the treatment site. The system has dynamic tracking software that can follow lesions in six dimensions (three translational and three rotational axes) to account and compensate for any patient movement. If any movement of the target during treatment is detected, the LINAC is repositioned to the new target location. Although the CyberKnife has the theoretical potential to create a dose plan by firing from an infinite number of radiation beams, in practice the CyberKnife uses 101 specific nodes in space, each with 12 approach angles, allowing for more than 1200 possible radiation beams. Because the CyberKnife can be used to treat extracranial targets, it is the most flexible of the commercially available radiosurgical devices.[78]

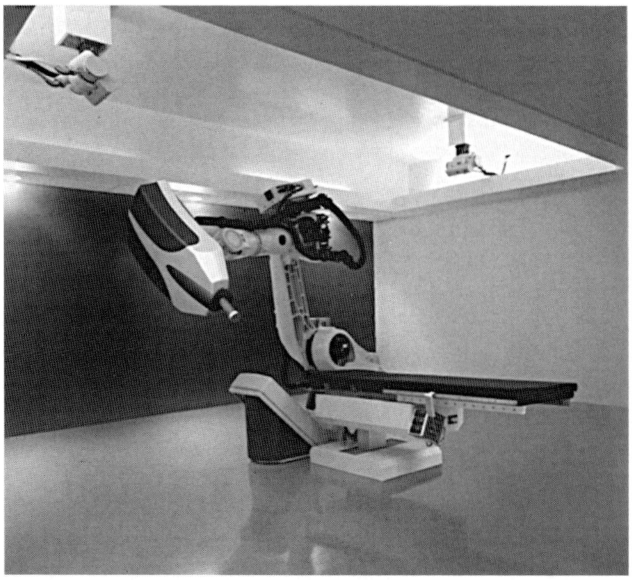

Figure 7-19. Photograph of the CyberKnife. (*Courtesy of Accuray, Sunnyvale, CA.*)

► CONCLUSION

Although this chapter serves only as an introduction to the basic principles of radiotherapy and radiosurgery, it provides a background for the chapters that follow that outline the role of different radiotherapy modalities (conventional radiotherapy, altered fractionation, particulate radiation, stereotactic radiotherapy, IMRT, brachytherapy, and radiosurgery) in the treatment of central nervous system tumors. As technology continues to improve and evolve, having a solid understanding of the basic principles of radiation will be even more important when making optimal treatment decisions.

REFERENCES

1. Rossi HH, Kellerer AM. Roentgen. Radiat Res 1995;144: 124–128.
2. Sherman AA. Translation of an historic paper. On a new, strongly radioactive substance, contained in pitchblende: by MP Curie, Mme P Curie and MG Bemont; presented by M Becquerel. J Nucl Med 1970;11:269–720.
3. Simpson FE. Radium in the treatment of cancer and various other diseases of the skin. JAMA 1916;67:1508.
4. Sowers ZT. The uses of radium. Am Med 1903;7:261.
5. Kelly HA, Burnam CF. Radium in the treatment of carcinoma of the cervix uteri and vagina. JAMA 1915;65:1874.
6. del Regato JA. Fractionation: a panoramic view. Int J Radiat Oncol Biol Phys 1990;19:1329–1331.
7. Kahn FM. The physics of radiation therapy, 2nd ed. Baltimore: Williams & Wilkins, 1994.
8. Joensuu H, Kankaanranta L, Seppala T, et al. Boron neutron capture therapy of brain tumors: clinical trials at the Finnish facility using boronophenylalanine. J Neurooncol 2003;62:123–134.
9. Barth RF. A critical assessment of boron neutron capture therapy: an overview. J Neurooncol 2003;62:1–5.
10. Miller DW. A review of proton beam radiation therapy. Med Phys 1995;22:1943–1954.
11. Krengli M, Liebsch NJ, Hug EB, et al. Review of current protocols for proton therapy in USA. Tumori 1998; 84:209–216.
12. Houlthusen H. The present status of dosage measurement. Radiology 1928;10:292.
13. Hall EJ, Astor M, Bedford J, et al. Basic radiobiology. Am J Clin Oncol 1988;11:220–252.
14. Munro TR. The relative radiosensitivity of the nucleus and cytoplasm of Chinese hamster fibroblasts. Radiat Res 1970;42:451–470.
15. Frankenberg-Schwager M. Review of repair kinetics for DNA damage induced in eukaryotic cells in vitro by ionizing radiation. Radiother Oncol 1989;14:307–320.
16. Thompson LH, Suit HD. Proliferation kinetics of x-irradiated mouse L cells studied with time-lapse photography. II. Int J Radiat Biol Rel Studies Phys Chem Med 1969:2;15:347–362.
17. McCarthy NJ, Hazlewood SA, Huen DS, et al. The Epstein-Barr virus gene BHRF1, a homologue of the cellular oncogene Bcl-2, inhibits apoptosis induced by gamma radiation

and chemotherapeutic drugs. Adv Exp Med Biol 1996; 406:83–97.
18. Potten CS, Merritt A, Hickman J, et al. Characterization of radiation-induced apoptosis in the small intestine and its biological implications. Int J Radiat Biol 1994;65:71–78.
19. Haas RL, Poortmans P, de Jong D, et al. High response rates and lasting remissions after low-dose involved field radiotherapy in indolent lymphomas. J Clin Oncol 2003; 21:2474–2480.
20. Thames HD, Bentzen SM, Turesson I, et al. Time-dose factors in radiotherapy: a review of the human data. Radiother Oncol 1990;19:219–235.
21. Hall EJ, Brenner DJ. The radiobiology of radiosurgery: rationale for different treatment regimes for AVMs and malignancies [comment]. Int J Radiat Oncol Biol Phys 1993;25:381–385.
22. Littman P, Rosenstock J, Gale G, et al. The somnolence syndrome in leukemic children following reduced daily dose fractions of cranial radiation. Int J Radiat Oncol Biol Phys 1984;10:1851–1853.
23. Freeman JE, Johnston PG, Voke JM. Somnolence after prophylactic cranial irradiation in children with acute lymphoblastic leukaemia. Br Med J 1973;4:523–525.
24. Armstrong CL, Hunter JV, Ledakis GE, et al. Late cognitive and radiographic changes related to radiotherapy: initial prospective findings [see comments]. Neurology 2002;59: 40–48.
25. DeAngelis LM, Delattre JY, Posner JB. Radiation-induced dementia in patients cured of brain metastases. Neurology 1989;39:789–796.
26. Constine LS, Woolf PD, Cann D, et al. Hypothalamic-pituitary dysfunction after radiation for brain tumors [comment] [erratum appears in N Engl J Med 1993;328(16):1208]. N Engl J Med 1993;328:87–94.
27. Parsons JT, Bova FJ, Fitzgerald CR, et al. Radiation optic neuropathy after megavoltage external-beam irradiation: analysis of time-dose factors. Int J Radiat Oncol Biol Phys 1994;30:755–763.
28. Marcus RB Jr, Million RR. The incidence of myelitis after irradiation of the cervical spinal cord. Int J Radiat Oncol Biol Phys 1990;19:3–8.
29. Sheline GE, Wara WM, Smith V. Therapeutic irradiation and brain injury. Int J Radiat Oncol Biol Phys 1980;6:1215–1228.
30. Shaw E, Arusell R, Scheithauer B, et al. Prospective randomized trial of low- versus high-dose radiation therapy in adults with supratentorial low-grade glioma: initial report of a North Central Cancer Treatment Group/Radiation Therapy Oncology Group/Eastern Cooperative Oncology Group study. J Clin Oncol 2002;20:2267–2276.
31. Saunders MI, Dische S, Grosch EJ, et al. Experience with CHART [erratum appears in Int J Radiat Oncol Biol Phys 1991;21(6):1683]. Int J Radiat Oncol Biol Phys 1991;21: 871–878.
32. Chadderton RD, West CG, Schuller S, et al. Radiotherapy in the treatment of low-grade astrocytomas. II. The physical and cognitive sequelae [erratum appears in Childs Nerv Syst 1995;11(12):715 Note: Schulz S (corrected to Schuller S)]. Childs Nerv Sys 1995;11:443–448.
33. Cappelli C, Grill J, Raquin M, et al. Long-term follow up of 69 patients treated for optic pathway tumours before the chemotherapy era. Arch Dis Childhood 1998;79:334–338.
34. Gregor A, Cull A, Traynor E, et al. Neuropsychometric evaluation of long-term survivors of adult brain tumours: relationship with tumour and treatment parameters. Radiother Oncol 1996;41:55–59.
35. Taylor BV, Buckner JC, Cascino TL, et al. Effects of radiation and chemotherapy on cognitive function in patients with high-grade glioma [see comments]. J Clin Oncol 1998;16:2195–2201.
36. Torres IJ, Mundt AJ, Sweeney PJ, et al. A longitudinal neuropsychological study of partial brain radiation in adults with brain tumors. Neurology 2003;60:1113–1118.
37. Surma-aho O, Niemela M, Vilkki J, et al. Adverse long-term effects of brain radiotherapy in adult low-grade glioma patients. Neurology 2001;56:1285–1290.
38. Curnes JT, Laster DW, Ball MR, et al. MRI of radiation injury to the brain. AJR 1986;147:119–124.
39. Scheibel RS, Meyers CA, Levin VA. Cognitive dysfunction following surgery for intracerebral glioma: influence of histopathology, lesion location, and treatment. J Neurooncol 1996;30:61–69.
40. Imperato JP, Paleologos NA, Vick NA. Effects of treatment on long-term survivors with malignant astrocytomas. Ann Neurol 1990;28:818–822.
41. Hammack JE, Shaw EG, Ivnik RJ, et al. Neurocognitive function in patients receiving radiation therapy (rt) for supratentorial low grade glioma (lgg): A North Central Cancer Treatment Group (NCCTG) prospective study [abstract no. 299]. Proc Am Soc Clin Oncol 1995;14:151.
42. Armstrong CL, Corn BW, Ruffer JE, et al. Radiotherapeutic effects on brain function: double dissociation of memory systems. Neuropsychiatry Neuropsychol Behav Neurol 2000;13:101–111.
43. Armstrong C, Ruffer J, Corn B, et al. Biphasic patterns of memory deficits following moderate-dose partial-brain irradiation: neuropsychologic outcome and proposed mechanisms. J Clin Oncol 1995;13:2263–2271.
44. Armstrong C, Mollman J, Corn BW, et al. Effects of radiation therapy on adult brain behavior: evidence for a rebound phenomenon in a phase 1 trial. Neurology 1993;43:1961–1965.
45. Vigliani MC, Sichez N, Poisson M, et al. A prospective study of cognitive functions following conventional radiotherapy for supratentorial gliomas in young adults: 4-year results. Int J Radiat Oncol Biol Phys 1996;35:527–533.
46. Glosser G, McManus P, Munzenrider J, et al. Neuropsychological function in adults after high dose fractionated radiation therapy of skull base tumors. Int J Radiat Oncol Biol Phys 1997;38:231–239.
47. Brown PD, Buckner JC, O'Fallon JR, et al. Effects of radiotherapy on cognitive function in patients with low-grade glioma measured by the Folstein Mini-Mental State Examination. J Clin Oncol 2003;21:2519–2524.
48. Laack N, Brown P, Furth A, et al. Neurocognitive function after radiotherapy (RT) for supratentorial low-grade gliomas (LGG): results of a North Central Cancer Treatment Group (NCCTG) prospective study [abstract 18]. Int J Radiat Oncol Biol Phys 2003;57:134.
49. Brown PD, Buckner JC, Uhm JH, et al. The neurocognitive effects of radiation in adult low-grade glioma patients. Neuro-Oncology 2003;5:161–167.

50. Verhey LJ. Immobilizing and positioning patients for radiotherapy. Semin Radiat Oncol 1995;5:100–114.
51. Khoo VS, Adams EJ, Saran F, et al. A comparison of clinical target volumes determined by CT and MRI for the radiotherapy planning of base of skull meningiomas. Int J Radiat Oncol Biol Phys 2000;46:1309–1317.
52. Ma L, Yu C, Sarfaraz M. A dosimetric leaf-setting strategy for shaping radiation fields using a multileaf collimator. Med Phys 2000;27:972–977.
53. Cardinale RM, Benedict SH, Wu Q, et al. A comparison of three stereotactic radiotherapy techniques; ARCS vs. noncoplanar fixed fields vs. intensity modulation. Int J Radiat Oncol Biol Phys 1998;42:431–436.
54. Kooy HM, Dunbar SF, Tarbell NJ, et al. Adaptation and verification of the relocatable Gill-Thomas-Cosman frame in stereotactic radiotherapy. Int J Radiat Oncol Biol Phys 1994;30:685–691.
55. Alheit H, Dornfeld S, Dawel M, et al. Patient position reproducibility in fractionated stereotactically guided conformal radiotherapy using the BrainLab mask system. Strahlenther Onkol 2001;177:264–268.
56. Verellen D, Linthout N, Bel A, et al. Assessment of the uncertainties in dose delivery of a commercial system for LINAC-based stereotactic radiosurgery. Int J Radiat Oncol Biol Phys 1999;44:421–433.
57. Mohan R, Podmaniczky KC, Caley R, et al. A computerized record and verify system for radiation treatments. Int J Radiat Oncol Biol Phys 1984;10:1975–1985.
58. Herman MG, Balter JM, Jaffray DA, et al. Clinical use of electronic portal imaging: report of AAPM Radiation Therapy Committee Task Group 57. Med Phys 2001;28:712–737.
59. Hatherly K, Smylie J, Rodger A. A comparison of field-only electronic portal imaging hard copies with double exposure port films in radiation therapy treatment setup confirmation to determine its clinical application in a radiotherapy center. Int J Radiat Oncol Biol Phys 1999;45:791–796.
60. Scott C, Curran WJ, Yung WK, et al. Long term results of RTOG 9006: a randomized trial of hyperfractionated radiotherapy (RT) to 72.0 Gy and carmustine vs standard RT and carmustine for malignant glioma patients with emphasis on anaplastic astrocytoma (AA) patients [abstract 1546]. Proc Am Soc Clin Oncol 1998;17:401.
61. Fisher PG, Donaldson SS. Hyperfractionated radiotherapy in the management of diffuse intrinsic brainstem tumors: when is enough enough? Int J Radiat Oncol Biol Phys 1999;43:947–949.
62. Mandell LR, Kadota R, Freeman C, et al. There is no role for hyperfractionated radiotherapy in the management of children with newly diagnosed diffuse intrinsic brainstem tumors: results of a Pediatric Oncology Group phase III trial comparing conventional vs. hyperfractionated radiotherapy. Int J Radiat Oncol Biol Phys 1999;43:959–964.
63. Laperriere NJ, Leung PM, McKenzie S, et al: Randomized study of brachytherapy in the initial management of patients with malignant astrocytoma. Int J Radiat Oncol Biol Phys 1998;41:1005–1011.
64. Selker RG, Shapiro WR, Burger P, et al. The Brain Tumor Cooperative Group NIH Trial 87–01: a randomized comparison of surgery, external radiotherapy, and carmustine versus surgery, interstitial radiotherapy boost, external radiation therapy, and carmustine. Neurosurgery 2002:51:343–355; discussion 355–357.
65. Leksell L. The stereotactic method and radiosurgery of the brain. Acta Chir Scand 1951;102:316–319.
66. Larsson B. The history of radiosurgery: the early years (1950–1970). In: Kondziolka D, ed. Radiosurgery. Basel: Karger, 1996:1–10.
67. Leksell L. Stereotactic radiosurgery. J Neurol Neurosurg Psychiatry 1983;46:797–803.
68. Lunsford LD, Flickinger J, Coffey RJ. Stereotactic gamma knife radiosurgery. Initial North American experience in 207 patients. Arch Neurol 1990:47:169–175.
69. Kondziolka D, Maitz AH, Niranjan A, et al. An evaluation of the Model C gamma knife with automatic patient positioning. Neurosurgery 2002:50:429–431; discussion 431–432.
70. Heifetz MD, Wexler M, Thompson R. Single-beam radiotherapy knife. A practical theoretical model. J Neurosurg 1984;60:814–818.
71. Betti OO, Galmarini D, Derechinsky V. Radiosurgery with a linear accelerator. Methodological aspects. Stereotac Funct Neurosurg 1991;57:87–98.
72. Colombo F, Benedetti A, Pozza F, et al. Stereotactic radiosurgery utilizing a linear accelerator. Appl Neurophysiol 1985;48:133–145.
73. Colombo F, Benedetti A, Pozza F, et al. Linear accelerator radiosurgery of three-dimensional irregular targets. Stereotac Funct Neurosurg 1990;54–55:541–546.
74. Hartmann GH, Schlegel W, Sturm V, et al. Cerebral radiation surgery using moving field irradiation at a linear accelerator facility. Int J Radiat Oncol Biol Phys 1985;11:1185–1192.
75. Winston KR, Lutz W. Linear accelerator as a neurosurgical tool for stereotactic radiosurgery. Neurosurgery 1988;22:454–464.
76. Friedman WA, Bova FJ. The University of Florida radiosurgery system. Surg Neurol 1989;32:334–342.
77. Adler JR Jr, Chang SD, Murphy MJ, et al. The CyberKnife: a frameless robotic system for radiosurgery. Stereotac Funct Neurosurg 1997;69:124–128.
78. Ryu SI, Chang SD, Kim DH, et al. Image-guided hypofractionated stereotactic radiosurgery to spinal lesions. Neurosurgery 2001;49:838–846.

CHAPTER 8

Principles of Chemotherapy

SANJAY P. AHUJA / REGINA I. JAKACKI

Chemotherapy is now considered part of the multimodality approach to the treatment of both adults and children with brain tumors. The addition of chemotherapy to the armamentarium of surgery and radiation therapy has resulted in improved survival for certain types of central nervous system (CNS) tumors, while its impact on others has been marginal at best. Tumors of different histologies vary tremendously in their response to cytotoxic drugs. Some tumors such as medulloblastomas, lymphomas, oligodendrogliomas, and germ cell tumors are remarkably chemosensitive. Even so, with few exceptions, none of these tumors can usually be successfully treated with chemotherapy alone. As is explained below, chemotherapy works best in the setting of minimal residual or microscopic disease and is usually administered following the completion of radiation therapy. Because of the deleterious effects of radiation therapy on the developing brain, the strategy of using chemotherapy to delay the need for, or to reduce the doses and/or fields of, radiation therapy is particularly relevant to pediatrics. For infants and young children, chemotherapy often becomes the primary treatment modality following surgical resection.

▶ PRINCIPLES OF CHEMOTHERAPY

Basic Concepts

The fundamental principles of chemotherapy emanated from research begun in the 1950s, much of which was done in murine tumor models. Despite the complexity of the human system and the tremendous advances in our knowledge base since that time, understanding these concepts is still valuable today.

Tumor Burden

The number of tumor cells present when a malignancy is first diagnosed is known as *tumor burden*. It is well-recognized that there is an inverse relationship between tumor burden and curability. Using a laboratory model of rodent leukemia, Skipper determined that the doubling time of proliferating tumor cells is constant, forming a straight line on a semilog plot (Fig. 8-1).[1] Death of the mouse resulted when the number of tumor cells reached a certain fraction of the body weight, demonstrating the functional relationship between survival and tumor burden. This relationship is not always relevant to brain tumors, however, where a very small tumor in a critical location can be deadly. In addition, other factors obviously complicate this simplistic "law" of tumor growth, and we now know that tumor growth more typically follows a Gompertzian growth curve.

Gompertzian Growth

The Gompertzian growth curves, which are derived from a mathematical model describing biologic growth

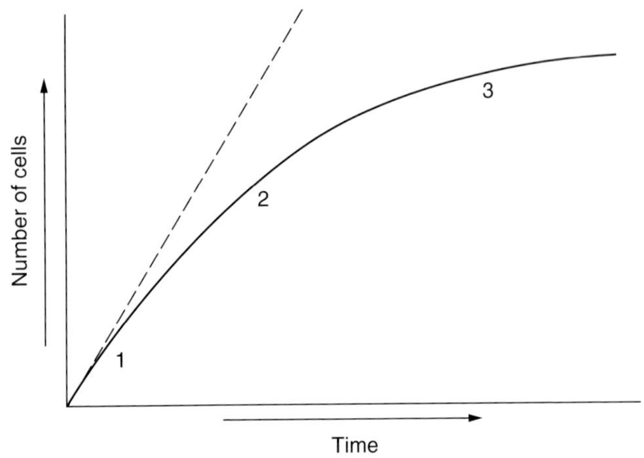

Figure 8-1. Comparison of the models describing patterns of tumor growth. The dashed line represents those with a constant doubling time; the solid line represents the mathematical model of Gompertzian growth.

in general,[2] are sigmoidal in shape rather than straight (see Fig. 8-1). This type of growth curve is more applicable to a heterogeneous population of tumor cells, some of which are actively proliferating, some of which are resting, and some of which are dying. As the tumor grows, the center of the tumor often loses its oxygen supply as a consequence of inadequate diffusion and the leading edge of the tumor outgrows its blood supply, leading to cell death and necrosis. This is a common occurrence in brain tumors, which are composed of both proliferating and nonproliferating cell populations, often with large areas of central necrosis.[3]

Cell Kill

Skipper also established that cytotoxic drugs kill tumor cells by first-order kinetics, i.e., a constant percentage, rather than an absolute number of cells are killed with each administration of drug.[4] The percentage of cells killed with each dose of drug remains constant regardless of the total body burden of tumor. For example, one log kill is defined as a 90% reduction in cell number or a reduction in cell number by a factor of 10. By first-order kinetics, if a drug kills 90% of the cancer cells at each administration, four cycles of the drug will result in a 99.99% reduction. However, this relatively simple picture is complicated in real life by many other factors, including the number of nonproliferating cells and the presence and appearance of drug-resistant clones (see "Drug Resistance" below). Brain tumors in particular are notoriously heterogeneous and have many cells that are either already resistant at the time of diagnosis or spontaneously develop resistance as they are treated.

Using the sigmoidal Gompertzian growth curve as a model to understand how tumors grow, the smallest tumors will have the largest growth fraction (point 1 on Fig. 8-1). Given what we know of the principles of cell kill and tumor burden, chemotherapy has the greatest chance of eradicating the tumor at this point. The other end of the curve (point 3 on Fig. 8-1) represents tumors that have grown large enough to outgrow their blood supply. At this point, the percentage of cells actually proliferating is low and are less likely to be eradicated by chemotherapy.[5]

Drug Resistance

The most common cause of treatment failure is the development of drug resistance. Drug resistance can be primary (i.e., present at the time of diagnosis before the tumor has received any treatment) or secondary (i.e., develops in response to chemotherapy exposure). In 1979, Goldie and Coldman[6] proposed a mathematical model showing that the probability of cure is a function of the spontaneous mutation rate, the inherent sensitivity of the tumor to the chemotherapy, and the size of the tumor at the time of diagnosis. Resistant clones develop spontaneously because of the genetic instability of the tumor cells resulting in frequent mutations, deletions, gene amplifications, translocations, and chromosomal rearrangements. Because cells are frequently mutating, more and more drug-resistant clones are constantly being generated. These resistant clones continue to grow exponentially unless they are exposed to an agent to which they are sensitive (Fig. 8-2). Consequently, multidrug therapy is theoretically more effective than single-drug therapy even for a tumor of small size.[7] Of note, normal cells never develop resistance to chemotherapeutic

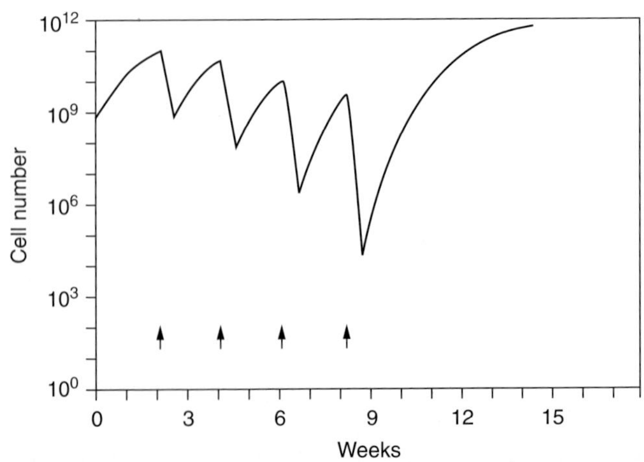

Figure 8-2. Log kill in tumor cells exposed to an agent to which they are sensitive (arrows), followed by the growth curve seen after the cells develop resistance.

agents, emphasizing the difference in the characteristics of normal and neoplastic cells.

The model also indicates that the likelihood of cure decreases with a delay in the initiation of treatment of even a couple of generation times. This has been extrapolated to the interval between treatment courses, in that delays theoretically result in time for the tumor to grow unhindered and/or develop resistant clones.

Cell-Cycle Specificity of Chemotherapy Agents

Assuming a tumor is sensitive to a particular chemotherapeutic agent, the response to chemotherapy will vary depending on where the individual cells are in the cell cycle. A cell cycle is defined as the interval between the midpoint of mitosis in the parent cell to the midpoint of mitosis in one of the daughter cells.[8] The cell cycle consists of five phases: G0, G1, S, G2, and M. Immediately after birth, a new cell has diploid chromosomes and is either in the G1 or G0 phase. G0 is the resting phase of the cell cycle; cells in G0 are not actively proliferating. In response to an environmental stimulus, cells will enter the G1 phase, where they prepare for mitosis. The next phase is the S phase, or DNA synthesis phase, during which the DNA undergoes doubling. The cells then enter a second gap, or G2 phase, where the final steps in the preparation for mitosis (M phase) are completed. It takes a normal mammalian cell about 2 to 4 days to complete the cell cycle.

Most chemotherapy agents work at multiple sites of the cell cycle and/or prevent the cells from progressing from one phase to another[8] (Fig. 8-3). Malignant cells are preferentially affected compared to normal cells as a result of the greater number of proliferating cells in the tumor.

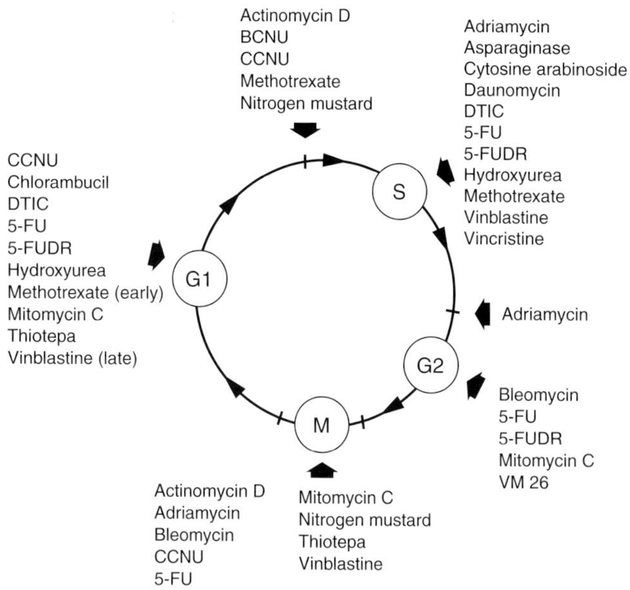

Figure 8-3. Phases of the cell cycle and the chemotherapy drugs that act at those sites.

Clinical Trials

Clinical trials provide the best means of making progress in the treatment of tumors by enrolling and treating patients in a homogeneous fashion, resulting in data that can be rigorously analyzed. A clinical trial seeks to answer a question about the effect of a therapeutic intervention on the outcome of a particular tumor. Clinical trials in oncology are categorized by the National Cancer Institute (NCI) drug development program into the following four types[9]:

- *Phase I trials* are primarily toxicity studies, evaluating new chemotherapy agents with the intent of establishing the maximum tolerated dose (MTD) using a given schedule or route of administration. The MTD is theoretically the dose that provides the best chance of a favorable therapeutic ratio.[10] For certain biologic response modifiers that have a specific measurable biologic effect, for example, inhibition of activity of a targeted enzyme, the desired effect can often be accomplished at doses below the MTD. Therefore, pushing the dose until there is intolerable toxicity is not necessary. In these cases, the end point of the study is to determine the biologically effective dose. Secondary aims of phase I trials include determining the toxicity profile of the drug, obtaining a preliminary assessment of efficacy, and performing pharmacokinetic sampling to determine how the drug is metabolized.
- *Phase II trials* seek to determine the effectiveness and side effects of a drug at a fixed dose, which is usually the MTD determined by the phase I study. Efficacy is usually defined by objective tumor responses and/or laboratory end points. Sometimes "time to progression" or "progression-free survival" at a predetermined end point is used. The results will often determine whether the treatment appears sufficiently active to be used in large-scale comparative studies.
- *Phase III trials* compare the effectiveness of the new treatment relative to the standard treatment, including a comparison of the incidence and severity of side effects. They may also involve a comparison of the new treatment to placebo or no treatment. Because of the large numbers of patients required to establish a statistically significant difference, most phase III trials are conducted in a multiinstitutional or cooperative group setting.

- *Phase IV trials* are used for after-marketing surveillance of a chemotherapeutic agent. This may occur even after regulatory approval has been obtained in order to evaluate toxicity on a larger scale, where less common side effects would surface.

Adjuvant Chemotherapy

Adjuvant chemotherapy is technically defined as chemotherapy administered in the setting of microscopic disease (i.e., no gross residual disease), usually after surgery or radiotherapy therapy, with the intent of destroying a low number of residual tumor cells and decreasing the risk of relapse, particularly at metastatic sites. According to the principles of Gompertzian growth, tumor burden, and cell kill, the small number of tumor cells remaining will theoretically have a high growth fraction and greater sensitivity to chemotherapy. Therefore, adjuvant chemotherapy should be started as soon as possible after surgery or radiation therapy, before the residual tumor cells increase in number. However, in neuro-oncology, the term *adjuvant chemotherapy* is generally applied to chemotherapy administered following the completion of radiation therapy, regardless of the amount of residual tumor. In patients who have received craniospinal radiation therapy, the start of adjuvant chemotherapy is usually delayed by 4 to 6 weeks to allow the large amount of bone marrow in the vertebral bodies to recover.

Several studies have evaluated the strategy of administering pre-irradiation chemotherapy, hypothesizing that delivery of chemotherapy to the tumor will be enhanced by surgically induced blood–brain barrier disruption and that radiation therapy will be potentially more effective if administered in the setting of as small a tumor burden as possible. In addition, chemotherapy given prior to large volume irradiation, particularly craniospinal irradiation, results in significantly less myelosuppression, allowing greater dose intensity, as well as less cisplatin-related ototoxicity. Studies in patients with medulloblastomas, however, have raised concern that this approach results in an unacceptable rate of early progression.[11,12] Given this, interest in pre-irradiation chemotherapy in those patients who are old enough to receive full doses of radiation therapy has waned. It is still occasionally used in a "window"-type setting in order to evaluate new agents and assess their response prior to the administration of radiation therapy.

Combination Therapy

Based on the basic concepts of cell kill and drug resistance, it follows that multidrug therapy should have a greater likelihood of eradicating tumor cells and effecting a cure. The use of multiple drugs theoretically reduces the probability that there will be cells present in the tumor that are resistant to all of the drugs administered. In addition, there may be additive or synergistic effects when agents working by different mechanisms are combined, and the prompt elimination of tumor cells (in chemosensitive tumors) reduces the likelihood of the emergence of resistant clones. Designing combination chemotherapy regimens requires a thorough knowledge of the pharmacology of each agent. The ideal combination regimen should use drugs that have demonstrated single-agent efficacy in phase II trials and have different mechanisms of action and nonoverlapping toxicities. Adequate cytotoxic doses of each agent should be able to be administered without resulting in inordinate delays between courses for recovery from toxicity.

In non-CNS tumors, the data are convincingly clear that combination therapy is superior to single-agent therapy.[13–16] However, the benefit of this strategy for brain tumors has never been proven. In fact, few randomized studies have shown a survival advantage with the use of combination regimens over that obtained with single agents. An older trial found that the combination regimen of PCV (procarbazine, CCNU [1,3-*cis*(2-chloroethyl)-1-nitrosoureal], and vincristine) was superior to single-agent BCNU (1,3-bis (2-chloroethyl)-1-nitrosourea) for patients with anaplastic gliomas.[17] However, a more recent prospective randomized trial found no difference in outcome between patients treated with radiation therapy alone versus those treated with radiation therapy and PCV.[18]

The "eight-drugs-in-1-day" regimen could be considered the ultimate combination regimen, using both lipid-soluble and water-soluble, cell-cycle-specific and nonspecific agents with different mechanisms of action for patients with brain tumors.[19] The chemotherapy agents include vincristine, lomustine (CCNU), procarbazine, hydroxyurea, cisplatin, ara-C (cytarabine), and either cyclophosphamide or dacarbazine (DTIC). Methylprednisolone was included as both an antiemetic and to ameliorate any treatment-related edema. Because of the number of agents administered over a short period of time, the dose intensity of each agent was relatively low. The regimen generated promising preliminary data in the phase II setting. However, when evaluated in a randomized Children's Cancer Group phase III trial for children with high-grade gliomas and in a separate phase III trial for medulloblastomas, there was either no benefit compared with CCNU, vincristine, and prednisone[20] or the results were inferior.[21] Similarly, in adults, there was no improvement in survival or time to progression with the "eight-drugs-in-1-day" regimen as compared with less toxic therapies.[22,23]

Another means of exploiting the potential therapeutic advantages of combination therapy is to administer chemotherapy concurrently with radiation therapy. Radiation can be modeled as a chemotherapeutic agent that is not cross-resistant with the drug component of the treatment protocol. The advantage to using chemotherapy concurrently with radiation therapy is the potential to achieve maximal tumor cell kill in the shortest period of time in tumors where radiation therapy is the most effective treatment modality. Chemotherapy can be used concurrently for its additional efficacy, and/or for its radiosensitizing properties. Radiosensitizing agents are chemical or pharmacologic compounds that, when administered in conjunction with radiation therapy, sensitize cells toward the lethal effects of radiation. Mechanisms of radiation enhancement include additive but independent cell killing, decrease in radiation-induced damage repair, prevention of accelerated repopulation of tumor cells that may occur once a tumor begins to respond to radiation therapy, and recruitment of cells in the resting phase into the more chemo- and radiosensitive proliferative phases.[24]

Dose Intensity

The concept of increasing dose intensity to maximize cell kill has been extensively evaluated for many different tumor types. Dose intensity is defined as the amount of drug delivered per unit time. Using this definition, increased dose intensity can be achieved by using higher drug doses, or by reducing the time between cycles, or both. Most chemotherapy drugs have a steep dose–response curve, which means that, at least in preclinical models, a small increase in the dose can significantly enhance therapeutic efficacy. In an osteosarcoma tumor model, Skipper[25] demonstrated that a 20% reduction in the dose of two effective cytotoxic agents lowered the cure rate by 50%. Response rate and survival correlate with dose intensity in both hematologic malignancies and several solid tumors.[26,27]

Historically, the treatment schedule and timing of chemotherapy was limited by neutrophil and platelet recovery. With the advent of cytokines (e.g., granulocyte colony-stimulating factor [G-CSF]) and stem cell support, the ability to intensify chemotherapy doses and shorten intervals has improved. Attempts to further increase dose intensity have resulted in the use of extremely high-dose chemotherapy with autologous bone marrow or peripheral blood stem cell rescue. The alkylating agents are the most appropriate class of drugs to be incorporated into these regimens as they have the steepest dose–response curves and are active at several stages of the cell cycle. In addition, in vitro data show that resistance of tumor cells to standard doses of chemotherapy can potentially be overcome by increasing the concentration of the drug.[28] Myelosuppression limits the ability to significantly escalate the doses of alkylating agents in the nontransplantation setting. The extreme myelosuppression resulting from high-dose chemotherapy can be mitigated by harvesting the bone marrow or peripheral blood stem cells (PBSCs) from the patient prior to administering the chemotherapy. The patient is then "rescued" by giving back the PBSCs after the chemotherapy is given. This approach has been explored for various newly diagnosed and recurrent childhood and adult CNS tumors, usually in a single-arm phase II setting. It has met with limited success in adults with malignant gliomas, and the toxicity has been substantial.[29,30] Clinical trials have shown no benefit to high-dose chemotherapy for patients with ependymomas and brainstem gliomas.[31] There has been heightened interest in this approach for very young pediatric patients with embryonal malignancies, such as primitive neuroectodermal tumors (PNETs) and atypical teratoid/rhabdoid tumors (AT/RTs), in an attempt to treat leptomeningeal disease more effectively and either thereby reduce the doses or avoid the need for craniospinal radiation therapy.[32,33] There are currently no data that undeniably prove this approach is superior to less aggressive regimens. The substantial treatment-related morbidity and mortality must be weighed against the potential benefits, and the approach in general is considered by most neuro-oncologists to be investigational and best used in the setting of a clinical trial. The patients who appear to be the best candidates for this approach are those with chemoresponsive tumors who go into transplant with minimal residual disease.

Attempts to increase dose intensity in the treatment of brain tumors have also included using peripheral blood stem cells to decrease the interval between treatment courses (time compression). The combination regimen of PCV has been used for malignant brain tumors since the 1970s and is considered by many to be standard chemotherapy for anaplastic astrocytomas. Myelosuppression is dose limiting for both CCNU and procarbazine,[34] and the nadir in blood counts occurs later with this regimen than with most other chemotherapeutic agents. The degree and duration of the blood count nadir becomes more severe with each subsequent course of chemotherapy. Through the use of peripheral blood stem cells, it was possible to nearly double the dose of procarbazine and CCNU in the PCV regimen as compared to the standard regimen. Chemotherapy was delivered on time in 80% of the courses with minimal toxicity.[35] Although responses were seen, the long-term outcome did not appear to be improved.

In summary, neither increased dose intensity nor combination chemotherapy is of proven benefit in the treatment of malignant brain tumors, although ongoing clinical trials continue to evaluate these concepts.

Mechanisms of Drug Resistance and Strategies to Overcome Them

Numerous mechanisms of chemotherapy resistance have been identified (Table 8-1).[36] Two mechanisms of resistance that may be particularly relevant to

TABLE 8-1. MECHANISMS OF CHEMOTHERAPY RESISTANCE

Class	Mechanism	Example
Transport-mediated resistance	Alterations in drug uptake or efflux across the tumor cell membrane or between the cytoplasm and the nucleus	Multidrug resistance (MDR)/P-glycoprotein
DNA repair-mediated resistance	Alterations in DNA repair processes	AGT and mismatch repair genes
Metabolic-mediated resistance	Alterations in activation or inactivation of drugs within the tumor cell	Glutathione-*S*-transferase
Drug target-mediated resistance	Alterations in the levels or affinity of enzymes that are the target for a specific chemotherapeutic drug	Topoisomerases
Apoptosis-mediated resistance	Alterations in the ability of tumor cells to execute programmed cell death or apoptotic pathways	bcl2, p53

AGT = alkylguanine-DNA alkyltransferase.

neuro-oncology and are the focus of ongoing clinical trials are discussed below.

Multidrug Resistance

P-glycoprotein (P-gp) is a membrane transport protein encoded by the "multidrug resistance" (*mdr*) gene *mdr1*.[37] Overexpression of P-gp confers cellular resistance to a variety of structurally unrelated chemotherapeutic agents by actively excreting them from the cell,[38,39] as well as acting as a permeability barrier in preventing certain substances from getting into the cell.[40] Tumors that are P-gp–positive tend to be more resistant to treatment and carry a worse prognosis than those that are P-gp–negative.[41–43] The multidrug resistance phenotype on tumor cells may be constitutively expressed or acquired in response to exposure to chemotherapeutic agents that are substrates for P-gp.[44,45] These chemotherapeutic agents include the vinca alkaloids (e.g., vincristine and vinblastine), anthracyclines (e.g., Adriamycin and daunomycin), epipodophyllotoxins (e.g., etoposide [VP16]), and the taxanes.

Many brain tumors are P-gp–positive at the level of the tumor cell itself.[46,47] Although only a minority of high-grade glioma cells express P-gp, 60% to 100% express P-gp in the endothelial cells of the tumor blood vessels.[48–51] This is noteworthy because normal capillary endothelial cells, with the exception of those in the brain and testes, do not express P-gp, and vascular endothelial staining for P-gp has not been demonstrated in tumors outside the CNS. In a study of CNS tumor of children and young adults, 35 of 50 tumors (70%) had P-gp detected in the blood vessel endothelium, 31% of which were positive in the majority of vessels.[52] Vascular endothelial staining for P-gp was seen in 17 of 23 high-grade gliomas and in 8 of 8 ependymomas. This suggests that the role of P-gp in the chemoresistance of brain tumors is potentially twofold: effluxing chemotherapy out of tumor cells in those that are P-gp–positive, as well as restricting drug entry into tumor cells that may or may not be P-gp–positive, that is, forming a blood–tumor barrier. Thus, chemotherapy resistance in CNS tumors may result not only from the characteristics of the tumor cells themselves, but also from the characteristics of the tumor vasculature, potentially explaining why some CNS tumors may be chemosensitive in vitro, but not in vivo.

P-gp is also an important contributor to both the blood–brain barrier[53,54] as well as the blood–cerebral spinal fluid (CSF) barrier created by the choroid plexus,[55] providing protection against toxic substances. Therefore, reversal of P-gp is a promising strategy to improve the treatment of chemotherapy-resistant brain tumors.

DNA Repair Enzymes

BCNU is a member of a class of compounds known as chloroethylalkylating agents, which produce cytotoxicity by causing the formation of covalent DNA interstrand cross-links. This covalent bond precludes DNA transcription and results in a lethal injury to the cell. However, if the tumor cell is capable of removing the alkyl group, no damage is sustained. The major repair pathway uses the protein moiety alkylguanine-DNA alkyltransferase (AGT). The alkylated form of AGT is unstable in mammalian cells and is rapidly degraded.[56] Once the enzyme is depleted, further repair by this mechanism requires de novo synthesis of the protein.

Tumor cell lines that lack AGT activity are generally exquisitely sensitive to alkylating agents in vitro.[56] Conversely, tumors that express high levels of alkyltransferase activity are typically resistant to alkylating agents.[57] Although endogenous AGT levels are known to vary by organ—even by cell type within a given organ—AGT levels in many tumors are much higher than what is seen in the corresponding normal tissue, suggesting that this protein can serve as an acquired mechanism of drug resistance. For example, normal brain tissue is known to express low to undetectable levels of the protein, whereas significant levels of expression have been observed in 73% of a series of 60 brain tumor specimens, often several orders of magnitude higher than normal baseline levels.[58] A high percentage of both pediatric and adult malignant gliomas have elevated AGT levels.[58,59] Several clinical trials have confirmed an adverse association between elevated AGT levels and therapeutic response to nitrosoureas in humans.[60,61] The strategy of blocking AGT activity with agents such as O^6-benzylguanine (O^6-BG) is now being evaluated in an attempt to improve the therapeutic responsiveness to agents such as the nitrosoureas (see "High-Grade Gliomas" below).

In Vitro Drug Sensitivity Testing

"Send this patient's tumor for culture and sensitivity." In this editorial published in the *New England Journal of Medicine* in 1983,[62] Daniel Von Hoff emphasized the theoretical importance of in vitro drug sensitivity testing (DST) for optimizing the treatment of patients with cancer. Since then, these techniques have been used both preclinically and clinically to select the most effective chemotherapy regimens for a given patient. Testing is similar to the in vitro sensitivity testing performed to determine the optimal antibiotic treatment. After surgical removal, the tumor cells are exposed to chemotherapeutic agents in vitro. To determine the sensitivity or resis-tance of the tumor, the survival of tumor exposed to drug is compared with that of tumor not exposed to drug. These assays are expensive and time-consuming, however, and their clinical benefit has not been deter mined. The ability to obtain adequate amounts of viable tumor tissue for in vitro testing is also problematic. A recent review identified 12 prospective studies that evaluated the benefit of chemotherapy selected by DST as treatment for various malignancies.[63] The response rates with the in vitro selected regimens appeared to be somewhat higher than with empiric regimens, although a survival benefit was documented in only 2 of the 12 studies. In a retrospective analysis of 40 patients with glioblastoma treated with individualized chemotherapy based on DST, patients treated with individualized chemotherapy had a favorable outcome compared with historical controls.[64] Of the 31 assessable patients, 8 patients (26%) achieved partial response, and 20 (65%) had stable disease. Results from such studies are encouraging, although prospective trials assessing response and survival are necessary to conclusively prove that this approach offers an advantage over standard empiric therapy.

Concept of the Cancer Stem Cell

An intriguing concept that is finding more and more support is that of the cancer stem cell. It appears that only a small number of tumor cells actually have unlimited proliferative potential, while the remainder have either limited or no proliferative potential.[65] Similar to the hematopoietic stem cells, these cancer stem cells give rise to a phenotypically heterogeneous population of cells with various degrees of differentiation. Medulloblastomas and gliomas contain self-renewing multipotent neural stem cells that have the capacity to produce neurons and glia.[66,67] Unlike normal neural stem cells, however, these tumor-derived progenitors have an increased capacity to proliferate and differentiate into abnormal cells. This concept has tremendous implications for optimizing therapy, and if borne out could potentially change the focus of therapy to the identification and selective eradication of only the cancer stem cells rather than attempting to kill all existing cancer cells.

▶ FACTORS INFLUENCING THE DELIVERY OF CHEMOTHERAPY TO THE BRAIN

The delivery of chemotherapy to brain tumors is affected by many factors, some of which are unique to the central nervous system.

The blood–brain barrier was first described by Paul Ehrlich in 1885, who observed that when certain vital dyes were injected intravenously into animals, all body tissues except the brain were stained.[68] It is now well established that the blood–brain barrier is a unique membranous barrier that tightly segregates the brain from the circulating blood.[69] In contrast to vessels elsewhere in the body, the endothelial cells of brain capillaries have tight interendothelial junctions, few pinocytic vesicles, and no fenestrations. Therefore, the principal route by which drugs cross the blood–brain barrier is by simple diffusion. Further contributing to the integrity of the barrier are the astrocytic foot processes, which are interposed between the capillaries and neurons and cover more than 95% of the endothelial basement membranes.[70] The impact of the blood–brain barrier on the ability to treat malignancies that can spread to the central nervous system has been highlighted by the experience in acute lymphoblastic leukemia (ALL). The relapse rate in the central nervous system when treatment for ALL does not include intrathecal chemotherapy is quite high, demonstrating that adequate concentrations of chemotherapy in the CNS cannot be achieved via the systemic route. Only un-ionized, low-molecular-weight lipophilic drugs can freely penetrate the blood–brain barrier.[71] The nitrosoureas are the chemotherapeutic agents that best fit these characteristics and, not surprisingly, are among the most commonly used drugs for brain tumors. Table 8-2 lists the ability of various chemotherapeutic agents to penetrate the blood–brain barrier.

Whereas the blood–brain barrier plays a major role in determining how much of a drug will get into the CSF, the permeability characteristics of the microvessel population within the tumor (i.e., the brain–tumor barrier) plays a major role in determining the ability of drugs to get into the tumor. These vessels are formed by angiogenic factors produced by the tumor and have varying degrees of permeability, as evidenced by the various degrees of gadolinium enhancement seen in different tumors. Histologically, brain tumor capillaries show thinning of the endothelial cells, aberrations in the basement membrane, increased surface area between vascular space and parenchyma, and even frank openings between endothelial cells,[72] which can contribute to edema formation. Therefore, many of the polar molecules that are excluded from normal brain have relatively unrestricted access to the intercellular spaces of the tumor itself. The permeability of the tumor blood vessels often vary throughout the tumor, so that some parts of the tumor will be exposed to systemic levels of drug, whereas others will be exposed to very low concentrations.[73] Tumor cells are known to infiltrate beyond the region of contrast enhancement[74] into the region of the brain adjacent to the tumor. Capillary permeability within the brain adjacent to the tumor may even be less than that of normal brain.[75] As a result of this differential permeability to polar agents, the growing edge of the tumor is often exposed to lower concentrations of these agents,[76] while drug concentrations of lipid-soluble agents that are able to cross the capillaries of both normal brain and tumor remain relatively constant in the tumor and the brain adjacent to the tumor.

▶ **TABLE 8-2.** CSF PENETRATION OF COMMONLY USED CHEMOTHERAPY DRUGS

Drug	CSF-to-Plasma Ratio (%)
Carboplatin	20–30
Carmustine (BCNU)	>90
Cisplatin	<10
Cyclophosphamide	
4-OH-cyclophosphamide	10–20
Parent	50
Dexamethasone	<10
Ifosfamide	30
Methotrexate	2–3
Prednisolone	<10
Temozolomide	30
Vincristine	<5

Blood flow to the tumor is another factor that affects drug delivery. Significant regional variation in blood flow to various parts of the tumor frequently exists, at least in part because of variations in tumor interstitial pressure, with the lowest rates of flow in the central necrotic areas.[77,78] Even chemotherapeutic agents that are highly lipid soluble and thus relatively easily able to cross the blood–brain barrier are less able to reach the center of the tumor because of the decreased blood flow to these areas.

In summary, multiple factors determine drug delivery to brain tumors. Given all the obstacles, less than 1% of any drug administered systemically will reach a brain tumor, regardless of the drug's permeability and/or degree of tumor capillary permeability,[79] essentially "wasting" the remainder and imposing significant limitations on the total dose of drug that can be given. Many strategies have been employed to attempt to overcome these barriers (see "Strategies for Overcoming Barriers to Drug Delivery" below).

Role of Steroids

Steroids play an important role in the management of patients with brain tumors, particularly those with bulky tumors and/or hydrocephalus. Dexamethasone has the best CNS penetration of any of the steroids and is therefore the most commonly used.[80] Steroids also appear to be able to decrease CSF production and cerebral blood flow. Weiss and Nulsen[81] found that CSF production decreased by 50% in dogs after administration of glucocorticoids. One of the most important roles of steroids in patients with brain tumors is to reduce the tumor-associated vasogenic edema and alleviate the symptoms of mass effect by decreasing the permeability of the abnormal capillaries within the tumor. Unfortunately, this effect results in a significant obstacle to the delivery of chemotherapy to the tumor. Therefore, steroids given in conjunction with chemotherapy can potentially adversely affect outcome. Survival in patients with poor-prognosis high-grade gliomas receiving high-dose methylprednisolone in addition to BCNU and radiation was inferior to those treated with BCNU and radiation without steroids.[82] In addition, dexamethasone has been shown to inhibit apoptosis in human astrocytoma cells even in the presence of chemotherapeutic agents, suggesting an additional mechanism of interference with the efficacy of chemotherapy.[83] For these reasons, the use of steroids as an antiemetic is contraindicated in patients receiving chemotherapy for brain tumors.

The assessment of response to treatment can also be affected by steroid use. Not only the degree of gadolinium enhancement, which is a surrogate measure of the leakiness of the tumor blood vessels, but the measurable volume of the tumor can be decreased by as much as 50% to 60% if the patient is receiving steroids.[84] Guidelines for determining responses to chemotherapy now mandate that the patient be on the same or a lower steroid dose as compared to baseline before declaring a response.[85]

▶ STRATEGIES FOR OVERCOMING BARRIERS TO DRUG DELIVERY

Intraarterial Chemotherapy

The principal advantage of delivering chemotherapy intraarterially is that the tissue perfused by that artery is exposed to higher plasma concentrations of the drug during the first passage through the circulation. This is particularly advantageous in the setting where the tumor blood flow is very low or where the chemotherapy agent is rapidly metabolized or excreted when given systemically. Mathematical modeling predicts that intraarterial infusion can produce as much as a 10-fold increase in peak drug concentrations.[86] Although higher concentrations of drug within the tumor can be achieved in human brain tumor xenograft models,[87] there are many practical drawbacks associated with this approach in humans, and no conclusive evidence that it results in increased efficacy. In a large, randomized phase III trial, patients with high-grade gliomas received either intraarterial or intravenous BCNU with or without 5-fluorouracil (5-FU). The study was closed early when an interim analysis found shorter survival times in patients receiving intraarterial BCNU.[88] Moreover, there were serious treatment-related toxicities in the intraarterial BCNU arm, including leukoencephalopathy (10%) and blindness ipsilateral to the infused carotid artery (15%).

Manipulating the Permeability of the Blood–Brain Barrier and Brain–Tumor Barrier

Various chemical agents have been used to modify the blood–brain barrier and/or brain–tumor barrier in an attempt to increase the drug concentration within the tumor. These barrier-modifying approaches are often used in conjunction with intraarterial chemotherapy. Hyperosmolar agents such as mannitol and vasoactive compounds such as bradykinin analogues have been the most extensively evaluated. Hyperosmolar solutions increase capillary permeability by temporarily opening the intercellular tight junctions of the brain endothelium, resulting in greater movement of water-soluble substances out of the blood vessels. The effect is greatest on the vessels in the normal brain (blood–brain barrier), with a variable effect on the vessels of the tumor, that is, the brain–tumor barrier. In a study of 13 patients with malignant astrocytomas, intraarterial hyperosmolar blood–brain barrier disruption prior to methotrexate administration increased the permeability of the vessels in the normal brain by 1000%, but only increased the permeability of the tumor vessels by 60%.[89] The Children's Cancer Group study CCG-9881 administered mannitol intravenously with etoposide in children with recurrent brain tumors. There was no benefit in terms of response or survival in the children who received mannitol compared with those who did not.[90] Intraarterial RMP-7, a bradykinin analogue, appears to have a greater effect on the permeability of the tumor blood vessels than the normal brain,[91] and studies evaluating the benefit of this agent are ongoing.

Intracerebrospinal Fluid Chemotherapy

Intra-CSF chemotherapy involves administration of drugs either into the lumbar subarachnoid space (i.e., intrathecal therapy) or into the lateral ventricle, usually through some form of surgically implanted subcutaneous device, such as an Ommaya reservoir.[92] Relatively small doses of chemotherapeutic agents given intrathecally can produce high concentrations within the CSF with minimal systemic toxicity. Intrathecal administration of methotrexate achieves drug levels 10-fold higher than what can be obtained with systemic administration.[93] Additional advantages include minimal enzymatic degradation of the drug and increased availability of the unbound or free drug in the CSF. When given through an Ommaya reservoir, methotrexate concentrations remain therapeutic for at least 24 hours.[93] However, for primary brain tumors, the utility of this approach is often limited by abnormal CSF flow and even complete obstruction related to tumor and/or scarring and inflammation from prior surgical interventions. For this reason, clinical trials evaluating new intrathecal agents generally require documentation of normal CSF flow prior to enrollment. Even when CSF flow is normal, there are numerous potential technical difficulties and sedation issues that may be encountered when performing serial lumbar punctures or Ommaya taps. In addition, intrathecal administration of chemotherapy is associated with increased risks of neurotoxicity and chemical meningitis.

Drugs administered intrathecally have virtually no penetration into the brain parenchyma itself, limiting usefulness to either treatment or prophylaxis of leptomeningeal disease. This approach is used routinely in patients with leukemia and lymphoma, but remains investigational for primary brain tumors. The drugs most commonly administered intrathecally for leukemia are methotrexate, ara-C, and steroids, which are not particularly useful for most CNS tumors. There are several agents being evaluated in phase I and phase II clinical trials for primary CNS tumors.

Wafers/Implants

This strategy has been used for high-grade gliomas, which predominantly recur locally. As mentioned above, only a small percentage of systemically administered chemotherapy actually gets to the brain tumor. The systemic toxicity prevents further dose escalation and limits the effectiveness of these agents. Repeated local administration of nitrosoureas through an Ommaya reservoir placed in the surgical resection cavity was associated with unacceptable brain edema, necrosis, and other pathologic changes.[94] However, the surgical implantation of solid-phase reagents effectively allows delivery of high concentrations and sustained levels of drug to the tumor site without significant systemic or local side effects. The most commonly used "wafer" is composed of a copolymer matrix with BCNU, which can be directly implanted into the tumor resection cavity at the time of surgical resection or debulking.[95] Clinical trials have shown very modest prolongation of survival with the use of the BCNU wafers, usually on the order of several weeks.[96,97]

▶ CHEMOTHERAPY FOR VARIOUS CNS TUMORS

Tables 8-3 and 8-4 list the most commonly used chemotherapy drugs and regimens, respectively, for primary CNS tumors.

Primary Central Nervous System Lymphomas

Primary CNS lymphomas (PCNSLs) belong to the family of non-Hodgkin lymphomas arising within and restricted to the central nervous system. PCNSLs are most commonly seen in immunosuppressed patients, where they almost universally arise from Epstein-Barr virus (EBV)-infected B lymphocytes.[98] There is no such association when PCNSL arises in immunocompetent patients.

Approximately 40% of PCNSLs are exquisitely sensitive to steroids with resultant rapid tumor lysis.[99] The use of steroids to reduce peritumoral edema and mass effect is typically initiated as soon as the magnetic resonance imaging (MRI) or computerized tomography (CT) scan is obtained. This frequently complicates or even eliminates the ability to make the diagnosis, as some tumors can completely disappear radiographically before a definitive diagnosis can be made.[100] Not surprisingly, the standard chemotherapy regimens used against non-Hodgkin lymphomas outside of the CNS fail to produce sustained remissions, as these agents have little ability to penetrate the blood–brain barrier. Initial responses are short-lived

▶ TABLE 8-3. COMMONLY USED CHEMOTHERAPEUTIC AGENTS FOR CNS TUMORS

Drug	Synonyms	Route	Mechanism of Action	Toxicities
Cyclophosphamide	Cytoxan, CTX	IV	Alkylation; cross-linking	M, N&V, A, cystitis, water retention, cardiac (HD)
Ifosfamide	IFOS, IFEX	PO, IV	Alkylation; cross-linking	M, N&V, A, cystitis, NT, renal, cardiac (HD)
Lomustine	CCNU	PO	Alkylation; cross-linking; carbamoylation	M, N&V, renal and pulmonary
Carmustine	BCNU	IV	Alkylation; cross-linking; carbamoylation	M, N&V, renal and pulmonary
Cisplatin	Platinol, CDDP	IV	Platination; cross-linking	M(Mild), N&V, A, renal, NT, ototoxicity, HSR
Carboplatin	CBDCA	IV	Platination; cross-linking	M(Plt), N&V, A, hepatic (mild), HSR
Temozolomide	TMZ	PO	Methylation	M, N&V
Procarbazine	Matulane, PCZ	PO	Methylation; free radical formation	M, N&V, NT, rash, mucositis
Methotrexate	MTX	PO, IM, SC	Interferes with folate metabolism	M, (mild), mucositis, rash, hepatic; renal, NT (HD)
Vincristine	Oncovin, VCR	IV	Mitotic inhibitor; blocks microtubule polymerization	NT, A, SIADH, hypotension, vesicant
Dexamethasone	Decadron, DEX	PO, IV	Receptor-mediated lympholysis	Increased risk of infection, hyperglycemia, osteoporosis, cushingoidism, hypertension

A = alopecia; HD = high dose; HSR = hypersensitivity reaction(s); M = myelosuppression; N&V = nausea and vomiting; NT = neurotoxicity; Plt = platelets; SIADH = syndrome of inappropriate antidiuretic drug hormone secretion.

▶ **TABLE 8-4.** FREQUENTLY USED CHEMOTHERAPY REGIMEN/AGENTS

Medulloblastoma/primitive neuroectodermal tumor	CCNU/cisplatin/vincristine Cyclophosphamide
Low-grade gliomas	Carboplatin/vincristine Temozolomide Vinblastine
High-grade gliomas	Temozolomide Procarbazine/CCNU/vincristine BCNU
Primary CNS lymphoma	Methotrexate
Meningioma	Hydroxyurea
Germ cell tumors	
Germinomas	Carboplatin or cisplatin/VP16 (etoposide)
Nongerminomas	Cisplatin/ifosfamide/VP16 (etoposide)
Oligodendrogliomas	Procarbazine/CCNU/vincristine Temozolomide
Infants with embryonal CNS malignancies	Cisplatin/cyclosphosphamide/vincristine Ifosfamide/carboplatin/VP16 (etoposide)

and soon overshadowed by the appearance of disease in new sites of the brain, including the leptomeninges.[101] The use of high-dose methotrexate has significantly impacted survival as doses greater than 3 g/m^2 achieve therapeutic drug concentrations in the CSF.[102] Methotrexate has now become the common denominator to all CNS lymphoma chemotherapeutic regimens, and is considered the most effective drug against PCNSL. As long as high-dose methotrexate is included in the chemotherapy regimen, chemoradiotherapy is superior to radiotherapy alone.[103,104] The optimal dose and schedule of methotrexate has yet to be defined. When given after cranial radiation, methotrexate is quite neurotoxic, causing a potentially severe leukoencephalopathy,[105,106] so that its use is limited to the neoadjuvant (i.e., pre-irradiation) setting. For elderly patients > 70 years of age who have an increased risk of radiation-related neurotoxicity, deferral of radiation therapy until relapse is often recommended.

Primitive Neuroectodermal Tumors

Primitive neuroectodermal tumors are densely cellular, highly malignant small, round, blue cell tumors of the CNS that have a propensity to disseminate throughout the neuraxis. They can arise anywhere within the central nervous system, although the posterior fossa, specifically the cerebellar vermis, is the most common primary site. These posterior fossa PNETs have retained the term *medulloblastoma*. Medulloblastomas account for less than 1% of CNS tumors in adults,[107] but are the most common CNS malignancy in children.[108] Dissemination throughout the cerebrospinal fluid, at least at the microscopic level, is assumed for all PNETs, and craniospinal radiation therapy is the mainstay of treatment, affording the best chance of long-term tumor control.

Medulloblastomas are quite chemosensitive and respond to a variety of cytotoxic drugs.[109] The most active agents include cisplatin, cyclophosphamide, carboplatin, and methotrexate. Because chemotherapy is generally administered after craniospinal radiation, the use of methotrexate has largely been abandoned outside of the infant population because of neurologic toxicity.[105] For newly diagnosed patients old enough to receive craniospinal radiation therapy (generally > 3 years of age), the incorporation of chemotherapy into the treatment regimen has increased the survival rates for "high-risk" patients[110] and has allowed the craniospinal dose to be reduced from 3600 cGy to 2340 cGy for standard-risk patients.[111] The platinum-based chemotherapy regimen developed by Packer and associates[112] is the most commonly used adjuvant chemotherapy regimen.

Central Nervous System Germ Cell Tumors

CNS germ cell tumors are a rare and heterogeneous group of tumors. These tumors are considered either germinomatous, which are slow growing and highly responsive to treatment, or nongerminomatous germ cell tumors (NGGCTs), which are typically rapid growing and less responsive to therapy. Because all malignant germ cell tumors have the potential to disseminate throughout the cerebrospinal fluid, the most conservative treatment consists of craniospinal radiation therapy. More than 90% of patients with pure germinomas are cured following treatment with craniospinal radiation therapy. However, because these tumors most commonly occur in children and adolescents, concern about the neurocognitive and growth-related sequelae of craniospinal radiation has led to attempts to reduce the dose and fields of radiation, with or without the use of chemotherapy. The use of pre-irradiation chemotherapy followed by reduced-dose involved-field radiation therapy to patients with localized disease has become quite popular.[113] Chemotherapy typically consists of two courses of carboplatin or cisplatin and VP16 (etoposide), followed by reduced doses of involved-field radiation therapy for those patients who demonstrate a complete radiographic response. Initial pilot study results were encouraging, although long-term followup data has raised concerns over the number of ventricular and subarachnoid metastases, particularly in patients with elevated levels of beta human chorionic gonadotropin (bhCG).[114]

In contradistinction to what is seen with germinomas, radiation therapy as the sole treatment modality for patients with nongerminomatous germ cell tumors results in long-term tumor control in a minority of patients. The addition of chemotherapy, particularly with the platinum-based regimens, has significantly improved the prognosis.[115] Chemotherapy is usually given prior to radiation in order to assess response and to minimize the risk of cisplatin-related ototoxicity. Second-look surgery to attempt to resect the residual mass is often recommended prior to radiation therapy.

High-Grade Gliomas

High-grade gliomas, for example, glioblastomas and anaplastic astrocytomas, are the most common primary brain tumors of adults.[116] Glioblastomas are notoriously resistant tumors that remain a therapeutic frustration despite increasingly aggressive treatment. Radiation therapy prolongs survival, yet only to a median of 35 weeks, compared with 14 weeks for supportive care alone.[117] The nitrosoureas have long been considered the most active chemotherapeutic agents against high-grade gliomas, initially of interest because of their lipid solubility and ability to cross the blood–brain barrier. The addition of single-agent BCNU following surgery and radiation therapy resulted in a statistically significant difference in the percentage of survivors at 18 months (19% for the combination vs. 4% for those treated with radiation therapy alone, $p < 0.01$).[117] A subsequent prospective randomized trial found that patients treated with postradiation BCNU had a significant increase in median survival, compared with those patients who were treated with postradiation methylprednisolone.[118] Studies showing that procarbazine[118] and vincristine[119] had activity against high-grade gliomas led to the combination regimen of PCV. The regimen is advantageous in that CCNU and procarbazine are both given orally with high bioavailability, and CCNU has less pulmonary toxicity than BCNU. One randomized trial showed a significant survival advantage (157 weeks for PCV vs. 82 weeks with BCNU alone) in patients with anaplastic astrocytomas.[17] Based on these results, PCV became the standard treatment for patients with anaplastic astrocytomas. A meta-analysis of the published randomized trials comparing radiation therapy alone to radiation plus adjuvant nitrosourea-based chemotherapy confirmed the results of the earlier studies, finding that adjuvant chemotherapy resulted in an increase in survival of 10.1% at 1 year and 8.6 % at 2 years.[120] However, a recent large randomized prospective trial involving 674 patients with high-grade gliomas found no difference between patients who were treated with radiation therapy alone versus radiation therapy followed by PCV chemotherapy.[18] In reviewing all the data, the most that can be said for adjuvant nitrosourea-based chemotherapy is that it appears to increase the proportion of patients surviving longer than 18 months by 5% to 15%.[117,120,121] It does not appear possible to predict who will benefit from chemotherapy, as a review of the characteristics of the long-term survivors from two randomized prospective Brain Tumor Study Group trials found neither age nor any other prognostic factor to be of value.[121] Results from recent pediatric trials have been similarly disheartening. In the Children's Cancer Group 945 trial, the 5-year progression-free survival was 16% ± 7% after excluding patients with discordant pathology.[20] There was no difference in outcome between patients randomized to receive vincristine, lomustine, and prednisone versus the eight-drugs-in-1-day regimen. Interestingly, children age 3 years and younger with high-grade gliomas actually appear to do as well, if not better, when treated with postoperative chemotherapy alone, than older children who are treated with both chemotherapy and radiation therapy.[122]

Many new agents, including various nitrosourea analogues, platinum compounds, and topoisomerase inhibitors have been evaluated in the search for new therapies. Phase II studies evaluating various chemotherapeutic agents in patients with recurrent high-grade gliomas not uncommonly report a 10% to 15% objective response rate, with responses of very short duration, usually on the order of weeks. The platinum compounds initially appeared to be of promise, and encouraging results were seen in the pilot studies combining BCNU and cisplatin.[123] However, a recent phase III study of neoadjuvant cisplatin-BCNU followed by radiotherapy versus radiotherapy with adjuvant BCNU, found no advantage to the neoadjuvant regimen but significantly more toxicity, suggesting a limited role for cisplatin.[124] A meta-review of the published clinical trials of adults with recurrent high-grade gliomas found that the nitrosoureas resulted in a statistically significant increase in time to tumor progression as compared with any other drug ($p = 0.018$).[125]

No new drugs were approved for the treatment of high-grade gliomas until temozolomide received FDA approval in 1999 for recurrent anaplastic astrocytomas. Temozolomide is a methylating agent with good oral bioavailability, and has shown significant activity against high-grade gliomas.[126,127] In preclinical pharmacokinetic studies, temozolomide penetrates well across the blood–CSF barrier with a CSF-to-plasma ratio of 30%.[128] It is generally extremely well tolerated, with no significant nonhematologic toxicity. Temozolomide given concurrently with radiation followed by adjuvant temozolomide is now considered the standard of care based on the results of a prospective randomized clinical trial in newly diagnosed patients with glioblastoma. Patients treated with chemotherapy and radiation therapy had a statistically significant improvement in median progression-free survival and 2-year overall survival.[127]

Both the nitrosoureas and temozolomide exert their effect on DNA by methylating guanine at the O^6-position. The resultant O^6-methylguanine can be repaired by the DNA repair protein, AGT, which confers resistance to these chemotherapeutic agents (see "Mechanisms of Drug Resistance" above). O^6-BG is a modulating agent that irreversibly inactivates and depletes AGT and can effectively reverse AGT-mediated resistance to alkylating agents in vitro.[129] In preclinical studies, O^6-BG potentiates the antitumor effects of temozolomide[130] and the nitrosoureas,[131] even in tumors with low levels of AGT. Clinical trials evaluating the combination of O^6-BG and either temozolomide or BCNU are ongoing.

There remains a tremendous need for effective treatment strategies for high-grade gliomas, and it is doubtful that variations of any of the previously tried methods will result in a "magic bullet." Most of these tumors are, or quickly become, increasingly resistant to the DNA-damaging effects of standard cytotoxic agents. The focus of clinical trials evaluating treatments for high-grade gliomas is now shifting away from the use of nonspecific cytotoxic agents. An increased understanding of cancer biology has led to the development of new classes of anticancer agents that act by completely different mechanisms. These cytostatic compounds are potentially capable of affecting more specific targets on the tumor cell that can block growth, inhibit tumor cell invasion, and suppress angiogenesis. Signal transduction pathways are now widely recognized as an important target for anticancer agents. The exceedingly complex interactions between pathways result in cascades of signals that are critical to the life cycle and biologic functions of the cell. These pathways can be stimulated by growth factors or other molecules that are mediated through surface receptors. There is extensive research ongoing in the development of compounds that bind to cell surface receptors and either compete with or block the normal substrates from binding. In tumors that are dependent on such pathways for growth, the use of these agents can potentially result in cell death. Many of these agents are now being evaluated in clinical trials for patients with brain tumors (Table 8-5). Patients should be encouraged to participate in ongoing clinical trials evaluating novel therapeutic approaches so that those with promise can be appropriately embraced or discarded.

Low-Grade Gliomas

Low-grade gliomas (LGGs) include a large number of histologic subtypes, all of which are classified by the World Health Organization (WHO) as either grade I or II. In pediatrics, the most common subtype is the grade I juvenile pilocytic astrocytoma (JPA), which is usually well-circumscribed and often curable without other intervention if amenable to gross total resection.[132] Grade I astrocytomas are uncommon in adults. The grade II, or fibrillary, astrocytoma is much more infiltrative than a grade I tumor, and is the most common LGG seen in adults. LGGs may be composed of more than one glial element, in which case they are termed *mixed gliomas*. In general, LGGs are slow growing, although some may demonstrate periods of rapid and/or erratic growth. They typically do not metastasize, although young children with hypothalamic tumors appear to have a higher likelihood of dissemination throughout the neuraxis than do tumors in other locations.[133]

Approximately 25% of adults with LGGs[134] are able to undergo a gross total or near gross total resection. Other than for those patients with well-circumscribed tumors that are completely resected (usually only grade I tumors), adjuvant therapy will almost always be necessary at some point. Radiation therapy typically results in tumor shrinkage and a decrease in mass effect,[135] often for long periods of time. A randomized study involving newly diagnosed adult patients with low-grade gliomas showed no benefit to the addition of adjuvant chemotherapy with procarbazine, CCNU, and vincristine following

▶ TABLE 8-5. BIOLOGIC RESPONSE MODIFIERS AND THEIR SPECIFIC TARGETS

STI-571 (Gleevec)	Platelet-derived growth factor receptor inhibitor
ZD1839 (Iressa)	Epidermal growth factor receptor inhibitor
OSI-774 (Tarceva)	Epidermal growth factor receptor inhibitor
R115777 (Zarnestra)	Farnesyltransferase inhibitor
Cilengitide	Antiangiogenesis agent
SCH66336	Farnesyltransferase inhibitor
Marimastat	Matrix metalloprotein inhibitor
Difluoromethylornithine (DFMO)	Polyamine inhibitor

postoperative radiation therapy.[136] Consequently, the use of chemotherapy in adults is generally reserved for patients whose tumors have recurred after radiation therapy. Responses to a variety of chemotherapeutic agents have been documented in patients with recurrent or progressive low-grade gliomas. In a phase II trial of temozolomide in patients with progressive or recurrent low-grade gliomas, radiographic responses were seen in 61% of patients, with an additional 35% of patients showing stable disease.[137] Median progression-free survival in the responders was only 22 months, however, with patients who had previously received radiation therapy or chemotherapy having the shortest duration of effect.

In pediatric patients, where the neurocognitive, endocrine, and vascular sequelae of radiation therapy to the developing brain can be severe if not prohibitive and the ability to delay radiation therapy for 2 to 3 years can make a big difference in the functional outcome of the patient, the upfront use of chemotherapy has become routine for those with unresectable tumors. Children with neurofibromatosis type 1 are at particular risk for developing low-grade gliomas involving the visual pathway.[138] Virtually all of these tumors are pilocytic astrocytomas (grade I). The reasons to avoid radiation therapy are manifold in these patients who (a) are at greater risk for radiation-induced second malignancies as well as severe vasculopathy (moyamoya); (b) have the potential for neoplastic foci to develop throughout the entire visual pathway; and (c) have a better prognosis than patients without neurofibromatosis.[139] The growth pattern of these tumors tends to be very erratic, and prolonged tumor stabilization without intervention is not uncommon and even spontaneous regressions have been reported.[140] Even harder to understand, neurofibromatosis-associated visual pathway tumors usually become inactive as the children get beyond the middle school years.

The first chemotherapeutic regimen to be evaluated in young patients with low-grade gliomas consisted of actinomycin D and vincristine. The results were surprisingly good, with 15 of 24 patients (62.5%) showing either objective radiographic responses or stable disease for a median of 4.3 years.[141] These encouraging results sparked interest in evaluating other chemotherapeutic agents with better-documented single-agent activity against low-grade gliomas. Subsequent clinical trials have documented the efficacy of carboplatin and vincristine given weekly with scheduled breaks, which has now replaced actinomycin D and vincristine as the most frequently used chemotherapeutic regimen for young children with progressive low-grade gliomas.[142] Figure 8-4 shows a low-grade glioma and its response to treatment with carboplatin and vincristine. One of the appealing features of this nonalkylator chemotherapy regimen is the lack of known long-term side effects, particularly important in a population of patients with a relatively

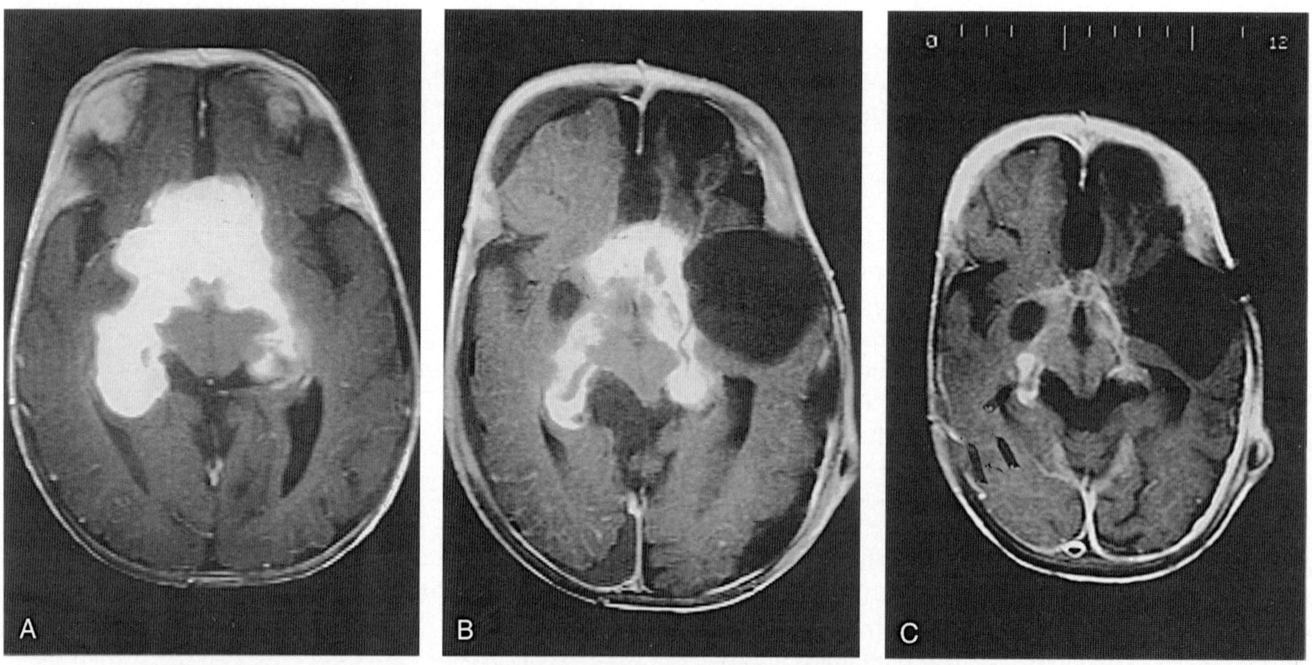

Figure 8-4. (A) Axial T_1-enhanced images of a large, enhancing glioma involving the entire visual pathway in an infant presenting with proptosis. (B) and (C) show the radiographic response to carboplatin/vincristine over the next several months.

long survival time. Alkylator-based chemotherapy carries a small but definite risk of developing a second malignancy, which may be even more of a risk in patients with neurofibromatosis, who by virtue of their disease already have an increased risk for developing malignancies. Unfortunately, anywhere from 10% to 30% of patients will develop severe and even life-threatening hypersensitivity reactions to the carboplatin, usually after the first few months of treatment,[143,144] which often necessitates discontinuing what is believed to be the most active agent of the two. Many other chemotherapeutic agents, either alone or in combination, have been or are being evaluated in this patient population, including temozolomide, vinblastine, and nitrosourea-based regimens. As experience with chemotherapy in this population of patients has increased, it has become clear that at least for patients without neurofibromatosis, the duration of response to chemotherapy is typically much shorter than what is seen with radiation therapy[145] and that although chemotherapy usually allows radiation therapy to be delayed, it can rarely be avoided.

Similar to what was seen in the adult randomized study,[136] there appears to be no benefit to chemotherapy given in addition to radiation therapy for newly diagnosed pediatric patients with low-grade gliomas. In the Children's Cancer Group's 945 study for patients with high-grade gliomas, 70 patients were reclassified as having low-grade gliomas on central pathologic review and accounted for the preponderance of long-term survivors. All patients received either eight-drugs-in-1-day chemotherapy or CCNU and vincristine in addition to involved-field radiation therapy. The overall survival of the patients with low-grade gliomas was no different from a contemporary group of patients with low-grade gliomas treated with chemotherapy alone.[146]

Oligodendrogliomas

Oligodendrogliomas account for approximately 4% of primary brain tumors,[147] although this number is probably an underestimate, because neoplastic oligodendroglial cells are often entrapped in a background of axons and reactive gliosis and the diagnosis can be difficult to make with confidence.[148] Oligodendrogliomas are distinguished from other gliomas by their often striking sensitivity to chemotherapy. This was first reported in 1988 when Cairncross and Macdonald[149] reported dramatic responses to chemotherapy in eight consecutive patients with recurrent anaplastic oligodendrogliomas. The PCV regimen emerged as the standard treatment after a cooperative group clinical trial found major durable responses in 75% of patients.[150] Subsequent studies have reported responses to many different alkylating agents, including temozolomide, which is usually extremely well-tolerated.[151] Responses to chemotherapy are also seen in low-grade oligodendrogliomas.[152]

Molecular genetic studies have revealed an association between radiographic responses and allelic loss of chromosome 1p, often in association with loss of chromosome 19q.[153] Patients with anaplastic oligodendrogliomas or anaplastic mixed gliomas with oligodendroglial morphology and 1p loss had a median survival in excess of 10 years, more than five times longer than for patients with malignant oligodendrogliomas without these cytogenetic abnormalities.[154] Although these cytogenetic abnormalities are most commonly observed in tumors with oligodendroglial features, even tumors in adults that lack these histologic features appear to have a more favorable prognosis if these genetic changes are present. This does not appear to be true in pediatric gliomas, even though deletion of 1p and 19q are found in approximately 20%.[155] Because oligodendrogliomas are so rare in pediatrics, the prevalence and significance of these cytogenetic abnormalities in this patient population is not clear.

Ependymomas

Ependymomas are uncommon in adults, but are the third most common brain tumor in children. They often occur in very young children, in whom the sequelae of radiation therapy is the most severe. Unfortunately, no study has shown an improvement in survival with the addition of chemotherapy to surgery and radiation therapy. A Children's Cancer Group study randomizing patients between postoperative radiation therapy versus radiation therapy plus adjuvant chemotherapy with CCNU, vincristine, and prednisone showed no benefit to chemotherapy.[156] Radiographic responses to chemotherapy are occasionally seen in phase II trials, and the platinums appear to have the greatest activity.[157,158] Chemotherapy is most commonly used for infants and young children with ependymomas in an attempt to delay the need for radiation therapy, although there is some concern that patients who receive chemotherapy prior to radiation therapy fare worse than those who receive immediate postoperative radiation therapy.[159]

Meningiomas

Meningiomas are the most common intracranial neoplasm in adults, with the vast majority histologically benign.[160] In children, meningiomas are typically related to prior radiation therapy. Various hormonal and biologic agents have been evaluated for the treatment of recurrent tumors that are not candidates for further surgery or radiotherapy. Hydroxyurea, a well-tolerated oral chemotherapeutic agent, has emerged as the only agent with promise, often resulting in at least stabilization of tumor growth.[161,162]

REFERENCES

1. Skipper HE. Laboratory models: the historical perspective. Cancer Treat Rep 1986;70:3–7.
2. Laird AK. Dynamics of growth in tumors and normal organisms. Natl Cancer Inst Monogr 1969;30:15–28.
3. Hoshino T, Wilson CB, Rosenblum ML, et al. Chemotherapeutic implication of growth fraction and cell cycle time in glioblastoma. J Neurosurg 1975;43:127–137.
4. Skipper HE, Schabel FM, Wilcox WS. Experimental evaluation of potential anticancer agents. XIII. On the criteria and kinetics associated with "curability" of experimental leukemia. Cancer Chemother Rep 1964;35:3–111.
5. Norton L, Simon R. The Norton-Simon hypothesis revisited. Cancer Treat Rep 1986;70:163–169.
6. Goldie JH, Coldman AJ. A mathematical model for relating the drug sensitivity of tumors to their spontaneous mutation rate. Cancer Treat Rep 1979;63:1727–1733.
7. Berenbaum MC. In vivo determination of the fractional kill of human tumor cells by chemotherapeutic agents. Cancer Chemother Rep 1972;56(5):563–571.
8. Hill B, Baserga R. The cell cycle and its significance for cancer treatment. Cancer Treat Rev 1975;2:159–175.
9. Muggia FM, Carter SK, Macdonald JS. The cancer therapy evaluation program of the National Cancer Institute. Semin Oncol 1981;8:394–402.
10. Pantiadosi S. Clinical trials as experimental designs. In: Pantiadosi S, ed. Clinical trials—a methodologic perspective. New York: Wiley-Interscience, 1997:79–86.
11. Mosijczuk AD, Nigro MA, Thomas PRM, et al. Pediatric chemotherapy in advanced medulloblastoma: a Pediatric Oncology Group Pilot Study. Cancer 1993;72:2755–2762.
12. Timmerman B, Kortmann RD, Kuhl J, et al. Role of radiotherapy in the treatment of supratentorial primitive neuroectodermal tumors in childhood: results of the prospective German Brain Tumor Trials HIT 88/89 and 91. J Clin Oncol 2002;20:842–840.
13. Frei E, Freireich E, Gehan E, et al. Studies of sequential and combination antimetabolite therapy in acute leukemia—6-mercaptopurine and methotrexate. Blood 1961;54:431–454.
14. Greenspan EM. Combination chemotherapy for advanced mammary carcinoma—a twelve-year experience. J Mt Sinai Hosp 1966;33:435–445.
15. Henderson EH, Samaha RJ. Evidence that drugs in combination have materially advanced the treatment of human malignancies. Cancer Res 1969;29:2272–2280.
16. DeVita VT, Serpick AA, Carbone PP. Combination chemotherapy in the treatment of advanced Hodgkin's disease. Ann Intern Med 1970;73:881–895.
17. Levin VA, Silver P, Hannigan J, et al. Superiority of post-radiotherapy adjuvant chemotherapy with CCNU, procarbazine and vincristine (PCV) over BCNU for anaplastic gliomas: NCOG final report. Int J Radiat Oncol Biol Phys 1990;18:321–324.
18. Medical Research Council Brain Tumor Working Party. Randomized trial of procarbazine, lomustine, and vincristine in the adjuvant treatment of high-grade astrocytoma: a Medical Research Council Trial. J Clin Oncol 2001;19(2):509–518.
19. Pendergrass TW, Milstein JM, Geyer R, et al. Eight drugs in one day chemotherapy for brain tumors: experience in 107 children and rationale for preradiation chemotherapy. J Clin Oncol 1987;5:1221–1231.
20. Finlay JL, Boyett JM, Yates AJ, et al. Randomized phase III trial in childhood high-grade astrocytoma comparing vincristine, lomustine, and prednisone with the eight-drugs-in-1-day regimen. J Clin Oncol 1995;13:112–123.
21. Zeltzer PM, Boyett JM, Finlay JL, et al. Metastasis stage, adjuvant treatment, and residual tumor are prognostic factors for medulloblastoma in children: conclusions from the Children's Cancer Group 921 randomized phase III study. J Clin Oncol 1999;17(3):832–845.
22. Boiardi A, Silvani A, Milanesi I, et al. Efficacy of "8-drugs-in-one-day" combination in treatment of recurrent GBM patients. J Neurooncol 1992;12:153–158.
23. Rozental JM, Robins HI, Finlay J, et al. "Eight-drugs-in-one-day" chemotherapy administered before and after radiotherapy to adult patients with malignant gliomas. Cancer 1989;63:2475–2481.
24. Wilkins DE, Heller DP, Raaphorst GP. Inhibition of potentially lethal damage recovery by cisplatin in a brain tumor cell line. Anticancer Res 1993;13:2137–2142.
25. Skipper HE. Data and analyses having to do with the influence of dose intensity and duration of treatment (single drugs and combinations) on lethal toxicity and the therapeutic response of experimental neoplasms. Birmingham, AL: Southern Research Institute, booklets 13, 1986, and 2–13, 1987.
26. Gurney H, Dodwell D, Thatcher N, et al. Escalating drug delivery in cancer chemotherapy: a review of concepts and practice. Part 2. Ann Oncol 1993;4:103–115.
27. Wood WC, Budman DR, Korzun AH, et al. Dose and dose intensity of adjuvant chemotherapy for stage II, node positive breast carcinoma. N Engl J Med 1994;330:1253–1259.
28. Doroshow JH. Pharmacological basis for high-dose chemotherapy. In: Thomas ED, Blume KG, Forman SJ, eds. Hematopoietic cell transplantation. Malden, MA: Blackwell Science, 1999:105–106.
29. Caincross G, Swinnen L, Bayer R, et al. Myeloablative chemotherapy for recurrent aggressive oligodendroglioma. J Neurooncol 2000;2(2):114–119.
30. Abrey LE, Rosenblum MK, Papadopoulos E, et al. High dose chemotherapy with autologous stem cell rescue in adults with malignant primary brain tumors. J Neurooncol 1999;44:147–153.
31. Dunkel IJ, Finlay JL. High-dose chemotherapy with autologous stem cell rescue for brain tumors. Crit Rev Oncol Hematol 2002;41:197–204.
32. Graham ML, Herndond JE, Casey JR, et al. High-dose chemotherapy with autologous stem cell rescue in patients with recurrent and high-risk pediatric brain tumors. J Clin Oncol 1997;15:1814–1823.
33. Dupuis-Girod S, Hartmann O, Benhamou E, et al. Will high-dose chemotherapy followed by autologous bone marrow transplantation supplant cranio-spinal irradiation in young children treated for medulloblastoma? J Neurooncol 1996;27:87–98.
34. Hoagland HC. Hematologic complications of cancer chemotherapy. In: Perry MC, ed. The chemotherapy

source book. Baltimore: Williams and Wilkins, 1992:498–502.

35. Jakacki RI, Jamison C, Mathews VP, et al. Dose-intensification of procarbazine, CCNU, vincristine (PCV) with peripheral blood stem cell support in young patients with gliomas. Med Pediatr Oncol 1998;31:483–490.
36. Arceci RJ. Can multidrug resistance mechanisms be modified? Br J Hematol 2000;110(2):285–291.
37. Riordan JR, Ling V. Genetic and biochemical characterization of multidrug resistance. Pharmacol Ther 1985;28:51–75.
38. Pastan I, Gottesman M. Multidrug resistance in human cancer. N Engl J Med 1987;316:1388–1393.
39. Ueda K, Cardarelli M, Gottesman MM, et al. Expression of a full-length cDNA for the human "MDR1" gene confers resistance to colchicine, doxorubicin and vinblastine. Proc Natl Acad Sci USA 1987;84:3004–3008.
40. Stein WD, Cardarelli C, Pastan I, et al. Kinetic evidence suggesting that the multidrug transporter differentially handles influx and efflux of its substrates. Mol Pharmacol 1994;45:763–772.
41. Campos L, Guyotat D, Archimbaud E, et al. Clinical significance of multidrug resistance P-glycoprotein expression on acute nonlymphocytic leukemia cells at diagnosis. Blood 1992;79:473–476.
42. Chan HS, Thorner PS, Haddad G, et al. Immunohistochemical detection of P-glycoprotein: prognostic correlation in soft tissue sarcoma of childhood. J Clin Oncol 1990;8:689–704.
43. Chan HS, Haddad G, Thorner PS, et al. P-glycoprotein expression as a predictor of outcome of therapy for neuroblastoma. N Engl J Med 1991;325:1608–1614.
44. Fojo AT, Ueda K, Salmon DJ, et al. Expression of a multidrug resistance gene in human tumors and tissues. Proc Natl Acad Sci USA 1987;84:265–269.
45. Goldstein LJ, Galski H, Fojo A, et al. Expression of a multidrug resistance gene in human cancers. J Natl Cancer Inst 1989;81:116–124.
46. Billson AL, Palmer JB, Walker DA, et al. Multidrug resistance gene (MDR1) expression in neuro-axial tumors of children and young adults. Br J Neurosurg 1994;8(5):585–591.
47. Regina A, Demeule M, Laplante A, et al. Multidrug resistance in brain tumors: roles of the blood–brain barrier. Cancer Metastasis Rev 2001;20(1–2):13–25.
48. Von Bossanyi P, Diete S, Dietzmann K, et al. Immunohistochemical expression of P-glycoprotein and glutathione S-transferases in cerebral gliomas and response to chemotherapy. Acta Neuropathol 1997;94:605–611.
49. Korshunov A, Golanov A, Sycheva R, et al. Prognostic value of the immunoexpression of chemoresistance-related proteins in cerebral glioblastomas: an analysis of 168 cases. Neuropathology 1999;19:143–149.
50. Nabors MW, Griffin CA, Zehbauer BA, et al. Multidrug resistance gene (MDR1) expression in human brain tumors. J Neurosurg 1991;75:941–946.
51. Henson JW, Cordon-Cardo CC, Posner JB. P-glycoprotein expression in brain tumors. J Neurooncol 1992;14:37–43.
52. Billson AL, Palmer JB, Walker DA, et al. Multidrug-resistance gene (MDR1) expression in neuro-axial tumors of children and young adults. Br J Neurosurg 1994;8:585–591.
53. Cordon-Cardo C, O'Brien JP, Casals D, et al. Multidrug resistance gene (P-glycoprotein) is expressed by endothelial cells at blood-brain barrier sites. Proc Natl Acad Sci USA 1988;86:695–698.
54. Tatsuta T, Natio M, Ohhara T, et al. Functional involvement of P-glycoprotein in blood-brain barrier. J Biol Chem 1992;267:20383–20391.
55. Rao VV, Dahlheimer JL, Bardgett ME, et al. Choroid plexus epithelial expression of MDR1 P glycoprotein and multidrug resistance-associated protein contribute to the blood-cerebrospinal fluid drug-permeability barrier. Proc Natl Acad Sci USA 1999;96:3900–3905.
56. Pegg AB. Mammalian O^6-alkylguanine-DNA alkyltransferase: regulation and importance in response to alkylating carcinogenic and therapeutic agents. Cancer Res 1990;50:6119–6129.
57. Brent TP, Houghton PJ, Houghton JA. O^6-alkylguanine-DNA alkyltransferase activity correlates with the therapeutic response of human rhabdomyosarcoma xenografts to 1-(2-chloroethyl)-3-trans-(4-methylcyclohexyl)-1-nitrosourea. Proc Natl Acad Sci USA 1985;82:2985–2989.
58. Silber JR, Mueller BA, Ewers TG, et al. Comparison of O^6-methylguanine-DNA methyltransferase activity in brain tumors and adjacent normal brain. Cancer Res 1993;53:3416–3420.
59. Hongeng S, Brent TP, Sanford RA, et al. O^6-methylguanine-DNA methyltransferase protein levels in pediatric brain tumors. Clin Cancer Res 1997;3:2459–2463.
60. Hotta T, Saito Y, Fujita H, et al. O^6-alkylguanine-DNA alkyltransferase activity of human malignant glioma and its clinical implications. J Neurooncol 1994;21:135–140.
61. Esteller M, Garcia-Foncillas J, Andion E, et al. Inactivation of the DNA-repair gene MGMT and the clinical response of gliomas to alkylating agents. N Engl J Med 2000;343:1350–1354.
62. Von Hoff DD. Send this patient's tumor for culture and sensitivity. N Engl J Med 1983;308:154–155.
63. Cortazar P, Johnson BE. Review of the efficacy of individualized chemotherapy selected by in vitro drug sensitivity testing for patients with cancer. J Clin Oncol 1999;17:1625–1631.
64. Iwadate Y, Fujimoto S, Namba H, et al. Promising survival for patients with glioblastoma multiforme treated with individualized chemotherapy based on in vitro drug sensitivity testing. Br J Cancer 2003;89:1896–1900.
65. Reya T, Morrison SJ, Clarke MF, et al. Stem cells, cancer, and cancer stem cells. Nature 2001;414:105–111.
66. Singh SK, Clarke ID, Terasaki M, et al. Identification of a cancer stem cell in human brain tumors. Cancer Res 2003;63(18):5821–5828.
67. Hemmati H, Nakano I, Lazareff J, et al. Cancerous stem cells can arise from pediatric brain tumors. Proc Nat Acad Sci USA 2003;100(25):15178–15183.
68. Ehrlich P. Das sauerstoff-bedurfnis des organismus: eine Farbenanalytlsche studie. Berlin: Hirschwald, 1885.
69. Begley DJ. The blood-brain barrier: principles for targeting peptides and drugs to the central nervous system. J Pharm Pharmacol 1996;48:136–146.
70. Engelhard JJ. Brain tumors and the blood–brain barrier. In: Bernstein M, Berger MS, eds. Neuro-oncology. The essentials. New York: Thieme Medical, 2000.

71. Rappaport SI, Ohno K, Pettigrew KD. Drug entry into the brain. Brain Res 1979;172:354–359.
72. Rall DP, Zubrod CG. Mechanisms of drug absorption and excretion: passage of drugs in and out of central nervous system. Ann Rev Pharmacol 1962;2:109–128.
73. Waggener JD, Beggs JL. Vasculature of neural neoplasms. Adv Neurol 1976;15:27–49.
74. Kelly PJ. Stereotactic histologic correlations of computed tomography- and magnetic resonance imaging-defined abnormalities in patients with glial neoplasms. Mayo Clin Proc 1987;62(6):450–459.
75. Stewart DJ. A critique of the role of the blood-brain barrier in the chemotherapy of human brain tumors. J Neurooncol 1994;20(2):121–139.
76. Levin VA, Freeman-Dove W, Landahl HD. Permeability characteristics of brain adjacent to tumors in rats. Arch Neurol 1975;32:785–791.
77. Oldendorf WH, Davson H. Brain extracellular space and the sink action of the CSF. Arch Neurol 1967;17:196–205.
78. Boucher Y, Salehi H, Witwer B, et al. Interstitial fluid pressure in intracranial tumors in patients and in rodents. Br J Cancer 1997;75(6):829–836.
79. Groothuis DR. The blood–brain and blood–tumor barriers: a review of strategies for increasing drug delivery. Neuro-oncology 2000;2:45–59.
80. Balis FM, Lester CM, Chrousos GP, et al. Differences in cerebrospinal fluid penetration of corticosteroids: possible relationship to the prevention of meningeal leukemia. J Clin Oncol 1987;5:202–207.
81. Weiss MH, Nulsen FE. The effect of glucocorticoids on cerebral spinal fluid flow in dogs. J Neurosurg 1970;32:452–458.
82. Green SB, Byar DP, Walker MD, et al. Comparisons of carmustine, procarbazine and high-dose methylprednisolone as additions to surgery and radiotherapy for the treatment of malignant glioma. Cancer Treat Rep 1983;67:1–12.
83. Gorman AM, Hirt UA, Orrenius S, Ceccatelli S. Dexamethasone pre-treatment interferes with apoptotic death in glioma cells. Neuroscience 2000;96(2):417–425.
84. Watling CJ, Lee DH, Macdonald DR, Cairncross G. Corticosteroid-induced magnetic resonance imaging changes in patients with recurrent malignant glioma. J Clin Oncol 1994;12:1886–1889.
85. Macdonald DR, Cascino TL, Schold SC, et al. Response criteria for phase II studies of supratentorial malignant glioma. J Clin Oncol 1990;8(7):1277–1280.
86. Fenstermacher JD, Cowles AL. Theoretic limitations of intracarotid infusions in brain tumor chemotherapy. Cancer Treat Rep 1977;61:518–526.
87. Neuwelt EA, Barnett PA, McCormick C, et al. Differential permeability of a human brain tumor xenograft in the nude rat: impact of tumor size and method of administration on optimizing delivery of biologically diverse agents. Clin Cancer Res 1998;4:1549–1556.
88. Shapiro WR, Green SB, Burger PC, et al. A randomized comparison of intra-arterial versus intravenous BCNU, with or without intravenous 5-florouracil for newly diagnosed patients with malignant glioma. J Neurosurg 1992;76:772–781.
89. Zunkeler B, Carson RE, Olson J, et al. Quantification and pharmacokinetics of blood-brain barrier disruption in humans. J Neurosurg 1996;85:1056–1065.
90. Kobrinsky NL, Packer RJ, Boyett JM, et al. Etoposide with or without mannitol for the treatment of recurrent or primarily unresponsive brain tumors: a Children's Cancer Group study, CCG-9881. J Neurooncol 1999; 45(1):47–54.
91. Black KL, Cloughesy T, Huang SC, et al. Intracarotid infusion of RMP-7, a bradykinin analog and transport of gallium-68 ethylenediamine tetraacetic acid into human gliomas. J Neurosurg 1997;86:603–609.
92. Ommaya AK. Subcutaneous reservoir and pump for sterile access to ventricular cerebro-spinal fluid. Lancet 1963; 2:983–984.
93. Shapiro R, Young DF, Mehta BM. Methotrexate distribution in cerebrospinal fluid after intravenous, ventricular and lumbar injections. N Engl J Med 1975;293:161–166.
94. Yamashima T, Yamashita J, Shoin K. Neurotoxicity of local administration of two nitrosoureas in malignant gliomas. Neurosurgery 1990;26:794–800.
95. Sipos E, Tyler B, Piantadosi S, et al. Optimizing interstitial delivery of BCNU from controlled release polymers for the treatment of brain tumors. Cancer Chemother Pharmacol 1997;39:383–389.
96. Westphal M, Hilt D, Bortey E, et al. A Phase III trial of local chemotherapy with biodegradable carmustine (BCNU) wafers (GLIADEL wafers) in patients with primary malignant gliomas. Neuro-Oncology 2003;5(2):79–88.
97. Valtonen S, Timonen U, Toivanen P, et al. Interstitial chemotherapy with carmustine-loaded polymers for high grade gliomas—a randomized, double-blind study. Neurosurgery 1997;1:44–49.
98. Bashir RM, Harris NL, Hochberg FH, Singer RM. Detection of Epstein-Barr virus in CNS lymphoma by in-situ hybridization. Neurology 1989;39:813–817.
99. Singh A, Strobos RJ, Singh BM, et al. Steroid-induced remissions in CNS lymphoma. Neurology 1982;32:1267–1271.
100. Geppert M, Ostertag CB, Seiztz G, et al. Glucocorticoid therapy obscures the diagnosis of cerebral lymphoma. Acta Neuropathol 1990;80:629–634.
101. Cher L, Glass J, Harsh GR, et al. Treatment of primary CNS lymphoma with methotrexate-based chemotherapy and deferred radiotherapy: preliminary results. Neurology 1996;46:1757–1759.
102. Pitman SW, Frei E III. Weekly methotrexate-calcium leucovorin rescue: effect of alkalinization on nephrotoxicity, pharmacokinetics in the CNS, and use in CNS non-Hodgkin's lymphoma. Cancer Treat Rep 1997;61:695–701.
103. DeAngelis LM, Seiferheld W, Schold SC, et al. Combination chemotherapy and radiotherapy for primary central nervous system lymphoma: Radiation Therapy Oncology Group Study 93–10. J Clin Oncol 2002;20:4643–4648.
104. Blay JY, Conroy T, Chevreau C, et al. High-dose methotrexate for the treatment of primary cerebral lymphomas: analysis of survival and late neurologic toxicity in a retrospective series. J Clin Oncol 1998;16:864–871.
105. Weiss H, Walker M, Wiernik P. Neurotoxicity of commonly used antineoplastic agents. N Engl J Med 1974;291:75–81, 127–133.
106. Allen J, Rosen G, Mehta B, et al. Leukoencephalopathy following high-dose IV methotrexate chemotherapy with leucovorin rescue. Cancer Treat Rep 1980;64: 1261–1273.

107. Hubbard JL, Scheithauer BW, Kispert DB, et al. Adult cerebellar medulloblastoma: the pathological, radiographic and clinical spectrum. J Neurosurg 1989;70:536–544.
108. Cohen ME, Duffner PK. Brain tumors in children: principles of diagnosis and treatment, 2nd ed. New York: Raven Press, 1994.
109. Friedman HS, Oakes WJ. The chemotherapy of posterior fossa tumors in childhood. J Neurooncol 1987;5:217–229.
110. Evans AE, Jenkin RDT, Sposto R, et al. The treatment of medulloblastoma: results of a prospective randomized trial of radiation therapy with and without CCNU, vincristine, and prednisone. J Neurosurg 1990;72:572–582.
111. Packer RJ, Goldwein J, Nicholson HS, et al. Treatment of children with medulloblastomas with reduced-dose craniospinal radiation therapy and adjuvant chemotherapy: a Children's Cancer Group Study. J Clin Oncol 1999; 17:2127–2136.
112. Packer RJ, Sutton LN, Elterman R, et al. Outcome for children with medulloblastoma treated with radiation and cisplatin, CCNU and vincristine chemotherapy. J Neurosurg 1994;81:690–698.
113. Sawamura Y, Shirato H, Ikeda J, et al. Induction chemotherapy followed by reduced-volume radiation therapy for newly diagnosed central nervous system germinoma. J Neurosurg 1998;88:66–72.
114. Aoyama H, Shirato H, Ikeda J, et al. Induction chemotherapy followed by low-dose involved field radiotherapy for intracranial germ cell tumors. J Clin Oncol 2002;20: 857–865.
115. Calaminus G, Bamberg M, Baranzelli MC, et al. Intracranial germ cell tumors: a comprehensive update of the European data. Neuropediatrics 1994;25:26–32.
116. Burger PC, Scheithauer BW, Vogel FS. Surgical pathology of the nervous system and its coverings, 3rd ed. New York: Churchill Livingstone, 1991:194–271.
117. Walker MD, Alexander E, Hunt WE, et al. Evaluation of BCNU and/or radiotherapy in the treatment of anaplastic gliomas. A cooperative clinical trial. J Neurosurg 1978; 49:333–343.
118. Green SP, Byar DP, Walker MD, et al. Comparison of carmustine, procarbazine and high-dose methylprednisolone as additions to surgery and radiotherapy for the treatment of malignant glioma. Cancer Treat Rep 1993;67:121–132.
119. Lassman LP, Pearce GW, Gang J. Sensitivity of intracranial gliomas to vincristine sulphate. Lancet 1965;1:196–198.
120. Fine HA, Dear KBG, Loeffler JS, et al. Meta-analysis of radiation therapy with and without adjuvant chemotherapy for malignant gliomas in adults. Cancer 1993;71:2585–2597.
121. DeAngelis LM, Burger PC, Green SB, et al. Malignant glioma: who benefits from adjuvant chemotherapy? Ann Neurol 1998;44:691–695.
122. Geyer JR, Finlay JL, Boyett JM, et al. Survival of infants with malignant astrocytomas. Cancer 1995;75:1045–1050.
123. Grossman SA, Wharam M, Sheidler V, et al. Phase II study of continuous infusion carmustine and cisplatin followed by cranial irradiation in adults with newly diagnosed high-grade astrocytoma. J Clin Oncol 1997;15(7):2596–2603.
124. Grossman S, O'Neill A, Grunnet M, et al. Phase III study comparing three cycles of infusional BCNU/cisplatin followed by radiation with radiation and concurrent BCNU for patients with newly diagnosed supratentorial glioblastoma multiforme: ECOG Group Trial 2394. J Clin Oncol 2003;21(8):1485–1491.
125. Huncharek M, Muscat J. Treatment of recurrent high grade astrocytoma: results of a systematic review of 1415 patients. Anticancer Res 1998;18:1303–1311.
126. Yung WKA, Prados MD, Yaya-Tur R, et al. Multicenter phase II trial of temozolomide in patients with anaplastic astrocytoma or anaplastic oligoastrocytoma at first relapse. J Clin Oncol 2000;17:2762–2771.
127. Stupp R, Mason WP, van den Bent MJ, et al. Radiotherapy plus concomitant and adjuvant temozolomide for glioblastoma. N Engl J Med 2005;352:987–996.
128. Patel M, McCully C, Godwin K, et al. Plasma and cerebrospinal fluid pharmacokinetics of intravenous temozolomide in non-human primates. J Neurooncol 2003; 61:203–207.
129. Dolan ME, Mitchell RB, Mummert C, et al. Effect of O^6-benzylguanine analogues on sensitivity of human tumor cells to the cytotoxic effects of alkylating agents. Cancer Res 1991;51:3367–3372.
130. Wedge SR, Newlands ES. O^6-benzylguanine enhances the sensitivity of a glioma xenograft with low O^6-alkylguanine-DNA alkyltransferase activity to temozolomide and BCNU. Br J Cancer 1996;73:482–490.
131. Mitchell RB, Moschel RC, Dolan ME. Effect of O^6-benzylguanine on the sensitivity of human tumor xenografts to 1,3-bis (2-choroethyl)-1-nitrosourea and on DNA interstrand cross-link formation. Cancer Res 1992;52; 1171–1175.
132. Pollack IF, Claassen D, Al-Shboul Q, et al. Low-grade gliomas of the cerebral hemispheres in children: an analysis of 71 cases. J Neurosurg 1995;82:536–547.
133. Mamelak AN, Prados MD, Obana WG, et al. Treatment options and prognosis for multicentric juvenile pilocytic astrocytoma. J Neurosurg 1994;81:24–30.
134. Phillippon JH, Clemenceau SH, Fauchon F, et al. Supratentorial low-grade astrocytomas in adults. Neurosurgery 1993;32:554–559.
135. Bauman G, Pahapill P, Macdonald D, et al. Low grade glioma: measuring radiographic response to radiation therapy. Can J Neurol Sci 1999;26(1):18–22.
136. Eyre HJ, Crowley JJ, Townsend JJ, et al. A randomized trial of radiotherapy versus radiotherapy plus CCNU for incompletely resected low-grade gliomas: a Southwest Oncology Group Study. J Neurosurg 1993;78:909–914.
137. Quinn JA, Reardon DA, Friedman AH, et al. Phase II trial of temozolomide in patients with progressive low-grade gliomas. J Clin Oncol 2003;21(4):646–651.
138. Listernick R, Louis DN, Packer RJ, et al. Optic pathway gliomas in children with neurofibromatosis type 1: consensus statement from the NF1 Optic Pathway Glioma Task Force. Ann Neurol 1997;41:143–149.
139. Deliganis AV, Geyer JR, Berger MS. Prognostic significance of type 1 neurofibromatosis (von Recklinghausen disease) in childhood optic glioma. Neurosurgery 1996;38:1114–1119.
140. Schmandt SM, Packer RJ, Vezine LG, Jane J. Spontaneous regression of low-grade astrocytomas in childhood. Pediatr Neurosurgery 2000;37:132–136.
141. Rosenstock JG, Packer RJ, Bilaniuk L, et al. Chiasmatic optic glioma treated with chemotherapy. A preliminary report. J Neurosurg 1985;63:862–866.

142. Packer RJ, Ater J, Allen J, et al. Carboplatin and vincristine chemotherapy for children with newly diagnosed progressive low-grade gliomas. J Neurosurg 1997;86:747–754.
143. Schiavetti A, Varrasso G, Maurizi P, et al. Hypersensitivity to carboplatin in children. Med Pediatr Oncol 1999; 32:183–185.
144. Yu DY, Dahl GV, Shames RS. Weekly dosing of carboplatin increases risk of allergy in children. J Pediatr Hematol Oncol 2001;23(6):349–352.
145. Fouladi M, Wallace D, Langston JW, et al. Survival and functional outcome of children with hypothalamic/chiasmatic tumors. Cancer 2003;97:1084–1092.
146. Fouladi M, Hunt D, Pollack IF, et al. Outcome of children with centrally reviewed low-grade gliomas treated with chemotherapy with or without radiotherapy on Children's Cancer Group high-grade glioma study CCG-945. Cancer 2003;98:1243–1252.
147. Mork SJ, Lindegaard KF, Halvorson TB, et al. Oligodendroglioma: incidence and biological behavior in a defined population. J Neurosurg 1985;63:881–889.
148. Coons SW, Johnson PC, Scheithauer BS, et al. Improving diagnostic accuracy and interobserver concordance in the classification and grading of primary gliomas. Cancer 1997;79:1381–1393.
149. Cairncross J, Macdonald DR. Successful chemotherapy for recurrent malignant oligodendroglioma. Ann Neurol 1988;23:360–364.
150. Cairncross J, Macdonald D, Ludwin S, et al. Chemotherapy for anaplastic oligodendroglioma. J Clin Oncol 1994;12: 2013–2021.
151. Chinot O, Honore S, Dufour H, et al. Safety and efficacy of temozolomide in patients with recurrent anaplastic oligodendrogliomas after standard radiotherapy and chemotherapy. J Clin Oncol 2001;19:2449–2455.
152. Mason WP, Krol GS, De Angelis LM. Low-grade oligodendroglioma responds to chemotherapy. Neurology 1996;46:203–207.
153. Cairncross JG, Ueki K, Zlatescu MC, et al. Specific genetic predictors of chemotherapeutic response and survival in patients with anaplastic oligodendrogliomas. J Natl Cancer Inst 1998;90:1473–1479.
154. Ino Y, Zlatescu MC, Sasaki H, et al. Long survival and therapeutic responses in patients with histologically disparate high-grade gliomas demonstrating chromosome 1p loss. J Neurosurg 2000;92:983–990.
155. Pollack IF, Finkelstein SD, Burnham J, et al. The association between chromosome 1p loss and outcome in pediatric malignant gliomas: results from the CCG-945 cohort. Pediatr Neurosurg 2003;39:114–121.
156. Evans AE, Anderson JR, Lefkowitz-Boudreaux IB, Finlay JL. Adjuvant chemotherapy of childhood posterior fossa ependymoma: craniospinal irradiation with or without adjuvant CCNU, vincristine and prednisone: a Children's Cancer Group study. Med Pediatr Oncol 1996;27:8–14.
157. Bertolone SJ, Baum ES, Krivit W, et al. A phase II study of cisplatin therapy in recurrent childhood brain tumors. A report from the Children's Cancer Study Group. J Neurooncol 1989;7:5–11.
158. Gaynon PS, Ettinger LJ, Baum ES, et al. Carboplatin in childhood brain tumors. A Children's Cancer Study Group Phase II trial. Cancer 1990;66:2465–2469.
159. Merchant TE, Jenkins JJ, Burger P, et al. Influence of tumor grade on time to progression after irradiation for localized ependymoma in children. Int J Radiat Oncol Biol Phys 2002;53:52–57.
160. Rorhinger M, Sutherland GR, Louw DR, et al. Incidence and clinicopathological features of meningioma. J Neurosurg 1989;71:665–672.
161. Schrell UM, Rittig MG, Anders M, et al. Hydroxyurea for treatment of unresectable and recurrent meningiomas. Decrease in the size of meningiomas in patients treated with hydroxyurea. J Neurosurg 1997;86:840–844.
162. Mason WP, Gentili F, MacDonald DR, et al. Stabilization of disease progression by hydroxyurea in patients with recurrent or unresectable meningioma. J Neurosurg 2002;97:341–346.

CHAPTER 9

Supportive Care

Herbert B. Newton

The modern treatment of brain tumor patients usually involves a team approach from a dedicated group of physicians, nurses, and support staff that specialize in various aspects of neuro-oncology.[1] Although the focus of the treatment team will be on therapeutic strategies to control tumor growth (e.g., surgical resection, radiotherapy, chemotherapy), many other facets of care are necessary and will involve patient support and symptom management in an effort to maintain quality of life. The challenge for the treatment team begins at the moment of diagnosis, when the bad news must be communicated to the patient and family. Recent research suggests there are several important factors that should be considered when imparting a new cancer diagnosis.[2] It is critical that the physician use simple, nontechnical language in a nonpatronizing manner, with a warm and caring tone. Every effort should be made to empathize with the emotions the patient is experiencing. The physician should sit close to the patient and maintain good eye contact. It is also permissible to initiate physical contact, in an effort to provide comfort. A quiet, private, and comfortable room should be used for the meeting, where interruptions and distractions can be minimized. Many patients also find it helpful when the physician gives some kind of warning that bad news is forthcoming and does not rush through the ensuing discussion.

The role of support is crucial for brain tumor patients and their families, and continues until the patient is cured or, more often, succumbs to disease.[3] The most important initial form of support is information and education about the diagnosis. At the moment the patient and family hear the words "brain tumor," they enter into a crisis mode and often feel a loss of control, fear of the unknown, and sense of helplessness. To regain some aspect of control of their lives, they need to learn as much as possible about the disease and form a partnership with their physician, taking an aggressive and active role in the plan for treatment and recovery. Informational brochures and other written materials are helpful, as are the web sites of organizations that provide services and resources for brain tumor patients and families, such as the North American Brain Tumor Coalition.[3] The Coalition is a network of charitable organizations dedicated to the cure of brain tumors, and includes the American Brain Tumor Association, the Brain Tumor Foundation for Children, the Brain Tumor Foundation of Canada, The Brain Tumor Society, The Children's Brain Tumor Foundation, the National Brain Tumor Foundation, the Pediatric Brain Tumor Foundation of the United States, and the Preuss Foundation. During the course of a devastating illness such as a brain tumor, the patient's family will usually be the greatest source of support and comfort, as well as active caregivers in the home setting.[3,4] In this context, family members often take on the role of information seekers and patient advocates. It is important to note that family caregivers are also at risk for depression and other signs of stress, and require a strong support network to function effectively in this role.[5] Other sources of support for the patient and caregivers include the nurses of the treatment team, oncologic social workers, chaplains affiliated with the hospital or from the private sector, and hospital-based support groups (brain tumor specific or general).

The remaining sections of this chapter review the various aspects of supportive care that may be necessary in the management of brain tumor patients.

▶ SEIZURES AND ANTICONVULSANT THERAPY

Seizure activity is a frequent complication in neuro-oncology patients and often compromises quality of life by the restriction of driving privileges, through seizure-related injuries, loss of time at work, and anxiety related to subsequent ictal events.[1,6–8] In addition, quality of life can be further affected by the side effects, drug interactions, and expenses incurred by the use of antiepileptic drugs (AEDs). Seizures occur at presentation in 20% to 50% of patients with primary (PBTs) and metastatic (MBTs) brain tumors.[1,6,9] It is important to note that more than 25% of adults between 25 and 64 years of age with newly diagnosed seizures will have an underlying brain tumor.[6] At the time of tumor progression, seizure activity often becomes more frequent and severe, affecting another 10% to 20% of patients. The overall incidence of seizures is highest in patients with PBTs of low histologic grade and slow growth potential, and becomes less frequent in those with high-grade PBTs and MBTs. For example, approximately 80% to 90% of patients with oligodendroglioma and ganglioglioma will have seizures, whereas patients with more malignant PBT, such as anaplastic astrocytoma and glioblastoma multiforme, carry a risk for seizure activity of 68% and 33%, respectively.[8] Younger patients (e.g., children and young adults) tend to have a higher incidence of seizure activity when the tumors are supratentorial in location. In general, supratentorial tumors are most likely to cause seizures, especially when located within or near the cortex. Multifocal or bihemispheric tumors are also known to cause frequent ictal events. Seizures are much less common with tumors that are deep-seated or confined to the white matter.

Patients with low-grade tumors typically manifest seizures that are equally divided among partial motor, partial complex, and secondarily generalized varieties.[6–8] For patients with high-grade gliomas or brain metastases, focal motor seizures are the predominant variety, with less common secondarily generalized and complex partial seizures. The neurologic examination tends to be relatively normal and nonfocal in patients with seizures from low-grade tumors. In contrast, patients with high-grade PBTs and MBTs are more likely to have seizure activity associated with focal neurologic deficits on examination.[6,7]

The pathophysiologic mechanisms underlying tumor-associated seizures (TASs) remain unclear.[8,10,11] Recent evidence using direct brain recordings of electrical activity suggest that TASs originate from intact, noninfiltrated, neural tissue adjacent to tumors, and not from within the tumor mass itself.[10] Histologically, epileptogenic regions of brain demonstrate gliosis and mild reactive astrocytosis, without evidence for tumor cells. It is now theorized that these peritumoral epileptogenic foci develop an imbalance between excitatory and inhibitory inputs, due to multifactorial alterations in the local milieu from the tumor. The intra- and extracellular pH is slightly alkaline in peritumoral tissues, which enhances excitatory neuronal pathways and induces a 30% reduction of activity in GABAergic inhibitory pathways.[10] In biopsy samples from peritumoral epileptic foci, the number of gamma-aminobutyric acid (GABA)- and somatostatin-containing neurons are decreased.[12] Similar biopsy studies have noted an elevated concentration of glutamine, the direct precursor of glutamate, in peritumoral epileptogenic foci.[13] Glutamine is taken up and secreted by normal glia and glioma cells, thus providing a large reservoir of precursor for peritumoral neurons to convert to glutamate. In addition, recent evidence suggests that glioma cells directly secrete glutamate, causing significantly increased, excitotoxic concentrations in peritumoral tissues.[14,15] In vitro experiments have demonstrated extensive *N*-methyl-D-aspartate (NMDA) and α-amino-3-hydroxy-5-methylisoxazole-4-propionic acid (AMPA) receptor stimulation and delayed Ca^{2+}-dependent cell death in exposed neurons. These reports suggest that exposure of peritumoral neurons to chronically elevated concentrations of glutamate could contribute to neuronal injury, abnormalities of neuronal circuitry, and the development of epileptiform activity. Other peritumoral alterations that may contribute to epileptogenic potential include increased extracellular Fe^{3+}, dysfunction of astrocytic syncytial gap junctions because of the infiltration of tumor cells, and the presence of proinflammatory cytokines (e.g., tumor necrosis factor [TNF]-α), which can increase membrane excitability.[8]

The diagnosis of a seizure in a brain tumor patient is usually a clinical diagnosis, based on the history and description of the symptom complex from the patient and family members.[1,6–8] Testing with routine electroencephalography (EEG) is not helpful in most patients, because only 25% to 33% of patients will demonstrate any focal interictal epileptiform activity. Prolonged EEG monitoring (with or without a video component) may be more helpful in diagnosing seizures in confusing or subtle cases. Of patients with a malignant PBT who have had a seizure, 50% to 75% will continue to have seizures.[7] In half of the active seizure group, ictal events will occur more than once per month, and another 25% will have events more than once per week, despite the use of an AED. The presence of seizure activity does not impact on the overall survival of brain tumor patients.[6] However, patients who present with a seizure or have long-standing seizures do have a more favorable prognosis. There are several explanations for this phenomenon, including the increased likelihood that the tumor will be an oligodendroglioma, which typically have longer survival times, and that seizures will often lead to a more prompt workup and earlier diagnosis, when the tumor is smaller and more amenable to surgical resection. Patients with chronic seizures that develop a new pattern, with frequent "breakthrough" activity, may relate to a change in the tumor such as bleeding or transformation into a more rapidly growing and more malignant lesion. It is also possible to have a "flare-up" of seizure activity in otherwise well-controlled patients at the onset of certain therapies that may cause irritation to surrounding brain, such as at the initiation of external beam radiotherapy and with certain forms of chemotherapy (e.g., Gliadel wafers, intraarterial cisplatin).

There is general consensus that any brain tumor patient with a well-documented, unequivocal seizure (generalized or focal) should be placed on an AED (Table 9-1).[1,6–10] For adult patients with generalized seizures, phenytoin, carbamazepine, and valproate have relatively equivalent efficacy for reducing seizure activity.[16,17] Similarly, all three drugs are effective for partial motor, partial sensory, and partial complex seizures. However, a comparative trial of carbamazepine and valproate demonstrated better control of complex partial seizure activity with carbamazepine.[18] Monotherapy with phenytoin, carbamazepine, or valproate should be the initial management approach in most patients.[1,16,17] In some patients, a second drug must be added if high therapeutic concentrations of several of the first-line drugs are unable to control seizure activity. Phenytoin or carbamazepine in combination with valproate is a common strategy. Alternatively, one of the new anticonvulsants

▶ **TABLE 9-1.** ANTIEPILEPTIC DRUGS COMMONLY USED FOR TREATMENT OF SEIZURES IN BRAIN TUMOR PATIENTS

Drug	Dose (mg/d)	Metabolism	Enzyme Inducing?	Mechanism	Bound Fraction (%)
Traditional AEDs					
Phenytoin	300–400	Hepatic +++	+++	Sodium channel	90–95
Carbamazepine	800–1600	Hepatic +++	+++	Sodium channel	75
Valproic acid	1000–3000	Hepatic +++	No; inhibitory	Sodium channel; enhanced GABA	80–90
Phenobarbital	90–180	Hepatic +++	+++	EAA antagonist; enhanced GABA	45
Newer AEDs					
Felbamate	2400–3600	Hepatic ++	+	EAA antagonist; enhanced GABA	25
Lamotrigine	100–500	Hepatic +++	None	Sodium channel	55
Gabapentin	1800–3600	Renal +++	None	Enhanced GABA	<5
Topiramate	200–400	Hepatic +	None	Sodium channel; EAA antagonist; enhanced GABA	9–17
Tiagabine	32–56	Hepatic +++	None	Enhanced GABA	95
Oxcarbazepine	600–1800	Hepatic +++	+	Sodium channel	40
Levetiracetam	1000–3000	Renal ++	None	?N-type calcium channels	<10
Zonisamide	100–400	Hepatic ++	None	Sodium and calcium channels; enhanced GABA	40

+ = mild; ++ = moderate; +++ = severe; AED = antiepileptic drug; EAA = excitatory amino acids; GABA = gamma-aminobutyric acid.
Source: Adapted from references 6, 10, 16, and 17.

(e.g., levetiracetam, gabapentin, topiramate, zonisamide) could be added to one of the first-line agents.[19–21] Levetiracetam may be an excellent choice, because initial experience suggests it is effective and well tolerated in brain tumor patients, and has minimal potential to interact with other drugs such as corticosteroids or chemotherapy agents.[21] Ongoing studies will determine if levetiracetam and other new agents might be appropriate for first-line use or as secondary, stand-alone agents. Serum drug concentrations must be monitored and optimized in all patients whenever possible (e.g., phenytoin, carbamazepine, valproate).

In the brain tumor population, seizures remain difficult to control despite the use of AEDs. Patients who present with seizures tend to be more refractory to therapy than those who develop seizures later in the course of their disease.[6,7] In general, recurrent seizure activity is common, despite aggressive anticonvulsant therapy. Patient compliance can contribute to this problem and is frequently suboptimal. In many patients with a recent seizure, anticonvulsant levels are subtherapeutic. Further complicating the situation is that brain tumor patients are more susceptible to AED toxicity and side effects, including cognitive impairment, hepatotoxicity, myelosuppression, skin rashes (including Stevens-Johnson syndrome), and interactions with concomitant medications.[6] Several of the AEDs (e.g., phenytoin, carbamazepine, phenobarbital) enhance hepatic microsomal P450-mediated metabolism of concomitant medications. This is especially problematic for patients receiving chemotherapy (e.g., nitrosoureas, temozolomide, irinotecan, paclitaxel, methotrexate), leading to lower tissue concentrations and reduced efficacy.[6,22] Some of the newer AEDs (e.g., levetiracetam, gabapentin) do not enhance the hepatic P450 system and may be better choices in selected patients.

Anticonvulsant drugs are frequently administered to brain tumor patients at the time of diagnosis or after craniotomy as prophylaxis for potential seizure activity.[6] This practice was given early support in the literature, despite the fact that the data in these reports were modest at best.[23,24] All subsequent reports on the use of AED prophylaxis do not support this practice, including a randomized, blinded, placebo-controlled trial of valproate in patients with newly diagnosed PBT and MBT.[25–29] In this study, the odds ratio for a seizure in the valproate arm relative to the placebo arm was 1.7 ($p = 0.3$).[29] Most authors would now recommend withholding implementation of AED in newly diagnosed patients until a seizure has been documented. This approach is supported by a recent meta-analysis by Glantz and associates for the American Academy of Neurology.[30] In addition, for patients who have not had a seizure and have received AED for craniotomy, tapering and discontinuing the AED after the first postoperative week is recommended.[30]

▶ CORTICOSTEROIDS

The use of corticosteroids is often necessary in PBT and MBT patients to control symptoms caused by increased intracranial pressure (e.g., headache, nausea and emesis, confusion, weakness).[1,9,31] Peritumoral edema is the principal cause of elevated intracranial pressure and is mediated through numerous mechanisms, including the leaky neovasculature associated with tumor angiogenesis, as well as increased permeability induced by factors secreted by the tumor and surrounding tissues, such as oxygen free radicals, arachidonic acid, glutamate, histamine, bradykinin, atrial natriuretic peptide, and vascular endothelial growth factor (VEGF).[32–34] Dexamethasone is the high-potency steroid used most often to treat the edema associated with brain tumors.[1,31] It has several advantages over other synthetic glucocorticoids, including a longer half-life, reduced mineralocorticoid effect, lower incidence of cognitive and behavioral complications, and diminished inhibition of leukocyte migration.[35] The mechanisms by which dexamethasone and other glucocorticoids reduce peritumoral edema remain unclear. It is known that both PBT and MBT have high concentrations of glucocorticoid receptors. The effects of these drugs on tumor-induced edema are most likely mediated through binding to these receptors, with subsequent transfer to the nucleus and the expression of novel genes.[34] In a recent magnetic resonance imaging (MRI) study, dexamethasone was able to induce a dramatic reduction in blood–tumor barrier permeability and regional cerebral blood volume, without significant alteration of cerebral blood flow or the degree of edema.[36] The inhibition of production and/or release of vasoactive factors secreted by tumor cells and endothelial cells, such as VEGF and prostacyclin, appears to be involved in this process.[33,34] In addition, glucocorticoids appear to inhibit the reactivity of endothelial cells to several substances that induce capillary permeability.

The exact dose of steroids necessary for each patient will vary depending on the histology (i.e., benign or malignant), size and location of the tumor, and amount of peritumoral edema. In general, most patients with malignant tumors will require between 8 and 16 mg of dexamethasone per day to remain clinically stable. The lowest dose of steroid that can control the patient's pressure-related symptoms should be used.[1,31] This approach minimizes some of the toxicity and complications that can arise from long-term corticosteroid usage, which includes hyperglycemia, peripheral edema, proximal myopathy, gastritis, infection, osteopenia, weight gain, bowel perforation, and psychiatric or behavioral changes (e.g., euphoria, hypomania, depression, psychosis, sleep disturbance).[1,37–42] Patients with dexamethasone-induced proximal myopathy will often improve when the dosage is reduced.[41,42] In addition, the proximal leg muscles can usually be strengthened if the patient is placed on a lower extremity exercise regimen. Some authors have also reported an improvement in the myopathy when dexamethasone is replaced by an equivalent dosage of prednisone or hydrocortisone.[41,42] The neuropsychiatric complications of steroids can often be improved by dosage reduction or discontinuation of the drug.[40] For those patients in whom continued steroid usage is necessary, symptomatic pharmacologic intervention is appropriate. For example, patients experiencing steroid-induced delirium or psychosis will often improve with low-dose haloperidol (0.5 to 1.0 mg PO, IM, or IV), titrated to control symptoms. Steroid-induced sleep disturbances often respond to dosage reduction or by eliminating any doses after dinner. In refractory cases, the use of a hypnotic medication at bedtime (e.g., triazolam 0.25 mg) is often beneficial. Corticosteroid-induced osteoporosis is a common problem, affecting 30% to 50% of patients receiving treatment for 1 year or longer.[37,43,44] Patients on long-term dexamethasone require a preventive program to minimize osteoporosis, including calcium and vitamin D supplements and weight-bearing exercises. These measures should be started early, because bone loss is greatest in the first 2 to 4 months of chronic steroid treatment. For patients on long-term steroid therapy (i.e., ≥3 months), or in those patients with established osteoporosis or evidence of an osteoporotic fracture, bisphosphonate therapy (e.g., risedronate 2.5–5.0 mg/d; alendronate 5–10 mg/d) should be added to the regimen of calcium and vitamin D supplements.[44]

Brain tumor patients can be immunosuppressed for a variety of reasons, including long-term steroid use, immunomodulatory factors secreted by the tumor, and the effects of chemotherapy.[35,37] Chronic steroid usage can lead to lymphopenia, mainly through a reduction in the concentration of CD4+ T cells, and an associated increased risk of systemic infection. Recent studies suggest that brain tumor patients on chronic steroids are at substantial risk for *Pneumocystis carinii* pneumonia (PCP), a serious infection with a 50% to 55% fatality rate. In a pair of reports that reviewed the Johns Hopkins experience over the past 20 years, Grossman and colleagues noted that the rate of PCP in primary brain tumor patients was less than 1.0%.[45,46] However, of all HIV-negative patients with PCP over the prior 5 years, the percentage with primary brain tumors had increased from 22% to 40% (half of which were primary central nervous system lymphoma [PCNSL]). In fact, it appears that patients with PCNSL are at particular risk for developing PCP, possibly as a result of the recent widespread use of methotrexate-based chemotherapy regimens, which can significantly reduce CD4+ T cell counts.[46] The authors did not recommend PCP prophylaxis for every brain tumor patient on long-term steroids or chemotherapy. Rather, they suggested careful monitoring of all patients for the onset of lymphopenia, including an assessment in high-risk cases of the concentration of CD4+ T cells. For those high-risk patients with lymphopenia and CD4 counts below 200 cells/mL, a prophylactic anti-PCP regimen should be instituted.[46] The most commonly used prophylactic antibiotic is trimethoprim-sulfamethoxazole (TMP-SMX, 160 + 800 mg), at a dose of 1 double-strength tablet per day. For patients with a sulfa allergy or deleterious interactions between TMP-SMX and other drugs (e.g., methotrexate), alternative prophylactic medications include pentamidine (300 mg/mo by nebulizer) and dapsone (100 mg/d PO).

▶ GASTRIC ACID INHIBITORS

Brain tumor patients on long-term dexamethasone are at increased risk for gastrointestinal complications (i.e., gastritis, ulceration, bowel perforation), although there remains some debate in the literature regarding ulcer formation.[31,37,39] A comprehensive review of the topic would suggest that ulcer prophylaxis is appropriate, because the incidence of ulcer formation is increased in patients with advanced malignant disease.[47] Patients at risk should be treated prophylactically with a gastric acid inhibitor such as ranitidine hydrochloride (150 mg PO bid), famotidine (20 mg po bid), or omeprazole (20–40 mg PO qd).[48,49] These medications can be discontinued after the patient has been completely tapered off dexamethasone.

▶ THROMBOEMBOLIC COMPLICATIONS AND ANTICOAGULATION

The risk of thromboembolism (i.e., deep venous thrombosis [DVT], pulmonary embolism [PE]) is high in cancer patients, with an antemortem incidence of symptomatic events approaching 15%.[50,51] However, at autopsy the incidence rates are much higher, between 45% and 50% in some series. For patients with brain tumors, the risk for DVT and PE appears to be even higher than the general cancer population.[51,53] In the perioperative period, the overall incidence of thrombosis after brain tumor resection was 45%, as detected by ^{125}I-labeled fibrinogen scans.[52] The incidence varied depending on the tumor type, and was 72%, 60%, and 20% for meningioma, glioblastoma multiforme (GBM), and MBT patients, respectively. The high incidence of thromboembolism in meningioma patients was unexpected, considering their generally benign natural history, and suggested that tumor biology may play a predominant role in risk for perioperative DVT and PE. Thromboembolic risk continues to remain high in brain tumor patients after the perioperative period (i.e., beyond 6 weeks). A meta-analysis of malignant glioma patients by Marras and colleagues noted a DVT incidence rate that ranged from 0.013 to 0.023 per patient-month of followup, corresponding to overall rates of 7% to 24%.[54] The only prospective study included in the analysis followed 75 patients until death and had a DVT incidence rate of 24% (0.015 DVT/ patient-month).[55] In addition to biologic factors related to individual tumor histology, several clinical factors are also associated with increased risk of DVT and PE, including arm paresis, leg paresis, history of prior DVT or PE before tumor diagnosis, longer operative time, and presence of GBM.[53,54,56] Other less important factors that may also be relevant are older age, larger tumor size, and the use of chemotherapy.

When patients with a PBT or MBT develop a thromboembolic event, should they be treated with conventional anticoagulation approaches, or is that too dangerous? Should they instead receive an inferior vena cava filter (VCF) without anticoagulation? The core of this dilemma is the risk of intratumoral hemorrhage while receiving anticoagulant therapy. This is a common problem for the neuro-oncology treatment team and continues to be studied in the literature. In general, the risk for symptomatic hemorrhage into a primary or metastatic brain tumor is quite low during conservative anticoagulation with heparin and Coumadin.[53,55–60] Most authors report a hemorrhage rate of 2% to 3% for PBT and 5% to 7% for MBT. To minimize the potential for intratumoral hemorrhage, the parameters for heparin and Coumadin therapy need to be very conservative, with partial thromboplastin time (PTT) and prothrombin time (PT) values in the 1.5 to 2.0 times control range.[56] Once the patient has shifted completely over to Coumadin, the international normalized ratio (INR) should be maintained between 1.5 and 2.5.[53,58]

A more recent approach to treating a thromboembolic event is to use a low-molecular-weight heparin (LMWH).[50,61] The LMWHs (e.g., enoxaparin, dalteparin) are composed of fragments of unfractionated heparin produced by controlled enzymatic or chemical depolymerization, yielding chains with an average molecular weight of 5000 daltons. In comparison to unfractionated heparin, LMWHs have a more predictable anticoagulant response because of better bioavailability, a longer half-life, and more dose-dependent clearance.[61] In addition, the LMWHs can be administered subcutaneously in the outpatient setting and do not require monitoring of coagulation status. When used in clinical trials of patients with DVT, LMWHs (e.g., enoxaparin, 100 U/kg BID) have proved as effective or more effective than unfractionated heparin, with a lower hemorrhage rate.[61] Meta-analyses of the clinical trial data conclude, in general, that LMWHs are more effective and safer than unfractionated heparin. However, the above-mentioned studies have not included brain tumor patients. Clinical trials specifically to evaluate the safety and efficacy of LMWH in brain tumor patients have not been completed.

The utility of VCF in brain tumor and other cancer patients remains controversial.[62] Several studies demonstrate a significant complication rate for VCF in primary and metastatic brain tumor patients (range: 40% to 62%) and suggest that biologic factors related to the tumor may be involved.[59,60] Complications after VCF placement include filter thrombosis, recurrent DVT, recurrent PE, and thrombosis of the inferior vena cava. Patients receiving anticoagulation had a lower recurrence rate of PE and DVT. Although most authors now suggest that acute and long-term anticoagulation is superior to VCF placement for brain tumor patients with DVT and/or PE, selected patients should still be considered for this approach. Patients with large regions of intratumoral hemorrhage, impaired neurologic function and excessive risk for falling episodes, and gastrointestinal bleeding should be evaluated for VCF placement instead of anticoagulation.

▶ DYSPHAGIA AND SWALLOWING DISORDERS

Dysphagia and swallowing disorders are common in patients with neurologic disease, and can be associated with stroke, multiple sclerosis, motor neuron disease, neurodegenerative disorders, and structural lesions such as a brain tumor.[63–69] Swallowing dysfunction can lead to serious morbidity from malnutrition, dehydration, and aspiration pneumonia. There remains a paucity of literature regarding the incidence and presentation of dysphagia in the brain tumor population. The best-described presentation involves dysfunction of the brainstem, either from compression to, or growth within, this region.[63,70,71] Tumors that can induce dysphagia in this manner include brainstem glioma, brainstem metastases, ependymoma, choroid plexus papilloma, large pineal region tumors (i.e., pinealoma, astrocytoma), and neoplasms of the cerebellopontine angle such as acoustic schwannoma and meningioma. Direct tumor compression causes impairment of the brainstem circuitry that underlies swallowing, including the nucleus tractus solitarius, ventromedial reticular formation, and cranial nerve motor efferents (V_3, VII, IX, X, XII, and ansa cervicalis).[72–74] Other reports contend that unilateral, supratentorial tumors can also cause dysphagia.[75,76] In a prospective analysis of dysphagia in PBT patients and a set of non–brain-tumor neurologic controls, Newton and colleagues noted that 17 of 117 (14.5%) tumor patients complained of swallowing problems.[76] Formal swallowing assessment of the symptomatic cohort revealed that most patients significantly underestimated their degree of dysfunction. It was also noted that symptomatic patients with decreased level of alertness (LOA) were more likely to have abnormalities during bedside and videofluoroscopic testing. Twelve of the 17 symptomatic patients (70.5%; 7 with GBM) had large and diffuse, unilateral, supratentorial lesions with surrounding edema and mass effect, often associated with decreased LOA. The neuroanatomic basis for dysphagia from a unilateral lesion remains unclear. However, it is probably a result of a combination of several factors, including reduced awareness of oral sensory feedback cues during mastication in patients with reduced LOA, contralateral weakness of the face and tongue, and oral apraxia with impaired motor programming ability for oral-lingual feeding behavior.

Based on the available literature, it would seem prudent to routinely screen all brain tumor patients for dysphagic symptoms, especially in the latter stages of their disease, with or without reduced LOA. All symptomatic patients should undergo a formal swallowing evaluation, even when the complaint seems trivial.[76] The initial bedside screening examination can assess oral and laryngeal function and identify patients at risk for aspiration.[77] In addition, bedside testing can allow modification of eating behavior to diminish the risk of aspiration. Further examination is often needed after the initial bedside evaluation to allow more detailed assessment of the swallowing mechanism, such as delays during the pharyngeal swallow, the degree of laryngeal elevation, pharyngeal symmetry, pooling or coating of pharyngeal recesses, and silent aspiration. The modified barium swallow is used for this assessment and can accurately reveal the abnormalities of the swallowing mechanism, the degree of aspiration, and how best to modify the diet.[76–79]

Management of dysphagic brain tumor patients can often be a complex issue. Patients must be able to demonstrate the necessary cognitive and communication skills to actively participate in a swallowing management program.[77,79] Tumor patients with diminished LOA or significant cognitive alterations may be unable to pursue complex rehabilitation strategies similar to those used for patients with other neurologic disorders (e.g., stroke). In those patients with adequate LOA, swallowing rehabilitation should be pursued. If compensatory techniques do not improve oral efficiency, an alternate route of nutrition may be required, such as a gastric feeding tube.

▶ PSYCHIATRIC ISSUES

There are several important psychiatric issues that must be assiduously screened for during the care of brain tumor patients and family members. These issues include depression, associated problems with sleep, and anxiety.[80–85] All cancer patients face numerous stressors during their illness, including fears of a painful death, disability, disfigurement, dependency, and separation from loved ones. The psychological impact of these stressors is quite variable, however, depending on differences in personality, coping mechanisms, social support structure, and medical factors. If cancer patients as a whole are screened using criteria of the *Diagnostic and Statistical Manual of Mental Disorders* IV (DSM-IV), between 50% and 55% will be shown to have adjusted adequately to the stresses of cancer without exhibiting a diagnosable psychiatric disorder.[81] However, approximately 45% will have a diagnosable psychiatric disorder, of which two thirds will be an adjustment disorder with reactive anxiety and/or depression, 13% a major depression, and 8% an organic mental disorder (e.g., delirium).

Depressive symptoms are common in cancer patients, with an overall incidence of major depression ranging from 20% to 25% in most studies.[80–82,84] Patients at more advanced stages of disease, or with severe disability and/or pain, are more likely to develop depression, with rates approaching 75% to 80%. At the time of initial diagnosis, patients usually enter a brief phase of shocked disbelief that lasts several days. The next phase is one of depressed mood, anxiety, anorexia, insomnia, irritability, and psychological malaise that may last 2 to 3 weeks. During this phase patients note a pervasive sense of sadness and uncertainty about the future, and are preoccupied with thoughts about their illness, death, and loss of loved ones. Activities of daily living may become difficult to perform, along with generally poor concentration and information processing. These symptoms are consistent with a reactive depression and are transient. The next phase is one of adaptation to the diagnosis, with renewed hope and optimism as the patient begins to implement the treatment plan with their physicians and treatment team. Symptoms of reactive depression do not require specific antidepressant therapy. However, reactive depression may recur during critical transition points in the illness, as the patient is made aware of bad news (e.g., progressive disease on MRI scan).

When is the presence of depressive symptoms severe enough to require treatment? Many of the symptoms of major depression are similar to those of reactive depression, but differ in their severity and persistence. Using criteria as outlined in the DSM-IV (Table 9-2), a major depressive episode can be diagnosed if five or more of the listed symptoms have been present for 2 weeks or more and represent a change from the baseline level of functioning.[86] At least one of the symptoms needs to be depressed mood or loss of interest in pleasurable activities (i.e., anhedonia). The symptoms need to be severe enough to cause significant distress to the patient and to impair social, occupational, or familial functioning. Patients with advanced stages of disease and poorly controlled pain are

▶ TABLE 9-2. DSM-IV CRITERIA FOR THE DIAGNOSIS OF MAJOR DEPRESSION

Five or more of the following symptoms have been present during the same 2-week period and represent a change from previous functioning. At least one of the symptoms is either depressed mood or loss of interest in pleasurable activities.

1. Depressed mood most of the day, nearly every day. Can be subjective report or observation by others.
2. Markedly diminished interest in pleasurable activities most of the day, nearly every day.
3. Significant weight loss when not dieting or weight gain (i.e., a change of more than 5% of body weight in a month), or a decrease or increase in appetite nearly every day.
4. Insomnia or hypersomnia nearly every day.
5. Psychomotor agitation or retardation nearly every day, which is observable by others and not just a subjective feeling of restlessness or being slowed down.
6. Fatigue or loss of energy nearly every day.
7. Feelings of worthlessness or excessive or inappropriate guilt (which may be delusional) nearly every day.
8. Diminished ability to think or concentrate, or indecisiveness, nearly every day.
9. Recurrent thoughts of death (not just a fear of dying), recurrent suicidal ideation without a specific plan, or a suicide attempt or a specific plan for committing suicide.

Source: Reproduced with permission from American Psychiatric Association. Diagnostic and Statistical Manual of Mental Disorders, 4th ed. Washington, DC: American Psychiatric Association, 1994:317–391.

usually the most severely depressed. For example, the Karnofsky performance status (KPS) is highly correlated with the occurrence of depression.[87] Major depression was noted in only 23% of patients with a KPS of 70 or higher, but was present in 77% of those patients with a KPS of less than 40. Many of the somatic symptoms of depression (e.g., fatigue, loss of energy, anorexia, weight loss, insomnia) overlap with the common symptoms of cancer patients, especially those undergoing treatment. Therefore, to correctly diagnose depression in brain tumor patients, it is important to focus on the psychological symptoms, including dysphoric mood, hopelessness, guilt, worthlessness, anhedonia, and suicidal ideation.

Patients with suicidal ideation should be questioned in more detail to assess suicide risk.[80–82,84] Cancer patients are at increased risk of suicide when compared with the general population, particularly in the advanced stages of disease. Suicidal ideation is noted in 15% to 20% of cancer patients with painful symptoms.[81] In half of the cohort with suicidal ideation, an adjustment disorder was present with anxious and depressive features, while in another 30% to 35% a major depression was noted. For most patients, suicidal ideation functions as a "steam valve" for thoughts and worries centered on issues of control of the cancer and of not being overwhelmed (i.e., "if things get too bad, I have a way out"). Patients most likely to act on thoughts of suicide have feelings of hopelessness and loss of control, in addition to depression. The physician should explore how serious the suicidal thoughts are and assess risk factors (e.g., prior suicide attempts, severe pain, poor performance status, severe depression, and hopelessness). It is important to determine if the patient has a plan in place and the means to carry it out. All patients considered at risk for a suicide attempt require a prompt psychiatric evaluation for suicide intervention. In general, most cancer patients are not at high risk for suicide. Early intervention, including treatment of depression and adequate pain control, will usually negate this option. Crisis intervention-oriented psychotherapy is often beneficial to the suicidal patient, and should include the patient's loved ones and social support system.

Once the patient has been diagnosed with major depression and contributing medical problems have been resolved, several treatment approaches are available.[80–82,84] Therapeutic options that are often helpful in combination with drug therapy include supportive psychotherapy and cognitive-behavioral techniques.[88,89] Psychotherapy, in the form of individual or group counseling, is effective at reducing depressive symptoms and psychological distress in cancer patients. Cognitive-behavioral interventions, such as relaxation techniques and positive imagery, have also been shown to improve depressive symptoms in patients with mild to moderate levels of depression. For most cancer patients with moderate to severe depression, the mainstay of therapy will be pharmacologic intervention with an antidepressant medication (Table 9-3). There are several classes of antidepressant drugs; comparative clinical trials suggest that the efficacy of drugs within each class and between classes is similar. Clinical improvement usually takes 2 to 3 weeks to become evident, with a peak effect at 4 to 6 weeks. The first depressive symptoms to improve are

▶ **TABLE 9-3.** ANTIDEPRESSANT DRUGS AVAILABLE FOR TREATMENT OF DEPRESSION IN BRAIN TUMOR PATIENTS

Drug	Anticholinergic	Sedation	Orthostatic Hypotension	Metabolism	Target Dose (mg/d)
Tricyclics					
Imipramine	++	++	+++	Liver	10–125
Amitriptyline	+++	+++	+++	Liver	10–125
Desipramine	+	+	++	Liver	25–125
Nortriptyline	++	++	+	Liver	25–125
Doxepin	++	+++	++	Liver	25–125
Amoxapine	+	++	+	Liver	100–150
Protriptyline	+++	+	++	Liver	30–60
Selective serotonin reuptake inhibitors					
Fluoxetine	+	+	+	Liver	20–60
Sertraline	0	+	+	Liver	50–150
Paroxetine	+	+	+	Liver	20–50
Fluvoxamine	+	+	+	Liver	150–200
Citalopram	+	+	+	Liver	20–60
Escitalopram	+	+	+	Liver	10–20
Other agents					
Bupropion	0	0	0	Liver	200–400
Maprotiline	+	+	++	Liver	100–225
Amoxapine	+	+	0	Liver	200–500
Trazodone	++	+++	++	Liver	200–600
Venlafaxine	+	++	+	Liver	75–375
Mirtazapine	+	++	+	Liver	15–60
Nefazodone	+	++	+	Liver	300–600

0 = negligible, + = mild, ++ = moderate, +++ = severe.
Source: Adapted from references 79–81 and 83.

mood, quality of sleep, appetite, and personal grooming. Renewed interest in activities and increased energy level occur soon afterwards. In general, depressed cancer patients tend to respond to lower doses of antidepressant medication than patients without cancer. If a patient does not respond to maximal dosing of one antidepressant, a drug from a different class should be attempted next.

Because antidepressant efficacy is fairly uniform, the choice of drug will mainly depend on the toxicity profile and potential interactions of a given agent in relation to a specific patient and their medical condition.[80–82,84] Depressed patients with agitation, anxiety, and poor sleep would benefit from an antidepressant with sedating effects such as amitriptyline, doxepin, trazodone, nefazodone, or mirtazapine. Patients with depression that manifests psychomotor slowing, fatigue, or sedation from other medications might benefit from an activating antidepressant that causes minimal sedation, such as desipramine or one of the serotonin selective reuptake inhibitors (SSRIs) such as fluoxetine, bupropion, or citalopram. Patients with stomatitis, slowed intestinal motility, or urinary retention should receive an antidepressant with minimal anticholinergic activity, such as desipramine, nortriptyline, or one of the SSRIs. The tricyclic antidepressants as a class have the potential for cardiotoxicity and should be given with caution to cancer patients with unrelated heart disease. In particular, these drugs should not be prescribed to patients with cardiac conduction abnormalities or bundle-branch block. For the majority of depressed cancer patients, the SSRIs (e.g., fluoxetine, sertraline, paroxetine, fluvoxamine, citalopram) will be the antidepressant drugs of choice.[82,84] The SSRIs are well tolerated, effective, and associated with less cardiotoxicity and anticholinergic side effects than the tricyclic class of antidepressants. In addition, they are safer in the setting of a depressed cancer patient who attempts suicide by overdose.

Anxiety is common in the cancer patient population, with an incidence of 10% to 30%, and often coexists with depression.[80,81,83] Several anxiety syndromes can be present and include reactive anxiety related to the stress of cancer and its treatment, anxiety that is a manifestation of a medical or physiologic problem associated with the cancer (organic anxiety disorder), and premorbid phobias or chronic anxiety disorders that are exacerbated by the illness. Reactive anxiety fluctuates during the course of the patient's illness, becoming more severe during critical moments of bad news. High levels of anxiety can disrupt the patient's ability to function normally, interfere with interpersonal relationships and activities at work, and may impair ability to comply with cancer therapy. The mainstay of treatment for anxiety is pharmacologic therapy with short-acting benzodiazepines such as alprazolam (0.25 to 2.0 mg TID to QID), oxazepam (10 to 15 mg TID to QID), or lorazepam (0.5 to 2.0 mg TID to QID). Patients who experience breakthrough anxiety or end-of-dose failure using a short-acting benzodiazepine may benefit by switching to a longer-acting drug such as diazepam (5 to 10 mg BID to QID) or clonazepam (0.5 to 2.0 mg BID to QID). An alternative drug is the nonbenzodiazepine anxiolytic buspirone, which is effective at doses of 5 to 10 mg TID. Neuroleptic drugs such as haloperidol (0.5 to 5 mg BID to QID) or thioridazine (10 to 25 mg TID) may be useful as adjunctive treatment for patients who do not respond well to benzodiazepines or who have psychotic features (e.g., hallucinations, delusions) that accompany the anxiety. The most common causes of an organic anxiety disorder in cancer patients are uncontrolled pain, medication effects (e.g., narcotic analgesics, corticosteroids), infection, and metabolic derangements. Treatment of the underlying medical condition and judicious use of benzodiazepines and/or low-dose antipsychotics are appropriate. In addition to pharmacologic approaches, behavioral interventions such as relaxation training, systematic desensitization, and positive imagery techniques can be beneficial for select patients.

▶ PAIN CONTROL ISSUES

Other than the fear of dying, pain is the most common concern of patients diagnosed with cancer.[90] Overall, pain occurs in 20% to 50% of cancer patients at diagnosis and in 75% to 90% at advanced stages of disease.[91,92] Many studies suggest that 10% to 30% of cancer patients with severe pain are inadequately treated.[91] It is imperative that the physician diagnose and treat pain aggressively. In the brain tumor population, the most common form of pain is headache (i.e., 60%–90% of patients) caused by elevation of intracranial pressure.[1,9] Dexamethasone, used in judicious doses, is the most effective pharmacologic treatment for brain tumor headache.[31] Less common pain syndromes in primary brain tumor patients include central pain from tumors that affect the integrity of the thalamus or its regulatory pathways, leptomeningeal spread of neoplasm causing nerve root irritation or damage, and extraneural metastases.[93–95] Similar pain syndromes can develop in patients with metastatic brain tumors, except that systemic involvement from the primary neoplasm (e.g., bone, lung, pleura, liver, brachial or lumbosacral plexopathy, leptomeningeal metastases, epidural spinal cord compression) is more frequent. During routine clinic visits and hospital stays, the physician should always include questions about pain control in the review of systems. Any neuro-oncology patient with an unexplained progressive pain problem (e.g., facial pain, arm pain, radiating leg pain) should immediately undergo a diagnostic investigation to ascertain the etiology.[96]

The current pharmacologic management of cancer-related pain is effective in most patients (Table 9-4).[91,92,97] In some cases, analgesics are used to augment pain relief provided by primary therapy (i.e., surgery, radiotherapy, chemotherapy). In others, analgesics form the mainstay of therapy. The three-step "analgesic ladder" provides a systematic approach to alleviating the patient's pain using analgesic pharmacotherapy.[92] In step 1, nonopioid analgesics (e.g., acetaminophen, aspirin, nonsteroidal antiinflammatory drugs) are used, possibly in combination with an adjuvant analgesic (e.g., antidepressants, anticonvulsants, local anesthetics), to treat mild pain. If this level of analgesia proves ineffective, step 2 proceeds with the use of opioids designed for mild to moderate pain (e.g., codeine, oxycodone, propoxyphene) in combination with nonopioid and adjuvant analgesics. In patients with moderate to severe pain, more potent opioid analgesics are selected for step 3 (e.g., morphine, fentanyl patch, oxycodone, hydromorphone), often in conjunction with nonopioid and adjuvant analgesics. The transdermal fentanyl patch is an excellent alternative to oral medication approaches, because it is available in a wide variety of doses (25, 50, 75, and 100 μg/h) and provides steady release of drug for 72 hours per patch.[98] For patients with severe pain that requires inpatient evaluation and treatment, many authors recommend a patient-controlled analgesia approach.[99] Short-acting narcotic analgesics such as morphine, hydromorphone, and fentanyl are used for this purpose and are usually administered by the intravenous, epidural, subcutaneous, or intrathecal route. In addition, short-acting narcotic analgesics are used for breakthrough pain that can occur intermittently in patients who are otherwise well controlled.[100] It is uncommon for brain tumor patients to have pain that is refractory to the stepwise application of systemic pharmacotherapy (in addition to primary treatment and dexamethasone). However, neuro-oncology patients with other types of pain syndromes, such as malignant plexopathy or spinal cord compression, may have severe pain that will only respond to step 3 analgesics. In rare cases of severe pain refractory to step 3 medications, neuro-oncology patients may require invasive analgesic techniques such as

▶ TABLE 9-4. ANALGESIC MEDICATIONS AVAILABLE FOR TREATMENT OF PAIN IN BRAIN TUMOR AND NEURO-ONCOLOGY PATIENTS

Drug	Route	Dose (mg/d)	Peak Effect (h)	Duration (h)
Analgesics for mild pain: Step 1				
Aspirin	Oral	1000–4000	0.25	4–6
Acetaminophen	Oral	1000–4000	0.25	4–6
NSAIDs (e.g., ibuprofen, ketorolac)	Oral	1200–4000	0.25	4–6
Steroids (e.g., dexamethasone)	Oral, IV, IM	4–16	2–4	6–8
Adjuvant analgesic medications				
Amitriptyline	Oral	10–100	—	qd; long-term
Mexiletine	Oral	150–900	—	qd; long-term
Carbamazepine	Oral	200–1200	—	qd; long-term
Baclofen	Oral	10–80	—	qd; long-term
Analgesics for moderate pain: Step 2				
Codeine	Oral, IM	60–240	0.5	3–6
Oxycodone	Oral	30–180	0.5	3–6
Hydrocodone	Oral	15–45	0.5	4–6
Propoxyphene	Oral	130–390	1.0	4–6
Analgesics for severe pain: Step 3				
Morphine	Oral, IM, IV	40–240 (oral) 10–40 (IV, IM)	1.5–2	4–6
Hydromorphone	Oral, IM, IV	10–48 (oral) 4–24 (IV, IM)	1–2	3–4
Meperidine	Oral, IM, IV	100–400	1–2	3–6
Fentanyl	TD	25–100 μ/h q 72 h	72	—
Methadone	Oral	10–60	0.5–1.5	4–6

NSAIDs = nonsteroidal antiinflammatory drugs; TD = transdermal.
Source: Adapted from references 90, 91, 96, and 99.

regional anesthesia, sympathetic blockade, somatic neurolysis, or cordotomy.[91,92]

Some physicians and nurses are reticent about aggressive analgesic pharmacotherapy because of fears that the patient may become addicted or could expire earlier from the treatment.[90] If one of the goals of the physician is to provide comfort and remove suffering, then it is morally and ethically proper to prescribe the amount of analgesia necessary to achieve these goals. If this action inadvertently hastens the time of death, a situation known as the *doctrine of double effect*, then the physician is still acting within proper ethical boundaries.[90] In this situation, the benefits to the patient far outweigh the burdens or risks.

▶ HOSPICE CARE AND END OF LIFE ISSUES

The hospice movement originated in England in the 1960s when Dr. Cicely Saunders founded the first multidisciplinary hospice to care for terminally ill patients.[101–103] The movement expanded and eventually spread to the United States in the 1970s. In England most of the hospice care was administered within inpatient facilities, whereas in the United States the care was shifted, whenever possible, to the home setting. Recent data suggest that the quality of hospice care is superior to the care available in the nonhospice setting for patients in the end stages of life.[104] The improved quality of care was equivalent whether the patient was in a hospital-based unit, inpatient non–hospital-based unit, or home hospice setting. Because of the success of the early hospice programs, Congress passed legislation resulting in the establishment of the Medicare Hospice Benefit in 1982.[102,103] The Medicare Hospice Benefit subsidizes care for terminally ill patients with a life expectancy of 6 months or less, as certified by their attending physician and the hospice medical director. In addition to the life-expectancy criteria, other qualifications for Medicare Hospice Benefit include eligibility for Medicare (i.e., at least 65 years of age or certified as disabled), foregoing further aggressive or "curative" therapy, being able to receive most care in the home, and having a primary caregiver present at home. The Medicare Hospice Benefit will continue to pay for patients who live longer than 6 months, as long as the attending physician continues to certify the patient is terminally ill. Most patients admitted to hospice do not live longer than the typical 6 months allowed by the Medicare Hospice Benefit. In fact, the majority of them die within 4 to 6 weeks, suggesting that physicians are not referring their patients to hospice care early enough.[103] Recent statistics show that more than half of all terminally ill cancer patients in the United States are not being offered hospice services at all or are entering hospice care too late to achieve maximal benefit.[102]

For brain tumor and other neuro-oncology patients in whom continued treatment is futile, the most important and critical step will be to broach the subject of hospice care and palliative symptom contro1.[90,105–107] Similar to when the physician first tells the patient the diagnosis, this must be done with the utmost compassion and sensitivity. Patients should be referred to hospice as soon as curative or stabilizing therapy has been discontinued and the primary goal becomes comfort. Hospice care works best when there is time for members of the hospice team to develop meaningful relationships with the patient and family (i.e., over weeks to months).

The purpose of hospice care is to provide medical, psychosocial, and spiritual support for terminally ill patients and their families.[101–107] This is an especially critical time when hope for cure is lost and anxiety about the future is overwhelming. Hospice care attempts to alleviate the physical and emotional suffering of the brain tumor patient. Hope for cure is shifted to hope for maximizing dignity, comfort, quality of life, and the process of enjoying each remaining day to its fullest. In addition, support is provided for the family members, who are also suffering and attempting to cope with the imminent loss of their loved one.[108] A very common fear about advanced incurable cancer is isolation from family and loved ones. The presence of the hospice care team, especially in the home setting, alleviates this fear and ensures that isolation and loneliness are minimized.

The use of hospice is an important aspect of the complete care of virtually all patients with malignant brain tumors and many with progressive, benign brain tumors. It should be offered to all patients in the terminal stages of their disease once efforts to halt the progression of the malignancy have ceased. In addition to expertise at treating many aspects of cancer-related pain, hospice physicians and nurses can also effectively manage some of the problems specific to brain tumor patients, such as swallowing difficulties and seizures.[109] During the terminal phases of disease, many patients cannot take oral anticonvulsants properly, either because of neurologic compromise of the swallowing mechanism or a reduced level of consciousness. It is often helpful for the hospice nurse to administer these medications rectally as a suspension (using a dose that is approximately 25% higher than the oral dose). Sublingual diazepam (Valium) drops can also be used, if needed, to augment seizure control. Patients with respiratory compromise and dyspnea may benefit from the use of opioids, with the dose depending on the level of prior exposure to this class of medications.[110]

▶ ETHICAL ISSUES

The care of brain tumor and other neuro-oncology patients is often complicated by numerous ethical dilemmas and discussions.[111–114] In no other subspecialty of medicine are there such large numbers of seriously ill patients in which the day-to-day care involves life and death decisions. These patients are not only adversely affected by their disease, but frequently suffer deleterious side effects and complications from treatment, which is often very intense and rigorous. Physicians caring for neuro-oncologic patients should be well versed in ethical principles and theory. This foundation will better prepare the physician for the many complex ethical predicaments that inevitably develop during the course of therapy and, in many cases, subsequent palliative care.

There are several basic ethical principles that require definition. The most important ethical principles are respect for autonomy, justice, beneficence, and nonmaleficence.[111–113] *Respect for autonomy* refers to recognition by the physician of the patient's right and ability to make his or her own decisions. These decisions are unique, are influenced by the patient's value system, and may differ from what is advised by the physician. *Justice* relates to fairness and what people are legitimately entitled to once they enter the medical system. In this context, justice demands that patients with brain tumors have access to care (e.g., treatment, pain control, nutritional support) equal to patients with other diseases that may have a less grave prognosis. *Beneficence* refers to actions by the physician toward the patient that will maximize positive outcomes and avoid unnecessary pain, injury, and suffering. These activities can include treatment of the cancer and extension of quality survival, control of pain and other disease-related symptoms, and interpersonal support. *Nonmaleficence* means that the physician should "do no harm" while providing care to the patient. This principle has a broad scope and can refer to many issues, including withholding relevant diagnostic or prognostic information, improper treatment of pain, inappropriate undertreatment, and persistent overtreatment.

Physicians usually have an ethical position or frame of reference that incorporates these basic ethical principles. In the most common ethical stance, the physician makes a decision based on an assessment of the good or bad consequences of each course of action. This ethical position, called *consequentialism* or *utilitarianism*, justifies a given decision by comparing probable good or benefit with potential harm or pain.[115] The second most common ethical position, *respect for persons*, relies heavily on the ethical principles of autonomy and respect.[111] This approach emphasizes the importance of allowing patients to be involved in all decisions about their care and treatment. An alternative to *respect for persons* is *paternalism*, in which the physician assumes that all decisions should be made for the good of the patient, without regard to his or her specific wishes or needs.[111–113,115]

It is often difficult to be honest with a patient when discussing a new diagnosis as devastating as cancer, especially when it is a brain tumor.[102–113,116,117] In fact, a survey of ethical issues in the oncology literature determined that *truth telling* was the most commonly debated subject.[115] Between 1961 and 1979, most physicians took the paternalistic approach and withheld information regarding diagnosis and prognosis in order to maintain hope and minimize psychological damage to their patients. Since 1979, attitudes have changed so that many physicians now prefer to reveal accurate information about their patient's diagnosis and prognosis.[116,117] This trend away from paternalism, toward a more "patient-oriented" or "respect for persons" approach when discussing diagnosis and prognosis, is important because the vast majority of patients want to know as much as possible about their disease, treatment options, and chances of survival.[117]

The physician caring for a brain tumor patient needs to balance the ethically appropriate duty to convey accurate information about diagnosis and prognosis with the equally important responsibility to nurture and maintain hope. However, it is now clear that a more honest and accurate diagnostic interview does not remove hope and is more likely to strengthen the physician–patient relationship.[117] The physician should explore what hope means to each patient, because it can represent many different things, some of which will be separate from the hope for cure or lengthy survival.

Ethical issues arise frequently during the design and administration of clinical trials for oncology patients. The moral cornerstone of any clinical trial is the concept and practice of valid informed consent.[117] Valid consent has three features: the provision of adequate information, the absence of coercion, and the competence of the patient. Adequate information must be provided about tests, procedures, and treatments inherent in any clinical trial. Significant risks and benefits, if any, must be outlined. All serious risks that are likely to occur should be included. Any risk of death beyond a trivial risk should also be included, because death is such a serious evil that the patient must be made aware of any chance that it may occur.[119] Rational alternative treatment to the clinical trial in question must be presented by the physician in an open, objective, and unbiased manner. Alternative treatments should include those offered at other medical centers. One duty of a physician is to inform the patient of the consequences and probable outcome with no treatment at all. The patient should know that the final decision concerning any clinical trial is his or hers alone to make. Competency, in this setting, implies that the patient understands the information provided during the consent process and appreciates that it applies to him or her at that particular point in time.

The protection of the patient's best interests falls squarely and heavily on the shoulders of the physician seeking participation in the clinical trial.[114] The physician must take into account the influence of personal beliefs, biases, and academic ambitions before embarking on such endeavors. The focus of the physician who designs and performs clinical trials must always be on the need for conclusive proof of efficacy. A study designed according to rigorous scientific and ethical criteria can accrue patients with confidence and good faith.

The decision to stop therapy is often very difficult for patients, family members, and the treatment team.[111–113,120,121] It signals the "beginning of the end," when all reasonable hope for cure or prolonged stabilization is gone and the patient's death is imminent. These decisions usually arise when the patient has just progressed through the latest protocol and has often suffered further neurological deterioration. In many cases, the neurologic status is quite poor, to a degree that functional ambulation, cognition, and verbal interaction are severely compromised. Although there are often other treatment options that could be offered, the physician must state clearly and honestly that further therapy will not significantly affect outcome. In this situation, it is critical to weigh the adverse effects of further therapy on quality of life against the potential benefits for improvement of quality of life and prolongation of survival, which would be extremely limited. The physician must reassure the patient and family that the termination of active treatment does not mean the physician will abandon them. Even though the focus of subsequent care will shift to comfort, pain relief, and symptom control, the physician will remain actively involved in the patient's care. In addition to questions about the potential for extension of survival, many patients and family members want to know if further treatment might improve neurologic function. In other words, could the patient's current neurologic status be reversed somewhat to enhance quality of life for the time the patient has left? Neurologic function is rarely restored or improved at these late stages of disease; it would be optimistic even to expect further therapy to stabilize the patient's condition.

Because quality of life is so subjective and the behavior of brain tumors can be so variable, the proper time to stop treatment differs from patient to patient. Some patients accustomed to a high level of function cannot tolerate living their life in a severely compromised fashion while suffering the rigors of treatment. For others, the alterations of function and lifestyle are more easily accepted, so that simple survival is adequate, with less regard for the quality of existence.

Is it ethically appropriate to terminate therapy? If the physician has explained the situation properly and is acting in accordance with the wishes of the patient or family, the decision would be consistent with the principles of respect for autonomy, beneficence, and nonmaleficence.[111–113,120–122] The physician would be acting to allow a more dignified, peaceful death without the rigors of active therapy. Active treatment is terminated to "promote the good," which is to let the patient die on the patient's own terms. It is ethically improper and contrary to the principle of nonmaleficence for the physician to coerce or force the patient into undergoing further therapy.

▶ CONCLUSION

Although the focus of the treatment team is on curative or stabilizing therapy for most patients, it is still very important for the treating physician to be aware of the many aspects of supportive care outlined above. Common problems related to seizure control, toxicity of anticonvulsants and corticosteroids, depression, prophylaxis and treatment of thromboembolic complications, and pain control must be assiduously monitored in every patient. As each patient enters the final stages of his or her disease, the physician must also be aware of end-of-life issues and the appropriate use of hospice resources. All of these aspects of care should be performed in the context of proper ethical conduct and under the principles of respect for autonomy and beneficence.

REFERENCES

1. Newton HB. Primary brain tumors: review of etiology, diagnosis, and treatment. Am Fam Phys 1994;49:787–797.
2. Ptacek JT, Ptacek JJ. Patients' perceptions of receiving bad news about cancer. J Clin Oncol 2001;19:4160–4164.
3. Feldman GB. The role of support in treating the brain tumor patient. In: Black PM, Loeffler JS, eds. Cancer of the nervous system. Cambridge, MA: Blackwell Science, 1997: 335–345.
4. Given BA, Given CW, Kozachik S. Family support in advanced cancer. CA Cancer J Clin 2001;51:213–231.
5. Nijboer C, Tempelaar R, Triemstra M, et al. The role of social and psychologic resources in caregiving of cancer patients. Cancer 2001;91:1029–1039.
6. Glantz M, Recht LD. Epilepsy in the cancer patient. In: Vecht CJ, ed. Handbook of clinical neurology, vol. 25 (69): neuro-oncology, part III. Amsterdam: Elsevier Science, 1997:9–18.
7. Moots PL, Maciunas RJ, Eisert DR, et al. The course of seizure disorders in patients with malignant gliomas. Arch Neurol 1995;52:717–724.
8. Elisevich K. Epilepsy and low-grade gliomas. In: Rock JP, Rosenblum ML, Shaw EG, Cairncross JG, eds. The practical management of low-grade primary brain tumors. Philadelphia: Lippincott Williams & Wilkins, 1999:149–169.
9. Newton HB. Neurological complications of systemic cancer. Am Fam Phys 1999;59:878–886.
10. Schaller B, Rüegg SJ. Brain tumor and seizures: pathophysiology and its implications for treatment revisited. Epilepsia 2003;44:1223–1232.
11. Ettinger AB. Structural causes of epilepsy: tumors, cysts, stroke, and vascular malformation. Neurol Clin 1994;12: 41–56.
12. Highland MM, Berger MS, Kunkel DD, et al. Changes in gamma-aminobutyric acid and somatostatin in epileptic cortex associated with low-grade gliomas. J Neurosurg 1992;77:209–216.
13. Bateman DE, Hardy JA, McDermott JR, et al. Amino acid neurotransmitter levels in gliomas and their relationship to the incidence of epilepsy. Neurol Res 1988;10:112–114.
14. Ye ZC, Sontheimer H. Glioma cells release excitotoxic concentrations of glutamate. Cancer Res 1999;59:4383–4391.
15. Behrens PF, Langemann H, Strohschein R, et al. Extracellular glutamate and other metabolites in and around RG2 rat glioma: an intracerebral microdialysis study. J Neurooncol 2000;47:11–22.
16. Brodie MJ, Dichter MA. Antiepileptic drugs. N Engl J Med 1996;334:168–175.
17. Britton JW, So EL. Selection of antiepileptic drugs: a practical approach. Mayo Clin Proc 1996;71:778–786.
18. Mattson RH, Cramer BS, Collins JF, et al. A comparison of valproate with carbamazepine for the treatment of complex partial seizures and secondarily generalized tonic-clonic seizures in adults. N Engl J Med 1992;327:765–771.
19. Dichter MA, Brodie MJ. New antiepileptic drugs. N Engl J Med 1996;334:1583–1590.
20. Rosenfeld WE. Topiramate: a review of preclinical, pharmacokinetic, and clinical data. Clin Ther 1997;19:1294–1308.
21. Wagner GL, Wilms EB, Van Donselaar CA, et al. Levetiracetam: preliminary experience in patients with primary brain tumours. Seizure 2003;12:585–586.
22. Vecht CJ, Wagner GL, Wilms EB. Interactions between antiepileptic and chemotherapeutic drugs. Lancet Neurol 2003;2:404–409.
23. North JB, Penhall RK, Hanieh A, et al. Phenytoin and postoperative epilepsy: a double-blind study. J Neurosurg 1983;58:672–677.

24. Boarini DJ, Beck DW, Van Gilder JC. Postoperative prophylactic anticonvulsant therapy in cerebral gliomas. Neurosurg 1985;16:290–292.
25. Cohen N, Strauss G, Lew R, et al. Should prophylactic anticonvulsants be administered to patients with newly-diagnosed cerebral metastases? A retrospective analysis. J Clin Oncol 1988;6:1621–1624.
26. Franceschetti S, Binelli S, Casazza M, et al. Influence of surgery and antiepileptic drugs on seizures symptomatic of cerebral tumours. Acta Neurochir 1990;103:47–51.
27. Shaw MDM. Post-operative epilepsy and the efficacy of anticonvulsant therapy. Acta Neurochir Suppl 1990;50: 55–57.
28. Foy PM, Chadwick DW, Rajgopalan N, et al. Do prophylactic anticonvulsant drugs alter the pattern of seizures after craniotomy? J Neurol Neurosurg Psychiatry 1992; 55:753–757.
29. Glantz MJ, Cole BF, Friedberg MH, et al. A randomized, blinded, placebo-controlled trial of divalproex sodium prophylaxis in adults with newly diagnosed brain tumors. Neurology 1996;46:985–991.
30. Glantz MJ, Cole BF, Forsyth PA, et al. Practice parameter: anticonvulsant prophylaxis in patients with newly diagnosed brain tumors: report of the Quality Standards Subcommittee of the American Academy of Neurology. Neurology 2000;54:1886–1893.
31. Newton HB, Turowski RC, Stroup TJ, et al. Clinical presentation, diagnosis, and pharmacotherapy of patients with primary brain tumors. Ann Pharmacother 1999;33: 816–832.
32. Ohnishi T, Sher PB, Posner JB, et al. Capillary permeability factor secreted by malignant brain tumor. Role in peritumoral edema and possible mechanism for anti-edema effect of glucocorticoids. J Neurosurg 1990;72:245–251.
33. Del Maestro RF, Megyesi JF, Farrell CL. Mechanisms of tumor-associated edema: a review. Can J Neurol Sci 1990;17:177–183.
34. Samdani AF, Tamargo RJ, Long DM. Brain tumor edema and the role of the blood–brain barrier. In: Vecht CJ, ed. Handbook of clinical neurology, vol. 23(67): Neuro-oncology, part I. Amsterdam: Elsevier Science, 1997;4:71–102.
35. Mukwaya G. Immunosuppressive effects and infections associated with corticosteroid therapy. Pediatr Infect Dis J 1988;7:499–504.
36. Østergaard L, Hochberg FH, Rabinov JD, et al. Early changes measured by magnetic resonance imaging in cerebral blood flow, blood volume, and blood-brain barrier permeability following dexamethasone treatment in patients with brain tumors. J Neurosurg 1999;90:300–305.
37. Lester RS, Knowles SR, Shear NH. The risks of systemic corticosteroid use. Dermatol Clin 1998;16:277–286.
38. Weissman DE, Dufer D, Vogel V, et al. Corticosteroid toxicity in neuro-oncology patients. J Neurooncol 1987;5:125–128.
39. Fadul CE, Lemann W, Thaler HT, et al. Perforation of the gastrointestinal tract in patients receiving steroids for neurologic disease. Neurology 1988;38:348–352.
40. Stiefel FC, Breitbart WS, Holland JC. Corticosteroids in cancer: neuropsychiatric complications. Cancer Invest 1989;7:479–491.
41. Dropcho EJ, Soong SJ. Steroid-induced weakness in patients with primary brain tumors. Neurology 1991; 41:1235–1239.
42. Batchelor TT, Taylor LT, Thaler HT, et al. Steroid myopathy in cancer patients. Neurology 1997;48:1234–1238.
43. Joseph JC. Corticosteroid-induced osteoporosis. Am J Hosp Pharm 1994;51:188–197.
44. McIlwain HH. Glucocorticoid-induced osteoporosis: pathogenesis, diagnosis, and management. Prev Med 2003;36: 243–249.
45. Mahindra AK, Grossman SA. Pneumocystis carinii pneumonia in HIV negative patients with primary brain tumors. J Neurooncol 2003;63:263–270.
46. Mathew BS, Grossman SA. Pneumocystis carinii pneumonia prophylaxis in HIV negative patients with primary CNS lymphoma. Cancer Treat Rev 2003;29: 105–119.
47. Ellershaw JE, Kelly MJ. Corticosteroids and peptic ulceration. Palliat Med 1994;8:313–319.
48. Garnett WR, Garabedian-Ruffalo SM. Identification, diagnosis, and treatment of acid-related diseases in the elderly: implications for long-term care. Pharmacotherapy 1997; 17:938–958.
49. Sachs G. Proton pump inhibitors and acid-related diseases. Pharmacotherapy 1997;17:22–37.
50. Lee AYY, Levine MN. Management of venous thromboembolism in cancer patients. Oncology (Huntingt) 2000; 14:409–421.
51. Gomes MPV, Deitcher SR. Diagnosis of venous thromboembolic disease in cancer patients. Oncology (Huntingt) 2003;17:126–139.
52. Sawaya R, Zuccarello M, Elkalliny M, et al. Postoperative venous thromboembolism and brain tumors: part I. Clinical profile. J Neurooncol 1992;14:119–125.
53. Hamilton MG, Hull RD, Pineo GF. Venous thromboembolism in neurosurgery and neurology patients: a review. Neurosurgery 1994;34:280–296.
54. Marras LC, Geerts WH, Perry JR. The risk of venous thromboembolism is increased throughout the course of malignant glioma: an evidence-based review. Cancer 2000; 89:640–646.
55. Brandes AA, Scelzi E, Salmistraro E, et al. Incidence and risk of thromboembolism during treatment of high-grade gliomas: a prospective study. Eur J Cancer 1997;33: 1592–1596.
56. Quevedo JF, Buckner JC, Schmidt JL, et al. Thromboembolism in patients with high-grade glioma. Mayo Clin Proc 1994;69:329–332.
57. Ruff RL, Posner JB. The incidence and treatment of peripheral venous thrombosis in patients with glioma. Ann Neurol 1983;13:334–336.
58. Altshuler E, Moosa H, Selker RG, et al. The risk and efficacy of anticoagulant therapy in the treatment of thromboembolic complications in patients with primary brain tumors. Neurosurgery 1990;27:74–77.
59. Levin JM, Schiff D, Loeffler JS, et al. Complications of therapy for venous thromboembolic disease in patients with brain tumors. Neurology 1993;43:1111–1114.
60. Schiff D, DeAngelis LM. Therapy of venous thromboembolism in patients with brain metastases. Cancer 1994;73: 493–498.
61. Weitz JI. Low-molecular-weight heparins. N Engl J Med 1997;337:688–698.

62. Dorfman GS. Evaluating the roles and functions of vena caval filters: will data be available before or after these devices are removed from the market? Radiology 1992;185:15–17.
63. Buchholz D. Neurologic causes of dysphagia. Dysphagia 1987;1:152–156.
64. Kirshner HS. Causes of neurogenic dysphagia. Dysphagia 1989;3:184–188.
65. Barer DH. The natural history and functional consequences of dysphagia after hemispheric stroke. J Neurol Neurosurg Psychiatry 1989;52:236–241.
66. Lieberman AN, Horowitz L, Redmond P, et al. Dysphagia in Parkinson's disease. Am J Gastroenterol 1980;74: 157–160.
67. Daly DD, Code CF, Anderson HA. Disturbances of swallowing and esophageal motility in patients with multiple sclerosis. Neurology 1962;59:250–256.
68. Robbins J. Swallowing in ALS and motor neuron disease. Neurol Clin 1987;5:213–229.
69. Buchholz D. Neurologic evaluation of dysphagia. Dysphagia 1987;1:187–192.
70. Frank Y, Schwartz SB, Epstein NE, et al. Chronic dysphagia, vomiting and gastroesophageal reflux as manifestations of a brain stem glioma: a case report. Pediatr Neurosci 1989;15:265–268.
71. Straube A, Witt TN. Oculo-bulbar myasthenic symptoms as the sole sign of tumour involving or compressing the brain stem. J Neurol 1990;237:369–371.
72. Cunningham ET, Donner MW, Jones B, et al. Anatomical and physiological overview. In: Jones B, Donner MW, eds. Normal and abnormal swallowing: imaging in diagnosis and therapy. New York: Springer-Verlag, 1991:7–32.
73. Dodds WJ, Stewart ET, Logemann JA. Physiology and radiology of the normal oral and pharyngeal phases of swallowing. AJR 1989;154:953–963.
74. Sessle BJ, Henry JL. Neural mechanisms of swallowing: neurophysiological and neurochemical studies on brain stem neurons in the solitary tract region. Dysphagia 1989;4:61–75.
75. Meadows JC. Dysphagia in unilateral cerebral lesions. J Neurol Neurosurg Psychiatry 1973;36:853–860.
76. Newton HB, Newton C, Pearl D, Davidson T. Swallowing assessment in primary brain tumor patients with dysphagia. Neurology 1994;44:1927–1932.
77. Emick-Herring B, Wood P. A team approach to neurologically based swallowing disorders. Rehabil Nurs 1990; 15:126–132.
78. Dodds WJ, Logemann JA, Stewart ET. Radiologic assessment of abnormal oral and pharyngeal phases of swallowing. AJR 1990;154:965–974.
79. Bloch AS. Nutritional management of patients with dysphagia. Oncology (Huntingt) 1993;7:127–137.
80. Levine SH, Jones LD, Sack DA. Evaluation and treatment of depression, anxiety, and insomnia in patients with cancer. Oncology (Huntingt) 1993;7:119–125.
81. Breitbart W. Psycho-oncology: depression, anxiety, delirium. Semin Oncol 1994;21:754–769.
82. Pirl WF, Roth AJ. Diagnosis and treatment of depression in cancer patients. Oncology (Huntingt) 1999;13:1293–1301.
83. Stark D, Kiely M, Smith A, et al. Anxiety disorders in cancer patients: their nature, associations, and relation to quality of life. J Clin Oncol 2002;20:3137–3148.
84. Schwartz L, Lander M, Chochinov HM. Current management of depression in cancer patients. Oncology (Huntingt) 2002;16:1102–1110.
85. Maguire P. Improving the recognition of concerns and affective disorders in cancer patients. Ann Oncol 2002; 13:177–181.
86. American Psychiatric Association. Diagnostic and statistical manual of mental disorders, 4th ed. Washington, DC: American Psychiatric Association, 1994:317–391.
87. Bukberg J, Penman D, Holland JC. Depression in hospitalized cancer patients. Psychosomatics 1984;46: 199–212.
88. Redd WH, Montgomery GH, DuHamel KN. Behavioral intervention for cancer treatment side effects. J Natl Cancer Inst 2001;93:810–823.
89. Newell SA, Sanson-Fisher RW, Savolainen NJ. Systematic review of psychological therapies for cancer patients: overview and recommendations for future research. J Natl Cancer Inst 2002;94:558–584.
90. Hammes BJ, Cain JM. The ethics of pain management for cancer patients: case studies and analysis. J Pain Symptom Manage 1994;9:166–170.
91. Grossman SA, Staats PS. Current management of pain in patients with cancer. Oncology 1994;8:93–107.
92. Cherny NI, Portenoy RK. Cancer pain management: current strategy. Cancer 1993;72:3393–3415.
93. Gonzales GR. Central pain: diagnosis and treatment strategies. Neurology 1995;45(Suppl 9):S11–S16.
94. Awad I, Bay JW, Rogers L. Leptomeningeal metastasis from supratentorial malignant gliomas. Neurosurgery 1986;19:247–251.
95. Hoffman HJ, Duffner PK. Extraneural metastases of central nervous system tumors. Cancer 1985;56:1778–1782.
96. Cherny NI, Hiller N. Diagnostic investigations in cancer pain. Cancer Invest 2000;18:651–663.
97. Grossman SA, Benedetti C, Payne R, et al. NCCN practice guidelines for cancer pain. Oncology (Huntingt) 1999; 13:33–45.
98. Breitbart W, Chandler S, Eagel B, et al. An alternative algorithm for dosing transdermal fentanyl for cancer-related pain. Oncology (Huntingt) 2000;14:695–705.
99. Ripamonti C, Bruera E. Current status of patient-controlled analgesia in cancer patients. Oncology (Huntingt) 1997; 11:373–384.
100. Patt RB, Ellison NM. Breakthrough pain in cancer patients: characteristics, prevalence, and treatment. Oncology (Huntingt) 1998;12:1035–1046.
101. Rhymes J. Hospice care in America. JAMA 1990;264: 369–372.
102. Kinzbrunner BM. Ethical dilemmas in hospice and palliative care. Support Care Cancer 1995;3:28–36.
103. Von Gunten CF, Neely KJ, Martinez J. Hospice and palliative care: program needs and academic issues. Oncology (Huntingt) 1996;10:1070–1074.
104. Finlay IG, Higginson IJ, Goodwin DM, et al. Palliative care in hospital, hospice, at home: results from a systematic review. Ann Oncol 2002;13:257–264.
105. Baile WF, Glober GA, Lenzi R, et al. Discussing disease progression and end-of-life decisions. Oncology (Huntingt) 1999;13:1021–1031.

106. von Gunten CF. Discussing hospice care. J Clin Oncol 2003;21:31s–36s.
107. Kahn MJ, Lazarus CJ, Owens DP. Allowing patients to die: practical, ethical, and religious concerns. J Clin Oncol 2003;21:3000–3002.
108. Brenner PR. Managing patients and families at the ending of life: hospice assumptions, structures, and practice in response to staff stress. Cancer Invest 1997;15:257–264.
109. D'Olimpio J. Contemporary drug therapy in palliative care: new directions. Cancer Invest 2001;19:413–423.
110. Thomas JR, Von Gunten CF. Treatment of dyspnea in cancer patients. Oncol 2002;16:745–750.
111. Latimer E. Ethical challenges in cancer care. J Palliat Care 1992;8:65–70.
112. Smith TJ, Bodurtha JN. Ethical considerations in oncology: Balancing the interests of patients, oncologists, and society. J Clin Oncol 1995;13:2464–2470.
113. Newton HB, Malkin MG. Ethical issues in neuro-oncology. Semin Neurol 1997;17:219–226.
114. Vick NA, Wilson CB. Total care of the patient with a brain tumor. With considerations of some ethical issues. Neurol Clin 1985;3:705–710.
115. Vanderpool HY, Weiss GB. Ethics and cancer: a survey of the literature. South Med J 1987;80:500–506.
116. Gert B, Culver CM. Moral theory in neurologic practice. Semin Neurol 1984;4:9–14.
117. Butow PN, Kazemi JN, Beeney LJ, et al. When the diagnosis is cancer. Patient communication experiences and preferences. Cancer 1996;77:2630–2637.
118. Gert B, Nelson WA, Culver CM. Moral theory and neurology. Neurol Clin 1989;7:681–696.
119. Culver CM, Gert B. Basic ethical concepts in neurologic practice. Semin Neurol 1984;4:1–8.
120. Thomasma DC. The ethics of caring for the older patient with cancer: defining the issues. Oncology (Huntingt) 1992;6:124–130.
121. Nelson WA, Bernat JL. Decisions to withhold or terminate treatment. Neurol Clin 1989;7:759–774.
122. Bernat JL, Goldstein ML, Viste KM. The neurologist and the dying patient. Neurology 1996;46:598–599.

CHAPTER 10

Neuropsychological Issues

ELANA FARACE / MARK E. SHAFFREY

Neuropsychological changes, such as decreases in short-term memory or attention, are frequently encountered in the course of living with a brain tumor. In fact, neurocognitive deficits are far more frequent than physical deficits in patients in neuro-oncology.[1–3] The degree of neuropsychological impairment can range from a barely detectable nuisance (e.g., forgetting a phone number) to significant deficits that prevent patients from being able to communicate their needs or control their behavior. Not only can individual patients experience improvement and decline over the course of the disease, but patients differ from one another both in terms of their objective deficits at any given time and the impact of those deficits on their overall quality of life (QOL).

Physicians and patients in neuro-oncology potentially must choose between trade-offs in quality and quantity of life. For example, because brain tumors frequently encompass functional cortex,[4] a choice is made for greater extent of surgical resection with higher risk of poor QOL versus limited resection and lower risk of poor QOL but potentially shorter survival. Awareness that QOL is at least as important as survival to patients is increasing in neuro-oncology.[5,6] QOL as a construct for brain tumor patients needs to include neurocognition. An improved understanding of neurocognitive sequelae has the potential to help physicians, patients, and families make informed choices bearing on QOL and survivorship, perhaps even including length of survival.

This chapter details what is currently known about neurocognition in patients with brain tumors and discusses the myriad influencing factors. In this chapter, "brain tumors" refers to primary brain tumors without regard to specific tumor grade or pathology, given that tumor pathology appears to be independent of neuropsychological sequelae,[7] unless otherwise specified. The terms "neurocognitive" and "neurocognition" refer to the cognitive functions (e.g., thinking, learning) closely linked to the function of particular areas or neural pathways of the brain. First, we discuss "quality of life" as a construct, its measurement challenges, and the contribution of neuropsychological information to understanding QOL. Next we discuss measurement issues in neuropsychology, and detail interactions with tumor variables (location, edema), treatment (surgery, radiation, and chemotherapy), and the patient's age. Because neurocognition is also influenced by other personal factors such as depression, mood, and pain, these issues are discussed in turn. The degree to which these neuropsychological factors affect QOL and potentially survival are discussed. Finally, suggestions to encourage "patient-oriented" research—information gained from detailed assessment of patients' behaviors—are discussed. Attention is given throughout to factors that may improve further research in this area.

▶ "QUALITY OF LIFE": MEASURING THE ELUSIVE

"Quality of life" is a construct that is typically understood to mean "one's overall enjoyment of life." Yet QOL is a complex, abstract, and multidimensional concept,[8] which makes it difficult to operationalize.[9–11] QOL itself comprises three main domains: (a) the *physical*, such as ability to perform activities of daily living (ADL) and specific disease symptom control; (b) the *psychological* dimension, which includes emotional and neurocognitive components; and (c) the *social* dimension, which includes the individual's roles and functions, and interpersonal relationships.[12] Other dimensions, such as spiritual QOL, have been proposed.[12] "Health-related" QOL (HR-QOL) refers to QOL outcomes specifically as they relate to the disease.[13] Common QOL measures used in oncology, such as the European Organization of Research and Treatment of Cancer (EORTC) QLQ-C30[14] and the Functional Assessment of Cancer Therapy (FACT),[15] attempt to incorporate the measurement of these multiple dimensions. However, often results are often tallied only in terms of global QOL (e.g., a question that asks, "Overall, how would you rate your quality of life?" See Osoba and associates[16] for discussion), highlighting the subjective nature of QOL and thus its measurement difficulties.

Dictionaries, for example, often define QOL as one's personal satisfaction (or dissatisfaction) with the cultural or intellectual conditions under which one lives (as distinct from material comfort).

It is important to keep in mind how individualistic QOL is in all people, but particularly in patients with brain tumors. This concept can be illustrated by application of the World Health Organization's system of understanding overall patient function.[17] This system defines patient function on three levels, which range from personal to global: *impairment,* or specific physical or neurocognitive deficits; *disability,* or how impairments affect activities of daily living; and *handicap,* how disability affects overall community participation. For example, if a patient has aphasia, a specific kind of impairment, this may affect the patient's level of disability (e.g., difficulty asking spouse for help with grooming) and cause a large handicap (e.g., inability to return to work).

QOL best relates to "handicap" not only as regards that person's community participation but also how this handicap affects that individual. Continuing the example of an aphasic patient, even if several persons had the identical specific degree of impairment from aphasia, some patients might be relieved not to return to work (relating to higher QOL), while others might find it devastating (relating to lower QOL) and many would fall in between. Indeed, an updated understanding of these three levels of function (renamed *body functions and structures, activities,* and *participation*) was recently included in the International Classification of Functioning, Disability, and Health (ICF) by the World Health Organization. This update incorporates the latest version of the Institute of Medicine's view of disability, in which handicap is viewed as "the *interaction* of the person with a potentially disabling condition with their environment, to determine the amount of *perceived* disability." This perceived disability has a significant effect on patients' subjective report of their own QOL.

▶ QUALITY OF LIFE ASSESSMENT

Given the complexity of QOL measurement, each method for the assessment and interpretation of QOL has strengths and weaknesses. Four measures have most commonly been used to measure QOL in neuro-oncology: Karnofsky Performance Status (KPS), the Short Form Health Survey (SF-36),[18] the EORTC QLQ-C30[19] usually with the Brain Cancer Module (BCM-20),[20] and the FACT[15] with the brain disease–specific subscale (BR).[21] The strengths and weaknesses of each of these measures are discussed next.

Karnofsky Performance Status

Patients' ability to perform their own ADL, such as dressing themselves, doing their own grooming, toileting appropriately, and the like has been the traditional measure of QOL in brain tumor patients.[22] Patients who are independent in their ADL at baseline, typically represented as KPS greater than or equal to 70, have better prognosis than do patients needing physical assistance.[23,24]

ADL measures such as KPS mostly assess the physical domain of QOL and are not sensitive to areas such as personality changes or neurocognitive impairment. KPS is a very gross scale that mixes impairments and disabilities.[17] Although functional independence is often equated with overall QOL,[25,26] direct investigation has shown that KPS is distinct from both QOL and neurocognitive function.[1,27] KPS is particularly insensitive to patient function in the higher end (90 to 100).[28] In fact, Whitton and associates found that in patients with KPS of 100, neurocognitive morbidity was reported in 65% of patients and pain in greater than 40%.[1] However, KPS is still the most commonly used marker of QOL in brain tumor research, perhaps because it is a very simple measure to determine from information available from a variety of sources.

Short Form Health Survey

The SF-36[18] is a 36-question "short form" originally developed to study to survey health status in the Medical Outcomes Study, a 2-year study of QOL in patients with chronic conditions. The SF-36 is now a very commonly used QOL measure. It was designed for use in clinical practice and research, health policy evaluations, and general population surveys. The survey was constructed for self-administration by persons 14 years of age and older, and for administration by a trained interviewer in person or by telephone.

The SF-36 includes one multi-item scale that assesses eight health concepts: (a) limitations in physical activities because of health problems; (b) limitations in social activities because of physical or emotional problems; (c) limitations in usual role activities because of physical health problems; (d) bodily pain; (e) general mental health (psychological distress and well-being); (f) limitations in usual role activities because of emotional problems; (g) vitality (energy and fatigue); and (h) general health perceptions. However, the SF-36 has been criticized for use in populations with neurocognitive impairment because it has a strong emphasis on patients' level of physical impairment, but tends to underrepresent the social, psychological, and neurocognitive domains of QOL unique to brain tumor patients.[29]

European Organization of Research and Treatment of Cancer QLQ-C30 with Brain Cancer Module

The health-related QOL of brain tumor patients can also be assessed with the EORTC QLQ-C30[19] plus the BCM-20.[20] These measures have been extensively validated in the North American population and are reliable and valid instruments in the setting of malignant brain tumors.[16,20] The EORTC QLQ-C30 contains 30 items that result in 5 functioning domains (physical, role, emotional, social, and neurocognitive), a global QOL domain, 3 symptom domains (fatigue, pain, nausea and vomiting), and 6 single items (dyspnea, diarrhea, constipation, anorexia, insomnia, and financial impact). The BCM-20 contains 20 items that result in 4 domains (future uncertainty, visual disorder, communication deficit, and motor dysfunction), and 7 single items (headache, seizure, drowsiness, hair loss, itching, weakness of both legs, and difficulty controlling bladder function). Some of these symptoms are related to toxicity from previous treatment with radiation therapy or chemotherapy (e.g., hair loss and itching), whereas the remainder are associated with recurrence in glioblastoma.[30] For the function scales and the global QOL scale, a higher score indicates better functioning, whereas for the symptoms scales, a higher score indicates more of the symptom of difficulty. The BCM-20 is scored in an analogous manner. The results of the EORTC are more meaningful in terms of patients' QOL than the KPS or SF-36, with understandable trade-offs for time to administer and complexity of the results.

Functional Assessment of Cancer Therapy with Brain Disease-Specific Subscale

The FACT-BR is a validated QOL instrument, comprising a general component (FACT-G) with 5 subscales (number of questions in parentheses): physical (8), social (8), emotional (3), functional (6), and relationship with doctor (3),[15] and a disease-specific subscale of 20 questions, designed to study brain cancer.[21] Like the EORTC, this measure is much better than the KPS or SF-36 for measuring QOL comprehensively; however, the administration, scoring, and interpretation are more complicated.

Interestingly, the generic forms of the FACT (the FACT-G) and the EORTC were compared in 244 patients with either breast cancer or Hodgkin disease.[31] The authors found that although there was some overlap, the measures investigated two markedly different aspects of QOL. The EORTC tends to measure constructs that are more directly observable, and thus overrepresents the physical domain (e.g., social role implications of the physical state). In contrast, the social and family well-being subscale of the FACT-G focuses on social support and emotional closeness. For example, on the emotional well-being subscales, the EORTC asks, "did you worry?" whereas the FACT asks about more existential problems: "I worry that my condition will get worse." Neither of these measures is superior to the other, but as researchers design a study they should give consideration to the type of QOL most relevant to the research. A comparison of these two QOL measures in brain tumor patients, including the brain tumor–related modules, would be helpful in this regard.

▶ CONTRIBUTION OF NEUROPSYCHOLOGY TO AN UNDERSTANDING OF QUALITY OF LIFE

Primary brain tumors are both life-threatening malignancies and neurodegenerative disorders.[32] Neuropsychological sequelae of brain tumors have an immediate impact on a patient beginning at diagnosis, regardless of whether the patient has any neurocognitive deficits or not. The psychological import on the patient after having been told she or he has a brain tumor can be particularly frightening because it carries an association with loss of mental capabilities, unlike other forms of cancer.[12] Neurocognitive deficits have a significant effect on patients' QOL.

The relationship between patients' neurocognitive impairment and QOL was tested in a study of 30 patients with malignant glioma undergoing a full neuropsychological battery; the more severe the neurocognitive impairment, the lower the patient QOL.[33] Impairments in language had the highest correlation with poor patient QOL. As Figure 10-1 illustrates, global patient QOL

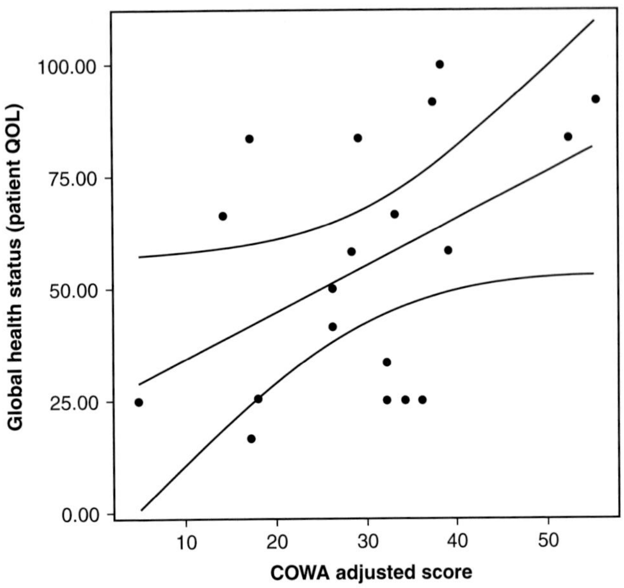

Figure 10-1. Global patient QOL is significantly negatively related to patients' deficits in verbal fluency (r = 0.43; R^2 = 0.18). Poor patient QOL was also significantly negatively related to patients' deficits in object naming (r = 0.45; R^2 = 0.20).

is significantly negatively related to patients' deficits in verbal fluency (r = 0.43; R^2 = 0.18). Poor patient QOL was also significantly negatively related to patients' deficits in object naming (r = 0.45; R^2 = 0.20). Executive function deficits, as measured by the Stroop test, a test of executive dysfunction often indicative of impulsivity and disinhibition, were also strongly correlated with poor patient QOL (r = –0.56; R^2 = 0.31).

These neurocognitive deficits have a similar impact on QOL to the impact on other neurologically impaired patient populations (e.g., Alzheimer disease[34,35] and acquired brain injury[36–38]). Low QOL in a neuro-oncologic population (transcallosal microsurgery for near-midline tumors) is directly related to neurocognitive impairments.[39] In brain tumor patients, deterioration in neurologic function is accompanied by significant deterioration in global QOL.[14] Thus, neurocognitive impairment appears to relate directly to poor global QOL.

"Return to work" is frequently used in health research as a marker of QOL and treatment success. However, neurocognitive impairment is a barrier to returning to work in almost all professional areas,[22] and is a likely explanation for the low number of brain tumor patients who return to work after their initial surgery. The Glioma Outcomes Registry (GO Project), a multicenter, longitudinal, observational registry designed to track patterns of clinical practice and outcomes among patients who undergo surgery for malignant glioma, collected data on 788 patients between December 1997 and December 2001. The GO Project data showed that only 12% of patients were working full-time at enrollment, with an additional 6% of patients working part-time, for a total of 18% of patients employed in some capacity. This low rate of employment likely reflects the older average age of patients with malignant glioma (e.g., many patients may be retired) but also likely reflects the immediate impact on a glioma on patients who were working prior to diagnosis. These percentages of employment were constant when patients were measured again within 3 months and within 6 months of their surgery. Although some patients may return to work at a later time, many patients who do return to work need to resign later because of increasing physical or neurocognitive impairment.[40] In one study of patients with astrocytomas who survived at least 1 year after surgery and radiotherapy (XRT), 13 patients were selected who had failed to return to premorbid levels of work or school.[41] All patients showed deficits in executive function, specifically in problem-solving and coping with novel situations. Vocational or educational performance was not found to be associated with tumor severity, psychiatric problems, or other medical illness, suggesting that these neurocognitive deficits were the crucial factor preventing patients from returning to work or school.

QOL and physical impairment tend to have a very poor correlation in studies of brain tumor patients. For example, in a study by Bampoe and associates, using the Toronto Measure of QOL, a linear-analogue self-assessment format in which patients are asked to rate their own QOL, essentially there was no correlation between KPS scores and global QOL (r = 0.0001).[42] Other researchers have also demonstrated this low correlation between KPS and ADL with QOL.[13,28] In one study of 30 patients with malignant glioma,[33] results showed not only that patients' global QOL was not correlated with ADL function (Barthel Index; r = 0.014), but also that global patient QOL was unrelated to direct measurement of fine motor skills (grooved pegboard test; r = 0.012). These results suggest that physical impairment is not a large component of global QOL in brain tumor patients. In clinical practice, minimizing physical impairment is stressed from surgical planning to rehabilitation. However, these results suggest that in this population, neurocognitive impairment will be a far more important predictor of patients' QOL.

Neurocognition in neuro-oncology is particularly complex because of the numerous mediators that affect an individual's abilities. For example, instead of a deficit occurring from a one-time injury, such as in traumatic brain injury, the injury to the brain from a solid brain tumor occurs over time with tumor growth and treatment. Although patients' neurocognitive abilities typically decline at some point, the pattern of decline is much more variable than in other neurologic disorders (e.g., dementia). Other patient-oriented factors, such as baseline intelligence, education level, affect, coping skills, and social support, are also likely mediators of neurocognitive ability.

Consequently, the remainder of this chapter familiarizes clinicians with the assessment, interpretation, and prognostic significance of neurocognition and QOL in the neuro-oncologic setting. Ideally, elucidation of these factors will improve decision making by patients, families, and the clinicians who care for them. The ultimate goal is to maximize both survival and QOL.

▶ MEASUREMENT OF NEUROCOGNITION AND QUALITY OF LIFE

A full description of the benefits and mechanics of a neuropsychological assessment is beyond the scope of this chapter. However, there are some attributes of neuropsychological assessment in this population that bear further consideration. For example, given the potentially fluctuating nature of a patient's neurocognitive status, repeated administrations are possible and in fact, recommended. This section details the particular considerations that should be given to neuropsychological assessment in a neuro-oncologic population. Given the complex nature of neurocognition, Osoba and associates recommend that detailed measures of neurocognitive status be a standard part of QOL assessment in these patients.[20]

Measurement of Neurocognitive Dysfunction

Measurement of patients' neurocognitive function in a neuro-oncology setting should occur along the same lines as neuropsychological assessment in other disease settings.[2] These assessments are provided by doctoral-level clinical psychologists with at least 2 years of additional training in neuropsychology following the doctorate. The tests themselves are sometimes administered by a technician (a "psychometrician"), but the neuropsychologist interprets the test results and melds them with the results of the diagnostic interview to provide conclusions about patient functioning.

Regarding the benefits of adding neuropsychological assessment to the neurologic assessment of brain tumor patients, Pahlson and associates[3] performed a study of 35 patients with low-grade glioma, in which patients were evaluated by both a neurologist and a neuroopsychologist to determine disability. The neurologist used a standardized neurologic assessment tool (the Edinburgh Functional Impairment Test) that measures both the physical and the neurocognitive domains. The neuropsychologist used a standardized battery of neuropsychological assessment tools. Patients were also asked to report on their own function. Results indicated that there was a much higher agreement between patients and neuropsychologists for estimations of severity of language and memory dysfunction than the neurologist's estimation. Indeed, the neurologist did not detect severe language or memory impairment in any patient, whereas the neuropsychologist and patients identified severe impariments in approximately 40% and approximately 30% of cases, respectively. The authors concluded that "this study demonstrates the usefulness of neuropsychological assessment as a complement to neurological examination to detect cogntive dysfunction."

The use of the Folstein Mini Mental Status Examination (MMSE) is not recommended for the assessment of neurocognitive impairment or change in neuro-oncology. Although the brevity and simplicity of the MMSE has made it attractive for inclusion in clinical trials (e.g., Choucair and associates,[43] Brown and associates[44]), the MMSE has a number of shortcomings in this population (see references 45 and 46 for a discussion). The MMSE is an inadequate measure because it is insensitive to small changes, while having a large practice effect.[46] The MMSE also lacks standardized norms for low education, and its scores are meaningless in the face of language dysfunction and/or motor impairment.[47] Because it lacks a timed component, the MMSE is also insensitive to psychomotor slowing from white matter changes, perhaps the most common neurocognitive symptom seen in brain tumors.[40]

Ideally, the selection of specific neuropsychological tests should include the following characteristics:

- Widely used standardized psychometric instruments.
- Published normative data that take into account age and, where appropriate, education and gender.
- Alternate forms to minimize the effects of repeated administration.
- Short administration times with stopping rules to prevent patients from becoming overwhelmed.

The neuropsychological battery should ideally give the psychologist the ability to:

- Assess specific neurocognitive impairment known to be affected by brain tumors and treatment.
- Measure a wide, minimally overlapping range of neurocognitive abilities.
- Use multiple measures to provide better sensitivity than any single test to identify the functions affected and degree to which they are affected.
- Distinguish between a cortical and a subcortical syndrome.
- Record potential changes from estimated premorbid function and baseline measures.

Administration time would ideally not be over 2 hours, with 30 minutes being an ideal assessment time that almost all patients can tolerate.

A sample neuropsychology battery that adheres to most of these suggestions is the following:

- *Premorbid IQ*: estimated using the Barona Index[48] (first assessment only), full-scale IQ
- *Visual scanning speed*: Trails A tests,[49] number of seconds to complete (maximum seconds = 300)
- *Divided attention*: Trails B tests,[49] number of seconds to complete (maximum seconds = 300), errors (range: 0–26)
- *Language*: Controlled Oral Word Association Test,[50] age- and sex-adjusted raw score (range: 0 to no upper limit)
- *Memory*: Hopkins Verbal Learning Test,[51] number of words recalled 3 times (maximum score = 36), number of words correctly recognized (maximum score = 12), and number of words recalled after delay (maximum score = 12)
- *Psychomotor speed*: Digit Symbol subtest of the Wechsler Adult Intelligence Scale (WAIS)-III[52] age-corrected subtest score (0–20).
- *Fine motor*: Grooved pegboard test,[53] number of seconds to complete (maximum seconds = 300)

A screening measure for depression ideally should also be included, given the high prevalence of depression in brain tumor patients.[54] Depression also is thought to impact patients' neuropsychological scores negatively on testing,[55] although recently this has been debated.[56,57]

Quality of Life Assessment Considerations

When QOL is explicitly measured in neuro-oncologic populations, whether for clinical or research purposes, there are extra factors to consider when asking patients to fill out these paper and pencil measures.

Compliance with Quality of Life Measures

Patient compliance in filling out QOL measures is very high in most oncologic populations. For example, one study of compliance in patients with malignant melanoma and breast cancer reported that more than 95% of the questionnaires were returned, and more than 99% of the questions were answered.[58] Concerns are occasionally raised about the motivation and ability of brain tumor patients to complete these measures given the potential for neurocognitive impairment. However, compliance in the brain tumor population has been reported at 100% at baseline and 88% at followup.[20] Another study reported compliance with QOL measures to only be 50% at 6 months, but found that in the vast majority of cases of noncompliance (70%), the cause was the researchers' own administrative failure.[59] In addition, KPS greater than or equal to 70 is a frequent inclusion criterion for outcome studies, and patients who are independent in their ADL functioning do not, in our experience, show neurocognitive impairment to the degree that they are unable to respond to the QOL assessment. Therefore, these concerns should not preclude the inclusion of a QOL measure in neuro-oncology clinical research.

Interaction with Neurocognition

In a repeated-measures design wherein patients will be tested at intervals over time, occasional concerns are expressed regarding patients' ability to fill out QOL questionnaires once their neurocognitive status has declined too far. Again, this important concern should not preclude QOL testing in this population. In fact, in one study of brain tumor patients who exhibited mental confusion, reliability measures (Cronbach's alpha) were higher in some QOL domains than for patients without mental confusion.[20] Thus, confused patients did not provide less reliable QOL information than did the nonconfused patients.

The use of caregivers or significant others as proxy raters has been proposed to help with measurement of QOL in patients with brain tumors. Sneeuw and colleagues[60] examined the reliability of simultaneous patient and proxy ratings of QOL. They found that ratings are generally similar in most domains, but are less so for more neurocognitively impaired patients. The conclusion is that proxy ratings are better than missing data, but they do not fully represent the QOL status of the patient. Of note, no studies have been performed with the use of testers trained in the objective administration of psychometric tests such as those used in neuropsychological testing. It may be that bias would be greatly reduced with the use of a neutral observer assisting the patient, rather than a caregiver who presumably has a significant amount of emotional investment in a patient's QOL. In our experience, psychometric testers trained in unbiased assessment who administer the neuropsychological battery can elicit responses from a patient with neurocognitive deficits who has some difficulty in completing the form (e.g., vision or motor impairment, or difficulty with speech).

▶ NEUROPSYCHOLOGICAL SEQUELAE

Neurocognitive impairment in brain tumor patients is frequent at baseline, with 91% of patients having at least one area of deficit compared to the normal population, and 71% demonstrating at least three deficits.[61] Although mental status changes are one of the most frequent symptoms of a brain tumor,[23,62] studies of neurocognitive sequelae of adult brain tumor patients are not common in the literature. The effects of many treatment choices (e.g., radiotherapy, chemotherapy, microsurgery, radiosurgery) on neurocognitive status are also not well defined. This section describes the incidence and causes of neurocognitive impairment in brain tumor patients. The causes of specific neurocognitive impairments are beyond the scope of this chapter, although this chapter does focus on the relationship of neurocognitive status to outcomes. At the end of this section, it should be clear that the inclusion of neurocognitive status is extremely important for QOL-based treatment decisions by physicians, patients, and their families.

Effects of Surgery and Tumor Location

The most common types of neurocognitive impairments are not location specific, and include fatigue, depression, and psychomotor slowing. Impairments of psychomotor speed, attention, and working memory are ubiquitous in brain tumor patients, largely as a result of the effects of the tumor and treatment on the frontal–brainstem–reticular system.[63,64] In a comparison of neuropsychological deficits between patients with brain tumors and patients with strokes, matched for lesion location, stroke patients were shown to have more severe neurocognitive deficits.[65] Rate of tumor growth is a predictor of degree of neurocognitive impairment: slow tumor growth may displace normal tissue slowly enough so as not to displace function too drastically,[65] whereas rapid tumor growth will cause more severe deficits.[66]

Specific areas of neurocognitive impairments caused by the tumor itself will vary from patient to patient with the site of the lesion.[2,22,67,68] For example, left hemisphere lesions tend to produce changes in language.[32] Third ventricle tumors tend to cause impairments in memory, executive function, and manual dexterity (interestingly, independent of the effects of surgery or hydrocephalus).[69] One study found that lesion location was the only significant predictor of postradiosurgery complications.[70] The size and location of the tumor at the time of diagnosis also impacts survival, given that tumors that arise in areas with a difficult surgical approach (e.g., deep tumors) or tumors in "eloquent cortex" are not so amenable to surgical resection.[6,23] There is also a risk for the surgical approach damaging healthy brain tissue, and the location of any bleeding will impact future neurocognitive status similar to that following a stroke.[22]

Effects of Edema

Computerized tomography (CT) and magnetic resonance imaging (MRI) often demonstrate peritumoral edema surrounding brain tumors. Peritumoral edema is thought to represent extravasated plasma water and proteins through a disrupted blood–brain barrier within the tumor.[71] It is often unclear whether neurocognitive impairment is related to the tumor mass alone, peritumoral edema, or both. Edema may be in large part responsible for the waxing and waning of neurocognitive impairment in patients. Peritumoral edema is frequently treated with glucocorticoids,[72] which commonly result in neurologic improvement for patients with brain tumors.[73] Length of survival for brain tumors patients has been correlated with response to steroids.[74] However, glucocorticoid therapy has been associated with neurobehavioral disturbance as well. Depression, hypomania, mood swings, anxiety, acute psychotic reactions, and even a case of obsessive-compulsive behavior disorder have been reported.[75] Although the literature supports a trend for neurologic improvement, psychometric testing cannot ignore possible behavioral effects of steroid medication.

Influence of Radiation

This topic is also reviewed in Chapter 32, but highlights are stressed here. Neurocognitive impairment following XRT is likely to be dose-dependent, and may occur from minutes to up to 30 years after completion of treatment.[76] The range of neurologic complications can include acute encephalopathy, somnolence syndrome, radiation necrosis, and radiation-induced tumors.[76] Radiation-induced progressive mental disturbance, dementia, ataxia, and death in the absence of tumor recurrence have all been described.[77–80] Some patients are diagnosed with definite radiation-induced dementia,[78] frequently termed *radiation encephalopathy*.[81] Neurocognitive impairment caused by XRT follows the known pattern of standard subcortical white matter dysfunction similar to the subcortical dementias.[82,83] Specifically, these neurocognitive impairments are in the areas of information processing, executive functioning, memory, attention, and motor coordination.[41,68,84–89] Thus, radiation-induced neurocognitive impairment can be discriminated from deficits caused by the tumor's structural effect on brain parenchyma using standardized neuropsychological testing, with comparison of the pattern of deficits to the normal population and preradiation treatment patterns of neurocognitive impairment.[2,82] Radiation necrosis, an irreversible condition (although it can be palliated with steroids), may also result in a focal lesion that further decrements specific neuropsychological performance.[23]

In general, the higher the dose of radiation, the greater the neurocognitive impairment. In one study of 19 pediatric patients with medulloblastoma, a significant negative correlation was found between IQ and whole-brain irradiation dose ($r = -0.72$).[90] In a recent study of adults undergoing radiation for treatment of skull base tumors,[91] neurocognitive impairment was related to the total dose of radiation delivered but not to the volume of brain irradiated, side of radiation boost, or chemotherapy treatment. This study is important because neurocognitive radiation effects are seen even though the brain was not the direct radiation target.

The relationship of increased neurocognitive impairment with increasing radiation dose[91] is of particular importance because in many brain tumor studies higher than standard radiation dose does not show a benefit in terms of survival. Therefore, higher radiation doses should be considered carefully in terms of potentially increasing neurocognitive impairment and decreasing QOL, particularly if radiation does not impart a survival benefit.

Influence of Chemotherapy

In adults, standard cancer chemotherapy has been related to neuropsychological deficits. Cytokines, interleukin-2, and corticosteroids have all been suggested to be agents that decrease neurocognitive status.[92] Potential complications include acute and chronic encephalopathy and cerebellar syndrome. Conventional chemotherapy for breast cancer has also been proposed to cause neurocognitive impairment.[93–99]

Combined radiotherapy and chemotherapy can also induce neurotoxicity at doses that alone would be safe.[76,100] Neurocognitive impairment has been reported in a trial of fractionated radiotherapy and chemotherapy.[101] It may be that chemotherapeutic agents attack the same targets as radiation, causing an additive effect, or that the chemotherapeutic agent acts as a radiosensitizer, or that radiotherapy alters the distribution of chemotherapy agents.[76] Therefore, information on concurrent chemotherapy in brain tumor patients is also important to analyze in neuropsychological neuro-oncology research.

A recent trend in chemotherapy protocols when QOL measures are included is to report a "QOL benefit" of chemotherapy. For example, one report noted simply that the use of paclitaxel did not lead to major QOL complications, as QOL was generally stable over time, although paclitaxel was of limited value in terms of response and survival.[34] Caution should be taken in the interpretation of these results, however. The lack of QOL decline while on chemotherapeutic treatment is a benefit, but it should be made clear to patients that this benefit will not mean that QOL is *improved* by the intervention.

Effect of Patient Age

Detailed analyses of the effect of age at diagnosis reveal that younger children have worse neurocognitive impairment and have more toxic reactions to radiation than do older children at the time of diagnosis.[90,102,103] Conversely, in adults, the older the patient, the more sensitive the patient is to neurotoxicity from radiation and chemotherapy.[104] The elderly appear to be more susceptible to radiation-induced brain atrophy and dementia.[105] In fact, in two separate studies, brain tumor survivors older than age 40[106] and 45[107] years showed a more rapid decline in clinical and neurocognitive status than did younger patients. Maire and associates[108] found that only 20% of patients younger than 30 years old showed neurocognitive impairment, whereas older patients had a significantly higher rate of impairment.

Treatment of Neurocognitive Sequelae

Methylphenidate (MPD) is a central nervous system stimulant that is FDA-approved for the treatment of attention deficit hyperactivity disorder and narcolepsy. It is often used off-label to treat neurocognitive deficits, fatigue, and mood in neurologic disorders. MPD is an inexpensive, commonly used medication in the United States, with more than 2 million Americans (mostly children) currently receiving treatment with this drug.[109] The complete mechanism by which MPD exerts its behavioral effects is unknown. The prevailing theory is that MPD influences hyperactivity and behavior largely via a direct effect on key dopaminergic areas of the brain.[110] However, MPD has appreciable effects on norepinephrine reuptake and also binds to the serotonin transporter.[111] The possibility that MPD causes its behavioral effects by influencing multiple neurotransmitters has been suggested.[112] Importantly, MPD exerts its actions with relatively few side effects.

Meyers and associates[113] examined the effect of MPD on patients with malignant brain tumors. In this study, MPD (20–60 mg/d) was administered to 30 patients with primary brain tumors, and the effect on mood, as well as on neurocognitive ability and functional status, was assessed. Significant improvements in neurocognitive function were observed at the 20 mg/d dose of MPD.[113] In particular, significant improvements were noted in psychomotor speed, memory, visual-motor function, executive function, and motor speed and dexterity. Importantly, in half of these patients, the improvement in cognition was observed despite ongoing neurologic injury as a consequence of disease progression or radiation therapy. In addition to effects on neurocognition, the majority of patients on the 20 mg/d dose of MPD experienced subjective improvements in their ability to function, whereas 100% of patients on the 60 mg/d dose reported improvement. These functional improvements included improved gait, increased stamina and motivation to perform activities, better concentration, and, in one case, increased bladder control. Adverse effects were minimal and immediately resolved when treatment was discontinued.[113]

▶ PSYCHIATRIC SEQUELAE

Approximately half of all cancer patients have a psychiatric disorder, typically an adjustment disorder with depression. Moreover depression is significantly correlated with increased mortality.[114] Brain tumor patients have been shown to develop de novo psychiatric symptoms.[55] A significant number of patients with low-grade infiltrating tumors and meningiomas are referred for psychiatric consultation before the recognition of the tumor.[23] Psychiatric symptoms may depend on the location of the tumor.[55,115] Hecaen[116] found that 67% of patients with frontal lobe tumors exhibited confused states and dementia. Patients with temporal lobe lesions tend to have marked personality changes and mood swings.[117] Patients with right hemisphere tumors may also show paranoid ideation, hallucinations, and agitation.[118] Localized damage to the hypothalamus, whether from tumor, surgery, or radiation damage, results in behavioral changes such as anxiety, depression, emotional lability, belligerence, recalcitrance, garrulousness, hypersexuality, anomia, apraxia, decreased attention and reasoning ability, and memory loss (see, e.g., reference 119). Both depression and pain will be further discussed below, given their significant impact on QOL.

Depression

Depression is one of the most common neurologic morbidities in brain tumor patients.[54,120] Rates of depression in malignant brain tumor patients vary as a result of differences in assessment methods (e.g., self-report vs. physician report), timing of assessment, and the like. Patients commonly present with depression at diagnosis.[115,121] According to a study analyzing data from the GO Project,[54,122] between 12% and 37% of glioma patients report depression, either at the initial evaluation or at the 3- or 6-month followup evaluation. One recent study of brain tumor patients (meningiomas and gliomas) found that 15% of patients had clinically significant levels of depression[123] by physician rating using the Hamilton Depression Scale, whereas Mackworth and colleagues[28] found that 50% of primary brain tumor patients reported depression.

The exact cause of depression in patients with brain tumors is not known. Explicit knowledge of the grim prognosis in patients with brain tumors has been proposed as an explanation for the degree of depression, under the assumption that depression is a normal reaction to a poor prognosis.[123] Conversely, psychological morbidity was not correlated with the extent to which the malignant brain tumor patients were aware of the nature of their disease,[123] or the manner in which information was conveyed to patients.[124] It is also possible that depression is related to physiologic brain changes secondary to the tumor, similar to what has been demonstrated in stroke patients.[125,126] In addition to the tumor itself, it is possible that treatments (surgery, radiation, chemotherapy) may also affect neurochemical function to cause depression, although the relationships among treatments and depression have never been tested. Some depressive symptoms overlap with symptoms of "somatization," and it has been proposed that high rates of true somatization symptoms (e.g., anxiety) create a falsely high impression of depression. However, when somatization factors are controlled for, differences in depression remain,[127] suggesting that depression is a separate construct.

The relationship between QOL and depression may be intuitive, as depression has frequently been shown to have a negative impact on QOL in cancer patients,[128] although they remain separate constructs.[129–131] In one study of QOL in patients with malignant brain tumors,[28] depression accounted for a majority of the variance in QOL scores in a multiple regression analysis ($p < 0.001$), and was independent of other common outcome predictors such as patient age. A similar study found that depression was the single most important predictor of patient QOL.[132]

Mood

Depression should also be considered as a separate construct from "mood," although both potentially impact QOL. A patient's various beliefs, assumptions, appraisals, and expectations concerning problems and problem-solving orientation impact the ability to adapt one's role to living with cancer.[133] Patients who have a positive affect are more optimistic about their future and have lower levels of anxiety and depressive symptoms,[134] whereas a negative affect or orientation is vulnerable to pessimism, negative emotional experiences, and clinical depression.[133] Role retention was significantly related to higher QOL, and negative mood was inversely related to role retention at a statistically significant level in a population of cancer patients who were bone marrow transplantation survivors.[135]

Pain

Pain has the potential for directly impacting QOL in brain tumor patients. Pain symptoms are thought to be far less common in brain tumors than in many other forms of cancer. However, in a study of 50 brain tumor patients given self-report measures, nearly 50% of participants reported pain.[1] QOL scores of patients with recurrent brain tumors have been reported to be similar to QOL scores in patients with advanced ovarian and lung cancer, except that patients with recurrent brain tumors reported worse neurocognitive functioning and less pain.[30]

▶ BEYOND SURVIVAL: NEUROCOGNITIVE PROGNOSIS AND QUALITY OF LIFE

Length of survival in neuro-oncology is primarily influenced by tumor grade, patient age, and degree of independence of ADL at baseline.[136–152] Prognosis is discussed extensively in other chapters, but the value of neurocognition, depression, and global QOL as additional prognostic factors is discussed in this section.

Neurocognition

Neurocognitive impairment is a significant predictor of survival in numerous other neurologic disorders such as multiple sclerosis[153] and dementia.[154] Both depression and neurocognitive impairment are independent predictors of mortality in medically ill older adults.[56] Even though mental status changes are one of the most common presenting signs of a brain tumor,[23] the degree and impact of these changes on prognosis is only beginning to be studied in neuro-oncology.[2]

Meyers and associates[2] showed that neurocognitive status (verbal memory performance) was independently and strongly related to survival in patients with recurrent glioma even after accounting for age, tumor grade, KPS, and time since diagnosis. An analysis of 445 patients with brain metastases found that decreasing baseline MMSE ($p = 0.003$) and primary site (breast vs. lung vs. other, $p = 0.032$) were highly associated with a terminal event, in a Cox proportional hazards model adjusting for age, gender, and KPS.[155] The benefit of neurocognitive information added to a prognostic model has also been shown in patients with leptomeningeal or parenchymal brain lesions.[156] Another study found a relationship between baseline neurologic deficits as an independent predictor of survival in patients with low-grade glioma,[157] although neuropsychological deficits were not directly tested.

Neurocognitive deficits are strong predictors of other health outcomes in neuro-oncology. For example, neurocognitive change (decline) has been shown to predict MRI evidence of tumor progression in low-grade[158] and high-grade gliomas,[22,47] and in patients with brain metastases.[159]

Depression

Emphasis has been given to the relationship between depression and survival in other cancers. For example, one recent study of depression following stem cell transplantation for malignancies found that depressed patients had a threefold greater risk of dying than did nondepressed patients, adjusting for other prognostic factors.[160] Depression is a risk factor for treatment noncompliance[161] and various psychoneuroendocrinologic explanations have been proposed.[114,162,163] Also, depression was suggested to predict response to chemotherapy in breast cancer.[164]

The GO Project included physician and patient ratings of QOL and depression, although, unfortunately, no neurocognitive information was collected. Using data from the GO Project, a recent paper showed depression as an independent predictor of survival in patients with malignant glioma.[54] In a multivariate, Cox proportional hazards model using backward, stepwise analysis, with known predictors of survival (tumor grade, patient age, baseline KPS) included as covariates, history of major depressive episode (2 weeks of significant depression within the past year) and recent major depressive disorder (within the past year feeling depressed or sad most of the time) were independent, significant predictors of length of survival ($p < 0.0001$ and $p < 0.049$, respectively). Interestingly, having felt sad or depressed most days for 2 years of your life or more (dysthymic disorder) was not an independent predictor of survival ($p = 0.253$). A postoperative complication of morbid depression was also a significant predictor of survival ($p < 0.008$). These results suggest that depression in the pre- or perioperative period is an independent predictor of shorter length of survival in patients with malignant gliomas, as was previously found in other neurologic diseases. It is unknown whether the etiology of depression is an adjustment reaction, or whether there is a physiologic basis for the depression.

Quality of Life

Baseline QOL has been shown to be a significant predictor of survival in non–central nervous system cancers.[165] A similar pattern is possible in brain tumor patients through complicated relationships among issues such as self-care, help-seeking behavior, social and caregiver support, and neurocognitive impairment of the patient.

A better understanding of the interaction between QOL and survival is crucial to guide ethical decision making by physicians and families, particularly end-of-life decisions. As medical practice improves, our ability to extend the length of survival improves. Thus, there may be a point at which survival and QOL become inversely related, wherein our ability to extend the quantity of life exceeds our ability to maintain quality of life.

In their report in the year 2000, the National Institutes of Health (NIH) Brain Tumor Progress Review Group characterized the problem as follows: "The end points of survival and disease-free survival, which traditionally have been used to assess outcome in patients with cancer, fall painfully short as measures of success in treating brain tumors. From the perspective of patients and families, 'outcome' is a multidimensional daily reality, and quality of life can be at least as important as survival."[166]

▶ FUTURE DIRECTIONS

After reviewing the information in this chapter, it should be clear that clinical research needs to include patient-oriented measures. Only in gaining this information can we improve the QOL and survivorship of people living with brain tumors.

Promote Patient-Oriented Outcomes Research in Neuro-Oncology

Patient-oriented research is rare in many forms of cancer, but is very rare in neuro-oncology. Traditional research has placed a great deal of emphasis on the process of care and technical measures of success, and little emphasis on patient-oriented measures, with few exceptions.[42,167,168] Neurosurgery as a field can be characterized as having enjoyed improvements in technology far in advance of developments in clinical outcomes research.[169] Clinical research in neurosurgery has historically focused on physical outcomes and survival[169] (for example, see reference 170), and traditional neurosurgical outcomes research has only been measured on a single scale[167] such as survival at a given point in time ("yes" or "no").

"Outcomes research" is the study of the effects of a treatment or prognostic factor on patients themselves (e.g., survival, QOL), rather than the study of measures removed from the patient (e.g., cell counts).[169] "Patient-oriented" research involves the *direct* measurement of a patient's function, performed either by the clinician or patient's self-report. Examples of patient-oriented outcomes include patients' report of pain, ADL, QOL, and satisfaction with treatment.[171] Cancer patients, including patients with malignant brain tumors, are likely underdiagnosed and undertreated for these patient-oriented symptoms, according to the June 19, 2001, Institute of Medicine report *Improving Palliative Care for Cancer*.[172]

For almost a century, clinicians reporting the treatment of patients with cancer have been analyzing the cancer, but not the patients.[173]

Although survival is almost always the primary goal in the treatment of a patient with a brain tumor, there is little debate that this single outcome measure cannot adequately describe the multifactorial patient-oriented outcomes in brain tumors.[167] In clinical neuro-oncology research, an improved understanding of outcomes beyond survival such as QOL is needed. Yet most clinical neuro-oncology research to date has only included medical outcomes (e.g., time-to-tumor progression, survival) rather than patient-oriented outcomes such as QOL. Given the typically poor prognosis of patients with malignant brain tumors, both the *quality* of survival, as well as the *length* of survival, deserve research attention.

An improved understanding of QOL in neuro-oncologic populations has the potential to improve clinical care. Clinical followup of brain tumor patients often does not routinely include patient-oriented QOL-based assessments, nor are patients' QOL scores routinely evaluated in clinical trials, although both practices are increasing in frequency. A paucity of information about QOL limits the ability for clinicians, patients, and families to weigh the risks and benefits of new therapies and to develop strategies to improve QOL-related outcomes.[166]

In recent years, an understanding of the need to improve the assessment and treatment of patient-oriented outcomes has emerged[168] and the importance of patient perspectives in treatment decisions and outcomes is now more frequently discussed.[167,174] For example, a recent survey of academically based Canadian oncologists found that the majority identified QOL as more appropriate than survival as an outcome measure for randomized controlled trials in cancer.[175] Yet a complete understanding of the interrelationships of variables that make up patients' QOL, their trajectory over time, and their prognostic value in brain tumors has not yet been developed.

Expand Survivorship Research in Neuro-Oncology

The National Cancer Institute (NCI) has taken a stand on the importance of cancer survivorship research. NCI's plan for fiscal year (FY) 2003, *NCI: The Nation's Investment in Cancer Research*, states that research on survivorship and end-of-life issues are a priority. Its FY 2002 plan stated: "...there should be a critical examination of whether, when, and how NCI-sponsored trials, which have been the backbone of the clinical discovery process in cancer, should give greater emphasis to patient-centered outcomes in addition to the important traditional endpoints of survival and tumor progression." This priority was also shown by the submission of the Cancer Survivorship Research and Quality of Life Act of 2002 to Congress.

The NCI has now declared that brain tumors are a top priority for patient-oriented research.[168] The NCI Brain Tumor Progress Review Group Report has stated that the research goal in this population is to predict the impact of the tumor and treatment on a patient's neurocognition and QOL to achieve the best possible outcome.[166] The report states that routine neurocognitive and QOL assessments and interventions are necessary, and should become the standard of care for patients with brain tumors.[166] According to this report, long-term studies of neurotoxicity are needed to develop quantitative QOL and neurocognitive measures and treatment strategies to improve neurocognition, as are further study on how the tumor itself may affect brain function.[166] Priorities include correlation of demographic characteristics, imaging, and neurocognitive/QOL assessments (Outcomes Priority 1); design and evaluation of innovative interventions to ameliorate undesirable symptoms and functional deficits, including empirical investigations of what works—pharmacologic, behavioral, neurocognitive, or a combination of these approaches (Outcomes Priority 2); and investigation of the epidemiology of neurotoxicity and other toxic effects of treatment, such as what makes some patients susceptible and what exerts a protective effect (Epidemiology Priority 3).

According to the NCI Planning Agenda for disease-specific research, "brain tumors pose unique challenges for researchers and patients.... We have to carefully weigh the potential benefit of every brain tumor surgery, chemotherapy, or radiation treatment against the risk of mental and functional damage." Clarification of the complex interrelationships between neurocognition, QOL, and survival needs to be performed for a complete understanding of the implications of this area of research.

REFERENCES

1. Whitton AC, Rhydderch H, Furlong W, et al. Self-reported comprehensive health status of adult brain tumor patients using the Health Utilities Index. Cancer 1997;80(2):258–265.
2. Meyers CA, Hess KR, Yung WKA, et al. Cognitive function as a predictor of survival in patients with recurrent malignant glioma. J Clin Oncol 2000;18(3):646–650.
3. Pahlson A, Ek L, Ahlstrom G, et al. Pitfalls in the assessment of disability in individuals with low-grade gliomas. J Neurooncol 2003;65(2):149–158.
4. Schiffbauer H, Ferrari P, Rowley HA, et al. Functional activity within brain tumors: a magnetic source imaging study. Neurosurgery 2001;49(6):1313–1320; discussion 1320–1321.
5. Laws ER. The decade of the brain: 1990–2000. Neurosurgery 2000;47(6):1257–1260.
6. Laws E, Shaffrey M. Surgical management of intracranial gliomas–biopsy resection or watchful waiting. Clin Neurosurg (in press).
7. Kayl AE, Meyers CA. Does brain tumor histology influence cognitive function? Neuro-oncol 2003;5(4):255–60.
8. Wilson IB, Cleary PD. Linking clinical variables with health-related quality of life. A conceptual model of patient outcomes. JAMA 1995;273(1):59–65.
9. Bergner M. Quality of life, health status, and clinical research. Med Care 1989;27(Suppl 3):S148–S156.
10. Cella DF. Quality of life: concepts and definition. J Pain Symptom Manage 1994;9(3):186–192.
11. Mast ME. Definition and measurement of quality of life in oncology nursing research: review and theoretical implications. Oncol Nurs Forum 1995;22(6):957–964.
12. Lovely MP. Quality of life of brain tumor patients. Semin Oncol Nurs 1998;14(1):73–80.
13. Osoba D, Brada M, Prados MD, et al. Effect of disease burden on health-related quality of life in patients with malignant gliomas. Neuro-oncology 2000;2:221–228.
14. Aaronson N, Ahmedzai S, Bergman V, et al. The European organization for research and treatment of cancer QLQ-C30: a quality of life instrument for use in international trials in oncology. J Natl Cancer Inst 1993;85:365–376.
15. Cella DF, Tulsky DS, Gray G, et al. The Functional Assessment of Cancer Therapy scale: development and validation of the general measure. J Clin Oncol 1993;11(3):570–579.
16. Osoba D, Aaronson NK, Muller M, et al. The development and psychometric validation of a brain cancer quality-of-life questionnaire for use in combination with general cancer-specific questionnaires. Qual Life Res 1996;5(1):139–150.
17. Wade D. Measurement in neurological rehabilitation. Oxford: Oxford University Press, 1992.
18. Ware JE Jr, Sherbourne CD. The MOS 36-item short-form health survey (SF-36). I. Conceptual framework and item selection. Med Care 1992;30(6):473–483.
19. Aaronson NK, Beckman J, eds. The quality of life for cancer patients. New York: Raven Press, 1987.
20. Osoba D, Aaronson NK, Muller M, et al. Effect of neurological dysfunction on health-related quality of life in patients with high-grade glioma. J Neurooncol 1997;34(3):263–278.
21. Weitzner MA, Meyers CA, Gelke CK, et al. The Functional Assessment of Cancer Therapy (FACT) scale. Development of a brain subscale and revalidation of the general version (FACT-G) in patients with primary brain tumors. Cancer 1995;75(5):1151–1161.
22. Meyers CA. Quality of life of brain tumor patients. In: Bernstein M, Berger MS, eds. Neuro-oncology: the essentials. New York: Thieme, 2000:466–472.
23. Packer RJ, Miller DC, Shaffrey MS, et al. Intracranial neoplasms. In: Rosenberg RN, Pleasure DE, eds. Comprehensive neurology. New York: John Wiley, 1998:187–243.
24. Abrahams JM, Torchia M, Putt M, et al. Risk factors affecting survival after brain metastases from non-small cell lung carcinoma: a follow-up study of 70 patients. J Neurosurg 2001;95(4):595–600.
25. Patchell R, Tibbs P, Walsh JW, et al. A randomized trial of surgery in the treatment of single metastases to the brain. N Engl J Med 1990;22:494–500.
26. Recht L, Glantz M, Chamberlain M, et al. Quantitative measurement of quality outcome in malignant glioma patients using an independent living score (ILS). Assessment of a retrospective cohort. J Neurooncol 2003;61(2):127–136.
27. Meyers C, Boake C, Levin V, et al. Symptom management, rehabilitation strategies, and improved quality of life for patients with brain tumors. In: Levin V, ed. Cancer in the nervous system. New York: Churchill Livingstone, 1996: 449–462.
28. Mackworth N, Fobair P, Prados M. Quality of life self-reports from 200 patients: comparisons with Karnofsky Performance Scale. J Neurooncol 1992;14:243–253.
29. Farace E, Marshall LF. Quality of life in acoustics. J Neurosurg 2003;99(5):807–808; discussion 808–809.
30. Osoba D, Brada M, Yung WK, et al. Health-related quality of life in patients treated with temozolomide versus procarbazine for recurrent glioblastoma multiforme. J Clin Oncol 2000;18(7):1481–1491.
31. Kemmler G, Holzner B, Kopp M, et al. Comparison of two quality-of-life instruments for cancer patients: the functional assessment of cancer therapy-general and the European Organization for Research and Treatment of Cancer Quality of Life Questionnaire-C30. J Clin Oncol 1999;17(9):2932–2940.
32. Hahn CA, Dunn RH, Logue PE, et al. Prospective study of neuropsychologic testing and quality-of-life assessment of adults with primary malignant brain tumors. Int J Radiat Oncol Biol Phys 2003;55(4):992–999.
33. Farace E, Shaffrey ME. Neurocognitive predictors of malignant brain tumor outcomes. Paper presented at the 14th International Conference on Brain Tumor Research and Therapy. Asheville, NC: 2001.

34. Zankd S, Leipold B. The relationship between severity of dementia and subjective well-being. Aging Ment Health 2001;5(2):191–196.
35. Demers L, Oremus M, Perrault A, et al. Review of outcome measurement instruments in Alzheimer's disease drug trials: introduction. J Geriatr Psychiatr Neurol 2000;13(4):161–169.
36. Riemsma RP, Forbes CA, Glanville JM, et al. General health status measures for people with cognitive impairment: learning disability and acquired brain injury. Health Technol Assess 2001;5(6):1–100.
37. DePalma JA. Measuring quality of life of patients of traumatic brain injury. Crit Care Nurs Q 2001;23(4):42–51.
38. Steadman-Pare D, Colantonio A, Ratcliff G, et al. Factors associated with perceived quality of life many years after traumatic brain injury. J Head Trauma Rehabil 2001;16(4): 330–342.
39. Hutter BO, Spetzger U, Bertalanffy H, et al. Cognition and quality of life in patients after transcallosal microsurgery for midline tumors. J Neurosurg Sci 1997;41(1): 123–129.
40. Meyers CA. Neurocognitive dysfunction in cancer patients. Oncology (Huntingt) 2000;14(1):75–79; discussion 79.
41. Hochberg FH, Slotnick B. Neuropsychologic impairment in astrocytoma survivors. Neurology 1980;30(2):172–177.
42. Bampoe J, Laperriere N, Pintile M, et al. Quality of life in patients with glioblastoma multiforme participating in a randomized study of brachytherapy as a boost treatment. J Neurosurg 2000;93:917–926.
43. Choucair AK, Scott C, Urtasun R, et al. Quality of life and neuropsychological evaluation for patients with malignant astrocytomas: RTOG 91–14. Radiation Therapy Oncology Group. Int J Radiat Oncol Biol Phys 1997;38(1):9–20.
44. Brown PD, Buckner JC, O'Fallon JR, et al. Effects of radiotherapy on cognitive function in patients with low-grade glioma measured by the Folstein Mini-Mental State Examination. J Clin Oncol 2003;21(13):2519–2524.
45. Klein M, Heimans JJ. The measurement of cognitive functioning in low-grade glioma patients after radiotherapy [comment]. J Clin Oncol 2004;22(5):966–967; author reply 967–968.
46. Meyers CA, Wefel JS. The use of the mini-mental state examination to assess cognitive functioning in cancer trials: no ifs, ands, buts, or sensitivity [comment]. J Clin Oncol 2003;21(19):3557–3558.
47. Meyers CA, Hess KR. Multifaceted end points in brain tumor clinical trials: cognitive deterioration precedes MRI progression. Neuro-oncol 2003;5(2):89–95.
48. Barona A, Reynolds CR, Chastain R. A demographically based index of premorbid intelligence for the WAIS-R. J Consult Clin Psychol 1984;52:885–887.
49. Partington JE, Leiter RG. Partington's pathway test. Psychol Serv Center Bull 1949;1:9–20.
50. Spreen O, Benton AL. Neurosensory Center Comprehensive Examination for Aphasia (NCCEA). Victoria, Canada: University of Victoria Neuropsychology Laboratory, 1969.
51. Benedict RHB, Schretlen D, Groninger L, et al. Hopkins verbal learning test—revised: normative data and analysis of inter-form and test-retest reliability. Clin Neuropsychol 1998;12(1):43–55.
52. Wechsler D. Wechsler adult intelligence scale-III. New York: Psychological Corporation, 1997.
53. Matthews CG, Klove H. Instruction manual for the adult neuropsychology test battery. Madison, WI: University of Wisconsin Medical School, 1964.
54. Litofsky NS, Farace E, Anderson F Jr, et al. Depression in patients with high-grade glioma: results of the Glioma Outcomes Project. Neuro-surgery 2004;54(2):358–366; discussion 366–367.
55. Lezak MD. Neuropsychological assessment. New York: Oxford University Press, 1995:650–685.
56. Arfken CL, Lichtenberg PA, Tancer ME. Cognitive impairment and depression predict mortality in medically ill older adults. J Gerontol Series A Biol Sci Med Sci 1999;54(3):M152–M156.
57. Rohling ML, Green P, Allen LM, et al. Depressive symptoms and neurocognitive test scores in patients passing symptoms validity tests. Arch Clin Neuropsychol 2002;17:205–222.
58. Sadura A, Pater J, Osoba D, et al. Quality-of-life assessment: patient compliance with questionnaire completion. J Natl Cancer Inst 1992;84(13):1023–1026.
59. Walker M, Brown J, Brown K, et al. Practical problems with the collection and interpretation of serial quality of life assessments in patients with malignant glioma. J Neurooncol 2003;63(2):179–186.
60. Sneeuw KC, Aaronson NK, Osoba D, et al. The use of significant others as proxy raters of the quality of life of patients with brain cancer. Med Care 1997;35(5):490–506.
61. Tucha O, Smely C, Preier M, et al. Cognitive deficits before treatment among patients with brain tumors. Neurosurgery 2000;47(2):324–333; discussion 333–334.
62. Klein M, Taphoorn MJB, Heimans JJ, et al. Neurobehavioral status and health-related quality of life in newly diagnosed high-grade glioma patients. J Clin Oncol 2001;19(20): 4037–4047.
63. Iversen LL. Dopamine receptors in the brain. Science 1975;188(4193):1084–1089.
64. Simon H, Scatton B, Moal ML. Dopaminergic A10 neurons are involved in cognitive functions. Nature 1980; 286(5769):150–151.
65. Anderson SW, Damasio H, Tranel D. Neuropsychological impairments associated with lesions caused by tumor or stroke. Arch Neurol 1990;47(4):397–405.
66. Hom J, Reitan RM. Neuropsychological correlates of rapidly vs. slowly growing intrinsic cerebral neoplasms. J Clin Neuropsychol 1984;6(3):309–324.
67. Farace E, Turkheimer E, Wilkniss S. Utility of analyzing lesion location in an outcome study of traumatic brain injury. Seattle, WA: International Neuropsychological Society, 1995.
68. Scheibel RS, Meyers CA, Levin VA. Cognitive dysfunction following surgery for intracerebral glioma: influence of histopathology, lesion location, and treatment. J Neurooncol 1996;30(1):61–69.
69. Friedman MA, Meyers CA, Sawaya R. Neuropsychological effects of third ventricle tumor surgery. Neurosurgery 2003;52(4):791–798; discussion 798.
70. Gelblum DY, Lee H, Bilsky M, et al. Radiographic findings and morbidity in patients treated with stereotactic radiosurgery. Int J Radiat Oncol Biol Phys 1998;42(2):391–395.

71. Andersen C, Astrup J, Gyldensted C. Quantitative MR analysis of glucocorticoid effects on peritumoral edema associated with intracranial meningiomas and metastases. J Comput Assist Tomogr 1994;18(4):509–518.
72. Routh A, Khansur T, Hickman BT, et al. Management of brain metastases: past, present, and future. South Med J 1994;87(12):1218–1226.
73. Vecht CJ, Hovestadt A, Verbiest HB, et al. Dose-effect relationship of dexamethasone on Karnofsky performance in metastatic brain tumors: a randomized study of doses of 4, 8, and 16 mg per day. Neurology 1994;44(4):675–680.
74. Lagerwaard FJ, Levendag PC, Nowak PJ, et al. Identification of prognostic factors in patients with brain metastases: a review of 1292 patients. Int J Radiat Oncol Biol Phys 1999;43(4):795–803.
75. Bick PA. Obsessive-compulsive behavior associated with dexamethasone treatment. J Nerv Mental Dis 1983; 171(4):253–254.
76. Keime-Guibert F, Napolitano M, Delattre JY. Neurological complications of radiotherapy and chemotherapy. J Neurol 1998;245(11):695–708.
77. DeAngelis LM. Management of brain metastases. Cancer Invest 1994;12(2):156–165.
78. DeAngelis LM, Delattre JY, Posnel JB. Radiation-induced dementia in patients cured of brain metastases. Neurology 1989;39(6):789–796.
79. Sundaresan N, Galicich JH, Deck MD, et al. Radiation necrosis after treatment of solitary intracranial metastases. Neurosurgery 1981;8(3):329–333.
80. Sheline GE, Wara WM, Smith V. Therapeutic irradiation and brain injury. Int J Radiat Oncol Biol Phys 1980; 6(9):1215–1228.
81. Crossen JR, Garwood D, Glatstein E, et al. Neurobehavioral sequelae of cranial irradiation in adults: a review of radiation-induced encephalopathy. J Clin Oncol 1994;12(3): 627–642.
82. Cummings J. Introduction. In: Cummings J, ed. Subcortical dementia. New York: Oxford University Press, 1990:3–16.
83. Roman GC, Tatemichi TK, Erkinjuntti T, et al. Vascular dementia: diagnostic criteria for research studies: report of the NINDS-AIREN International Workshop. Neurology 1993;43(2):250–260.
84. Archibald YM, Lunn D, Ruttan LA, et al. Cognitive functioning in long-term survivors of high-grade glioma. J Neurosurg 1994;80(2):247–253.
85. Imperato JP, Paleologos NA, Vick NA. Effects of treatment on long-term survivors with malignant astrocytomas [see comments]. Ann Neurol 1990;28(6):818–822.
86. Lieberman AN, Foo SH, Ransohoff J, et al. Long-term survival among patients with malignant brain tumors. Neurosurgery 1982;10(4):450–453.
87. Salander P, Karlsson T, Bergenheim T, et al. Long-term memory deficits in patients with malignant gliomas. J Neurooncol 1995;25(3):227–238.
88. Taphoorn MJ, Schiphorst AK, Snoek FJ, et al. Cognitive functions and quality of life in patients with low-grade gliomas: the impact of radiotherapy. Ann Neurol 1994; 36(1):48–54.
89. Surma-aho O, Niemela M, Vilkki J, et al. Adverse long-term effects of brain radiotherapy in adult low-grade glioma patients [see comments]. Neurology 2001;56(10):1285–1290.
90. Yang TF, Wong TT, Cheng LY, et al. Neuropsychological sequelae after treatment for medulloblastoma in childhood—the Taiwan experience. Childs Nerv Syst 1997;13(2):77–80; discussion 81.
91. Meyers CA, Geara F, Wong PF, et al. Neurocognitive effects of therapeutic irradiation for base of skull tumors. Int J Radiat Oncol Biol Phys 2000;46(1):51–55.
92. Baile WF. Neuropsychiatric disorders in cancer patients. Curr Opin Oncol 1996;8(3):182–187.
93. Olin JJ. Cognitive function after systemic therapy for breast cancer. Oncology (Huntingt) 2001;15(5):613–618; discussion 618, 621–624.
94. Bender CM, Paraska KK, Sereika SM, et al. Cognitive function and reproductive hormones in adjuvant therapy for breast cancer: a critical review. J Pain Symptom Manage 2001;21(5):407–424.
95. Paganini-Hill A, Clark LJ. Preliminary assessment of cognitive function in breast cancer patients treated with tamoxifen. Breast Cancer Res Treat 2000;64(2):165–176.
96. Brezden CB, Phillips KA, Abdolell M, et al. Cognitive function in breast cancer patients receiving adjuvant chemotherapy. J Clin Oncol 2000;18(14):2695–2701.
97. Schagen SB, van Dam FS, Muller MJ, et al. Cognitive deficits after postoperative adjuvant chemotherapy for breast carcinoma. Cancer 1999;85(3):640–650.
98. van Dam FS, Schagen SB, Muller MJ, et al. Impairment of cognitive function in women receiving adjuvant treatment for high-risk breast cancer: high-dose versus standard-dose chemotherapy. J Natl Cancer Inst 1998;90(3):210–218.
99. Ganz PA. Cognitive dysfunction following adjuvant treatment of breast cancer: a new dose-limiting toxic effect [letter; comment]? J Natl Cancer Inst 1998;90(3):182–183.
100. Ahles TA, Silberfarb PM, Herndon J II, et al. Psychologic and neuropsychologic functioning of patients with limited small-cell lung cancer treated with chemotherapy and radiation therapy with or without warfarin: a study by the Cancer and Leukemia Group B. J Clin Oncol 1998;16(5):1954–1960.
101. Groves MD, Maor MH, Meyers C, et al. A phase II trial of high-dose bromo-deoxyuridine with accelerated fractionation radiotherapy followed by procarbazine, lomustine, and vincristine for glioblastoma multiforme. Int J Radiat Oncol Biol Phys 1999;45(1):127–135.
102. Dennis M, Spiegler BJ, Hetherington CR, et al. Neuropsychological sequelae of the treatment of children with medulloblastoma. J Neurooncol 1996;29:91–101.
103. Cervoni L, Cantore G. Medulloblastoma in pediatric age: a single-institution review of prognostic factors. Childs Nerv Syst 1995;11:80–85.
104. Cortes J, Kantarjian H, O'Brien S, et al. Result of interferon-alpha therapy in patients with chronic myelogenous leukemia 60 years of age and older. Am J Med 1996;100(4): 452–455.
105. Asai A, Matsutani M, Kohno T, et al. Subacute brain atrophy after radiation therapy for malignant brain tumor. Cancer 1989;63(10):1962–1974.
106. Stylopoulos LA, George AE, de Leon MJ, et al. Longitudinal CT study of parenchymal brain changes in glioma survivors. AJNR 1988;9(3):517–522.
107. Trojanowski T, Peszynski J, Turowski K. Quality of survival of patients with brain gliomas treated with post-operative CCNU and radiation therapy. J Neurosurg 1989;70:18–23.

108. Maire JP, Coudin B, Guerin J, et al. Neuropsychologic impairment in adults with brain tumors. Am J Clin Oncol 1987;10(2):156–162.
109. Diller LH. The run on Ritalin: attention deficit disorder and stimulant treatment in the 1990s. Hastings Cent Rep 1996;26:12–18.
110. Seeman PMBK. Anti-hyperactivity medication: methylphenidate and amphetamine. Mol Psychiatr 1998;3: 386–396.
111. Challman TDL JJ, Methylphenidate: its pharmacology and uses. Mayo Clin Proc 2000;75(7):711–721.
112. Volkow ND, Wang GJ, Gatley SJ, et al. Temporal relationships between the pharmacokinetics of methylphenidate in the human brain and its behavioral and cardiovascular effects. Psychopharmacology (Berl) 1996;123:26–33.
113. Meyers CA, Weitzner MA, Valentine AD, et al. Methylphenidate therapy improves cognition, mood, and function of brain tumor patients. J Clin Oncol 1998;16(7):2522–2527.
114. Spiegel D. Cancer and depression. Br J Psychiatry Suppl 1996(30):109–116.
115. Irle E, Peper M, Wowra B, et al. Mood changes after surgery for tumors of the cerebral cortex. Arch Neurol 1994;51(2):164–174.
116. Hecaen H. Clinical symptomatology in right and left hemisphere lesions. In: Mountcastle VB, ed. Interhemispheric relations and cerebral dominance in man. Baltimore, MD: Johns Hopkins University Press, 1962;215–243.
117. Heilman KM, Bowers D, Valenstein E. Emotional disorders associated with neurological diseases. In: Heilman KM, Valenstein E, eds. Clinical neuropsychology. New York: Oxford University Press, 1993;461–497.
118. Price BH, Mesulam M. Psychiatric manifestations of right hemisphere infarctions. J Nerv Ment Dis 1985;173:610– 614.
119. Mechanick JI, Hochberg FH, LaRocque A. Hypothalamic dysfunction following whole-brain irradiation. J Neurosurg 1986;65(4):490–494.
120. Weitzner MA. Psychosocial and neuropsychiatric aspects of patients with primary brain tumors. Cancer Invest 1999;17(4):285–291; discussion 296–297.
121. Barclay LL, Blass JP, Lee RE. Cerebral metastases mimicking depression in a "forgetful" attorney. J Am Geriatr Soc 1984;32(11):866–867.
122. Burton M, Parker R. Psychological aspects of cancer surgery: surgeon's attitudes and opinions. Psychooncology 1997;6:47–64.
123. Anderson SI, Taylor R, Whittle IR. Mood disorders in patients after treatment for primary intracranial tumours. Br J Neurosurg 1999;13(5):480–485.
124. Ziemer MM. Effects of information on postsurgical coping. Nurs Res 1983;32(5):282–287.
125. Gainotti G, Antonucci G, Marra C, et al. Relation between depression after stroke, antidepressant therapy, and functional recovery. J Neurol Neurosurg Psychiatry 2001;71(2): 258–261.
126. Berg A, Palomaki H, Lehtihalmes M, et al. Poststroke depression in acute phase after stroke. Cerebrovasc Dis 2001;12(1):14–20.
127. D'Antonio LL, Long SA, Zimmerman GJ, et al. Relationship between quality of life and depression in patients with head and neck cancer. Laryngoscope 1998;108(6): 806–811.
128. Barge-Schaapveld DQ, Nicolson NA, Berkhof J, et al. Quality of life in depression: daily life determinants and variability. Psychiatr Res 1999;88(3):173–189.
129. Dodd MJ, Dibble S, Miaskowski C, et al. A comparison of the affective state and quality of life of chemotherapy patients who do and do not develop chemotherapy-induced oral mucositis. J Pain Symptom Manage 2001;21(6):498–505.
130. Skarstein J, Aass N, Fossa SD, et al. Anxiety and depression in cancer patients: relation between the Hospital Anxiety and Depression Scale and the European Organization for Research and Treatment of Cancer Core Quality of Life Questionnaire. J Psychosom Res 2000;49(1):27–34.
131. Weitzner MA, Meyers CA, Stuebing KK, et al. Relationship between quality of life and mood in long-term survivors of breast cancer treated with mastectomy. Support Care Cancer 1997;5(3):241–248.
132. Pelletier G, Verhoef MJ, Khatri N, et al. Quality of life in brain tumor patients: the relative contributions of depression, fatigue, emotional distress, and existential issues. J Neurooncol 2002;57(1):41–49.
133. Nezu AM, Nezu CM, Friedman SH, et al. Helping cancer patients cope: a problem solving approach. Washington, DC: American Psychological Association, 1998.
134. Cohen L, de Moor C, Amato RJ. The association between treatment-specific optimism and depressive symptomatology in patients enrolled in a phase I cancer clinical trial. Cancer 2001;91(10):1949–1955.
135. Baker F, Curbow B, Wingard JR. Role retention and quality of life of bone marrow transplant survivors. Soc Sci Med 1991;32(6):697–704.
136. Kowalczuk A, Macdonald RL, Amidei C, et al. Quantitative imaging study of extent of surgical resection and prognosis of malignant astrocytomas [see comments]. Neurosurgery 1997;41(5):1028–1036; discussion 1036–1038.
137. Andreou J, George AE, Wise A, et al. CT prognostic criteria of survival after malignant glioma surgery. AJNR 1983;4(3):488–490.
138. Anonymous. Medical Research Council Brain Tumour Working Party: prognostic factors for high-grade malignant glioma: development of a prognostic index. J Neurooncol 1990;9:47–55.
139. Cohadon F, Aouad N, Rougier A, et al. Histologic and non-histologic factors correlated with survival time in supratentorial astrocytic tumors. J Neurooncol 1985;3(2):105–111.
140. Duncan GG, Goodman GB, Ludgate CM, et al. The treatment of adult supratentorial high grade astrocytomas. J Neurooncol 1992;13(1):63–72.
141. Fischbach AJ, Martz KL, Nelson JS, et al. Long-term survival in treated anaplastic astrocytomas. A report of combined RTOG/ECOG studies. Am J Clin Oncol 1991;14(5): 365–370.
142. Ganju V, Jenkins RB, O'Fallon JR, et al. Prognostic factors in gliomas. A multivariate analysis of clinical, pathologic, flow cytometric, cytogenetic, and molecular markers. Cancer 1994;74(3):920–927.
143. Halperin EC, Herndon J, Schold SC, et al. A phase III randomized prospective trial of external beam radiotherapy, mitomycin C, carmustine, and 6-mercaptopurine for the treatment of adults with anaplastic glioma of the brain. CNS Cancer Consortium. Int J Radiat Oncol Biol Phys 1996;34(4):793–802.

144. Kinsella TJ, Collins J, Rowland J, et al. Pharmacology and phase I/II study of continuous intravenous infusions of iododeoxyuridine and hyperfractionated radiotherapy in patients with glioblastoma multiforme. J Clin Oncol 1988;6(5):871–879.
145. Miller PJ, Hassanein RS, Giri PG, et al. Univariate and multivariate statistical analysis of high-grade gliomas: the relationship of radiation dose and other prognostic factors. Int J Radiat Oncol Biol Phys 1990;19(2):275–280.
146. Nazzaro JM, Neuwelt EA. The role of surgery in the management of supratentorial intermediate and high-grade astrocytomas in adults [see comments]. J Neurosurg 1990;73(3):331–344.
147. Prados MD, Gutin PH, Phillips TL, et al. Highly anaplastic astrocytoma: a review of 357 patients treated between 1977 and 1989. Int J Radiat Oncol Biol Phys 1992;23(1):3–8.
148. Quigley MR, Maroon JC. The relationship between survival and the extent of the resection in patients with supratentorial malignant gliomas. Neurosurgery 1991;29(3):385–388; discussion 388–389.
149. Watne K, Hannisdal E, Nome O, et al. Prognostic factors in malignant gliomas with special reference to intra-arterial chemotherapy. Acta Oncol 1993;32(3):307–310.
150. Weir B. The relative significance of factors affecting postoperative survival in astrocytomas, grades 3 and 4. J Neurosurg 1973;38(4):448–452.
151. Wood JR, Green SB, Shapiro WR. The prognostic importance of tumor size in malignant gliomas: a computed tomographic scan study by the Brain Tumor Cooperative Group. J Clin Oncol 1988;6(2):338–343.
152. Diener-West M, Dobbins TW, Phillips TL, et al. Identification of an optimal subgroup for treatment evaluation of patients with brain metastases using RTOG study 7916. Int J Radiat Oncol Biol Phys 1989;16(3):669–673.
153. Peyser JM, Rao SM, LaRocca NG, et al. Guidelines for neuropsychological research in multiple sclerosis. Arch Neurol 1990;47(1):94–97.
154. Jelic V, Johansson SE, Almkvist O, et al. Quantitative electroencephalography in mild cognitive impairment: longitudinal changes and possible prediction of Alzheimer's disease. Neurobiol Aging 2000;21(4):533–540.
155. Murray KJ, Scott C, Zachariah B, et al. Importance of the mini-mental status examination in the treatment of patients with brain metastases: a report from the Radiation Therapy Oncology Group protocol 91–04. Int J Radiat Oncol Biol Phys 2000;48(1):59–64.
156. Meyers CA, Mehta MP, Rodrigus P, et al. Motexafin gadolinium (MGD) delays neurocognitive progression in patients with brain metastases from lung cancer: results of a randomized phase III trial. Neuro-oncol 2002;4:372.
157. Pignatti F, van den Bent M, Curran D, et al. Prognostic factors for survival in adult patients with cerebral low-grade glioma. J Clin Oncol 2002;20(8):2076–2084.
158. Armstrong CL, Goldstein B, Shera D, et al. The predictive value of longitudinal neuropsychologic assessment in the early detection of brain tumor recurrence. Cancer 2003; 97(3):649–656.
159. Meyers CA, Smith JA, Bezjak A, et al. Neurocognitive function and progression in patients with brain metastases treated with whole-brain radiation and motexafin gadolinium: results of a randomized phase III trial. J Clin Oncol 2004;22(1):157–165.
160. Loberiza FR Jr, Rizzo JD, Bredeson CN, et al. Association of depressive syndrome and early deaths among patients after stem-cell transplantation for malignant diseases. J Clin Oncol 2002;20(8):2118–2126.
161. DiMatteo MR, Lepper HS, Croghan TW. Depression is a risk factor for noncompliance with medical treatment: meta-analysis of the effects of anxiety and depression on patient adherence. Arch Intern Med 2000;160(14): 2101–2107.
162. Capuron L, Ravaud A, Gualde N, et al. Association between immune activation and early depressive symptoms in cancer patients treated with interleukin-2-based therapy. Psychoneuroendocrinology 2001;26(8):797–808.
163. Tashiro M, Itoh M, Kubota K, et al. Relationship between trait anxiety, brain activity and natural killer cell activity in cancer patients: a preliminary PET study. Psychooncology 2001;10(6):541– 546.
164. Walker LG, Heys SD, Walker MB, et al. Psychological factors can predict the response to primary chemotherapy in patients with locally advanced breast cancer. Eur J Cancer 1999;35(13):1783–1788.
165. Dancey J, Zee B, Osoba D, et al. Quality of life scores: an independent prognostic variable in a general population of cancer patients receiving chemotherapy. The National Cancer Institute of Canada Clinical Trials Group. Qual Life Res 1997;6(2):151–158.
166. BTPRG. Report of the Brain Tumor Progress Review Group (BTPRG). Baltimore, MD: National Institutes of Health, 2000.
167. Deen HG. Outcomes research: a review [letter; comment]. Neurosurgery 1999;44(4):919–920.
168. Haines SJ, Olson NO. An agenda for clinical research in neurosurgery. Chicago: Congress of Neurological Surgeons, 1997:5–9.
169. Gerszten PC. Outcomes research: a review [see comments]. Neurosurgery 1998;43(5):1146–1156.
170. Yasargil MG. A legacy of microneurosurgery: memoirs, lessons, and axioms. Neurosurgery 1999;45(5):1025–1092.
171. Liang MH, Andersson G, Bombardier C, et al. Strategies for outcome research in spinal disorders. An introduction. Spine 1994;19(Suppl 18):2037S–2040S.
172. Foley KM, Gelband H. Improving palliative care for cancer. Washington, DC: National Cancer Policy Board, Institute of Medicine and National Research Council, 2001:64.
173. Feinstein AR. On classifying cancers while treating patients [editorial]. Arch Intern Med 1985;145(10):1789–1791.
174. Deyo RA, Andersson G, Bombardier C, et al. Outcome measures for studying patients with low back pain. Spine 1994;19(Suppl 18):2032S–2036S.
175. Bezjak A, Taylor KM, Ng P, et al. Quality-of-life information and clinical practice: the oncologist's perspective. Cancer Prevent Control 1998;2(5):230–235.

CHAPTER 11

Clinical Trial Design in Neuro-Oncology

Judith R. O'Fallon / Jan C. Buckner

Although observational studies based on databanks and case series gleaned from medical records can provide useful information for developing hypotheses about therapeutic performance and disease processes, only clinical trials can provide solid evidence to address these hypotheses scientifically. This chapter outlines sound principles of clinical trial development, presenting the perspectives of both the clinical researcher and the statistician. Although the issues discussed are relevant to clinical research in general, we also highlight design considerations that are unique to neuro-oncology research.

▶ BASIC CONCEPTS AND DEFINITIONS

The following three definitions form the basis for our discussion:

- A clinical trial is a planned experiment to study human beings forward in time (i.e., prospectively) to gain information about the behavior of disease processes and/or treatments.
- For clinical trial purposes, the term *treatment* includes the use of single-modality therapies (e.g., surgery, radiation therapy, chemotherapy, hormonal therapy, vaccination), multimodality regimens, placebos, and careful observation without any sort of therapeutic intervention.
- Because clinical trials are planned experiments, they require protocols. A protocol is a written document that carefully (a) defines the study goals, (b) defines the end points and analyses to be used to measure those goals, (c) specifies the patient population(s) to be studied, and (d) describes in detail the procedures to be used to conduct the investigation in a scientifically sound manner.

Basic Concepts

Consent Form

Because the study subjects are human beings, clinical trials are highly regulated. In particular, every study subject (or his or her guardian) must sign a consent form that fully describes in lay language the key components of the trial before the subject can participate in the trial.

Trial Oversight

The design and conduct of the trial itself must be carefully monitored from initial protocol development until the last patient enrolled in the trial has completed the study requirements. Such monitoring is usually performed by pertinent government agencies, funding sources, Institutional Review Boards at the sites where patients are enrolled, and appropriately constituted Data Monitoring Committees (DMCs).

Data Monitoring Committee

Regulations now require that most clinical trials be monitored by suitably constituted DMCs while patients are being accrued, treated, and evaluated. DMCs are responsible for safeguarding the rights of patients and preserving study integrity and credibility. Specific DMC duties are to (a) provide ethical and scientific support for trial goals and design and (b) make definitive recommendations to trial sponsor(s) about decisions affecting trial conduct, such as whether to stop the trial early or make crucial design changes. Essentially, DMCs must balance responsibilities toward three groups of patients: patients now in the trial, patients who will enroll in the trial in the future, and patients outside the trial whose treatment at some future time will be influenced by the results of this clinical trial. To meet their responsibilities appropriately, the DMC for a given trial or set of related trials must (a) include representatives of all relevant disciplines involved in the trial(s); (b) exclude personnel with substantial conflicts of interest, be they financial, scientific, or regulatory; and (c) periodically review and thoroughly discuss detailed status reports based on clean, complete, current data for each trial.

Clinical Study Team

Clinical trials are generally complex studies, often addressing multiple research questions and involving multimodality treatments. Thus, they usually require regular input from investigators with several types of expertise (e.g., different medical and laboratory specialties). Moreover, clinical trials may require long periods of time to complete. Therefore, to provide dependable, consistent leadership, a *study team* is needed to design, conduct, analyze, and report each clinical trial appropriately.

- The study team for a clinical trial is the group of investigators with overall responsibility for the trial who collectively possess the key areas of expert knowledge (e.g., medical specialties, laboratory specialties, biostatistics, epidemiology) required to design, conduct, analyze, and report the trial appropriately.
- The *principal investigator* (PI) is the leader of the study team.

Site Principal Investigator

Clinical trials are necessarily collaborative studies as they rarely can be performed properly and completed in timely fashion by one clinician working alone. Medical personnel who enroll patients in the trial must be able to treat and evaluate their patients whenever they return according to defined schedules specified by protocol. To do so generally requires the participation of a medical team at the site to provide appropriate backup. Furthermore, patient accrual generally cannot be completed in timely fashion unless several medical investigators—often at diverse sites—participate in the accrual process. Thus, multisite clinical trials require a principal investigator at each site.

- The site PI for a given site is the leader of the medical team at that site who takes primary responsibility for insuring that the trial is conducted properly at that site.

▶ TYPES OF CLINICAL TRIALS

There are six major types of clinical trials conducted in clinical settings:

- *Observational trials*, which are designed to describe interesting features of a disease or treatment, for example, the natural history of a disease or condition or the pharmacokinetics or other physiologic effects of a treatment in the body.
- *Phase I trials*, which are designed to determine appropriate dose levels of new treatments, characterize adverse events patterns, and obtain preliminary evidence of therapeutic activity.
- *Pilot trials*, which are small trials designed to assess the tolerability and/or feasibility of a previously evaluated treatment prior to its widespread use in a specified group of patients.
- *Phase II trials*, which are designed to characterize—but not to compare—specific outcomes in one or more patient groups and decide whether the treatment administered to a given group merits further study in subsequent trials.
- *Phase III trials*, which are designed to compare specific outcomes in two or more patient groups.
- *Phase IV trials*, which are large studies performed after a therapy has been approved for marketing in order to assess more precisely the efficacy and adverse events profile in the overall population treated.

▶ ESSENTIAL ELEMENTS OF CLINICAL TRIAL DESIGN

Well-designed clinical trials require careful attention to several issues: (a) one or more clinically and scientifically important question(s); (b) sound rationale supported by preclinical and clinical observations; (c) precisely stated study goals; (d) end points appropriate to assess the study goals; (e) carefully chosen and well-defined patient population(s) to be studied; (f) well-designed interventions that minimize risk to patient and maximize likelihood of therapeutic benefits; and (g) a statistical design appropriate for the goals.

Significance of the Question

Regardless of the design of a clinical trial, if the question being asked is neither clinically nor scientifically important or interesting, the study will not be useful. Although it may appear self-evident that only important questions should be addressed, it is worth stating explicitly. Given the multitude of potential questions to be addressed, and the limited subject and infrastructure resources, prioritization of concepts to be developed is a key feature of successful clinical trial design. Often prioritization may be difficult, given competing interests among involved parties including patients, clinical investigators, laboratory collaborators, and governmental and industry interests. Consequently, choosing the appropriate question to be addressed, taking into consideration the interests of all parties, may well be the most important factor determining the success of the trial.

Scientific Rationale

Once the scientific question has been defined, it is important to examine carefully the scientific rationale for the proposed study. The background section of the protocol sets the stage for all that follows. Careful review of literature of published reports relevant to the study question, exposition of preliminary unpublished data, and logical explanation of theoretical and laboratory or clinical extrapolations constitute the essential rationale for both the clinical and translational study goals to be addressed. Both supporting data and contradictory data relevant to the study goals should be included with explanations of the reasons for going forward with the trial in the face of known or potential contraindications. Often, preparations of the background section of a protocol will require multidisciplinary input from the relevant clinical disciplines involved in the protocol, as well as collaborators from laboratories, epidemiology, and social sciences. Describing the strengths and weaknesses of the planned study assures that the subsequent detailed trial design is adequate to address design concerns.

Study Goals

The study goals should flow naturally from the background section of the protocol. There is usually a primary study goal that states the overarching reason for proceeding with the trial. This goal defines the essential reason to do the study. There may also be one or more secondary goals that provide supportive and ancillary information important in the interpretation of the primary goal or important information to obtain in order to generate hypotheses for future trials. For example, if the primary goal is to determine the benefit of a particular novel therapeutic intervention, the secondary goals may be to assess the toxicities of that intervention, the impact of the intervention on quality of life, the association of tumor tissue or serum markers of the disease with outcomes to be observed in the trial, or physiologic consequences of the intervention on the tumor or normal physiologic parameters.

Study goals must be precisely stated because they uniquely determine the type of clinical trial to be performed and identify appropriate end points and study designs for the trial. The following statements are too vague to convey precisely what the study team wishes to do: "To compare treatment A versus treatment B" and "To assess the activity of treatment A." More detailed statements such as "To compare survival distributions in patients who are treated with treatment A versus treatment B" and "To assess the objective response rate and adverse event patterns in patients treated with treatment A" convey vital information about the intended purpose(s) of the trial.

Study goals uniquely identify the appropriate type of clinical trial for the study. For example: If the goal is "to determine a safe and tolerable treatment combination of radiotherapy + agent X," a phase I trial is needed. If the goal is "to assess the response rate and adverse event patterns of regimen A and to decide whether it merits further study," a phase II trial is needed. If the goal is "to compare the survival distributions of patients treated with regimen A versus regimen B," a phase III trial is needed.

End Points

Several end points may be appropriate to address a specific study goal. For example, phase I trials evaluating cytotoxic agents often use the three end points of maximum tolerated dose, dose-limiting toxicity, and response rate, whereas phase I trials evaluating cytostatic agents may use time-to-disease-progression and/or changes in relevant biologic processes such as target molecule concentrations. Similarly, phase II and phase III trials may assess efficacy using relevant clinical end points or surrogate end points.

Clinical Versus Surrogate End Points

These end points are defined as follows:

- *Clinical end points* are measures of the patient's length or quality of life, for example, survival, disease-free survival, incidence of disease progression or recurrence, or performance scores, cognitive function scores, quality of life scores, at specific points in time following start of treatment.
- *Surrogate end points* measure short-term changes in biologic activity such as response (e.g., tumor shrinkage) or changes in laboratory or physical measures of relevant biologic processes.

In general, patients and their physicians tend to assess therapeutic efficacy using clinical end points such as longer survival, improved cognitive function, or improved quality of life. Nonetheless, surrogate end points are often chosen as the primary end point for trials because they are expected to reduce the sample size and/or the trial duration and hence reduce the cost of the trial. However, surrogate end points often give misleading or incorrect answers. There are several reasons for this unfortunate fact, including (a) biologic processes are imperfectly measured by surrogates; (b) prognosis may depend on other biologic processes besides the one of primary interest; (c) most treatments have many mechanisms of action; and (d) treatments may be chosen for study based on expected effects upon the surrogate.[1]

The Cardiac Arrhythmia Suppression Trial reported in 1991[2] provides a notorious example of surrogate end point problems. This randomized, double-blind, placebo-controlled trial in patients who had recently experienced a myocardial infarction was designed to assess the efficacy of two agents (encainide and flecainide) that had been shown to reduce ventricular arrhythmias, a well-known risk factor for sudden death in cardiac patients. The primary study goal was to determine whether either agent reduced the incidence of death as a consequence of arrhythmia compared with placebo. The agents were chosen for study based on prior information about their beneficial effects on a surrogate end point, that is, ventricular arrhythmias, whereas the primary study goal was defined to be a clinical end point, that is, death or cardiac arrest as a consequence of arrhythmia. When 1500 patients had been enrolled in the trial, the independent DMC for the trial recommended that both drugs be discontinued because interim analyses revealed that the death rates in both drug groups were more than double those of their respective placebo groups and that the rates of death or cardiac arrest as a consequence of arrhythmias were nearly triple the placebo rates. Thus, observed beneficial effects on the surrogate end point not only failed to translate into clinical benefits, but the treatment may actually have been harmful as measured by the clinical end point of postinfarction survival.

Choosing End Points for Neuro-Oncology Trials

In phase II trials, the usual goals are to screen for clinical activity in a defined group of patients and to assess the toxicities of that therapeutic intervention in a specified target group of patients. Potential end points include response rate as assessed by either neuroimaging modalities or clinical evaluations, or both; and event-time measures such as time to progression (TTP), progression-free survival (PFS), and overall survival. The choice of the end point is often determined by the nature of the intervention and by the patient population under study.

Response or Regression Rates

Definition

The response "rate" is the percentage of all patients receiving the intervention who experience a "successful outcome," as defined by protocol. In neuro-oncology, "successful outcome" often means that there is imaging evidence of benefit.

Imaging Issues

The criteria defined by Macdonald and associates are the most commonly used.[3] Simply stated, neuroimaging must demonstrate at least a 50% reduction in the product of perpendicular diameters of a contrast-enhancing mass using computed tomography (CT) or magnetic resonance imaging (MRI) scans compared with baseline in order to consider the treatment a success. More recently, the National Cancer Institute proposed that a 30% reduction in the largest single diameter of the contrast-enhancing mass is appropriate to consider the treatment a success.[4] The study that assessed the performance of these criteria, called RECIST (Response Evaluation Criteria in Solid Tumors) involved the evaluation of only 31 brain tumor patients. Therefore, Galanis and associates[5] performed a study to compare several strategies for measuring success using scan measurements in nearly 100 brain tumor patients. This study confirmed that the unidimensional measurement of contrast-enhancement is as good as bidimensional measurement, confirming the initial claims for RECIST. These criteria provide a useful starting point for assessing benefits.

There are some limitations to the use of either RECIST or the Macdonald criteria in brain tumors, however. For example, the criteria take into account only contrast-enhancing portions of the tumor. It is well-known that tumor cells extend well beyond the contrast-enhancing component apparent on a CT or MRI scan. Consequently, there could be improvement in nonenhancing portions of the tumor as reflected in decreasing T_2-signal abnormality on an MRI scan or decreased mass effect while there is minimal change in the contrast-enhancing mass. Conversely, there could be reduction in the contrast enhancement, representing improvement in blood–brain barrier breakdown, without any impact upon non–contrast-enhancing tumor cells. The Galanis study could not confirm the reliability of changes in contrast-enhancement volume, but changes in T_2-signal area and volume appear to be reliable predictors of outcome. While these theoretical problems may not materialize, it is certainly possible in the advent of new targeted therapies that imaging assessment by conventional criteria may be insufficient to determine benefits of therapy. Similarly, other imaging techniques such as positron emission tomography (PET), magnetic resonance spectroscopy, dynamic contrast enhancement, and measures of cerebral blood flow by MRI may provide new methods of assessing the benefit of interventions.

The clinical utility of these methods is still undergoing refinement at the present time.

Factors Affecting Response Rates

The assessment of response rate is also complicated by factors other than the treatment intervention. For example, corticosteroids are known to reduce T_2-signal abnormality and the extent of contrast enhancement on MRI.[6] Consequently, a well-designed trial in which response rate or evidence of tumor progression as assessed by neuroimaging modalities will account for this variable in some manner. If it is possible to maintain patients on a stable dose of corticosteroids 1 to 2 weeks prior to the baseline scan and to monitor corticosteroid usage throughout the course of the trial, interpretation of changes on neuroimaging studies will be more reliable.

Distinguishing tumor shrinkage or growth from surgical changes and radiation effects is a major consideration in assessing interventions using methods that depend upon interpretation of radiographic changes. Surgical changes may occur in the few days following surgical intervention and may persist for months.[7] Consequently, stating in the protocol the manner in which surgical changes may impact the end point will be important. Moreover, delayed radiation effects may mimic tumor progression. Those effects may subside spontaneously over time, without intervention. Figure 11-1 demonstrates one such case of delayed radiation effect, which resolved spontaneously without any intervention. At the present time, there is no foolproof technology that can discern late radiation changes from tumor progression. Thus, radiation effects may lead the investigator to conclude the

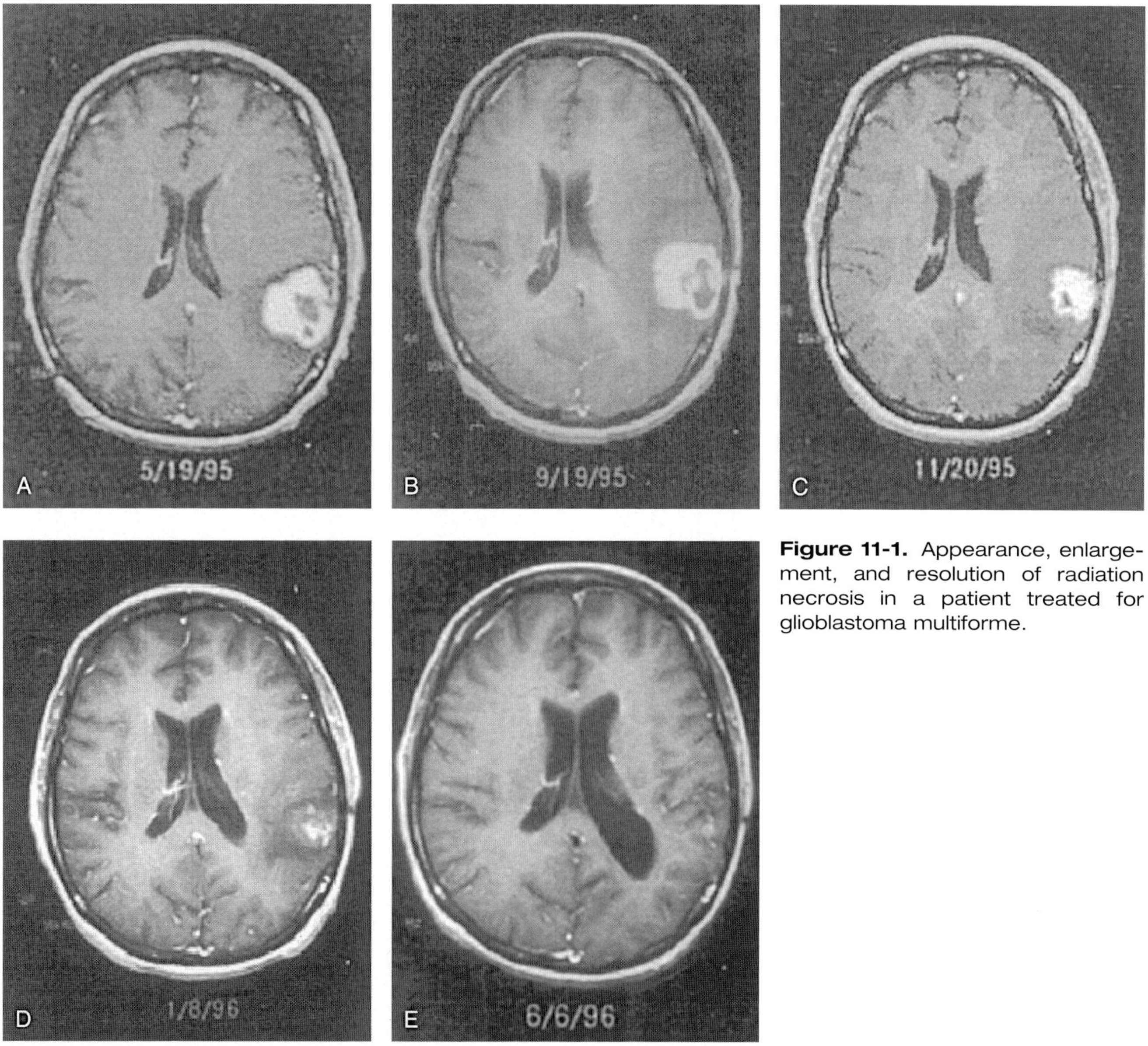

Figure 11-1. Appearance, enlargement, and resolution of radiation necrosis in a patient treated for glioblastoma multiforme.

intervention is either ineffective or effective when in reality the patient may not have experienced any impact of the intervention whatsoever. The frequency of this phenomenon is not clear, but even if it were in the range of 5% to 15% of patients, given the response rate to many current agents, this magnitude of variability could confound interpretation of clinical trial results.

Scan technique may also impact response rate as an end point. For example, if patients sequentially undergo different types of imaging such as CT or MRI, interpretation of results may be difficult. Thus, maintaining the same scanning technique throughout the protocol improves the confidence in the results. Moreover, there may be interobserver variability in scan interpretation. For example, in one trial assessing the impact of procarbazine, 1,3-*cis*(2-chloroethyl)-1-nitrosourea (CCNU), and vincristine in low-grade glioma patients, there is a significant discordance between the interpretation of benefit as assessed by the clinician and the neuroradiology reviewer.[8] In this example, there is good concordance in interpreting differences in contrast enhancement, but relatively poor concordance between clinicians and neuroradiologists in assessing changes in T_2-signal abnormality changes. Consequently, prospective standards for quality control of scan interpretation enhance the value of a trial in which radiographic end points are used to assess either tumor shrinkage or tumor growth.

Event-Time Variables

Time to Progression and Progression-Free Survival

Many of the factors that affect interpretation of response rate as an end point also affect the time to progression and progression-free survival end points, whenever progression is defined by radiographic results.

- *Time to progression* is the time from the date that study therapy started until the date that evidence of progression is documented.
- *Progression-free survival* is the time from the date that study therapy started until the last date when there is documented evidence that progression has not occurred.
- PFS at a specific point in time is a yes/no variable that is scored "yes" if the patient has documented evidence that progression has not occurred at that time point and "no" otherwise. For example, PFS at 6 months measures the proportion of patients who had documented evidence that their disease had not worsened during the 6 months after starting protocol intervention.

Both TTP and PFS may be affected by frequency of observation, nontreatment variables largely related to inherent biologic variability among patients within the study, missing or censored data, and imaging interpretation. For example, both TTP and PFS can be estimated more precisely when scans are obtained every 2 months rather than every 4 months. Such small differences may or may not be important clinically, depending upon the natural history of the disease. In studies in which small differences compared with historical experience are sought, it becomes more important to define the time to progression for each patient most precisely.

Using PFS evaluated at a particular point in time (e.g., 1 year) as an end point may be influenced by exactly the same factors as described as for time to progression. In addition, this measure may not predict the benefits of an intervention at either earlier or later time points. Nevertheless, PFS at a particular point in time may well be an appropriate surrogate for overall survival.[9]

There are several advantages for using TTP or PFS as a primary end point. Because TTP requires agreement on the definition of progression and PFS requires agreement on what is not progression, both depend on imaging techniques to some extent. However, these are less problematic than using the regression end point, which requires agreement on definitions of what constitutes clinically important tumor shrinkage as well as what constitutes tumor progression. In addition, neither TTP nor PFS is affected by therapies administered subsequent to the interventional therapy. In disease settings in which there are clearly beneficial therapies that may be administered subsequent to the interventional therapy, TTP and PFS are most appropriate. In settings in which there are no clearly beneficial therapies to be administered subsequent to the experimental intervention, survival is the most precise and reliable end point.

Survival

- *Survival* is the time from the date that treatment starts until the date of death or, if death has not yet occurred, the most recent date when the person was known to be alive.

Survival as an end point is generally unambiguous, precise, and is not dependent on frequency of observation. Survival may also account both for efficacy and serious toxicities. Consequently, for most phase III trials in neuro-oncology, survival remains an important end point, not only as a primary end point, but also as a secondary one.

Choosing End Points

Defining end points in the clinical trial is extremely important. In the trial illustrated in Fig. 11-2, patients with recurrent glioblastoma multiforme were randomized between temozolomide and procarbazine. Three of the end points—median progression-free survival, 6-month progression-free survival, and 6-month survival—demonstrated statistically significant differences between

End point	*P*-value
6-month PFS	0.008
Median PFS	0.006
6-month survival	0.019
Overall survival	0.330
PR	NS

PR = partial response
NS = not significant
PFS = progression-free survival

Figure 11-2. Variability in significance of end points in a randomized phase II trial of temozolomide versus procarbazine in recurrent glioblastoma multiforme patients.

the two treatment groups. Two end points were not statistically significant, including overall survival and partial response rate. Multivariate analysis identified Karnofsky performance scale (KPS) as the only statistically significant variable associated with progression-free survival, whereas both KPS and age were associated with survival. Treatment was not identified as a variable associated with either progression-free survival or overall survival. One could legitimately interpret these results to favor temozolomide or not to favor temozolomide, depending on one's assessment within the context of the particular clinical trial.[10] Consequently, end point selection is context-specific and must be done carefully, taking into account the patient population to be studied and the intervention to be administered.

Primary Variables

- *Primary variables* are numerical quantities that are used to measure the primary end points.

Frequently, there are several variables that can be used to measure a given end point. The choice of primary variables determines appropriate analyses for the trial and thereby can substantially affect the sample size requirements for the trial. For example, survival, time to progression, and other event-time end points are often measured by either (a) the number of days between the start of treatment and the date when the event occurred or, if it hasn't yet occurred, the date of the most recent followup examination, or (b) a success/failure variable defined to be a "success" if the event has not yet occurred at a specific time point such as 365 days and "failure" if the event occurred before the specified time point, for example, in fewer than 365 days. Continuous event-time variables like the one described in (a) are usually estimated and compared using censored time-to-event methods that include Kaplan-Meier curves and logrank tests, whereas success/failure variables are estimated and compared using binomial methods that include chi-squared tests. Similarly, an adverse event end point can be measured by a yes/no incidence variable or a categorical severity variable scored as, say, ranging from 0 = none to 5 = lethal. Incidence variables are often analyzed using chi-squared tests and other methods developed for binomial variables, whereas severity variables are usually analyzed with Wilcoxon signed-rank tests or other methods suitable for ordered multinomial variables.

There are several issues to be considered when choosing the primary variable for a specific primary goal of the trial. Two key considerations are total sample size and trial duration. The sample size needed to provide an excellent chance to detect clinically meaningful differences in the values of the primary variable between different treatment groups may be substantially larger if a censored event-time variable such as (a) is chosen rather than a binomial variable such as (b). However, if the patient accrual rate is quite rapid and the time-point used to define "success" for a binomial variable such as (b) requires patients to be monitored for several years after treatment starts, then the total duration of the trial may be longer using the binomial variable than a censored event-time variable.

Patient/Subject Selection

It has been said that "selection is the silent partner of success" (source unknown). There may be considerable variability in outcomes among patients with a given disease. In the cases in which sources of the variability are known, accounting for these variables is critical to defining the appropriate population to enter the trial and for subsequent statistical design and analysis. In neuro-oncology these may be patient variables, tumor variables, treatment variables, and time variables.

Prognostic Variables in Brain Tumors

Patient variables that confer a better prognosis in brain tumor patients include younger age, better performance score, and better cognitive performance.[11] Known glioma variables include the histologic diagnosis, including both cell type (e.g., astrocytoma versus oligodendroglioma) and grade (e.g., grade 3 vs. grade 4). Some studies suggest that tumor variables may include tumor size,[12] as well as genetic alterations such as epidermal growth factor receptor (EGFR) amplification or mutation, phosphatase tensin homologue (PTEN) deletion,[13] and 1p and 19q deletions in patients with oligodendroglioma.[14,15] Prior and concurrent treatment variables that might affect outcomes include the extent of surgery, presence or absence of prior radiation therapy, prior radiation dose, corticosteroid use, and the use of concurrent medications, especially enzyme-inducing anticonvulsants.[16] Finally, there may be time variables that are important as well, including the year of the study and duration of disease prior to entering the clinical trial.[17]

Figure 11-3 illustrates the impact of patient selection variables. If one looks at the median survival time and the standard deviation bars, it would appear that the intervention used in protocol 88-72-51 adversely affected patient outcomes, whereas treatment on 86-72-53 was highly successful. In fact, when multiple variable analysis was performed on this large set of recurrent glioma patients enrolled in clinical trials, there was no treatment effect.[17]

Patient condition at the time of trial entry is another baseline factor that can strongly affect trial outcomes. Trials that permit patients in poor condition to be enrolled can lead to the wrong conclusions. For example, if the primary end point will be assessed on scans or specimens taken 3 months after treatment begins, then patients who die within 3 months will necessarily contribute missing values to the primary analysis. Consequently, to achieve the sample size needed to meet design specifications, additional patients will have to be enrolled to replace those who died in less than 3 months. On the other hand, if the primary clinical end point is survival measured by a success/failure variable with success defined to be alive 3 months after start of treatment, then patients who die within 3 months will necessarily be classified as failures. If patients whose life expectancy is clearly less than 3 months are enrolled (perhaps for compassionate reasons), they reduce the success rate for the trial and make the study treatment look worse than it really is.

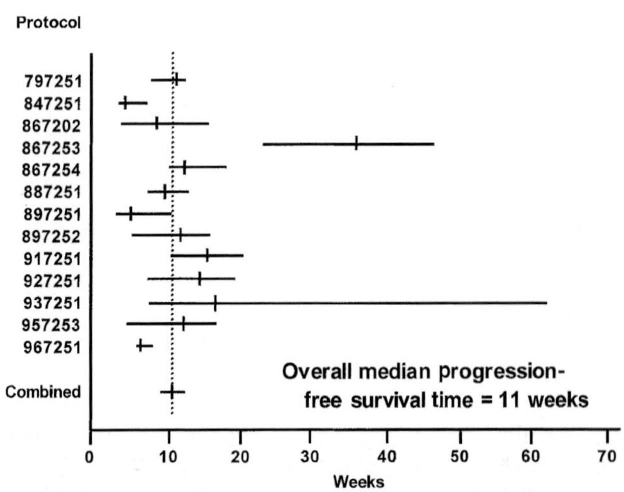

Figure 11-3. Median survival and standard deviation in a series of phase II trials in patients with recurrent glioma.

Broad versus Restrictive Eligibility Criteria

Given the considerations discussed above, there are lively debates in the medical research community about the relative merits of restrictive versus broad eligibility criteria for defining patient populations for trials. With restrictive eligibility criteria, patients who are relatively homogeneous tend to be accrued, whereas with broad criteria, patients who are relatively diverse tend to be accrued. Measurements made on homogeneous groups tend to have less variability than those measured on diverse groups, so primary trial end points can be measured more precisely with smaller sample sizes in homogeneous groups than in diverse groups. On the other hand, the pool of patients who satisfy restrictive eligibility criteria is necessarily smaller than the pool of patients who satisfy broad criteria. Thus, it usually takes more time to accrue homogeneous groups than diverse groups. Moreover, results obtained in homogeneous patient groups may not be considered as generalizable as those obtained in more diverse patient groups.

Statistical Designs

There are several useful designs available for each type of clinical trial, although there may be only one that is suitable for a particular type of primary variable. Historically, different designs have arisen from different strategies used to try to minimize the number of patients exposed to ineffective therapies and to control the chance of obtaining false-positive results whenever (as is customary with clinical trials) the data are analyzed several times during the trial. Each design has performance characteristics that should be carefully considered in choosing the design for a particular trial.

Phase I Designs

Phase I trial designs include (a) the "standard" groups-of-three design, (b) continual reassessment designs based on statistical models, and (c) accelerated titration designs that permit dose escalation within patients. Option (a) is the most cautious of the three types of phase I designs; consequently, it may take a long time to find the "optimum" dose level and may allow many patients to be treated at suboptimal dose levels in the process. Option (b) is likely to find the "optimum" dose level more quickly, that is, using fewer patients, if the assumed model is reasonably correct, but it has a greater chance of treating patients at too-high doses. Option (c) requires fewer patients and ensures that no patient is undertreated, but because its goal is to find the maximum tolerable dose for each patient, it has a greater chance of treating patients at too-high doses.

Phase II Designs

Phase II trial designs include (a) multistage accrual designs that accrue patients in well-defined batches, suspend accrual after each batch is enrolled, and provide rules for using data measured on the enrolled patients to decide whether to accrue the next batch, and (b) one-stage accrual designs that do not suspend accrual but do specify that interim analyses be performed and provide associated stopping rules that permit patient accrual to be promptly stopped if an interim analysis detects strong evidence of excessive toxicity and/or poor or exceptionally good therapeutic activity.

Multistage designs tend to minimize the number of patients needed to achieve the study goals. However, one-stage designs are increasingly favored because they avoid the procedural hassles involved in repeatedly closing and reopening accrual. Furthermore, they can achieve study goals in less time whenever the primary variable is a success/failure variable that requires several months to evaluate because the suspension time between batches for corresponding multistage designs is necessarily lengthy. But if the total accrual goal is likely to be achieved before the first interim analysis can be performed, a one-stage design may not be a wise choice because it cannot reduce the number of patients exposed to the treatment if it proves to be a poor one.

The term *randomized phase II designs* applies not to special designs but to trials that use randomization (see "Randomization and Stratification" below) to allocate patients among two or more independent phase II trials, each of which is designed to assess the efficacy and adverse events profile of a different treatment regimen of interest in a specific patient population. The individual component trials may have any of the phase II designs discussed above. In general, there are too few patients enrolled in each component trial to have much chance to detect clinically interesting differences in outcome among the regimens.

Phase III Designs

Phase III trial designs include (a) single-factor designs that are appropriate whenever the trial has one and only one primary goal and (b) multifactor designs that are appropriate whenever the trial has two or more primary goals.

Single-Factor Designs

Like the phase II designs discussed above, the single-factor phase III designs can be grouped into multistage accrual designs that suspend accrual between batches and single-stage accrual designs that do not suspend accrual but do specify that interim analyses be performed and provide associated stopping rules that permit patient accrual to stop promptly whenever an interim analysis gives sufficiently strong evidence that the primary question has been answered.

Multifactor Designs

The multifactor designs most often used are multiple-comparison designs, factorial designs, and crossover designs.

Multiple-comparison designs are generally used to answer questions about the comparative effectiveness of distinct treatments that cannot be combined, for example, two new separate chemotherapy agents and a placebo or active control. Such designs divide the patients among the treatment groups and perform pairwise comparisons among the groups. For example, to answer the questions, "Does experimental regimen #1 produce better survival than the standard regimen?" and "Does experimental regimen #2 produce better survival than the standard regimen?", a multiple-comparison design divides the patients among three treatment groups (A = experimental regimen #1, B = experimental regimen #2, C = standard) and compares the survival distributions in group A versus group C to answer the first question and compares the survival distributions in group B versus group C to answer the second question.

Factorial designs are used to answer questions about the effectiveness of two or more treatments that can be combined, for example, radiation therapy (RT) and chemotherapy (chemo). Such designs divide the patients among treatment groups consisting of all possible combinations of these treatments and answer each question by comparing suitably pooled groups. For example, to answer the questions, "Does aggressive RT produce better survival than standard RT?" and "Does aggressive chemo produce better survival than standard chemo?", a 2 × 2 factorial design divides the patients among the following four treatment groups: A = standard RT + standard chemo, B = standard RT + aggressive chemo, C = aggressive RT + standard chemo, and D = aggressive RT + aggressive chemo. To answer the RT question, the survival distributions are compared between the standard RT groups (A+B) and the aggressive RT groups (C+D). To answer the chemo question, the survival distributions are compared between the standard chemo groups (A+C) and the aggressive chemo groups (B+D). Factorial designs can provide valuable evidence regarding treatment interactions.

- A *treatment interaction* between two treatments exists whenever the effect of one treatment depends on the level of the other treatment. For example, if aggressive chemo is beneficial in patients receiving standard RT but detrimental in patients receiving aggressive RT, there is a treatment interaction between chemo and RT.

In the absence of treatment interactions, factorial designs are very efficient, permitting two (or three) questions to be answered with half (or a third) of the patients required for separate trials. If treatment interactions are present, however, the results of pooled analyses are very difficult to interpret, and the sample sizes available for unpooled analyses are too small to detect all but very large differences. Thus, choosing factorial designs is a gamble.

Crossover designs require patients to undergo a series of treatments comprising all of the study therapies in the trial. Such designs divide the patients into treatment groups defined by the distinct sequences of the study treatments, administer each of the treatments to each patient for the same length of time in the order specified by the treatment group assignment, and compare treatment effects using the differences in outcomes observed within each patient. For example, if there are three agents (X, Y, and Z) to be assessed in the trial, three treatment periods are needed in order for each patient to receive all three of the agents, and there are six distinct treatment groups defined by the six distinct sequences in which the agents can be administered; that is, XYZ, XZY, YXZ, YZX, ZXY, and ZYX.

Whenever they are appropriate, crossover designs require very small samples because they reduce variability by comparing each patient to him-/herself. Moreover, they are attractive to both patients and physicians because they assure that each patient receives each of the study treatments. However, crossover designs are rarely appropriate in neuro-oncology because they require that (a) none of the treatments can have long-lasting effects, (b) all of the treatments can be administered appropriately in the same length of time, (c) patients must be in relatively stable condition throughout the trial, and (d) patients must be willing and able to finish the entire series of treatments. Patients who drop out before they complete the whole treatment series cannot be used in the final analysis and thereby damage the comparability of the original treatment groups in addition to reducing the sample size substantially. Furthermore, it may be difficult to assure that patients will be in comparable shape at the beginning of each treatment period because there might be period (time) effects (e.g., psychological changes, deterioration as a consequence of disease, "learning curves," increasing unwillingness to cooperate or comply with treatment) or carryover effects from earlier treatment (e.g., "cure," long-lasting improvement, persistent toxic effects).

Randomization and Stratification

There are treatment assignment issues that need to be considered when developing the design for a specific trial. Some trials require treatment groups to be as similar as possible at study entry so that it is valid to conclude that differences in outcome can be attributed to differences in treatment. Phase III trials designed to compare two or more different treatments obviously belong to this class of trials, but so do phase II trials designed to characterize the performance of several different treatments in the same patient population and decide whether any of them is worth future investigation.

Treatment Assignment Issues

Good treatment allocation systems are characterized by the following features: (a) the treatment assignment remains unknown to the patient, attending medical personnel, and all other clinic personnel until it is needed to begin treatment; (b) future assignments cannot be predicted from past assignments; (c) the order of treatment allocations is reproducible; (d) the process provides a clear audit trail; (e) departures from the proper sequence of assignments can be detected; (f) the process used for generating the treatment assignment has known mathematical properties; and (g) methods for generating and administering the assignment schedule are documented.

Treatment groups tend to become dissimilar in important characteristics whenever treatments are chosen by either the patient or the attending physician because their allocation procedures are consciously or unconsciously biased by personal preferences, and these differences among the resulting treatment groups make it difficult to assess differences caused by treatments.

- In general, a *bias* is a tendency to deviate systematically from the truth. Procedures are biased if they introduce systematic error by selecting or encouraging one outcome or answer over others. An estimator is biased if its expected value deviates systematically from the quantity that it is supposed to estimate.

For example, when a clinical trial was designed to compare surgery versus radiation therapy in patients with early-stage breast cancer, most eligible patients insisted on choosing their treatments instead of accepting the results of a randomized treatment allocation process. Because the patients who preferred radiation differed substantially from those who preferred surgery, treatment differences would be difficult to distinguish from the differential effects of prognostic factors in the groups. Thus, the trial had to be abandoned as unfeasible. Similarly, attending physicians have been known to prefer that strong, vigorous patients receive aggressive treatments and fragile patients receive less toxic treatments. With treatment groups unbalanced according to baseline patient condition, distinguishing treatment differences from differences caused by initial patient condition would be difficult.

Consequently, randomization is used to balance the distributions of both known and unknown prognostic factors among treatment arms and thereby to guarantee the validity of statistical tests. In addition, stratification may help to insure that treatment arms are well balanced with respect to important known baseline prognostic factors.

- In clinical trials, *randomization* is a controlled distribution of treatment assignments in such a way as to simulate a random (or chance) distribution and yield unbiased data from which a generalized conclusion can be drawn.
- *Stratification* is a process used to insure that treatment groups are well balanced with respect to specific factors, generally chosen from among the currently recognized baseline prognostic factors.

The major reason for choosing to stratify is that it tends to prevent chance imbalances that can (a) diminish the power of the planned statistical analyses and (b) require sophisticated analysis techniques to overcome, potentially reducing the credibility of the final analyses. The major reasons for choosing not to stratify are (a) the trial is so large that randomization alone provides adequate balance; (b) the prognostic factors are not well known; or (c) the prognostic factors are too complex or too difficult to measure dependably prior to randomization.

Randomization Procedures

There are four types of randomization strategies that are widely used in clinical trials. Each has different advantages and disadvantages.

Unstratified Randomization

The two major types of unstratified randomization are simple unrestricted randomization and random permuted blocks.

- *Simple unrestricted randomization* is an allocation procedure by which each patient has an equal chance of being assigned to each treatment group. Examples include (a) flipping a fair coin to assign the patient to one of two treatment groups and (b) rolling a fair die to assign the patient to one of three or six treatment groups.

Simple unrestricted randomization procedures are simple, easy to use, easy to understand, and unpredictable. However, they can easily produce treatment groups with seriously unequal numbers of patients, thus diminishing the ability of the planned analyses to detect treatment differences of clinical interest. For this reason, the random permuted blocks method is often used instead.

- *Random permuted blocks* denotes an allocation procedure that ensures that the number of patients in every treatment group is exactly the same at key points in the accrual process. This is done by specifying a block size that is a multiple of the number of treatment groups available and then choosing a treatment allocation scheme that insures that all treatment groups get an equal number of patients in each block.

For example, if there are 3 treatment groups in the trial, the block size must be a multiple of 3 (e.g., 3, 6, 9, 12). Using a block size of six will assure that all three treatment groups will have exactly the same number of patients when the 6th, 12th, 18th, and so on, patient has been enrolled. This can be done by randomly assigning the initial patients in the block to treatment groups until two have been assigned to one group, then randomly assigning the remainder in the block of six to the other two treatment groups until another group has two patients, then assigning the rest of the patients in the block to the third group. Random permuted blocks are relatively easy to construct, simple to use, and assure balanced treatment groups, but they can be predictable. Thus, blocks of different sizes should be used, and the pattern of block sizes should be kept secret.

Stratified Randomization

The two major types of stratified randomization are random permuted blocks within strata and dynamic allocation.

- *Random permuted blocks within strata* is a stratified randomization procedure that uses a random permuted blocks procedure to assign treatments to patients classified by strata.

For example, suppose a trial designed to compare three treatment groups has two stratification factors, for example, sex (male vs. female) and age (younger than 40 years vs. 40 to 60 years vs. older than 60 years). These define six distinct strata (young males, young females, middle-aged males, middle-aged females, old males, old females). If the desired block size is three, then the first three patients classified as young males will be divided equally among the three treatment groups in some order, and the next three young males will be divided equally among the treatment groups, usually in a different order, and so on. Similarly, the first three young females will be divided equally among the treatment groups in some order, and the next three young females will be divided equally among the treatment groups, probably in a different order, and so on. Patients classified in each of the remaining four strata will be divided among the three treatment groups in similar fashion.

The random permuted blocks within strata procedure is relatively simple to develop and use, but it can produce treatment groups of substantially unequal sizes whenever there are not enough patients in specific strata to "fill up" a block. Moreover, future treatment assignments may be predictable in some situations. Dynamic allocation constitutes a different approach to stratified randomization.

- *Dynamic allocation* is a stratified randomization procedure designed to assure that all treatment groups have the same distribution of patients with each stratification factor, but it does not assure that the treatment groups have the same number of patients in each of the strata. It uses a relatively simple computational procedure to calculate the treatment assignment for a given patient based on (a) the patient's own stratification factor values, (b) the stratification factor values of all the patients who enrolled in the trial before this patient, and (c) the treatment assignments for all the previously enrolled patients.

For example, for the three-treatment, six-strata example described above, dynamic allocation assures that (a) females comprise 40% of each treatment group if 40% of all patients enrolled in the trial are females and (b) patients younger than age 40 years comprise 25% of each treatment group if 25% of all patients enrolled in the trial are younger than age 40 years, but it will not assure that females younger than age 40 years comprise 15% of each treatment group whenever 15% of all patients enrolled in the trial belong to the young females stratum.

Dynamic allocation produces treatment groups of nearly equal size and assures that they have nearly equal distributions of each stratification factor—even when there are several stratification factors. Its treatment assignments are generally unpredictable and can be calculated quickly with pencil and paper if the total sample size is less than 100. However, manual calculations are rarely necessary because the calculations have been successfully computerized. The major criticism of this method is that it is not a truly random process, except insofar as the stratification factor values of the patients entering the trial tend to occur in unpredictable, random order.

Treatment Blinding/Masking

Another key study design issue is whether to blind (or mask) the treatments.

- *Blinding* or *masking* designates methods used to make the study treatments appear identical so that neither the patient nor his/her medical evaluator knows which treatment the patient is receiving.

The motivation for blinding is to help assure that patient and physician attitudes toward the expected benefits are similar in all treatment groups, thereby minimizing three types of bias: (a) psychological bias on the part of the patient, (b) assessment bias on the part of the medical personnel who evaluate the patient's response to treatment, and (c) treatment management bias on the part of medical personnel who manage the patient's care.

- *Psychological bias* denotes differences in the patient's expectations about the different treatments in the trial that can lead to marked differences in the patient's attitude toward the patient's assigned treatment. For example, patients who expect a new treatment to be more promising than any of the current standard treatments are likely to have positive attitudes if assigned to receive the new treatment, and negative attitudes if assigned to receive a standard treatment; such positive/negative attitudes can influence their physical condition and clinical outcomes.
- *Assessment bias* denotes differences in the medical evaluator's expectations about the different treatments in the trial that can lead to marked differences in his or her evaluation of patient response and adverse events. For example, the evaluator may unconsciously tend to regard small improvements as real if the patient is receiving a treatment that the evaluator expects to be effective but negligible if the patient is receiving a treatment that the evaluator expects to perform poorly.
- *Treatment management bias* denotes differences in attending medical personnel's expectations about the importance of adverse events between treatment groups that can lead to marked differences in the ways that adverse events are managed. For example, patients who present with severe anemia may be hospitalized for aggressive management if they are receiving a new treatment, but may be treated less intensively if they are receiving a standard treatment. Such differences in management could affect patient outcomes.

Pertinent Issues

Several ethical and feasibility issues need to be considered before blinding is chosen for a trial: (a) use of masked treatments should not harm patients or increase their risk; (b) the magnitude and/or severity of bias if masking is not used must be sufficiently large to warrant the added expenses associated with blinding; and (c) blinding may not be feasible. Feasibility of masked administration requires that (a) medical personnel can care for the patient properly without knowing the precise treatment the patient is receiving and (b) all treatment regimens can be given in identical fashion, a requirement that often can be satisfied using placebo medications. For example, if one treatment is a red pill scheduled to be given at mealtimes and the other is a green liquid scheduled to be given before breakfast and at bedtime, then if realistic red placebo pills and green placebo liquid can be produced, it will be possible to administer to each patient both red pills and green liquid on the proper schedule without revealing which contains active agents and which contains placebo agents.

Placebo Control

Still another major design issue is whether to incorporate a placebo control arm into the trial. Placebo control arms may help investigators to assess the amount of benefit that patients experience from a positive attitude. Over the years, placebo-controlled trials have repeatedly demonstrated that even when the treatment is irrelevant (as with placebo controls), the patient's attitude toward his or her illness—and possibly the illness itself—may be improved by a feeling that something is being done about it. Moreover, the power of suggestion should not be underestimated in a large variety of symptomatic conditions.

▶ SAMPLE-SIZE CALCULATIONS

After the study team has made key decisions about study end points, primary variables, and the patient population(s) to be studied, it is ready to calculate the sample size for the trial. Their objective is to determine sample size(s) that can provide sufficiently precise estimates of important population parameters and/or provide adequate power to detect differences of genuine interest in key population parameters without increasing the significance level for the trial above acceptable levels.

Key Concepts

A *population parameter* is a measurable characteristic of the target population. Examples often encountered in clinical trials are the mean and median to measure the central values of the characteristic, the variance and range to measure the spread of its values, and the percentage of its values that are classified as "successes."

A *point estimator* is a numerical measurement that is calculated from a sample and produces a single number that is expected to be close in value to its related population parameter.

A *test* is a numerical procedure for using sample data to decide whether or not to reject a prespecified null hypothesis about a population parameter and thereby accept a prespecified alternative hypothesis about that population parameter.

The *significance level of a test* is the probability that the test will produce a false-positive result, that is, will lead to rejection of the null hypothesis when, in fact, it is true.

The *power of a test* is the probability that the test will produce a true-positive result, that is, will lead to rejection of the null hypothesis when, in fact, the alternative hypothesis is true.

It is important for clinical investigators to realize that the analysis results obtained from a specific clinical trial—that is, the estimates and test values calculated using measurements made on the patients enrolled in that trial—are based on a single sample from the target population and that, if the trial were repeated in the same target population with exactly the same protocol, different results would be obtained because they would be calculated on different samples from the target population. For example, the percentage of "successes" observed in a series of trials conducted with exactly the same protocol in the same target population might range from 5% to 25%. In effect, then, the result of a specific analysis obtained in a specific clinical trial is really only one value in a whole range of values that would be obtained for that analysis if the trial were repeated hundreds of times. One estimator that is frequently used to estimate a range of parameter values that are consistent with the results observed in this specific clinical trial is the confidence interval.

A *95% (or 90% or some other percentage) confidence interval* estimator of a specific population parameter is a range of values calculated in such a way that the probability that it contains the true value of the population parameter is 95% (or 90% or the designated percentage).

Confidence intervals tend to estimate population parameters better than point estimates do because they (a) identify a range of values for the population parameter that are very likely to occur and (b) provide information about the size of the sample used to calculate the confidence interval. There are entertaining classroom exercises that quickly demonstrate that the range of values obtained for a specific measurement such as the sample mean calculated for each of several samples drawn from the target population depends on the size of the sample. Specifically, if the sample size is relatively small (e.g., N = 10), the range of values obtained for the sample mean will be relatively large; but if the sample size is large (e.g., N = 100), the range of values obtained for the sample mean will be much smaller. Therefore, if it is important to obtain a fairly precise estimate of some population parameter, it will be necessary to use a large sample for the trial.

Importance of Appropriate Sample Sizes

Realistic estimates of treatment benefit based on sample sizes large enough to detect the anticipated benefit are critical for assessing a proposed intervention adequately. For example, the benefit of adjuvant therapy in gliomas has remained controversial in part because several initial trials produced inconsistent results based on relatively small numbers of patients that provided only modest chances of detecting the modest benefits to be expected[18,19] from available chemotherapeutic agents. Subsequently, meta-analyses[20,21] were performed using data from several trials to determine if there was evidence of a small but definite benefit from treatment. Both meta-analyses concluded that adjuvant alkylator-based therapy is beneficial.

Calculating Sample Sizes

Sample size calculations for clinical trials depend on the answers to certain specific questions, which must be supplied by the study team.

1. *Estimation question*: "What is the width you want for your confidence interval?"
   - Typical answer: "We'd like to estimate the true (i.e., population) percentage of successes within 10%."
2. *Testing question*: "What is your null hypothesis (H_0), that is, the conclusion that you hope to reject?"
   - Typical answer #1 (single-sample trial): "Currently, the success rate for treatments in this population is 25% or less. We're hoping to show that the success rate for our new treatment is better than that. So H_0 must be that the success rate for the new treatment is 25% or less."
   - Typical answer #2 (comparative trial): "We're hoping to identify a treatment group that has better survival, so H_0 must be that the survival distributions are the same for all the treatment groups."
   - Typical answer #3 (comparative trial): "We're hoping to show that patients who receive our gentler treatment live just as long as or possibly just a bit less than those who receive the tough standard treatment. So our H_0 must be that the survival of patients on the gentler treatment is substantially worse than that of patients on the standard treatment."
3. *Testing question*: "What is your alternative hypothesis (H_A), that is, the conclusion you would like to find if it is true?"
   - Typical answer #1 (single-sample trial): "We want to find out if the success rate for our new treatment is better than 25%. So H_A is that the success rate for our new treatment is more than 25%."
   - Typical answer #2 (comparative trial): "We want to determine which of these current treatments for this disease produces better survival. So H_A is that the survival distributions are significantly different among the treatment groups." This H_A identifies a two-sided superiority trial, that is, a superiority trial with a two-sided alternative hypothesis.
   - A *superiority trial* is a comparative clinical trial designed to determine which treatment is superior.
   - A *two-sided alternative hypothesis* is a statement that the treatments are different without specifying which one is superior.
   - Typical answer #3 (comparative trial): "We want to know if our new treatment produces better survival than the current standard treatment. So H_A is that patients receiving our new treatment live longer than patients receiving the standard treatment." This H_A identifies a one-sided, active-controlled, superiority trial, that is, a superiority trial with a one-sided alternative hypothesis and a standard treatment serving as the active control.
   - A *one-sided alternative hypothesis* is a statement that one specific treatment is superior.
   - Typical answer #4 (comparative trial): "We want to know if our new treatment has any efficacy, that is, is better than placebo treatment. So H_A is that patients receiving our new treatment live longer than patients receiving placebo treatment." This H_A identifies a one-sided, placebo-controlled, superiority trial.
   - Typical answer #5 (comparative trial): "We want to know if the survival curves are about the same for all of the treatment groups. So H_A is that the survival differences among treatment groups are very small." This H_A identifies an equivalence trial.
   - An *equivalence trial* is a comparative clinical trial designed to determine whether the treatments are approximately the same in terms of specific measures of effectiveness and/or adverse events.
   - Typical answer #6 (comparative trial): "We want to know if this kinder, gentler treatment is not too much worse than the tough standard treatment. So H_A is that the survival of patients receiving the gentler new treatment is as good as or perhaps only slightly less than that of patients receiving the standard treatment." This H_A identifies a noninferiority trial.
   - A *noninferiority trial* is a comparative clinical trial designed to determine whether a "nicer" new treatment is as good as or only slightly worse than a standard treatment.

Sample-size calculations depend on H_0, H_A, and several numerical quantities that must be supplied by the study team. In general, there are three that pertain to trials of all types: (a) the minimum difference in values of the primary variable that will be considered clinically meaningful to detect; this quantity helps define H_A more precisely; (b) the desired significance level, that is, the probability of reaching a false-positive conclusion; and (c) the desired power, that is, the probability of reaching a true-positive conclusion when the minimum difference is true. Additionally, if the primary variable (e.g., age) has a bell-shaped distribution, an estimate of its variance is needed for the sample-size calculations. If the primary variable is a censored event-time variable such as survival, estimates of the median survival for one treatment group, the expected accrual time, and the minimum time that all patients will be followed must be specified because the power of the primary analysis in this case depends on the number of deaths observed during the trial, not on the number of patients enrolled in the trial.

It should be noted that the clinically meaningful minimum difference defined above must be much smaller for equivalence and noninferiority trials than for superiority trials because the former are looking for very small differences between the treatments whereas the latter are looking for convincingly large differences. Because it takes much larger sample sizes to detect small differences, equivalence and noninferiority trials necessarily require larger sample sizes than do superiority trials. For example, one national trial (93-72-51) was designed to answer two questions in patients with newly diagnosed glioblastoma: (a) a noninferiority query, "Is the survival of patients who receive a twice-daily RT regimen the same as or not much worse than that of patients who receive standard once-daily RT?" and (b) a superiority query, "Is the survival of patients who receive an aggressive new combination chemotherapy better than that of patients who receive the standard one-agent chemotherapy?" The study team defined the clinically meaningful minimum difference to be a 25% reduction in median survival for the RT question and a 50% increase in median survival for the chemotherapy trial. The resulting sample sizes required to provide approximately 82% power for these tests were 400 patients for the RT question and 200 patients for the chemotherapy question. Therefore, to provide the desired power to answer both questions the total sample size for the trial had to be 400.

The total sample size required for a trial must be large enough to satisfy the desired power and precision specifications for (a) each of the primary goals of the trial and (b) every subset that will be analyzed separately in the final analysis. For example, in evaluating a treatment expected to have greater effect in patients with a specific chromosome abnormality, the study team may wish to assess it separately in patients with and without the abnormality. Moreover, the study team must decide whether to perform the final analysis using the Intent to Treat sample or the Per Protocol subsample.

- The *Intent to Treat sample* (ITT) contains all patients enrolled in the trial (with the possible exception of those who failed to satisfy certain eligibility criteria) and classifies them according to their assigned treatments regardless of errors or compliance problems.
- The *Per Protocol subsample* (PP) contains all eligible patients who were properly enrolled and whose treatment satisfied certain standards and classifies them according to the treatment they actually received.

When PP analyses are performed in phase II and phase III trials, treatment outcomes may appear better than they really are because the patients most likely to fail quickly are often removed from analysis calculations. Moreover, PP analyses compare treatment groups that are no longer truly comparable because the treatment assignments obtained by unbiased randomization procedures have been changed and are likely to reflect patient and/or physician preferences. ITT analyses protect the integrity of the treatment groups. However, in equivalence and noninferiority trials with procedural errors, ITT analyses may lead to incorrect conclusions because substantial treatment differences may be obscured by those procedural errors and thus not be detected.

▶ FEASIBILITY ASSESSMENT

Finally, the study team must assess the feasibility of the trial. To do so, they must estimate the time needed to complete each of the three major phases of clinical trial conduct: (a) accruing patients into all major subsets involved in the final analysis, (b) treating all enrolled patients per protocol specifications, and (c) evaluating all patients and collecting all data required for the final analysis. Study feasibility depends on the estimated total duration of the trial, the financial and personnel costs associated with all three phases, and the available funding. Trials are not feasible if they cost too much money, absorb too many personnel resources, or take so long to complete that all interest in the answers they provide vanishes.

▶ SUMMARY

Clinical trials remain the primary means by which we assess benefits of diagnostic, preventive, and therapeutic strategies in neuro-oncology. They require interdisciplinary participation from the relevant clinical, laboratory, and biostatistical collaborators. Phase I, phase II, and phase III trials each address a series of specific hypotheses to be tested and require designs appropriate to those hypotheses. To be successful, each trial should address a significant question as supported by sound scientific rationale. The study goals should be specific enough to be associated with an appropriate trial design. Selection of appropriate end points to assess the study goals requires an understanding of the disease entity under investigation, as well as the pros and cons of the various end points available to assess the impact of the intervention. In neuro-oncology, it is particularly important to address the strengths and limitations of neuroimaging assessments, including the impact of scan frequency and technique, as well as confounding variables including corticosteroids, prior radiation therapy, and prior surgery. The primary variable selected to assess the primary end point determines the appropriate analysis methods for the trial and so should be chosen carefully. Patient or subject selection can substantively influence—either favorably or unfavorably—the interpretation of trial outcomes. Consequently, careful definition of patient selection criteria is important. The statistical design, including randomization and stratification methods, chosen for the trial is extraordinarily important in defining the sample size for the trial appropriate for detecting scientifically and clinically meaningful results implicit in the statistical design. Additionally, collaboration between the clinical and biostatistical collaborators is critical in addressing the magnitude of clinical benefit that would warrant adoption of a new intervention into clinical practice and defining an acceptable chance that any observed differences will occur as a result of chance alone. Careful sample-size calculations ensure that enough patients will be studied to provide sufficient power to detect the desired amount of benefit. Finally, after the study design is complete, it is important to assess the feasibility of the trial in terms of the financial and personnel costs required to complete the trial.

REFERENCES

1. Fleming TR, DeMets DL. Surrogate endpoints in clinical trials: are we being misled? Ann Intern Med 1996;125:605–613.
2. Echt DS, Liebson PR, Mitchell LB, et al. Mortality and morbidity in patients receiving encainide, flecainide or placebo: the Cardiac Arrhythmia Suppression Trial. N Engl J Med 1991;324:781–788.
3. Macdonald DR, Cascino TL, Schold SC Jr, et al. Response criteria for phase II studies of supratentorial malignant glioma. J Clin Oncol 1990;8(7):1277–1280.
4. Therasse P, Arbuck SG, Eisenhauer EA, et al. New guidelines to evaluate the response to treatment in solid tumors. J Natl Cancer Inst 2000;92(3):205–216.
5. Galanis E, Maurer MJ, Ballman KV, et al. Validation of neuroradiologic response assessment in gliomas: RECIST (1D) vs 2D measurements vs computer-assisted tumor area vs volume [abstract 423]. Cur Proc Am Soc Clin Oncol 2003;22:106.
6. Watling CJ, Lee DH, Macdonald DR, et al. Corticosteroid-induced magnetic resonance imaging changes in patients with recurrent malignant glioma. J Clin Oncol 1994;12(9): 1886–1889.
7. Cairncross JG, Pexman JH, Rathbone MP, et al. Postoperative contrast enhancement in patients with brain tumor. Ann Neurol 1985;17(6):570–572.
8. Buckner JC, Gesme D, O'Fallon JR, et al. Phase II trial of procarbazine, lomustine, and vincristine as initial therapy for patients with low-grade oligodendroglioma or oligoastrocytoma: efficacy and associations with chromosomal abnormalities. J Clin Oncol 2003;21(2):251–255.
9. Hess KR, Wong ET, Jaeckle KA, et al. Response and progression in recurrent malignant glioma. Neuro-oncol 1999; 1(4):282–288.
10. Yung WK, Albright RE, Olson J, et al. A phase II study of temozolomide vs. procarbazine in patients with glioblastoma multiforme at first relapse. Br J Cancer 2000;83(5): 588–593.
11. Buckner JC. Factors influencing survival in high-grade gliomas. Semin Oncol 2003;30(6 Suppl 19):10–14.
12. Pignatti F, van den Bent M, Curran D, et al. Prognostic factors for survival in adult patients with cerebral low-grade glioma. J Clin Oncol 2002;20(8):2076–2084.
13. Smith JS, Tachibana I, Passe SM, et al. PTEN mutation, EGFR amplification and outcome in patients with anaplastic astrocytoma and glioblastoma multiforme. J Natl Cancer Inst 2001;93:1246–1256.
14. Cairncross JG, Ueki K, Zlatescu MC, et al. Specific genetic predictors of chemotherapeutic response and survival in patients with anaplastic oligodendrogliomas. J Natl Cancer Inst 1998;90:1473–1479.
15. Reifenberger J, Reifenberger G, Liu L, et al. Molecular genetic analysis of oligodendroglial tumors shows preferential allelic deletions on 19q and 1p. Am J Pathol 1994; 145:1175–1190.
16. Grossman SA, Hochberg F, Fisher J, et al. Increased 9-aminocamptothecin dose requirements in patients on anticonvulsants. NABTT CNS Consortium. The new approaches to brain tumor therapy. Cancer Chemother Pharmacol 1998;42(2);118–126.
17. Buckner JC, O'Fallon JR, Novotny P, et al. Determinants of time to progression and overall survival of patients in clinical trials for recurrent glioma [abstract 30]. Neuro-oncol 2000;2:276.
18. Walker MD, Alexander E Jr, Hunt WE, et al. Evaluation of BCNU and/or radiotherapy in the treatment of anaplastic gliomas. J Neurosurg 1978;49:333–343.
19. Walker MD, Green SB, Byar DP, et al. Randomized comparisons of radiotherapy and nitrosoureas for the treatment of malignant glioma after surgery. N Engl J Med 1980;303:1323–1329.
20. Fine HA, Dear KBG, Loeffler JS, et al. Meta-analysis of radiation therapy with and without adjuvant chemotherapy for malignant gliomas in adults. Cancer 1993;71: 2585–2597.
21. Stewart LA. Chemotherapy in adult high-grade glioma: a systemic review and meta-analysis of individual patient data from 12 randomised trials. Lancet 2002;359:1011–1018.

CHAPTER 12

The Phakomatoses

DAVID H. GUTMANN / CYNTHIA WETMORE / BRIAN PATRICK O'NEILL

In 1933 van der Hoeve classified five hereditary neurocutaneous conditions as "phakomatoses" (phakos [Gr] = "mother spot") because they were associated with hamartoma formation.[1] Now the term neurocutaneous syndrome *refers collectively to a set of genetically determined disorders that preferentially involve the skin and the nervous system. Eponyms such as von Recklinghausen disease (neurofibromatosis type 1 [NF1]) and Bourneville disease (tuberous sclerosis complex [TSC]) are historically important and their alternative names are sometimes descriptive of their malignant potential (e.g., multiple endocrine neoplasia [MEN]).*

Each of these syndromes has a well-defined genetic abnormality, and, in each case, the responsible gene and gene product has been identified. According to Rust,[1] only those conditions with potential for tumor development should be considered phakomatoses. The phakomatoses' importance far outweighs the impact of their numbers. Tumors of the nervous system typically occur in a sporadic fashion without a preexisting familial predisposition. The genes that are linked to hereditary cancer syndromes are almost invariably important in fundamental cellular processes such as cell division, apoptosis, and DNA repair.[2] Thus, the uncommon tumors that arise in the context of a tumor predisposition syndrome can provide valuable insights into the critical genetic events important for tumorigenesis in the nervous system. Table 12-1 lists the conditions, the genetic abnormality, the gene product, and the associated conditions and neoplasms.

All these disorders share the following commonalities: autosomal dominant inheritance; variable expressivity; spontaneous mutation potential; neurologic disorders; ectodermally derived abnormalities, most commonly skin; and potential for nervous system and, sometimes, systemic malignancies. Furthermore, the degree and rate of evolution are likely influenced by multiple factors such as age, hormonal status, environment, medication, and the state of tissue development.[1] This chapter reviews the most common of these conditions that predispose to nervous system malignancies. Special emphasis is given to those neurocutaneous conditions for which there are robust mouse models. Additionally, two rare neurocutaneous syndromes could be considered phakomatoses. MEN comprises tumors of hormone-producing tissues. MEN type 1 tumors affect mostly the pituitary gland (and parathyroid and pancreas). Neurocutaneous melanosis patients are patients who have large congenital melanocytic nevi (LCMN) and associated leptomeningeal melanocytosis with or without central nervous system melanomas. Conditions that are not strictly phakomatoses (e.g., Li-Fraumeni syndrome and Turcot syndrome) are discussed elsewhere in this volume. For in-depth discussion of these topics the interested reader is referred to references 1 to 7.

▶ **TABLE 12-1.** THE FIVE COMMON PHAKOMATOSES

Syndrome	Gene	Gene Product (Function)	Nervous System Neoplasms
NF1	*NF1* (17q)	Neurofibromin (GTPase-activating protein	Neurofibroma, malignant peripheral nerve sheath tumor, optic glioma
NF2	*NF2* (22q)	Merlin (cytoskeletal protein)	Schwannoma, ependymoma meningioma
TSC	*TSC 1* (9q)	Tuberin (GTPase-activating protein)	Astrocytoma
VHL	*VHL* (3p)	pVHL (modulator of mRNA elongation)	Hemangioblastoma (retina, cerebellum, cord)
NBCCS	*PTCH* (9q)	PTH (developmental regulator)	Medulloblastoma

NBCCS = nevoid basal cell carcinoma syndrome; NF = neurofibromatosis; TSC = tuberous sclerosis complex; VHL = von Hippel-Lindau.

▶ NEUROFIBROMATOSIS TYPES 1 (VON RECKLINGHAUSEN DISEASE) AND 2

Neurofibromatosis type 1 (NF1) and neurofibromatosis type 2 (NF2) are autosomal dominant disorders characterized by an increased susceptibility to both benign and malignant tumors. NF1 is far more common than NF2, estimated to represent more than 75% of all neurofibromatosis cases. The genes responsible for NF1 (neurofibromin) and NF2 (merlin/schwannomin) were identified by positional cloning and encode proteins that function as negative growth regulators. Although there have been studies that suggest differences in the histopathologic appearance of NF-associated and sporadic tumors, there are no conclusive data to support such claims. In general, the tumor types seen in NF1 and NF2 are relatively indistinguishable from those that arise in the general population. Distinguishing features of NF-associated tumors include the number of tumors, the age at presentation, and the clinical context in which they arise.[3,4]

The *NF1* gene on the long arm of chromosome 17 was identified by positional cloning and spans over 350 kilobases (kb) of genomic DNA.[8] The *NF1* gene encodes an mRNA of 11 to 13 kb with at least 60 exons and a protein of 2818 amino acids. Neurofibromin, the 220-kilodalton (kDa) *NF1* gene product, is most abundantly expressed in neurons, oligodendrocytes, and Schwann cells, but is also expressed in astrocytes, leukocytes, and the adrenal medulla.[9] Neurofibromin expression is more widespread during embryonic development, suggesting a role as a negative growth regulator in developing tissues.[10]

Sequence analysis has revealed homology between neurofibromin (exons 20 to 27a) and a family of molecules, termed *guanosine triphosphatase* (GTPase)-*activating proteins* (GAPs), involved in the downregulation of RAS activity (Fig. 12-1). RAS is a low-molecular-weight GTPase protein involved in stimulating cell growth and promoting tumor formation. RAS exists in an active form when bound to guanosine triphosphate (GTP) and in an inactive form when guanosine diphosphate (GDP)-bound. GAP proteins, like neurofibromin, inhibit RAS by stimulating its intrinsic GTPase activity and accelerating the conversion of GTP-bound active RAS to the inactive GDP-bound form.[11] Failure to inactivate RAS, resulting

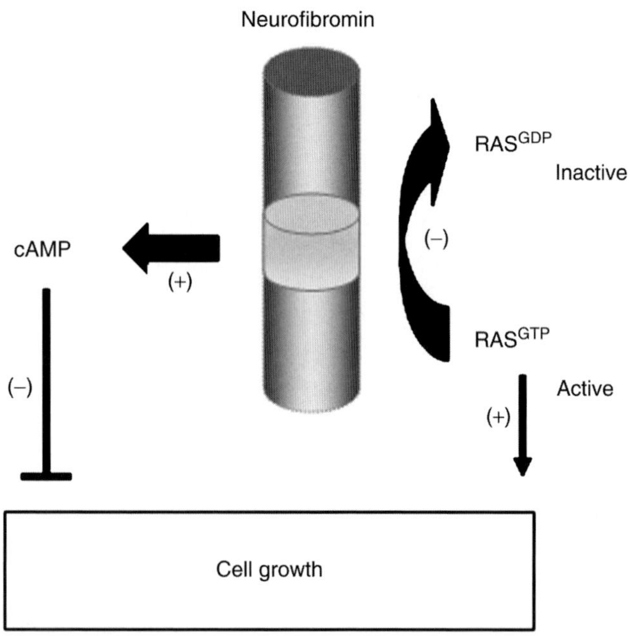

Figure 12-1. Neurofibromin functions as both a negative regulator of RAS and a positive regulator of intracellular cyclic adenosine monophosphate (cAMP). The GTPase-activating domain (GAP) domain of neurofibromin accelerates the conversion of active RAS-GTP to its inactive cytidine diphosphate (CDP)-bound form. Active RAS leads to increased cell growth. In addition, neurofibromin increases intracellular cAMP generation, which, in turn, leads to reduced cell growth. Loss of neurofibromin results in increased cell growth secondary to both increased RAS activation and reduced cAMP levels.

from loss of neurofibromin function as a consequence of *NF1* gene inactivation, leads to increased cell proliferation and tumor formation.[12]

NF1 mutational analyses have not demonstrated a correlation between the mutation type or location and the phenotype of an affected individual.[13] There is relatively little clustering of *NF1* gene mutations, with the exception of exons 10 and 37, where 30% of germline mutations have been identified.[14] Most mutations are unique to a single family. Aside from specific mutations within the GAP domain, most mutations are thought to result in a truncated or nonfunctional protein.

The *NF2* gene was identified by positional cloning in 1993 and is located on the long arm of chromosome 22.[15,16] The *NF2* gene encodes a 2.2-kb messenger RNA and a 595-amino-acid protein named merlin (or schwannomin). Merlin is expressed in neurons, lens fibers, blood vessels, leptomeningeal cells, astrocytes, gonadal tissue, and Schwann cells, but similar to neurofibromin, there is more widespread expression during embryonic development.[14] Merlin is a member of the protein 4.1 family whose members link the actin cytoskeleton to cell surface glycoproteins. Merlin consists of an amino terminal protein 4.1, ezrin, radixin, ezrin (FERM) domain followed by a predicted α-helical region, both of which are conserved in the ERM (ezrin, radixin, and moesin) subclass of protein 4.1 molecules (Fig. 12-2). However, merlin is the only ERM protein known to function as a tumor suppressor.[17]

Similar to ERM proteins, merlin binds to cell surface glycoproteins through its conserved amino terminal (FERM) domain. Notably, merlin associates with CD44, a transmembrane receptor involved in cell–cell and cell–matrix signaling, to modulate cell growth.[18] In the growth-permissive state, merlin is phosphorylated, perhaps by Rac1,[19] and resides in an inactive, "open"

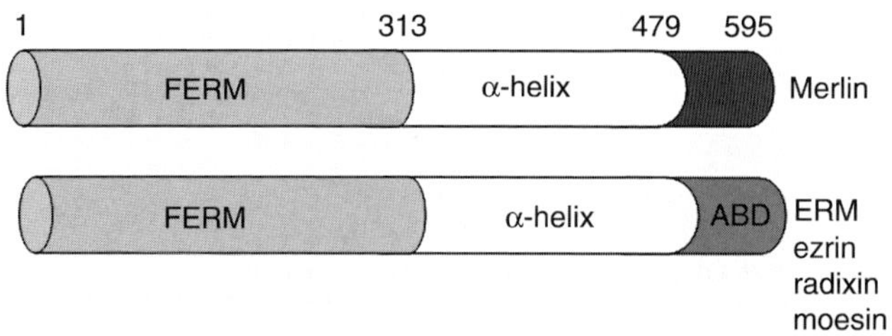

Figure 12-2. Merlin is structurally related to the protein 4.1 molecules. Merlin contains three predicted structural domains, including a 4.1, ezrin, radixin, ezrin (FERM) domain, a predicted α-helical region, and a unique carboxyl terminal domain. Unlike ERM proteins, which contain an actin-binding domain (ABD), merlin's association with the actin cytoskeleton requires residues in the aminoterminal region of the protein. The numbers denote the merlin amino acid residues.

conformation. Dephosphorylation of merlin permits merlin folding and activation, permitting merlin to bind to the cytoplasmic tail of CD44 and abrogate the CD44-mediated growth signal. The mechanism by which merlin transduces its growth suppressor message is not known. However, studies have suggested that merlin interacts with a number of potential effector molecules important for Schwann cell proliferation such as hepatocyte growth factor-regulated tyrosine kinases receptor substrate (HRS[20]). Further studies will be required to determine whether they are required for merlin growth suppression.

Like NF1, a majority of the mutations associated with NF2 represent new mutations. A significant percentage of patients (20%) without a family history have localized disease and are mosaic for an *NF2* gene mutation. Germline mutations in NF2 patients are heterogeneous, involving frequent deletions, splice-site mutations, nonsense mutations, and, less commonly, missense mutations.[21] An early onset and more severe clinical phenotype is often associated with mutations that result in early protein truncation (e.g., frameshift mutations). Single-strand conformation polymorphism (SSCP) analysis has been used to screen patients and can identify mutations in about two-thirds of all patients with NF2.[22]

Both NF1 and NF2 are considered tumor suppressor disorders. The mechanism by which autosomal dominant tumor suppressor genes result in the formation of tumors is explained by the Knudson "two-hit" hypothesis, whereby affected individuals start life with a germline mutation in the *NF1* (or *NF2*) gene in all cells of their bodies.[23] Random somatic mutation in the one remaining functional *NF1* or *NF2* gene, the "second hit," is then required for loss of *NF1* or *NF2* tumor suppressor function and tumor formation. These second mutations are stochastic and may be affected by other genetic factors, resulting in differential expression of the disorder, even in individuals within the same family. Thus, while the disorder is inherited as an autosomal dominant trait, tumor formation is autosomal recessive at the cellular level, because both genes need to be inactivated to result in dysregulated cell growth.[24]

Further support for the "two-hit" hypothesis has been provided by studies demonstrating loss of either neurofibromin or merlin expression in tumor specimens from patients with NF1 and NF2, respectively. Loss of *NF1* gene expression and therefore loss of neurofibromin protein has been demonstrated in malignant peripheral nerve sheath tumors, pheochromocytomas, myeloid leukemia cells, plexiform neurofibromas, cutaneous neurofibromas, and pilocytic astrocytomas in patients with NF1.[25] In support of the role of neurofibromin as a negative regulator (inhibitor) of RAS, studies have demonstrated increased levels of activated RAS in tumor cells from NF1 patients with malignant tumors.[26]

Consistent with the lack of pathologic and clinical differences between sporadic and NF2-associated meningiomas and schwannomas, the molecular basis of these tumors is also remarkably similar. Similar to that described for NF1-associated tumors, loss of *NF2* expression has been reported in vestibular schwannomas and meningiomas from patients with NF2. In addition, mutations in the *NF2* gene and loss of merlin expression are also seen in 30% to 70% of sporadic meningiomas and nearly all sporadic schwannomas.[27] This suggests that merlin is an indispensable negative growth regulator for leptomeningeal cells and Schwann cells. A description of the clinical features of NF1 and NF2 follows.

Neurofibromatosis Type 1

NF1 is a relatively common autosomal dominant disorder with an incidence of 1 in 3500 individuals worldwide.[28] NF1 has the highest spontaneous mutation rate of the phakomatoses. Nearly half of newly diagnosed patients have no known relative with NF1 and are considered new mutations. There is no known racial or ethnic predilection. While many of the organ systems involved in this disorder arise from neural crest cells (i.e., Schwann cells, peripheral nerves, melanocytes, adrenal medulla, and select skull bones), the clinical manifestations are not limited to these cell types. Blood vessels, bone, connective tissue, and the gastrointestinal tract are examples of nonectodermally derived tissues that are frequently affected in NF1.[29]

Most individuals with NF1 present in infancy or early childhood with hyperpigmented lesions such as café-au-lait macules, skinfold freckling, or Lisch nodules (iris hamartomas). Table 12-2 lists the diagnostic criteria for NF1, which were originally formulated by the National Institutes of Health Consensus Panel.[3] For an individual to be given the diagnosis of NF1, two of these seven diagnostic criteria must be present. Other characteristic features are short stature, with 13% of all patients being more than 2 standard deviations below the mean, and macrocephaly, with more than 24% being more than 2 standard deviations above the mean. Nontumor phenotypes include cognitive deficits, renal and cerebral artery stenosis, and bony abnormalities, including sphenoid wing dysplasia, distinctive bony lesions, and scoliosis.

Café-au-lait macules occur in more than 90% of individuals with NF1 and are frequently the earliest manifestation of the disorder. While it is not uncommon for one or two café-au-lait macules to be seen in unaffected individuals in the general population, patients with NF1 have many more such café-au-lait macules. These macules are frequently noted at birth, or shortly thereafter, but sometimes they are so indistinct as to be overlooked. Café-au-lait macules tend to increase in number during the first 2 years of life, and rarely increase in number or size after that time. Typically, these macules have smooth regular borders and demonstrate homogeneous pigmentation. Often, café-au-lait macules fade in adults with NF1, making the diagnosis of NF1 difficult in an adult in whom the childhood history is lacking. Histopathologically, café-au-lait macules are associated with increased numbers of large melanosomes (macromelanosomes).

Like café-au-lait macules, intertriginous freckling is also an early diagnostic sign and is seen in 80% of children by age 6 years. Freckling typically occurs in regions where there is frequent skin friction, such as the axilla, inguinal region, and beneath the chin. In women, freckling may be seen under the breasts. Lisch nodules are benign pigmented nodules of the iris that are not clinically significant, other than being useful for diagnostic purposes. Lisch nodules do not interfere with vision. Although only approximately 30% of NF1 patients have Lisch nodules by age 6 years, nearly all do so by adulthood. Slit lamp examinations are usually required to identify these lesions accurately.

The most common tumor seen in individuals with NF1 is the benign neurofibroma, composed of Schwann cells, fibroblasts, and mast cells (see Chapter 5). These

► TABLE 12-2. DIAGNOSTIC CRITERIA FOR NEUROFIBROMATOSIS TYPE 1 (NF1)

Two or more of the following features must be present for an individual to be diagnosed with NF1:

- Six or more café-au-lait spots with diameters greater than 0.5 mm before puberty or 1.5 cm after puberty
- Two or more neurofibromas or a single plexiform neurofibroma
- Freckling in the axillary and inguinal regions (Crowe sign)
- Optic pathway tumor
- Lisch nodules (hamartomas of the iris)
- A distinctive bony lesion: dysplasia of the sphenoid bone or dysplasia/thinning of long bone cortex
- A first-degree relative diagnosed with NF1

Source: Reproduced with permission from Gutmann DH, Aylsworth A, Carey JC, et al. The diagnostic evaluation and multidisciplinary management of neurofibromatosis 1 and neurofibromatosis 2. JAMA 1997;278:51–57.

tumors may appear as defined cutaneous or subcutaneous lesions or as larger more extensive tumors involving multiple nerves (plexiform neurofibromas). The number of dermal neurofibromas typically increases as a function of age, with tumors first appearing around the time of puberty. They may increase abruptly during pregnancy and may be preceded by a tender, pruritic, violaceous area. Discrete neurofibromas are always benign tumors and harbor no risk of malignant transformation. Cutaneous neurofibromas may be a source of skin irritation when they occur in particular locations and may become a major cosmetic problem when abundant. Subcutaneous neurofibromas may be located in any portion of a peripheral nerve or sympathetic ganglia and may range in size from a few millimeters to several centimeters (or larger). Those located in the paraspinal region may expand centripetally and lead to nerve root compression but rarely compromise the spinal cord (Fig. 12-3A).

Plexiform neurofibromas likely represent congenital lesions, found in approximately 25% of patients with NF1. They may grow anywhere along the length of major peripheral nerves and may result in bony abnormalities or functional impairment. In contrast to the dermal neurofibroma, these tumors involve multiple nerve fascicles. Although often considered congenital lesions present in infancy, they may arise from deeper structures and remain clinically silent until later in life (Fig. 12-3B). Plexiform neurofibromas may be extensive and involve multiple tissues, including skin, fascia, muscle, bone, and internal organs. Their presence may stimulate underlying bone growth to result in leg length discrepancy or scoliosis. Orbital plexiform neurofibromas may be associated with sphenoid wing dysplasia, often resulting in intracranial extension and exophthalmos. Surgical removal of plexiform neurofibromas may be difficult, as these tumors cross tissue planes and are nearly impossible to resect completely. In addition, plexiform neurofibromas often exhibit significant vascularity and may result in tremendous blood loss during surgery.

Unlike the discrete neurofibroma, plexiform neurofibromas may transform into aggressive malignant peripheral nerve sheath tumors (MPNSTs) in approximately 10% of patients.[30] The two most predictive clinical signs suggestive of malignant transformation are pain and new neurologic deficit. Unfortunately, reliable signs of malignant transformation are lacking. Individuals with clinical signs suspicious for malignancy require prompt and aggressive management. These often appear at limb–trunk junctions and are firm, tender, and globoid. Recent studies have evaluated the role of [^{18}F]fluorodeoxyglucose positron emission tomography (FDG-PET) for distinguishing malignant from benign peripheral nerve sheath tumors.[31] Based on these preliminary observations, FDG-PET might become an adjunct diagnostic tool in the evaluation of an NF1 patient in whom MPNST is suspected (see Fig. 12-3B). Most MPNSTs are highly malignant neoplasms and have the propensity for distant metastasis to bone and lung. New onset of bone pain or fracture in an NF1 patient with an MPNST warrants a search for metastases. MPNSTs are not typically sensitive to conventional chemotherapy and radiation. Local radiotherapy after wide surgical excision of an MPNST may delay the time to local recurrence, but does not improve the overall long-term survival. The 5-year survival rate after aggressive resection is less than 5 years.[32]

The second most frequent tumor in NF1 is the optic pathway glioma, occurring in 15% of individuals. These tumors are almost entirely restricted to childhood, with a mean age at presentation of 4.2 years. The optic pathway glioma in NF1 is almost always a low-grade (World Health Organization [WHO] grade I) pilocytic astrocytoma. These tumors may arise anywhere along the length of the optic pathway from the retrobulbar optic nerve to the postchiasmatic optic radiations. They may also extend into the hypothalamus to cause neuroendocrine dysfunction, such as precocious puberty. Many of these tumors are detected incidentally on brain magnetic resonance imaging (MRI), and only about one-third of these are clinically symptomatic. Some NF1-associated optic pathway gliomas have been reported to regress even without treatment. Clinical surveillance includes annual ophthalmologic evaluations in the first decade of life to identify visual impairment resulting from these tumors.[33] Routine brain imaging in asymptomatic individuals is not recommended, as the decision to treat is based on clinical symptoms. NF1-associated gliomas may also involve the brainstem. Compared to the brainstem gliomas seen in individuals without NF1, NF1-associated brainstem tumors are more likely to be located in the medulla (Fig. 12-3C), but are less likely to progress clinically or radiographically. While sporadic brainstem gliomas carry a poor prognosis, NF1-associated brainstem tumors are more often low-grade lesions with lower morbidity and mortality.[34]

Gliomas have sometimes been misdiagnosed in individuals with NF1 who have other intracranial signal abnormalities uniquely found in NF1 patients on brain MRI (Fig. 12-3D). High-signal-intensity lesions on T_2-weighted images are seen in more than half of NF1 children. These nonenhancing lesions are most often found in the brainstem, thalamus, cerebellum, and basal ganglia.[35] Pathologically, these lesions may represent regions of vacuolar or spongiotic change, although clear clinicopathologic correlates are lacking. They have no known potential for neoplastic degeneration, but may enlarge and are then misdiagnosed as low-grade gliomas. Multiple studies have investigated a potential correlation between the number of these lesions and cognitive deficits yet no consensus has been reached regarding their clinical significance.[36]

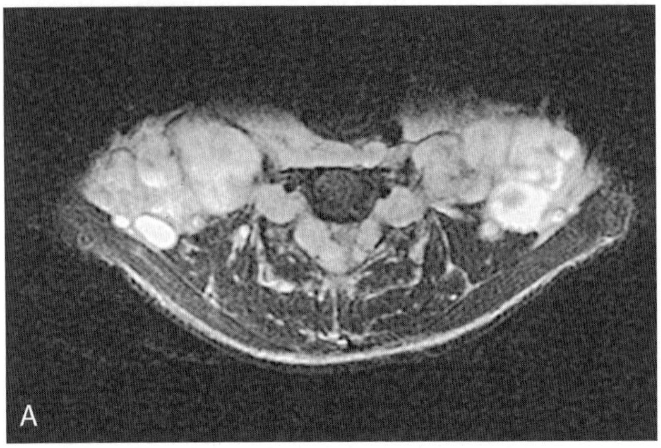

Figure 12-3. (A) Centripetal extension of multiple paraspinal neurofibromas causing spinal cord compression. (B) Plexiform neurofibroma of left pelvis (left). Aggressive surgical resection was carried out after positron emission tomography (PET) scan (middle) demonstration of hypermetabolic state. Modern neuroimaging and peripheral nerve surgery allow aggressive resections without sacrificing function. This patient had relief of symptoms with no new neurologic deficit after surgery (right). (C) Likely low-grade astrocytoma of left medulla in NF1. (D) Indeterminate left temporal lobe process, stable over more than a decade, in 47-year-old man with NF1.

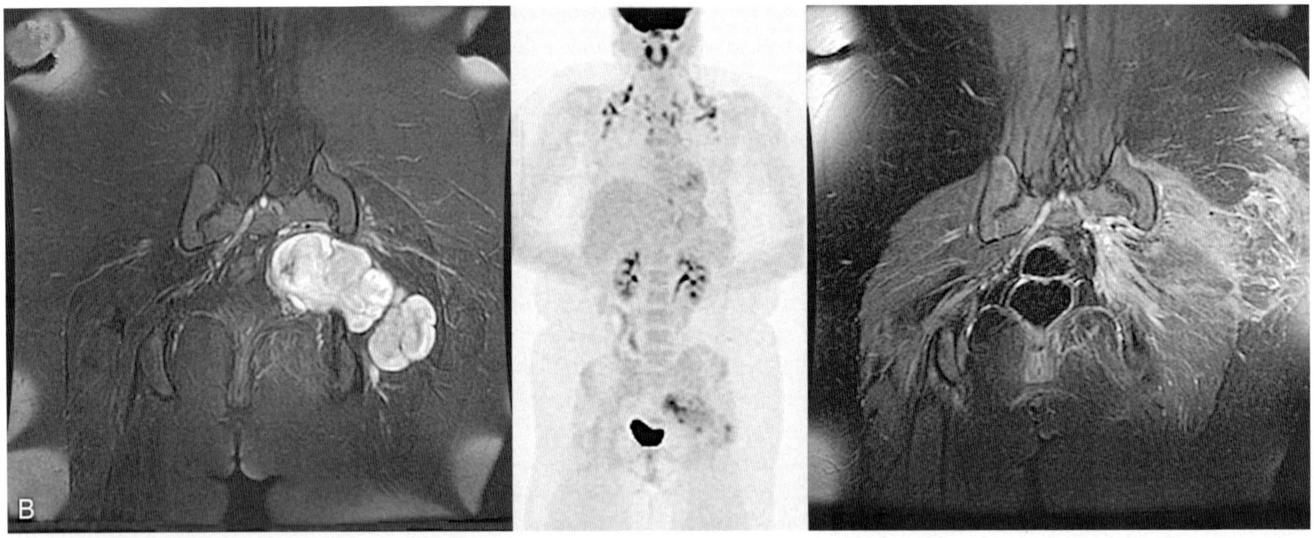

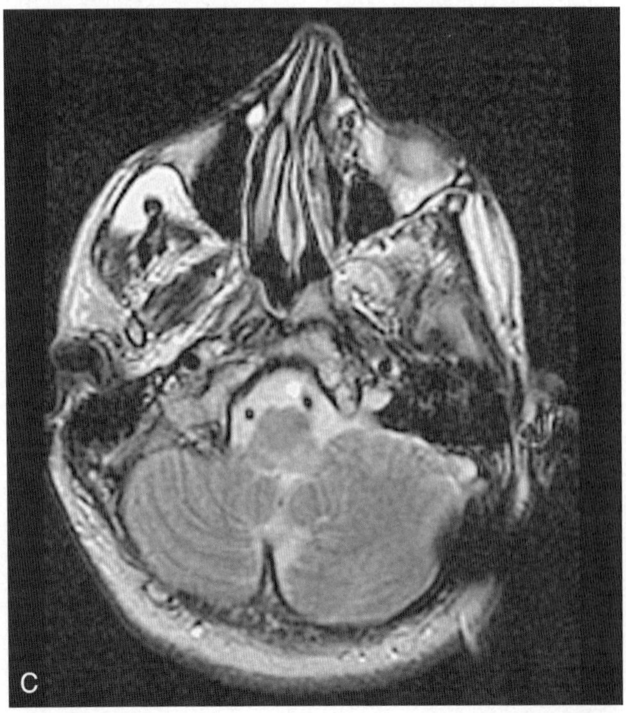

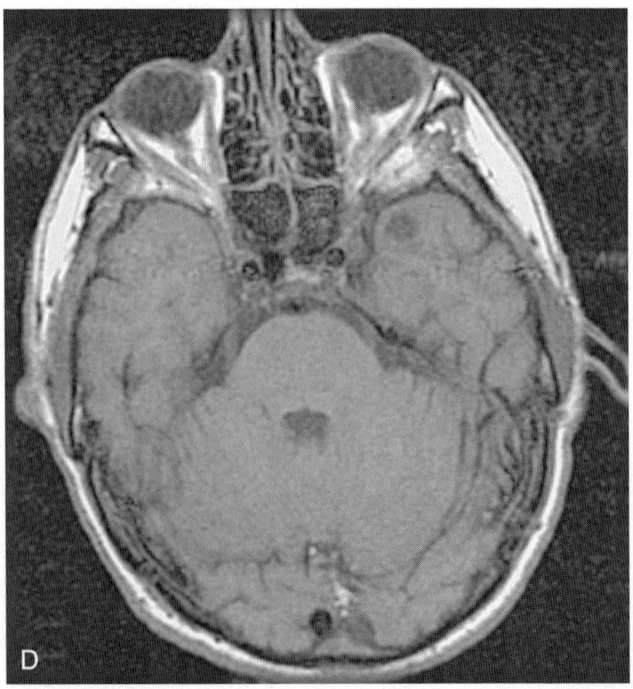

NF1 patients are also at higher risk for specific bony and vascular abnormalities, as well as rare tumors. Scoliosis occurs in 10% to 20% of patients with NF1.[37] The scoliosis in children with NF1 may resemble the idiopathic form, or may present earlier when related to vertebral dysplasia or secondary to paravertebral neurofibromas. Scoliosis resulting from a paravertebral neurofibroma or spinal cord tumor may manifest with a dramatic abrupt angle curvature (dystrophic scoliosis), unusual for non–NF1-associated cases. Tibial pseudarthrosis and sphenoid wing dysplasia are both osseous lesions that are quite specific to patients with NF1. These distinctive bony lesions typically are obvious in early infancy. Bowing of the long bones may be the result of cortical thinning or dysplastic bony changes and may lead to pathologic fracture in NF1.[38] Repeated fracture and incomplete healing produces the appearance of a "false joint" or pseudarthrosis. Early recognition is essential to avoid limb amputation. Sphenoid wing dysplasia will usually manifest as an orbital deformity. Patients may have unilateral exophthalmus which may be pulsatile. Skull bone radiographs should readily identify this bony defect. Vascular abnormalities, including renal artery stenosis, which may cause hypertension, and moyamoya, a cerebral vessel abnormality that can result in stroke, are unusual complications of NF1, found in less than 1% of patients.[39] NF1 patients are also at a higher risk for other malignancies, including pheochromocytoma, Wilms tumor and juvenile chronic myeloid leukemia.[14]

A hallmark feature of NF1 is phenotypic variability. There is typically as much difference in the spectrum of clinical features between individuals within a single family who all harbor an identical germline *NF1* mutation as there is between individuals from different families. Parents with few clinical features of NF1 (e.g., café-au-lait macules and skinfold freckles) can have children with more clinically serious manifestations (e.g., MPNSTs and optic pathway gliomas). This variability suggests that other factors besides the germline *NF1* mutation determine the clinical expression of the disorder. Some studies implicate injury as an inciting stimulus for tumor formation in NF1. For example, cutaneous neurofibromas sometimes grow at sites of previous wounds or skin grafts. Further work will be required to determine what effects these factors have on tumor formation and growth in NF1.

Rare individuals have been identified with segmental NF1, affecting only a single region of the body.[40] Some of these patients are genetically mosaic for mutations in *NF1* gene and therefore are known to harbor the mutation in only a subset of their cells. Mosaicism, resulting from a somatic mutation occurring at a later stage in fetal development, is more likely to affect fewer cells and result in a more restricted somatic distribution of clinical abnormalities. Given that mosaicism could also potentially affect the gonadal tissues, the probability of transmission of NF1 may be as high as 50%, as seen in typical cases of NF1, but generally is lower. Although the parent may have a mosaic or segmental pattern of NF1, affected offspring will have the generalized NF1 phenotype, as they would have inherited a germline NF1 mutation in all cells.

The diagnosis of NF1 can be made accurately and early based on clinical exam findings and history alone (see Table 12-2). Although only 26% of sporadic patients meet criteria by age 1 year, almost all (97%) meet criteria for diagnosis by age 8 years because many of the cutaneous signs develop during early childhood.[6] Although *NF1* gene mutation analysis is available for diagnostic purposes, it is only useful in families with known mutations, and is costly and time-consuming, given the large size of the gene and lack of mutation clustering.[3,41] For this reason, the diagnosis of *NF1* remains a clinical one.

Routine management of patients with NF1 involves annual ophthalmologic assessments to evaluate for visual abnormalities suggestive of a symptomatic optic pathway glioma in children younger than age 10 years. If deficits are demonstrated on ophthalmologic evaluation, cranial magnetic resonance imaging is indicated. Any other abnormal neurologic symptom, sign, or examination finding should likewise prompt radiographic evaluation. Plexiform neurofibromas should be closely monitored for the development of sudden pain, new neurologic deficit, or rapid growth. Scoliosis should be screened for clinically and tibial bowing should be referred to an experienced orthopedic surgeon. Routine determinations of blood pressure are recommended to recognize potential complications including renal artery stenosis and pheochromocytoma. Growth should be followed and signs of precocious puberty should be identified and further evaluated. A child's school performance should be monitored for signs of learning disabilities.

Tumors in patients with NF1 deserve special attention. Presently, the mainstay of NF1 treatment is anticipatory management. Careful examination of patients at risk for specific age-dependent features and the prompt recognition of specific signs and symptoms is required in order to identify those patients who require treatment. Multidisciplinary teams including neurologists, surgeons, ophthalmologists, dermatologists, oncologists, and radiologists with experience with these disorders are mandatory to avoid unnecessary treatment and to identify problems early. Given the natural history of many NF1-associated tumors, a conservative approach with close clinical and radiographic surveillance is recommended. The indolent nature of most of these, the uncertainty around the neoplastic nature of brainstem lesions, and the potential risk of developing secondary tumors after treatment of patients argue for this "watch and wait" approach.

Nevertheless, some patients require treatment. The modality chosen is situation specific. For example, some plexiform neurofibromas are removed secondary to compression. Chemotherapy is reserved for selective optic nerve gliomas that progress.[42] Radiation therapy is usually recommended against in glioma patients with NF1 because major sequelae are encountered.[43] Radiation therapy is typically employed in the adjuvant treatment of surgically resected MPNSTs.[44] Decisions regarding shunting, ventriculostomy, and decompressive surgery are similarly an individual decision between the patient and family and the responsible physician. For example, some patients have benefitted from cervical laminectomy to decompress "kissing" neurofibromas causing intradural extramedullary spinal cord compression (see Fig. 12-3A).

With an improved and detailed understanding of the molecular biologic mechanisms that underlie NF1-associated neoplasms, the development of targeted and rational therapeutic strategies becomes possible. Although comparatively less is known about how merlin regulates cell proliferation, the identification of the *NF1* gene and the discovery that it may function as a tumor suppressor by inactivating RAS has opened the door to clinical trials aimed at RAS inactivation. Several clinical trials are presently underway using farnesyltransferase inhibitors to block the addition of a farnesyl group to RAS, a posttranslational modification required for RAS membrane translocation and activation. Other therapeutic approaches will likely result from additional basic science research. One such therapy is pirfenidone, an antifibrotic agent that targets important pathways in fibroblast metabolism.[45] Studies are underway to determine its usefulness in plexiform neurofibromas.

Neurofibromatosis Type 2

NF2 is much less common than NF1 and has an estimated incidence of 1 in 40,000.[28] Like NF1 there is no ethnic or racial predilection, and as many as three-quarters of cases represent new mutations. NF2 is characterized by the early development of multiple schwannomas affecting cranial, spinal, and peripheral nerves. Table 12-3 lists the diagnostic criteria for NF2. In contrast to NF1, the large tumor burden often results in a diminished life expectancy. Nearly all individuals with NF2 will develop schwannomas and, in about half of affected patients, meningiomas and ependymomas. Astrocytomas involving the brain and spinal cord are considerably less common and optic nerve gliomas do not occur. In addition to nervous system tumors, common ocular findings include posterior subcapsular lenticular opacities (cataracts). Although NF2 is often referred to as a neurocutaneous disorder, the presence of cutaneous features is much less common than in NF1. Fusiform subcutaneous schwannomas may be palpated in patients with NF2, but are never present in the hundreds, as may occur with cutaneous neurofibromas in NF1.

Bilateral acoustic schwannomas are the most common manifestation of NF2 (Fig. 12-4A). The majority of adult patients with NF2 present with unilateral hearing loss, often associated with imbalance and tinnitus. This may relate to the common imaging observation that one tumor tends to be considerably larger than the other. Left undiagnosed (or in the rare aggressive form) a full "cerebellar–pontine angle (CPA) syndrome" of V, VII, and VIII cranial neuropathies and brainstem compression may develop. Children, who have more serious disease because of an early onset and more rapidly progressive clinical course, are more likely to present with tumors involving other cranial and peripheral nerves. In some families with NF2, the onset and severity are similar in all affected individuals, suggesting a relationship between the phenotype and the underlying genetic mutation.[22]

The most common tumor found in NF2 is the schwannoma, which comprises neoplastic Schwann cells.

TABLE 12-3. DIAGNOSTIC CRITERIA FOR NEUROFIBROMATOSIS TYPE 2 (NF2)

Confirmed (definite) NF2

- Bilateral vestibular schwannomas (VS) or
- Family history of NF2 (first degree family relative) plus:
  - Unilateral VS at <30 years old, or
  - Any two of the following: meningioma, glioma, schwannoma, juvenile posterior subcapsular lenticular opacities/juvenile cortical cataract

Individuals with the following clinical features should be evaluated for NF2 (presumptive or probable NF2):

- Unilateral VS at <30 years old, plus at least one of any of the following: meningioma, glioma, schwannoma, juvenile posterior subcapsular lenticular opacities/juvenile cortical cataract
- Multiple meningiomas (two or more) plus unilateral VS at <30 years old, or
- Any one of the following: glioma, schwannoma, juvenile posterior subcapsular **lenticular** opacities/juvenile cortical cataract

Source: Reproduced with permission from Gutmann DH, Aylsworth A, Carey JC, et al. The diagnostic evaluation and multidisciplinary management of neurofibromatosis 1 and neurofibromatosis 2. JAMA 1997;278:51–57.

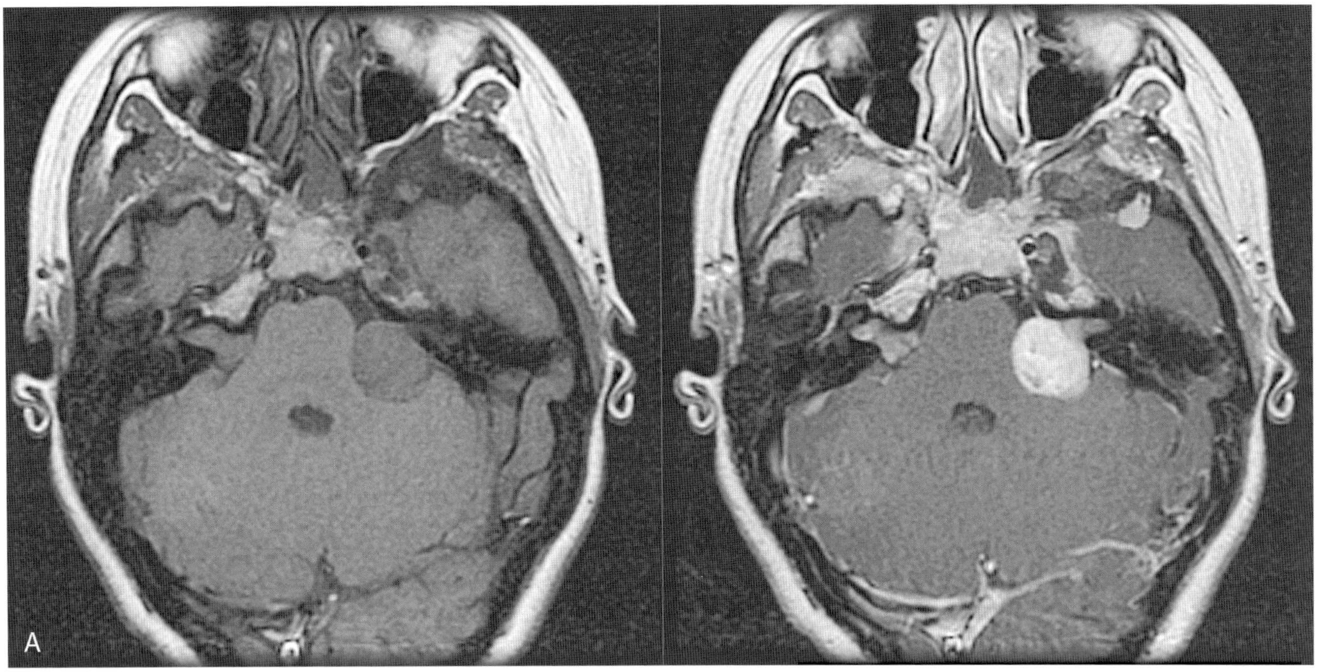

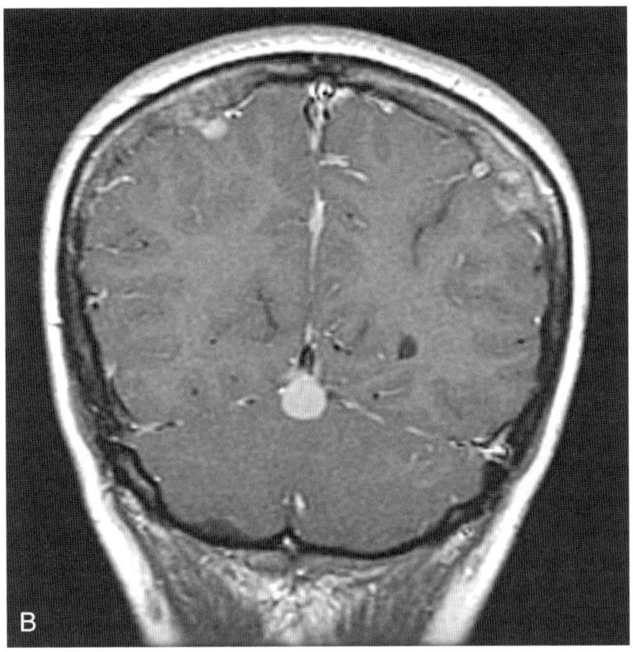

Figure 12-4. (A) Bilateral but asymmetric acoustic schwannomas in NF2; without (L) and with contrast (R). (B) NF2 patient with multiple meningiomas. Patient presented at age 18 years with foramen magnum meningioma.

Clinically, schwannomas from individuals with NF2 are not different from their sporadic counterparts, except that they are often multiple and typically occur at an earlier age. Despite the misnomer "acoustic neuroma," schwannomas most frequently affect the vestibular branch of the eighth cranial nerve, although other cranial nerves may be affected. Similarly, extramedullary spinal schwannomas may arise at any vertebral level. Vestibular schwannomas are so common in NF2 patients that they are required for a definite diagnosis of the disorder.[3] Likewise, spinal schwannomas are identified in nearly 80% to 90% of individuals with NF2 by using gadolinium-enhanced MRI.

Meningioma is the second most common tumor in NF2 and occurs both intracranially and within the spinal cord (Fig. 12-4B). Most are supratentorial, occurring in the parasagittal region, cerebral convexities, or sphenoid ridge. They may also occur at the foramen magnum. Like schwannomas, meningiomas are also common sporadic tumors; however, only 1% of individuals with a single meningioma meet criteria for NF2. The recognition of multiple meningiomas in a child or young adult should prompt a search for other signs of NF2, as meningiomas are typically found in older adults in the general population.

The initial diagnostic workup for patients at risk for NF2 includes full cranial[46] and spinal[47] MRI to evaluate for schwannomas, meningiomas, and intramedullary tumors. Brain MRI, neurologic examinations, and audiologic assessments are recommended and should be dictated by clinical findings.[42] Brainstem auditory-evoked responses may also be helpful in assessing eighth nerve function. Brain MRI also serves as an effective screening exam for asymptomatic individuals, as a normal MRI scan at age 30 years makes a diagnosis of NF2 extremely unlikely.[22]

Because of the difficulty involved in identifying *NF2* gene mutations as a rapid screening test for NF2, clinical examination and history remain the standard for diagnosis. Mutation scanning, using SSCP followed by direct sequencing, reveals about 65% of causative mutations. Linkage studies can also be performed on families with multiple affected individuals.[48]

Schwannomatosis is a rare disorder defined by multiple noncranial schwannomas in the absence of meningiomas, ependymomas, or astrocytomas.[49] These patients tend to develop schwannomas later in life and therefore have a longer life expectancy. In contrast to patients with NF2, these individuals do not harbor germline mutations in the *NF2* gene, but their schwannomas contain somatic mutations in both *NF2* alleles. Another subset of patients with NF2 has disease-related tumors restricted to one region of the nervous system, such as localized meningiomas and unilateral vestibular schwannomas.[40] These patients have segmental or mosaic NF2, characterized by somatic mutations in the *NF2* gene occurring later during fetal development, much as described above for segmental NF1. Mosaicism is much more common in NF2 than in NF1, accounting for up to 20% of patients with no previous family history.[50]

Management of NF2 patients requires close surveillance for cranial and spinal tumors. Complete cranial and spinal magnetic resonance imaging is indicated at diagnosis. Annual physical examinations and repeat cranial and spinal imaging studies are recommended to identify and follow tumors as clinically indicated. Audiometry and brainstem auditory evoked responses aid in the detection of clinically significant vestibular schwannomas. Patients are best followed in established centers that have a multidisciplinary team familiar with NF2. Some individuals may benefit from hearing aids, cochlear implants, or brainstem implants, depending on the particular situation.

Tuberous Sclerosis Complex (Bourneville Disease)

TSC is an autosomal dominant tumor predisposition syndrome that affects approximately 1 in 7500 individuals worldwide.[51] Approximately two-thirds of cases are new mutations. TSC is characterized by benign, hamartomatous growths in multiple organs, including the kidney, skin, retina, lung, and brain. Rarely, malignant tumors, including renal cell carcinoma, may develop. Characteristic skin lesions and epilepsy are the most common presentations among new cases. TSC is usually diagnosed by clinical criteria (Table 12-4).

Linkage studies have identified two distinct loci that undergo mutational inactivation in individuals with TSC.[52] The clinical TSC phenotype occurs when inactivating mutations occur in one of the two genes, *TSC1* or *TSC2*. The *TSC1* gene is located on chromosome 9q34. The gene contains 23 exons and encodes the 130-kDa hamartin protein.[53] Hamartin has little sequence homology to other known proteins. The *TSC2* gene on chromosome 16p13 encodes the 180- to 200-kDa tuberin protein.[54] Tuberin contains a small region with sequence similarity to proteins with GTPase-activating protein function (see discussion under NF1, page 234). Both hamartin and tuberin contain predicted coiled-coil domains that mediate their interaction to form the tuberin–hamartin protein complex (THC) (Fig. 12-5).[55,56] The formation of this complex is critical for tuberin and hamartin functions and *TSC* gene-associated mutations frequently disrupt this interaction and render the THC functionally inactive.

TABLE 12-4. DIAGNOSTIC CRITERIA FOR THE TUBEROUS SCLEROSIS COMPLEX (TSC)

Consensus diagnostic criteria for tuberous sclerosis*
Major features
Cortical tubers
Subependymal glial nodules
Three or more typical hypomelanotic macules
Retinal phakomas (peripapillary retinal hamartomas or "pseudodrusen")
Midfacial ("adenoma sebaceum") or ungual/periungual angiofibromas/fibromas
Multiple renal angiomyolipomas
Cardiac rhabdomyomas
Pulmonary lymphangiomyomatosis
Shagreen patch
Minor features
Fibrous forehead or scalp plaques
Gingival fibromas
Wedge-shaped cortical or subcortial brain calcification
Multiple subcortical changes: hypodense by CT, high signal T_2-weighted MRI
Renal cysts
Dental enamel pits
Bone cysts
Hamartomatous rectal polyps
First-degree relative with TS

*Diagnosis by consensus criteria: one major and first-degree relative with tuberous sclerosis or one major and two minor. One major and one minor = probable. One major and two or more minor = possible.

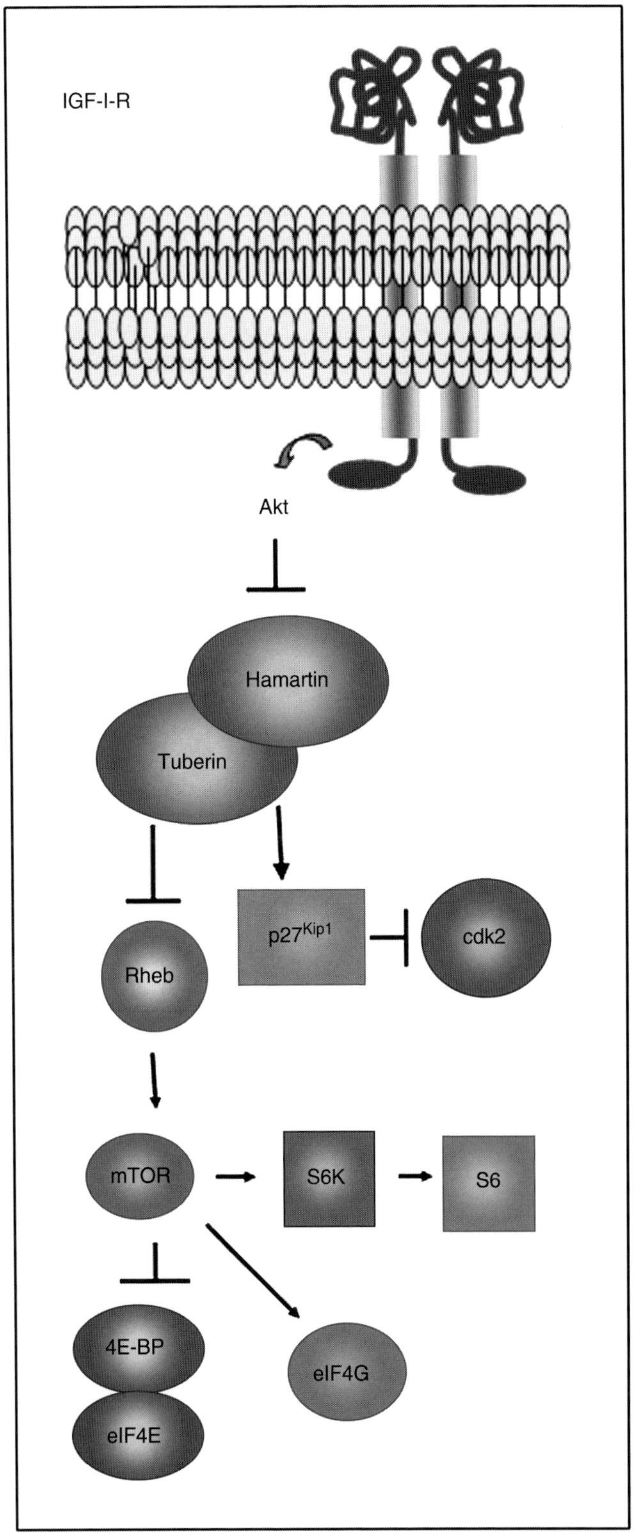

Figure 12-5. Tuberin–hamartin complex (THC) regulation of intracellular signaling. Activation of the insulin-like growth factor receptor (IGF-R) results in activation of Akt, which phosphorylates tuberin to inactivate the THC. The THC negatively regulates Rheb by converting Rheb from its active GTP-bound conformation to its inactive GDP-bound form. Rheb-GTP, in turn, activates mammalian target of rapamycin (mTOR), which results in a cascade of activation (phosphorylation) events involving S6K and its downstream target, ribosomal S6. Hyperactivation of S6 results in protein translation and increased cell size. In addition, mTOR increased eIF4E activity by phosphorylating the 4E-binding protein (4E-BP) as well as activating eIF4G by phosphorylation. 4E-BP phosphorylation results in release of eIF4E inhibition and allows eIF4E and eIF4G to form a complex with eIF4A to promote protein translation. Lastly, the THC positively regulates p27Kip1 through an unknown mechanism to result in inhibition of cdk2 activity. In this regard, THC inactivation results in reduced p27Kip1 expression, increased cdk2 activity, and increased cell size and growth.

Identified *TSC* gene mutations include missense and nonsense mutations, in-frame deletions, and large deletions.[57] Although familial cases of TSC have an approximately equal distribution of families with *TSC1* and *TSC2* mutations, *TSC2* mutations are approximately four times more common in sporadic cases.[58] Because two-thirds of all TSC patients have sporadic mutations, the high frequency of *TSC2* mutations may reflect a higher intrinsic mutation rate for the *TSC2* gene.

The observation that individuals who are born with a mutated copy of the *TSC1* or *TSC2* gene in all cells of their bodies are predisposed to develop tumors in several different organs, including the central nervous system (CNS), suggested that these genes act as tumor suppressors. Tumors develop in these individuals when one or more somatic cells undergo a "second hit" and the remaining, wild-type *TSC* gene is inactivated.[59] This loss of *TSC1* or *TSC2* expression results in abnormal cell growth and proliferation. Indeed, hamartomas from patients with both familial and sporadic forms of the disease have shown loss of a normal copy of *TSC1* or *TSC2*, termed *loss of heterozygosity* (LOH), indicating that these genes act as classical tumor suppressors.[60] In vitro studies have also supported the role of these genes as tumor suppressors. When either tuberin or hamartin is overexpressed in cultured cells, the cells undergo growth arrest. Similarly, downregulation of *TSC2* expression in cultured fibroblasts by antisense inhibition resulted in increased cell proliferation.[61–63]

Tuberin and hamartin are highly expressed in the CNS of humans and mice in both neurons and glial cells.[64] Tuberin and hamartin appear to be required for CNS development and tuberin may be required for neuronal differentiation.[65] Similar to other organs, these proteins likely act as tumor suppressors in the CNS as tuberin expression is reduced or absent in 30% of sporadic astrocytomas.[66] There are conflicting reports as to whether somatic mutations of the wild-type *TSC1* or *TSC2* allele in a precursor cell is required for cortical tuber formation in patients who have only one normal copy of one of the two *TSC* genes.[67] Because these lesions are composed of many different cell types, it may be difficult to identify the subset of cells that have undergone a second mutational event. In support of the hypothesis that two genetic "hits" are required for TSC-associated tuber formation, recent evidence suggests that, in mice, neuroepithelial cell progenitors that lack *TSC2* expression have many features of the giant cells found in cortical tubers.[68]

Clinically, the CNS complications of TSC are the most disabling. Cortical tubers are the pathognomonic lesions that characterize TSC. Pathologic evidence suggests that cortical tubers represent areas of abnormal neuronal differentiation and migration. Surrounding areas of cortex are not disrupted (Fig. 12-6A). Tubers are formed early in development and have been identified as early as 20 weeks of gestation.[68] Tubers contain dysmorphic neurons, increased numbers of astrocytes, and "giant" cells. Tubers are detected as high intensity signals on T_2-weighted MRI images that are often located at the junctions between the gray and white matter. The size and location of cortical tubers has been suggested to correlate with the major CNS manifestations of TSC: seizures, mental retardation, and autism.[69,70] The number and location of cortical tubers, as well as the age of seizure onset, are highly correlated with neurologic outcome. Individuals who experience seizures at an earlier age have poorer cognitive outcomes.[71]

Epilepsy occurs in approximately 80% of affected individuals. TSC-affected children commonly present with partial motor seizures or infantile spasms within the first year of life.[72] An increase in seizure frequency and severity is common during early childhood. Epileptogenic foci identified by electroencephalography (EEG) frequently correlate with cortical tubers visualized by MRI.[73,74] In addition, the progression from infantile spasms to other seizure types may reflect the formation of tubers at different times during cortical development. Thus, tubers in areas of the brain that become functionally mature earlier (e.g., temporal or occipital regions) may become epileptogenic before tubers located in brain regions that mature more slowly, including the frontal lobes. Because clinicians cannot accurately visualize each of these lesions, predicting the progression of epilepsy in TSC patients is difficult. TSC-associated seizures are often refractory to conventional pharmacologic therapies. Improved seizure control has been achieved using the gamma-aminobutyric acid (GABA) agonist vigabatrin in some TSC patients.[75] Surgical treatment may be helpful for select patients, especially those who have a single epileptogenic tuber.[76]

TSC-affected individuals develop low-grade astrocytic neoplasms (see Chapter 14). Subependymal nodules (SENs) are benign, proliferative lesions that line the surface of the lateral ventricles. Unlike the cortical tubers, these lesions are often asymptomatic but can develop into SEGAs.[77] While not frankly malignant, SEGAs can cause ventricular obstruction and hydrocephalus that require neurosurgical intervention. In addition to glial cells, SENs and SEGAs may also contain giant cells. These lesions, like cortical tubers, are thought to develop early in life and have been identified as early as 27 weeks of gestation.[78] Like cortical tubers (Fig. 12-6A), these lesions are thought to arise from abnormal development of precursor cells during brain development. Whether cortical tubers can develop into astrocytomas is still not settled.

Hypopigmented macules ("ash-leaf" spot) is the most prevalent TSC finding (see Fig. 12-6B). Although as many as 5% of otherwise normal individuals may have one such spot, TSC patients have multiple lesions over the trunk and buttocks. Although they tend to fade with

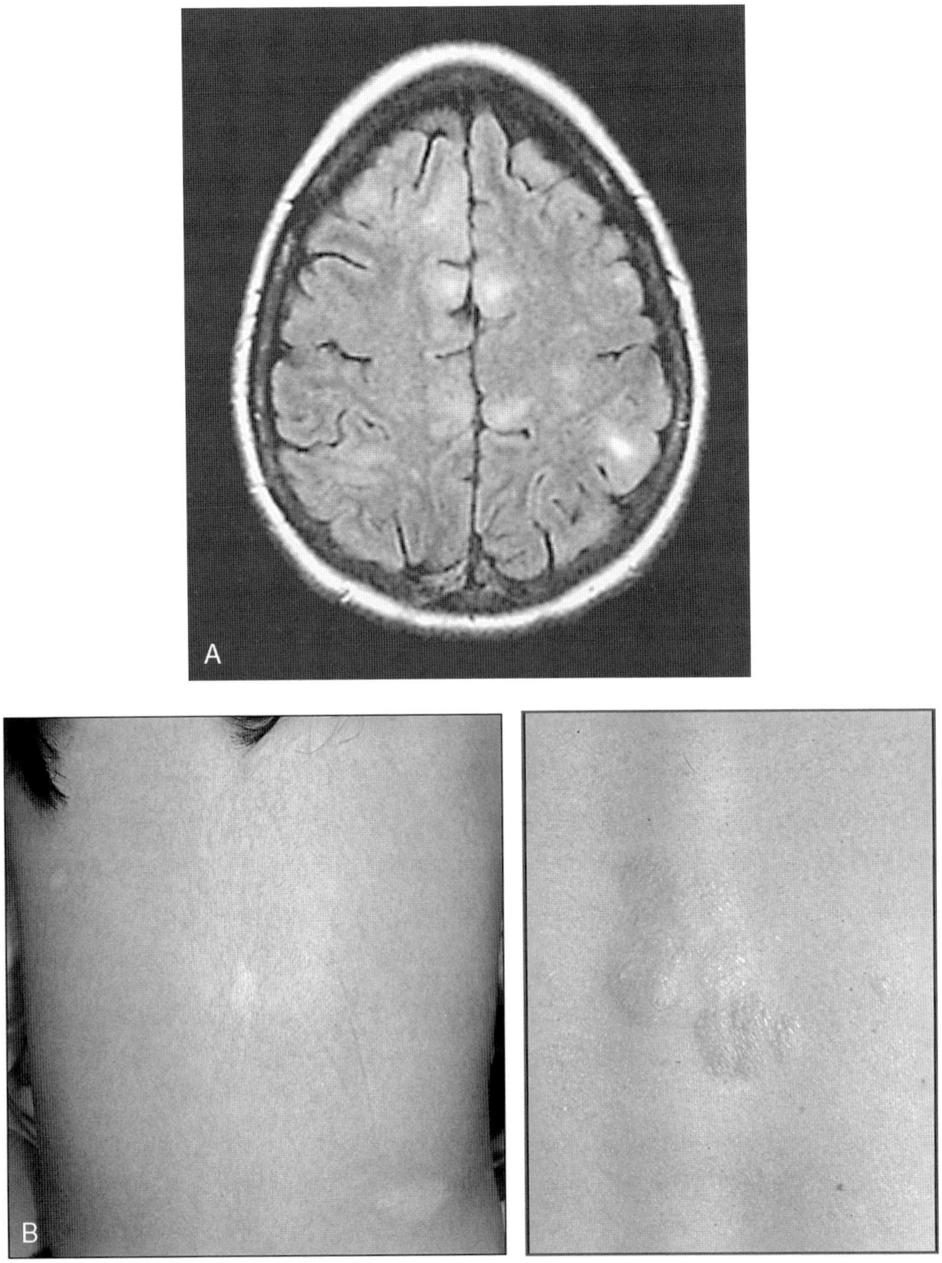

Figure 12-6 (PLATE 43). (A) Multiple subcortical tubers. (B) "Ash leaf" depigmentation (left) and Shagreen patch (right) in TSC (*courtesy of Dusica Babovic MD, DSc, Department of Human Genetics, Mayo Medical School, Rochester MN 55905*). (*Continued*)

age they can be easily demonstrated with the use of a Wood lamp. Other skin lesions, such as angiofibromata, Shagreen patches, and subungual fibromas, are caused by faulty cellular differentiation (see Fig. 12-6B). Facial angiofibromata were previously known as "adenoma sebaceum." Certainly the identification of such a skin lesion in a child with epilepsy should prompt a thorough investigation for TSC.

Renal disease is secondary only to CNS disease in terms of TSC morbidity and mortality. The renal lesions seen in TSC include renal cell carcinoma, oncocytoma, renal cyst, angiolipoma, and polycystic kidney.[79] Angiomyolipomas (Fig. 12-6C) are the most common of these and at least 60% are asymptomatic; renal cysts are next most common. Clinical manifestations include hypertension (from renal artery compression) and hematuria.

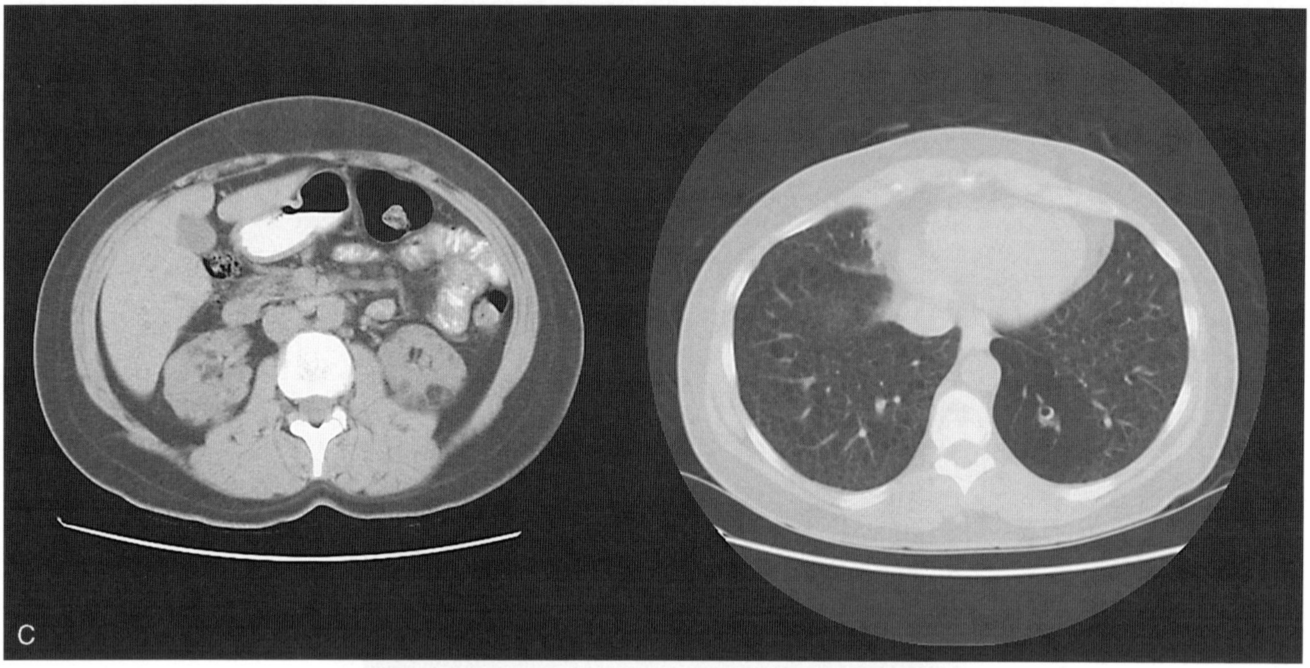

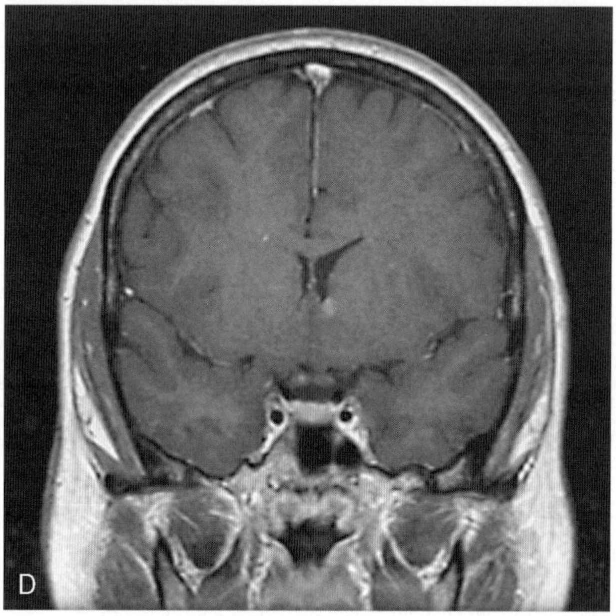

Figure 12-6. (*Continued*) (C) Multiple angiomyolipomas and cysts in kidneys (left) and lungs (right) typical of TSC. (D) Subependymal giant cell astrocytoma (SEGA). Lesion (arrow) is small with no ventricular enlargement. Lesion found on routine screening and will serve as baseline for comparison to subsequent imaging.

Renal cell carcinomas tend to occur at a younger age, are more likely to remain localized, and grow more slowly than the sporadic counterparts.[80] Whether they arise de novo, from renal cysts or angiomyolipomas is still unresolved.[81] Overall, renal pathology is the main cause of death in patients older than age 30 years.[79] Other manifestations include retinal hamartomas (which are present in nearly half of TSC patients), liver angiomyolipomas (which are invariably associated with renal angiomyolipomas in TSC patients), pulmonary lymphangiomyolipomas (seen in approximately 5% of TSC patients, predominantly women), cardiac rhabdomyomas, and unusual vascular lesions, including aneurysms of carotid, axillary, and renal arteries.[82]

Management of TSC is largely symptomatic and anticipatory. Once TSC is suspected (or diagnosed) appropriate scanning should be performed of chest, abdomen, and pelvis for evidence of occult neoplasms or preneoplastic lesions (Fig. 12-6C demonstrates multiple lesions in chest and abdominal viscera). Presently computerized tomography (CT) scanning is sufficient to detect most angiolipomas. Head imaging with high-quality MRI scanning (including fluid-attenuated inversion recovery [FLAIR] sequences) is essential to detect early SEGA development so that ventricular obstruction does not go undetected (Fig. 12-6D). Neurosurgical management consists of resection. A medical genetics consultation is appropriate to screen other family members to define penetrance. Routine genetic testing is not available. Molecular genetic testing has been used to define genotype–phenotype correlations.[83] As is true with the other phakomatoses, the spontaneous mutation rate is high. Cosmetic surgery is usually not necessary in the majority of patients.

von Hippel-Lindau Disease

von Hippel-Lindau (VHL) disease is an autosomal dominant tumor predisposition syndrome with a predilection for tumors of the eye, kidney, adrenals, brain, and spinal cord.[6,84] VHL is caused by a mutation of a tumor suppressor gene located on chromosome 3p25, which is a region of the genome that is frequently deleted in sporadic (nonhereditary) kidney cancer.[85] The gene is relatively small, consisting of three exons, and is conserved in rodents, flies, and worms. Its incidence is approximately 1 in 35,000 (one-tenth the incidence of NF1[86]). The incidence of new mutations is not known. Unlike NF1, somatic mutations do not appear to transmit the abnormal gene. As with the other phakomatoses there is no ethnic predisposition. Although considered a "phakomatosis," VHL is not strictly a neurocutaneous syndrome as skin manifestations are rare. The "phakoma" in this instance is in the eye.

The VHL tumor suppressor gene conforms to the "two-hit" model.[23] Individuals with VHL disease have typically inherited a defective *VHL* allele from one of their parents. Pathology, such as the development of cysts or tumors, is linked to the somatic inactivation or loss of the remaining wild-type *VHL* allele.[87] Essentially all individuals who have been clinically diagnosed with VHL disease can be shown to possess a *VHL* mutation. *VHL* inactivation is also a common feature of sporadic clear-cell carcinomas and hemangioblastomas.[88] Some genotype–phenotype correlations are emerging in VHL. Most striking is the fact that VHL families with a high risk of pheochromocytoma (so-called type 2 VHL disease) almost invariably harbor a *VHL* missense mutation.[89] The tumors in these patients differ from those in sporadic cases because they occur in younger patients and are often bilateral, multiple, and extraadrenal.[90] Somatic *VHL* mutations are rare in sporadic pheochromocytomas.

VHL messenger RNA (mRNA) encodes a protein of 213 amino-acid residues with an apparent molecular weight of 24 to 30 kDa. A second protein isoform, with an apparent molecular weight of 19 kDa, is produced as a result of internal translation initiation from an in-frame adenine-thymine-guanine (ATG) at codon 54.[91] This smaller form of the *pVHL* protein seems to predominate in many tissues. At present, it is not known why cells make two forms of the p*VHL* protein; additionally, the two isoforms behave fairly similarly in the biochemical and functional assays performed so far.[92] For simplicity, the term *pVHL* is used when referring to these two proteins generically. Biochemical fractionation and immunohistochemical studies indicate that *pVHL* shuttles back and forth between the cytosol and nucleus, with most of the protein located in the cytosol. The primary sequence of *pVHL* neither closely resembles other known proteins nor reveals obvious structural motifs that might provide clues as to its function.[6]

Because skin manifestations are rare, VHL is diagnosed either when a signature lesion is identified in a new patient or a new member of a known kindred is screened.[93] These manifestations are frequently a neoplastic one. VHL is the most robust tumor predisposition disorder among the phakomatoses. Associations of tumors within VHL have been described; for example, approximately 20% of VHL patients with retinal hemangioblastoma develop cerebellar hemangioblastoma.[94] Presumably these associations are mutation specific. However the only established genotype–phenotype correlation is with pheochromocytoma.[90]

Hemangioblastomas are uncommon benign central nervous system tumors. Nearly half of those encountered are in VHL patients. The remainder represent somatic mutations.[95] Hemangioblastomas typically occur in the retina and in the cerebellum in approximately equal frequency.[84] Each usually presents either as a mass lesion or as parenchymal hemorrhage (or both). Tumors are often multiple, and the mean age of VHL patients at diagnosis of hemangioblastomas is considerably younger than that of patients with sporadic cases.[96] The primary age range of VHL patients who present with CNS lesions is 25 to 40 years, although CNS lesions can occur in children.

In the cerebellum, small tumors appear solid on MRI or CT scan, whereas larger ones typically are thin-walled cystic structures with a mural nodule (Fig. 12-7A). Both the nodule and the cyst wall are neoplastic tissue. Hemangioblastomas occasionally presents as a compressive lesion following an increase in the cystic component. The cerebellar lesions are usually located in the paramedian cerebellum and may be multiple (Fig. 12-7A). The midline location facilitates obstructive hydrocephalus and herniation. This represents a neurosurgical emergency.

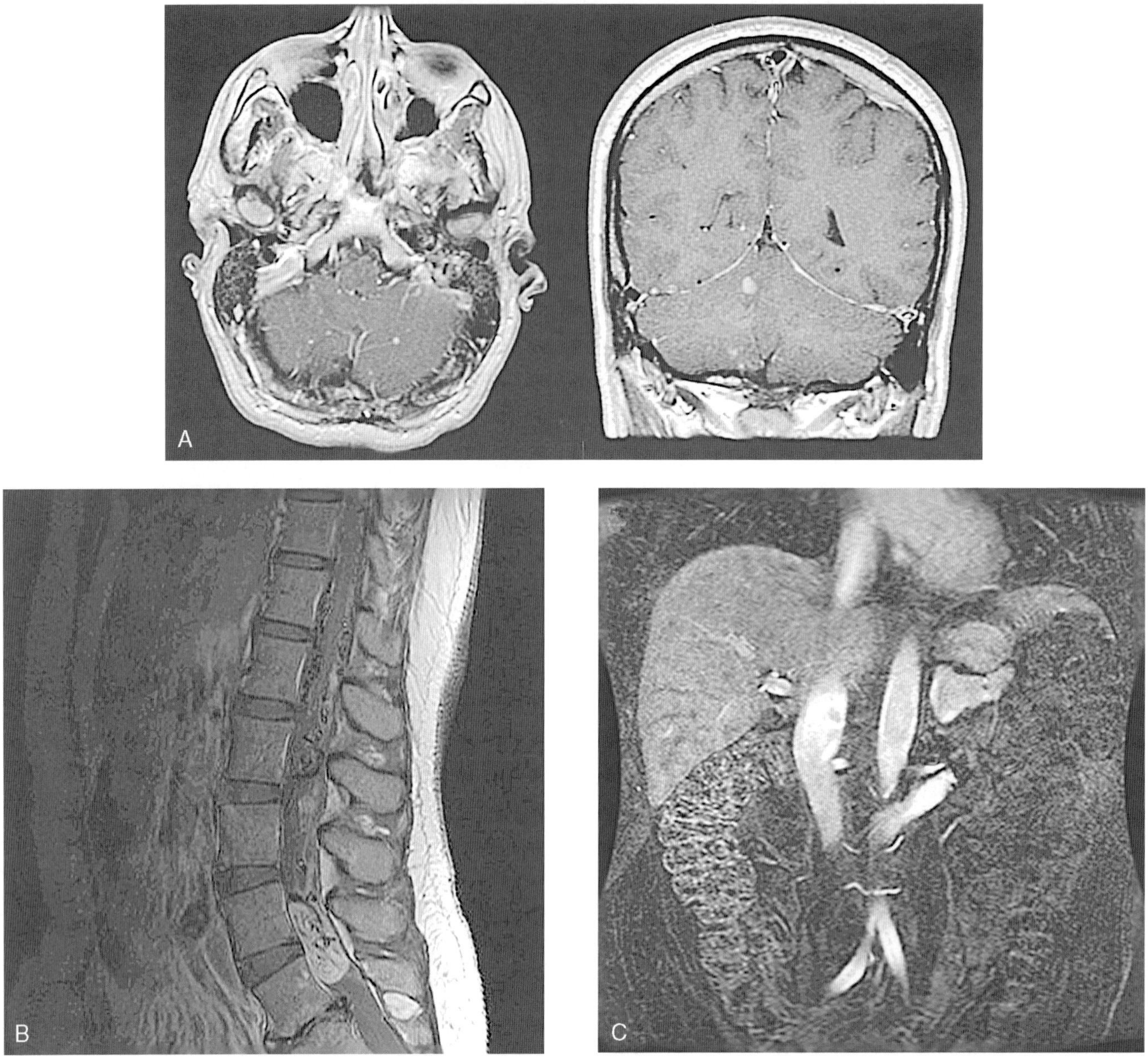

Figure 12-7. (A) Several small hemangioblastoma lesions (left) noted on surveillance scahning in a patient who presented with a hemorrhagic tumor mass in the left cerebellar hemisphere. The largest remaining lesion is in the characteristic paramedian location (right). (B) Hemangioblastoma of spinal root. (C) Tiny, enhancing nodule at junction of body and tail of the pancreas (closed arrow) identified on routine screening of patient whose two sons had pheochromocytomas. Next to the nodule is a small pancreatic cyst (open arrow).

Small and asymptomatic lesions are now being managed by stereotactic radiosurgery with excellent results.[97]

The next most common location is in the cervical spinal cord followed by medulla and pons. The imaging features are similar to those of cerebellar hemangioblastomas described above. A not infrequent presentation is cervical hematomyelia following trauma caused by hemorrhage into an occult cord lesion. The true nature of the lesion is determined only after pathologic examination of the tissue around the hemorrhage. Rare cases of hemangioblastomas are described involving spinal nerve roots (Fig. 12-7B).[98]

Retinal angiomas (hemangioblastomas) are present in more than half of all patients with VHL.[99] These benign tumors are often multiple, bilateral, and recurrent. If untreated, they may cause retinal detachment and hemorrhage, leading to blindness. Retinal presentations can occur at any age including in later life. However, most angiomas are found in the second and third decades of life, with a mean age at diagnosis of 25 years.[99] Retinal lesions in known VHL patients are usually detected on screening.[100] Often, there are no clinical symptoms until serious damage occurs as a consequence of hemorrhage, retinal detachment, or other complications. Detection of these lesions is by ophthalmoscopic examination, with the classic finding being a reddish spherical tumor of variable size with a dilated feeding artery and a draining vein. Most small lesions are peripheral and difficult to treat. Treatment of small lesions is by laser coagulation and cryotherapy, usually with few complications.[101]

Systemic malignancies are critical elements of the syndrome. Hypernephroma or renal cell carcinoma (RCC) is the third most common manifestation of VHL, and, in some series, the most common cause of death.[6,102] RCC may exist as a single lesion, as multiple lesions in one kidney or as bilateral tumors.[103] Elevation in total red blood cells due to erythropoietin stimulation may occur in either RCC or hemangioblastomas. Recognition of its significance can lead to an early diagnosis of either tumor. Pheochromocytomas are the next most common malignancy in VHL and comprise the bulk of familial pheochromocytomas.[104] Pancreatic islet cell tumors are less common.[90] Benign cysts of kidneys, pancreas, adrenal glands, and endolymphatic sacs are also typical of VHL (Fig. 12-7C).

Minimal diagnostic criteria for patients with a known family history of VHL include the presence of a single retinal or cerebellar hemangioblastoma, RCC, or pheochromocytoma (Table 12-5). In an isolated case, the clinical diagnosis of VHL can be made in a person who has two or more retinal or CNS hemangioblastomas or a single hemangioblastoma and a characteristic visceral tumor.[84] De novo mutations tend to be underrecognized compared with mutations in a familial setting. A diagnosis of VHL should be considered in any patient with a retinal or CNS hemangioblastoma, especially if onset is at an early age and there are familial, early onset, or bilateral clear-cell RCC; familial or bilateral pheochromocytoma; and bilateral endolymphatic sac tumors.

▶ **TABLE 12-5.** DIAGNOSTIC CRITERIA FOR VON HIPPEL-LINDAU DISEASE (VHL)

If positive family history, one of the following:
- Single retinal or cerebellar hemangioblastoma
- Renal cell carcinoma
- Pheochromocytoma
- Multiple pancreatic cysts

If no family history, one of the following:
- Two or more retinal or cerebellar hemangioblastomas
- One hemangioblastoma and one visceral tumor (renal clear cell or pheochromocytoma)

Nevoid Basal Cell Carcinoma Syndrome (Gorlin Syndrome)

Nevoid basal cell carcinoma syndrome (NBCCS), also known as Gorlin syndrome, is an autosomal dominant disorder with an incidence of approximately 1 in 60,000.[105,107] There is no known ethnic predisposition. Approximately 60% of patients have no affected family member with at least half of these representing new mutations. NBCCS defines a syndrome characterized by multiple developmental anomalies and a predisposition to the development of early onset neoplasms, particularly in the skin (basal cell carcinoma) and nervous system (medulloblastoma[107,108]). Table 12-6 defines the diagnostic criteria for NBCCS.

The genetic basis of NBCCS is a germline mutation of the human homologue of *Patched* (*Ptc*), a segment polarity gene originally described in *Drosophila*

▶ **TABLE 12-6.** DIAGNOSTIC CRITERIA FOR NEVOID BASAL CELL CARCINOMA SYNDROME (GORLIN SYNDROME)

Major criteria*
- More than two or one basal cell carcinoma diagnosed in patients younger than age 20 years
- Odontogenic keratocyst of the jaw proven by histology
- Three or more palmar or plantar pits
- Bilamellar calcification of the falx cerebri
- Bifid, fused, or markedly splayed ribs
- First-degree relative with NBCCS

Minor criteria*
- Macrocephaly determined after adjustment for height
- Congenital malformations: cleft lip or palate, frontal bossing, coarse face, moderate or severe hypertelorism
- Other skeletal abnormalities: Sprengel deformity, marked pectus deformity, marked syndactyly of the digits
- Radiologic abnormalities: bridging of the sella turcica, vertebral anomalies such as hemivertebrae, fusion, or elongation of the vertebral bodies, modeling defects of the hands and feet, and flame-shaped lucencies of the hands or feet
- Ovarian fibroma
- Medulloblastoma

*A diagnosis is made when two major or one major and two minor criteria are present.

melanogaster.[108,109] The human homologue, *PTCH*, is located on the long arm of chromosome 9 (9q22.3-q31). *PTCH* encodes a large protein that contains 13 membrane-spanning domains and serves, together with *Smoothened* (*SMO*), as a receptor and signal transduction complex for the secreted mitogen, *sonic hedgehog*.[110] *PTCH* serves to repress the constitutive activity of *SMO* in transducing the proliferative *sonic hedgehog* signal, and thereby, restricts the activation of *sonic hedgehog*–induced targets.[111] Mutations in *PTCH* are believed to alter the interaction between *PTCH* and *SMO* and allow for persistent, and often inappropriate, proliferative signals to be propagated within cells of the skin and nervous system.[109] Loss of the wild-type allele commonly occurs but is not required for tumor formation in the skin or nervous system, as tumors have developed with persistent expression of *PTCH* in both humans[112–114] and mice.[115,116] While haploinsufficiency of *PTCH* clearly has a broad range of phenotypic effects, the mechanism by which *PTCH* loss contributes to malignant transformation remains to be elucidated.

Because medulloblastoma is covered in Chapter 20, only those areas that relate to the neurocutaneous component are reviewed here. Developmental manifestations include characteristic facies with frontoparietal bossing and hypertelorism, palmoplantar pits, jaw cysts, rib and vertebrae abnormalities, macrocephaly, and dural calcifications. Neoplastic manifestations are primarily skin basal cell carcinoma, and medulloblastoma (MB). Rhabdomyosarcomas have not been documented to occur as a component of NBCCS as originally described in humans[107,108]; however, soft-tissue sarcomas are reported to occur with increased frequency in mice carrying a germline mutation of *PTCH*.[115,117,118]

Although only approximately 5% of NBCCS patients develop medulloblastoma, there are distinct clinical differences between them and the typical sporadic form,[105,119,120] including an earlier age of onset, a higher incidence of the desmoplastic variant, and better outcome (see Chapter 20). In a recent review of 76 consecutive patients with medulloblastoma, the incidence of NBCCS was 4% overall.[105] After inclusion of the age variable, the incidence of NBCCS was 10.7% for patients younger than 5 years old and 25% for patients younger than 2 years old. The incidence of NBCCS among patients with the desmoplastic subtype was 20%, and, after inclusion of age, the incidence of NBCCS in this subtype was 60% for patients younger than 5 years old and 100% for patients younger than 2 years old. Because medulloblastoma is almost always the first manifestation of NBCCS the syndrome is recognized when the patient develops multiple nevoid carcinomas in the irradiated field (Fig. 12-8). Patients with NBCCS syndrome are hypersensitive to ionizing radiation and are prone to develop numerous basal cell nevi in the field of radiation.[121–123] The mechanism of increased sensitivity of cells of NBCCS patients to therapeutic doses of ionizing radiation is not well understood even though first noted two decades ago.[124,125] As medulloblastoma may be the first manifestation of NBCCS, evaluation of the young child (<4 years of age) for stigmata supportive of a diagnosis of NBCCS should be done prior to initiating radiation therapy.

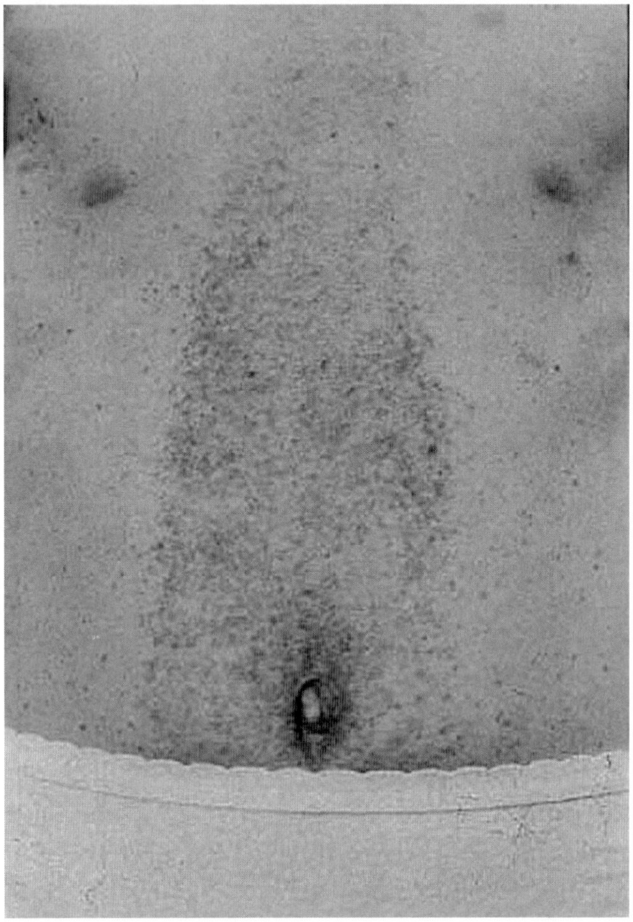

Figure 12-8 (PLATE 44). Subsequent development of nevoid basal cell carcinomas in treatment field of medulloblastoma patient who received neuraxis irradiation.

Management is principally expectant in persons known to have the gene defect. Periodic examination of the skin and MRI scans of the brain are reasonable. Current recommendations are for MRI scans at least yearly to age 10 years. Cardiac and abdominal ultrasonography are similarly recommended for cardiac and uterine fibromas, respectively. Uterine ultrasonography is recommended at 19 weeks of gestation in known NBCCS women. Currently, it is not recommended to do gene mutation screening in every new medulloblastoma patient. However, every newly diagnosed NBCCS patient should then lead to an examination of family members at risk for the gene.

▶ MOLECULAR GENETICS AND THE ROLE OF MOUSE MODELS

In an effort to learn more about the molecular pathogenesis of the clinical features and to develop preclinical models for the phakomatoses, a number of research groups have generated mice with targeted disruptions of the putative tumor suppressor genes. Not only do transgenic mice allow for analysis of disruption or overexpression of single genes but these mice can be interbred to assess the effects of multiple genetic changes. In this way, these genetically engineered mice can serve as useful preclinical models for the study of disease pathophysiology and potential therapies. Robust models now exist for NF1, NF2, TSC, and NBCCS.

Neurofibromatosis

Early studies demonstrated that homozygous deletion of the *NF1* gene resulted in embryonic lethality by gestational day 14. However, mice heterozygous for a mutation in the *Nf1* gene (*Nf1*+/− mice) exhibit normal development but manifest deficits in specific learning and memory paradigms.[126] By age 18 to 24 months, *Nf1*+/− mice developed two malignancies associated with *NF1*—myeloid leukemia and pheochromocytoma. *Nf1*+/− mice do not develop neurofibromas or astrocytomas, the two most common tumor types seen in patients with NF1.

To develop more refined models of NF1-associated tumors, several different approaches have been taken. First, mice have been generated by varying the percentage of *Nf1* null embryonic stem cells in the developing blastocyst. These models bypassed the inherent lethality of complete absence of neurofibromin during development and ensured the presence of some neurofibromin-expressing cells during development. Some of these chimeric mice developed plexiform neurofibromas, histologically similar to their human counterparts.[127] The initiating event in the pathogenesis of plexiform neurofibromas in these mice therefore appears to be the complete absence of neurofibromin in specific tissues at an early stage of development. Likewise, plexiform neurofibromas in humans are also thought to be congenital lesions, suggesting *NF1* inactivation in specific cells during fetal development.

Other investigators bypassed the known lethality of *Nf1* null mice by selectively ablating the gene in specific cell types. Selective ablation of the *Nf1* gene in neurons resulted in mutant mice with growth retardation and cerebral astrogliosis, but no tumor formation.[128] Astrocyte-specific *Nf1* conditional knockout mice show increased astrocyte proliferation, supporting a role for neurofibromin in regulation of astrocyte proliferation. Interestingly, while the *Nf1*+/− mouse did not develop astrocytic tumors, conditional deletion of *Nf1* in cells destined to become astrocytes did result in tumorigenesis when the conditional mutant was bred onto an *Nf1*+/− genetic background.[106] Similar results were obtained with Schwann cell–specific *NF1* inactivation and neurofibroma formation.[129] These experiments elegantly demonstrate the extensive interaction between tumor and host cells and allude to the complexities of intracellular and extracellular signaling in malignant transformation.[130]

To determine what additional genetic events are required for the development of malignant tumors, mice heterozygous for *Nf1* inactivation were mated with mice heterozygous for a targeted mutation in *p53*, a tumor suppressor gene mutated in many sporadic tumors, including brain tumors and MPNSTs. Depending on the genetic background, these *Nf1*+/−; *p53*+/− mice developed MPNSTs, high-grade sarcomas, and glioblastomas as a result of loss of heterozygosity at both *p53* and *Nf1* loci.[131] These findings corroborate observations on human tumors, in which some NF1-associated MPNSTs harbor mutations in the *p53* gene. However, compared to the glioblastomas in the mouse model, NF1-associated pilocytic astrocytomas lack p53 mutations and only rarely become clinically aggressive tumors. Further studies will likely identify the genes responsible for the phenotypic differences seen between mice of different backgrounds with identical *p53* and *Nf1* mutations.

Mice in which both copies of the *Nf2* gene are inactivated die by embryologic day 7 as a consequence of failure to complete gastrulation as a result of an abnormal extra embryologic ectoderm. These findings argue that merlin (like neurofibromin) plays an important role in embryonic development. *Nf2*+/− mice develop highly malignant and metastatic cancers during the second year of life, including malignant sarcomas, hepatocellular carcinomas, and fibrosarcoma.[24] Loss of the wild-type *Nf2* allele was noted in nearly all of these tumors, again indicating that the *Nf2* gene functions as a classic tumor suppressor gene. Nevertheless, similar to *Nf1*+/− mice, the tumors that develop in the *Nf2*+/− mice are not the typical tumors identified in human NF2. To facilitate development of a more phenotypically accurate mouse model of NF2, mice were created by homozygous disruption of *Nf2* gene only in Schwann cells. These mice developed tumors characteristic of NF2, including schwannomas, suggesting that loss of merlin is sufficient for schwannoma development.[20]

Of note, conditional deletion of *Nf2* in cells of the arachnoid was permissive for the development of meningiomas in 30% of the mice that were phenotypically similar to those that arise in humans. However, in contrast to the acceleration of high-grade sarcomas and glioblastomas in Nf1+/−p53+/− mice, the development of meningioma in these mice was not further accelerated by crossing the *Nf2* conditional knockout mice onto a *p53* hemizygous background.[132] Recent reports suggest that epigenetic factors also modulate gene expression in inbred strains of mice and can influence the tumor phenotype.[133]

Tuberous Sclerosis Complex

The two abnormal cellular phenotypes in TSC involve an increase both in cell proliferation and in cell size. Insights into how the THC might regulate these processes first came from studies in *Drosophila* linking the insulin signaling pathway to the regulation of cell growth and proliferation.[134] In support of this hypothesis, overexpression of *TSC1* or *TSC2* rescued lethality in *Drosophila* mutants in which the insulin receptor was nonfunctional and reversed the cell proliferation defects of flies that overexpressed the insulin receptor.[135,136] Additional studies indicated that the THC functions in the insulin-like growth factor (IGF) receptor pathway downstream of phosphotidylinositide-3 kinase (PI3K) and Akt (see Fig. 12-7). This pathway is known to regulate both cell proliferation and cell size. Akt phosphorylate tuberin, resulting in its dissociation from hamartin and inactivation of the THC.[137–139] The functional THC normally inhibits the activity of the mammalian target of rapamycin (mTOR).[140,141] However, when the THC is inactivated by Akt-mediated phosphorylation of tuberin, mTOR inhibition is relieved. Activation of mTOR results in an increase in protein synthesis and, ultimately, cell growth. In cells where the THC is permanently inactivated as a consequence of genetic mutation, unregulated cell growth occurs. This effect can be blocked by treatment with rapamycin, a drug that inhibits mTOR.[142]

Initial attempts to recapitulate the human TSC phenotype in mice were performed using conventional knockout mice in which germline expression of *Tsc1* or *Tsc2* was inactivated. Mice homozygous for loss of *Tsc1* or *Tsc2* die in mid-embryogenesis of apparent cardiac malformations and liver hypoplasia.[143,144] In the CNS of $Tsc2^{+/-}$ and $Tsc1^{+/-}$ mice, the numbers of astrocytes increased, suggesting that hamartin and tuberin are important astrocyte growth regulators.[145] However, when grown in vitro, $Tsc2^{+/-}$ astrocytes did not demonstrate a cell-autonomous growth advantage. In addition, compound heterozygotes that lack one copy of both *Tsc1* and *Tsc2* had further increases in the number of astrocytes. Together, these observations support the role of tuberin and hamartin as regulators of cell growth and proliferation in the CNS.

The observations that reduced expression of tuberin or hamartin resulted in abnormal astrocyte proliferation, that TSC-affected individuals frequently develop astrocytic tumors (SEGAs), and that *TSC2* expression is reduced or absent in 30% of high-grade sporadic astrocytomas suggested that *TSC* gene expression in astrocytes may be of particular importance to the CNS defects that characterize this disease.[146] Because conventional knockout mice for either of these two genes die before brain development is complete, it is not possible to study astrocyte defects in these animals. To circumvent this, a conditional knockout (cKO) approach was used to inactivate *Tsc1* in astrocytes. Although these *Tsc1* cKO mice do not have frank cortical tubers, brains from these animals have an increased number of immunoreactive astrocytes by 3 weeks of age and four times as many actively proliferating astrocytes at 6 weeks of age.[145] The hippocampus exhibited the most pronounced enlargement in these animals and demonstrates significant architectural disorganization. Astrocytes from *Tsc1* cKO mice grown in vitro exhibit a growth advantage at confluence, suggesting that the normal inhibitory cues that trigger cells to stop dividing when they become too densely packed are defective in hamartin-deficient astrocytes. In addition to an increased number of astrocytes, *Tsc1* cKO mice exhibit electroencephalographically documented seizures after 4 weeks of age and begin to die at 3 to 4 months of age.[145] The underlying defect is thought to be the decreased expression of glutamate transporter and decrease in glutamate current in the *Tsc1* mutant astrocytes.[147]

▶ GENETIC TESTING IN ROUTINE CLINICAL PRACTICE

This chapter's sections discussed practical management for each of the phakomatoses. For each of the described phakomatoses the responsible gene and the gene product were identified (see Table 12-1). DNA tests are now available for NF1, NF2, TSC, and VHL (limitations are discussed in each section). Clinical screening can be limited to people who have an inherited predisposition. However, as DNA-based tests can indicate genotype but cannot predict phenotype, there is no consensus on what exactly needs to be done and at what age. More evidence is needed to document that screenings diminish the rate of severe complications and improve outcome.

REFERENCES

1. Rust RS. Neurocutaneous disorders. In: Noseworthy JH, ed. Neurological therapeutics: principles and practice. New York: Martin Dunitz, 2003:1646–1680.
2. Rose VM. Neurocutaneous syndromes. Mol Med 2004;101: 112–116.
3. Gutmann DH, Aylsworth A, Carey JC, et al. The diagnostic evaluation and multidisciplinary management of neurofibromatosis 1 and neurofibromatosis 2. JAMA 1997;278:51–57.
4. MacCollin M, Mautner VF. The diagnosis and management of neurofibromatosis 2 in childhood. Semin Pediatr Neurol 1998;5:243–252.
5. Gomez MR, Sampson JR, Whittemore VH. Tuberous sclerosis, 3rd ed. New York: Oxford University Press, 1999.
6. Kaelin WG Jr. Molecular basis of the VHL hereditary cancer syndrome. Nat Rev Cancer 2002;2:673–682.

7. Wetmore CJ. Sonic hedgehog in normal and neoplastic proliferation: insight gained from human tumors and animal models. Curr Opin Genet Dev 2003;13:34–42.
8. Marchuk DA, Saulino AM, Tavakkol R, et al. cDNA cloning of the type 1 neurofibromatosis gene: complete sequence of the *NF1* gene product. Genomics 1991;11:931–940.
9. Daston MM, Scrable H, Norlund M, et al. The protein product of the neurofibromatosis type 1 gene is expressed at highest abundance in neurons, Schwann cells and oligodendrocytes. Neuron 1992;8:415–428.
10. Xu GF, O'Connell P, Viskochil D, et al. The neurofibromatosis type 1 gene encodes a protein related to GAP. Cell 1990;62:599–608.
11. Bollag G, McCormick F. Regulators and effectors of *ras* proteins. Ann Rev Cell Biol 1991;7:601–632.
12. Wittinghofer A. Signal transduction via ras. Biol Chem 1998;379:933–937.
13. Messiaen LM, Callens T, Mortier G, et al. Exhaustive mutation analysis of the NF1 gene allows identification of 95% of mutations and reveals an increased frequency of unusual splicing defects. Hum Mutat 2000;15:541–545.
14. Reed N, Gutmann DH. Tumorigenesis in neurofibromatosis: new insights and potential therapies. Trends Mol Med 2001;7:157–162.
15. Rouleau GA, Merel P, Lutchman M, et al. Alteration in a new gene encoding a putative membrane-organizing protein causes neuro-fibromatosis type 2. Nature 1993;363:515–521.
16. Xie YG, Han FY, Peyrard M, et al. Cloning of a novel, anonymous gene from a megabase-range YAC and cosmid contig in the neurofibromatosis type 2/meningioma region on human chromosome 22q12. Hum Mol Genet 1993;2:1361–1368.
17. Sherman L, Xu HM, Geist RT, et al. Interdomain binding mediates tumor growth suppression by the NF2 gene product. Oncogene 1997;15:2505–2509.
18. Morrison H, Sherman LS, Legg J, et al. The NF2 tumor suppressor gene product, merlin, mediates contact inhibition through interactions with CD44. Genes Dev 2001;15: 968–980.
19. Shaw RJ, Paez JG, Curto M, et al. The NF2 tumor suppressor, merlin, functions in rac-dependent signaling. Dev Cell 2001;1:63–72.
20. Giovannini M, Robanus-Maandag E, van der Valk M. Conditional biallelic *Nf2* mutation in the mouse promotes manifestations of human neurofibromatosis type 2. Gene Dev 2000;14:1617–1630.
21. Evans DG, Trueman L, Wallace A, et al. Genotype/phenotype correlations in type 2 neurofibromatosis (NF2): evidence for more severe disease associated with truncating mutations. J Med Genet 1998;35:450–455.
22. Parry DM, MacCollin M, Kaiser-Kupfer MI, et al. Germ-line mutations in the neurofibromatosis 2 gene correlation with disease severity and retinal abnormalities. Am J Hum Genet 1996;59:529–539.
23. Knudson AG. Mutation and cancer: a statistical study of retinoblastoma. Proc Natl Acad Sci USA 1971;68:820–823.
24. McClatchey AI, Saotome I, Mercer K. Mice heterozygous for a mutation at the NF2 tumor suppressor locus develop a range of highly metastatic tumors. Gene Dev 1998;12: 1121–1133.
25. Feldkamp MM, Lau N, Provias JP, et al. Acute presentation of a neurogenic sarcoma in a patient with neurofibromatosis type 1: a pathological and molecular explanation. J Neurosurg 1996;84:867–873.
26. Bollag G, Clapp DW, Shih S, et al. Loss of NF1 results in activation of the *ras* signaling pathway and leads to aberrant growth in haematopoietic cells. Nat Genet 1996;12:144–148.
27. Ueki K, Wen-Bin C, Navita Y, et al. Tight association of loss of merlin expression with loss of heterozygosity at chromosome 22q in sporadic meningiomas. Cancer Res 1999; 59:5995–5998.
28. Friedman JM, Gutmann DH, MacCollin M, et al. Neurofibromatosis: phenotype, natural history and pathogenesis, 3rd ed. Baltimore, MD: Johns Hopkins Press, 1999.
29. DeClue JE, Cohen BD, Lowy DR. Identification and characterization of the neurofibromatosis type 1 protein product. Proc Natl Acad Sci USA 1991;88:9914–9918.
30. King AA, DeBaun MR, Riccardi VM, et al. Malignant peripheral nerve sheath tumors in neurofibromatosis 1. Am J Med Genet 2000;93:388–392.
31. Cardona S, Schwarzbach M, Hinz U, et al. Evaluation of F18-deoxyglucose positron emission tomography (FDG-PET) to assess the nature of neurogenic tumours. Eur J Surg Oncol 2003;29:536–541.
32. Huang JH, Zaghloul K, Zager EL. Surgical management of brachial plexus region tumors. Surg Neurol 2004;61: 372–378.
33. Listernick R, Louis DN, Packer RJ, et al. Optic pathway gliomas in children with neurofibromatosis 1: consensus statement from the NF1 optic pathway glioma task force. Ann Neurol 1997;41:143–149.
34. Pollack IF, Shultz B, Mulvihill JJ. The management of brainstem gliomas in patients with neurofibromatosis 1. Neurology 1996;46:1652–1660.
35. Fortman BJ, Kuszyk BS, Urban BA, et al. Neurofibromatosis type 1: a diagnostic mimicker. Radiographics 2001;21: 601–612.
36. DiPaola DP, Zimmerman RA, Rorke LB, et al. Neurofibromatosis type 1: pathologic substrate of high-signal intensity foci in the brain. Radiology 1995;195:721–724.
37. Virdis R, Street ME, Bandello MA, et al. Growth and pubertal disorders in neurofibromatosis type 1. J Pediatr Endocrinol Metab 2003;16(Suppl 2):289–292.
38. North K. Neurofibromatosis type 1. Am J Med Genet 2000; 97:119–127.
39. Hamilton SJ, Friedman JM. Insights into the pathogenesis of neurofibromatosis 1 vasculopathy. Clin Genet 2000;58: 341–344.
40. Ruggieri M, Huson S. The clinical and diagnostic implications of mosaicism in the neurofibromatoses. Neurology 2001;56:1433–1443.
41. Shen MH, Harper OS, Upadhyaya M. Molecular genetics of neurofibromatosis type 1 (NF1). J Med Genet 1996;33:2–17.
42. Mantadakis E, Raissaki M, Danilatou V, et al. Remission of a chiasmatic glioma in a non-NF1 patient after brief chemotherapy with vincristine and carboplatin: case report and literature review. J Neurooncol 2004;67:95–100.
43. Cappelli C, Grill J, Raquin M, et al. Long-term follow up of 69 patients treated for optic pathway tumours before the chemotherapy era. Arch Dis Child 1998;79:334–338.

44. Robertson TC, Buck DA, Schmidt-Ullrich R, et al. Isolated plexiform neurofibroma: treatment with three-dimensional conformal radiotherapy. Laryngoscope 2004;114:1139–1142.
45. Babovic-Vuksanovic D, Petrovic L, Knudsen BE, et al. Survival of human neurofibroma in immunodeficient mice and initial results of therapy with pirfenidone. J Biomed Biotechnol 2004;2:79–85.
46. Parry DM, Eldridge R, Kaiser-Kupfer MI, et al. Neurofibromatosis 2 (NF2): clinical characteristics of 63 affected individuals and clinical evidence for heterogeneity. Am J Med Genet 1994;52:450–461.
47. Patronas NJ, Courcoutsakis N, Bromley CM, et al. Intramedullary and spinal canal tumors in patients with neurofibromatosis 2: MR imaging findings and correlation with genotype. Radiology 2001;218:434–442.
48. Evans DGR, Trueman L, Wallace A, et al. Genotype/phenotype correlations in type 2 neurofibromatosis (NF2): evidence for more severe disease associated with truncating mutations. J Med Genet 1998;35:450–455.
49. MacCollin M, Woodfin W, Kronn D, et al. Schwannomatosis: a clinical and pathologic study. Neurology 1996;46: 1072–1079.
50. Kluwe L, Mautner V, Heinrich B, et al. Molecular study of frequency of mosaicism in neurofibromatosis 2 patients with bilateral vestibular schwannomas. J Med Genet 2003; 40:109–114.
51. Roach ES, Gomez MR, Northrup H. Tuberous sclerosis complex consensus conference: revised clinical diagnostic criteria. J Child Neurol 1998;13:624–628.
52. Povey S, Burley MW, Attwood J, et al. Two loci for tuberous sclerosis: one on 9q34 and one on 16p13. Ann Hum Genet 1994;58:107–127.
53. van Slegtenhorst M, de Hoogt R, Hermans C, et al. Identification of the tuberous sclerosis gene TSC1 on chromosome 9q34. Science 1997;277:805–808.
54. Identification and characterization of the tuberous sclerosis gene on chromosome 16. European Chromosome 16 Tuberous Sclerosis Consortium. Cell 1993;75:1305–1315.
55. van Slegtenhorst M, Nellist M, Nagelkerken B, et al. Interaction between hamartin and tuberin, the TSC1 and TSC2 gene products. Hum Mol Genet 1998;7:1053–1057.
56. Plank TL, Yeung RS, Henske EP. Hamartin, the product of the tuberous sclerosis 1 (TSC1) gene, interacts with tuberin and appears to be localized to cytoplasmic vesicles. Cancer Res 1998;58:4766–4770.
57. Hodges AK, Li S, Maynard J, et al. Pathologic mutations in TSC1 and TSC2 disrupt the interaction between hamartin and tuberin. Hum Mol Genet 2001;159:217–224.
58. Cheadle JP, Reeve MP, Sampson JR, et al. Molecular genetic advances in tuberous sclerosis. Hum Genet 2000;107: 1135–1138.
59. Kwiatkowski DJ. Tuberous sclerosis: from tubers to mTOR. Ann Hum Genet 2003;67:87–96.
60. Niida Y, Stemmer-Rachamimov AO, Logrip M. Survey of somatic mutations in tuberous sclerosis complex (TSC) hamartomas suggests different genetic mechanisms for pathogenesis of TSC lesions. Am J Hum Genet 2001;69: 493–503.
61. Benvenuto G, Li S, Brown SJ, et al. The tuberous sclerosis-1 (TSC1) gene produce hamartin suppresses cell growth and augments the expression of the TSC2 product tuberin by inhibiting its ubiquitination. Oncogene 2000;19:6306–6316.
62. Miloloza A, Rosner M, Nellist M, et al. The TSC1 gene product, hamartin, negatively regulates cell proliferation. Hum Mol Genet 2000;9:1721–1727.
63. Soucek T, Pusch O, Wienecke R, et al. Role of the tuberous sclerosis gene-2 product in cell cycle control. Loss of the tuberous sclerosis gene-2 induces cells to enter S phase. J Biol Chem 1997;272:29301–29308.
64. Gutmann DH, Zhang Y, Hasbani MJ, et al. Expression of the tuberous sclerosis complex gene products, hamartin and tuberin, in central nervous system tissues. Acta Neuropathol 2000;5:276–286.
65. Park SH, Pepkowitz SH, Kerfoot C, et al. Tuberous sclerosis in a 20-week gestation fetus: immunohistochemical study. Acta Neuropathol 1997;94:180–186.
66. Wienecke R, Guha A, Maize JC Jr, et al. Reduced TSC2 RNA and protein in sporadic astrocytomas and ependymomas. Ann Neurol 1997;15:1611–1616.
67. Ramesh V. Aspects of tuberous sclerosis complex (TSC) protein function in the brain. Biochem Soc Trans 2003;31: 579–583.
68. Onda H, Crino PB, Zhang H, et al. TSC2 null neuroepithelial cells are a model for human tuber giant cells and show activation of an mTOR pathway. Mol Cell Neurosci 2002;21:561–574.
69. Asano E, Chugani DC, Muzik O, et al. Autism in tuberous sclerosis complex is related to both cortical and subcortical dysfunction. Neurology 2001;51:1269–1277.
70. Bolton PF, Park RJ, Higgins JN, et al. Neuro-epileptic determinants of autism spectrum disorders in tuberous sclerosis complex. Brain 2002;125:1247–1255.
71. Joinson C, O'Callaghan FJ, Osborne JP, et al. Learning disability and epilepsy in an epidemiological sample of individuals with tuberous sclerosis complex. Psychiatr Med 2003;33:335–344.
72. Curatolo P, Seri S, Verdecchia M, et al. Infantile spasms in tuberous sclerosis complex. Brain Dev 2001;23:502–507.
73. Cusmai R, Chiron C, Curatolo P, et al. Topographic comparative study of MRI and EEG in 34 children with tuberous sclerosis. Epilepsia 1990;31:747–755.
74. Goodman M, Lamm SH, Engel A, et al. Cortical tuber count: a biomarker indicating neurologic severity of tuberous sclerosis complex. J Child Neurol 1997;12:85–90.
75. Hancock E, Osborne JP. Vigabatrin in the treatment of infantile spasms in tuberous sclerosis: literature review. J Child Neurol 1999;41:123–126.
76. Bebin EM, Kelly PJ, Gomez MR. Surgical treatment for epilepsy in cerebral tuberous sclerosis. Epilepsia 1993;34: 651–657.
77. Shepherd CW, Scheithauer BW, Gomez MR, et al. Subependymal giant cell astrocytoma: a clinical, pathologic, and flow cytometry study. Neurosurgery 1991;38:864–868.
78. Mirkin LD, Ey EH, Chaparro M. Congenital subependymal giant cell astrocytoma: case report with prenatal ultrasonogram. Pediatr Radiol 1999;29:776–780.
79. Karumanchi SA, Merchan J, Sukhatme VP. Renal cancer: molecular mechanisms and newer therapeutic options. Curr Opin Nephrol Hypertens 2002;11:37–42.

80. Tello R, Blickman JG, Buonomo C, et al. Meta analysis of the relationship between tuberous sclerosis complex and renal cell carcinoma. Eur J Radiol 1998;27:131–138.
81. Martignoni G, Pea M, Rigaud G, et al. Renal angiomyolipoma with epithelioid sarcomatous transformation and metastases: demonstration of the same genetic defects in the primary and metastatic lesions. Am J Surg Pathol 2000;24:889–894.
82. Beltramello A, Puppini G, Bricolo A, et al. Does the tuberous sclerosis complex include intracranial aneurysms? A case report with a review of the literature. Pediatr Radiol 1999;29:206–211.
83. Dabora SL, Jozwiak S, Franz DN. Mutational analysis in a cohort of 224 tuberous sclerosis patients indicates increased severity of TSC2, compared with TSC1, disease in multiple organs. Am J Hum Genet 2001;68:64–80.
84. Couch V, Lindor NM, Karnes PS, et al. Von Hippel-Lindau disease. Mayo Clin Proc 2000;75:265–272.
85. Yao M, Latif F, Orcutt ML, et al. von Hippel-Lindau disease: identification of deletion mutations by pulsed-field gel electrophoresis. Hum Genet 1993;92:605–614.
86. Maher ER, Iselius L, Yates JR, et al. Von Hippel-Lindau disease: a genetic study. J Med Genet 1991;28:443–447.
87. Karsdorp N, Elderson A, Wittebol-Post D, et al. Von Hippel-Lindau disease: new strategies in early detection and treatment. Am J Med 1994;97:158–168.
88. Wizigmann-Voos S, Breier G, Risau W, et al. Up-regulation of vascular endothelial growth factor and its receptors in von Hippel-Lindau disease-associated and sporadic hemangioblastomas. Cancer Res 1995;55:1358–1364.
89. Chen F, Kishida T, Yao M, et al. Germline mutations in the von Hippel-Lindau disease tumor suppressor gene: correlations with phenotype. Hum Mutat 1995;5:66–75.
90. Neumann HP, Berger DP, Sigmund G, et al. Pheochromocytomas, multiple endocrine neoplasia type 2, and von Hippel-Lindau disease. N Engl J Med 1993;329:1531–1538.
91. Latif F, Tory K, Gnarra J, et al. Identification of the von Hippel-Lindau disease tumor suppressor gene. Science 1993;260:1317–1320.
92. Richards FM, Schofield PN, Fleming S, et al. Expression of the von Hippel-Lindau disease tumour suppressor gene during human embryogenesis. Hum Mol Genet 1996;5:639–644.
93. Melmon KL, Rosen SW. Lindau's disease: review of the literature and study of a large kindred. Am J Med 1964;36:595–617.
94. Huson SM, Harper PS, Hourihan MD, et al. Cerebellar hemangioblastomas and von Hippel-Lindau disease. Brain 1986;109:1297–1310.
95. Richard S, Martin S, David P, et al. Von Hippel-Lindau disease and central nervous system hemangioblastoma. Progress in genetics and clinical management. Neurochirurgie 1998;44:258–266.
96. Neumann HP, Eggert HR, Weigel K, et al. Hemangioblastomas of the central nervous system. A 10-year study with special reference to von Hippel-Lindau syndrome. J Neurosurg 1989;70:24–30.
97. Pan L, Wang EM, Wang BJ, et al. Gamma knife radiosurgery for hemangioblastomas. Stereotact Funct Neurosurg 1998;70(Suppl 1):179–186.
98. Roessler K, Dietrich W, Haberler C, et al. Multiple spinal "miliary" hemangioblastomas in von Hippel-Lindau (vHL) disease without cerebellar involvement. A case report and a review of the literature. Neurosurg Rev 1999;22:130–134.
99. Ridley M, Green J, Johnson G. Retinal angiomatosis: the ocular manifestations of von Hippel-Lindau disease. Can J Ophthalmol 1986;21:276–283.
100. Moore AT, Maher ER, Rosen P, et al. Ophthalmological screening for von Hippel-Lindau disease. Eye 1991;5:723–728.
101. Welch RB. Von Hippel-Lindau disease: the recognition and treatment of early angiomatosis retinae and the use of cryosurgery as an adjunct to therapy. Trans Am Ophthalmol Soc 1970;68:367–424.
102. Linehan WM, Walther MM, Zbar B. The genetic basis of cancer of the kidney. J Urol 2003;170(6 Pt 1):2163–2172.
103. Bodmer D, van den Hurk W, van Groningen JJ, et al. Understanding familial and non-familial renal cell cancer. Hum Mol Genet 2002;11:2489–2498.
104. Richard S, Chauveau D, Chretien Y, et al. Renal lesions and pheochromocytoma in von Hippel-Lindau disease. Adv Nephrol Necker Hosp 1994;23:1–27.
105. Amlashi SF, Riffaud L, Brassier G, et al. Nevoid basal cell carcinoma syndrome: relation with desmoplastic medulloblastoma in infancy. A population-based study and review of the literature. Cancer 2003;98:618–624.
106. Bajenaru ML, Hernandez MR, Perry A, et al. Optic nerve glioma in mice requires astrocyte Nf1 gene inactivation and Nf1 brain heterozygosity. Cancer Res 2003;63:8573–8577.
107. Manfredi M, Vescovi P, Bonanini M, et al. Nevoid basal cell carcinoma syndrome: a review of the literature. Int J Oral Maxillofac Surg 2004;33:117–124.
108. Bale AE. The nevoid basal cell carcinoma syndrome: genetics and mechanism of carcinogenesis. Cancer Invest 1997;15:180–186.
109. Bale AE. Hedgehog signaling and human disease. Annu Rev Genomics Hum Genet 2002;3:47–65.
110. Ingham PW, McMahon AP. Hedgehog signaling in animal development: paradigms and principles. Gene Dev 2001;15:3059–3087.
111. Taipale J, Cooper MK, Maiti T, et al. Patched acts catalytically to suppress the activity of *Smoothened*. Nature 2002;418:892–897.
112. Vorechovsky I, Tingby O, Hartman M, et al. Somatic mutations in the human homologue of *Drosophila* patched in primitive neuroectodermal tumours. Medulloblastomas of the desmoplastic variant carry mutations of the human homologue of *Drosophila* patched. Sporadic medulloblastomas contain PTCH mutations. Oncogene 1997;15:361–366.
113. Pietsch T, Waha A, Koch A, et al. Medulloblastomas of the desmoplastic variant carry mutations of the human homologue of *Drosophila* patched. Sporadic medulloblastomas contain PTCH mutations. Cancer Res 1997;57:2085–2088.
114. Raffel C, Jenkins RB, Frederick L, et al. Sporadic medulloblastomas contain PTCH mutations. Cancer Res 1997;57:842–845.

115. Wetmore C. Sonic hedgehog in normal and neoplastic proliferation: insight gained from human tumors and animal models. Curr Opin Genet Dev 2003;13:34–42.
116. Wetmore C, Eberhart DE, Curran T. The normal patched allele is expressed in medulloblastomas from mice with heterozygous germ-line mutation of patched. Cancer Res 2000;60:2239–2246.
117. Goodrich LV, Scott MP. Hedgehog and patched in neural development and disease. Neuron 1998;21:1243–1257.
118. Hahn H, Wojnowski L, Miller G, et al. The patched signaling pathway in tumorigenesis and development: lessons from animal models. J Mol Med 1999;77:459–468.
119. Kimonis VE, Goldstein AM, Pastakia B, et al. Clinical manifestations in 105 persons with nevoid basal cell carcinoma syndrome. Am J Med Genet 1997;69:299–308.
120. Shanley S, Ratcliffe J, Hockey A, et al. Nevoid basal cell carcinoma syndrome: review of 118 affected individuals. Am J Med Genet 1994;50:282–290.
121. Dezawa M, Fujii K, Kita K, et al. Increase in nucleoli after x-radiation of fibroblasts of patients with Gorlin syndrome. J Lab Clin Med 1999;134:585–591.
122. Frentz G, Munch-Petersen B, Wulf HC, et al. The nevoid basal cell carcinoma syndrome: sensitivity to ultraviolet and x-ray irradiation. J Am Acad Dermatol 1987;17:637–643.
123. O'Malley S, Weitman D, Olding M, et al. Multiple neoplasms following craniospinal irradiation for medulloblastoma in a patient with nevoid basal cell carcinoma syndrome. Case report. J Neurosurg 1997;86:286–288.
124. Ringborg U, Lambert B, Landergen J, Lewensohn R. Decreased UV-induced DNA repair synthesis in peripheral leukocytes from patients with the nevoid basal cell carcinoma syndrome. J Invest Dermatol 1981;76:268–270.
125. Stefanini M, Lagomarsini P, Berardesca E, et al. Normal sensitivity to mutagens, spontaneous chromosome breakage, and mutation frequency in nevoid basal cell carcinoma syndrome. Arch Dermatol Res 1988;280(Suppl):S19–S23.
126. Costa RM, Federov NB, Kogan JH, et al. Mechanism for the learning deficits in a mouse model of neurofibromatosis type 1. Nature 2002;415:426–430.
127. Cichowski K, Shih TS, Schmitt E, et al. Mouse models of tumor development in neurofibromatosis type 1. Science 1999;286:2172–2176.
128. Costa RM, Yang T, Huynh DP, et al. Learning deficits, but normal development and tumor predisposition, in mice lacking exon 23a of Nf1. Nat Genet 2001;27:399–405.
129. Zhu Y, Parada LF. The molecular and genetic basis of neurological tumours. Nat Rev Cancer 2002;2:616–626.
130. Zhu Y, Ghosh P, Charnay P, et al. Neurofibromas in NF1: Schwann cell origin and role of tumor environment. Science 2002;296:920–922.
131. Zhu Y, Romero MI, Ghosh P, et al. Ablation of NF1 function in neurons induces abnormal development of cerebral cortex and reactive gliosis in the brain. Genes Dev 2001;15:859–876.
132. Reilly KM, Loisel DA, Bronson RT, et al. Nf1;Trp53 mutant mice develop glioblastoma with evidence of strain-specific effects. Nat Genet 2000;26:109–113.
133. Reilly KM, Tuskan RG, Christy E, et al. Susceptibility to astrocytoma in mice mutant for Nf1 and Trp53 is linked to chromosome 11 and subject to epigenetic effects. Proc Natl Acad Sci USA 2004;101:13,008–13,013.
134. Stocker H, Hafen E. Genetic control of cell size. Curr Opin Genet Dev 2000;10:529–535.
135. Gao X, Pan D. TSC1 and TSC2 tumor suppressors antagonize insulin signaling in cell growth. Gene Dev 2001;5:1383–1392.
136. Huang H, Potter CJ, Tao W, et al. PTEN affects cell size, cell proliferation, and apoptosis during Drosophila eye development. Development 1999;126:5365–5372.
137. Dan HC, Sun M, Yang L, et al. Phosphatidylinositol-3-kinase/Akt pathway regulates tuberous sclerosis tumor suppressor complex by phosphorylation of tuberin. J Biol Chem 2002:277:35364–35370.
138. Noki K, Li Y, Zhu T, et al. TSC2 is phosphorylated and inhibited by Akt and suppresses mTOR signaling. Nat Cell Biol 2002;4:648–657.
139. Tee AR, Fingar DC, Manning BD, et al. Tuberous sclerosis complex-1 and 2 gene products function together to inhibit mammalian target of rapamycin (mTOR)-mediated downstream signaling. Proc Natl Acad Sci USA 2002;99:13,571–13,576.
140. Potter CJ, Pedraza LG, Xu T. Akt regulates growth by directly phosphorylating Tsc2. Nat Cell Bio 2002;4:658–665.
141. Gao X, Zhang Y, Arrazola P, et al. Tsc tumor suppressor proteins antagonize amino acid-TOR signaling. Nat Cell Biol 2002;4:699–704.
142. Castro AR, Rebhun JF, Clark GJ, et al. Rheb binds TSC2 and promotes S6 kinase activation in a rapamycin and farnestylation-dependent manner. J Biol Chem 2003;278:32,493–32,496.
143. Kobayashi T, Minowa O, Kuno J, et al. Renal carcinogenesis, hepatic hemangiomatosis, and embryonic lethality caused by a germ-line Tsc2 mutation in mice. Cancer Res 1999;59:1206–1211.
144. Kobayashi T, Minowa O, Sugitani Y, et al. A germ-line Tsc1 mutation causes tumor development and embryonic lethality that are similar, but not identical to, those caused by Tsc2 mutation in mice. Proc Natl Acad Sci USA 2001;98:8762–8767.
145. Uhlmann EJ, Wong M, Baldwin RL, et al. Astrocyte-specific TSC1 conditional knockout mice exhibit abnormal neuronal organization and seizures. Ann Neurol 2002;52:285–296.
146. Wienecke R, Guha A, Maize JC Jr, et al. Reduced TSC2 RNA and protein in sporadic astrocytomas and ependymomas. Ann Neurol 1997;15:1611–1616.
147. Wong M, Ess KC, Uhlmann EJ, et al. Impaired glial glutamate transport in a mouse tuberous sclerosis epilepsy model. Ann Neurol 2003;54:251–256.

PART II

Specific Tumors

CHAPTER 13

High-Grade Astrocytomas

JOHN F. DE GROOT / KENNETH D. ALDAPE / HOWARD COLMAN

Although not one of the most common cancers, high-grade astrocytomas are among the most feared and devastating human tumors because of their almost uniformly poor clinical outcome and the symptoms they produce. They are particularly deadly because of their invasive nature, resistance to treatment, and high rates of morbidity and mortality. Despite significant investigation and progress in the realms of neurosurgery, radiation therapy, and chemotherapy, the median survival for the highest-grade astrocytomas, glioblastoma (GBM), remains approximately 1 year, with relatively few long-term survivors. Partly as a result of the disappointing efficacy of standard therapies for these tumors, extensive effort has been expended to better understand the genetic and molecular alterations responsible for tumor initiation, progression, and treatment resistance. Although these advances have yet to translate into significant therapeutic improvements, promising molecular targets have been identified and various novel therapies are in development or being assessed in clinical trials.

▶ EPIDEMIOLOGY

Incidence

Recent estimates define the yearly incidence of primary brain tumors in the United States as approximately 35,000 new cases[1] (reviewed in references 2 and 3). Of these, high-grade astrocytomas account for the majority, with GBM accounting for approximately 47% of all primary brain tumors, and more than 80% of all diffuse astrocytomas.[1,2] Although the incidence of some primary brain tumors such as medulloblastoma and circumscribed gliomas is highest in the pediatric age group and declines at older ages, the overall incidence of primary brain tumors, and high-grade astrocytomas in particular, generally increases with age, with the peak incidence for GBM occurring around age 70 years.[3] There is a male predominance, with gliomas affecting 40% more males than females.[1] There is also a strong age-dependent effect on survival in GBM; although the 2-year survival approaches 30% in patients younger than age 20 years and in the 20- to 44-year-old age groups, it plummets to less than 10% in patients 45 to 64 years old and approximately 2% in patients older than age 65 years.[3] It is not entirely clear whether the prognostically significant influence that age has on survival is related to underlying molecular and genetic differences of tumors in different age groups; this is an area of current investigation.[2,4,5]

Causative and Risk Factors for High-Grade Astrocytoma

A number of genetic, environmental, and therapeutic factors are implicated as, or hypothesized to be, risk factors for the development of primary brain tumors, including high-grade astrocytomas. However, in many cases, these potential links are difficult to verify, resulting in significant controversy in both the scientific and popular press. Nonetheless, consensus does exist regarding several of these factors, and ongoing investigation continues into many others.

Genetic Predisposition

As more is understood about the molecular genetics of high-grade astrocytoma, additional genetic factors will likely be identified as important in the oncogenesis of tumors in individual patients or groups of patients. However, specific genetic syndromes are currently known to account for only a very small percentage of cases.[6]

Li-Fraumeni Syndrome

As discussed below in the p53 pathway section the TP53 tumor suppressor gene is a key factor in the initiation of several human tumors, including gliomas. Inherited mutations in the TP53 gene have been identified in some families with the Li-Fraumeni syndrome, which is associated with an increased incidence of multiple cancers, including breast, soft tissue, bone, adrenal, leukemia, and brain cancer, encompassing both gliomas and medulloblastomas.[7] However, this syndrome is an uncommon cause of glioma, with germline mutation in TP53 observed in only a minority of cases of gliomas harboring p53 alterations.[8,9] In addition, in families with an increased incidence of glioma, but not other primary cancers, the incidence of germline TP53 mutation is low.[10–12]

Other Hereditary Syndromes

Several additional hereditary syndromes are associated with the formation of primary brain tumors. While not the predominant type of brain tumors seen in these syndromes, high-grade astrocytomas or GBM have also been described in association with neurofibromatosis types 1 and 2, Turcot syndrome, tuberous sclerosis, and Ollier disease (reviewed in references 2 and 3). Interestingly, mutations of the particular gene involved in these syndromes has generally not been observed in sporadic gliomas, suggesting that these genetic lesions are not part of the typical molecular ontology of malignant gliomas.

Environmental Factors

Ionizing Radiation

There is consensus that prior exposure to therapeutic doses of ionizing radiation is a significant risk factor for high-grade gliomas.[13,14] Studies have identified an increased risk of gliomas associated with varying doses of radiation used to treat numerous conditions, including tinea capitis, skin hemangiomas, adenoid hypertrophy, childhood leukemia, and other cancers (see reference 3 for a review). In one study, even low intracranial radiation doses resulting from the treatment of hemangiomas were associated with an average excess relative risk of all brain tumors (including benign lesions) of 2.7/Gy. However, this relationship declined rapidly with age, and the excess relative risk was 0.4/Gy if the treatment was given after 7 months of age.[15] Data are sparse regarding the specific relative risk of malignant gliomas related to higher doses of cranial radiation at older ages, but some studies report a high prevalence (17%) of prior radiation in patients with GBM,[13] and one study found a 22-fold excess of secondary brain tumors in children who received radiation for treatment of acute leukemia.[16] Currently, there does not seem to be an increased risk of glioma associated with diagnostic X-rays.[17] Some studies found a small increased risk of brain tumors related to occupational exposure of nuclear facility workers to radiation,[18] although the contribution of other confounding factors remains a possibility.

Electromagnetic Fields and Cellular Telephones

Concern over an increased risk of brain tumors associated with a high exposure to electromagnetic fields stems from several studies that found a positive association between brain tumors and high-current residential wiring,[19,20] and occupational exposure in electrical workers.[21,22] Other studies found no relationship between electromagnetic fields and an increased risk of brain tumors in either the residential[23,24] or occupational settings.[25,26] These differences may result from methodological issues, confounding variables, or other factors.[3] However, at present, the potential association between electromagnetic fields and risk of brain tumors remains controversial.

Another epidemiologic controversy erupted in the popular press around the possible connection between cellular telephone use and its associated radio frequency electromagnetic fields and the development of brain tumors. Several studies have either identified an overall increased risk of brain tumors associated with analog cellular phone usage,[27] or a higher incidence of tumors on the side of the head on which cell phones were used in some patients.[27–29] However, other large studies examined the risk of cell phone usage and brain tumors and found no increased risk.[30–35] Thus, the evidence to date is contradictory, but does not support a strong overall increase in the risk of primary brain tumors, particularly astrocytomas, associated with cellular phone usage.

Diet and Other Factors

Several studies suggest that there is an association between dietary intake of nitrosamines, present in cured foods, and brain tumor risk,[36–38] although other studies report conflicting data (reviewed in reference 39). There are also diverse findings regarding the risk of brain tumors associated with patient or maternal pesticide exposure.[40] Additional factors such as smoking, alcohol, virus exposure, and other dietary and environmental exposures have been investigated as potential risks for brain tumor formation (see reference 3 for a review), but so far none have been conclusively linked to gliomagenesis.

▶ GENETICS AND MOLECULAR BIOLOGY

One aspect of glioma biology that has become increasingly clear is that the degree of molecular and genetic alterations in these tumors is extensive and complex, involving multiple changes at the DNA, RNA, protein, and cellular levels. Such alterations affect key cellular processes and pathways that have been implicated in the pathogenesis of a number of human cancers. Investigators have referred to some of these key pathways as "hallmarks of cancer."[41] Modifications in these pathways affect fundamental cellular processes that, in some ways, define the differences between normal and cancerous cells. These properties include unlimited cellular proliferation, invasion, maintained growth stimulation and lack of response to antigrowth signals, avoidance of cell death, and angiogenesis. Although many human tumors share these characteristics and fundamental mechanisms, the specific alterations that are involved often differ among tumor types. As discussed below, our understanding of several of the key genetic and molecular mechanisms in high-grade astrocytomas is increasing.

It has also become clear that a more detailed molecular understanding of these tumors is important for improved classification, prognostication, and tailoring specific treatments to individual tumor types or patients. High-grade astrocytomas are currently defined by histopathologic features (see "Histopathology of High-Grade Astrocytic Tumors" below). However, it has becoming readily apparent that even though some tumors share similar histopathologic features, they actually represent multiple distinct molecular phenotypes.[42–45] Furthermore, these distinct molecular profiles are potentially clinically relevant in relation to prognosis or response to specific treatment modalities. Examples of how specific molecular alterations affect treatment response have been identified in other gliomas, namely anaplastic oligodendroglioma[46,47] and nonneural tumors.[48,49] While a similarly dramatic link between a specific genetic alteration and clinical response to treatment has not been identified in high-grade astrocytomas, evidence is accruing that particular molecular markers may define specific prognostic groups or molecular subtypes of tumors within the broader categories of anaplastic astrocytoma (AA) and GBM.[42–45,47,50–55]

It remains to be determined whether these differences reflect the existence of diverse developmental and/or molecular origins of these tumors, or differences in mechanisms of tumor maintenance or progression. An improved understanding of these disparities will almost certainly impact the ability to better diagnose, classify, and predict the response of these tumors to specific treatments. Thus, a hope of researchers in the field is that a more complete understanding of the genetic and molecular alterations that distinguish high-grade astrocytomas will lead to more effective and specific treatments—a major focus in neuro-oncology.

Cell of Origin

It is perhaps surprising that although high-grade gliomas were first classified pathologically by Bailey and Cushing in 1926,[56] the specific cell or cells of origin for these tumors remains unknown. The current pathologic classifications divide high-grade gliomas into astrocytoma, oligodendroglioma, or mixed oligoastrocytoma, based on histopathology and immunohistochemical evidence of expression of glial markers for astrocytes or oligodendrocytes.[57] But whether astrocytes or oligodendrocytes are the ultimate cells of origin of astrocytomas and oligodendrogliomas, respectively, is not clear. In fact, high-grade astrocytomas share multiple cellular and molecular features of both glial precursors and neural stem cells. This commonality has led to the hypothesis that gliomas could arise directly from stem cells or glial precursors, or involve dedifferentiation of mature astrocytes or oligodendrocytes.[58–62] Indeed, mouse models of glioma formation have demonstrated tumor formation both from astrocytes and neural stem cells, with a lower threshold for oncogenic transformation in the stem cells.[58–62] However, whether these same predispositions hold true in the adult human brain remains unproven. As the molecular alterations within a given category of brain tumor are diverse, it is also possible that the spectrum of tumors defined as high-grade astrocytomas may actually represent several tumor types, with different cells of origin, and distinct genetic and molecular pathways underlying tumor formation and progression.

Molecular Alterations Associated with Primary and Secondary Glioblastoma

The distinction drawn between primary and secondary GBM demonstrates the concept that there are distinct subtypes of high-grade astrocytomas with unique molecular alterations and clinical features, but a common histopathology.[52,63–65] Distinct molecular phenotypes parallel the distinct natural histories of these two types of GBM.

Secondary glioblastomas are thought to arise through progression of preexisting lower grade gliomas, and are most commonly seen in younger patients.[52,57,65] The most common molecular alteration observed in both the low- and high-grade tumors in these patients is mutation of the TP53 gene.[63,65,66] This multifunctional tumor suppressor gene plays a central role in many human tumors, acting through several key pathways to maintain genomic integrity and cell viability. Alterations in the TP53 gene—by chromosomal alteration, gene mutation, or both—are seen in approximately one-third of low-grade astrocytomas and in a similar percentage of AAs and secondary GBMs.[67,68]

In contrast to secondary GBMs, primary GBMs have no identified lower-grade precursor and appear to arise de novo as a high-grade lesion, predominantly in older adults.[52,57,65] These tumors have a high frequency of amplification of the epidermal growth factor receptor (EGFR).[52,65] Additionally, primary GBMs also have a low rate of the TP53 gene mutation.[63] At the cytogenetic level, primary GBMs have a high frequency of loss of the long arm of chromosome 10.[52,65,69] Gains of all or portions of chromosome 7 are a feature of both low-grade and higher-grade astrocytomas.[70,71] These findings led to the hypothesis that, although sharing identical histopathologic features, primary and secondary GBMs have distinct, and potentially mutually exclusive, molecular ontologies.[63] However, using alternate methods to look at EGFR amplification within different regions of GBM samples, a study by Okada and associates[72] found that 4 of 6 tumors with TP53 mutation actually had isolated EGFR-amplified cells in different regions.[72] The authors argue that while TP53 mutation and EGFR amplification are not mutually exclusive, the presence of TP53 mutation does not favor the selection of cells with EGFR amplification. These new findings raise the possibility that while certain alterations may be primary, or more numerous, in one molecular subtype or tumor, molecular heterogeneity within a tumor may mirror the cellular heterogeneity that is often observed. In addition, it is important to note that although specific molecular alterations may be more common in particular tumor types, many of these alterations target common pathways or effectors, suggesting that these pathways may be essential to glioma oncogenesis. The recent findings of lack of mutual exclusivity of TP53 and EGFR alterations suggest that the distinction of primary from secondary GBM may not be as clear-cut as once thought. Nevertheless, it is clear that there are subtypes of infiltrating astrocytomas, and that a further understanding of the molecular signatures of these tumors will likely lead to a more robust subclassification of these tumors. Furthermore, these novel molecular classifications may have important clinical implications for prognosis and targeted therapies (see "Molecular Classification and Marker of Prognosis").

Molecular and Genetic Changes Associated with Astrocytoma Progression

Eventual progression of lower-grade gliomas (World Health Organization [WHO] grade II astrocytoma and WHO grade III anaplastic astrocytoma) to GBM occurs in the majority of patients. Studies of the genetic, cytogenetic, and molecular alterations observed in these different grades of tumors have led to a general hypothesis that certain common alterations are associated with or necessary for tumor progression (Fig. 13-1) (see references 57 and 62 for reviews). As discussed below, these alterations occur at different molecular levels and appear to converge on several key regulators of oncogenesis in high-grade gliomas, including the p53 pathway, the retinoblastoma protein (Rb) pathway, and growth factor receptor signaling pathways.

Key Genetic and Molecular Pathways in High-Grade Astrocytomas

In high-grade gliomas, specific alterations affecting growth signals, invasion, angiogenesis, and apoptosis have been identified in several key pathways. Some of these perturbations appear to contribute to tumor formation, others to tumor maintenance or treatment resistance, and others to tumor progression. Our understanding of these molecular alterations results from combined observations of the predisposition to tumorigenesis on the basis of specific inherited genetic changes, as well as genetic and molecular analyses of both low- and high-grade gliomas. The number and diversity of these alterations in gliomas is impressive, suggesting that these tumors can develop, in some cases, via multiple molecular routes to the same functional endpoint. This mechanistic diversity may explain, in part, the extreme treatment resistance of these tumors. Nonetheless, advances in understanding these molecular alterations have led to the development of numerous pharmacologic inhibitors and modulators currently being tested in gliomas and other human cancers in clinical trials[73] (see "Targeted and Individualized Therapy"). The hope is that these targeted therapies, specific for the dysregulated pathways in these tumors, will have a significant effect, alone or in combination with other agents, in the clinical treatment of this disease.

The p53 Pathway

The tumor suppressor gene TP53, located on chromosome 17p13.1, is a key regulator in numerous human cancers. The mutation of one of the two chromosomal copies of the TP53 gene in humans, which encodes the p53 protein, is one of the germ line alterations that occur in the familial cancer syndrome Li-Fraumeni. Patients with Li-Fraumeni syndrome are at increased risk for a number of tumor types, including gliomas.[74]

As the multiple roles of p53 have been discovered, it has become clear that this pathway acts as one of the major "guardians of the genome."[75] This multifunctional molecule plays an important role in multiple cellular processes related to oncogenesis, including cellular response to DNA damage, cell cycle regulation, and cell

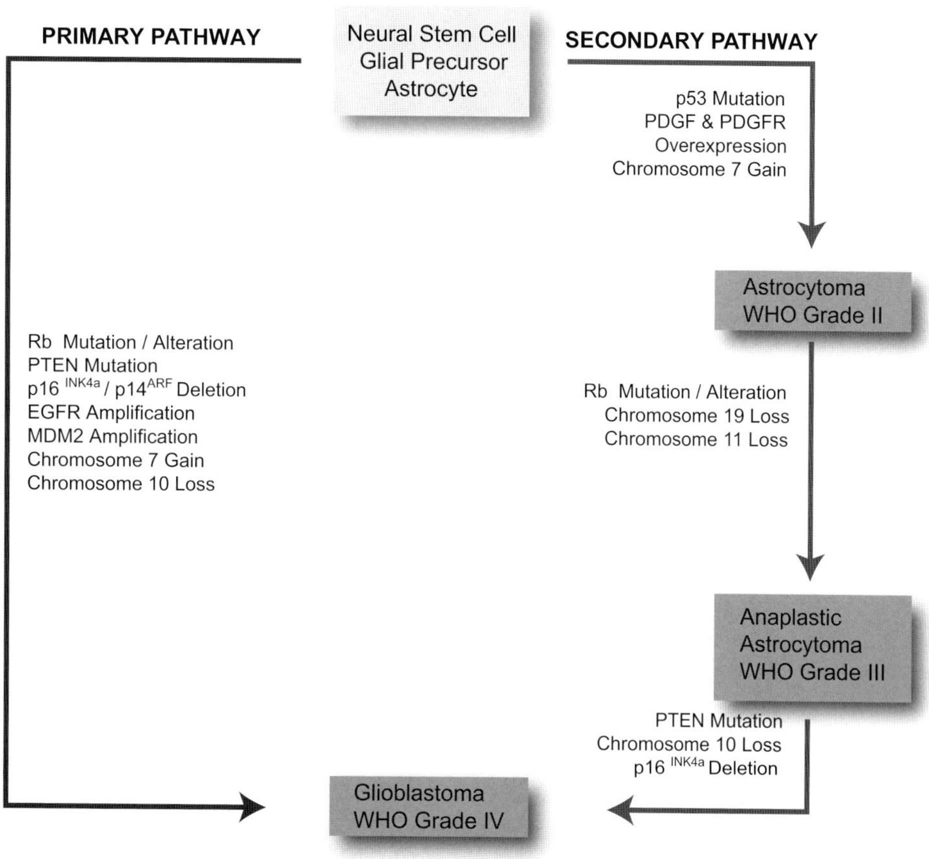

Figure 13-1. Molecular and genetic alterations associated with development of glioblastoma through the primary and secondary pathways.

death (apoptosis) (see reference 76 for a review). Acting as a sensor in normal cells, p53 inhibits cellular proliferation and, in some cases, induces cell death, in response to DNA damage. This prevents the accumulation of potentially oncogenic DNA alterations. Cells without an intact p53 pathway are thus prone to genomic instability and cancer formation. Mutations in the p53 gene itself are observed primarily in AAs and secondary GBMs and are seen at significantly lower frequencies in primary GBMs.

The p53 pathway has many different components, however, and alterations in other portions of the p53 pathway have been observed in many types and grades of gliomas, including primary GBM. The MDM2 gene is both a downstream target of p53 and an inhibitor of the p53 protein via direct binding to p53 and the subsequent promotion of its degradation. Thus, these genes form a feedback loop that regulates both p53 and MDM2 expression and function. Amplification of MDM2 has been observed in approximately 10% of GBMs,[77] and overexpression of the protein has been seen in as many as 50% of primary GBMs.[78]

Another modulator of p53 is the tumor suppressor $p14^{ARF}$ protein, which acts by binding and inhibiting the effects of MDM2 on p53. $p14^{ARF}$ is located on chromosome 9p and results from an alternate reading frame of the cyclin-dependent kinase N2A (CDKN2A) locus that also encodes the p16 protein (see "The Rb Pathway"). Frequent deletions of this region are seen in AAs and GBMs.[79,80] Loss of $p14^{ARF}$ through genomic deletion results in increased activity of MDM2, and increased inhibition of p53. This mechanism provides an additional pathway for interrupting normal p53 pathway functioning in high-grade astrocytomas. A primary function of the p53 pathway is to maintain cellular and DNA integrity by abrogating cell proliferation and, if necessary, inducing cell death in response to DNA damage. The multiple alterations in this pathway observed in astrocytomas suggest that the interruption of these functions may be central to the initiation and progression of high-grade gliomas.

Additionally, specific genetic or protein alterations of the p53 pathway are seemingly mutually exclusive in any given tumor,[81] signifying that multiple alternative routes converge in these tumors on a common functional endpoint. Some of the primary components of the p53 pathway and their alterations in high-grade astrocytomas are schematized in Fig. 13-2.

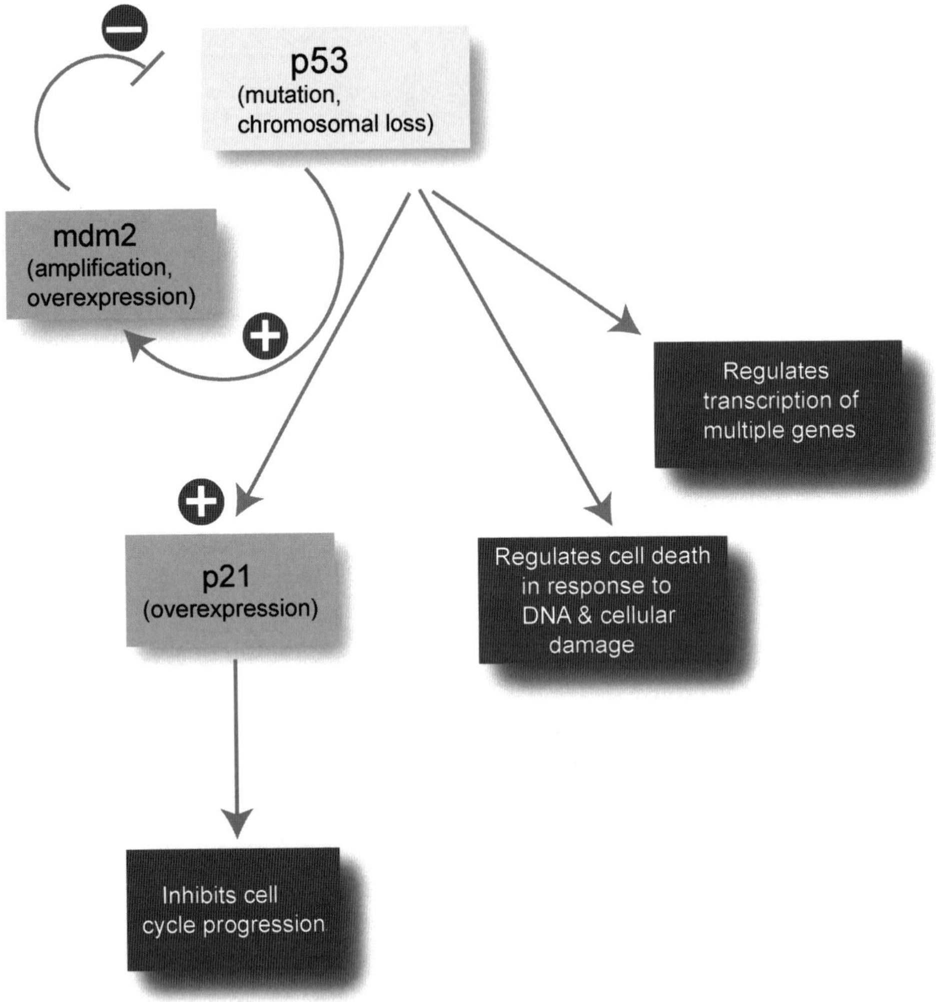

Figure 13-2. p53 Pathway alterations in astrocytomas. The functional interactions and consequences of several key molecules in the p53 pathway are shown. The most common alterations of these molecules observed in high-grade astrocytomas are in parentheses.

The Rb Pathway

Like TP53, the RB1 (retinoblastoma) gene is an important tumor suppressor gene in the formation and/or progression of various human tumors, including gliomas. The Rb protein plays a central role in regulating cellular proliferation and cell-cycle progression. The Rb protein binds the E2F transcription factor. Phosphorylation of Rb leads to release of E2F, which can then activate the transcription of multiple genes that are involved in cell proliferation.[82] As a result, alterations that result in lesser amounts or modified function of Rb can decrease the regulation and control of cell-cycle progression.

Various components of the Rb and cell-cycle regulation pathways are altered in high-grade astrocytomas. Analogous to the situation with the p53 pathway, many of these alterations are apparently mutually exclusive.[83,84] Because most (or all) high-grade astrocytomas exhibit some form of dysregulation of this pathway, it is likely that the Rb pathway is central to the initiation or progression of these tumors.[84] The potential role of the Rb pathway in gliomagenesis is supported by several mouse models of tumor formation.[59–61,85,86]

Mutations in the RB1 gene itself have been identified in a subset (approximately 30%) of high-grade astrocytomas.[87] Alterations affecting a number of other genes and proteins in this pathway have also been observed. The CDKN2A and CDKN2B genes together encode several products, including p16 and p15. Inactivation of this chromosomal locus, often by deletion, is observed in a majority of high-grade gliomas resulting in decreased expression of both p15 and p16.[79] Deletions in this region also affect the p14 protein, which results from an alternative reading frame.

Both p15 and p16 negatively regulate cyclin-dependent kinase (CDK) 4 (CDK4) and CDK6, which normally act in combination with cyclin D to phosphorylate Rb. As expected, loss of p15 and p16 results in increased CDK4 and CDK6 activity, causing increased Rb phosphorylation, release of E2F, and resulting cell cycle progression. In addition to deletion of p15 and p16, amplification and overexpression of CDK4[80,88] and CDK6[89] have also been observed in high-grade gliomas. These observations suggest that the vast majority of high-grade gliomas harbor alterations in the Rb/CDK/cyclin pathway.[83,84,90] Figure 13-3 summarizes the Rb pathway alterations observed in high-grade astrocytomas.

Growth Factor Pathways in High-Grade Astrocytomas

Growth factors, acting primarily through receptor tyrosine kinases, are implicated in a multitude of normal and pathologic processes in the nervous system. Several of these growth factors are central to normal neural development, including maintenance and expansion of neural stem cells, and regulation of cellular growth and differentiation. In addition, these growth factor receptors are implicated in the initiation and progression of multiple cancers, including gliomas (see references 57, 60, and 62 for reviews). Some of these growth factors are cellular homologues of viral oncogenes and have the ability to transform several cell types. Although differences in signaling exist among different growth factors, most act through specific membrane-bound receptor tyrosine kinases and share several common downstream targets and effectors, including the ras/raf/mitogen-activated protein kinase (MAPK) and phosphatidylinositol 3-kinase (PI3K) pathways, phospholipase C (PLC), Jak-Stat, and others. Evidence suggests that in gliomas the growth factors and their receptors have potential roles in processes as diverse as cellular proliferation, treatment resistance, cellular migration, and angiogenesis.[57,60,62] These diverse functions have made these growth factors and associated pathways a central focus, both in deepening the understanding of glioma biology, and in the search for novel therapeutic targets and agents.

Platelet-Derived Growth Factor

Platelet-derived growth factor (PDGF) is an important growth factor in neural development, particularly in the oligodendrocyte differentiation pathway.[91] PDGF is the cellular homologue of the v-sis oncogene and transforms several cell types.[92] The potential role of PDGF in astrocytoma initiation is highlighted by the observation that both the ligand (PDGF) and the receptor (PDGFR) are overexpressed in low-grade gliomas, potentially establishing an autocrine loop that enables constitutive activation.[93] In fact, along with p53 mutation, the overexpression of PDGF and PDGFR are the most common molecular alterations observed in low-grade astrocytomas.[93] Furthermore, overexpression of PDGF and PDGFR are seen in approximately equal percentages of low- and high-grade astrocytomas, suggesting that this pathway is important in the initiation, although probably not the progression, of astrocytomas.[94]

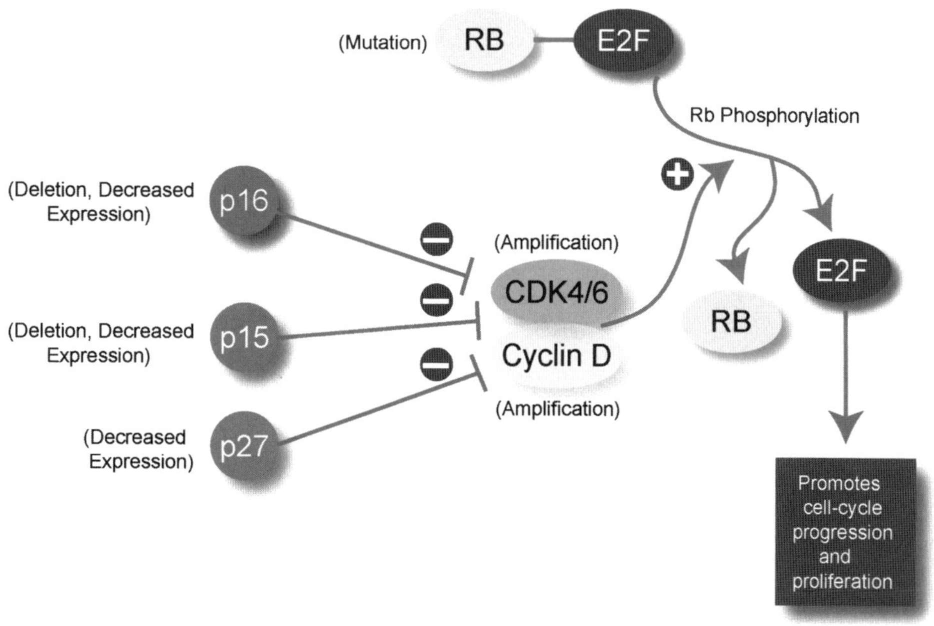

Figure 13-3. Rb pathway alterations in astrocytomas. The functional interactions and consequences of several key molecules in the Rb pathway active in gliomas are shown. The most common alterations of these molecules observed in high-grade astrocytomas are in parentheses.

Epidermal Growth Factor Receptor

EGFR is a receptor tyrosine kinase that binds both EGF and tumor growth factor-α (TGF-α). Like PDGF, EGFR and its ligands are important in the normal development of the nervous system. EGFR signaling has been demonstrated to be crucially important in both the maintenance and expansion of neural stem cells, as well as in the generation of early glial precursors.[95] In fact, EGF/EGFR signaling is a major mitogen for neural stem cells in vivo[96] and in vitro.[97] Interestingly, EGFR is the cellular homologue of the viral oncogene vErbB, highlighting its potential role in oncogenesis, which is supported by mouse models of glioma formation.[61,86]

This receptor has been a central focus of study in the biology of high-grade astrocytomas, both because of its potential role in proliferation and transformation, and because of the high frequency of alterations in this pathway in GBM. In fact EGFR is the most commonly amplified gene in these tumors.[98–101]

Activation of the EGF/EGFR pathway in GBMs occurs through diverse mechanisms. First, the tumors express both the ligands (EGF, TGF-α) and the receptor (EGFR),[102] creating the potential for autocrine loops and resultant constitutive activity of the receptor and downstream pathways. Second, approximately 40% of GBMs have amplification of the EGFR gene.[100,101] This amplification typically occurs on extrachromosomal pieces of DNA called *double minutes*.[103] Third, in approximately half of the cases of GBM with EGFR amplification, exons 2 to 7 of the EGFR are mutated by genomic deletion, resulting in a mutant receptor referred to as EGFRvIII, delta-EGFR, or de2–7EGFR.[104,105] This mutant form of the receptor lacks part of the extracellular domain, resulting in constitutive activity of the receptor (although at lower levels than the normal receptor).[106] The mutant receptor is also less susceptible to internalization and degradation.

EGFR activation and downstream signaling have been linked to a number of potentially important cellular processes in GBM. Some of the major pathways and intracellular second messengers involved in EGFR and other receptor tyrosine kinase signaling include the Ras/Raf/MAPK pathway, PI3K/AKT, PLC, and Jak-Stat. EGFR activation and signaling have been implicated in increased tumor cell proliferation,[107] increased cellular migration and invasion,[108] increased resistance to chemotherapy, and decreased cell death.[109]

Growth Factor Receptor Signaling and Downstream Effectors

Activation of receptor tyrosine kinases, whether through binding of appropriate ligands or constitutive activation from mutation, affects a number of intracellular signaling cascades. Although many of the details of these pleiotropic signals in gliomas remain to be elucidated, and differences in effects and mediators exist between receptors, there appear to be several key common pathways activated by a number of these receptors (Fig. 13-4).

Ras

Ras is an important downstream effector of the receptor tyrosine kinases.[110,111] Although itself an oncogene, with mutated forms of the Ras gene observed in a number of cancers, no activating mutations of Ras have been identified in gliomas.[112] Rather, increased Ras activity has been observed in a high proportion of GBM samples studied.[113] This increased activity appears to be at least partially due to activation of the receptor tyrosine kinases. Ras, in turn, activates a number of downstream molecules, including Rac and Raf, resulting in activation of several MAPKs. These pathways are implicated in promoting cell proliferation and cell-cycle progression.[114]

PI3K/AKT/PTEN

PI3K is also activated, in part, by activation of receptor tyrosine kinases.[110,111] PI3K acts through a complex second messenger signaling cascade by creating phosphatidylinositol (3,4,5) triphosphate (PIP3), causing translocation to the cell membrane and activation of several molecules, including AKT.[115] Activated AKT has been found to have several potential effects in tumor cells, including inhibiting cell death, promoting cell cycle progression, increasing cellular metabolism, and activation of additional downstream targets, including mammalian target of rapamycin (mTOR).[115]

An important inhibitor of the PI3K/AKT pathway is PTEN (phosphatase and tensin homologue). Also called MMAC1 (mutated in multiple advanced cancers-1), PTEN was originally identified as a candidate tumor suppressor gene based on its high rate of mutation in gliomas and several other high-grade cancers.[116,117] One effect of PTEN is dephosphorylation of PIP3, with a resulting decrease in activation of AKT. Loss of PTEN correlates with higher PIP3 and activated AKT levels in glioma cells.[118] The PTEN gene is located on the long arm of chromosome 10. One copy of this chromosomal region is lost in a high percentage (>75%) of high-grade astrocytomas.[52,65,69] Mutations in the other copy of the PTEN gene are also observed in a significant percentage (30%–40%) of these tumors.[119,120] Loss of chromosome 10q and PTEN mutation are also associated with the progression from anaplastic astrocytoma to GBM, and thus loss or mutation of PTEN appears to be an important feature of both primary and secondary GBMs.

Vascular Endothelial Growth Factor and Angiogenesis

Vascular endothelial growth factor (VEGF) is an additional growth factor that also acts through tyrosine kinase receptors, and has been implicated in vascular

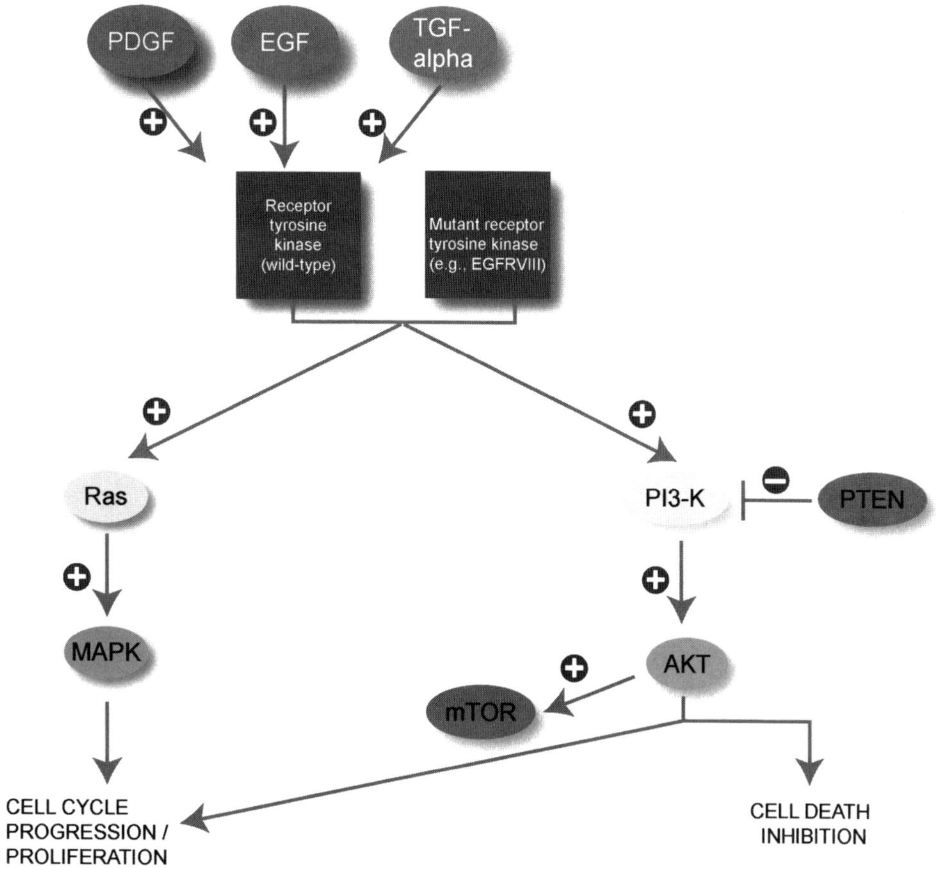

Figure 13-4. Receptor tyrosine kinase signaling in astrocytomas. Binding of ligand (PDGF, EGF, TGF-α) or activating mutation of the receptor tyrosine kinases in gliomas can activate a number of downstream targets including the Ras/MAPK pathway and the PI-3/AKT/mammalian target of rapamycin (mTOR) pathway.

development and proliferation in high-grade astrocytomas (see reference 121 for a review). Vascular proliferation is one of the pathologic criteria used for differentiating GBM from lower-grade astrocytomas.[57] Evidence suggests that VEGF, acting through its tyrosine kinase receptors (VEGF receptor-1 [Flt-1], VEGF receptor-2 [Flk-1], and VEGF receptor-3 [Flt-4]), is central to the initial stages of endothelial proliferation and early vessel formation.[122–126] Levels of VEGF expression are highest in the pseudopalisading cells around areas of necrosis in GBM, and VEGF expression is induced by hypoxia, suggesting that hypoxia may be a driving force for neovascularization in GBM.[127,128] In addition, VEGF has been implicated in increasing vascular permeability in GBM, potentially mediating both peritumoral edema[122,129] and response to steroids.[130,131] Additional important mediators of angiogenesis in GBM are PDGF,[93] the angiopoietins (1 and 2) and their receptor (Tie-2).[132] Because of the prominent role of angiogenesis in GBM, there continues to be enthusiasm over the potential for antiangiogenic therapies, and several agents are in clinical trials (see reference 73 for a review).

Molecular Classification and Markers of Prognosis

One of the goals of understanding the molecular biology and genetics of high-grade gliomas is to classify and grade these tumors with more accuracy, as well as to deduce the prognosis and best treatment for an individual patient. The current pathologic classification and grading system for gliomas is based on histopathology alone. Although these classes and grades are a general predictor of treatment response and survival, there is growing evidence that a variety of molecular markers have the potential to improve both the classification and prognostication of these tumors.

Various approaches have been used to identify molecular markers that correlate with tumor grade and prognosis in AA and GBM. At the level of cytogenetics and chromosomal aberrations, loss of heterozygosity of chromosomal arm 10q has been associated with worse prognosis for both AA and GBM.[51,133,134] In another study examining differences in long- and short-term surviving patients with GBM, loss of the chromosomal arms 6q, 10q, and the gain of 19q were associated with short-term survival, and loss of 19q was associated with long-term survival.[54] Combined loss of chromosome 1p and 19q is a powerful predictor of treatment response and survival in anaplastic oligodendrogliomas,[46,135] and is correlated with certain clinical and radiographic features.[136] Some studies have extended the association of chromosome 1p/19q loss and improved survival to astrocytic tumors and GBM.[32,51] However, other studies have failed to show such an association.[137]

At the level of individual genes, several candidates associated with survival differences have been identified. Mutation of the PTEN gene on chromosome 10q, which is also involved in cytogenetic changes at this locus, is associated with poor prognosis in AA.[5] Loss or mutation of PTEN is also associated with progression to GBM, so it remains possible that these alterations may be identifying a set of tumors that are histopathologically AA based on the available tissue and current criteria, but are actually closer to GBMs on the molecular level.

The interpretation of the importance of several other genes on prognosis in GBM has been difficult as a consequence of the confounding factor of patient age. Older patients are more likely to have primary GBMs, with a high frequency of EGFR amplification. Secondary GBMs, with a high frequency of TP53 mutations, are more common in younger patients. Because age is routinely one of the independent variables associated with better survival in the vast majority of high-grade glioma studies, this raises the question of whether the effects of age and molecular phenotype are independent predictors of survival, or just highly correlated.

Several studies have attempted to control for the effects of age when examining molecular correlates of survival. In one study of GBMs comparing a long-term surviving group (≥3 years) with a short-term surviving group (<1.5 years), nuclear p53 expression was independently associated with improved survival, after age, performance status, and other factors were included in the multivariate analysis.[45] This study also found that overexpression of MDM2 (a negative regulator of p53) was independently associated with poor survival, but no significant association between p53 mutation and survival was observed.[45] Other studies have found a positive association of p53 mutation with improved survival, but this lost significance when age was factored in.[5,55,138–141] The interpretation of the association of EGFR status and prognosis is also complicated by the confounding variable of patient age. One study found that EGFR amplification was an independent predictor of prolonged survival in patients older than 60 years of age, but was also associated with a trend towards worse survival in patients who were age 60 or younger.[5] However, other authors found that EGFR amplification was an overall significant independent predictor of poor survival in a group of 87 GBM patients, although the significance was higher in patients younger than 60 years of age.[142] A recent study by Batchelor and associates,[4] found that the prognostic effects of p53 mutation, EGFR amplification, CDKN2A/p16 alterations, and chromosome 1p loss were all significantly associated with patient age.[4] The authors conclude that the tumorigenic pathways to GBM vary with age, and that the prognostic effects of these alterations may thus also be age dependent.[4]

New technologies, such as gene expression array chips, have enabled investigators to look at the patterns of expression of thousands of genes in individual tumors to try to identify individual genes or patterns of gene expression that are correlated with clinical factors, including survival. In high-grade gliomas, a combination of supervised learning and cross-validation approaches was used to develop a model for classification of tumors based on expression patterns.[50] These authors found that these expression patterns or "clusters" were a better predictor of patient survival than pathologic classification in GBM and anaplastic oligodendroglial tumors with nonclassic histopathologic features.[50] Similar approaches were used to identify clusters of genes that differentiate gliomas of different grades and histologies based on expression profiles alone.[43,44–53,143] Gene expression profiling has also been used to identify molecular subtypes of GBMs that differ in expression levels of EGFR.[53]

Targeted and Individualized Therapy

In addition to more accurate tumor classification and prediction of treatment response and survival, an ultimate goal of "molecular medicine" is to design or identify molecular targets in specific diseases that are amenable to therapeutic intervention. Hope for devising such an approach for the treatment of gliomas remains high, in part because of the overall disappointing efficacy of "nonspecific" therapies like external beam radiation and cytotoxic chemotherapy in this disease. The significant association between chromosome 1p and 19q loss and treatment response in anaplastic oligodendroglioma[46,135] has enforced this hope in glioma research. In addition, recent studies have identified specific mutations of the EGFR receptor in non–small-cell lung cancer patients that correlate with treatment response to the EGFR inhibitor gefitinib (Iressa).[48,49] While similar mutations have not been identified in GBM so far, this finding has reinforced the idea that understanding and identifying the fundamental molecular and genetic alterations in high-grade gliomas will eventually lead to improved, and possibly patient-specific, treatment options.

▶ HISTOPATHOLOGY OF HIGH-GRADE ASTROCYTIC TUMORS

Classification and Grading

The classification of high-grade astrocytomas into grade III astrocytoma (AA) and grade IV astrocytoma (GBM) is based primarily on histologic appearance during routine sectioning. Hypercellularity, the presence of more than the usual number of nuclei per unit area, is the most common histologic finding that signals an abnormality. Once it is established that the histology of the sections represent abnormal tissue, verification that the disease process represents a neoplastic rather than reactive process is sought. Finding that the abnormal cells represent a single cell type, rather than a mix (e.g., glial cells, macrophages, inflammatory cells), is evidence in favor of a neoplasm. Macrophages are especially important to identify, because their presence in large numbers warrants careful consideration of an infarct or demyelinating process rather than a neoplasm. The pattern of glial cell proliferation is also important. Hypertrophic glial cells that are spaced relatively evenly apart, without clustering of glial nuclei, favor the diagnosis of a gliosis rather than a neoplasm. Disordered/haphazardly arranged astrocytic cells without an obvious pattern is evidence in favor of a diagnosis of astrocytoma.

A nearly universal feature of infiltrating gliomas, usually seen in generously sampled lesions, is evidence of infiltration of surrounding central nervous system (CNS) parenchyma. A gradual decrease in cellularity, in which atypical astrocytic cells are present in a background of normal cellular constituents, is a typical picture as one moves from the central to peripheral aspects of the lesion. Identification of the relationship of the tumor to surrounding parenchyma (e.g., an infiltrative vs. noninfiltrative border) is a key feature in the diagnosis of CNS neoplasms. Metastatic tumors (most often carcinoma and melanoma) tend to infiltrate as groups or nests, especially along vessels (Virchow-Robin spaces) compared to the single-cell infiltration of diffuse gliomas. This feature is often diagnostically helpful in the intraoperative setting. In addition, some astrocytic tumors, such as pilocytic astrocytoma and pleomorphic xanthoastrocytoma, are noninfiltrating. Distinguishing these entities from the more common diffuse gliomas is important because they exhibit a different clinical and biologic behavior from infiltrating gliomas.

Tumors are assigned grades according to their most anaplastic region, as it is assumed that this region will determine overall biology and clinical course. For this reason small biopsy specimens, if not derived from the center of the lesion, can occasionally lead to undergrading a tumor (i.e., the histologic features present permit making a diagnosis of a lower grade tumor than the tumor that the patient actually has). Occasional tumors appear to have no "center" and can correlate with the clinicopathologic picture of gliomatosis. However, these are the exception rather than the rule, and finding tumor cells against a background of normal neuropil should prompt consideration of whether the center of the lesion has been sufficiently sampled. This concern is most important with respect to accurately grading astrocytomas.

Historically, the grading of astrocytomas has been accomplished using different grading schemes. The most widely accepted and currently used is the WHO grading system.[144] Pilocytic tumors and other astrocytomas that are considered to be noninfiltrating are designated as grade I, whereas infiltrating astrocytomas are divided into grades II, III, and IV. Grade II astrocytomas are hypercellular and have nuclear atypia without significant mitotic activity. Grade III astrocytomas have the additional feature of mitotic activity, but lack tumor necrosis and microvascular proliferation, features reserved for making a diagnosis of GBM (grade IV astrocytomas). In the current WHO classification scheme, the presence of either microvascular proliferation or necrosis in the setting of an infiltrating astrocytic tumor is sufficient for arriving at a diagnosis of GBM. In practice, both characteristics are usually seen in generously resected GBM specimens, although one or the other of them may be absent in biopsy specimens.

As with all tumor-grading schemes, it is important to realize that designating tumor types as discrete grades is a somewhat artificial categorization of what is really a biologic continuum. As such, it is inevitable that some cases fit easily within the categorization, whereas others are borderline. This is of particular concern when differentiating grade II from grade III astrocytomas, because in some centers this distinction determines whether the patient will receive treatment (e.g., with radiation therapy) or be observed only via serial imaging studies. In practical terms, drawing this distinction often rests upon the identification of more than one mitotic figure in a diffuse astrocytoma. Because this scenario can be affected by factors such as tumor sampling and potentially technical issues such as tissue processing, it is clear that the WHO system, which is generally meaningful, could be imperfect for accurately diagnosing the occasional borderline case. It is hoped that as we arrive at a better understanding of the molecular events that drive the aggressive and clinically refractory behavior of these tumors, genetic analysis may serve to improve our ability to better predict outcome and treatment response for patients with infiltrating astrocytic tumors.

Within the category of diffusely infiltrating gliomas, the distinction between astrocytoma and oligodendroglioma must be made. In general, astrocytic tumors have a relatively patternless architecture as visualized on low-power microscopy, and exhibit more variation in nuclear size and shape than oligodendrogliomas. The nuclei of astrocytomas tend to be elongate or cigar-shaped, although this feature can be seen in conjunction with round nuclei in the same tumor. Oligodendroglial tumors tend to appear monomorphic on low-power microscopy, with one area appearing nearly identical or very similar to the next. The nuclei tend to be rounder and more uniform than seen in astrocytomas, although grade III oligodendrogliomas can demonstrate significant nuclear pleomorphism. Nuclei tend to be surrounded by "haloes," which are thought to be an artifact of tissue processing. Focal calcifications may be present. In practice, distinguishing among astrocytomas and oligodendrogliomas can be difficult in some cases, since none of the histologic features that distinguish one from the other are absolute. Classic examples of each exist, but many cases have features that are intermediate rather than strictly astrocytic or oligodendroglial.

Different approaches are taken toward the differential diagnosis of astrocytomas versus oligodendrogliomas. One approach is to label indeterminate cases as mixed oligoastrocytomas, which may or may not reflect an actual dual differentiation as much as our inability to distinguish one from the other. Another strategy is to err on the side of making a diagnosis of the more treatment-amenable oligodendroglial tumor so as to provide an opportunity to the patient for obtaining therapy to which the patient may respond.

The recent interest in the relationship between loss of chromosome 1p/19q loci in oligodendroglioma and treatment response magnifies the interest and importance of making this distinction. However, because oligodendroglial tumors with a loss of 1p/19q tend to have the classic oligodendroglial histology,[145] it is likely that most infiltrating gliomas with indeterminate astrocytic-oligodendroglial features will be less responsive to therapy. Accordingly, our approach is to reserve the classification of tumors as oligodendroglial only when they are unequivocal, with as many of the others as possible being classified as having an astrocytic histology. We use the designation of mixed oligoastrocytoma or anaplastic oligoastrocytoma only as a last resort. In the future, studies comparing molecular signatures in astrocytomas, oligodendrogliomas, and mixed gliomas will likely resolve the issue as to whether and to what extent mixed gliomas represent an entity distinct from astrocytic and oligodendroglial tumors.

Once a tumor has been assigned to the category of infiltrating astrocytoma, grading is performed by taking into account various histologic features, including cellularity (the degree of increased cellular crowding compared with normal CNS parenchyma) nuclear atypia, mitotic activity, microvascular proliferation, and necrosis. Grade II astrocytomas show only minimal increases in cellularity, often exhibit only slightly atypical nuclei, and either no or minimal evidence of mitotic activity (a common interpretation of the WHO guidelines is that one mitotic figure is "allowed" within a grade II astrocytoma).

Histopathology of AAs

Grade III astrocytomas demonstrate a corresponding increase in cellularity, with increased mitotic activity. Smear preparations, often used for intraoperative consultation, reveal oval to elongate nuclei, and mitoses can frequently be appreciated (Fig. 13-5A). Eosinophilic refractile processes are sought to confirm astrocytic differentiation (Fig. 13-5B). In general, mitotic activity is required (Fig. 13-5C to F) and more than one mitotic figure is found in these tumors. However, for small-needle biopsy specimens, it may be impractical to require the presence of multiple mitoses in a specimen that has relatively low numbers of tumor cells available for examination. The rule may be relaxed in this circumstance. The morphology of neoplastic astrocytes may be in the form of so-called gemistocytes (Fig. 13-5G and H), with a defined eosinophilic cytoplasm and an eccentric nucleus. Such gemistocytic astrocytomas often reveal perivascular cuffs of lymphocytes (Fig. 13-5I). This appearance contrasts with the more classical fibrillary forms that evidence cytoplasmic processes (Fig. 13-5J). While in the absence of mitoses some neuropathologists upgrade gemistocytic astrocytomas to grade III tumors, the WHO guidelines do not permit this, although it is acknowledged that such tumors may behave more aggressively than fibrillary grade II astrocytomas. Care must be taken not to overinterpret as an oligodendroglioma the occasional astrocytic tumor that demonstrates perinuclear haloes (Fig. 13-5K). The variation in nuclear size and shape is a feature of astrocytic tumors. Additionally, the presence of perivascular structuring in an astrocytic tumor (Fig. 13-5L) is a regular feature, and should not be interpreted as being a perivascular pseudorosette, a characteristic of ependymoma.

GBM Histopathology

Glioblastomas share many histologic features with anaplastic astrocytomas and have a tendency to be more cellular, although this is not always the case. They also exhibit tumor necrosis (Fig. 13-6A), often with an arrangement of tumor nuclei around the area of necrosis, which is designated as pseudopalisading (Fig. 13-6B). Pseudopalisading is best appreciated on low-power microscopy examination. Additionally, the vasculature is proliferative, so that there is a larger number of cells than is normally seen in small vessels (Fig. 13-6C and D). This microvascular proliferation sometimes appears to be similar to the glomerulus in the kidney and is known as glomeruloid microvascular proliferation (Fig. 13-6E). Direct evidence of microvascular proliferation can occasionally be identified by a finding of mitotic activity within the vasculature (Fig. 13-6F). Although the WHO grading system requires either tumor necrosis or microvascular proliferation to be present for a diagnosis of GBM, most cases show both features. However, the infrequent case, especially biopsy samples, may demonstrate only one. Occasional bizarre cells are often seen (Fig. 13-6G), and in the extreme, compose the entire tumor, such as in giant cell GBM (Fig. 13-6H). On the other hand, small-cell GBM is a recognized subtype, with a distinct molecular

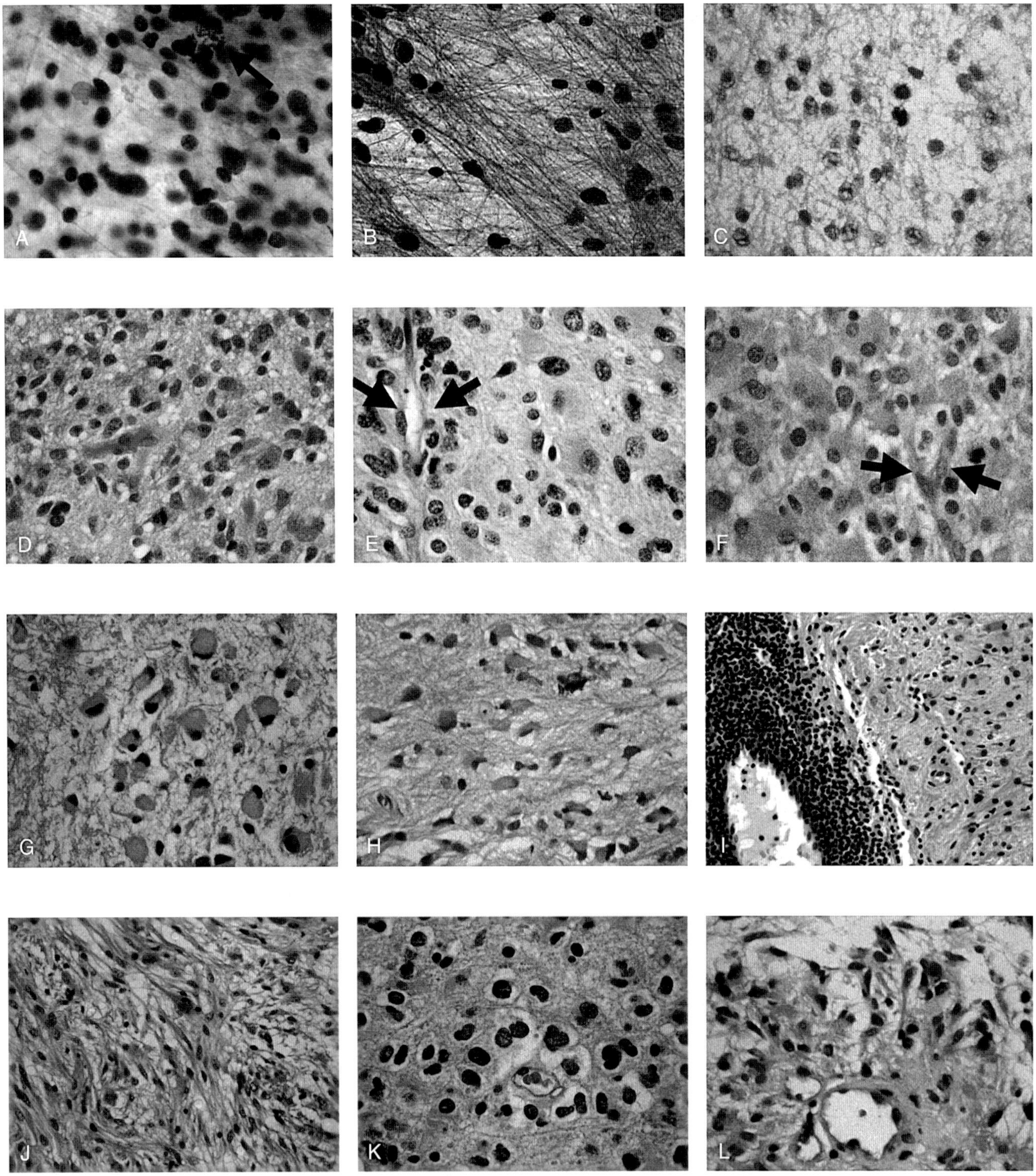

Figure 13-5 (PLATE 45). Histopathology of anaplastic astrocytoma. (A and B) Smear preparations. Smears are often useful for intraoperative consultation in conjunction with a frozen section. On this smear, note the mitotic activity (A, arrowhead) and the eosinophilic astrocytic processes (B). (C to F) Representative examples of AA. Each example shows mitoses, moderate to high cellularity, but with delicate, nonproliferative vasculature (E and F, arrows). (G to I) Gemistocytic astrocytoma. Tumor cells with defined eosinophilic cytoplasm. This is often accompanied by perivascular lymphocytic cuffing (I). An example of fibrillary anaplastic astrocytoma (J) is shown for comparison. (K and L) Diagnostic mimics. Occasional examples can show perinuclear haloes (K) or perivascular structuring (L). Although reminiscent of oligodendroglioma (K) or ependymoma (L), the cytologic features are more consistent with an astrocytic tumor.

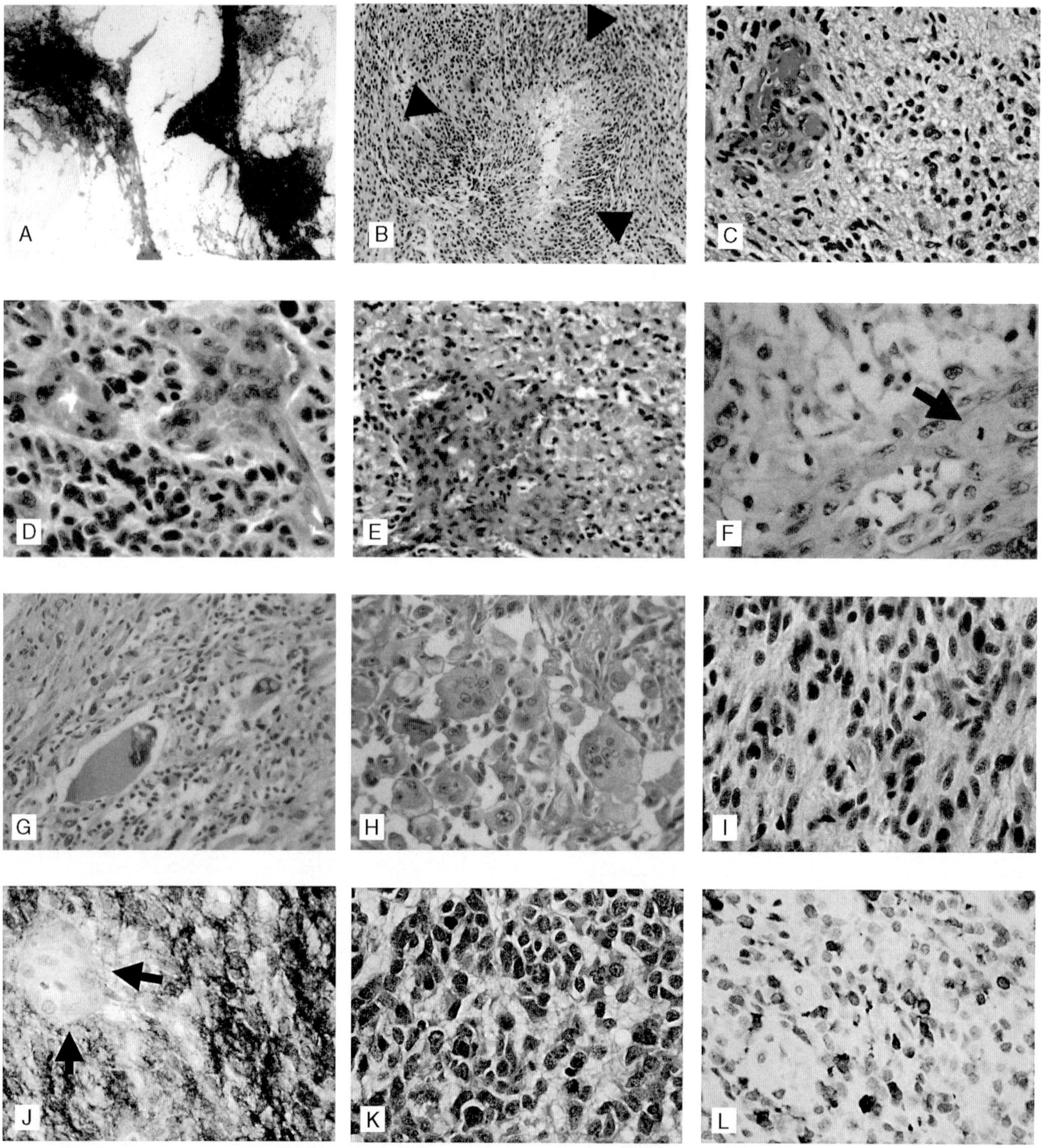

Figure 13-6 (PLATE 46). Histopathology of GBM. (A) A smear preparation of GBM typically shows viable tumor (right) in association with acellular necrotic material (left). (B) Pseudopalisading around necrotic areas is typical (arrowheads). (C to F) Microvascular proliferation. Piling-up of cells within vascular structures is another hallmark. The vascular structure in (E) resembles the glomerulus of the kidney, and is referred to as "glomeruloid" microvascular proliferation. Mitotic activity within the vessel is seen in (F, arrow), highlighting the proliferation of cells within vessels. Occasional large bizarre cells are seen (G), which when they compose the majority of the tumor, are called giant-cell GBM (H). (I and J) Small-cell GBM. Tumors with small minimally atypical nuclei which are also highly proliferative (note mitoses) are seen in approximately 10% of cases. Most of these tumors overexpress EGFR, as shown in the positive, predominately membrane, immunostaining using an anti-EGFR antibody (J). Note the lack of staining in the vessel (arrows), which serves as an internal negative control. (K and L) Use of tumor markers to supplement histology. Some specimens are highly cellular, but lack tumor necrosis or microvascular proliferation (K). By strict criteria, a glioblastoma diagnosis cannot be made. Staining for EGFR vIII (L) confirms that this tumor is best regarded as GBM.

profile, marked by a high rate of EGFR amplification/overexpression[146] (Fig. 13-6I and J). While, as mentioned above, microvascular proliferation or necrosis is required to make a diagnosis of GBM, some tumors (particularly biopsy specimens) are highly cellular and mitotically active, but lack the necessary features for an absolute diagnosis (Fig. 13-6K). Additional analyses will likely help to correctly classify inadequately sampled tumors. For example, the presence of EGFR vIII, which is essentially restricted to GBM (Fig. 13-6L), can be used for diagnostic purposes to supplement histologic features.

▶ CLINICAL PRESENTATION

Presenting Signs and Symptoms

The neurologic signs and symptoms of malignant glioma depend on the location of the tumor and its rate of growth. Tumor location determines, in part, if signs and symptoms are generalized or focal. Malignant gliomas most frequently involve the frontal lobes followed in frequency by the temporal lobes, parietal lobes, and, least frequently, the occipital lobes.[147] High-grade gliomas involving the posterior fossa and brainstem are infrequent. Because high-grade astrocytomas are fast-growing neoplasms often associated with significant edema, there is usually a shorter duration of symptoms prior to diagnosis than in lower grade gliomas. Table 13-1 outlines the most common symptoms at presentation.

Generalized Symptoms

Malignant gliomas frequently present with generalized symptoms that are caused by diffuse tumor infiltration, cerebral edema, and increased intracranial pressure (ICP). The most common clinical presentations caused by increases in ICP are headache, seizures, mental disturbances, nausea, and vomiting. Headache is the most frequent initial symptom reported by patients with malignant glioma, occurring in 20% to 40% of patients. At diagnosis and throughout the course of the illness, as many as 70% of patients complain of headaches, which on average are present for more than 4 months before diagnosis.[147]

▶ TABLE 13-1. MOST FREQUENT SYMPTOMS AT PRESENTATION

Headache	78%
Seizure	30%
Cognitive dysfunction	43%
Motor weakness	43%
Aphasia	30%

Source: Adapted from Roth JG, Elvidge AR. Glioblastoma multiforme: a clinical survey. J Neurosurg 1960;17:736–750; and Frankel SA, German WJ. Glioblastoma multiforme: review of 219 cases with regard to natural history, pathology, diagnostic methods, and treatment. J Neurosurg 1958;15(5);489–503.

Focal Symptoms

Focal deficits are caused by localized disruption of normal brain function and vary depending on tumor location. Approximately 3% to 5% of malignant gliomas are multifocal tumors and can present with multiple neurologic deficits. Tumor growth causing mass effect, infiltration of tumor into normal tissue, vasogenic edema, and even tissue infarction (stroke) can result in both reversible and irreversible deficits. Rapid worsening of symptoms can be related to tumor progression, focal ischemia, or hemorrhage. It is important to distinguish among these states, although it can be difficult to tell them apart either clinically or radiographically.

Duration and Onset of Symptoms

GBM and AA generally have symptoms of shorter duration prior to diagnosis than do low-grade tumors because of high proliferation rates and extensive invasion into normal brain. Subacute presentations are common. On average, the duration of symptoms prior to the time of histologic diagnosis is approximately 3 to 5 months.[148] Rarely, a patient will have a prior history of seizures, raising the possibility that an occult lower-grade tumor dedifferentiated into a higher-grade glioma. Headaches that are severe, with an acute onset, are most likely related to intracranial hemorrhage or increased ICP. As a presenting symptom, hemorrhage into a tumor is an uncommon event seen in only approximately 4% to 6% of patients.[149]

Seizures

Seizures are the second most common initial symptom of malignant astrocytomas. Throughout the course of illness, seizures occurred in 25% to 30% of patients in older studies[147,148] but now are recognized to affect 40% to 50% of patients. Tumors that involve the cerebral cortex and are fast growing are most likely to produce seizures. Frontal, parietal, and temporal lobes are associated with the highest incidence of seizures.

Cognitive Dysfunction

Although deficits in thinking, memory, and attention are less common as presenting complaints, cognitive dysfunction or changes in mental status are prevalent symptoms, occurring in more than 70% of patients with malignant brain tumors prior to treatment.[150] Careful attention to cognitive function is thus important. For example, at the time of GBM recurrence, tests of cognitive function such as verbal memory are independently related to survival after controlling for age, Karnofsky performance status (KPS), histology, and time since diagnosis.[150]

Brainstem and Cerebrospinal Fluid Involvement

At autopsy as many as 20% of patients have evidence of meningeal involvement, which is manifested at some time during their illness in approximately two-thirds.[151] Meningeal dissemination typically occurs with tumors in the basal ganglia, thalamus, and cerebellum. Symptoms of cerebral spinal fluid (CSF) involvement include back pain with radicular symptoms, headache, cranial nerve palsies, cauda equine syndrome, and mental status changes.

Fewer than 2% of primary brain tumors in adults originate within the brainstem. Patients who have brainstem tumors usually present with unilateral facial or abducens cranial nerve palsies, and nausea and hydrocephalus when the upper medulla is involved. Long tract signs, including unilateral weakness or limb apraxia, may be present.

Diagnostic Evaluation

Radiographic Imaging

Once a brain tumor is suspected, contrast-enhanced magnetic resonance imaging (MRI) imaging is the modality of choice to delineate tumor location in relation to normal anatomy, tumor size and associated edema, and degree of contrast enhancement (Fig. 13-7). If MRI cannot be performed, computerized tomography (CT) imaging with and without contrast is an acceptable choice and can provide similar information, although with less anatomic detail. Table 13-2 summarizes the imaging characteristics of AA and GBM. Tumor imaging characteristics typically include hypointensity on T_1-weighted imaging with inhomogeneous enhancement following contrast administration, and increased signal on T_2-weighted images (see Fig. 13-7). AAs are poorly circumscribed lesions with inhomogeneous tissue density. AA may be nonenhancing, or may have small foci of faintly enhancing tissue or a subtle rim of enhancement surrounding the tumor.[152] Glioblastoma are more heterogeneous, exhibiting mixed-signal intensity with necrosis or cyst formation. Strong but heterogeneous enhancement is common in GBM images. Ring-like enhancement is characteristic of GBM but is not

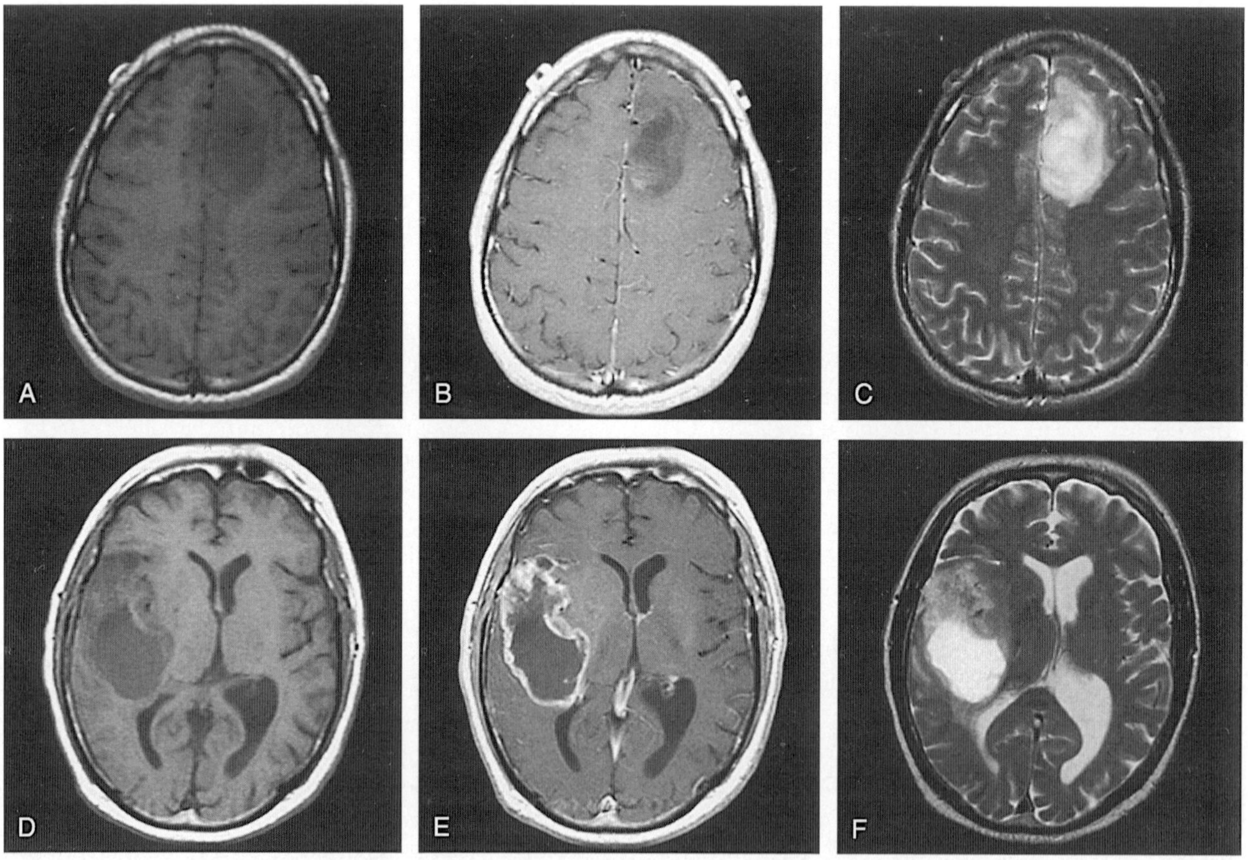

Figure 13-7. Magnetic resonance imaging (MRI) scan of AA and GBM tumors. The AA on the top series of images from the same patient illustrates typical MRI characteristics. A heterogeneous mass is shown in T_1-weighted images (A) with a subtle rim of peripheral enhancement after gadolinium contrast administration (B). T_2-weighted image from the same tumor (C) highlights the area of tumor and surrounding edema and brain-around-tumor (BAT). The bottom series of images shows MRI imaging characteristics from a patient with a GBM. The T_1-weighted image (D) shows a large area of hypodensity and central area of necrosis and a characteristic ring of enhancement following contrast (E). The T_2-weighted image (F) illustrates an extensive region of abnormality.

▶ **TABLE 13-2.** IMAGING CHARACTERISTICS: AA AND GBM

AA	GBM
Mixed density mass	Thick rim of tissue with necrotic center
Some edema	Significant edema
No or subtle rim of peripheral enhancement	Ring-like enhancement
	High vascularity

pathognomonic. Astrocytomas are infiltrative tumors that invade through the extracellular space along white matter tracts. Fluid-attenuated inversion recovery (FLAIR) and T_2-weighted images highlight surrounding edema, which is admixed with infiltrative tumor cells. Tumor cells can be found outside the area of contrast enhancement and T_2 signal abnormalities.[153] Preoperative meningeal contrast enhancement suggests meningeal dissemination of tumor (Fig. 13-8), and CSF cytology can confirm gliomatous involvement of the leptomeninges.

Definitive Diagnosis

Although radiographic characteristics in the appropriate clinical setting are often strongly indicative of a diagnosis of high-grade glioma, other tumor types and some non-neoplastic processes can mimic high-grade glioma. Additional diagnoses to consider include infarction, demyelination, infection with abscess formation, and non-glial tumors such as systemic metastases and primary CNS or systemic lymphoma (Table 13-3). Neuroimaging techniques that can be useful in distinguishing tumor from non-neoplastic processes include magnetic resonance spectroscopy (MRS) and positron emission tomography with fluorodeoxyglucose (FDG-PET). A definitive diagnosis and tumor grading can only be made by pathologic examination of tissue obtained from surgical specimens.

Newer neurosurgical techniques permit safe resection of what were historically considered to be "inoperable" tumors. As a result of these improvements, and the potential for other diagnoses, biopsy or resection of a suspected glioma is indicated in all but the most unusual circumstances in adults. The issue of whether to attempt stereotactic biopsy, open biopsy, partial resection, or complete resection is complex, with a number of diagnostic and therapeutic considerations. Stereotactic biopsy has the risk of sampling error because of tumor heterogeneity, and has been found to be inaccurate in determining the correct diagnosis in some cases (38% of the time in one study[154]). In addition, as described in "Role of Surgical Resection," a greater extent of resection may have a beneficial influence on symptom alleviation and survival in some patients. However, the potential benefits of radical resection have to be weighed against the risk of increased postoperative deficits and morbidity, and thus, more limited biopsy may be reasonable based on individual circumstances.

Treatment of Anaplastic Astrocytomas and Glioblastoma

The mainstays in the treatment of malignant astrocytomas are surgical resection followed by radiotherapy and chemotherapy. Surgery effectively and rapidly decreases tumor burden. Following surgery, patients are treated with external beam radiation. Radiation has proved to be the single most effective treatment in the management of malignant astrocytomas. In contrast, results of phase III trials with cytotoxic chemotherapy have generally been disappointing, with a modest survival benefit seen only in selected populations. Adjuvant chemotherapy is often given following irradiation when tumor burden is low. Young patients with a favorable KPS and those with AA, rather than GBM, appear to respond best to systemic chemotherapy. New data with the oral alkylator temozolomide, discussed on page 280, appear likely to overthrow

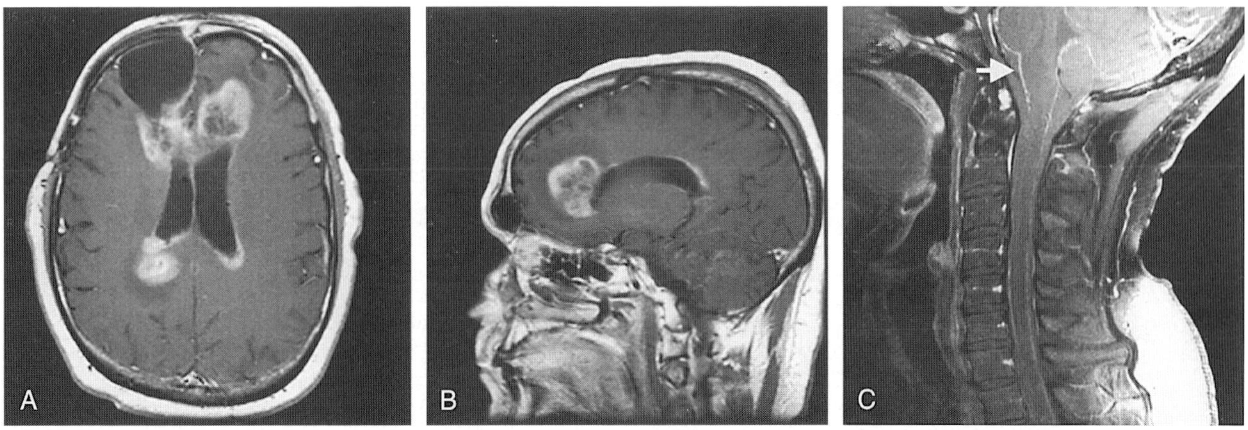

Figure 13-8. Leptomeningeal dissemination. These sagittal and axial postcontrast T_1-weighted images show a patient with extensive leptomeningeal involvement from a GBM.

▶ TABLE 13-3. RADIOGRAPHIC DIFFERENTIAL DIAGNOSIS

Nonneoplastic processes
Cerebral infarction
Demyelination
Infection/abscess formation
Nonastrocytic neoplasms
Systemic metastasis
CNS lymphoma

these historical tenets. The use of recursive partitioning analysis to determine combinations of factors associated with prognosis from the large Radiation Therapy Oncology Group (RTOG) database resulted in the identification of discrete classes of patients with different survivals.[155,156] Figure 13-9A presents a treatment algorithm for newly diagnosed patients; Fig. 13-9B shows management guidelines for patients with recurrent disease. The general principles outlined are meant as guidelines supported by data presented in the text.

Role of Surgical Resection

Neurosurgical management of brain tumors is the cornerstone of the initial treatment of malignant astrocytomas. Surgical intervention has at least three goals: (a) definitive diagnosis, (b) reduction of neurologic symptoms and mass effect, and (c) cytoreduction to improve outcome.

Because high-grade tumors are heterogeneous, stereotactic biopsy alone has the potential risk of sampling error, and may be insufficient in some circumstances to provide adequate tumor tissue for accurate histologic diagnosis. Although biopsy may be the only option for some tumors, such as deep thalamic or brainstem lesions, more complete resection reduces the sampling errors encountered with biopsy alone.[154] Fortunately, a number of technologic advances have increased the neurosurgeon's

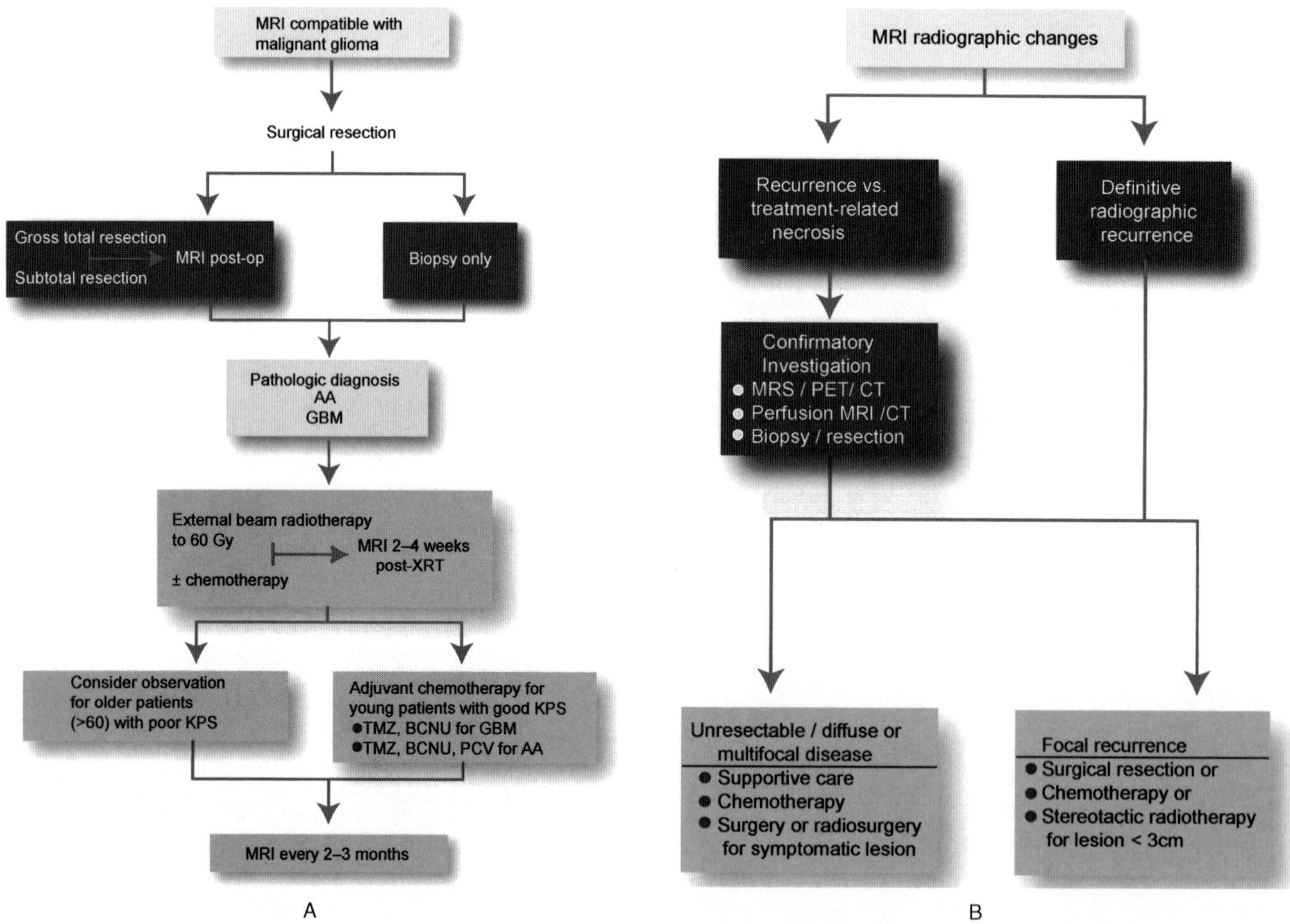

Figure 13-9. (A) Treatment algorithm for adult patients with newly diagnosed AA and GBM. BCNU = carmustine; MRI = magnetic resonance imaging; PCV = procarbazine, CCNU (or lomustine) and vincristine; TMZ = temozolomide; XRT = external beam radiation therapy. (B) Treatment algorithm for patients with recurrent AA or GBM. CT = computed tomography; MRI = magnetic resonance imaging; MRS = magnetic resonance spectroscopy; PET = positron emission tomography. Emerging data with TMZ may alter these traditional guidelines.

ability to resect tumor tissue and have reduced procedural morbidity and mortality. Intraoperative ultrasonography and image-guided systems with real-time MRI are examples of new technologies that have profoundly influenced the safety with which maximal tumor volume can be resected without damaging important brain structures. In addition, awake craniotomies with cortical mapping and somatosensory evoked potentials are valuable tools for aggressive tumor removal in and around eloquent brain tissue.

High-grade gliomas cause a great deal of morbidity and diminished quality of life for patients because of symptoms related to increased ICP and mass effect on tissue surrounding the tumor. Maximal removal of tumor tissue is often effective in improving neurologic symptoms related to mass effect and edema.[157] Reduction of mass effect can also allow lower doses to be given or steroid therapy to be discontinued following a postoperative steroid taper.

Despite the fact that maximal surgical resection has potential diagnostic and symptomatic benefits, the diffusely infiltrating nature of malignant gliomas means that macroscopic surgical resection alone is never curative. Surgical advances notwithstanding, as many as 80% of recurrences will occur within 2 to 3 cm of the site of the original tumor.[158] Nonetheless, the effectiveness of radiation and adjuvant chemotherapy may be enhanced when there is minimal residual tumor burden following aggressive surgical resection.

The effect of the extent of surgical resection on survival has been a point of long-term controversy. Extent of resection has been identified as an independent variable associated with improved survival in a number of prospective randomized and retrospective studies evaluating the efficacy of various radiation and chemotherapy modalities. Median survival after gross total resection was 10.4 months, compared with 6.6 months with biopsy alone, in one study.[159] However, other studies show no benefit.[160,161] A recent large retrospective analysis found that gross total resection was associated with longer survival, especially in patients with prognostically favorable characteristics, such as younger age.[162] In many studies, known prognostic variables such as age, tumor histology and KPS were more strongly associated with survival than extent of resection. Nonetheless, maximal resection of tumor remains a foundation in the treatment of primary brain tumors with a goal of minimizing morbidity and improving outcome.

Surgical Resection for Tumor Recurrence

Tumor recurrence or diagnostic exigencies may make a second surgical resection necessary following initial surgery, radiation, and chemotherapy. Patients should be evaluated as they were before their first surgical procedure. A second resection provides the chance to reevaluate tumor histology. For recurrent tumor, treatment changes may be needed. Alternatively, radiation necrosis may be misdiagnosed as tumor recurrence and should not be considered as a treatment failure. For malignant astrocytomas at recurrence, the most predictive variable of survival was a preoperative KPS greater than 60.[163] Other important prognostic factors include young age (younger than 50 years), the presence of seizures, a long interval between surgeries, circumscribed lesions, and the availability of different treatment options after surgery. Median survival for patients with GBM following a second surgery ranges from 14 to 36 weeks. Given the generally poor survival for patients with GBM, which is approximately 1 year, extending survival 14 to 36 weeks is not a trivial amount of time. However, it is important to note that this is a highly selected group of patients, as only those patients with adequate performance status and other variables will be candidates for additional surgery. In contrast, the median survival for patients with AA after a second surgery ranges from 56 to 88 weeks.[164–166]

In summary, surgical resection remains a cornerstone of treatment for malignant glioma. Extensive surgical resection likely offers a survival advantage in selected patients. New surgical techniques offer the opportunity to remove a maximal amount of tumor while minimizing patient morbidity. Reoperation of malignant gliomas may offer an improved survival for carefully chosen patients.

Role of Radiation

Despite the high percentage of eventual recurrences following radiation therapy, external beam irradiation has been shown to be the single most effective therapy in the treatment of high-grade gliomas. Randomized controlled trials in the 1970s and 1980s using whole-brain irradiation demonstrated an increased survival from 5 months to 9 months.[167–169] Involved field treatment that includes the area of T_2-weighted imaging abnormality and a variable margin has supplanted whole-brain irradiation for the treatment of gliomas because it has equivalent efficacy with less neurotoxicity.[170,171] Interestingly, in one study whole-brain irradiation did not change the typical pattern of recurrence, usually within 2 to 3 cm of the original tumor.[158] The optimal dose of radiation in the treatment of high-grade gliomas has long been debated, with several large cooperative trials using different dosages. A dose–response relationship was found in a randomized clinical trial that enrolled patients with high-grade gliomas. The study results were that 60 Gray (Gy) was superior to 45 Gy, increasing survival by 3 months.[172,173] Doses of radiation up to 70 Gy and higher have not, however, proved to be more effective.[174] Radiation has a greater effect on survival in young patients; the benefit of irradiation to patients older than age 70 years, has not been demonstrated.

Three-dimensional reconstruction of tumor within the cranial vault using standard CT and MRI images facilitates radiation treatment planning. Conformal radiation fields are selected to optimize treatment of the tumor while minimizing irradiation of surrounding normal brain. Conformal techniques have been estimated to decrease the dose of normal brain irradiation as much as 50%.[175,176] Standard practice is to administer 58 to 60 Gy in 1.8 to 2.0 Gy fractions 5 days a week for 30 to 35 fractions. Forty Gy is generally administered as a focal dose to the area of tumor plus surrounding edema, with an addition 20 Gy boost given to the enhancing tumor plus a 1- to 2-cm margin.[177] Corticosteroids are usually given for several days before radiation therapy is begun to control local edema. Several weeks into treatment steroids can often be tapered and discontinued. Investigation of other treatment schemes, including hyperfractionation, chemical modifiers to enhance radiosensitivity, and interstitial brachytherapy using radioactive 125-iodine, is ongoing. Recent data combining temozolomide chemotherapy with radiation has shown promising results.[178] Tumor progression during radiation is a poor prognostic indicator and occurs in approximately 20% of patients with high-grade gliomas.

Median survival for patients with AA who have received radiation therapy is approximately 3 years. For patients with GBM, median survival is approximately 8 to 12 months, with few long-term survivors. Elderly patients (over 65 years old) can expect a survival of only 4 to 6 months.

Neurotoxicity and radiation necrosis can arise following standard doses of irradiation. In adults, neuropsychological deficits, including impairments in recent memory, learning abilities, and problem solving, can occur.

Radionecrosis is a late effect of irradiation, usually occurring at least 9 months after irradiation, although shorter time intervals have been reported. Imaging features suggestive of radiation necrosis include a focal, poorly demarcated area of contrast enhancement at a distance from the primary tumor, which usually involves subcortical white matter. However, it is often difficult to differentiate necrosis from tumor recurrence on MRI. Metabolic imaging using [^{18}F]fluorodeoxyglucose positron emission tomography (FDG-PET) or magnetic resonance spectroscopy (MRS) can help distinguish necrosis from tumor, although surgical debulking is often necessary to make the diagnosis because these imaging techniques are not perfect.[179] With proton MRS, areas of tumor typically have high levels of choline and reduced levels of N-acetylaspartate (NAA), whereas areas of necrosis have low levels of both choline and NAA. Figure 13-10 shows an example of MRS images from two separate patients; the top panel shows a FLAIR image (A) from a patient with a recurrent GBM, whereas the bottom panel shows a different patient who has treatment-related necrosis. Radiation necrosis can be treated symptomatically with steroids or surgical debulking but the tissue damage is irreversible. There are anecdotal data for the use of hyperbaric oxygen or anticoagulation to treat radiation necrosis, but definitive data for improved outcome are lacking.[180,181]

Stereotactic Radiosurgery

Stereotactic radiosurgery is a technique that delivers high doses of ionizing radiation to small areas of tumor recurrence, usually less than 3 cm in diameter. Linear accelerator-based, gamma knife, and proton beam radiosurgery are varied methods used to deliver a large, single fraction of radiation. The results from single institution trials suggest that there is a survival benefit when stereotactic radiosurgery is given as an adjuvant boost following conventional external beam irradiation or when directed to a focal recurrence. Median survival when radiosurgery is used as a boost is approximately 19 months, and 10 months when it is given for a local recurrence.[182,183] These studies are, however, methodologically flawed in that patients who are eligible for radiosurgery are a prognostically favorable subgroup with a good performance status and a small tumor volume. A recently completed phase III trial of newly diagnosed GBM patients treated with or without stereotactic radiosurgery prior to conventional radiation therapy and chemotherapy failed to support the role of stereotactic radiosurgery in the treatment of patients with malignant astrocytomas.[183a]

Interstitial Brachytherapy

Interstitial brachytherapy has been tried as an adjunct to traditional radiation therapy in an attempt to boost the dose of radiation administered to the tumor bed. Interstitial brachytherapy involves placement of encapsulated radioactive sources into the surgical cavity in an effort to maximize the dose of radiation to tumor without exposing normal brain to toxic doses of radiation. For newly diagnosed GBM, two phase III clinical trials have been completed to date, but neither study was able to demonstrate a survival benefit in patients whom received radioactive 125-iodine implants.[184,185] Interstitial brachytherapy has also been evaluated for the treatment of recurrent high-grade astrocytomas, but there are currently no randomized phase III clinical trials. A new delivery technology, GliaSite, an inflatable balloon catheter that acts as an 125-iodine radiation reservoir, was recently approved by the FDA for delivery of local radiation into tumor beds after resection. A study examining the safety and performance of this device for recurrent malignant gliomas has been done,[186] but no efficacy trials have been published to date.

Radiation therapy remains one of the backbones of malignant glioma treatment. External beam irradiation dramatically improves survival, particularly in young patients (<50 years old). Technologic advances in neuroimaging paired with conformal and stereotactic radiation

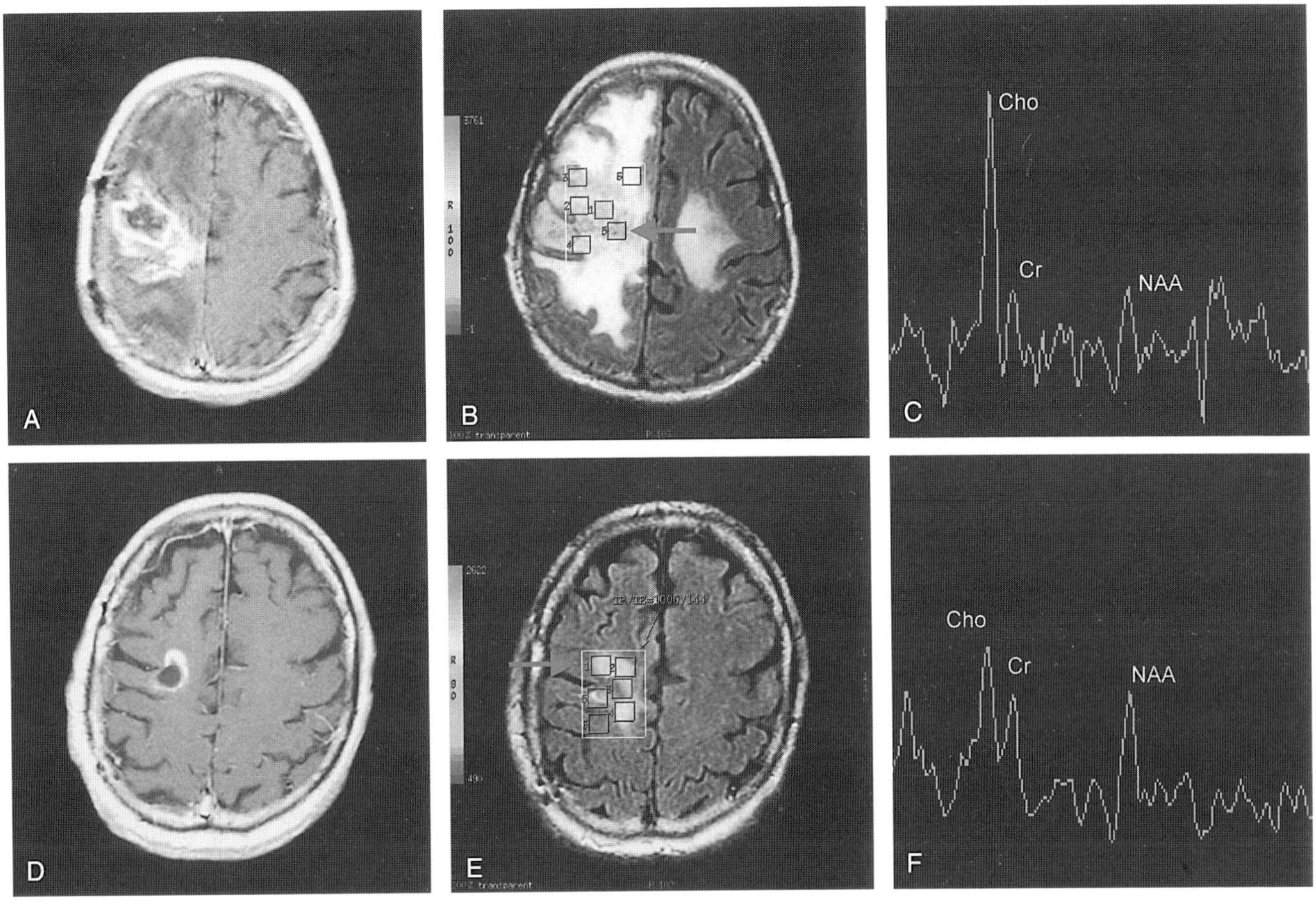

Figure 13-10. Magnetic resonance spectroscopy (MRS) image from a patient with prior history of GBM. Radiographic changes seen on T_1-weighted postcontrast (A) and FLAIR (B) images were suggestive of tumor recurrence. Multiple voxels overlay the regions of interest. Within individual voxels, the size of the choline (Cho), creatine (Cr), and N-acetyl-aspartate (NAA) peaks are compared. The MR spectrum demonstrating a high level of Cho and low levels of NAA (C) is suggestive of tumor recurrence. The T_1-weighted post-contrast (D) and FLAIR (E) images from a different patient represent treatment-related changes. The MR spectrum caused by tumor necrosis (F) is characterized by low levels of both Cho and NAA.

techniques minimize toxicity to normal brain. Radiation necrosis remains a diagnostic challenge even when using current noninvasive techniques and often requires surgical resection to confirm the diagnosis. Local recurrence of radioresistant glioma within the area of prior radiation treatment is a particular conundrum.

Role of Chemotherapy

The goal of systemic chemotherapy is to increase cell kill after surgery and radiation have removed the bulk of tumor cells. Despite intensive efforts to identify more successful agents or therapy combinations, the overall efficacy of chemotherapy in improving median survival has been disappointing. In general, chemotherapy effects a modest benefit, primarily for young patients with GBM and all patients with AA. The agents most commonly used to treat malignant astrocytomas have been the nitrosoureas (BCNU and CCNU), alone or in combination with procarbazine and vincristine (PCV), and, more recently, temozolomide.

Single-Agent Regimens

The nitrosoureas have historically been the most commonly used single agents for the chemotherapeutic treatment of malignant astrocytomas, although several large randomized studies have demonstrated only a small benefit of single-agent adjuvant chemotherapy with nitrosoureas.[168,187] Treatment with BCNU following radiotherapy resulted in an 8% increase in survivors at 6 months, a 10% increase in absolute survival at 1 year, and an increased median survival of 4.5 weeks.[172] Additional studies comparing procarbazine or BCNU to steroid-only treatment also showed a survival advantage at 1 year, extending survival in the procarbazine group by 2 weeks, and by 9 weeks in the BCNU group.[187]

Newer agents have been developed in an attempt to improve these results. Most notably, the oral alkylating agent temozolomide received FDA approval in 1999 for the treatment of AA based on the results of a phase II single-arm clinical trial. In patients at first relapse who had received radiation, some of whom had also received chemotherapy, there was a 35% response rate, which included the 22% of patients who had nitrosourea-resistant tumors.[188] Because its toxicity profile is more favorable than other alkylating agents, temozolomide is rapidly becoming a first-line therapy for patients with malignant gliomas.

Recent data suggest that postoperative single-agent temozolomide given with radiation followed by adjuvant temozolomide for 6 months is superior to surgery plus radiation alone.[178] In a phase III randomized trial, patients who received concurrent temozolomide with radiation followed by adjuvant temozolomide for 6 months had an increase in median survival of 2.4 months from 12 months in the control group to 14.4 months in the treatment arm. The overall survival at 2 years increased from 10% to 26.6%. Other drugs that have been used as single agents with variable results include platinum compounds, procarbazine, etoposide, tamoxifen, paclitaxel, and irinotecan.

Multiagent Regimens

While multidrug treatment regimens may demonstrate superior efficacy over single-agent therapy for patients with AA, the same is not true for patients with GBM. In a small phase III clinical trial comparing single-agent BCNU with PCV,[189] a post hoc analysis demonstrated the superiority of PCV with a doubling of the time to progression and survival for patients with AA who had a KPS greater than 70, had completed radiation therapy, and had at least one course of chemotherapy. It is likely that this benefit was largely a result of procarbazine, which has produced partial responses in some patients who have progressed while taking BCNU. In contrast, another retrospective study suggested there was no difference between single-agent BCNU and PCV for patients with AA.[190]

Overall Benefit of Chemotherapy: Results of Two Meta-Analyses

Apart from the recent trial of temozolomide during and after radiation therapy,[178] individual chemotherapy clinical trials have failed to show an increase in the median survival of patients treated with adjuvant chemotherapy. However, when data from patients enrolled in many different clinical trials were pooled and scrutinized in two meta-analyses, a modest benefit of adjuvant chemotherapy was identified for malignant gliomas. A meta-analysis of 16 randomized chemotherapy clinical trials involving 3000 patients demonstrated a 10% increase in survival at 1 year and 8.6% increase at 2 years. This benefit extended to patients with both AA and GBM treated with either BCNU or CCNU.[191] A more recent meta-analysis of 12 randomized controlled clinical trials demonstrated a modest, but significant, increase in median survival of approximately 2 months for patients treated with chemotherapy.[192] This increase in median survival translated to an overall boost in survival of 6% at 1 year, increasing the number of patients alive from 40% to 46% at 1 year. The 2-year survival rate of patients with GBM increased from 9% to 13% and from 31% to 37% in patients with AA. There was no evidence that the effect of chemotherapy differed on the basis of histology, age, sex, performance status, or extent of tumor resection.

Prediction of Response and Prognosis

Unlike the situation with 1p/19q-deleted oligodendrogliomas, no molecular markers, histologic hallmarks, or tumor-related characteristics currently allow prediction of the response to chemotherapy for patients with AA or GBM. Investigators are, however, actively seeking to identify molecular markers specific to individual tumors whose presence forecasts prognostic benefit. As a rule, patients with AA have a longer survival than patients with GBM, but there is no evidence that this survival benefit is associated with chemosensitivity. Careful analysis of patient responders in individual trials and meta-analyses suggests that in general, patients younger than 40 years of age with minimal residual disease after surgery and radiation, and patients with a good KPS are the most likely to respond favorably to chemotherapy (Table 13-4). A retrospective analysis[193] demonstrated the importance of age on response to chemotherapy. Nitrosoureas produced a partial response in 40% of patients younger than age 40 years, a 15% response in patients between the ages of 40 and 59 years, and only 5% in patients older than age 60 years. At the start of chemotherapy, median survival was 43 weeks for patients younger than age 60 years and 24 weeks for patients older than age 60 years. Importantly, patients older than age 60 years are much more likely (35% vs. 16%) to have myelotoxicity requiring hospitalization than are younger patients. This lower response rate and high risk of toxicity should prompt cautious use of toxic chemotherapy regimens in

▶ TABLE 13-4. PROGNOSTIC FACTORS PREDICTING LONGER SURVIVAL FOR PATIENTS WITH MALIGNANT GLIOMAS

Age
Histologic diagnosis: AA > GBM
Karnofsky performance status >70
Duration of symptoms
Extent of surgical resection

patients older than age 60 years. Additionally, one retrospective study correlated the size of residual tumor at the initiation of chemotherapy with response to chemotherapy in patients with GBM but not AA.[194] The extent of response and speed of achieving a response[195] have not been correlated with the duration of response.

Chemotherapy at Tumor Recurrence

The utility of chemotherapy at the time of tumor recurrence has not been defined. At the time of tumor recurrence, many patients have significant neurologic impairments that are not responsive to steroids. Patients have usually progressed despite treatment with traditional agents such as temozolomide, BCNU, or PCV. Other agents that are commonly used include platinum-based compounds such as carboplatin or cisplatin, irinotecan, procarbazine, cyclophosphamide, and etoposide. Differentiating agents that influence malignant cells to become more normal, such as retinoids, have less toxicity and may be used in elderly patients (age > 65) with a low KPS. As previously mentioned, temozolomide is a well-tolerated oral alkylating agent with activity shown in some patients with malignant astrocytomas. Because it is easy to administer via an oral route and usually does not cause significant myelotoxicity, it is a rational choice for the treatment of elderly patients and potentially as "maintenance" therapy for long-term survivors.

Because the results of clinical trials using traditional cytoreductive chemotherapy agents have generally been disappointing, newer approaches to the treatment of malignant astrocytomas are being explored. These have included neoadjuvant chemotherapy, intraarterial chemotherapy with or without blood–brain barrier disruption, and high-dose chemotherapy with stem cell rescue. So far, however, these have not improved the outcome of standard treatment with nitrosoureas or temozolomide.

Interstitial chemotherapy using biodegradable BCNU-impregnated wafers inserted into the surgical cavity at the time of surgery achieves very high local concentrations of BCNU with minimal or no systemic toxicity. Phase III trials demonstrated a survival benefit of approximately 2 to 3 months in patients receiving BCNU wafers compared with patients implanted with placebo.[196,197] The effectiveness of carmustine (Gliadel) wafers implanted in the surgical cavity of newly diagnosed patients with high-grade glioma was assessed in a phase III international, randomized, placebo-controlled clinical trial.[198] The median survival increased from 11.6 to 13.9 months in patients treated with Gliadel. Trials combining interstitial chemotherapy with systemic chemotherapy are ongoing.

Newer Chemotherapeutic Agents

As the molecular mechanisms of glioma are deciphered, there is increasing interest in targeting the specific pathways that lead to aberrant cell growth. Several studies have combined cytotoxic agents with newer cytostatic treatments with some promising results.[199–203] Most malignant astrocytomas rely on growth factor stimulation for growth and invasion and express the receptors for several different growth factors, including PDGF, VEGF, and EGF. New targeted therapies aim to inhibit these growth factor receptors and their tyrosine kinase-based intracellular signaling pathways. Currently, many such drugs are being tested in phase I and phase II clinical trials for the treatment of glioma (see reference 73 for a review). New blood vessel formation or angiogenesis is another target of glioma treatment and has been an active area of research for many years. There is renewed interest in taking an antiangiogenesis approach, as drugs that specifically target tumor blood vessel endothelium are being developed. Gene therapy trials have so far been disappointing, although new vectors designed to target more than one gene are being developed. The lack of efficiency of current delivery systems for targeted therapies has been a long-standing impediment in taking a molecular approach. Mechanisms that will improve transfection efficiency are being developed and this area of research is promising. Table 13-5 shows some of the newest agents being tested for the treatment of malignant glioma.

Symptomatic Treatments

Despite aggressive treatment, high-grade astrocytomas are not curable with current therapies. The main goal of treatment is to prolong life with careful attention directed to improving neurologic symptoms while maintaining patient quality of life. Minimizing the use of steroids and avoiding unnecessary treatment with anticonvulsants are important aspects of this approach to patient care. Additionally, a poor prognosis should not prevent aggressive physical rehabilitation, which may be necessary following surgery or radiation therapy to improve strength and endurance. Mood disturbances frequently accompany the diagnosis of cancer and should be treated with antidepressants. Patients can also benefit from psychotherapeutic interventions. Treatment of brain tumor patients with methylphenidate can improve cognitive function, attention, and motivation to impact overall quality of life in a positive manner.[204]

At the time of tumor diagnosis, symptomatic treatment with corticosteroids is usually necessary to control tumor-associated edema and to improve neurologic symptoms. Steroids ameliorate the symptoms associated with vasogenic edema by restoring the integrity of the blood–brain barrier. Dexamethasone is a high-potency steroid commonly used to treat tumor-related edema. Long-term use of steroids should be avoided to prevent complications associated with chronic steroid use such as myopathy, mood changes, infection, hyperglycemia,

▶ **TABLE 13-5.** NEW THERAPIES IN BRAIN TUMOR TREATMENT

Class of Drugs	Target	Agent(s)	Clinical Phase in Glioma
Targeted therapies	EGFR	Gefitinib	II
		Erlotinib	II
		AEE788	I/II
	PDGFR	Imatinib mesylate	II
		SU6668	I
	VEGFR	PTK787	II
		SU5416	I
	Ras	Tipifarnib	I/II
		Lonafarnib	I
	mTOR	Rapamycin	I/II
		CCI-779	I/II
		RAD001	I/II
	PKC	Tamoxifen	II
		LY317615	II
	HDAC	13-cis-retinoic acid	II
		LAQ824	Preclinical
Angiogenesis inhibitors	Tumor blood vessels	Everolimus	I
		Thalidomide	II
Oncolytic viruses		Delta-24	Preclinical
		ONYX-015	I
		HSV1716	I

EGFR = epidermal growth factor receptor; HDAC = histone deacetylase inhibitor; mTOR = mammalian target of rapamycin; PDGFR = platelet-derived growth factor receptor; PKC = protein kinase C; VEGFR = vascular endothelial growth factor receptor.
Source: Adapted from Rich JN, Bigner DD. Development of novel targeted therapies in the treatment of malignant glioma. Nat Rev Drug Discov 2004;3(5):430–446.

weight gain, hypertension, and gastrointestinal distress. Steroids also reduce blood vessel leakiness, which, in theory, could potentially reduce the permeability to drugs.

The routine use of prophylactic anticonvulsants for patients who do not have a history suggestive of seizures is controversial, because there is no current evidence that prophylactic anticonvulsants will prevent seizures from developing. Anticonvulsants have many potential harmful side effects, including altering the effectiveness of systemic chemotherapy. Several studies reveal that anticonvulsants that activate the liver cytochrome P450 system—phenytoin, carbamazepine, and phenobarbital—accelerate the systemic metabolism of some cytotoxic chemotherapy agents.[205] Because systemic chemotherapy must be delivered across the blood–brain barrier, lower systemic levels theoretically translate into lower doses of drug being delivered to the tumor. Most current clinical trials take anticonvulsant use into account when determining the proper chemotherapy dose to administer. Phenytoin and carbamazepine are the most effective agents in treating generalized seizures. Carbamazepine, oxcarbazepine, and valproic acid are commonly used to treat partial seizures. Newer antiepileptic drugs, such as levetiracetam and gabapentin do not activate the cytochrome P450 system or interfere with chemotherapy regimens and show promise for the treatment of seizures in patients with malignant astrocytomas.[206]

Venous thromboses, consisting of deep venous thrombosis in the lower extremities and pulmonary embolism, are a significant risk in malignant glioma patients.[207] No definitive data exist regarding the relative benefits of routine prophylaxis, or the potential increased risk of hemorrhage with anticoagulation in these patients. The use of low-molecular-weight heparins for prophylaxis in high-risk patients may be a consideration based on individual patient situation. Treatment of deep venous thrombosis or pulmonary embolism with low-molecular-weight heparins, warfarin, and/or inferior vena cava filter placement, are all reasonable options.

Terminal Care

Most patients with malignant astrocytomas die from progressive disease. A decision to discontinue additional treatments is made either because of family wishes or the futility of additional treatments. During the terminal stages of the disease, special attention to comfort care and avoiding prolonged suffering for the patient and family is needed. Consultation with social workers, psychiatry, and palliative care services can facilitate transitioning a patient to hospice care where end-of-life concerns are best addressed. There are also many support network groups that can be accessed through national brain tumor associations and foundations.

REFERENCES

1. CBTRUS. Statistical report: primary brain tumors in the United States 1992–1997. Chicago: Central Brain Tumor Registry of the United States, 2000.
2. Aldape KD, et al. Molecular epidemiology of glioblastoma. Cancer J 2003;9(2):99–106.
3. Wrensch M, et al. Epidemiology of primary brain tumors: current concepts and review of the literature. Neuro-oncol 2002;4(4):278–299.
4. Batchelor TT, et al. Age-dependent prognostic effects of genetic alterations in glioblastoma. Clin Cancer Res 2004; 10(1 Pt 1):228–233.
5. Smith JS, et al. PTEN mutation, EGFR amplification, and outcome in patients with anaplastic astrocytoma and glioblastoma multiforme. J Natl Cancer Inst 2001; 93(16): 1246–1256.
6. Grossman SA, et al. Central nervous system cancers in first-degree relatives and spouses. Cancer Invest 1999; 17(5):299–308.
7. Nichols KE, et al. Germ-line p53 mutations predispose to a wide spectrum of early-onset cancers. Cancer Epidemiol Biomarkers Prev 2001;10(2):83–87.
8. Kyritsis AP, et al. Germline p53 gene mutations in subsets of glioma patients. J Natl Cancer Inst 1994;86(5): 344–349.
9. Chen P, et al. Constitutional p53 mutations associated with brain tumors in young adults. Cancer Genet Cytogenet 1995;82(2):106–115.
10. Paunu N, et al. Analysis of p53 tumor suppressor gene in families with multiple glioma patients. J Neurooncol 2001;55(3):159–165.
11. van Meyel DJ, et al. Absence of hereditary mutations in exons 5 through 9 of the p53 gene and exon 24 of the neurofibromin gene in families with glioma. Ann Neurol 1994;35(1):120–122.
12. Tachibana I, et al. Investigation of germline PTEN, p53, p16(INK4A)/p14(ARF), and CDK4 alterations in familial glioma. Am J Med Genet 2000;92(2):136–141.
13. Hodges LC, et al. Prevalence of glioblastoma multiforme in subjects with prior therapeutic radiation. J Neurosci Nurs 1992;24(2):79–83.
14. Wrensch M, et al. Environmental risk factors for primary malignant brain tumors: a review. J Neurooncol 1993; 17(1): 47–64.
15. Karlsson P, et al. Intracranial tumors after exposure to ionizing radiation during infancy: a pooled analysis of two Swedish cohorts of 28,008 infants with skin hemangioma. Radiat Res 1998;150(3):357–364.
16. Neglia JP, et al. Second neoplasms after acute lymphoblastic leukemia in childhood. N Engl J Med 1991; 325(19):1330–1336.
17. Wrensch M, et al. Are prior head injuries or diagnostic X-rays associated with glioma in adults? The effects of control selection bias. Neuroepidemiology 2000;19(5):234–44.
18. Alexander V, DiMarco JH. Reappraisal of brain tumor risk among US nuclear workers: a 10-year review. Occup Med 2001;16(2):289–315.
19. Wertheimer N, Leeper E. Magnetic field exposure related to cancer subtypes. Ann N Y Acad Sci 1987;502:43–54.
20. Meinert R, Michaelis J. Meta-analyses of studies on the association between electromagnetic fields and childhood cancer. Radiat Environ Biophys 1996;35(1):11–18.
21. Kheifets LI, et al. Occupational electric and magnetic field exposure and brain cancer: a meta-analysis. J Occup Environ Med 1995;37(12):1327–1341.
22. Savitz DA, et al. Case-cohort analysis of brain cancer and leukemia in electric utility workers using a refined magnetic field job-exposure matrix. Am J Ind Med 2000; 38(4): 4417–4425.
23. Wrensch M, et al. Adult glioma in relation to residential power frequency electromagnetic field exposures in the San Francisco Bay area. Epidemiology 1999;10(5):523–527.
24. Kheifets LI, Sussman SS, Preston-Martin S. Childhood brain tumors and residential electromagnetic fields (EMF). Rev Environ Contam Toxicol 1999;159:111–129.
25. Floderus B, Stenlund C, Persson T. Occupational magnetic field exposure and site-specific cancer incidence: a Swedish cohort study. Cancer Causes Control 1999;10(5):323–332.
26. Johansen C, Olsen JH. [Risk of cancer among Danish electricity workers: a cohort study.] Ugeskr Laeger 1999; 161(14):2079–2085.
27. Hardell L, Mild KH, Carlberg M. Further aspects on cellular and cordless telephones and brain tumours. Int J Oncol 2003;22(2):399–407.
28. Hardell L, et al. Use of cellular telephones and the risk for brain tumours: a case-control study. Int J Oncol 1999; 15(1):113–116.
29. Muscat JE, et al. Handheld cellular telephone use and risk of brain cancer. JAMA 2000;284(23):3001–3007.
30. Rothman KJ, et al. Overall mortality of cellular telephone customers. Epidemiology 1996;7(3):303–305.
31. Dreyer NA, Loughlin JE, Rothman KJ. Cause-specific mortality in cellular telephone users. JAMA 1999;282(19): 1814–1816.
32. Inskip PD, et al. Cellular-telephone use and brain tumors. N Engl J Med 2001;344(2):79–86.
33. Johansen C, et al. Cellular telephones and cancer—a nationwide cohort study in Denmark. J Natl Cancer Inst 2001;93(3):203–207.
34. Morgan RW, et al. Radiofrequency exposure and mortality from cancer of the brain and lymphatic/hematopoietic systems. Epidemiology 2000;11(2):118–127.
35. Elwood JM. Epidemiological studies of radio frequency exposures and human cancer. Bioelectromagnetics 2003;Suppl 6:S63–S73.
36. Berleur MP, Cordier S. The role of chemical, physical, or viral exposures and health factors in neurocarcinogenesis: implications for epidemiologic studies of brain tumors. Cancer Causes Control 1995;6(3):240–256.
37. Preston-Martin S, et al. Maternal consumption of cured meats and vitamins in relation to pediatric brain tumors. Cancer Epidemiol Biomarkers Prev 1996;5(8): 599–605.
38. Lee M, Wrensch M, Miike R. Dietary and tobacco risk factors for adult onset glioma in the San Francisco Bay Area (California, USA). Cancer Causes Control 1997;8(1):13–24.
39. Blot WJ, Henderson BE, Boice JD Jr. Childhood cancer in relation to cured meat intake: review of the epidemiological evidence. Nutr Cancer 1999;34(1):111–118.

40. Daniels JL, Olshan AF, Savitz DA. Pesticides and childhood cancers. Environ Health Perspect 1997;105(10):1068–1077.
41. Hanahan D, Weinberg RA. The hallmarks of cancer. Cell 2000;100(1):57–70.
42. Louis DN, Gusella JF. A tiger behind many doors: multiple genetic pathways to malignant glioma. Trends Genet 1995;11(10):412–415.
43. Godard S, et al. Classification of human astrocytic gliomas on the basis of gene expression: a correlated group of genes with angiogenic activity emerges as a strong predictor of subtypes. Cancer Res 2003;63(20):6613–6625.
44. Shai R, et al. Gene expression profiling identifies molecular subtypes of gliomas. Oncogene 2003;22(31):4918–4923.
45. Burton EC, et al. Aberrant p53, mdm2, and proliferation differ in glioblastomas from long-term compared with typical survivors. Clin Cancer Res 2002;8(1):180–187.
46. Cairncross JG, et al. Specific genetic predictors of chemotherapeutic response and survival in patients with anaplastic oligodendrogliomas. J Natl Cancer Inst 1998; 90(19):1473–1479.
47. Ino Y, et al. Long survival and therapeutic responses in patients with histologically disparate high-grade gliomas demonstrating chromosome 1p loss. J Neurosurg 2000; 92(6):983–990.
48. Paez JG, et al. EGFR mutations in lung cancer: correlation with clinical response to gefitinib therapy. Science 2004;304(5676):1497–1500.
49. Lynch TJ, et al. Activating mutations in the epidermal growth factor receptor underlying responsiveness of non-small-cell lung cancer to gefitinib. N Engl J Med 2004;350(21):2129–2139.
50. Nutt CL, et al. Gene expression-based classification of malignant gliomas correlates better with survival than histological classification. Cancer Res 2003;63(7):1602–1607.
51. Schmidt MC, et al. Impact of genotype and morphology on the prognosis of glioblastoma. J Neuropathol Exp Neurol 2002;61(4):321–328.
52. von Deimling A, et al. Subsets of glioblastoma multiforme defined by molecular genetic analysis. Brain Pathol 1993;3(1):19–26.
53. Mischel PS, et al. Identification of molecular subtypes of glioblastoma by gene expression profiling. Oncogene 2003;22(15):2361–2373.
54. Burton EC, et al. Genetic aberrations defined by comparative genomic hybridization distinguish long-term from typical survivors of glioblastoma. Cancer Res 2002; 62(21): 6205–6210.
55. Simmons ML, et al. Analysis of complex relationships between age, p53, epidermal growth factor receptor, and survival in glioblastoma patients. Cancer Res 2001;61(3): 1122–1128.
56. Bailey P, Cushing H. A classification of tumors of the glioma group on a histogenetic basis with a correlation study of prognosis. Philadelphia: Lippincott, 1926.
57. Kleihues P, Cavenee W, eds. WHO classification of tumours: pathology and genetics of tumours of the nervous system. Lyon, France: IARC Press, 2000.
58. Holland EC. Progenitor cells and glioma formation. Curr Opin Neurol 2001;14(6):683–688.
59. Dai C, et al. PDGF autocrine stimulation dedifferentiates cultured astrocytes and induces oligodendrogliomas and oligoastrocytomas from neural progenitors and astrocytes in vivo. Genes Dev 2001;15(15):1913–1925.
60. Holland EC. Gliomagenesis: genetic alterations and mouse models. Nat Rev Genet 2001;2(2):120–129.
61. Bachoo RM, et al. Epidermal growth factor receptor and Ink4a/Arf: convergent mechanisms governing terminal differentiation and transformation along the neural stem cell to astrocyte axis. Cancer Cell 2002;1(3):269–277.
62. Maher EA, et al. Malignant glioma: genetics and biology of a grave matter. Genes Dev 2001;15(11):1311–1333.
63. Watanabe K, et al. Overexpression of the EGF receptor and p53 mutations are mutually exclusive in the evolution of primary and secondary glioblastomas. Brain Pathol 1996;6(3):217–223; discussion 223–224.
64. Benjamin R, Capparella J, Brown A. Classification of glioblastoma multiforme in adults by molecular genetics. Cancer J 2003;9(2):82–90.
65. Lang FF, et al. Pathways leading to glioblastoma multiforme: a molecular analysis of genetic alterations in 65 astrocytic tumors. J Neurosurg 1994;81(3):427–436.
66. Watanabe K, et al. Incidence and timing of p53 mutations during astrocytoma progression in patients with multiple biopsies. Clin Cancer Res 1997;3(4):523–530.
67. Louis DN. The p53 gene and protein in human brain tumors. J Neuropathol Exp Neurol 1994;53(1):11–21.
68. Sidransky D, et al. Clonal expansion of p53 mutant cells is associated with brain tumour progression. Nature 1992; 355(6363):846–847.
69. Fults D, Pedone C. Deletion mapping of the long arm of chromosome 10 in glioblastoma multiforme. Genes Chromosomes Cancer 1993;7(3):173–177.
70. Hirose Y, et al. Grade II astrocytomas are subgrouped by chromosome aberrations. Cancer Genet Cytogenet 2003; 142(1):1–7.
71. Nishizaki T, et al. Investigation of genetic alterations associated with the grade of astrocytic tumor by comparative genomic hybridization. Genes Chromosomes Cancer 1998;21(4):340–346.
72. Okada Y, et al. Selection pressures of TP53 mutation and microenvironmental location influence epidermal growth factor receptor gene amplification in human glioblastomas. Cancer Res 2003;63(2):413–416.
73. Rich JN, Bigner DD. Development of novel targeted therapies in the treatment of malignant glioma. Nat Rev Drug Discov 2004;3(5):430–446.
74. Malkin D, et al. Germ line p53 mutations in a familial syndrome of breast cancer, sarcomas, and other neoplasms. Science 1990;250(4985):1233–1238.
75. Carson DA, Lois A. Cancer progression and p53. Lancet 1995;346(8981):1009–1011.
76. Sherr CJ. Principles of tumor suppression. Cell 2004; 116(2):235–246.
77. Reifenberger G, et al. Amplification and overexpression of the MDM2 gene in a subset of human malignant gliomas without p53 mutations. Cancer Res 1993;53(12):2736– 2739.
78. Biernat W, et al. Amplification and overexpression of MDM2 in primary (de novo) glioblastomas. J Neuropathol Exp Neurol 1997;56(2):180–185.

79. Jen J, et al. Deletion of p16 and p15 genes in brain tumors. Cancer Res 1994;54(24):6353–6358.
80. Nishikawa R, et al. Loss of P16INK4 expression is frequent in high grade gliomas. Cancer Res 1995;55(9):1941–1945.
81. Fulci G, et al. p53 gene mutation and ink4a-arf deletion appear to be two mutually exclusive events in human glioblastoma. Oncogene 2000;19(33):3816–3822.
82. Serrano M, Hannon GJ, Beach D. A new regulatory motif in cell-cycle control causing specific inhibition of cyclin D/CDK4. Nature 1993;366(6456):704–707.
83. Ichimura K, et al. Human glioblastomas with no alterations of the CDKN2A (p16INK4A, MTS1) and CDK4 genes have frequent mutations of the retinoblastoma gene. Oncogene 1996;13(5):1065–1072.
84. Ueki K, et al. CDKN2/p16 or RB alterations occur in the majority of glioblastomas and are inversely correlated. Cancer Res 1996;56(1):150–153.
85. Uhrbom L, et al. Ink4a-Arf loss cooperates with KRas activation in astrocytes and neural progenitors to generate glioblastomas of various morphologies depending on activated Akt. Cancer Res 2002;62(19):5551–5558.
86. Holland EC, et al. A constitutively active epidermal growth factor receptor cooperates with disruption of G1 cell-cycle arrest pathways to induce glioma-like lesions in mice. Genes Dev 1998;12(23):3675–3685.
87. Henson JW, et al. The retinoblastoma gene is involved in malignant progression of astrocytomas. Ann Neurol 1994;36(5):714–721.
88. Reifenberger G, et al. Amplification of multiple genes from chromosomal region 12q13–14 in human malignant gliomas: preliminary mapping of the amplicons shows preferential involvement of CDK4, SAS, and MDM2. Cancer Res 1994;54(16):4299–4303.
89. Costello JF, et al. Cyclin-dependent kinase 6 (CDK6) amplification in human gliomas identified using two-dimensional separation of genomic DNA. Cancer Res 1997;57(7):1250–1254.
90. Biernat W, et al. Alterations of cell cycle regulatory genes in primary (de novo) and secondary glioblastomas. Acta Neuropathol (Berl) 1997;94(4):303–309.
91. Pringle N, et al. Platelet-derived growth factor in central nervous system gliogenesis. Ann N Y Acad Sci 1991;633:160–168.
92. Ross R, Raines EW, Bowen-Pope DF. The biology of platelet-derived growth factor. Cell 1986;46(2):155–169.
93. Hermanson M, et al. Platelet-derived growth factor and its receptors in human glioma tissue: expression of messenger RNA and protein suggests the presence of autocrine and paracrine loops. Cancer Res 1992;52(11): 3213–3219.
94. Westermark B, Heldin CH, Nister M. Platelet-derived growth factor in human glioma. Glia 1995;15(3):257–263.
95. Carraway KL 3rd, Burden SJ. Neuregulins and their receptors. Curr Opin Neurobiol 1995;5(5):606–612.
96. Burrows RC, et al. Response diversity and the timing of progenitor cell maturation are regulated by developmental changes in EGFR expression in the cortex. Neuron 1997;19(2):251–267.
97. Reynolds BA, Weiss S. Clonal and population analyses demonstrate that an EGF-responsive mammalian embryonic CNS precursor is a stem cell. Dev Biol 1996; 175(1): 1–13.
98. Libermann TA, et al. Amplification, enhanced expression and possible rearrangement of EGF receptor gene in primary human brain tumours of glial origin. Nature 1985; 313(5998):144–147.
99. Libermann TA, et al. Amplification and overexpression of the EGF receptor gene in primary human glioblastomas. J Cell Sci Suppl 1985;3:161–172.
100. Wong AJ, et al. Increased expression of the epidermal growth factor receptor gene in malignant gliomas is invariably associated with gene amplification. Proc Natl Acad Sci U S A 1987;84(19):6899–6903.
101. Fuller GN, Bigner SH. Amplified cellular oncogenes in neoplasms of the human central nervous system. Mutat Res 1992;276(3):299–306.
102. Ekstrand AJ, et al. Genes for epidermal growth factor receptor, transforming growth factor alpha, and epidermal growth factor and their expression in human gliomas in vivo. Cancer Res 1991;51(8):2164–2172.
103. Sauter G, et al. Patterns of epidermal growth factor receptor amplification in malignant gliomas. Am J Pathol 1996;148(4):1047–1053.
104. Sugawa N, et al. Identical splicing of aberrant epidermal growth factor receptor transcripts from amplified rearranged genes in human glioblastomas. Proc Natl Acad Sci U S A 1990;87(21):8602–8606.
105. Wong AJ, et al. Structural alterations of the epidermal growth factor receptor gene in human gliomas. Proc Natl Acad Sci U S A 1992;89(7):2965–2969.
106. Nishikawa R, et al. A mutant epidermal growth factor receptor common in human glioma confers enhanced tumorigenicity. Proc Natl Acad Sci U S A 1994;91(16):7727–7731.
107. Nagane M, et al. A common mutant epidermal growth factor receptor confers enhanced tumorigenicity on human glioblastoma cells by increasing proliferation and reducing apoptosis. Cancer Res 1996;56(21):5079–5086.
108. El-Obeid A, et al. Cell scattering and migration induced by autocrine transforming growth factor alpha in human glioma cells in vitro. Cancer Res 1997;57(24):5598–5604.
109. Nagane M, et al. Drug resistance of human glioblastoma cells conferred by a tumor-specific mutant epidermal growth factor receptor through modulation of Bcl-XL and caspase-3-like proteases. Proc Natl Acad Sci U S A 1998; 95(10):5724–5729.
110. Schlessinger J, Bar-Sagi D. Activation of Ras and other signaling pathways by receptor tyrosine kinases. Cold Spring Harb Symp Quant Biol 1994;59:173–179.
111. Kapoor GS, O'Rourke DM. Receptor tyrosine kinase signaling in gliomagenesis: pathobiology and therapeutic approaches. Cancer Biol Ther 2003;2(4):330–342.
112. Burgart LJ, et al. Oncogene abnormalities in astrocytomas: EGF-R gene alone appears to be more frequently amplified and rearranged compared with other protooncogenes. Mod Pathol 1991;4(2):183–186.
113. Guha A, et al. Proliferation of human malignant astrocytomas is dependent on Ras activation. Oncogene 1997; 15(23):2755–2765.
114. Bredel M, Pollack IF. The p21-Ras signal transduction pathway and growth regulation in human high-grade gliomas. Brain Res Brain Res Rev 1999;29(2–3):232–249.

115. Vivanco I, Sawyers CL. The phosphatidylinositol 3-kinase AKT pathway in human cancer. Nat Rev Cancer 2002; 2(7):489–501.
116. Li J, et al. PTEN, a putative protein tyrosine phosphatase gene mutated in human brain, breast, and prostate cancer. Science 1997;275(5308):1943–1947.
117. Steck PA, et al. Identification of a candidate tumour suppressor gene, MMAC1, at chromosome 10q23.3 that is mutated in multiple advanced cancers. Nat Genet 1997; 15(4):356–362.
118. Knobbe CB, Merlo A, Reifenberger G. PTEN signaling in gliomas. Neuro-oncol 2002;4(3):196–211.
119. Wang SI, et al. Somatic mutations of PTEN in glioblastoma multiforme. Cancer Res 1997;57(19):4183–4186.
120. Teng DH, et al. MMAC1/PTEN mutations in primary tumor specimens and tumor cell lines. Cancer Res 1997;57(23): 5221–5225.
121. Machein MR, Plate KH. VEGF in brain tumors. J Neurooncol 2000;50(1–2):109–120.
122. Plate KH, Breier G, Risau W. Molecular mechanisms of developmental and tumor angiogenesis. Brain Pathol 1994; 4(3):207–218.
123. Plate KH, et al. Vascular endothelial growth factor and glioma angiogenesis: coordinate induction of VEGF receptors, distribution of VEGF protein and possible in vivo regulatory mechanisms. Int J Cancer 1994;59(4):520–529.
124. Plate KH, et al. Vascular endothelial growth factor is a potential tumour angiogenesis factor in human gliomas in vivo. Nature 1992;359(6398):845–848.
125. Cheng SY, et al. Suppression of glioblastoma angiogenicity and tumorigenicity by inhibition of endogenous expression of vascular endothelial growth factor. Proc Natl Acad Sci U S A 1996;93(16):8502–8507.
126. Kim KJ, et al. Inhibition of vascular endothelial growth factor-induced angiogenesis suppresses tumour growth in vivo. Nature 1993;362(6423):841–844.
127. Shweiki D, et al. Vascular endothelial growth factor induced by hypoxia may mediate hypoxia-initiated angiogenesis. Nature 1992;359(6398):843–845.
128. Chan AS, et al. Expression of vascular endothelial growth factor and its receptors in the anaplastic progression of astrocytoma, oligodendroglioma, and ependymoma. Am J Surg Pathol 1998;22(7):816–826.
129. Weindel K, et al. Detection and quantification of vascular endothelial growth factor/vascular permeability factor in brain tumor tissue and cyst fluid: the key to angiogenesis? Neurosurgery 1994;35(3):439–448; discussion 448–449.
130. Heiss JD, et al. Mechanism of dexamethasone suppression of brain tumor-associated vascular permeability in rats. Involvement of the glucocorticoid receptor and vascular permeability factor. J Clin Invest 1996;98(6):1400–1408.
131. Machein MR, et al. Differential downregulation of vascular endothelial growth factor by dexamethasone in normoxic and hypoxic rat glioma cells. Neuropathol Appl Neurobiol 1999;25(2):104–112.
132. Stratmann A, Risau W, Plate KH. Cell type-specific expression of angiopoietin-1 and angiopoietin-2 suggests a role in glioblastoma angiogenesis. Am J Pathol 1998;153(5): 1459–1466.
133. Balesaria S, et al. Loss of chromosome 10 is an independent prognostic factor in high-grade gliomas. Br J Cancer 1999;81(8):1371–1377.
134. Tada K, et al. Analysis of loss of heterozygosity on chromosome 10 in patients with malignant astrocytic tumors: correlation with patient age and survival. J Neurosurg 2001;95(4):651–659.
135. Ino Y, et al. Molecular subtypes of anaplastic oligodendroglioma: implications for patient management at diagnosis. Clin Cancer Res 2001;7(4):839–845.
136. Zlatescu MC, et al. Tumor location and growth pattern correlate with genetic signature in oligodendroglial neoplasms. Cancer Res 2001;61(18):6713–6715.
137. Smith JS, et al. Alterations of chromosome arms 1p and 19q as predictors of survival in oligodendrogliomas, astrocytomas, and mixed oligoastrocytomas. J Clin Oncol 2000; 18(3):636–645.
138. Leenstra S, et al. Genetic sub-types of human malignant astrocytoma correlate with survival. Int J Cancer 1998; 79(2):159–165.
139. Newcomb EW, et al. Survival of patients with glioblastoma multiforme is not influenced by altered expression of p16, p53, EGFR, MDM2 or Bcl-2 genes. Brain Pathol 1998;8(4): 655–667.
140. Shiraishi S, et al. Influence of p53 mutations on prognosis of patients with glioblastoma. Cancer 2002;95(2):249–257.
141. Rasheed A, et al. Molecular markers of prognosis in astrocytic tumors. Cancer 2002;94(10):2688–2697.
142. Shinojima N, et al. Prognostic value of epidermal growth factor receptor in patients with glioblastoma multiforme. Cancer Res 2003;63(20):6962–6970.
143. Kim S, et al. Identification of combination gene sets for glioma classification. Mol Cancer Ther 2002;1(13): 1229–1236.
144. Kleihues P, et al. The WHO classification of tumors of the nervous system. J Neuropathol Exp Neurol 2002;61(3): 215–225; discussion 226–229.
145. Sasaki H, et al. Histopathological-molecular genetic correlations in referral pathologist-diagnosed low-grade "oligodendroglioma." J Neuropathol Exp Neurol 2002;61(1):58–63.
146. Burger PC, et al. Small cell architecture—a histological equivalent of EGFR amplification in glioblastoma multiforme? J Neuropathol Exp Neurol 2001;60(11):1099–1104.
147. Roth JG, Elvidge AR. Glioblastoma multiforme: a clinical survey. J Neurosurg 1960;17:736–750.
148. Frankel SA, German WJ. Glioblastoma multiforme; review of 219 cases with regard to natural history, pathology, diagnostic methods, and treatment. J Neurosurg 1958;15(5):489–503.
149. Kondziolka D, et al. Significance of hemorrhage into brain tumors: clinicopathological study. J Neurosurg 1987;67(6): 852–857.
150. Meyers CA, et al. Cognitive function as a predictor of survival in patients with recurrent malignant glioma. J Clin Oncol 2000;18(3):646–650.
151. Yung WA, Horten BC, Shapiro WR. Meningeal gliomatosis: a review of 12 cases. Ann Neurol 1980;8(6):605–608.
152. Ginsberg LE, et al. The significance of lack of MR contrast enhancement of supratentorial brain tumors in adults:

histopathological evaluation of a series. Surg Neurol 1998;49(4):436–440.
153. Earnest F 4th, et al. Cerebral astrocytomas: histopathologic correlation of MR and CT contrast enhancement with stereotactic biopsy. Radiology 1988;166(3):823–827.
154. Jackson RJ, et al. Limitations of stereotactic biopsy in the initial management of gliomas. Neuro-oncol 2001;3(3):193–200.
155. Curran WJ Jr, et al. Recursive partitioning analysis of prognostic factors in three Radiation Therapy Oncology Group malignant glioma trials. J Natl Cancer Inst 1993;85(9): 704–710.
156. Shaw EG, et al. Reexamining the radiation therapy oncology group (RTOG) recursive partitioning analysis (RPA) for glioblastoma multiforme (GBM) patients. Int J Radiat Oncol Biol Phys 2003;57(Suppl 2):S135–S136.
157. Salcman M. Surgical resection of malignant brain tumors: who benefits? Oncology (Huntingt) 1988;2(8):47–56, 59–60, 63.
158. Wallner KE, et al. Patterns of failure following treatment for glioblastoma multiforme and anaplastic astrocytoma. Int J Radiat Oncol Biol Phys 1989;16(6):1405–1409.
159. Simpson JR, et al. Influence of location and extent of surgical resection on survival of patients with glioblastoma multiforme: results of three consecutive Radiation Therapy Oncology Group (RTOG) clinical trials. Int J Radiat Oncol Biol Phys 1993;26(2):239–244.
160. Kowalczuk A, et al. Quantitative imaging study of extent of surgical resection and prognosis of malignant astrocytomas. Neurosurgery 1997;41(5):1028–1036; discussion 1036–1038.
161. Sandberg-Wollheim M, et al. A randomized study of chemotherapy with procarbazine, vincristine, and lomustine with and without radiation therapy for astrocytoma grades 3 and/or 4. Cancer 1991;68(1):22–29.
162. Lacroix M, et al A multivariate analysis of 416 patients with glioblastoma multiforme: prognosis, extent of resection, and survival. J Neurosurg 2001;95(2):190–198.
163. Young B, et al. Reoperation for glioblastoma. J Neurosurg 1981;55(6):917–921.
164. Ammirati M, et al. Reoperation in the treatment of recurrent intracranial malignant gliomas. Neurosurgery 1987; 21(5):607–614.
165. Harsh GR, et al. Reoperation for recurrent glioblastoma and anaplastic astrocytoma. Neurosurgery 1987;21(5):615–621.
166. Landy HJ, et al. Retreatment of intracranial gliomas. South Med J 1994;87(2):211–214.
167. Andersen AP. Postoperative irradiation of glioblastomas. Results in a randomized series. Acta Radiol Oncol Radiat Phys Biol 1978;17(6):475–484.
168. Walker MD, et al. Evaluation of BCNU and/or radiotherapy in the treatment of anaplastic gliomas. A cooperative clinical trial. J Neurosurg 1978;49(3):333–343.
169. Walker MD, et al. Randomized comparisons of radiotherapy and nitrosoureas for the treatment of malignant glioma after surgery. N Engl J Med 1980;303(23):1323–1329.
170. Leibel SA, Sheline GE. Radiotherapy for the treatment of cerebral astrocytomas. In: Thomas DG, ed. Neuro-oncology: primary malignant brain tumors. Baltimore: Johns Hopkins University Press, 1990, p93.
171. Levin VA, et al. Phase II study of accelerated fractionation radiation therapy with carboplatin followed by vincristine chemotherapy for the treatment of glioblastoma multiforme. Int J Radiat Oncol Biol Phys 1995;33(2):357–364.
172. Walker MD, Strike TA, Sheline GE. An analysis of dose-effect relationship in the radiotherapy of malignant gliomas. Int J Radiat Oncol Biol Phys 1979;5(10):1725–1731.
173. Bleehen NM, Stenning SP. A Medical Research Council trial of two radiotherapy doses in the treatment of grades 3 and 4 astrocytoma. The Medical Research Council Brain Tumour Working Party. Br J Cancer 1991;64(4):769–774.
174. Chang CH, et al. Comparison of postoperative radiotherapy and combined postoperative radiotherapy and chemotherapy in the multidisciplinary management of malignant gliomas. A joint Radiation Therapy Oncology Group and Eastern Cooperative Oncology Group study. Cancer 1983; 52(6):997–1007.
175. Thornton AF Jr, et al. Three-dimensional treatment planning of astrocytomas: a dosimetric study of cerebral irradiation. Int J Radiat Oncol Biol Phys 1991;20(6):1309–1315.
176. Ten Haken RK, et al. A quantitative assessment of the addition of MRI to CT-based 3-D treatment planning of brain tumors. Radiother Oncol 1992;25(2):121–133.
177. Garden AS, et al. Outcome and patterns of failure following limited-volume irradiation for malignant astrocytomas. Radiother Oncol 1991;20(2):99–110.
178. Stupp R, Mason WP, van den Bent MJ, et al. Radiotherapy plus concomitant and adjuvant temozolomide for glioblastoma. N Engl J Med 2005;352:987–996.
179. Kumar AJ, et al. Malignant gliomas: MR imaging spectrum of radiation therapy- and chemotherapy-induced necrosis of the brain after treatment. Radiology 2000;217(2): 377–384.
180. Glantz MJ, et al. Treatment of radiation-induced nervous system injury with heparin and warfarin. Neurology 1994; 44(11):2020–2027.
181. Chuba PJ, et al. Hyperbaric oxygen therapy for radiation-induced brain injury in children. Cancer 1997;80(10): 2005–2012.
182. Shrieve DC, et al. Comparison of stereotactic radiosurgery and brachytherapy in the treatment of recurrent glioblastoma multiforme. Neurosurgery 1995;36(2):275–282; discussion 282–284.
183. Shrieve DC, et al. Treatment of patients with primary glioblastoma multiforme with standard postoperative radiotherapy and radiosurgical boost: prognostic factors and long-term outcome. J Neurosurg 1999;90(1):72–87.
183a. Souhami L, Seiferheld W, Brachman D, et al. Randomized comparison of stereotactic radiosurgery followed by conventional radiotherapy with carmustine to conventional radiotherapy with carmustine for patients with glioblastoma multiforme: report of Radiation Therapy Oncology Group 93-05 protocol. Int J Radiat Oncol Biol Phys 2004;60:853–860.
184. Selker RG, et al. The Brain Tumor Cooperative Group NIH Trial 87–01: a randomized comparison of surgery, external radiotherapy, and carmustine versus surgery, interstitial radiotherapy boost, external radiation therapy, and carmustine. Neurosurgery 2002;51(2):343–355; discussion 355–357.
185. Laperriere NJ, et al. Randomized study of brachytherapy in the initial management of patients with malignant astrocytoma. Int J Radiat Oncol Biol Phys 1998;41(5):1005–1011.

186. Tatter SB, et al. An inflatable balloon catheter and liquid ^{125}I radiation source (GliaSite Radiation Therapy System) for treatment of recurrent malignant glioma: multicenter safety and feasibility trial. J Neurosurg 2003;99(2):297–303.
187. Green SB, et al. Comparisons of carmustine, procarbazine, and high-dose methylprednisolone as additions to surgery and radiotherapy for the treatment of malignant glioma. Cancer Treat Rep 1983;67(2):121–132.
188. Yung WK, et al. Multicenter phase II trial of temozolomide in patients with anaplastic astrocytoma or anaplastic oligoastrocytoma at first relapse. Temodal Brain Tumor Group. J Clin Oncol 1999;17(9):2762–2771.
189. Levin VA, et al. Superiority of post-radiotherapy adjuvant chemotherapy with CCNU, procarbazine, and vincristine (PCV) over BCNU for anaplastic gliomas: NCOG 6G61 final report. Int J Radiat Oncol Biol Phys 1990;18(2):321–324.
190. Prados MD, et al. Procarbazine, lomustine, and vincristine (PCV) chemotherapy for anaplastic astrocytoma: a retrospective review of radiation therapy oncology group protocols comparing survival with carmustine or PCV adjuvant chemotherapy. J Clin Oncol 1999;17(11):3389–3395.
191. Fine HA, et al. Meta-analysis of radiation therapy with and without adjuvant chemotherapy for malignant gliomas in adults. Cancer 1993;71(8):2585–2597.
192. Stewart LA. Chemotherapy in adult high-grade glioma: a systematic review and meta-analysis of individual patient data from 12 randomised trials. Lancet 2002;359(9311):1011–108.
193. Grant R, et al. Age influences chemotherapy response in astrocytomas. Neurology 1995;45(5):929–933.
194. Grant R, et al. Imaging response to chemotherapy with RMP-7 and carboplatin in malignant glioma: size matters but speed does not. J Neurooncol 2002;57(3):241–245.
195. Grant R, et al. Chemotherapy response criteria in malignant glioma. Neurology 1997;48(5):1336–1340.
196. Walter KA, et al. Intratumoral chemotherapy. Neurosurgery 1995;37(6):1128–1145.
197. Brem H, et al. Placebo-controlled trial of safety and efficacy of intraoperative controlled delivery by biodegradable polymers of chemotherapy for recurrent gliomas. The Polymer-Brain Tumor Treatment Group. Lancet 1995; 345(8956):1008–1012.
198. Westphal M, et al. A phase 3 trial of local chemotherapy with biodegradable carmustine (BCNU) wafers (Gliadel wafers) in patients with primary malignant glioma. Neuro-oncol 2003;5(2):79–88.
199. Jaeckle KA, et al. Phase II evaluation of temozolomide and 13-cis-retinoic acid for the treatment of recurrent and progressive malignant glioma: a North American Brain Tumor Consortium study. J Clin Oncol 2003;21(12):2305–2311.
200. Levin VA, et al. Phase III randomized study of postradiotherapy chemotherapy with combination alpha-difluoromethylornithine-PCV versus PCV for anaplastic gliomas. Clin Cancer Res 2003;9(3):981–990.
201. Groves MD, et al. Phase II trial of temozolomide plus the matrix metalloproteinase inhibitor, marimastat, in recurrent and progressive glioblastoma multiforme. J Clin Oncol 2002;20(5):1383–1388.
202. Baumann F, et al. Combined thalidomide and temozolomide treatment in patients with glioblastoma multiforme. J Neurooncol 2004;67(1–2):191–200.
203. Parney IF, Chang SM. Current chemotherapy for glioblastoma. Cancer J 2003;9(3):149–156.
204. Meyers CA, et al. Methylphenidate therapy improves cognition, mood, and function of brain tumor patients. J Clin Oncol 1998;16(7):2522–2527.
205. Grossman SA, et al. Increased 9-aminocamptothecin dose requirements in patients on anticonvulsants. NABTT CNS Consortium. The New Approaches to Brain Tumor Therapy. Cancer Chemother Pharmacol 1998;42(2):118–126.
206. Vecht CJ, Wagner GL, Wilms EB. Treating seizures in patients with brain tumors: Drug interactions between antiepileptic and chemotherapeutic agents. Semin Oncol 2003;30(6 Suppl 19):49–52.
207. Marras LC, Geerts WH, Perry JR. The risk of venous thromboembolism is increased throughout the course of malignant glioma: an evidence-based review. Cancer 2000; 89(3):640–646.

CHAPTER 14

Low-Grade Astrocytomas

WARREN P. MASON

Gliomas, a large and heterogeneous group of central nervous system neoplasms, account for approximately 30% to 60% of all primary brain tumors.[1,2] Like all intrinsic brain tumors, gliomas are believed to arise from glial cells or their precursors.[3,4] Tumors of glial origin can be described as diffuse to the extent that they infiltrate normal brain structures, or focal, with fairly discrete boundaries. Low-grade diffuse astrocytomas, including tumors of mixed histology, predominate in younger populations, and represent between 21% and 45% of gliomas in children and between 10% and 15% of gliomas in adults.[1,5–8] Although low-grade astrocytomas are indolent tumors, they are not benign and, with the exception of the completely resected pilocytic astrocytoma, account for considerable morbidity and mortality for most afflicted individuals.

The management of low-grade astrocytomas is one of the most controversial areas in neuro-oncology. Many aspects of the treatment of low-grade astrocytomas are debated, including the optimal timing of surgery and radiotherapy, the benefit of extensive surgery, and the impact of these variables on the natural history of these smoldering but ultimately incurable tumors.[9–11] Uncertainties surrounding the natural history of these tumors, difficulties in reliable tumor grading, and reliance on retrospective and often biased studies on which treatment recommendations are based have all hindered consensus on optimal management of these neoplasms. Patients with low-grade gliomas are clinically more heterogeneous than those with malignant gliomas, and many patients can have event-free survivals lasting a decade or more.[12] Moreover, the widespread availability of magnetic resonance imaging has made earlier diagnosis more likely, producing this shift in patient demographics toward younger patients who, having fewer symptoms and often normal neurologic examinations, do not appear to require immediate intervention. Consequently, the toxicities of radiotherapy and chemotherapy, and the potential morbidity of surgery, are very real concerns. Fortunately, recently published results of several large multicenter trials addressing the timing and dose of radiotherapy have provided solid evidence for delayed and reduced-dose irradiation.[5,13,14] These studies have also confirmed prognostic variables that can be used to guide the management of individual patients.[15] Importantly, the recognition that as many as two-thirds of low-grade gliomas have histologic or molecular genetic features consistent with oligodendroglial lineage, and the established chemosensitivity of oligodendroglial tumors, have raised new issues surrounding the potential value of chemotherapy for low-grade gliomas.[16]

▶ EPIDEMIOLOGY

Low-grade astrocytomas cluster in younger age groups. Although these tumors likely afflict males and females equally, males have been reported to constitute 55% to 65% of all patients with low-grade glial tumor.[17,18] Low-grade fibrillary and protoplasmic astrocytomas and mixed tumors are similar in their epidemiologic features, presenting in patients with a median age of 35 years.[19–22] Pilocytic astrocytomas are common in the second and third decades of life, with a median age at diagnosis of 14 years.[23,24]

Low-grade fibrillary astrocytomas generally arise in the cerebral hemispheres in young to middle-aged (aged 18–45 years) adults, and in the brainstem of children (<18 years old). Occasionally they arise in other regions of the neuraxis, such as the spinal cord or cerebellum. In the cerebral hemispheres, these tumors are distributed in a manner proportional to the cerebral mass. Thus, most fibrillary astrocytomas arise in the frontal and temporal lobes.[25,26] Protoplasmic tumors are also likely to arise in the cerebral hemispheres, but these tumors tend to arise in the superficial cortical regions. They, like fibrillary astrocytomas, are also prone to malignant dedifferentiation.[2] Pilocytic astrocytomas typically arise within the visual system (optic nerve and chiasm), hypothalamus and third ventricular region, cerebellum, and occasionally cerebral hemispheres.[27] Pilocytic astrocytomas that arise in the cerebral hemispheres tend to do so in older individuals, and appear to have a slight but discernible temporal lobe predominance.[18] Pilocytic astrocytomas of the cerebral hemispheres can arise in superficial cortical regions, or occupy intraventricular spaces. Cerebellar pilocytic astrocytomas, although identical histologically and radiographically to cerebral counterparts, present most frequently during the second decade of life.[28]

▶ GENETICS AND MOLECULAR BIOLOGY

The genetic events that drive the development of gliomas remain unclear, but an understanding is emerging based in part on advances in genomics, gene expression analysis, and mouse tumor models. Genetic derangements that lead to a glioma affect two key cellular functions: regulation of the cell cycle and activation or overexpression of growth factor–mediated signal transduction. The key genetic alterations that transform a glial cell or progenitor into a low-grade astrocytoma are elusive in part because no preneoplastic lesions are associated with gliomas. However, the most common chromosomal abnormality seen in low-grade astrocytomas is the deletion of chromosome band 17p13.1 and mutations of the tumor suppressor gene p53 (TP53), which is found in this region.[4,29–32] TP53 is responsible for transactivation of proapoptotic genes and inhibitors of the cell cycle in response to DNA damage. In so doing, TP53 induces cell-cycle arrest and apoptosis in cells that have sustained genetic damage that could lead to neoplastic transformation. The loss of TP53 probably is important in glioma formation to the extent that it interferes with apoptosis and establishes the potential for the accumulation of additional genetic abnormalities eventually leading to a tumor. Approximately 65% of low-grade astrocytomas harbor p53 mutations.[32] Interestingly, people with the Li-Fraumeni syndrome who carry germline p53 mutations have an increased risk of developing gliomas.

There is accumulating evidence that alterations of Ras-mediated signaling may be involved in the formation of low-grade astrocytomas. Mutations of Ras are distinctly uncommon in astrocytic tumors.[29] Thus the overactivity of this oncogenic pathway is likely mediated by overexpression of upstream components of the Ras pathway. Overexpression of platelet-derived growth factor (PDGF) and its receptor (PDGFR) are common in events in all grades of astrocytoma, and this may be activating the Ras pathway of low-grade astrocytoma. Although the mechanism responsible for the overexpression of PDGF and its receptor is unknown, predominantly the A-chain of the ligand and the α-chain of the receptor are overexpressed, suggesting an autocrine stimulatory loop.

Allelic loss of chromosome 22q occurs in approximately one-third of low-grade astrocytomas, suggesting a tumor suppressor gene at this locus.[29] This putative gene remains elusive; the neurofibromatosis 2 gene (NF2) resides at this site, but has been excluded as the responsible gene.

Advances in our understanding of the molecular biology of oligodendrogliomas have identified allelic losses of chromosomes 1p and 19q as early events in the formation of these tumors.[16] Approximately 60% to 70% of oligodendroglial tumors carry these genetic deletions, and recent reports associating this distinct genetic signature with response to chemotherapy and radiotherapy, and improved outcome have made the determination of 1p and 19q loss of heterozygosity an important clinical tool in the evaluation of all oligodendroglial tumors.[33–35] Because some oligodendroglial tumors appear histologically similar to astrocytomas, it is interesting that approximately 11% of tumors classified as astrocytomas by histologic criteria have allelic loss of chromosomes 1p and 19q.[16]

Pilocytic astrocytomas appear to have no distinct genetic profile. In contrast to low-grade fibrillary astrocytomas, p53 mutations do not appear to be common in these tumors, although a recent study detected p53 mutations in 7 of 35 evaluated pilocytic astrocytomas.[36,37] Cytogenetic studies of pilocytic astrocytomas demonstrated abnormal karyotypes in 50% of tumors, with structural and numeric abnormalities noted most frequently in chromosomes 7, 8, and 11.[38] Pilocytic astrocytomas can be a feature of neurofibromatosis 1. However, only exceptionally do sporadic tumors show loss of chromosome 17q, the region encoding the NF1 gene.

▶ RADIOLOGIC FEATURES

Low-grade gliomas have characteristic radiographic features that usually suggest the diagnosis before pathologic confirmation by surgical resection or biopsy. Nevertheless, the considerable variation in the radiographic appearance of low-grade gliomas, in part as a result of differing histology, makes pathologic confirmation of all suspicious lesions mandatory before treatment is administered. Table 14-1 presents a differential diagnosis of a radiographic lesion consistent with a low-grade astrocytoma.

▶ **TABLE 14-1.** DIFFERENTIAL DIAGNOSIS OF A MAGNETIC RESONANCE SCAN LESION CONSISTENT WITH A LOW-GRADE ASTROCYTOMA

Neoplastic lesions		
	Glial tumors	Low-grade astrocytoma
		Oligodendroglioma or oligoastrocytomas
		Ependymomas
		Others (pleomorphic xanthoastrocytoma, astroblastoma)
	Nonglial tumors	Lymphoma
		Metastases
		Neuronal tumors (ganglioglioma)
	Nonneoplastic lesions	Cerebral infarction/hemorrhage
		Demyelination
		Abscess

Computerized Tomography and Magnetic Resonance Imaging Scans

Although most low-grade gliomas can be identified by computerized tomography (CT) scans, the superior capacities of magnetic resonance imaging (MRI) have made this the imaging modality of choice for brain tumors (Fig. 14-1).[39] MR scans are more sensitive at detecting small tumors, and may disclose a lesion when a CT scan is apparently normal.[40] Fibrillary low-grade astrocytomas usually present as ill-defined, nonenhancing, and hypodense lesions on CT scans. Low-grade fibrillary gliomas usually appear as discrete areas of hypo- or isointensity on unenhanced T_1-weighted images, and usually more circumscribed hyperintense lesions

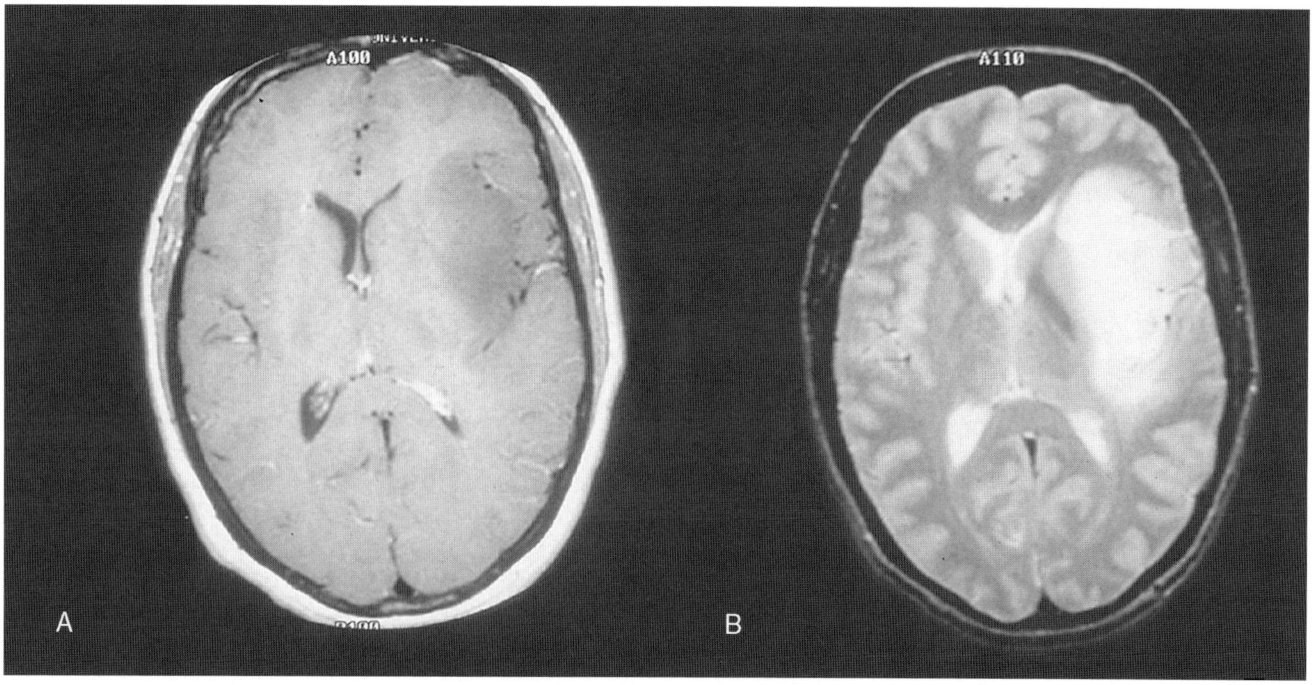

Figure 14-1. Typical appearance of a low-grade astrocytoma of the left frontal lobe on (A) T_1-weighted contrast-enhanced and (B) T_2-weighted axial images. The tumor is nonenhancing and hypointense on T_1 images, and sharply demarcated and hyperintense on T_2 images.

on T_2-weighted images.[39,41] Typically, low-grade gliomas appear larger on MRI than CT images. Often the appearance of a low-grade fibrillary glioma can remain unchanged over a period of many years. On both CT and MR images, low-grade fibrillary astrocytomas typically do not enhance following intravenous contrast administration. Contrast enhancement within a tumor represents disruption of the blood–brain barrier, and new enhancement usually but not always denotes transformation of a glioma to a more malignant grade.[42–44] However, imaging features alone cannot predict the grade of a presumed glial neoplasm. For instance, as many as 50% of nonenhancing tumors on CT will prove to be anaplastic at the time of pathologic grading.[45] For definitive diagnosis before therapy, biopsy must be performed to establish an accurate diagnosis.[46]

Fibrillary and pilocytic low-grade gliomas are easily distinguished on CT and MR images.[47] Pilocytic astrocytomas appear as sharply demarcated and smooth lesions with no or minimal edema (Fig. 14-2). On unenhanced MRI, they appear hypo- or isointense on T_1-weighted images, and hyperintense on T_2-weighted images, as do

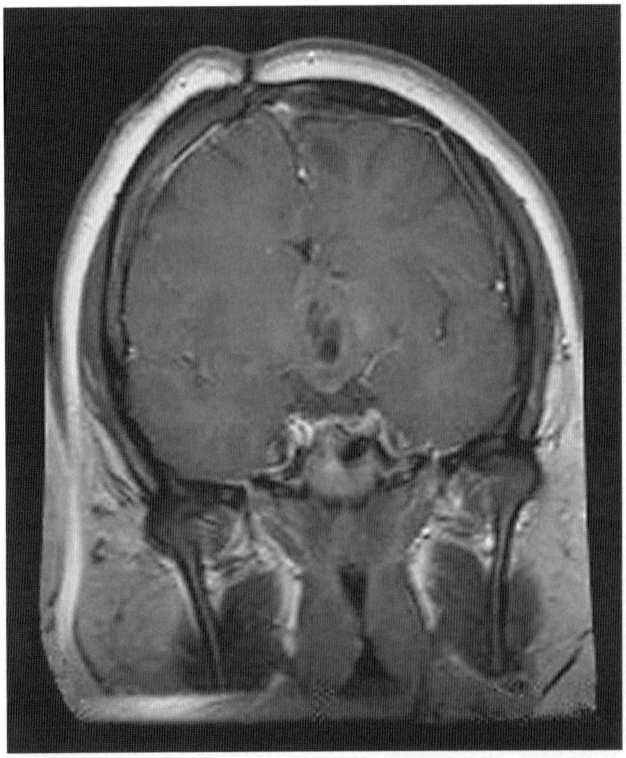

Figure 14-2. T_1-weighted contrast-enhanced coronal image of a young woman with a hypothalamic pilocytic astrocytoma. The tumor is diffuse and contrast-enhancing. The patient was a young woman who presented with headaches, hyperphagia, and endocrine dysfunction. Treatment consisted of insertion of a ventriculoperitoneal shunt and chemotherapy with subsequent clinical improvement and disease stabilization.

fibrillary gliomas. However, following contrast administration, pilocytic astrocytomas demonstrated marked and uniform enhancement. Furthermore, cyst formation and calcification are commonly noted. To some extent, the location of a pilocytic astrocytoma determines the radiographic features. A pilocytic astrocytoma arising in the optic pathway is often fusiform in shape, and in the cerebellum usually cystic with an enhancing mural nodule. A presurgical diagnosis of a pilocytic astrocytoma can be established with some certainty by coupling radiographic features with tumor location.

Positron Emission Tomography

Positron emission tomography (PET) can be helpful in the evaluation of patients with diffuse low-grade astrocytomas prior to biopsy.[48,49] A PET scan performed with [^{18}F]fluorodeoxyglucose can evaluate the metabolic activity of a brain tumor. Typically, low-grade gliomas appear hypometabolic on [^{18}F]fluorodeoxyglucose PET images. However, the appearance of a hypermetabolic region within an otherwise hypometabolic tumor can signify the malignant transformation of a low-grade astrocytoma, even in the absence of change or enlargement on CT or MRI scans.[50] Furthermore, a [^{18}F]fluorodeoxyglucose PET scan can, by identifying hypermetabolic regions within a low-grade tumor, select regions within a tumor that can be biopsied stereotactically, thereby leading to an accurate histologic grading of the neoplasm.

Magnetic Resonance Spectroscopy

Magnetic resonance spectroscopy is an emerging technique that may help distinguish astrocytomas from other brain lesions, and play a role in the noninvasive determination of tumor grade.[51,52] This technique remains experimental, and conclusions surrounding the clinical usefulness of this technology remain preliminary.

▶ PATHOLOGY

Low-grade astrocytomas presumably arise from astrocytes or their precursors. On gross inspection, most low-grade astrocytomas appear yellow or gray, and may have a gritty texture as a result of the presence of calcifications.[2] If cyst formation is present, a gelatinous appearance may be noted. Most low-grade gliomas diffusely infiltrate brain, and for this reason a blurring of the gray–white matter border may be present. Microscopically, these neoplasms may infiltrate brain several centimeters away from the bulk of the tumor.[41] Table 14-2 presents the World Health Organization's classification of low-grade astrocytic gliomas.

The grading of these neoplasms is based on classic morphologic criteria, and a variety of grading systems

▶ TABLE 14-2. WORLD HEALTH ORGANIZATION (WHO) CLASSIFICATION OF LOW-GRADE ASTROCYTIC GLIOMAS

Astrocytic gliomas
Astrocytoma
Fibrillary astrocytoma
Protoplasmic astrocytoma
Gemistocytic astrocytoma
Pilocytic astrocytoma
Pleomorphic xanthoastrocytoma
Subependymal giant cell astrocytoma
Subependyoma
Mixed gliomas
Oligoastrocytoma

exist to segregate astrocytic tumors into discrete groups with distinct prognoses and treatment recommendations. Features that are used to distinguish low- from high-grade astrocytomas include cellular and nuclear pleomorphism, increased cellularity, mitoses, neovascularization, and necrosis. Two grading systems for astrocytomas are in common use. The World Health Organization (WHO) uses a four-tiered system, where grade I tumors are pilocytic astrocytomas and grade II tumors are low-grade fibrillary astrocytomas.[53] The St. Anne-Mayo grading system is also a four-tiered system and is designed specifically for fibrillary astrocytic gliomas; low-grade gliomas can be grade 1 or 2. Grade 1 tumors are rare, making the St. Anne-Mayo system similar to the WHO system and essentially three-tiered: astrocytoma, anaplastic astrocytoma, and glioblastoma multiforme.[54] For this chapter, low-grade fibrillary astrocytomas are equivalent to the grade 2 astrocytoma of the St. Anne-Mayo classification and the grade II astrocytoma of the WHO classification.

Pilocytic astrocytomas appear grossly as well-circumscribed neoplasms with solid and cystic components.[28] They consist of areas of compact and loosely organized astrocytes with Rosenthal fibers, eosinophilic granular bodies, or both. These tumors are, as a rule, highly vascular, but unlike other astrocytomas, hypervascularity does not signify a malignant phenotype. These tumors typically arise in the optic nerve and its radiations (optic glioma), hypothalamus and third ventricular region, and cerebellum.

Fibrillary astrocytomas are the most common low-grade gliomas, and are well-differentiated infiltrative neoplasms of fibrillary astrocytes. These tumors typically arise in the cerebral hemispheres, where they expand and distort the regions from which they arise. Microscopically, these tumors are characterized by mild to moderate nuclear pleomorphism, but aggressive features are absent. The presence of microcysts can help distinguish a very indolent low-grade astrocytoma from reactive gliosis, which is the main differential diagnosis for very low-grade neoplasms. The gemistocytic variant of diffuse fibrillary astrocytoma is notable for the presence of abundant plump gemistocytes, which morphologically resemble reactive astrocytes, scattered throughout the tumor. Gemistocytic low-grade astrocytomas have traditionally been regarded as clinically aggressive neoplasms, and treated as anaplastic astrocytomas.[2,55] However, recent reports have documented survival figures and prognostic determinants similar to fibrillary low-grade astrocytomas in general, suggesting that gemistocytic astrocytomas do not behave exclusively in a malignant way.[56]

Protoplasmic astrocytomas are rare low-grade glial neoplasms consisting of cells that resemble protoplasmic astrocytes that are found in the gray matter.[2] These tumors are often cystic masses, and have a propensity for the cerebral cortex. They are moderately cellular, and consist of poorly fibrillated cells and prominent microcysts. It is important to distinguish these tumors from pilocytic astrocytomas and oligodendrogliomas.

▶ PRESENTING CLINICAL SIGNS AND SYMPTOMS

The spectrum of clinical presentations of low-grade gliomas is largely dependent on tumor histology. Patients with pilocytic astrocytomas have different clinical features from those who develop low-grade fibrillary astrocytomas.

Intrinsic tumors of the central nervous system produce symptoms and signs on the basis of two mechanisms: (a) increased intracranial pressure as a consequence of the expanding tumor or obstruction of the cerebrospinal fluid flow; and (b) infiltration and compression of adjacent neural structures. Increased intracranial pressure accounts for such symptoms as headaches, nausea and vomiting, and diffuse cerebral dysfunction causing memory impairment and personality change, and for signs such as papilledema. Infiltration or compression of brain accounts for lateralizing findings that vary with the site of neuraxis involvement. These focal abnormalities may be episodic, such as partial or generalized seizures, or progressive and include such neurologic deficits as weakness, sensory change, ataxia, and aphasia.

The most common presenting symptom for a patient with a low-grade astrocytoma is seizures, which are reported by 50% to 90% of all patients before diagnosis.[15,21,25,57–59] The advent of readily available CT and MRI has shortened the duration and reduced the severity of symptoms in patients with low-grade gliomas. Laws and associates,[25] summarizing their experience with 461 patients with low-grade gliomas diagnosed between 1915 and 1975, documented the following most common presenting features: motor weakness (53%), headache (47%), papilledema (47%), and seizures (42%). The median duration of symptoms before diagnosis was between 6 and 11 years. More recent studies are notable in that more patients appear to be presenting with seizures, and fewer with fixed neurologic deficits. For example, McCormack and associates[21] reported in their series of 53 adult patients with supratentorial low-grade astrocytomas the following presenting symptoms: seizures (68%), headache (13%), focal motor deficit (9%), visual changes (4%), nausea and vomiting (4%), and unspecified symptoms (17%). In this series, the median duration of symptoms before definitive diagnosis was only 6 months. Leighton and associates[60] reported presenting symptoms in 167 adults with supratentorial low-grade gliomas (89 astrocytoma, 78 oligodendroglioma/mixed glioma) diagnosed between 1979 and 1995. In this series, 78% had seizures at presentation, 31% focal neurologic deficits, 29% headache, 11% cognitive or behavioral change, and 9% papilledema. The median interval duration between symptom onset and first imaging was 2 months. Apparently, the ready availability of CT and MRI, leading to a shorter duration of symptoms before definitive diagnosis, has altered the demographics of patients with low-grade gliomas. Consequently, patients diagnosed today with low-grade astrocytomas are likely to present with isolated seizures, have less symptomatology, and have normal interictal examinations. Moreover, the widespread availability of imaging has extended the apparent natural history of the disease. For example, in 1984, Laws and associates[25] reported a median survival of 4 years in their series of patients with low-grade gliomas. In contrast, more recent studies conducted by Vertosick and associates[58] and McCormack and associates[21] reported median survivals of 8.2 years and 7.2 years, respectively. These discrepancies likely represent a lead-time bias made possible by modern imaging techniques, and not improvement in the outcome of this disease by therapeutic intervention.

▶ NATURAL HISTORY

The natural history of low-grade astrocytomas remains unclear for several reasons: widespread availability of CT and MRI have made earlier diagnosis more likely, thereby extending the apparent natural history of the disease; histologic, genetic, and behavioral heterogeneity of low-grade gliomas; the inclusion of pilocytic gliomas in large retrospective studies; and the unknown impact of therapeutic interventions at the time of diagnosis or at progression on the natural history of these tumors.

As with all neoplasms, the natural history of low-grade astrocytomas is one of progressive growth and eventual malignant degeneration. When patients with initially low-grade gliomas expire from tumor progression, the tumor at the time of death is usually an anaplastic astrocytoma or glioblastoma multiforme. Patients with an initial diagnosis of a low-grade astrocytoma seldom die of progressive low-grade disease. A number of recent studies have shed light on the natural history of these neoplasms. In a series reported by Leighton and associates,[60] 90 of 167 patients (54%) with supratentorial low-grade gliomas progressed within a median of 50 months from diagnosis. Seventy-one/90 (79%) had a tissue diagnosis at recurrence, and 36/71 (51%) had a dedifferentiated malignant glioma. An earlier review conducted by Muller and associates[61] documented a 31.5-month median time to progression for 57 patients with an initial pathologic diagnosis of low-grade glioma. At recurrence, 14% had pathologically low-grade astrocytomas, 55.5% had anaplastic astrocytomas, and 30.5% had glioblastomas. Given the high incidence of cryptic anaplastic foci in tumors classified as low-grade, this study suggests that most low-grade astrocytomas ultimately degenerate into more malignant astrocytomas.

Survival data for untreated patients with low-grade gliomas can only be inferred from published series because most patients eventually receive treatments that probably alter the natural history of the disease. Moreover, older historic series report survival data worse than the improved outcomes of recent series conducted in the era of modern neuroimaging and neurosurgical techniques. Van Wagenen[62] reported, in 1934, a median survival of less than 3 years for 13 patients undergoing surgery by Cushing in 1925. Gol,[63] reporting his experience with 194 patients diagnosed before 1960, reported a median survival of 2 months following biopsy alone. More recent series, such as one reported by Vertosick and associates,[58] reported a median survival of 8.2 years for 25 patients with well-differentiated cerebral astrocytomas after biopsy or resection and early or delayed radiotherapy. Moreover, a study conducted by Recht and associates[64] projected a median survival of 84 months for 26 patients who presented with transient neurologic events and radiographic evidence suggestive of a low-grade primary supratentorial neoplasm and were observed without specific intervention until neurologic or radiographic deterioration.

Estimates of overall and progression-free survival for untreated patients with low-grade gliomas can be extracted from modern studies where patients received deferred therapy or minimal intervention in the form of biopsy for diagnostic purposes. For example, Mundinger and Weigel[65] have reported 5- and 10-year survival rates of 17% and 6% for patients with low-grade glioma following limited biopsies, and Soffietti and associates[57] have published 5- and 10-year survival rates of 21% and 0% for 13 patients who had partial resections. These somewhat dismal survival statistics derived from small series contrast with a published European trial where 311 patients with low-grade gliomas were randomized to early versus deferred radiotherapy. They reported 66% overall survival and 37% time to progression estimates at 5 years for the arm that had irradiation delayed.[14]

▶ PROGNOSTIC FEATURES

A number of retrospective and a few prospective series have evaluated variables of potential prognostic significance in patients with low-grade astrocytomas. These studies suffer from a number of limitations, including investigator bias, patient heterogeneity, and variability of treatment offered. Nevertheless, a number of features relating to patient characteristics, tumor morphology, and treatment have consistently been identified as prognostic indicators for patients with low-grade gliomas.

Tumor-Related Prognostic Features

Tumor Characteristics

Tumor histology is of considerable prognostic significance. For instance, patients with pilocytic histology have a much better prognosis than those with fibrillary, protoplasmic, or mixed low-grade tumors. Shaw and associates[18] reported a 5-year survival estimate of 85% for 41 patients with pilocytic astrocytomas, and 50% for 126 patients with astrocytomas or mixed oligoastrocytomas. The influence of tumor grade on survival is unclear and controversial, with many studies finding no difference between Kernohan grade I or II astrocytoma, or Dumas-Duport grade I or II astrocytoma.[25,66] Other studies attribute improved survival for patients with grade I or grade II astrocytomas.[20] Additional histologic characteristics, such as the presence of gemistocytes within a tumor (gemistocytic astrocytoma), may confer a particularly poor prognosis.[67]

Flow Cytometry, Proliferative Markers, and Molecular Genetic Markers

Because histologic grading of brain tumors is inexact, efforts to refine diagnostic accuracy and to predict tumor behavior have led to the use of flow cytometry and labeling studies using bromo-uridine deoxyribose (BUdR), the antibody MIB-1 to Ki-67, and proliferating cell nuclear antigen (PCNA) as a means of predicting the proliferative activity of gliomas.[68,69] Cytokinetic data appear to have considerable prognostic significance, and thus will likely be used with increasing frequency to guide treatment in future studies. Molecular genetic abnormalities, such as p53 mutations or overexpression, are common in gliomas, but have been inconsistently correlated to prognosis. A majority of patients with oligodendroglial tumors harbor allelic losses on chromosomes 1p and 19q, and these genetic derangements predict for a favorable response to chemotherapy and prolonged survival.[33] There is recent evidence that a significant minority of patients with astrocytic low-grade gliomas also have these mutations, and that these genetic characteristics may also predict chemosensitivity, radiosensitivity and favorable outcome for low-grade astrocytomas.[35]

Cyst Formation

Historical studies emphasized the presence of a tumor cyst as being a favorable prognostic factor for long-term survival, but more recent studies fail to corroborate this observation.[18,57] Tumor cysts are associated with younger populations and with pilocytic histology, and it is believed that these last two features are likely responsible for the favorable outcomes in this subpopulation.

Magnetic Resonance Imaging and Computerized Tomography Scan Features

Tumor size at diagnosis has been demonstrated in a number of recent publications as having prognostic significance, with diminishing progression-free and overall survival as tumor size increases.[70] These data also support the variable observation of midline shift on radiographic images as a poor prognostic feature, and improved survival with more aggressive surgical resection.[71,72] Although the presence of contrast enhancement within a tumor is generally considered an unfavorable prognostic factor, contrast enhancement of a histologically low-grade neoplasm may not confer a worse prognosis.

Patient-Related Prognostic Features

Age

With the exception of histology, age is the most important and consistent prognostic factor for survival.[13,73,74] It is sometimes difficult to separate the influence of histology on age, because younger patients are more likely to have favorable gliomas such as pilocytic astrocytomas, but studies that have excluded patients with such tumors from analysis have found age to be a highly significant and independent favorable prognostic factor for patients with low-grade astrocytomas.

Sex

Sex does not appear to influence outcome and overall survival for patients with low-grade astrocytomas. Nonetheless, there are a few studies that have suggested a modest but consistent and statistically significant survival advantage for females.

Performance Status

Preoperative and, to a lesser extent, postoperative performance status correlate positively with prognosis in patients with low-grade astrocytomas.[13,15,57,60] Laws and associates,[25] who documented poor survival in patients with evidence of increased intracranial pressure, impaired consciousness and personality change, first noted this observation. In contrast, Soffietti and associates,[57] in 1989, found that patients with a fixed focal deficit as a first symptom still enjoyed a favorable rate of survival. They suggested that the increasing use of CT scans made an earlier diagnosis of a brain tumor possible, thereby accounting for the apparent improved survival. Consequently, the widespread availability of CT and MRI has probably contributed to the diminishing significance of performance status on outcome because few patients now present with severe and life-threatening neurologic deficits at the time of initial diagnosis.

Seizures

Seizures are the most common initial symptom of patients with low-grade astrocytomas.[59,60] A history of seizures has been cited as a good prognostic factor for patients with low-grade astrocytomas.[73] Seizures are a powerful prognostic factor on univariate analysis, but because seizures are common in younger patients, in those with good performance status, and in those with slow-growing tumors, the significance of seizures on outcome diminishes but remains positive when multivariate analyses are performed. Seizures in patients with low-grade astrocytomas are typically simple partial seizures, alone or in association with complex partial or generalized tonic–clonic seizures. Seizures in patients with low-grade astrocytomas are often refractory to standard anticonvulsants, but seizures can diminish in intensity and frequency following surgery, or following treatment with radiotherapy and chemotherapy in responding patients. Conversely, tumor progression can manifest as a return of seizures, or a change in their frequency or morphology.

▶ SURGICAL MANAGEMENT

Surgery is essential to the diagnosis and management of low-grade gliomas. Nonetheless, the timing and optimal extent of surgical resection for low-grade astrocytomas are some of the most contentious issues in clinical neuro-oncology.[10] Furthermore, although surgery can alleviate tumor-related symptoms, whether it prolongs survival is also controversial. Although randomized clinical trials would be needed to answer these questions definitively, a number of studies have retrospectively analyzed the consequences of surgical resection on outcome and survival, and these results do provide some insight into the role of surgery for low-grade astrocytomas, despite significant methodological shortcomings that include heterogeneous patient populations, variable followup and subsequent treatments, and difficulties in assessing extent of surgical resection by pre- and postoperative imaging.

Surgery remains necessary for the pathologic diagnosis of a suspected low-grade astrocytoma; CT or MRI characteristics alone are inadequate for reliable diagnosis. CT- or MRI-guided stereotactic biopsy is an excellent means of obtaining a firm diagnosis of small lesions that exert no or minimal mass effect or lesions situated in deep structures. The small size of a stereotactic biopsy specimen is a potential drawback, making possible a misdiagnosis or inaccurate (and underestimated) tumor grading. Stereotactic biopsies are usually safe procedures, but are not without complications. A recent series reported the worsening of neurologic deficit in approximately 5% of patients as a consequence of hemorrhage, and, for patients with glioblastoma multiforme, a mortality rate of approximately 2%.[75] Serial biopsies are likely to increase surgical morbidity and mortality.

Craniotomy with maximal surgical resection of a low-grade astrocytoma can often reduce tumor-related morbidity, but its impact on survival is not clear. Maximal surgical resection of tumors in locations that make them amenable to extensive surgical resection can be performed with acceptable morbidity and mortality. Ciric and associates[76] examined the relationship between extent of resection and immediate postoperative results for 42 patients with cerebral gliomas. Gross-total or near-total resections were achieved in 85% of patients, and none of these patients suffered permanent neurologic deterioration. At discharge, 55% of all patients were neurologically stable, and 41% were improved. This and other studies have provided convincing evidence that whenever possible maximal surgical resection has fewer neurologic complications, and no greater risk of neurologic compromise than biopsy or less extensive resections.[77] Increasingly, maximal surgical resection is the goal of surgery for patients with low-grade astrocytomas, and advances in neurosurgical techniques such as CT- or MRI-guided stereotactic surgery or intraoperative MRI permit more extensive tumor resection without increased morbidity and mortality.[44]

For adults with malignant gliomas, and for children with both malignant and low-grade gliomas, the extent of surgery appears to correlate positively with survival, with more complete resections appearing to prolong life without compromise of postoperative neurologic function. The prognostic significance of extent of resection has been examined retrospectively in low-grade glioma as well, and with a few notable exceptions, aggressive surgery appears beneficial for patients with low-grade astrocytomas, having a favorable influence on patient survival.[72,78–80] These studies may be biased, however, as tumors that are easily and extensively resected may differ in their biologic behavior from inaccessible tumors, and patients with easily resected tumors may have other characteristics that favor prolonged survival. Multivariate analysis of several large retrospective single-institution series shows a survival advantage for gross-total resection. For instance, Soffietti and associates[57] reported 5-year survivals of 51%, 24%, and 0% for 85 adults with nonpilocytic low-grade gliomas who had gross total resection, subtotal resection, or biopsy, respectively. Similarly, Laws and associates[81] analyzed outcome for 461 patients with supratentorial low-grade (grade 1 or 2) astrocytomas and noted statistically significant 5-year survival differences of 61%, 44%, and 32% for patients having total, radical subtotal, and subtotal resections or biopsies, respectively. Karim and associates,[13] in a prospective study designed to determine optimal radiation dose for 379 adults with low-grade gliomas, found a statistically significant ($p = 0.006$) increase in survival with more aggressive surgical resections. This observation supports an earlier study conducted by Berger and associates[82] who noted that patients with large low-grade gliomas had reduced rates of malignant transformation and recurrence when maximal surgery was performed.

Although it is increasingly clear that patients with low-grade gliomas should have maximal surgical resections when the decision to operate is made, the appropriate timing of cytoreductive surgery is largely unanswered. Surgery can reduce or eliminate neurologic morbidity from large tumors, and for patients with such tumors, early surgery seems appropriate for symptom alleviation. Moreover, large tumors are more likely to have anaplastic foci, and for this reason, early surgical intervention may delay progression, and ultimately prolong overall survival.[82] The optimal surgical management of patients with small low-grade astrocytomas that are asymptomatic, or have seizures as their sole manifestation, remains controversial. Some investigators favor early resection for all patients with presumed low-grade gliomas. Interestingly, Recht and associates[64] reported, in 1992, a retrospective review of 46 patients with radiographic evidence of low-grade gliomas. Twenty patients had early surgical intervention and treatment, and 26 had pathologic diagnosis and treatment deferred. No difference in the rate of malignant transformation, survival, and quality of life could be detected between these two groups. This experience, along with other studies, suggests that early stereotactic biopsy to establish pathologic diagnosis can be delayed until there is clinical or radiographic evidence of progression without adversely affecting the outcome for patients with presumed low-grade astrocytomas.

Pilocytic Astrocytomas

Pilocytic astrocytomas of the cerebrum and cerebellum represent a distinct subset of low-grade astrocytomas for a variety of reasons. These enhancing, solid, and cystic tumors are relatively noninfiltrative and well-demarcated from surrounding normal brain. Total or near-total resection of these tumors is often possible, and can result in cure or protracted recurrence-free survival without the need for further immediate therapy.[24,27] For this reason, aggressive resection of pilocytic astrocytomas is recommended. For cystic lesions, all enhancing components, including the cyst wall, should be resected to avoid recurrence. However, because cyst walls are pathologically gliotic, they need not be extirpated completely to achieve a surgical cure. Pilocytic astrocytomas located deep within the cerebrum are not usually completely resectable without the risk of unacceptable morbidity and mortality. However, when resection is complete, cure is possible, with reported 10-year survivals for both children and adults approaching 100% without further therapy.[24] Subtotal resection of pilocytic astrocytomas can also result in prolonged recurrence-free survival even without subsequent radiotherapy or chemotherapy. In the series reported by Forsyth and associates[24] 10-year survivals for patients with subtotal resections was 74%. Nevertheless, patients with subtotal resections require close and prolonged postoperative surveillance for recurrence.[24]

▶ ROLE OF RADIOTHERAPY

Radiotherapy has been a standard treatment for low-grade astrocytomas for decades where it has been administered to patients postoperatively as a means of improving otherwise disappointing outcomes. Although low-grade astrocytomas can respond to radiotherapy with as much as a 50% reduction in tumor area on CT or MRI, there is no statistically significant association between radiographic response and symptom alleviation and progression-free survival (Fig. 14-3).[83] Until recently, all recommendations for postoperative radiotherapy for low-grade astrocytomas had been based on retrospective reviews of patients. On balance, most retrospective series evaluating radiotherapy for low-grade gliomas are flawed for several reasons: inclusion of cerebellar pilocytic tumors with low-grade fibrillary astrocytomas; use of variable grading systems; inclusion of patients treated before the megavoltage era; variable treatment fields, schedules and doses; and confounding patient-related factors that influenced outcome. Despite these limitations, however, these studies are informative and support the use of postoperative radiotherapy, particularly for incompletely resected symptomatic supratentorial astrocytomas. These retrospective series do suggest the value of postoperative radiotherapy for low-grade astrocytomas where 5- and 10-year survival rates were reported at 48% and 26%, respectively.[17] These statistics contrast sharply with 5- and 10-year survivals of 26% and 12%, respectively, following surgery without irradiation.[82] Leibel and associates[17] have provided some of the most convincing data in support of postoperative irradiation following incomplete resection of low-grade gliomas. In their series of 108 patients with residual low-grade astrocytoma following surgery, 71 received postoperative radiotherapy while 37 did not. Most patients had fibrillary

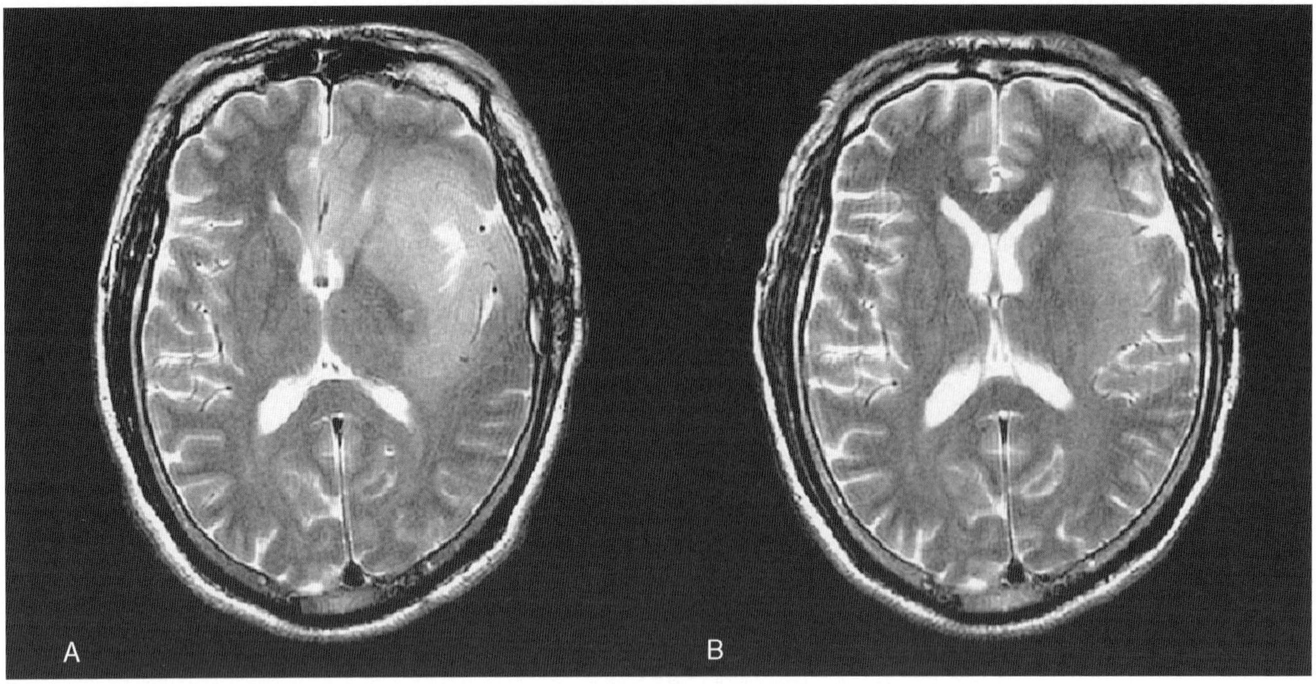

Figure 14-3. T_2-weighted axial MR images of a patient with a low-grade astrocytoma of the left frontal lobe before (A) and 6 months after cranial irradiation (B), demonstrating marked improvement of T_2-weighted signal abnormality.

tumors, and the two groups were balanced in terms of prognostic features. Patients receiving irradiation had 5-year survival rate of 32% while those who had surgery had a 5-year survival rate of only 10%. At 20 years followup, all nonirradiated patients had expired, whereas 23% of patients receiving radiotherapy were alive and free of progressive disease.

The role of postoperative irradiation for completely resected supratentorial fibrillary low-grade astrocytomas is controversial. The impact of radiotherapy for these patients probably underestimates survival because many patients who have complete surgical resections are not referred for radiotherapy. Following gross-total or radical subtotal resection of low-grade astrocytoma, 5-year survival has been reported ranging from 52% to 90%.[17,57,60,66,84] For this reason, many investigators have advocated observation without postoperative irradiation for patients who have had complete surgical resection of their low-grade tumors. However, others have advocated early postoperative radiotherapy for all patients with non-pilocytic low-grade tumors, citing similar survival data and recurrence patterns regardless of the extent of surgical resection. For example, Shaw and associates[18] reported similar 5- and 10-year survival rates of 52% and 23%, respectively, for patients undergoing gross-total, radical subtotal, or subtotal resection, and biopsy only. In this series, 19 patients who had no further therapy following complete or radical subtotal resection of a low-grade astrocytoma had a 10-year survival rate of only 11%.[18]

The benefits of radiotherapy appear to increase with advancing age. In fact, many series have demonstrated a survival advantage following radiotherapy only for patients age 35 to 40 years or older. For patients older than age 35 years, Shaw and associates[18] reported 5- and 10-year survival rates of 67% and 45%, respectively. For patients of a similar age receiving low-dose radiotherapy (less than 5300 cGy) or no radiotherapy, 5- and 10-year survival rates were reduced significantly to 37% and 5%, respectively. For patients younger than age 35 years, survival was not influenced by postoperative radiotherapy.

Historically, whole-brain radiotherapy was administered for patients with low-grade gliomas. However, the increasing recognition of the deleterious effects of cranial irradiation on neurocognitive function, and the overwhelming tendency of treatment failure to occur at the site of the primary tumor, have led to development of localized radiotherapy for these neoplasms. Current recommendations for treatment are partial brain radiotherapy to the CT or MRI scan-defined tumor volume and a 2-cm margin of normal tissue.[84] Recent refinements in delivering highly focused radiotherapy to the tumor while sparing normal surrounding brain have involved multiple complex three-dimensional treatment fields (three-dimensional conformal radiotherapy). This technique is effective to the extent that radiotherapy can be administered to a very precise irregular volume of tumor without increasing the frequency of recurrence outside the limited treatment field, but the impact on cognitive preservation has not yet been documented.

The optimal dose of radiotherapy for low-grade gliomas remains controversial, but doses between 45 and 65 Gy are commonly used, with most authorities recommending doses between 50 and 55 Gy in daily fractions between 1.8 and 2.0 Gy at 5 fractions per week. There is evidence, however, to support lower doses, as some investigators have noted poor survival with higher doses of radiation. For instance, Soffietti and associates[57] reported a 5-year survival rate of 25% for patients receiving less than 40 Gy, and a 9% 5-year survival rate for those receiving more than 40 Gy. Conversely, Shaw and associates[18] reported 5-year survival rates of 68% for patients receiving greater than 53 Gy and 47% for patients receiving less than 53 Gy. A significant recent study, conducted by the European Organization for the Research and Treatment of Cancer (EORTC Study 2284) reported the results of a prospective randomized trial to determine the existence of a dose-response curve of low-grade glioma. Between 1985 and 1991, 379 patients with a variety of low-grade gliomas were randomized to receive irradiation postoperatively with either 45 Gy in 5 weeks, or 59.4 Gy in 6.6 weeks.[13] After a median followup of greater than 6 years, results demonstrated no survival difference between the treatment arms. The 5-year survival rates were 59% and 58% for patients randomized to the high-dose arm and low-dose arm, respectively. An update from this study that examined the quality-of-life issues demonstrated that patients receiving the lower dose of radiotherapy had significantly higher quality-of-life indices than did those receiving the higher dose of radiotherapy.[15] A second, large, randomized intergroup study conducted by the North Central Cancer Treatment Group, Radiation Therapy Oncology Group, and Eastern Cooperative Oncology Group adds further support for lower doses of radiotherapy for low-grade glioma.[5] This study randomized 203 patients to either a high-dose radiotherapy arm of 64.8 Gy in 36 fractions, or to a low-dose arm where 50.4 Gy in 28 fractions was administered. Data from this study were recently analyzed, and after a median followup of 6.4 years, survival at 2 and 5 years is nonsignificantly better with low-dose radiotherapy. Specifically, survival at two and five years was 94% and 72%, respectively, with low-dose radiotherapy, and 85% and 64%, respectively, with high-dose radiotherapy. Moreover, toxicity was greater for patients receiving high-dose radiotherapy: the 2-year actuarial incidence of grades 3 to 5 radiation necrosis was 2.5% with low-dose radiotherapy, and 5% with high-dose radiotherapy. Thus, from the cumulative data from these two large, multiinstitutional, randomized trials from the modern era, it appears that lower doses of radiotherapy are as efficacious as and less toxic than higher doses.

The timing of radiotherapy has been a contentious issue for patients with low-grade astrocytomas. While the early application of radiotherapy for patients with low-grade gliomas and neurologic impairment, tumor progression, or malignant transformation is indicated, the routine use of early postoperative radiotherapy for all patients remains controversial. Moreover, although radiotherapy has been shown to reduce seizure frequency in patients with intractable epilepsy due to low-grade gliomas, radiotherapy is not a standard treatment for these patients who are more typically referred for seizure surgery. Leighton and associates[60] reported a retrospective study of 167 adults with supratentorial low-grade gliomas. Eighty (48%) had immediate postoperative radiotherapy and 87 (52%) had treatment delayed until tumor progression (40 received delayed radiotherapy at a median time to progression from surgery of 52 months). By univariate analysis the delayed radiotherapy group had significantly improved overall 5- and 10-year survival rates (84% and 70%, respectively) compared with the immediate radiotherapy group (62% and 35%, respectively), but no difference by multivariate analysis as a result of more favorable prognostic features in the delayed radiotherapy group. The question of timing of radiotherapy was addressed by a second EORTC study conducted between 1986 and 1997 that randomized 311 adult patients with low-grade gliomas after surgery to radiotherapy or observation until tumor progression.[14] The dose of radiation chosen for this study was 54 Gy over 6 weeks. After a median follow-up of 5 years, the 5-year estimates for time to progression were 44% and 37% for the treated and control arms, respectively. Five-year overall survival estimates were 63% and 66% for the treated and control arms, respectively. The differences were statistically significant only for the time-to-progression estimates. Thus, early radiotherapy appeared to extend time to progression, but not overall survival, for patients with low-grade gliomas. While this study could be interpreted to support early radiotherapy for this patient population, detailed quality-of-life assessments were not performed, and the delayed toxicities of radiotherapy were not documented. Consequently, an equally compelling interpretation of this study, given no difference in survival between the treated and control arms, would be to recommend withholding radiotherapy for patients with low-grade gliomas until there is evidence of radiographic or clinical progression.

Postoperative radiotherapy is not indicated for cystic pilocytic astrocytomas of the cerebrum or cerebellum, where surgical cure is expected, and reported 5- and 10-year survival rates without radiotherapy approach 100%.[24,27] Although recurrence following incomplete resection of these tumors is not uncommon, progression-free survival can be protracted, and radiotherapy can safely be deferred until recurrence is documented.

Postoperative radiotherapy for children with low-grade astrocytomas is not routinely indicated, where irradiation causes unacceptable toxicities. Reports of 5-year survival rates in the range of 80% to 95% for children with low-grade gliomas treated without radiotherapy suggest that a policy of withholding radiotherapy for children with these neoplasms until there is evidence of disease progression is reasonable. Nevertheless, radiotherapy remains an appropriate therapeutic modality for children with low-grade gliomas and symptomatic residual postoperative disease, and for progressive or recurrent disease following surgical and chemotherapeutic failure.

Attempts have been made to enhance the effects of radiotherapy without any evidence of added benefit. Interstitial brachytherapy has been employed in selected patients with small low-grade gliomas.[85,86] Reported 5-year survival estimates are identical to survival rates for patients treated with conventional external beam radiotherapy. Radiosurgery has also been used for these tumors, at doses ranging from 16 to 50 Gy in one or two fractions for tumors less than 4 cm in diameter.[87] Although some patients have had radiographic responses, no improvement in overall survival has been documented. Similarly, radiosensitizers have not extended survival for patients with low-grade gliomas who receive radiotherapy.

The toxicities of radiotherapy are not completely documented. The possibility of cognitive decline or dementia following radiotherapy is a very real concern for patients with low-grade gliomas, where median survival is likely in excess of 5 years (Fig. 14-4).[88] Recent studies of patients with low-grade gliomas treated with partial brain irradiation have not demonstrated a significant deleterious effect on neurocognitive function for most patients, at least for relatively short follow-up intervals in the range of 2 to 4 years following radiotherapy.[89–91] North and associates[92] evaluated performance status at 1 to 2 years following radiotherapy, and at last follow-up, between 2 and 12 years postoperatively. In a cohort of 46 patients, 80% of short-term survivors and 67% of long-term survivors were intellectually intact, and no patients developed radionecrosis. However, more recent imagings suggest that radiotherapy is damaging to normal brain. Although methionine or glucose uptake as measured by PET imaging is not affected in low-grade astrocytomas by radiotherapy, normal brain does demonstrate reduction of glucose and methionine uptake following radiation exposure, suggesting damage that may be subclinical, or perhaps not detectable by neuropsychological tools in current use.[93,94] Radiation necrosis appears to be infrequent when standard dosing and fields are applied. For instance, Leibel and associates[17] noted no cases of radionecrosis in their series of 147 patients, and Shaw and associates[18] reported an incidence of radionecrosis of 2% following external beam radiotherapy for low-grade gliomas. Occasional reports have suggested that radiotherapy can induce a second neoplasm in the treatment field, or accelerate the malignant transformation of a low-grade glioma. These reports are exceptional, and there is no convincing evidence that irradiation plays a significant role in the malignant dedifferentiation of a low-grade glial neoplasm.

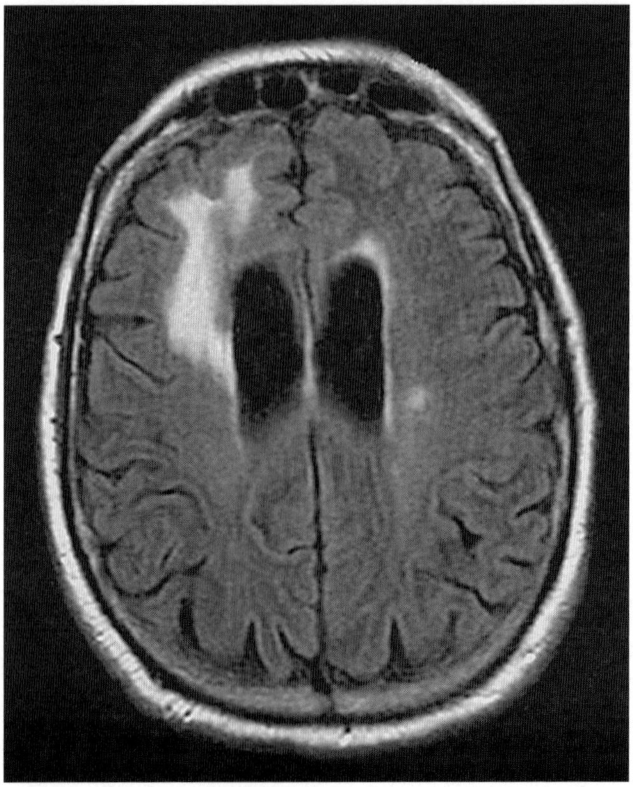

Figure 14-4. T_2-weighted axial MR image of a patient who developed memory impairment 5 years after receiving cranial irradiation for a low-grade astrocytoma of the right frontal lobe. The MR image demonstrates atrophy of the right frontal lobe, and frontal lobe and periventricular white matter changes consistent with radiation-induced leukoencephalopathy.

▶ ROLE OF CHEMOTHERAPY

Low-Grade Fibrillary Astrocytoma

Although the role of chemotherapy in the management of low-grade astrocytomas is poorly defined, there is increasing interest in using chemotherapy as initial treatment for low-grade glial neoplasms (Fig. 14-5).[95] For patients with low-grade astrocytomas, there are several advantages to an approach that avoids or delays cranial irradiation: chemotherapy may be more effective when administered as initial therapy; the central nervous system (CNS) toxicities of radiotherapy, namely dementia or radiation necrosis, can be avoided or postponed; and chemotherapy may result in substantial reduction in tumor volume, thereby reducing the size of radiotherapy fields when irradiation is

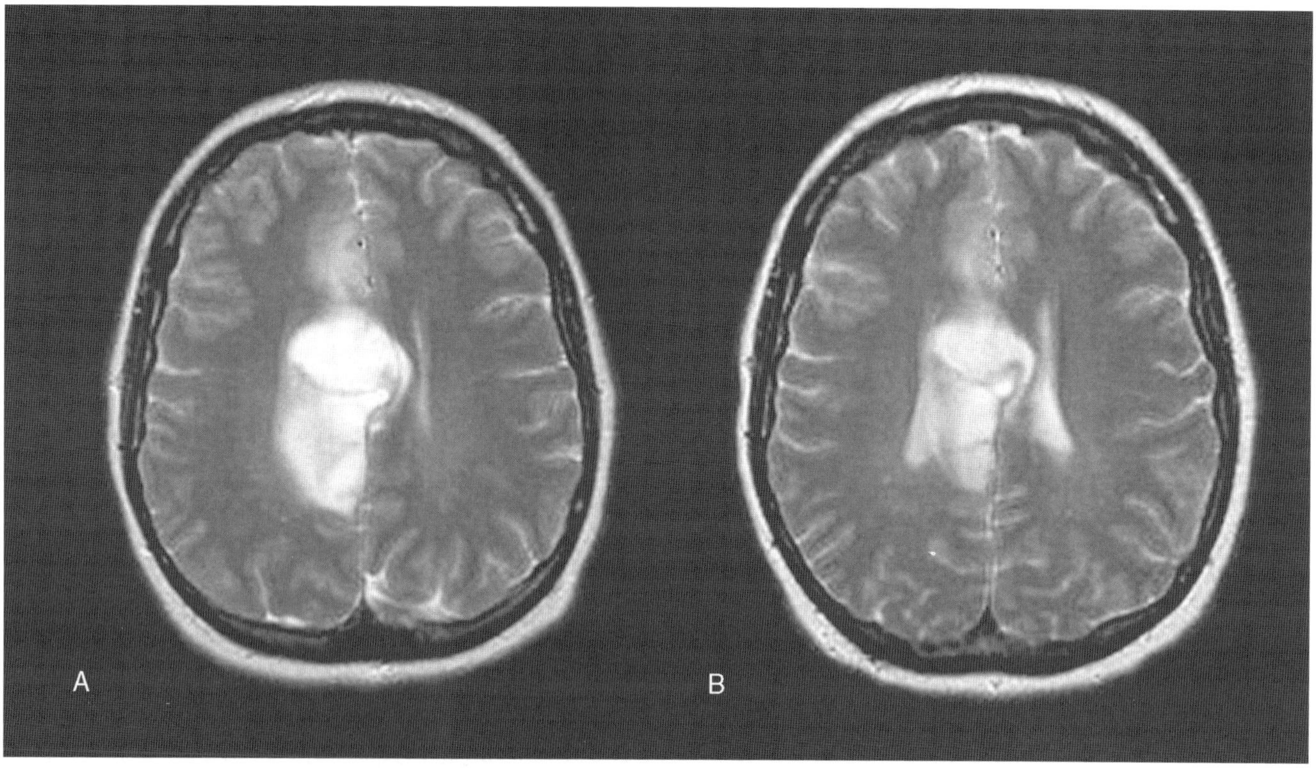

Figure 14-5. (A) T_2-weighted axial MR image of a young woman with a low-grade astrocytoma of the right frontal lobe. At the time of radiographic progression, her family declined radiotherapy because she would need daily anesthesia to ensure accurate delivery of her treatment. She was instead treated with temozolomide chemotherapy, and after 6 months of treatment a T_2-weighted image (B) demonstrated a partial radiographic response.

required. However, there are also significant risks associated with the use of chemotherapy in a population with indolent tumors and a survival that is typically measured in years. These risks include acute toxicities of chemotherapy such as myelosuppression, but also delayed toxicities such as the risk of irreversible organ damage, second malignancies, and the diminished options for further chemotherapy at recurrence or malignant transformation.

Most early studies evaluating chemotherapy for low-grade astrocytomas have been in young children, for whom the toxicities of radiotherapy are too great for this modality to be a reasonable therapeutic option.[96,97] Packer and associates[98] used a regimen consisting of vincristine and carboplatin to treat 60 children with newly diagnosed and recurrent low-grade gliomas. Radiographic responses were seen in 35 children, although most of these likely had pilocytic tumors. These investigators reported responses in four patients, and stabilization of disease in 11. Levin and associates,[99] using bromodeoxyuridine during radiation therapy followed by chemotherapy with procarbazine, lomustine, and vincristine (PCV chemotherapy) in 22 patients with low-grade astrocytoma, reported a 6-year survival of 79%. In contrast, another randomized study using adjuvant chemotherapy with lomustine following irradiation for patients with low-grade astrocytomas found no survival benefit from the addition to chemotherapy, highlighting the problems of conducting a therapeutic trial for this disease, where the natural history is long, and patient accrual slow because of the rarity of the tumor.[100]

Unlike low-grade astrocytomas, recent reports of successful chemotherapy for low-grade oligodendrogliomas have resulted in the increasing use of chemotherapy as initial treatment for tumors of oligodendroglial histology.[101] Chemosensitivity in anaplastic oligodendroglioma is linked to a specific tumor-associated genetic derangement where there is loss of heterozygosity of chromosomes 1p and 19q.[33] There is suggestive preliminary evidence that this genetic derangement occurs early in tumorigenesis, and is present in the majority of low-grade oligodendrogliomas where it predicts for a favorable response to chemotherapy and improved overall prognosis.[16] Moreover, approximately 11% of tumors that appear histologically as low-grade astrocytomas have allelic losses of chromosomes 1p and 19q, suggesting an oligodendroglial lineage at the genetic level. The increasing use of chemotherapy for oligodendroglial tumors, and the recent observation that a subset of astrocytic low-grade tumors has genetic features of oligodendrogliomas, has stimulated the use of chemotherapy for low-grade astrocytomas. Brada and associates[102] administered temozolomide chemotherapy as initial treatment to a series of patients with symptomatic, enlarging low-grade gliomas. Objective radiographic responses and stabilization of tumor growth was seen in patients with oligodendroglial and astrocytic pathology, with improvement in seizures in those with epilepsy, and modest improvement in quality of life. Furthermore, Quinn and associates[103] reported their results of a multicenter trial where temozolomide chemotherapy was administered to 46 patients with progressive low-grade gliomas that were predominantly of astrocytic histology. Although 14 patients had received prior radiotherapy and chemotherapy, complete and partial radiographic responses were seen in 61% of 46 patients. Moreover, a median progression-free survival of 22 months, and a 12-month progression-free survival of 76% were reported for the entire cohort. These striking results suggest an expanding role for temozolomide chemotherapy as initial treatment for symptomatic or enlarging low-grade astrocytomas.

Pilocytic Astrocytoma

Chemotherapy is usually not administered systematically as initial treatment for patients with pilocytic astrocytomas. Typically chemotherapy is administered for progressive disease after surgical and radiotherapeutic failure, or as a means of deferring irradiation in young children who require treatment for residual postoperative disease.[24,27] When chemotherapy has been administered for management of pilocytic astrocytomas, the tumors have usually been hypothalamic or chiasmatic, occasionally with leptomeningeal dissemination.[8,96,97,104] The most common agents have been the nitrosoureas, alone or in combination with platinum analogues, other alkylating agents, and vinca alkaloids.

▶ MANAGEMENT AT RECURRENCE

Following complete resection, pilocytic astrocytomas are unlikely to recur. However, most gliomas, including partially resected pilocytic astrocytomas, recur over a period of years following initial resection. Approximately 50% of low-grade astrocytomas recur as malignant gliomas (Fig. 14-6).[18,25,57,60] At recurrence, a number of therapeutic options are available, including surgery, radiotherapy, and chemotherapy. Surgery is indicated for large symptomatic tumors, where a debulking procedure can alleviate symptoms and provide a revised pathologic diagnosis. Following resection, radiotherapy is indicated for those who have had this treatment deferred. For those who have already received conventional radiotherapy, further irradiation is possible if stereotactic radiosurgery or brachytherapy is planned. Chemotherapy is a reasonable treatment for patients with recurrent pilocytic astrocytomas and for patients whose low-grade astrocytomas have recurred as

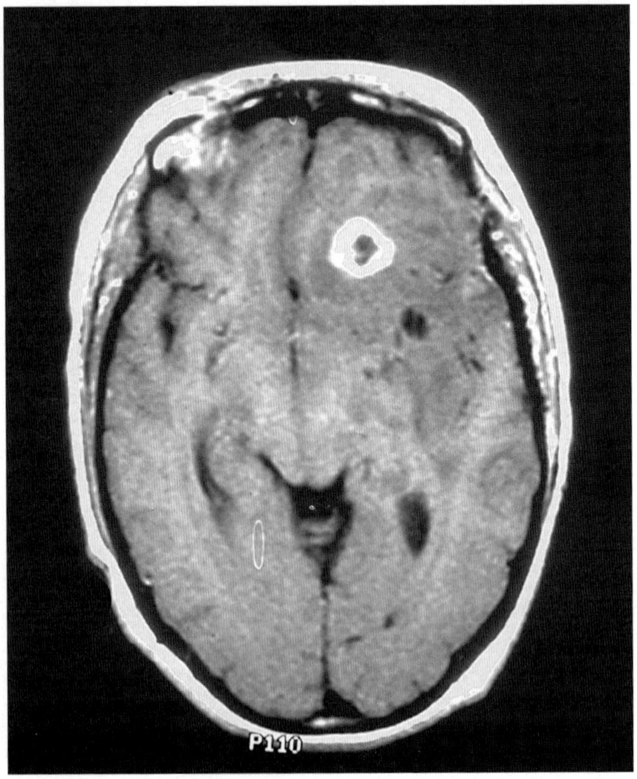

Figure 14-6. T_1-weighted contrast-enhanced MR image of a young woman with a diffuse fibrillary astrocytoma. She presented 3 years earlier with seizures, was treated only with anticonvulsants, and received frequent surveillance MRI. This image demonstrates the development of a central area of contrast enhancement and necrosis. Biopsy revealed a glioblastoma multiforme.

malignant gliomas. Suitable first-line chemotherapeutic agents include the nitrosoureas and temozolomide. There is some evidence that patients with malignant transformation of low-grade astrocytomas have enhanced responses to standard chemotherapy. Moreover, there is increasing use of chemotherapy as initial therapy for symptomatic or progressive recurrent low-grade astrocytomas, particularly with temozolomide. Unfortunately, responses to chemotherapy at recurrence are typically transient and brief, although dramatic responses and prolonged survival are occasionally observed.

▶ LESS COMMON LOW-GRADE ASTROCYTOMAS

Cerebellar Pilocytic Astrocytomas

Cerebellar pilocytic astrocytomas represent a distinct subtype of pilocytic tumors.[27,28] They usually present in children and young adults, and have distinct radiographic characteristics that suggest the pathologic diagnosis (Fig. 14-7).

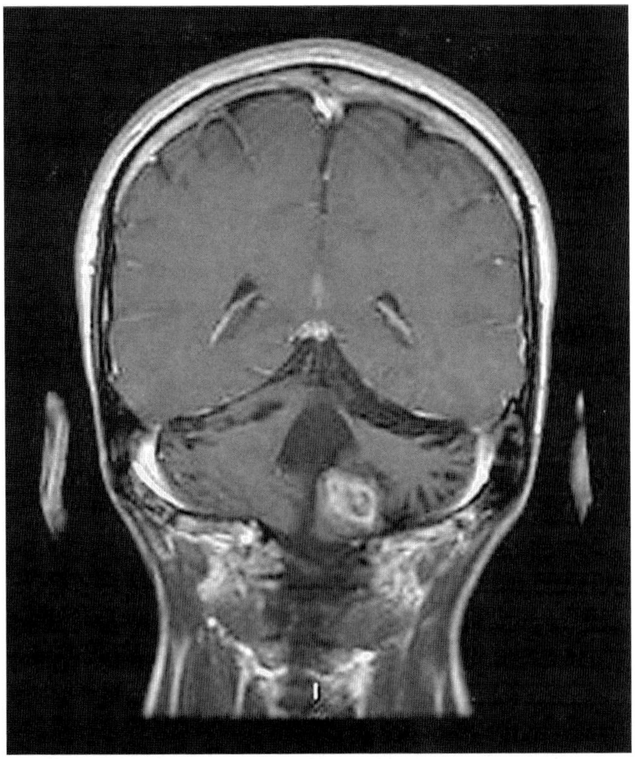

Figure 14-7. T_1-weighted contrast-enhanced coronal MR image of a young man with a cerebellar pilocytic astrocytoma. He presented 10 years earlier with headaches and ataxia. Following incomplete surgical resection, he received no further therapy, and most recent imaging reveals stable, contrast-enhancing residual disease.

Although these tumors appear discrete radiographically and on gross inspection, they often infiltrate surrounding white matter and leptomeninges. These tumors are often located in areas where gross resection is possible, and in these cases, cure can be achieved without postoperative radiotherapy. Moreover, even of patients who have subtotal resections of cerebellar astrocytomas, postoperative radiotherapy can be deferred as 5- and 10-year survival rates following surgery alone have been reported in the range of 80%.[24] For patients with incompletely resected pilocytic astrocytomas, regular radiographic surveillance is warranted as late recurrences are not uncommon. At recurrence these tumors tend to retain their benign pilocytic histology, although malignant transformation has rarely been reported.

Astroblastoma

Astroblastomas are rare primary brain tumors that were first described in 1930 by Bailey and Bucy, and formally defined as a distinct entity by Bonin and Rubenstein in 1989.[105] These tumors are well-demarcated, extraventricular, or superficial neoplasms of the cerebrum and posterior fossa. Histologically, these tumors are characterized by perivascular pseudorosettes and marked vascular hyalinization, and can further be classified as low-grade or high-grade on the basis of anaplastic features.

These tumors are obscure, and knowledge of their clinical behavior is limited for this reason. These tumors generally present in children and young adults who present with symptoms of increased intracranial pressure, focal neurologic deficits, or seizures. Symptoms usually precede the diagnosis by months, although occasionally patients have symptoms for years before a firm diagnosis is established. For patients with low-grade astroblastoma, prolonged survival following complete resection is typical. For patients with anaplastic astroblastomas, a favorable outcome after resection of a high-grade tumor is less certain, with early relapse, usually as glioblastoma, common. Postoperative radiotherapy is recommended for anaplastic astroblastoma.

Pleomorphic Xanthoastrocytoma

Pleomorphic xanthoastrocytomas are distinct low-grade astrocytomas that arise in the superficial temporal and occasionally parietal lobes of young people.[106,107] These tumors appear as well-circumscribed, enhancing, solid, or cystic masses on MRI scans, and usually demonstrate marked leptomeningeal involvement. The superficial location of these tumors makes surgical resection feasible, but these tumors are not encapsulated, and do often exhibit macroscopic infiltration of underlying brain without an apparent cleavage plane. Microscopically, these tumors demonstrate prominent cellular pleomorphism, pericellular reticulin positivity, vascular sclerosis, and occasional perivascular lymphocytic infiltration. Furthermore, in addition to areas that appear pleomorphic, this tumor also harbors regions where astrocytes appear more regular and have features more suggestive of low-grade astrocytomas. Despite the bizarre appearance of this tumor, mitoses are infrequent and necrosis is absent. Moreover, because these tumors characteristically behave in an indolent way, it is important to distinguish them from anaplastic astrocytomas, malignant tumors that require aggressive management. No characteristic genetic abnormalities have been identified; some tumors harbor p53 mutations, and others have EGFR amplification.

Because these tumors usually involve cortical areas, patients usually present with seizures, often for many years before the diagnosis is established. The treatment of this tumor is surgical. Complete or near-total resection is possible, with most patients surviving for years and often decades. The role of postoperative radiotherapy is unclear, with most patients receiving irradiation after incomplete initial resection or at recurrence. However, in view of the generally favorable prognosis for patients with pleomorphic xanthoastrocytomas, immediate postoperative radiotherapy should be deferred if initial resection is complete. Nonetheless, these tumors do occasionally recur, and sometimes seed the leptomeninges. A high mitotic rate and atypical mitoses may predict for recurrence. Generally, however, the prognosis is good, with recurrence-free survival rates of 72% at 5 years and 61% at 10 years. Overall survival at 10 years is 70%.[106]

Subependymal Giant Cell Astrocytoma

Subependymal giant cell astrocytomas are intraventricular tumors found in the region of the foramen of Monro.[108] These tumors consist of large astrocytic cells, and arise almost exclusively in patients with tuberous sclerosis. The behavior of these tumors is benign, although histologically they can demonstrate frequent mitoses and prominent areas of necrosis. These tumors likely arise from hamartomatous subependymal nodules, and usually present with symptoms of increased intracranial pressure, or as asymptomatic lesions on MRI scans of patients with tuberous sclerosis. Treatment is surgical, and following resection long-term survival is excellent, although recurrence and death have been reported.

Ganglioglioma

These low-grade tumors consist of neoplastic neurons and glial cells. These are rare tumors perhaps accounting for 1% of intracranial neoplasms, and cluster in children and young adults, although all age groups are affected.[109,110] The tumors are usually low-grade, but the potential for anaplastic transformation of the glial element is possible.[111] These tumors can be found anywhere in the nervous system, but there is a proclivity for superficial cortical regions, usually of the temporal lobe. Pathologically, gangliogliomas are composed of large pleomorphic neurons and glial cells embedded within a collagen-rich matrix with foci of infiltrating lymphocytes.[112] The neural elements can be abundant or sparse. Mitotic figures are uncommon, and MIB-1 labeling index varies from 1% to 3%. Clinically, most patients present with partial or generalized seizures.[113] Tumors located within midline structures usually present with signs and symptoms of hydrocephalus, and tumors located within the brainstem present with cranial neuropathies or ataxia. Most tumors are hypointense on T_1-weighted MR images and hyperintense on T_2-weighted MR images.[110] A cystic component and calcifications are common, but hemorrhage, mass effect, and edema are rare. The treatment of this disease is surgical, and in most cases is curative. Complete or even incomplete resection often results in improvement or disappearance of seizures. Sixty percent to 80% of patients become seizure-free after surgery.[114,115] Following resection, regardless of extent of tumor removal, no further treatment is required. Four-year progression-free survival has been reported at 78% for complete resection, and 63% for subtotal resection.[116] If recurrence occurs, reoperation followed by radiotherapy is recommended. There is no defined role for chemotherapy, but patients whose tumors recur as anaplastic gangliogliomas or glioblastoma are often treated with conventional chemotherapeutic agents.

Desmoplastic Infantile Ganglioglioma

This is an extremely rare tumor that usually arises in children who are younger than 2 years of age.[117–119] Desmoplastic infantile gangliogliomas (DIGs) are massive cystic tumors that preferentially arise in the supratentorial compartment and have large cysts with a clear attachment to the overlying dura. The lack of obtundation in affected children suggests a very indolent growth pattern and possible congenital origin. Typical symptoms associated with these tumors include increasing head circumference, bulging fontanelle, sunset sign, hemiparesis, and seizures. MRI features include a large cystic or multicystic mass with an enhancing solid peripheral component. Histologically, these tumors are characterized by a dense desmoplastic stroma and mixture of neoplastic astrocytes and neurons. Generally, mitotic activity is very low and there is no evidence of necrosis. When present, however, areas of brisk mitotic activity and areas of necrosis occur in areas of poorly differentiated cells, and in this context are not considered evidence of anaplastic transformation. The management of DIGs is surgical, and complete surgical resection is often possible and curative. Following incomplete resection, adjuvant chemotherapy or radiotherapy is often administered, with objective tumor responses and favorable survival.[118] However, recent reports have suggested that the outcome for patients with incomplete surgical resection can be good without the need of further treatment.[117,119,120] At progression, surgery is usually recommended, with or without postoperative chemotherapy or radiotherapy.

Dysembryoplastic Neuroepithelial Tumor

Dysembryoplastic neuroepithelial tumor (DNT) is another rare tumor that preferentially affects children and young adults.[121,122] This tumor has a predilection for temporal lobe, where it is cortically based, but rarely it can be found in other areas, including the posterior fossa. Patients usually present with intractable seizures, and the diagnosis is established during investigations for epilepsy surgery. The seizures usually begin in childhood, but cases have been reported where seizure onset was in adulthood. Most seizures are partial, with or without secondary generalization. MRI findings include a well-defined cystic mass that is hypointense on T_1 images and hyperintense on T_2 images.[123] Contrast enhancement, calcifications and hemorrhage are common. The tumor exerts mass effect that in long-standing cases may deform overlying bone, but edema is typically absent. These tumors are of mixed glial and neuronal origin, and pathologically have been classified as three types: simple, complex, and nonspecific. The simple DNT consists of glioneuronal elements aligned perpendicular to the cortical surface, with bundles of axons and associated mature glial cells creating columns between which neurons appear to float within an interstitial fluid. The complex form has additionally neoplastic astrocytes and oligodendrocytes with foci of cortical dysplasia. The third form cannot be distinguished from other gliomas pathologically, but the diagnosis is made by clinical and MR features.[122] This last subtype is controversial because of the absence of a distinct pathologic appearance and consequently may not be a valid entity. Treatment is surgical with no additional therapy required following complete resection, and the tumor does not recur unless resection is incomplete.[124] Control of tumor growth and seizures is possible with incomplete resection. At 5 years following surgery, 60% of DNT patients are seizure-free.[114]

Gliomatosis Cerebri

Gliomatosis cerebri, often shortened to gliomatosis, refers to diffuse infiltration of multiple lobes of the brain by a glioma that does not have an epicenter or discrete focal lesion. Typically, the neoplastic glial cells resemble astrocytes, although occasional cases suggest oligodendroglial origin. Mitoses are sometimes seen but endothelial proliferation is generally absent. By definition the process must involve more than two lobes, and at times the entire brain is diffusely enlarged with small ventricles and sulcal effacement.

Gliomatosis is a relatively rare disorder, with fewer than 300 patients reported.[125,126] The median age at diagnosis is approximately 50 years, and change in mental status or dementia the most common symptom. Headaches, seizures, hemiparesis, gait ataxia, and papilledema are also common. MRI, particularly fluid-attenuated inversion recovery (FLAIR) sequences, strongly suggests the diagnosis; stereotactic biopsy confirms it (Fig. 14-8).

The rarity of gliomatosis cerebri has led to a dearth of prospective clinical trials to optimize therapy. The diffuse nature of the disorder precludes debulking and creates difficulties for the radiotherapist given the large radiation ports required and the risk of producing leukoencephalopathy. Radiation has been used, but median survival has generally been less than 2 years.[125,127] Nonetheless, there is wide variability in patient outcome. Recent reports suggest that response rates to alkylator-based chemotherapy (temozolomide or PCV) are in the 30% to 40% range, which is similar to the range in low-grade glioma.[126,128] Using chemotherapy as an initial approach may allow some patients to defer fractionated radiotherapy, thereby minimizing the risk of treatment-related neurotoxicity.

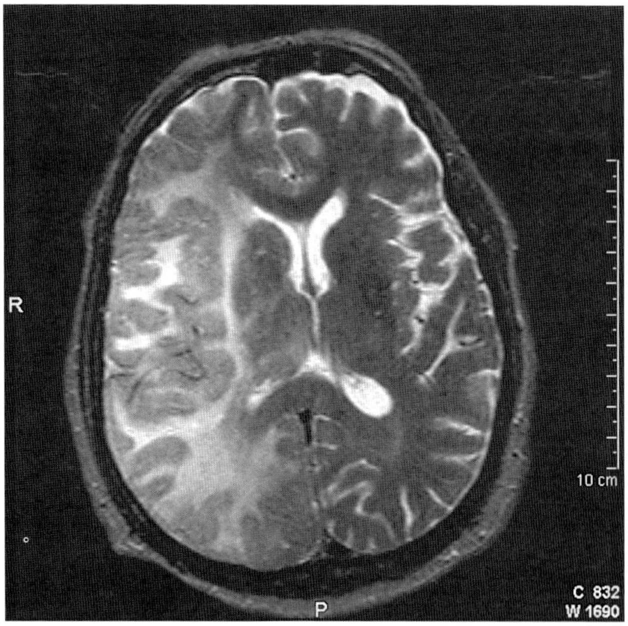

Figure 14-8. This 74-year-old man was followed for a T_2-hyperintense, nonenhancing right hemisphere signal abnormality for 3 years; it was initially detected when he underwent clipping of an aneurysm. He gradually developed hemiparesis and a seizure disorder. Stereotactic biopsy revealed low-grade oligodendroglioma. He succumbed to comorbid medical conditions shortly after starting temozolomide.

▶ FUTURE DIRECTIONS

The management of a patient with a diffuse low-grade astrocytoma is difficult, but tentative guidelines can be drawn from the considerable body of literature on the natural history and treatment response of these neoplasms. At this time, it appears reasonable to offer early and maximal surgical resection to patients with large tumors, or tumors causing persistent symptoms. Moreover, the need for immediate surgical intervention appears to increase with increasing age. The management of younger asymptomatic patients with small tumors is most challenging and controversial, but in the absence of disease progression, deferred treatment would not seem unreasonable given the well-documented long-term survival of this cohort.

A number of important conclusions regarding the postoperative management of low-grade gliomas can be drawn from the preliminary results of recent randomized studies exploring the role of radiotherapy for this disease. Significantly, it would appear that a lower dose, perhaps no greater than 50 Gy, should be administered to patients with this disease. Moreover, it appears to be safe to withhold radiotherapy until there is evidence of tumor progression. Both of these treatment strategies would reduce the toxicity and delayed neurocognitive sequelae associated with cranial irradiation.

The increasing use of chemotherapy for low-grade gliomas, and the possible association of chemosensitivity in low-grade glioma with oligodendroglial molecular markers, represent an opportunity to incorporate chemotherapy in the initial management of this disease and thereby further delay irradiation. At least two randomized intergroup studies incorporating chemotherapy for low-grade glioma are being planned. The Radiation Therapy Oncology Group is conducting a trial with the North Central Cancer Treatment Group, the Eastern Cooperative Oncology Group, and the Southwest Oncology Group for high-risk patients with supratentorial low-grade glioma. Patients are randomized to receive radiation alone at a dosage of 54 Gy in 30 fractions or radiotherapy followed by six courses of PCV chemotherapy. This protocol is aggressive because high-risk patients are being selected for treatment; consequently, a dose higher than recent studies would support and a chemotherapy regimen conventional for anaplastic gliomas are being administered. The European Organization for the Research and Treatment of Cancer with the National Cancer Institute of Canada are planning a trial where patients with symptomatic and progressive low-grade gliomas will be randomized to receive radiation at a dosage of 50 Gy or temozolomide chemotherapy. This study will address directly the role of chemotherapy for this disease, and temozolomide has been selected because it can be administered chronically with minimal cumulative toxicity.

The current management of low-grade gliomas is being refined by large clinical trials designed to address important therapeutic controversies. Nonetheless, the approach to a patient with a low-grade glioma is complex and must be individualized, and must take into account a number of important variables including tumor histology and genetics, tumor location, patient prognostic features and symptoms, and toxicities of available treatment modalities. These complexities mandate frank discussions with patients before embarking on a treatment plan because available treatments are not curative, and are associated with toxicities and sequelae that may impact unfavorably on quality of life. Fortunately, the medical community has recognized the limitations of current therapies, and efforts are presently directed at maximizing benefits while minimizing toxicities of available treatments for this intractable disease.

REFERENCES

1. Burger P, Scheithauer B. Tumors of the central nervous system. Washington, DC: Armed Forces Institute of Pathology, 1994.
2. Russell D, Rubinstein L. Pathology of tumors of the central nervous system. Baltimore, MD: Williams & Wilkins, 1989.
3. Linskey M. Glial ontogeny and glial neoplasia: the search for closure. J Neurooncol 1997;34:5–22.
4. Holland E. Gliomagenesis: genetic alterations and mouse models. Nat Rev Genet 2001;2:120–129.
5. Shaw E, Arusell R, Scheithauer B, et al. Prospective randomized trial of low- versus high-dose radiation therapy in adults with supratentorial low-grade glioma: initial report of a North Central Cancer Group/Radiation Therapy Oncology Group/Eastern Cooperative Oncology Group study. J Clin Oncol 2002;20:2267–2276.
6. CBTRUS. Statistical report: primary brain tumors in the United States, 1992–1997. Central Brain Tumor Registry of the United States, 2000.
7. Radhakrishnan K, Mokri B, Parisi J, et al. The trends in incidence of primary brain tumors in the population of Rochester, Minnesota. Ann Neurol 1995;37:67–73.
8. Freeman C, Farmer J-P, Montes J. Low-grade astrocytomas in children: evolving management strategies. Int J Radiat Oncol Biol Phys 1998;41:979–987.
9. Peterson K, DeAngelis L. Weighing the benefits and risks of radiation therapy for low-grade glioma. Neurology 2001;56:1255–1266.
10. Bampoe J, Bernstein M. The role of surgery in low-grade gliomas. J Neurooncol 1999;42:259–269.
11. Cairncross J, Laperriere N. Low-grade gliomas: to treat or not to treat? Arch Neurol 1990;47:1139–1140.
12. Buatti J, Meeks S, Ryken T, et al. Low-grade gliomas: answering one question in a myriad of new questions. J Clin Oncol 2002;20:2223–2224.
13. Karim A, Matt B, Hatlevoli R, et al. A randomized trial: no dose-response in radiation therapy of low-grade cerebral glioma: European Organization for Research and Treatment of Cancer (EORTC) study 22844. Int J Radiat Oncol Biol Phys 1996;36:549–556.
14. Karim A, Afra D, Cornu P, et al. Randomized trial on the efficacy of radiotherapy for cerebral low-grade glioma in the adult: European Organization for Research and Treatment of Cancer study 22845 with the Medical Research Council study BR04: an interim analysis. Int J Radiat Oncol Biol Phys 2002;52:316–324.
15. Pignatti F, van den Bent M, Curran D, et al. Prognostic factors for survival in adult patients with cerebral low-grade glioma. J Clin Oncol 2002;20:2076–2084.
16. van den Bent M, Chinot O-L, Cairncross J. Recent developments in the molecular characterization and treatment of oligodendroglial tumors. Neuro-oncol 2003;5:128–138.
17. Leibel S, Sheline G, Wara W, et al. The role of radiation therapy in the treatment of astrocytomas. Cancer 1975;35: 1551–1557.
18. Shaw E, Dumas-Duport C, Scheithauer B, et al. Radiation therapy in the management of low-grade supratentorial astrocytomas. J Neurosurg 1989;70:853–861.
19. Shaw E, Scheithauer B, O'Fallon J, et al. Mixed oligoastrocytomas: a survival and prognostic factor analysis. Neurosurgery 1994;34:577–582.
20. Philippon J, Clemenceau S, Fauchon F, et al. Supratentorial low-grade astrocytomas in adults. Neurosurgery 1993;32: 554–559.

21. McCormack B, Miller D, Budzilovich G, et al. Treatment and survival of low-grade astrocytoma in adults—1977–1988. Neurosurgery 1992;31:636–642.
22. Hart M, Petito C, Earle K. Mixed gliomas. Cancer 1974; 1:134–140.
23. Clark G, Henry J, McKeever P. Cerebral pilocytic astrocytoma. Cancer 1985;56:1128–1133.
24. Forsyth P, Shaw E, Scheithauer B, et al. Supratentorial pilocytic astrocytomas. A clinicopathologic, prognostic, and flow cytometric study of 51 patients. Cancer 1993; 72:1335–1342.
25. Laws E, Taylor W, Clifton M, et al. Neurosurgical management of low-grade astrocytoma of the cerebral hemispheres. J Neurosurg 1984;61:665–673.
26. Patronas N, Dichiro D, Kufta C, et al. Prediction of survival in glioma patients by means of positron emission tomography. J Neurosurg 1985;67:816–822.
27. Morreale V, Ebersold M, Quast L, et al. Cerebellar astrocytoma: experience with 54 cases surgically treated at the Mayo Clinic, Rochester, Minnesota, from 1978 to 1990. J Neurosurg 1997;87:257–261.
28. Pencalet P, Maixner W, Sainte-Rose C, et al. Benign cerebellar astrocytoma in children. J Neurosurg 1999;90:265–273.
29. Louis D. A molecular genetic model of astrocytoma histopathology. Brain Pathol 1997;7:755–764.
30. Louis DN. The p53 gene and protein in human brain tumors. J Neuropathol Exp Neurol 1994;53:11–21.
31. Louis D, von Deimling A, Chung R, et al. Comparative study of p53 gene and protein alterations in human astrocytomas. J Neuropathol Exp Neurol 1993;52:31–38.
32. Kitange G, Templeton K, Jenkins R. Recent advances in the molecular genetics of primary gliomas. Curr Opin Oncol 2003;15:197–203.
33. Cairncross JG, Ueki K, Zlatescu MC, et al. Specific genetic predictors of chemotherapeutic response and survival in patients with anaplastic oligodendrogliomas. J Natl Cancer Inst 1998;90:1473–1479.
34. Ino Y, Betensky R, Zlatescu M, et al. Molecular subtypes of anaplastic oligodendroglioma: implications for patient management at diagnosis. Clin Cancer Res 2001;7: 839–845.
35. Smith JS, Perry A, Borell TJ, et al. Alterations of chromosome arms 1p and 19q as predictors of survival in oligodendrogliomas, astrocytomas, and mixed oligoastrocytomas. J Clin Oncol 2000;18:636–645.
36. Ishii N, Sawamumura Y, Tada M, et al. Absence of p53 gene mutations in a tumor panel representative of pilocytic astrocytoma diversity using a p53 functional assay. Int J Cancer 1998;76:797–800.
37. Hayes V, Dirven C, Dam A, et al. High frequency of TP53 mutations in juvenile pilocytic astrocytomas indicates role of TP53 in the development of these tumors. Brain Pathol 1999;9:463–467.
38. Zattara-Cannoni H, Gambarelli D, Lena G, et al. Are juvenile pilocytic astrocytomas benign tumors? A cytogenetic study in 24 cases. Cancer Genet Cytogenet 1998;104:157–160.
39. Stack J, Antoun N, Jenkins J, et al. Gadolinium-DTPA as a contrast agent in magnetic resonance imaging of the brain. Neuroradiology 1988;30:145–154.
40. Brotchi J, Baleriaux D, Delecluse F. MRI and surgical treatment of low grade gliomas. IMBO/JIOC 1986:211–215.
41. Kelly P, Dumas-Duport C, Scheithauer B, et al. Stereotactic histologic correlations of computed tomography- and magnetic resonance imaging-defined abnormalities in patients with glial neoplasms. Mayo Clin Proc 1987;62:450–459.
42. Kilgore D, Breger R, Daniels D, et al. Cranial tissues: normal MR appearance after intravenous injection of Gd-DTPA. Radiology 1986;160:757–761.
43. Piepmeier J. Observations on the current treatment of low-grade astrocytic tumors of the cerebral hemispheres. J Neurosurg 1987;67:177–181.
44. Kelly P. Volumetric stereotactic surgical resection of intra-axial brain mass lesions. Mayo Clin Proc 1988;63:1186–1198.
45. Chamberlain M, Murovic J, Levin V. Absence of contrast enhancement on CT brain scans of patients with supratentorial malignant gliomas. Neurology 1988;38:1371–1374.
46. Kondziolka D, Lunsford L, Martinez A. Unreliability of contemporary neurodiagnostic imaging in evaluating suspected adult supratentorial (low-grade) astrocytoma. J Neurosurg 1993;79:533–536.
47. Lee Y-Y, Tassel P, Bruner J, et al. Juvenile pilocytic astrocytomas: CT and MR characteristics. Am J Radiol 1989; 152:1263–1270.
48. Byrne T: Imaging of gliomas. Semin Oncol 1994;21: 162–171.
49. Kaschten B, Stevenaert A, Sadzot B, et al. Preoperative evaluation of 54 gliomas by PET with fluorine-18-deoxyglucose and/or carbon-11-methionine. J Nucl Med 1998;39:778–785.
50. Francavilla T, Miletich R, Dichiro G, et al. Positron emission tomography in the detection of malignant degeneration of low-grade gliomas. Neurosurgery 1989;24:1–5.
51. Vigneron D, Bollen A, McDermott M, et al. Three-dimensional magnetic resonance spectroscopic imaging of histologically confirmed brain tumors. Magn Reson Imaging 2001;19:89–101.
52. Hwang J, Egnaczyk G, Ballard E, et al. Proton MR spectroscopic characteristics of pediatric pilocytic astrocytomas. Am J Neuroradiol 1998;19:535–540.
53. Kleihues P, Cavanee W. World Health Organization Classification of tumors: tumors of the nervous system—pathology and genetics. Lyon, France: IRAC Press, 2000.
54. Dumas-Duport C, Scheithauer B, O'Fallon J, et al. Grading of astrocytomas. A simple and reproducible method. Cancer 1988;62:2152–2165.
55. Garcia D, Fulling K, Marks J. The value of radiation therapy in addition to surgery for astrocytomas of the adult cerebrum. Cancer 1985;55:919–927.
56. Whitton A, Bloom H. Low grade glioma of the cerebral hemispheres in adults: a retrospective analysis of 88 cases. Int J Radiat Oncol Biol Phys 1990;18:783–786.
57. Soffietti R, Chio A, Giordana M, et al. Prognostic factors in well-differentiated cerebral astrocytoma in the adult. Neurosurgery 1989;24:686–692.
58. Vertosick F, Selker R, Arena V. Survival of patients with well-differentiated astrocytomas diagnosed in the era of computed tomography. Neurosurgery 1991;28: 496–501.

59. Liigant A, Haldre S, Oun A, et al. Seizure disorders in patients with brain tumors. Eur Neurol 2001;45:46–51.
60. Leighton C, Fisher B, Bauman G, et al. Supratentorial low-grade glioma in adults: an analysis of prognostic factors and timing of radiation. J Clin Oncol 1997;15:1294–1301.
61. Muller W, Afra D, Schroeder R. Supratentorial recurrences of gliomas. Morphological studies in relation to time intervals with astrocytomas. Acta Neurochir (Wien) 1977;37:75–91.
62. van Wagenen W. Verified brain tumors. End results of one-hundred and forty-nine cases eight years after operation. JAMA 1934;102:1454–1458.
63. Gol A. The relatively benign astrocytomas of the cerebrum: a clinical study of 194 verified cases. J Neurosurg 1961;18:501–506.
64. Recht L, Lew R, Smith T. Suspected low-grade glioma: is deferring treatment safe? Ann Neurol 1992;31:431–436.
65. Mundinger F, Weigel K. Considerations in the usage and results of curietherapy. In: Lunsford L, ed. Modern stereotactic neurosurgery. Boston: Martinus Nijhoff, 1988: 245–258.
66. Medbery C, Strauss K, Steinberg S, et al. Low-grade astrocytomas: treatment results and prognostic variables. Int J Radiat Oncol Biol Phys 1988;15:837–841.
67. Kosel S, Scheithauer B, Graeber M. Genotype-phenotype correlation in gemistocytic astrocytomas. Neurosurgery 2001;48:187–193.
68. Giannini C, Scheithauer B, Burger P, et al. Cellular proliferation in pilocytic and diffuse astrocytomas. J Neuropathol Exp Neurol 1999;58:46–53.
69. Litofsky N, Mix T, Baker S, et al. Ki-67 (clone MIB-1) proliferation index in recurrent glial neoplasms: no prognostic significance. Surg Neurol 1998;50:579–585.
70. Kreth F, Faist M, Rossner R, et al. Supratentorial World Health Organization Grade 2 astrocytomas and oligoastrocytomas. A new pattern of prognostic factors. Cancer 1997;79:370–379.
71. Janny P, Cure H, Mohr M, et al. Low grade supratentorial astrocytomas. Cancer 1994;73:1937–1945.
72. Scerrati M, Roselli R, Iacoangeli M, et al. Prognostic factors in low grade (WHO grade II) gliomas of the cerebral hemispheres: the role of surgery. J Neurol Neurosurg Psychiatry 1996;61:291–296.
73. van Veelen M, Avezaat C, Kros J, et al. Supratentorial low grade astrocytoma: Prognostic factors, dedifferentiation, and the issue of early versus late surgery. J Neurol Neurosurg Psychiatry 1998;64:581–587.
74. Lote K, Egeland T, Hager B, et al. Survival, prognostic factors, and therapeutic efficacy in low-grade glioma: a retrospective study in 379 patients. J Clin Oncol 1997; 15:3129–3140.
75. Bernstein M, Parrent A. Complications of CT-guided stereotactic biopsy of intra-axial brain lesions. J Neurosurg 1994;81:165–168.
76. Ciric I, Ammirati M, Vick N, et al. Supratentorial gliomas: surgical considerations and immediate postoperative results. Gross total resection versus partial resection. Neurosurgery 1987;21:21–26.
77. Fadul C, Wood J, Thaler H, et al. Morbidity and mortality of craniotomy for excision of supratentorial gliomas. Neurology 1988;38:1374–1379.
78. Salcman M, Scholtz H, Kaplan RS, et al. Long-term survival in patients with malignant astrocytoma. Neurosurgery 1985;34:213–220.
79. Vecht C, Avezaat C, Putten W, et al. The influence of the extent of surgery on the neurological function and survival in malignant glioma. A retrospective analysis of 243 patients. J Neurol Neurosurg Psych 1990;53:466–471.
80. Ammirati M, Vick N, Liao Y, et al. Effect of extent of surgical resection on survival and quality of life in patients with supratentorial glioblastomas and anaplastic astrocytoma. Neurosurgery 1987;21:201–206.
81. Laws E, Taylor W, Bergstralh E, et al. The neurosurgical management of low-grade astrocytoma. Clin Neurosurg 1986;61:665–673.
82. Berger M, Deliganis A, Dobbins J, et al. The effect of extent of resection on recurrence in patients with low grade cerebral hemisphere gliomas. Cancer 1994;74:1784–1791.
83. Bauman G, Pahapill P, Macdonald D, et al. Low grade glioma: measuring radiographic response to radiotherapy. Can J Neurol Sci 1999;26:8–22.
84. Wara W. Radiation therapy for brain tumors. Cancer 1985; 55:2291–2295.
85. Mundinger F, Ostertag C, Birg W, et al. Stereotactic treatment of brain lesions. App Neurophysiol 1980;43:198–204.
86. Szikla G, Schlienger M, Bond S. Interstitial and combined interstitial and external irradiation of supratentorial gliomas—results of 61 cases treated 1973–1981. Acta Neurochir 1984;33(Suppl):355–362.
87. Pozza F, Colombo F, Chierego G, et al. Low-grade astrocytomas: treatment with unconventionally fractionated external beam stereotactic radiation therapy. Radiology 1989;171:565–569.
88. Surma-Aho O, Niemela M, Vilkki J, et al. Adverse long-term effects of brain radiotherapy in adult low-grade glioma patients. Neurology 2001;56:1285–1290.
89. Taphoorn M, Schiphorst A, Snoek F, et al. Cognitive functions and quality of life in patients with low-grade gliomas: the impact of radiotherapy. Ann Neurol 1994;36:48–54.
90. Vigliani M-C, Sichez N, Poisson M, et al. A prospective study of cognitive functions following conventional radiotherapy for supratentorial gliomas in young adults: 4-year results. Int J Radiat Oncol Biol Phys 1996;35:527–533.
91. Kiebert G, Curran D, Aaronson N, et al. Quality of life after radiation therapy of cerebral low-grade gliomas of the adult: results of a randomized phase III trial on dose response (EORTC trial 22844). EORTC Radiotherapy Cooperative Group. Eur J Cancer 1998;34:1902–1909.
92. North C, North R, Epstein J, et al. Low-grade cerebral astrocytomas. Survival and quality of life after radiation therapy. Cancer 1989;66:6–14.
93. Roelcke U, von Ammon K, Hausmann O, et al. Operated low grade astrocytomas: a long-term PET study on the effect of radiotherapy. J Neurol Neurosurg Psychiatry 1999;66:644–647.
94. Bruehlmeier M, Roelcke U, Amsler B, et al. Effects of radiotherapy on brain glucose metabolism in patients operated on for low grade astrocytoma. J Neurol Neurosurg Psychiatry 1999;66:648–653.
95. Mason W. Chemotherapy for low-grade gliomas. FORUM Trends Exp Clin Med 2000;10:95–104.

96. Gropman A, Packer R, Nicholson H, et al. Treatment of diencephalic syndrome with chemotherapy: growth, tumor response, and long term control. Cancer 1998;83: 166–172.
97. Kato T, Sawamura Y, Tada M, et al. Cisplatin/vincristine chemotherapy for hypothalamic/visual pathway astrocytomas in young children. J Neurooncol 1998;37:263– 270.
98. Packer R, Lange B, Ater J, et al. Carboplatin and vincristine for recurrent and newly diagnosed low-grade gliomas of childhood. J Clin Oncol 1993;11:850–856.
99. Levin V, Prados M, Wara W, et al. Radiation therapy and bromodeoxyuridine chemotherapy followed by procarbazine, lomustine, and vincristine for the treatment of anaplastic gliomas. Int J Radiat Oncol Biol Phys 1995; 32:75–83.
100. Eyre H, Crowley J, Townsend J, et al. A randomized trial of radiotherapy versus radiotherapy plus CCNU for incompletely resected low-grade gliomas: a Southwest Oncology Group study. J Neurosurg 1993;78:909–914.
101. Mason WP, Krol GS, DeAngelis LM. Low-grade oligodendroglioma responds to chemotherapy. Neurology 1996; 46:203–207.
102. Brada M, Viviers L, Abson C, et al. Phase II study of primary temozolomide chemotherapy in patients with WHO grade II gliomas. Ann Oncol 2003;24:1715–1721.
103. Quinn J, Reardon DA, Friedman AH, et al. Phase II trial of temozolomide in patients with progressive low-grade glioma. J Clin Oncol 2003;21:646–651.
104. Tamura M, Zama A, Kurihara H, et al. Management of recurrent pilocytic astrocytoma with leptomeningeal dissemination in childhood. Childs Nerv Syst 1998;14:617– 622.
105. Bonnin J, Rubinstein L. Astroblastomas: a pathological study of 23 tumors, with a postoperative follow-up in 13 patients. Neurosurgery 1989;25:6–13.
106. Giannini C, Scheithauer B, Burger P, et al. Pleomorphic xanthoastrocytoma: what do we really know about it? Cancer 1999;85:2033–2045.
107. Tonn J, Paulus W, Warmuth-Metz M, et al. Pleomorphic xanthoastrocytoma: report of six cases with special consideration of diagnostic and therapeutic pitfalls. Surg Neurol 1997;47:62–69.
108. Shepherd C, Scheithauer B, Gomez M, et al. Subependymal giant cell astrocytoma: a clinical, pathological, flow cytometric study. Neurosurgery 1991;28:864–868.
109. Lang F, Epstein F, Ransohoff J, et al. Central nervous system gangliogliomas. Part 2: clinical outcome. J Neurosurg 1993;79:867–873.
110. Zentner J, Wolf H, Ostertun B, et al. Gangliogliomas: clinical, radiological, and histopathological findings in 51 patients. J Neurol Neurosurg Psychiatry 1994;57:1497–1502.
111. Kurian N, Nair S, Radhakrishnan V. Anaplastic ganglioglioma: case report and review of the literature. Br J Neurosurg 1998;12:277–280.
112. Miller D, Lang F, Epstein F. Central nervous system gangliogliomas. Part 1: pathology. J Neurosurg 1993;79:859–866.
113. Blumcke I, Wiestler O. Gangliogliomas: an intriguing tumor entity associated with focal epilepsies. J Neuropathol Exp Neurol 2002;61:575–584.
114. Aronica E, Leenstra S, van Veelen C, et al. Glioneuronal tumors and medically intractable epilepsy: a clinical study with long-term follow-up of seizure outcome after surgery. Epilepsy Res 2001;43:179–191.
115. Morris H, Matkovic Z, Estes M, et al. Ganglioglioma and intractable epilepsy: clinical and neurophysiologic features and predictors of outcome after surgery. Epilepsia 1998;39:307–313.
116. Selch M, Goy B, Lee S, et al. Gangliogliomas: experience with 34 patients and review of the literature. Am J Clin Oncol 1998;21:557–564.
117. Bachli H, Avoledo P, Gratzl O, et al. Therapeutic strategies and management of desmoplastic infantile ganglioglioma: two case reports and literature overview. Childs Nerv Syst 2003;19:359–366.
118. Duffner P, Burger P, Cohen M, et al. Desmoplastic infantile gangliogliomas: an approach to therapy. Neurosurgery 1994;34:583–589.
119. Tamburrini G, Colosimo C, Giangaspero F, et al. Desmoplastic infantile ganglioglioma. Childs Nerv Syst 2003;19:292–297.
120. Takeshima H, Kawahara Y, Hirano H, et al. Postoperative regression of desmoplastic infantile gangliogliomas: report of two cases. Neurosurgery 2003;53:979–984.
121. Cabiol J, Acebes J, Isamat F. Dysembryoplastic neuroepithelial tumor. Crit Rev Neurosurg 1999;9:116–125.
122. Dumas-Duport C, Varlet P, Bacha S, et al. Dysembryoplastic neuroepithelial tumors: nonspecific histological forms—a study of 40 cases. J Neurooncol 1999;41:267–280.
123. Lee D, Chung C, Hwang Y, et al Dysembryoplastic neuroepithelial tumor: radiologic findings (including PET, SPECT, and MRS) and surgical strategy. J Neurooncol 2000; 47:167–174.
124. Prayson R, Morris H, Estes M, et al. Dysembryoplastic neuroepithelial tumor: a clinicopathologic and immunohistochemical study of 11 tumors including MIB1 immunoreactivity. Clin Neuropathol 1996;15:47–53.
125. Vates GE, Chang S, Lamborn KR, et al. Gliomatosis cerebri: a review of 22 cases. Neurosurgery 2003;53: 261–271.
126. Sanson M, Cartalat-Carel S, Taillibert S, et al. Initial chemotherapy in gliomatosis cerebri. Neurology 2004;63: 270–275.
127. Jennings MT, Frenchman M, Shehab T, et al. Gliomatosis cerebri presenting as intractable epilepsy during early childhood. J Child Neurol 1995;10:37–45.
128. Levin N, Gomori JM, Siegal T. Chemotherapy as initial treatment in gliomatosis cerebri: results with temozolomide. Neurology 2004;63:354–356.

CHAPTER 15

Oligodendroglioma and Mixed Gliomas

MARTIN J. VAN DEN BENT / JOHAN M. KROS

In the 1920s, Bailey described and classified glial brain tumors in a number of papers. Some of these, he maintained, were composed of neoplastic oligodendroglia. This assumption was based on the morphologic resemblance between oligodendroglia and the cells within those oligodendroglial tumors.[1] Until about 1990, this diagnosis had few clinical implications, although it was clear that oligodendroglial tumors had a more favorable outcome than astrocytic tumors of similar histologic grade. This changed with the recognition of the marked sensitivity to procarbazine, CCNU, and vincristine (PCV) chemotherapy of oligodendroglial tumors by Cairncross and Macdonald.[2,3] It is now generally accepted that the histologic diagnosis of oligodendroglial tumors has clear clinical implications; consequently, chemotherapy with either PCV or temozolomide is part of the standard treatment of oligodendroglial tumors. The clinical need to distinguish this tumor with a favorable prognosis from astrocytoma did have a side effect: it has resulted in a change in the histologic criteria for oligodendroglial tumors, with a significant increase in incidence of oligodendroglial tumors.[4] This evolution has blurred the distinction between astrocytoma and oligodendroglioma, a situation not helped by the absence of specific oligodendroglial tumor markers and the existence of so-called mixed oligoastrocytomas. The latter tumors are tumors in which areas with astrocytic morphology are intermingled with areas resembling oligodendroglioma.

An important advance in the characterization of oligodendroglial tumors was the identification of loss of the short arm of chromosome 1 (1p) and the long arm of chromosome 19 (19q) as the most characteristic genetic lesions of oligodendroglial tumors.[5,6] Subsequent studies identified oligodendroglial tumors with this genotype as the chemotherapy-responsive oligodendroglioma. It is now well established that virtually all oligodendroglial tumors with combined loss of 1p/19q are responsive to chemotherapy.[7,8] This responsiveness, as well as specific clinical features, suggests that the oligodendroglial tumor with loss of 1p/19q is an entirely distinct clinical entity. Still, more than 80 years after the first description of oligo dendroglial tumors, the cause and the precursor cells of oligodendroglial tumors remain unknown. Often the pluripotent O-2A stem cell is assumed to give rise to oligodendroglial tumors, but this has not been proven. Despite the recent molecular biologic developments, the diagnosis of oligodendroglial tumor still rests on microscopic characteristics and encompasses a group of tumors with considerable clinical and molecular heterogeneity.

▶ EPIDEMIOLOGY

Older studies estimated that oligodendroglial tumors constituted approximately 5% of all glial tumors.[9] In more recent studies this figure has increased to 20%, which is probably a result of changing criteria for the diagnosis of oligodendroglial tumors.[4] Oligodendroglial tumor is predominantly a tumor of adulthood, with a peak incidence between the fourth and sixth decade of life. Low-grade oligodendroglial tumors tend to arise in slightly younger patients. In some series a slight preponderance of males has been observed.[9,10]

▶ GENETICS AND MOLECULAR BIOLOGY

Genetic Lesions in Oligodendroglioma

The most constant chromosomal lesions in low-grade oligodendroglial tumors are allelic loss of the 1p and 19q loci.[5,11] The incidence of either 1p or 19q chromosomal deletions in oligodendroglial tumors is approximately 75%; the combined loss of 1p and 19q is observed in 60% to 70% of all oligodendroglial tumors.[6,12] In comparison to low-grade oligodendroglial tumors, anaplastic oligodendroglioma (AOD) usually have additional chromosomal deletions. In particular, loss of heterozygosity for 9p and/or deletion of the cyclin-dependent kinase N2A (*CDKN2A*) gene occurs in 33% to 42% of AOD, and deletions on chromosome 10 occurs in 19% to 25% of cases.[11] Tumor suppressor gene *p53* (*TP53*) mutations and phosphatase tensin homologue (*PTEN*) mutations are rare in oligodendroglioma.[5,13] Loss of 10q is more frequent in oligodendroglial tumors than are *PTEN* mutations, which suggests that 10q carries another oligodendroglial tumor-related tumor suppressor gene.[14]

Oligoastrocytoma have morphologic elements of both oligodendroglioma and astrocytoma. Genetically, oligoastrocytoma fall into two categories: those that have 1p and 19q deletions, which are typical of oligodendroglial tumors, and those that have *TP53* mutations, which are typical of astrocytoma.[15] This suggests that one group is of oligodendroglial lineage, and the other of astrocytic lineage. A similar inverse relationship has been observed in oligodendroglial tumors. Approximately 30% to 40% of oligodendroglial tumors do not have combined loss of 1p/19q. Although *TP53* mutations do occur in tumors with oligodendroglial morphology, these are usually tumors that do not have loss of 1p/19q.[16] Furthermore, in AOD, both the loss of 10q and the amplification of epidermal growth factor receptor (EGFR) are found inversely related to 1p/19q loss.[17–19]

The mutually exclusive occurrence of 1p/19q loss in one set of tumors and *TP53* mutations, EGFR amplification, 10q loss, or *PTEN* mutations in other tumors suggests that these tumors are either derived from different precursor cells or have a different causal mechanism of disease. Several clinical and morphologic features support the notion that classical oligodendroglial tumors with combined loss of 1p/19q are a distinct clinicopathologic entity:

- Oligodendroglial tumors with a classical histologic appearance (perinuclear halo, chicken-wire vascular pattern) are associated with the loss of 1p/19q, whereas atypical oligodendroglial tumors usually show other chromosomal abnormalities (e.g., *TP53* mutations, 10q deletions).[8,16,19,20]
- Oligodendrogliomas with loss of 1p/19q rarely arise in the temporal lobe and are often located bilaterally in the frontal lobes. Similarly, oligoastrocytomas located solely within the temporal lobe have significantly more frequent *TP53* mutations without 1p/19q loss.[21–23]
- Virtually all oligodendroglial tumors with combined loss of 1p/19q respond to chemotherapy, and the genotype appears to be a better predictor of response to chemotherapy than the morphology of the tumor.[7,8,24]
- The prognosis of oligodendroglial tumors is much better if there is loss of 1p either as a single aberration or in combination with loss of 19q.[12,25]
- Oligodendrogliomas with loss of 1p/19q tend to present with seizures of long-standing duration.[8]
- Oligodendrogliomas with loss of 1p/19q tend to have a more homogeneous enhancing pattern, in contrast to a ring-like enhancement in non–1p/19q-loss tumors.[7]

However, none of these relations is absolute. Although these observations show that the genotyping of oligodendroglial tumors may result in a different tumor entity, it is at present unclear what clinical implications that would have.

Molecular Biology

Although deletion studies have identified several regions of interest mapping in particular to the regions 1p36 and 19q13, no candidate genes in these areas have yet been identified.[14] Furthermore, the initiating event, the cell of origin, and the pathogenetic mechanism of oligodendroglial tumors are still unknown.

From the earliest observation of the morphologic similarity between oligodendroglia and oligodendroglial tumors it has been assumed that oligodendrocytes give rise to oligodendroglial tumors. Recent research has focused on a glial progenitor cell, the oligodendrocyte-2 astrocyte progenitor (O-2A) cell. Depending on external growth factors (in particular the platelet-derived growth factor [PDGF] and basic fibroblast growth factor [bFGF]), these normal glial precursor cells can either differentiate into astrocytes or oligodendrocytes, or remain in their pluripotent state.[26,27] Both O-2A progenitor cells and oligodendroglioma express the combination of NG2 chondroitin proteoglycan sulfate and PDGF-α—a combination observed neither in glioblastoma multiforme nor in normal brain.[28]

A number of studies have investigated the potential role of the growth factor PDGF in oligodendroglial tumors. PDGF has a strong mitogenic effect on these glial progenitor cells.[29] The induction of PDGF expression in cell cultures of astrocytes and glial progenitor cells increased the proliferation rate and converted differentiated astrocytes into glial precursor-like cells.[30] Induction of PDGF expression by intracranial gene transfer of progenitor cells in mice induced the formation of oligodendrogliomas or oligoastrocytomas in a transgenic mice model.[30] A potential role of PDGF in oligodendroglial tumors is suggested by the expression of PDGF A and B, as well as both the PDGF-α and -β receptors by virtually all oligodendroglial tumors, suggestive of an autocrine loop.[31,32] PDGF-α and platelet-derived growth factor receptor (PDGFR)-A are more frequently expressed in oligodendroglial tumors than in astrocytic tumors.[28,32] However, PDGFR gene mutations are rare in oligodendroglial tumors, raising questions of the pathogenetic significance of PDGF signaling in oligodendroglial tumors.[33] The issue is whether PDGFR upregulation or abnormalities in the PDGF pathway are the driving force behind oligodendroglial tumors, or only secondary events in an already malignant transformed glial cell type. Indeed, to what extent laboratory experiments and gene transfer mimic the "real life" tumorigenesis of oligodendroglial tumors is uncertain. For example, the transfer of other oncogenes such as the middle T antigen into glial fibrillary acidic protein (GFAP)-expressing cells (thus exhibiting an astrocytic phenotype) also gave rise to tumors with oligodendroglial features.[34] This oncogene induces aberrant signal transduction pathways downstream of the tyrosine kinase receptors EGFR and PDGFR. In view of the potential role of PDGF-dependent signaling pathways in oligodendroglial tumors, clinical trials with PDGFR blocking agents such as imatinib mesylate (Gleevec) have been initiated, but results are not yet available.

Oligodendroglioma can be induced in rats by intrauterine exposure to nitrosoureas. This led to the hypothesis that these cells are "by nature" sensitive to alkylating agents, through a deficiency in repairing DNA damage caused by alkylating agents.[35] Such a deficiency would also explain the increased sensitivity of oligodendroglial tumors to alkylating agents. The enzyme alkyltransferase is the primary mechanism that protects the cell against alkylating agents. In vivo research revealed differences in alkyltransferase gene expression between astrocytes, O-2A progenitor cells, and oligodendrocytes, the latter being the most sensitive to the alkylating agent BCNU.[36] This might explain an increased sensitivity for alkylating agents for oligodendrocytes and tumors arising from them. No differences were found, however, in the methylation status of the promoter of the alkyltransferase gene in oligodendrogliomas and in astrocytomas.[16] To conclude, the driving molecular force(s) between oligodendroglial tumors and the explanation of chemotherapy sensitivity remains to be elucidated.

▶ CLINICAL PRESENTATION

Most oligodendroglial tumors arise in the supratentorial compartment, predominantly in the frontal lobes; but all cerebral lobes can give rise to these tumors. Oligodendroglial tumors located in the posterior fossa are rare. Similar to other glioma, the presenting signs and symptoms of oligodendroglial tumors are nonspecific and depend on the localization and rate of progression of the tumor. Patients may present with partial or complex seizures, increased intracranial pressure, cognitive deficits, or focal deficits. Low-grade oligodendroglial tumors tend to present with partial or generalized seizures, whereas patients with high-grade tumors often present with focal deficits, increased intracranial pressure, cognitive deficits, mood disturbances, and behavioral abnormalities early in the course or their disease. Similar to other gliomas, oligodendroglial tumors tend to remain localized to the central nervous system (CNS). Extra-CNS metastases (especially bone metastases) have been described but are very rare and if they occur, do so in later stages of the disease. Leptomeningeal spread is far from rare but usually does not develop until the time of recurrence. It may cause symptoms and signs at other levels of the neuraxis (e.g., nausea, lumbar pain). Rare cases of primary leptomeningeal oligodendroglioma have been reported.[37,38] Many patients with an oligodendroglial tumor initially present with a low-grade tumor, which becomes transformed to a more malignant phenotype with additional chromosomal losses at the time of recurrence.

▶ DIAGNOSTIC EVALUATION

Neuroimaging

On computed tomography (CT), low-grade oligodendroglial tumors typically appear as nonenhancing low-density masses that may exhibit calcifications (Fig. 15-1A and B). Although intratumoral calcification is common,

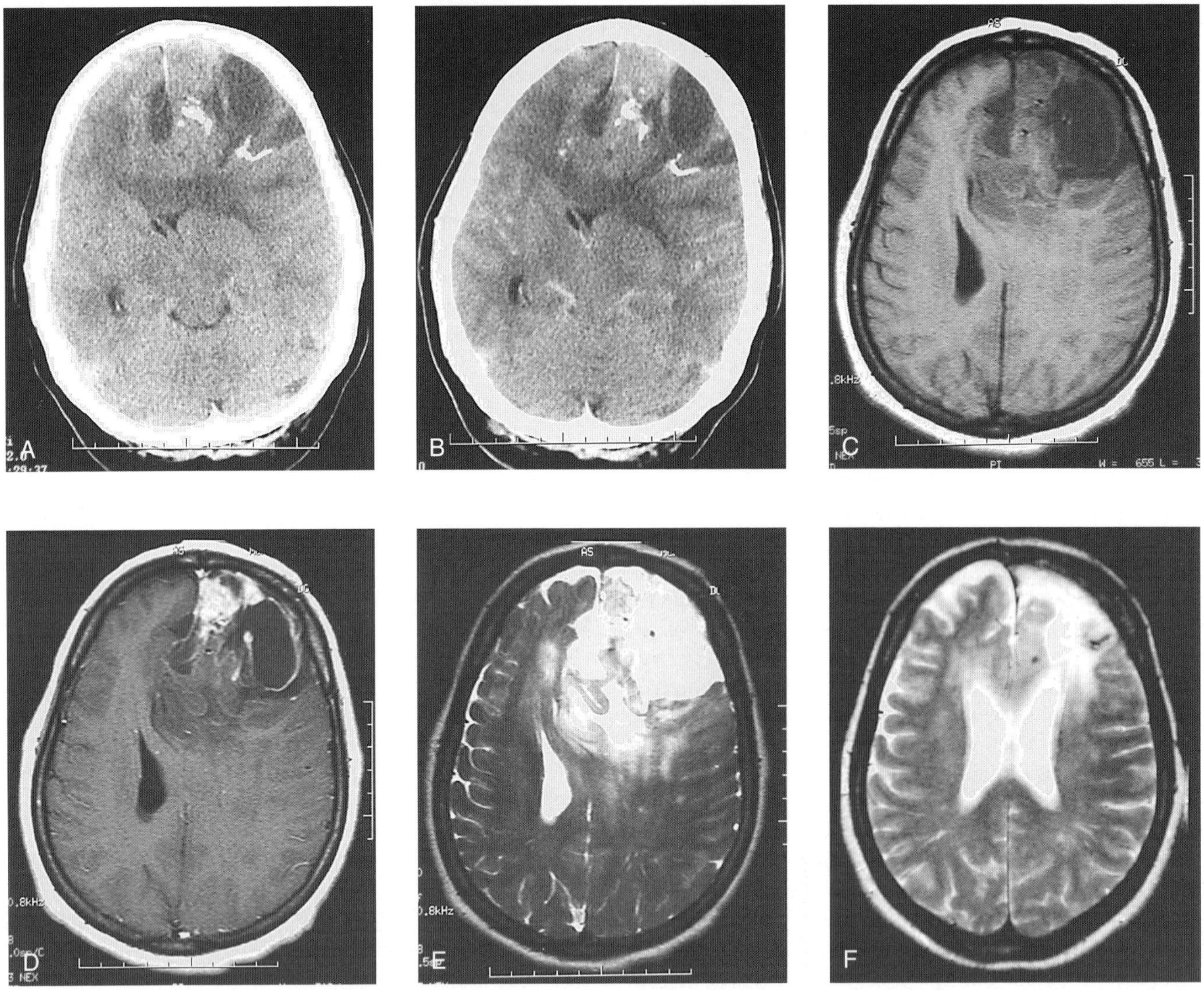

Figure 15-1. A 59-year-old female with an anaplastic oligodendroglioma and a 2-year history of progressive loss of initiative, behavioral changes, and memory disturbances, with weakness of the left arm and seizures of recent onset. CT before (A) and after (B) contrast administration, showing a large, space-occupying lesion with calcifications and minimal contrast uptake. T_1-weighted MR image of the same patient before (C) and after (D) contrast administration, followed by T_2-weighted images (E), gave a better delineation of the tumor, clear contrast enhancement, and a clear depiction of the cystic part of the tumor. (F) T_2-weighted MR images of this patient after radiotherapy, after which she made an excellent recovery to her prior level of functioning. No chemotherapy was given.

the presence of calcifications is not specific for oligodendroglial tumors. On magnetic resonance imaging (MRI), oligodendroglial tumors show increased signal intensity on T_2-weighted images without enhancement.[39] In general, MRI provides a much better delineation of brain tumors than does CT scan (Fig. 15-1C to E), and presently MRI is the imaging method of choice of brain tumors. The tumor border may be either distinct or vague. Mass effect may be absent but can be prominent with a significant midline shift. At times, only limited clinical signs and symptoms are present in patients with large lesions with mass effect, suggestive of a very slow growth rate. Cysts and areas with hemorrhage may be present. Calcifications are more easily appreciated on CT scan.

Most AODs are characterized by enhancement on CT/MRI. This enhancement is the "macroscopic" equivalent of microvascular proliferation, with breakdown of the normal blood–brain barrier. However, the absence of enhancement does not rule out the possibility of an anaplastic tumor.[40,41] At times the enhancement is hardly visible on CT, while clearly present on MRI (see Fig. 15-1B and D). The final histologic diagnosis and grading can only be made with microscopic examination of tumor tissue. None of the imaging findings are specific.

In cases with leptomeningeal spread this feature is usually readily recognized by the presence of distant tumor nodules along the ventricles or in the subarachnoid space, and sometimes by enhancement of cerebral sulci (Fig. 15-2A and B). A staging procedure, such as craniospinal axis imaging or cerebral spinal fluid (CSF) sampling, is only indicated in the presence of clinical signs and symptoms suggestive of leptomeningeal involvement. In patients with recurrent disease, the presence of leptomeningeal spread may alter treatment options.

MR spectroscopy and positron emission tomography (in particular ^{11}C-methionine PET scanning) are useful for the differentiation between the various types of glial tumors and nontumoral intracerebral lesions.[42,43] ^{11}C-methionine PET scanning shows a higher uptake in oligodendrogliomas than in astrocytomas, and the uptake is increased in anaplastic tumors as compared with low-grade tumors. Because of the limited specificity of these imaging modalities they do not play a role in the diagnosis of glial tumors, but they may be helpful in differentiating between tumor recurrence and radiation necrosis.

Genotyping of Oligodendroglioma

In most oligodendroglial tumors with loss at 1p and 19q, the entire short arm of chromosome 1 and the long arm of chromosome 19 are missing. The genotype of oligodendroglioma can be determined by comparative genomic hybridization (CGH), loss of heterozygosity studies (preferably with constitutional DNA, e.g., from leukocytes), and fluorescent in situ hybridization (FISH) with locus-specific probes. The latter technique is very laborious, but allows the assessment of the genetic lesions in archival specimens. Loss of heterozygosity (LOH) requires many specialized steps and blood DNA. With CGH small mutations at 1p and 19q may be missed, and this technique is rather complicated. In oligodendroglial tumors, FISH and LOH for loss of 1p36 and 19q13 showed a good concordance, and these are currently the most widely used methods.[6] Newer techniques like quantitative polymerase chain reaction (PCR) (which does not require blood samples) may offer an alternative but require optimization. The experience of

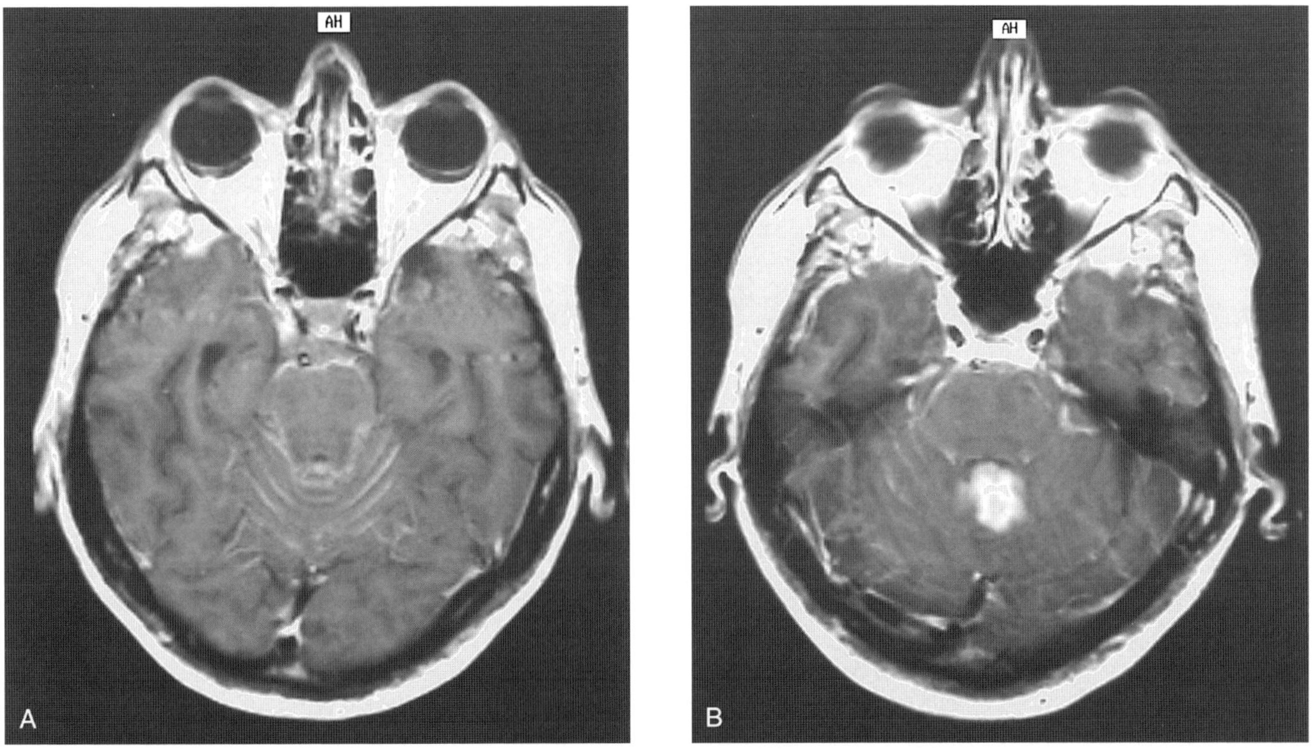

Figure 15-2. Leptomeningeal metastases: T_1-weighted MR images after contrast administration showing enhancement of the sulci of the cerebellar cortex and around the brainstem (A) and an enhancing tumor deposit in the fourth ventricle (B) in a patient previously operated on for a frontal oligodendroglioma.

the laboratory and the clinical setting should determine which technique is preferred.[14] At present the clinical implications of genotyping of oligodendroglial tumors are not clear; prospective comparative studies that incorporated information about 1p/19q status for clinical decision making are not yet available.

▶ HISTOPATHOLOGY

The current World Health Organization (WHO) definition of oligodendroglioma is "a well-differentiated, diffusely infiltrating tumor of adults, typically located in the cerebral hemispheres and composed predominantly of cells morphologically resembling oligodendroglia." The WHO definition for anaplastic oligodendroglioma is "An oligodendroglioma with focal or diffuse histologic features of malignancy and a less favorable prognosis" (Fig. 15-3A).[44] Mixed oligoastrocytoma tumors have morphologic characteristics of both astrocytic tumors and of pure oligodendroglial tumors.

Coons and associates suggested that the classic histologic features described above are insufficient for the diagnosis of oligodendroglial tumors and, therefore, oligodendroglial tumors may often be misdiagnosed as anaplastic astrocytoma (AA) or glioblastoma multiforme (GBM).[4] They suggested that when using histologic features to diagnose oligodendroglial tumors, special emphasis should be given to identifying other signs, such as microgemistocytes, gliofibrillary oligodendrocytes, and protoplasmic astrocytes, which all may suggest that the tumor is of oligodendroglial origin. The changes and widening of criteria proposed by these and other authors has greatly increased the percentage of tumors that are considered oligodendroglial. Nevertheless, a loosening of the histologic criteria for an oligodendroglial tumor diagnosis will result in a more heterogeneous tumor population in terms of genetic lesions and, more importantly, their sensitivity to

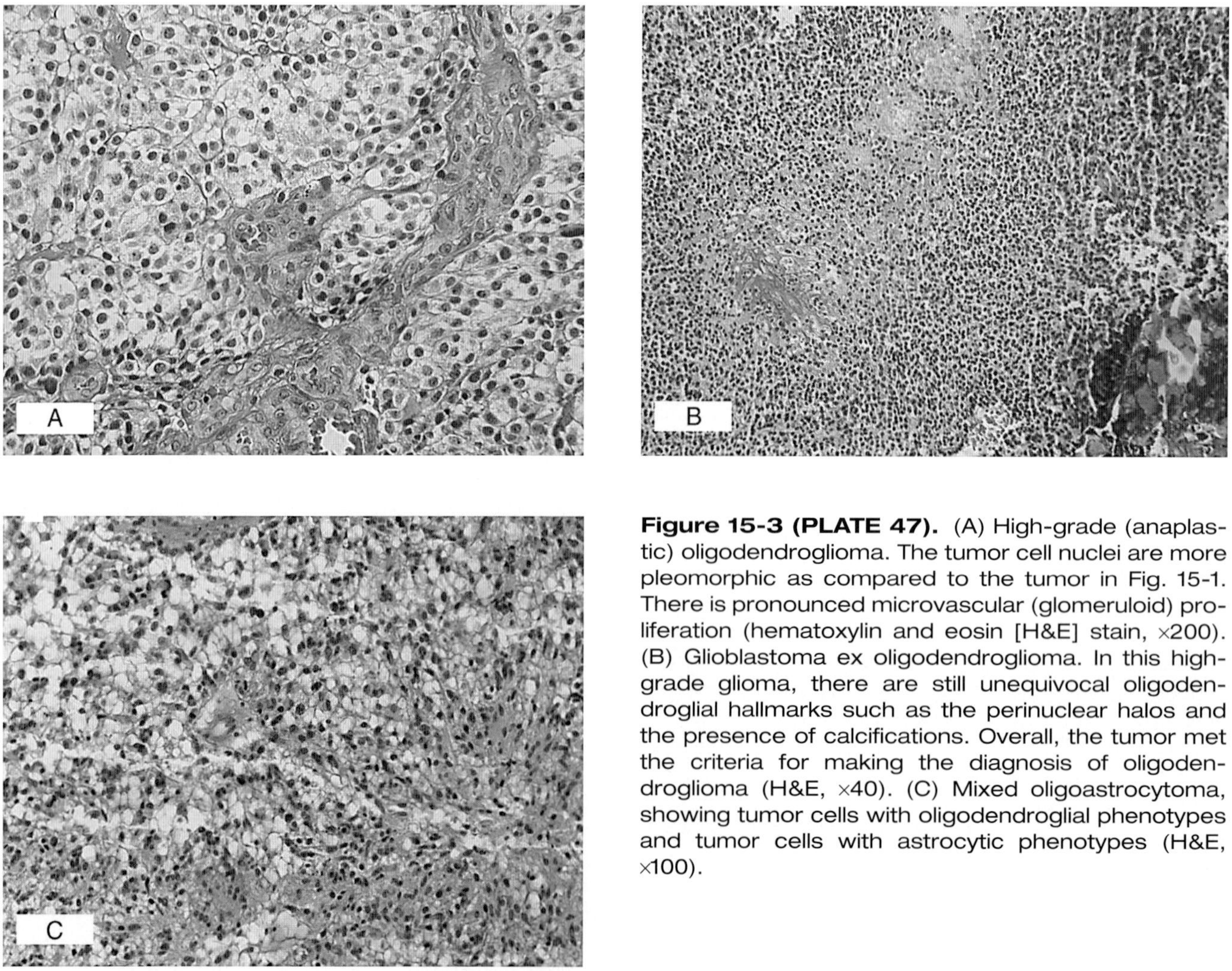

Figure 15-3 (PLATE 47). (A) High-grade (anaplastic) oligodendroglioma. The tumor cell nuclei are more pleomorphic as compared to the tumor in Fig. 15-1. There is pronounced microvascular (glomeruloid) proliferation (hematoxylin and eosin [H&E] stain, ×200). (B) Glioblastoma ex oligodendroglioma. In this high-grade glioma, there are still unequivocal oligodendroglial hallmarks such as the perinuclear halos and the presence of calcifications. Overall, the tumor met the criteria for making the diagnosis of oligodendroglioma (H&E, ×40). (C) Mixed oligoastrocytoma, showing tumor cells with oligodendroglial phenotypes and tumor cells with astrocytic phenotypes (H&E, ×100).

treatment. When reading articles on oligodendroglial tumors, one should realize that the histologic criteria for distinguishing oligodendroglial tumors from astrocytomas are subjective, with a significant interobserver variability.[12]

Histopathologic Features

Oligodendrogliomas may arise anywhere in the brain and spinal cord, with the hemispheric white matter and the frontal lobes as predilection sites. The putative derivation of oligodendroglioma was suggested by the monotonous round nuclei of this glioma subtype in its classic form, and the arrangement of the cells in regular rows or small lobules. The classic oligodendroglioma is the tumor with the "honeycomb" appearance (see Fig. 15-3A) caused by artificial perinuclear shrinkage of the cytoplasm, which is brought about by delayed fixation. Immediate placement of the specimen in fixative will yield a microscopic picture lacking the perinuclear halos, but with some faint staining in the cytoplasm instead. Another typical feature is the chicken wire–like arrangement of the microvasculature. These vessels encircle compartments of tumor cells of variable sizes. The presence of calcifications is yet another classic feature. The calcifications may be present well within the tumor tissue, but may characteristically also be noticed in relatively unaffected cerebral tissue around the tumor, where the arrangement is usually parallel to the pial surface. The presence of calcifications by itself is nonspecific and does not warrant the diagnosis of oligodendroglioma. Microcysts may be present in low-grade oligodendrogliomas, but are not an invariable or specific feature. The nuclei of oligodendroglial tumor cells are usually much larger than those of normal glial cells, and the chromatin pattern coarser.

The tumor delineation of oligodendrogliomas from normal cerebral tissue can be as gradual as usually seen in astrocytomas, but may also be rather abrupt, with formation of pushing borders. It is important to realize that in areas with diffuse infiltrating cells usually a significant astrocytic component is present, suggesting a diffuse astrocytoma. Oligodendroglial tumor cells tend to crowd along the pial surface of the brain and invade the subarachnoidal space relatively easy. However, exclusive localization in the arachnoidal space (leptomeningeal oligodendroglioma or "oligodendrogliomatosis") is extremely rare. Distant metastases have been described in bone and lungs, but this is a very rare phenomenon.

There are several histologic variations within the spectrum of oligodendroglioma. Oligodendroglial tumor tissue may undergo mucoid degeneration. Rarely, extensive areas with signet ring cells are seen. Another degenerative phenomenon is the formation of eosinophilic granular cells in these tumors, usually present in the areas of mucoid degeneration. Some tumors may display areas with cells of remarkable spindle cell morphology. A rather common tendency is the alignment of the tumor cell nuclei in rows of parallel arranged nuclei ("pseudopolar spongioblastoma"). Yet another histologic variant harbors rhabdoid tumor cells. These histopathologic presentations, sometimes very different from the classic picture, are still acknowledged as oligodendroglial because they are coexistent with tumor parts with unequivocal oligodendroglial histopathology. A particular form of anaplastic oligodendroglioma consists of scattered giant cells embedded in a glioma with otherwise features reminiscent of classic oligodendroglioma. This "polymorphous oligodendroglioma" is no longer considered a particular subtype.

Grading

Oligodendrogliomas belong to the group of diffusely infiltrating gliomas and usually evolve from low-grade into high-grade malignancy. Characteristically, this evolution takes more time in oligodendrogliomas than in astrocytic tumors. One should recognize that high-grade, anaplastic oligodendrogliomas have started as low-grade tumors, and thus both entities are basically the same tumor but present at a different stage of tumorigenesis. The histology of the low-grade oligodendrogliomas changes over time. This is witnessed in patients who undergo more than one surgery. The cell density increases over time, the tumor cell nuclei become more hyperchromatic and pleomorphic, the number of mitoses increases, microvasculature becomes hyperplastic and more extensive, and areas of necrosis appear as the result of vascular insufficiency. Several histopathologic grading schemes have been developed for oligodendrogliomas. The identification of the relevant histologic features for grading of oligodendrogliomas has proven to be difficult, however. Similar to the situation in the astrocytic tumors, the proposed schemes often lack a clear outline such as how to attribute scores to the features and how to define the respective grades. The grading scheme of Smith and associates[45] was univocal in scoring the features (and used a minimum of features), but the definition of the grades was imperfect. The St. Anne-Mayo scheme, developed for astrocytomas, has been adapted for use in oligodendrogliomas, with a reduction of the four respective grades to only two: low-grade and high-grade malignancy.[46] In the WHO classification of CNS tumors, the presence of high cell density, cytologic atypia, and high mitotic index within an oligodendroglial tumor are considered sufficient for the diagnosis of a high-grade oligodendroglial tumor, but the evaluation of these features is subject to large interobserver variation and no cut-off score for the mitotic index is provided.[44] The presence of microvascular proliferation and necrosis in oligodendroglial tumors warrants the attribution of a high-malignancy grade; both features were repeatedly identified as the most significant factors for survival.

Immunohistochemical staining for the proliferating cell antigen Ki-67 (by the MIB-1 monoclonal antibody) is very useful for estimating proliferation, but is not officially incorporated in any grading scheme. Another controversial issue is the delineation of anaplastic oligodendroglioma from glioblastoma, particularly in cases of glioblastoma in which oligodendroglial parts may be discerned (see Fig. 15-3B).

Mixed Oligoastrocytomas and Oligodendrogliomas Containing Glial Fibrillary Acidic Protein (GFAP)-Positive Cells

Approximately half of oligodendrogliomas contain GFAP-positive cells. These cells may be classic gemistocytic cells, that is, cells with voluptuous cytoplasm and few, short, and inconspicuous cell processes, with a somewhat flattened, eccentric placed nucleus. Miniature forms of these cells were named "mini-gemistocytes," and these cells usually have a somewhat more round nucleus. Together with the gliofibrillary oligodendrocytes, that is, neoplastic oligodendrocytes with a small rim of cytoplasm immunopositive for GFAP, these cells are called *transitional cells*: cells that are considered oligodendrocytic in nature, but with astrocytic differentiation as revealed by GFAP immunopositivity.[47] Although there is no serious objection in calling tumors with transitional cells mixed oligoastrocytomas, most authors consider tumors with transitional cells as pure oligodendrogliomas, unless there is another neoplastic astrocytic component in addition to the neoplastic oligodendrocytes. Most of the (otherwise classic) oligodendrogliomas harboring transitional cells are tumors in which the characteristic loss of 1p is found. Mixed oligoastrocytomas are considered tumors consisting of neoplastic oligodendrocytes and neoplastic astrocytes (see Fig. 15-3C). In the majority of these cases this mixture is diffuse; that is, cells of both lineages are intermingled. Tumors with completely separate fields of oligodendroglial and astrocytic cells are encountered rarely. This variant was designated as "compact type" of mixed oligoastrocytoma.[48] It is obvious that the delineation of the pure gliomas from a mixed glioma is subject to large interindividual differences. Attempts have been made to provide cut-off values for an oligodendroglial component in cases of mixed gliomas.[49–51] A considerable intratumoral variation in composition of the tumor, individual tumor cells with ambiguous morphologic characteristics, sampling errors, and interobserver variation are responsible for skepticism in the practical usefulness of such criteria. Not surprisingly, incidence figures of mixed oligoastrocytomas are hard to provide, and one should realize that papers addressing mixed tumors vary considerably in inclusion criteria of the tumors that were the subject of study. From recent data on genetic characteristics of oligodendroglioma (i.e., allelic losses of 1p and 19q) on the one hand, and those of astrocytoma (i.e., losses of chromosome 10, gains on 17, and p53 mutations) on the other hand, it is much more likely that the mixed oligoastrocytomas do not exist as a clinical entity. Genetically, oligoastrocytomas fall apart into two different groups, with either typical oligodendroglial chromosomal lesions or typical astrocytic chromosomal lesions.[15]

Differential Diagnosis

The differential diagnosis of oligodendroglioma includes basically all tumors in which clear cells are present. A pitfall in the diagnosis is the oligodendroglioma appearance of edematous white matter in which normal oligodendrocytes have obtained perinuclear halos. As to the delineation of oligodendroglioma from other neoplasms, there are mimics within and outside the glioma group. Metastases of clear-cell carcinomas of renal origin can be relatively easily differentiated by using immunohistochemistry for cytokeratins. Within the group of glial tumors, oligodendrogliomas may morphologically be confused with clear-cell ependymomas, central neurocytomas, and with clear cells in pilocytic astrocytomas. The delineation of the central neurocytoma is made with anti-synaptophysin antibodies. Nevertheless, some have discerned neuronal differentiation in oligodendrogliomas, blurring the differential diagnosis. The oligodendroglioma tumor cells inconsistently express proteins of developing oligodendrocytes. The results of practical use of antibodies against such antigens as myelin basic protein (MBP), myelin-associated glycoprotein (MAG), and galactocerebroside (GALC) have been variable.[52–54] Other oligodendroglia-progenitor cell markers, PDGFR, NG2, and proteolipid protein (PLP), have not proven to be useful in pathology practice because of lack of specificity. In a minority of tumors, Olig-1 and Olig-2, encoding basic helix-loop-helix transcription factors expressed in developing oligodendrocytes, were reported to be specific for oligodendrogliomas.[55,56] A recent study, however, observed that the expression of oligodendrocyte lineage gene (*OLIG*)-*1* and *OLIG2* is not limited to oligodendroglioma.[57] In particular pilocytic astrocytomas were found to express high levels of *OLIG* genes.

The ultrastructure of oligodendrogliomas is rather nonspecific, although in some cases crystalline structures have been discovered. Presently, electron microscopy as a tool in the determination of tumors is scarcely used.

▶ PROGNOSIS

Prognosis in the "Pregenetic" Era

The recognition of a classical oligodendroglioma, or of an oligodendroglial component in the case of a mixed tumor, has prognostic implications for the patient: In general, oligodendroglial tumors have a better outcome than astrocytic tumors of comparable malignancy. The prognosis of mixed oligoastrocytoma falls in between those of the pure gliomas. Still, even low-grade oligodendroglial tumors with a median survival time of 10 years or more have, apart from the occasional exception, a fatal outcome.[50,58–61] These tumors should thus never be considered "benign." A few data from selected studies provide an indication of patient prognosis:

- In a prospective study of low-grade glioma, the median survival in low-grade oligodendroglial tumors or oligoastrocytoma was 8.2 years, in contrast to 5.0 years in astrocytoma ($p = 0.011$; Fig. 15-4).[59]
- Retrospective studies on low-grade glioma patients reported a longer overall survival with low-grade oligodendroglial tumors or oligoastrocytomas compared with patients with low-grade astrocytomas (13 vs. 7.5 years, $p = 0.003$); 5-year survival rate in low-grade oligodendroglial tumors was approximately 75%.[46,62]
- Studies on supratentorial anaplastic glioma reported that patients with AOD had the longest median survival time (5.3 years) and a higher 5-year survival rate (approximately 40%) compared with patients with glioblastoma multiforme (8 months) or anaplastic astrocytoma and anaplastic oligoastrocytoma (13–14 months; Fig. 15-5).[63,64]
- Median survival for mixed anaplastic oligoastrocytomas was twice as long as the median survival of anaplastic astrocytoma (7.3 vs. 3.0 years).[58]

These data also show the influence of the tumor grade on the prognosis of oligodendroglial tumors. The tumor grade was the single most important prognostic factor for progression-free and overall survival before the prognostic significance of chromosomal lesions on the outcome of oligodendroglial tumors became established. Various anaplastic histologic features, including cell density, the number of mitoses (including Ki-67 labeling index), the presence of endothelial hyperplasia, necrosis, and the presence of pleomorphism are independent prognostic factors for AOD.[65,66] The current WHO classification divides oligodendroglial tumors into low-grade oligodendroglioma and anaplastic oligodendroglioma, but studies suggest that this dichotomy may actually obscure relevant prognostic differences. In anaplastic oligodendroglial tumors with endothelial proliferation and necrosis (formerly also designated Smith D), the prognosis is almost as bad as GBM, with a median survival time of about 18 months![45,67] The intermediate prognosis for low-grade mixed oligoastrocytoma and anaplastic oligoastrocytoma is explained by the observation that these tumors are genetically either of astrocytic or of oligodendroglial lineage (see below).

Known clinical prognostic factors are patient age, the performance status, and the type of presentation (seizures vs. focal deficits or increased intracranial pressure). The presence of enhancement on neuroimaging studies is also of prognostic significance, and probably reflects endothelial proliferation.[66] High uptake of the radioactively labeled ligand ^{11}C-methionine as measured with PET was found related to the prognosis and tumor grade.[42,68] Although these data suggest that ^{11}C-methionine

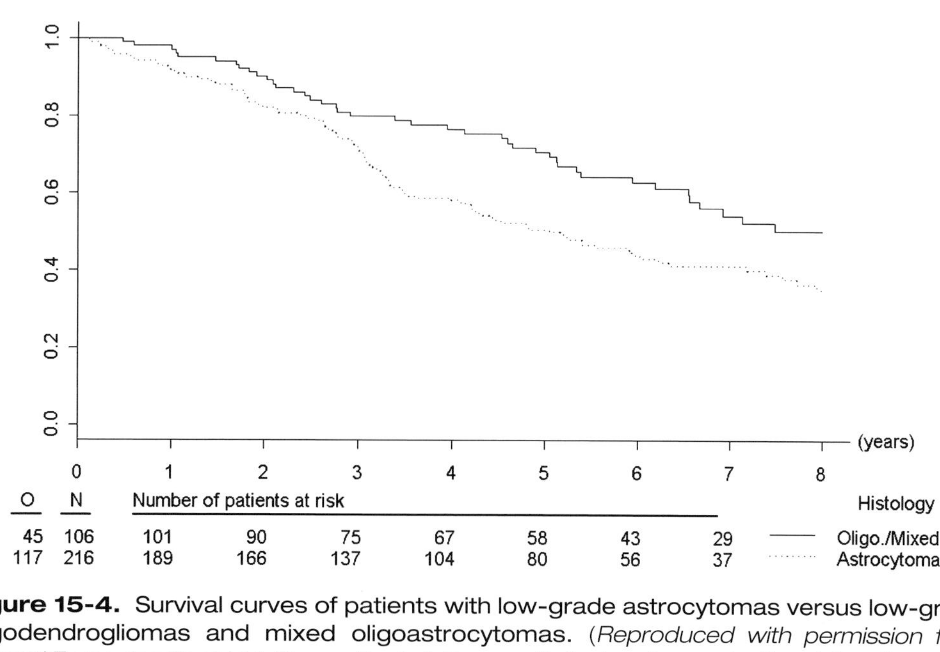

Figure 15-4. Survival curves of patients with low-grade astrocytomas versus low-grade oligodendrogliomas and mixed oligoastrocytomas. (*Reproduced with permission from Pignatti F, van den Bent MJ, Curran D, et al. Prognostic factors for survival in adult patients with cerebral low-grade glioma. J Clin Oncol 2002;20:2076–2084.*)

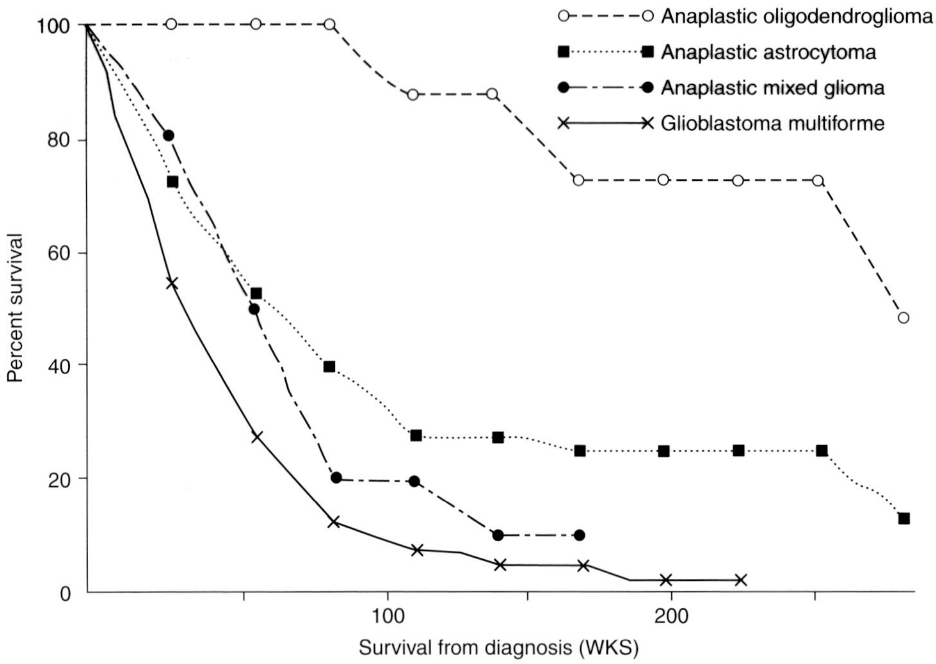

Figure 15-5. Survival curves for patients with anaplastic oligodendroglioma, anaplastic astrocytoma, anaplastic mixed glioma, and glioblastoma multiforme. (*Reproduced with permission from Winger MJ, Macdonald DR, Cairncross JG. Supratentorial anaplastic gliomas in adults. J Neurosurg 1989;71:487–493.*)

PET scanning could be of use to select patients for treatment, the overlap between low- and high-grade tumors combined with the absence of prognostic studies of sufficient size and the few sites with access to this technique limit the usefulness of this technique for everyday practice. Radioactive-labeled glucose [^{18}F]fluorodeoxyglucose positron emission tomography (FDG-PET) scanning is of limited usefulness in gliomas because of the high glucose metabolism of the normal cortex. Thallium single-photon emission computed tomography (SPECT) scanning is usually negative in low-grade gliomas.

Prognosis and Genotype

For oligodendroglial tumors, combined loss of 1p and 19q is a more important prognostic factor than either histology or clinical characteristics.[12,69] Virtually all oligodendroglial tumors with combined loss of 1p and 19q respond to PCV chemotherapy, and the presence of 1p deletions in oligodendroglial tumors is associated with longer progression-free survival after radiotherapy or chemotherapy.[8,24,25] Furthermore, oligodendroglial tumors with 1p/19q loss tend to have a more indolent behavior before initiation of treatment compared with tumors without 1p/19q loss.[7,8] In contrast, the presence of EGFR amplification, loss of 10q, *PTEN* mutations, and *CDKN2A* are associated with a worse prognosis.[7,13,18,24] These findings have been confirmed in oligoastrocytomas.[23] The picture that emerges from these observations is that there are two different sets of tumors with oligodendroglial morphology:

- One set with combined loss of 1p/19q, with, in general, a more typical oligodendroglial tumor morphology, a better prognosis, and better response to treatment
- A second set with genetic lesions that are more characteristic of tumors of astrocytic lineage, less sensitive to treatment, more often located in the temporal lobe, and have a prognosis resembling that of astrocytic tumors[11,17]

Because all the evidence points out that the genotype characterizes these tumors better than conventional histology, genotyping of tumors with oligodendroglial elements is likely to become a standard diagnostic procedure.[14] A first example of the potential value of the molecular diagnostics in oligodendroglial tumors is the recently published study by Nutt and associates.[70] This study showed that gene expression profiling using microarrays of a set of histologically nonclassical glioma proved superior in predicting prognosis in comparison to classical pathology.[70] Gene expression profiling could also distinguish low-grade from high-grade oligodendroglioma.[71] Although this is a rapidly developing field of research that promises tailored treatment in the long run, it is still in its infancy and the treatment implications of the genotype of oligodendroglial tumors for individual patients are still far from clear. The established treatment modalities for oligodendroglial tumors are still limited to surgery, radiotherapy, and chemotherapy ("cut, burn, and poison"), but this holds for all glial tumors, irrespective of their genetic background. Prospective studies in which treatment decisions were based on the genotype of the tumors have not been done. Until those are available it remains entirely speculative whether one, for example, should prefer chemotherapy above radiation therapy in oligodendroglial tumors with 1p/19q loss.

▶ TREATMENT

Until recently, randomized phase III trials on the treatment of glial tumors combined both astrocytic and oligodendroglial tumors. Trials that investigated the role of chemotherapy in newly diagnosed oligodendroglioma were not started until 1994–1995, and results are not yet available. Consequently, most data on the treatment of oligodendroglial tumors are derived from retrospective surveys with all their inherent pitfalls. The exceptions are the many chemotherapy studies devoted to oligodendroglial tumors, which are mainly uncontrolled single-arm studies. The initial treatment decisions depend on the mode of clinical and radiological presentation: young patients with "low-grade glioma-like lesions" presenting with seizures only are approached differently by many clinicians.

Treatment in Low-Grade Glioma/Oligodendroglioma

The best treatment policy for young patients with presumed low-grade glioma on neuroradiologic imaging who present with seizures only constitutes an ongoing controversy. The MRI findings suggestive of low-grade glioma are nonspecific; such lesions may be nonneoplastic or may harbor an anaplastic tumor. Because many of these patients may remain stable for a protracted period of time without any treatment, many physicians tend to defer treatment until clinical or radiological progression. An important rationale for the deferral of radiotherapy (XRT) is the concern that XRT may contribute to the cognitive deficits in patients with low-grade glioma.[61,72] A large Dutch study recently questioned this assumption, finding that only a large XRT fraction size (>2 Gy) and the use of antiepileptic drugs were associated with cognitive deficits in low-grade glioma patients.[73] Whether XRT to "limited fields" in fractions of 1.5 to 1.8 Gy increases long-term cognitive deficits in low-grade glioma patients is at present unclear.

Advocates of early intervention in patients with presumed low-grade glioma question whether it is safe to refrain from histologic verification of the presumed tumor. Retrospective studies show that up to 30% of patients with nonenhancing low-grade glioma-like lesions carry an anaplastic tumor. Thus, they recommend obtaining histologic proof in case of a presumed low-grade glioma.[40,41,74] An alternative approach is to repeat the MRI investigation within 2 to 3 months after the first MRI suggestive of a presumed low-grade glioma, which will readily detect early progression. There is general agreement that in patients with enhancing lesions, evidence of mass effect, focal neurologic signs or symptoms, or signs of increased intracranial pressure, treatment should be initiated without delay. Whether ^{11}C-methionine PET scanning is useful for the selection of patients that require treatment is undetermined.[68]

Surgical Management

Surgery for glioma serves three goals: verification of the nature of the lesion, relief of signs and symptoms in patients suffering from a lesion with mass effect or producing seizures, and improvement of the prognosis. The relevance of the first two are generally acknowledged, but so far no trial has given evidence beyond reasonable doubt that extensive surgery improves survival compared to less extensive resections. All available data for both low- and high-grade glioma come from retrospective or post hoc analysis; no randomized controlled trial has evaluated the effect of resection on survival in glioma as the primary end point—let alone of oligodendroglial tumors. A drawback of these retrospective studies is that superficial and small tumors are more likely candidates for extensive resections. In contrast, deep-seated lesions, large tumors, or tumors with growth into midline structures may confer a worse prognosis regardless of the extent of resection. Such patients will never undergo near-complete resections.[59] This raises the question whether the observed improved outcome after a more extensive resection is a result of patient selection or an effect of the surgical intervention.

One uncontrolled study found that complete resection in low-grade oligodendroglial tumors is associated with long disease-free intervals.[75] In another study, patients who underwent subtotal resection had improved survival, although many of these patients were young and had low-grade tumors (which are favorable prognostic factors).[10,60,76] In contrast, other studies have shown that gross total resection in patients with oligodendroglial tumors provided no survival benefit.[66,77] Nonetheless, given the potential clinical benefits, it is considered standard treatment to resect glioma regardless of histology and tumor grade as extensively as is safely possible once it is decided to start treatment.

Role of Radiotherapy

Randomized trials in high-grade glioma have demonstrated that adjuvant XRT provides significant, albeit modest, improvements in survival.[78] In low-grade glioma, the benefit of early radiation therapy, as compared with XRT at the time of progression, resulted in a modest improvement of time to progression without affecting overall survival.[79] Again, no trial specifically addressed low-grade or anaplastic oligodendroglial tumors. Some retrospective studies support postoperative XRT for oligodendroglial tumors, particularly in cases of neurologic deficits or limited surgery.[80,81] Other studies have

▶ TABLE 15-1. PCV AND PCV-I (INTENSIFIED) CHEMOTHERAPY*

Drug		Standard Intensity PCV	Intensified PCV
CCNU	day 1	110 mg/m² orally	130 mg/m² orally
Vincristine	days 8 and 29	1.4 mg/m² IV; cap at 2 mg	1.4 mg/m² IV
Procarbazine	days 8–21	60 mg/m² orally	75 mg/m² orally

*Cycles to be repeated every 6–8 weeks, for a maximum of six cycles.

reported no benefit of postoperative XRT in the treatment of oligodendroglial tumors at all.[10,46,82,83] In the absence of specific XRT trials on oligodendroglial tumors, it seems reasonable to use the available trials on low-grade and high-grade gliomas for treatment decisions.

In the absence of randomized trials, one may withhold XRT in younger patients (i.e., below 45 years of age) with low-grade oligodendroglial tumors whose clinical condition is good and who have undergone a complete or almost complete resection until progression. In contrast, patients with large, unresectable, or incompletely resected tumors; focal deficits; anaplastic tumors; or enhancing lesions should be given treatment that includes XRT without delay. Following the randomized dose-finding European Organization of Research and Treatment of Cancer (EORTC) and North Central Cancer Treatment Group (NCCTG) trials, in low-grade oligodendroglial tumors, a cumulative dose of 50 to 54 Gy should be given in fractions of 1.8 Gy to limit long-term cognitive and other late sequelae.[84–86] In high-grade oligodendroglial tumors, 60 to 65 Gy in 30 to 35 fractions should be given. Nowadays, some clinicians tend to replace XRT with upfront chemotherapy. Clinical data to support this change are not available (see Fig. 15-1F; also see "Upfront Chemotherapy" below).

Role of Chemotherapy

Chemotherapy for Recurrent Oligodendroglial Tumors

Most data on chemotherapy in oligodendroglial tumors have been obtained in studies on recurrent tumors after radiotherapy. Initially, most studies investigated chemotherapy consisting of PCV (Table 15-1), whereas more recent publications focus on the new alkylating agent temozolomide. No clear explanation is yet available for the favorable response to chemotherapy of oligodendroglial tumors as compared to astrocytic tumors. There are indications that the nuclear enzyme alkyltransferase, which mediates at least a part of the cell resistance to alkylating agents, is less expressed in oligodendroglial tumors.[36] In contrast, there is no difference in methylation status of the promoter of the gene for alkyltransferase between oligodendroglioma and astrocytoma.[16] At present it seems unlikely that differences in expression of alkyltransferase accounts for the entire difference in sensitivity to chemotherapy between astrocytic tumors and oligodendroglial tumors. It also does not explain why oligodendroglial tumors with combined loss of 1p and 19q, in particular, are sensitive to chemotherapy.

First-Line Chemotherapy in Recurrent Oligodendroglial Tumors

Two regimens have been systemically investigated in first-line chemotherapy: PCV and (to a much lesser extent) temozolomide (Table 15-2). Because of the satisfactory response rates with PCV and, subsequently, with temozolomide, these regimens have become the treatments of choice. Other regimens have only been investigated as second- (or third-) line interventions. Approximately two-thirds of patients achieve a complete or partial response to PCV chemotherapy (see Table 15-2, Fig. 15-6A to D). The time to progression in these patients is, in general, 12 to 18 months, but may occasionally be longer than 24 months.[2,3,87] Because the initial publications on the chemoresponsiveness of oligodendroglial tumors used

▶ TABLE 15-2. RESPONSE RATES (%), MEDIAN TIME TO PROGRESSION, AND 12-MONTH PROGRESSION-FREE SURVIVAL (IN MONTHS) IN STUDIES OF PCV OR TEMOZOLOMIDE CHEMOTHERAPY IN RECURRENT OR NEWLY DIAGNOSED OLIGODENDROGLIAL TUMORS

Reference	Regimen	n	CR	PR	SD	MTP	12-Mo PFS
van den Bent, et al.[3]	PCV	52	17%	46%	19%	10	42%
Soffietti, et al.[87]	PCV	26	12%	50%	31%	24	80%
Cairncross, et al.[2]	PCV	24	38%	38%	17%	16	NS
EORTC 26971[89]	Temozolomide	38	26%	26%	32%	10.1	39%

CR = complete response; MTP = median time to progression; NS = not stated; PCV = procarbazine, lomustine, and vincristine; PFS = progression-free survival; PR = partial response; SD = stable disease.

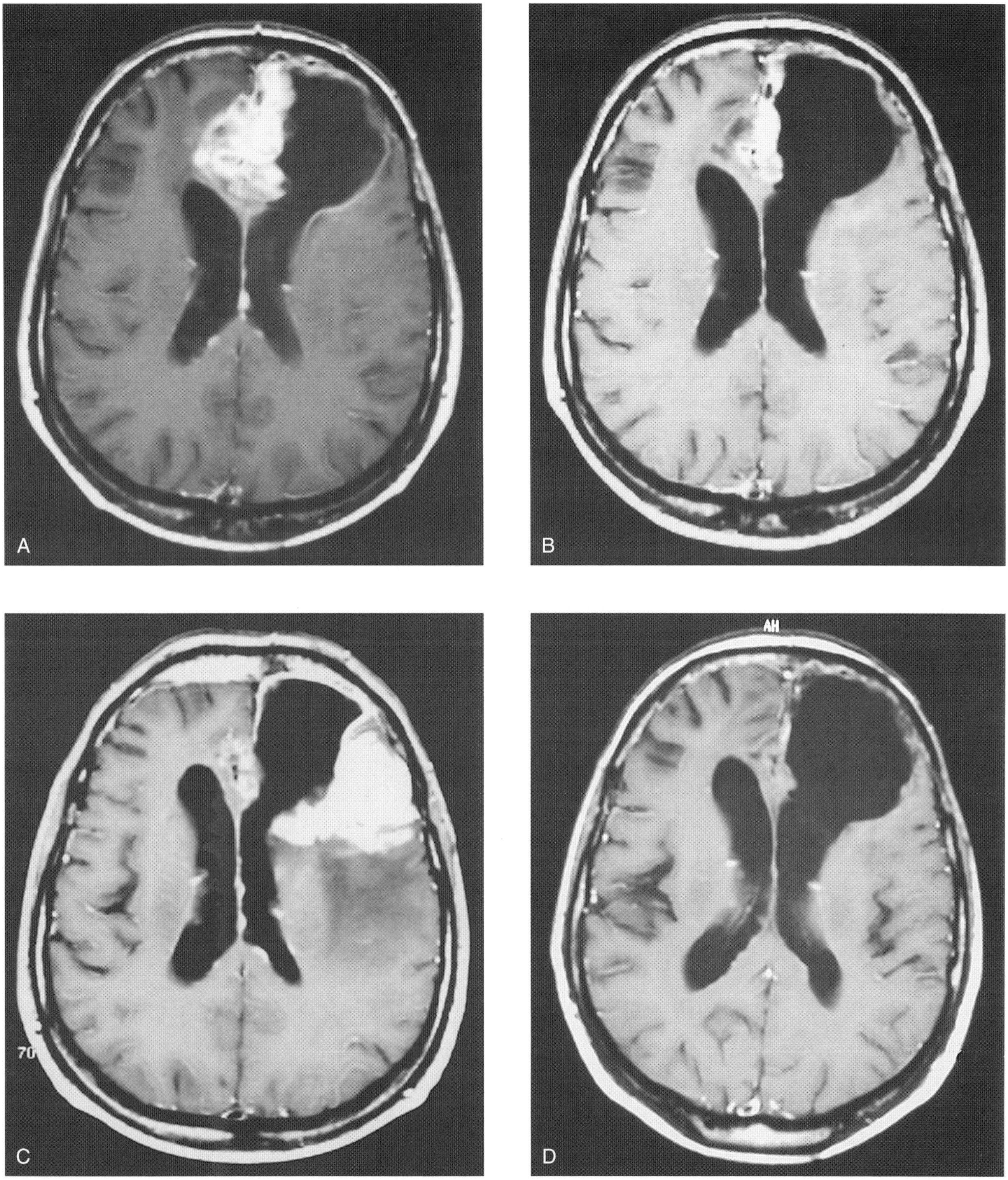

Figure 15-6. T_1-weighted images showing response to first- and second-line PCV in a 45-year-old male patient with a recurrent and leptomeningeal metastasized anaplastic oligodendroglioma with combined loss of 1p/19q. (A) Before PCV chemotherapy; (B) a partial response after six cycles; (C) recurrent tumor 15 months after the start of PCV; (D) repeated PCV chemotherapy induced a second partial response that lasted for another 6 months.

the PCV schedule, this regimen became the mainstay of treatment until the arrival of temozolomide. Although PCV is usually well tolerated, the cumulative hematologic toxicity, gastrointestinal side effects, skin toxicity, and fatigue associated with standard PCV often limit the duration and intensity of its administration. In some studies, the intensified PCV regimen was explored and was found to be considerably more toxic (especially hematologic and general side effects, including malaise and weight loss) without evidence of superior results.[2,3,88] Consequently, the intensified PCV regimen cannot be recommended. Several of these studies reported that oligoastrocytoma are less responsive to PCV, presumably because of the lower frequency of combined 1p/19q loss in oligoastrocytoma.

So far, only one prospective trial investigated first-line temozolomide in recurrent oligodendroglial tumors.[89] This trial reported a 54% response rate with 39% of patients free from progression at 12 months (Fig. 15-7). This outcome is in the lower range of the response rate, median survival, and progression-free survival at 12 months obtained in historical series with the PCV regimen. Treatment with temozolomide is well tolerated, the main side effects being (a) a short-lasting and reversible myelosuppression with thrombocytopenia and leukopenia, and (b) nausea and vomiting, which are usually easily controlled with modern 5-hydroxytryptamine (5HT)-antagonists.

This latter trial and the good results with temozolomide in recurrent anaplastic astrocytomas have raised the question of whether PCV or temozolomide is to be preferred as the first-line treatment.[90] No results of head-to-head comparisons of PCV and temozolomide are yet available. A major advantage of temozolomide is the good tolerability of this drug; in this respect, temozolomide compares favorably to the PCV regimen. Ultimately, all patients treated with either regimen relapse; even patients with a complete response usually relapse after 18 to 24 months (Fig. 15-8).

Second-Line Chemotherapy

After the introduction of temozolomide, several studies were performed that evaluated second-line temozolomide following prior PCV (Table 15-3). Twenty percent

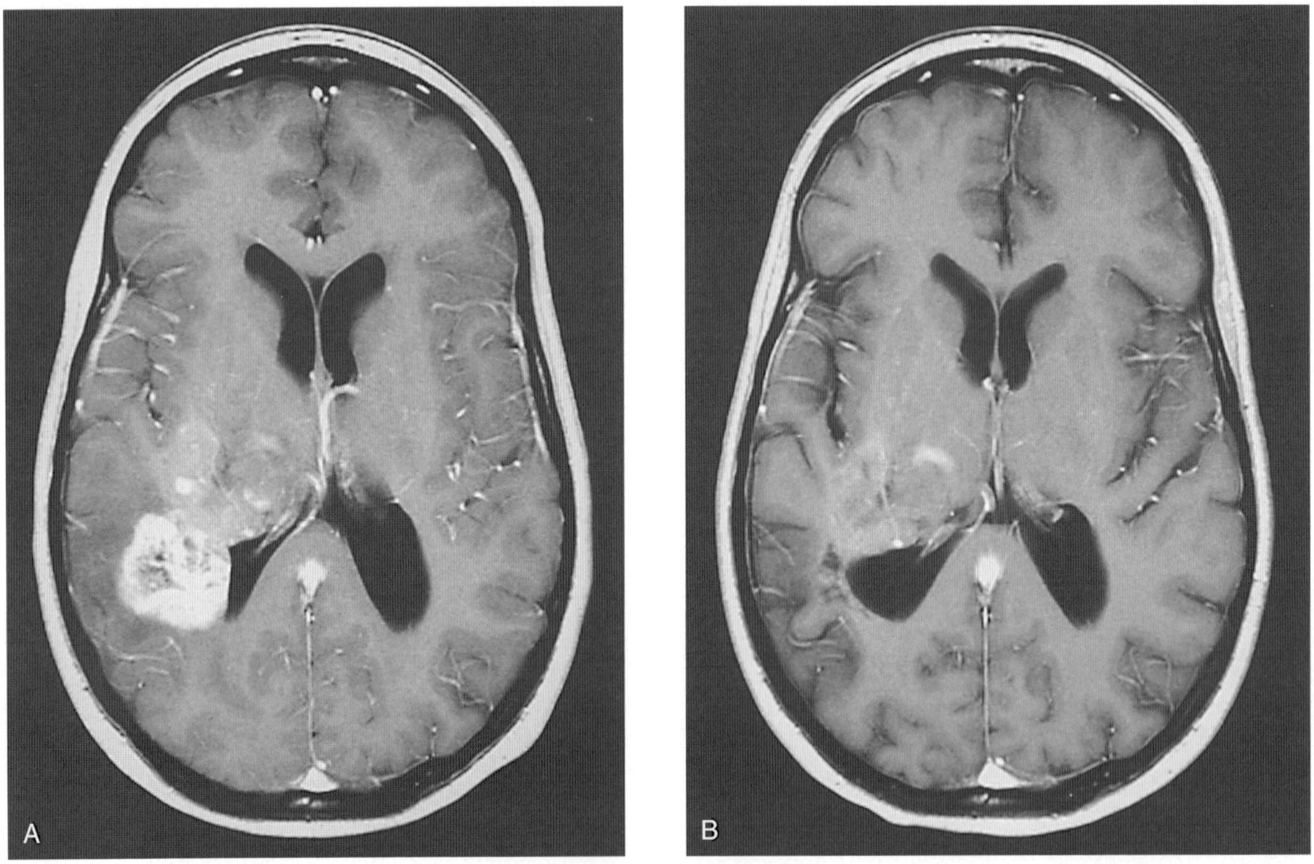

Figure 15-7. T_1-weighted images of a 31-year-old female with a recurrent oligoastrocytoma without loss of 1p/19q, showing the beginning of a necrotic center within the enhancing area (A). Despite the absence of combined loss of 1p/19q, she had an almost complete response to temozolomide (B), which lasted for 9 months. She had no response to second-line PCV chemotherapy.

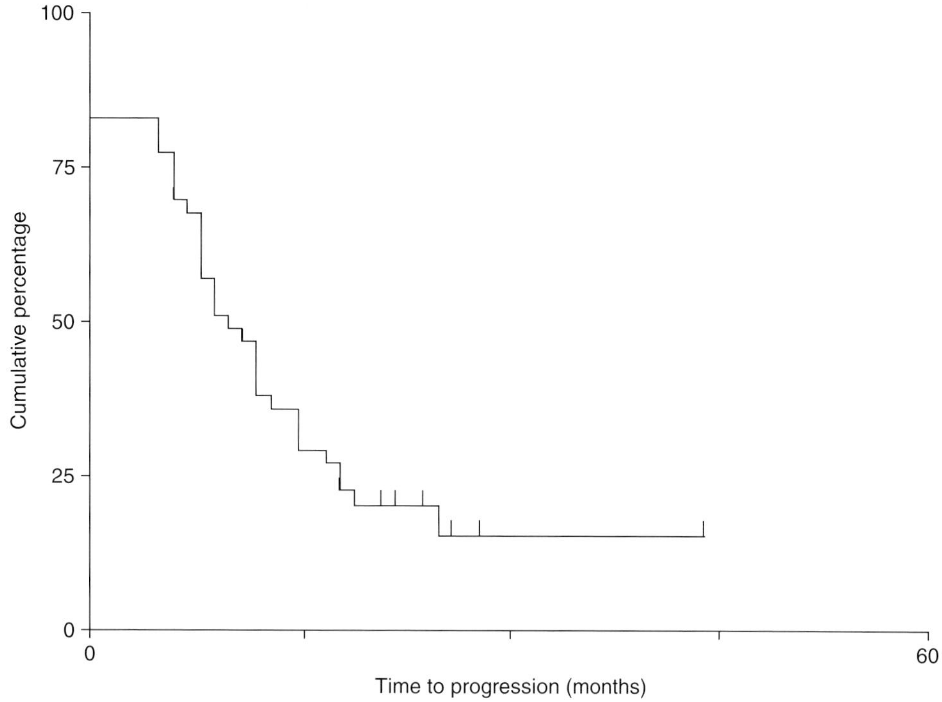

Figure 15-8. Kaplan-Meier survival curve of a group of 52 patients treated with PCV chemotherapy for recurrent and enhancing oligodendroglial tumors. (*With permission from van den Bent MJ, Kros JM, Heimans JJ, et al. Response rate and prognostic factors of recurrent oligodendroglioma treated with procarbazine, CCNU and vincristine chemotherapy. Neurology 1998;51:1140–1145.*)

to 30% of patients progressing after prior PCV chemotherapy (either given adjuvant or at first recurrence) respond to temozolomide, with 30% to 50% and 10% to 30% of patients free from progression at 6 and 12 months, respectively.[91–93] A fourth trial predominantly accrued patients who had responded favorably to PCV (response rate to first-line PCV: 83%).[94] In this trial, the objective response rate to temozolomide was 44%, with 50% and 25% of patients free from progression at 6 and 12 months. The key message of this trial is that better patient selection results in a more favorable outcome. In all series, temozolomide was well tolerated, even in patients who discontinued PCV for toxicity.

Limited data are now also available on the reverse sequence: PCV after first-line temozolomide. In 24 patients treated with second-line PCV for recurrent oligodendroglial tumors after prior temozolomide, 17% of patients achieved an objective response, and 50% of

▶ **TABLE 15-3.** RESULTS OF SECOND-LINE CHEMOTHERAPY WITH EITHER TEMOZOLOMIDE OR PCV IN RECURRENT OLIGODENDROGLIOMA FOLLOWING FIRST-LINE OR ADJUVANT TREATMENT WITH THE OTHER AGENT

Study	n	Second-Line TMZ/PCV	Response in First-Line	OR (%)	SD (%)	Median PFS (Mo)	6-Mo PFS (%)	12-Mo PFS (%)
van den Bent, et al.[91]	27	TMZ	38%	26	30	4	44	27
EORTC 26972[92]	28	TMZ	50%	28	30	3.7	29	11
Constanza, et al.[93]	34	TMZ	50%	26	44	6	48	30
Chinot, et al.[94]	48	TMZ	83%	44	40	6.7	50	25
Triebels, et al.[95]	24	PCV	54%	17	46	6	NS	21

OR = objective response (complete or partial response); PFS = progression-free survival; SD = stable disease; TMZ/PCV = regimen in second-line, either PCV or temozolomide.

patients remained free from progression for at least 6 months.[95] The median time to progression in the 15 responding and stabilized patients was 10 months, implying that PCV is an option for failures after first-line temozolomide. However, 25% of patients had to discontinue second-line PCV because of toxicity, in particular, delayed hematologic recovery. No severe acute toxicities were seen.

These studies on second-line temozolomide and PCV for progression after prior treatment with the other regimen show that whatever sequence of treatment is used, the response rate of the second-line is limited. Both regimens apply alkylating drugs, and these findings suggest cross-resistance.

Other Second-Line Chemotherapy After Prior PCV or Temozolomide Chemotherapy

Second-line therapies following first-line PCV or temozolomide have only moderate response rates and low percentages of patients remaining free from progression at 6 and 12 months. Apart from temozolomide, paclitaxel, CPT-11 (irinotecan), carboplatin, etoposide plus cisplatin, and topotecan have been investigated for second-line chemotherapy in AOD (Table 15-4).[96–100] Of 20 patients previously treated with surgery, XRT, and PCV, three (15%) obtained a partial response and seven (35%) achieved stable disease when treated with paclitaxel.[97] Median duration of response and stable disease in these patients was 9 months (range: 4–10 months). All patients had progressive disease at 12 months. Toxicity was primarily hematologic; 10% of patients had grade 3 anemia, and 30% and 15% of patients experienced grade 3 or 4 thrombocytopenia and neutropenia, respectively. Similarly, 2 of 15 (13%) treated patients responded to CPT-11, and 33% of patients remained free from disease progression at 6 months.[98] Likewise, 3 of 23 (13%) patients treated with second-line carboplatin 560 mg/m^2 once every 4 weeks achieved a response.[99] Only one of the responding patients was free from progression at 12 months. Myelosuppression was severe, with a grade 3 or 4 thrombocytopenia in 60% of patients and grade 3 or 4 granulocytopenia in 48% of patients. No responses were observed in 16 patients on second-line topotecan 1.5 mg/m^2 on days 1 to 5 in 3-week cycles, resulting in premature discontinuation of the study.[100] Grade 3 or 4 granulocytopenia was observed in 15 of these patients, requiring dose reductions in half of the cycles.

Four of 10 patients treated with cisplatin and etoposide as second-line chemotherapy after first-line PCV experienced an overall response; however, none of the responding patients was progression-free at 12 months.[96] Brandes and associates[101] investigated carboplatin 350 mg/m^2 on day 1 and teniposide 50 mg/m^2 on days 1 to 3 in 4-week cycles in patients with recurrent disease after both PCV and temozolomide. Two partial responses were observed, and 35% of patients were free from progression at 6 months. At this dosage of carboplatin only two patients required 25% dose reductions because of hematologic toxicity.

A considerable drawback of some of these agents (paclitaxel, CPT-11) is that they are metabolized through the hepatic cytochrome CYP 3A4, which implies that their metabolism may have been induced by enzyme-inducing antiepileptic agents (particularly phenytoin, carbamazepine, and phenobarbital). This limits the activity of many cytotoxic agents in glial tumors (which may also have affected the observed activity in the above-mentioned trials).

High-Dose Chemotherapy with Autologous Bone Marrow Rescue

Based on a single case report, high-dose thiotepa myeloablative chemotherapy with autologous stem cell support has been investigated both in newly diagnosed

▶ TABLE 15-4. THE OUTCOME TO SECOND-LINE (*AND THIRD-LINE) CHEMOTHERAPY AT FAILURE OF PCV IN PATIENTS WITH ANAPLASTIC OLIGODENDROGLIOMA AND OLIGOASTROCYTOMA

Study	Previous Treatment	Agent	N	OR, n (%)	SD, n (%)	MTP, months	6-Mo PFS, %	12-Mo PFS, %
Chamberlain, et al.[97]	PCV	Paclitaxel	20	3 (15)	7 (35)	4	35	0
Chamberlain[98]	PCV	CPT-11	15	2 (13)	5 (33)	—	33	—
Soffietti, et al.[99]	PCV	Carboplatin	23	3 (13)	10 (43)	3	35	9
Peterson, et al.[96]	Various	VP16 + cisplatin	10	3 (30)	1 (10)	—	20	0
Bélanger, et al.[100]		Topotecan	16	0	11 (68)	3.8	NS	NS
Brandes, et al.*[101]	PCV, temozolomide	Carboplatin + VM26	23	2 (9)	12 (52)	4.2	34.8	NS

*Third-line chemotherapy after prior PCV and temozolomide.
MTP = median time to progression; OR = overall response (either complete or partial); PCV = procarbazine, lomustine, and vincristine; PFS = progression-free survival; SD = stable disease.

oligodendrogliomas and in recurrent disease. Patients eligible for these studies had a prior response to PCV chemotherapy; these studies were thus limited to a subset of chemotherapy-sensitive disease. In patients with recurrences after prior radiotherapy, this approach was considered too toxic.[102] Although some durable responses were observed (20 of 38 patients were treated with the high-dose regimen, 6 of whom remained free from progression at 2 years), the authors concluded that this was a disappointing strategy with a median overall progression-free survival of 20 months. In newly diagnosed patients, this approach appears better tolerated, with an estimated median progression-free survival of 69 months.[103] Of 69 patients, 39 participated in the high-dose chemotherapy part of the study; in those patients, radiotherapy was deferred until progression. Thus far 12 transplantation patients have relapsed. Persistent nonenhancing tumor correlated with relapse. The median hospital stay for the transplantation procedure was 20 days. The obvious limitation of this study design is its uncontrolled nature. In the absence of a comparator arm, no conclusions can be drawn except for the expected feasibility of the approach. In view of the generally limited role of myeloablative chemotherapy in solid tumors, small phase II studies with their inherent selection bias will not establish the value of this approach. Until randomized studies have been done, myeloablative chemotherapy in oligodendroglial tumors must be considered experimental.

Adjuvant Chemotherapy

The value of adjuvant chemotherapy in high-grade glioma was finally shown in a large meta-analysis that showed that it increases the 1- and 2-year survival rate by approximately 5%, from 40% to 46% and from 15% to 20%, respectively.[104] As this benefit is rather small and no data exist on the influence on the quality of life of adjuvant chemotherapy, the clinical value of adjuvant chemotherapy in high-grade glioma remains a matter of debate. The sensitivity to chemotherapy of recurrent oligodendroglioma has renewed the interest in the role of adjuvant chemotherapy for this subset of glial tumors. Subgroup analysis of studies on adjuvant chemotherapy in anaplastic glioma failed to show evidence of increased survival after adjuvant chemotherapy in the subset of patients with oligodendroglial tumors.[105] In a chemotherapy-sensitive tumor one would expect a larger benefit from adjuvant chemotherapy, but this may not be the case if effective salvage treatment is available. Under these circumstances adjuvant chemotherapy may prolong progression-free survival without improving overall survival. Theoretically, it may well be more a matter of the best timing of the chemotherapy: the adjuvant setting or at recurrence. An often forgotten advantage of reserving chemotherapy until the time of recurrence and the presence of measurable disease is that this allows the discontinuation of treatment if the tumor proves to be chemotherapy-resistant. This avoids the useless continuation of an inactive treatment. At present two ongoing trials (EORTC and Radiation Therapy Oncology Group [RTOG]) are investigating the value of adjuvant or early chemotherapy in oligodendroglial tumors.

Upfront Chemotherapy in Newly Diagnosed Anaplastic Oligodendroglioma

A novel development is the treatment of newly diagnosed oligodendroglial tumors with upfront chemotherapy strategies, with or without subsequent XRT.[106] Although this may seem appealing in a chemotherapy-sensitive tumor, in the absence of randomized trials no conclusions can be drawn from the limited data published. The key issues here are the toxicities of treatment: Why should a local treatment delivered with modern XRT techniques be abandoned for a treatment with systemic toxicity? It is clear that with upfront PCV or temozolomide chemotherapy good responses are obtained, but whether the overall outcome is as good as following XRT is unknown. It is also unclear whether in case of a good response to chemotherapy XRT should be withheld. In view of the expected long overall survival in oligodendroglial tumors, these questions may be more a matter of side effects and of active salvage regimens than of progression-free survival. Phase III trials are needed to answer these questions.

Upfront Chemotherapy in Low-Grade Oligodendroglial Tumors

The clinical data on the use of chemotherapy in newly diagnosed low-grade oligodendroglial tumors are limited, but suggest that these tumors are as sensitive as their anaplastic counterparts.[88,107–109] A practical problem is that radiologic favorable responses are very infrequent. This is presumably a result of the similar MRI appearance of active tumor to reactive gliosis within a tumor that responds to chemotherapy. However, the clinical improvement and improved seizure control often outweigh the marginal MRI scan improvement.[107,109] From this perspective, the time to progression is more meaningful than radiographic response as an outcome measurement, but is less practical for the management of individual patients or for phase II studies. There is evidence that metabolic imaging (e.g., ^{11}C-methionine PET imaging) may be of use to assess response in low-grade oligodendroglioma (Fig. 15-9).

Both the PCV regimen and temozolomide have been investigated in low-grade oligodendroglial tumors.[88,107–109] Even tumors without loss of 1p/19q and mixed oligoastrocytoma may respond, and responses may last for a considerable period of time. In the absence of comparative trials, upfront chemotherapy may be a particularly appropriate choice for patients with large oligodendroglial tumor lesions (oligodendroglial "gliomatosis cerebri") so as to avoid whole-brain XRT in

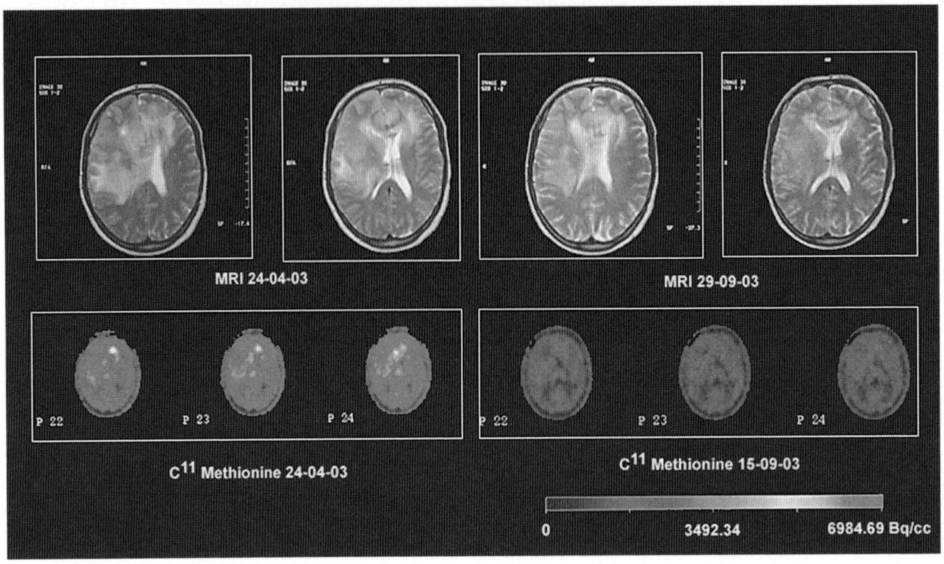

Figure 15-9 (PLATE 48). PCV chemotherapy in low-grade oligodendroglioma: T_2-weighted MR images and ^{11}C-methionine positron emission tomography scan before (left) and after (right) two cycles of PCV chemotherapy in a patient with gliomatosis cerebri with oligodendroglial morphology (1p/19q status unknown). Although there is some improvement of the MRI abnormalities, this does not qualify for a partial response according to Macdonald's criteria. In contrast, there is a marked reduction of the abnormal uptake of ^{11}C-methionine. During treatment, behavioral abnormalities that had been present for 2 years normalized.

patients with a favorable prognosis for long-term disease-free survival. Whether this is also useful in patients with smaller lesions who are candidates for XRT with limited fields is a matter of side effects. As noted above (see "Upfront Chemotherapy"), it is questionable whether it is rational to try to avoid limited-field XRT of a small brain lesion delivered by modern irradiation techniques by replacing it with prolonged systemic chemotherapy.

▶ FUTURE DIRECTIONS

Some 15 years after the initial observation of the sensitivity of oligodendroglial tumors to PCV chemotherapy, it is now clear that the chemotherapy-sensitive oligodendroglial tumor is characterized by a specific genotype showing combined loss of 1p and 19q. Although this allows better identification of treatment-sensitive tumors, no real outcome improvement has been achieved since the initial discovery of the sensitivity to the PCV regimen, and all patients still die from recurrent disease. The introduction of temozolomide does not improve treatment efficacy, its real advantage being better tolerability by patients. The obvious conclusion is that with a superior identification of treatment-sensitive tumors we still lack more active treatments and a more fundamental knowledge of the driving force behind the oligodendroglial tumor. With presently available knowledge of the genetic alterations of oligodendroglial tumors, we are better able to predict response to treatment. At the same time, it appears that the incidence of oligodendroglial tumors with combined loss of 1p/19q is in the same range as the incidence of oligodendroglial tumors in historical papers on histologically typical oligodendroglial tumors: 4% to 5% of all glial tumors. We are dealing again with an uncommon disease that requires multiinstitutional trials to achieve further progress. Further improvements in outcome must be derived from a better knowledge of the cellular abnormalities that characterize an oligodendroglial tumors. Gene array studies and proteomics may provide the knowledge required for this progress.

REFERENCES

1. Bailey P, Bucy PC. Oligodendrogliomas of the brain. J Pathol 1929;32:735–751.
2. Cairncross G, Macdonald D, Ludwin S, et al. Chemotherapy for anaplastic oligodendroglioma. J Clin Oncol 1994;12: 2013–2021.
3. van den Bent MJ, Kros JM, Heimans JJ, et al. Response rate and prognostic factors of recurrent oligodendroglioma treated with procarbazine, CCNU and vincristine chemotherapy. Neurology 1998;51:1140–1145.

4. Coons SW, Johnson PC, Scheithauer BW, et al. Improving diagnostic accuracy and interobserver concordance in the classification and grading of primary gliomas. Cancer 1997;79:1381–1391.
5. Reifenberger J, Reifenberger G, Liu L, et al. Molecular genetic analysis of oligodendroglial tumors shows preferential allelic deletions on 19q and 1p. Am J Pathol 1994;145:1175–1190.
6. Smith JS, Alderete B, Minn Y, et al. Localization of common deletion regions on 1p and 19q in human gliomas and their association with histological subtype. Oncogene 1999;18:4144–4152.
7. Cairncross JG, Ueki K, Zlatescu MC, et al. Specific genetic predictors of chemotherapeutic response and survival in patients with anaplastic oligodendrogliomas. J Natl Cancer Inst 1998;90:1473–1479.
8. van den Bent MJ, Looijenga LHJ, Langenberg K, et al. Chromosomal anomalies in oligodendroglial tumors are correlated with clinical features. Cancer 2003;97:1276–1284.
9. Mork SJ, Lindegaard K-F, Halvorsen TB, et al. Oligodendroglioma: incidence and biological behavior in a defined population. J Neurosurg 1985;63:881–889.
10. Celli P, Nofrone I, Palma L, et al. Cerebral oligodendroglioma: prognostic factors and life history. Neurosurgery 1994;35:1018–1035.
11. Bigner SH, Matthews MR, Rasheed BKA, et al. Molecular genetic aspects of oligodendrogliomas including analysis by comparative genomic hybridization. Am J Pathol 1999;155:375–386.
12. Smith JS, Perry A, Borell TJ, et al. Alterations of chromosome arms 1p and 19q as predictors of survival in oligodendrogliomas, astrocytoma, and mixed oligoastrocytomas. J Clin Oncol 2000;18:636–645.
13. Sanson M, Leuraud P, Aguirre-Cruz L, et al. Analysis of loss of chromosome 10q, DMBT1 homozygous deletion, and PTEN mutations in oligodendrogliomas. J Neurosurg 2002;97:1397–1401.
14. Reifenberger G, Louis DN. Oligodendroglioma: toward molecular definitions in diagnostic neuro-oncology. J Neuropathol Exp Neurol 2003;62:111–126.
15. Maintz D, Fiedler K, Koopmann J, et al. Molecular genetic evidence for subtypes of oligoastrocytomas. J Neuropathol Exp Neurol 1997;56:1098–1104.
16. Watanabe T, Nakamura M, Kros JM, et al. Phenotype versus genotype correlation in oligodendrogliomas and low-grade diffuse astrocytomas. Acta Neuropathol (Berl) 2002;103(3):267–275.
17. Hoang-Xuan K, Huguet S, Mokhtari K, et al. Molecular heterogeneity of oligodendrogliomas suggests alternative pathways in tumor progression. Neurology 2002;57:1278–1281.
18. Sasaki H, Zlatescu MC, Betensky RA, et al. PTEN is a target of chromosome 10q loss in anaplastic oligodendrogliomas and PTEN alterations are associated with poor prognosis. Am J Pathol 2001;159:359–367.
19. Ueki K, Nishikawa R, Nakazato Y, et al. Correlation of histology and molecular genetic analysis of 1p, 19q, 10q, TP53, CDK4, and CDKN2A in 91 astrocytic and oligodendroglial tumors. Clin Cancer Res 2002;8:196–201.
20. Sasaki H, Zlatescu MC, Betensky RA, et al. Histopathological-molecular genetic correlations in referral pathologist-diagnosed low-grade "oligodendroglioma." J Neuropathol Exp Neurol 2002;61:58–63.
21. Zlatescu MC, Tehrani Yazdi A, Sasaki H, et al. Tumor location and growth pattern correlate with genetic signature in oligodendroglial neoplasms. Cancer Res 2001;18:6713–6715.
22. Mueller W, Hartmann C, Hoffmann A, et al. Genetic signature of oligoastrocytomas correlates with tumor location and denotes distinct molecular subsets. Am J Pathol 2002;161:313–319.
23. Bissola L, Eoli M, Pollo B, et al. Association of chromosome 10 losses and negative prognosis in oligoastrocytomas. Ann Neurol 2002;52:842–845.
24. Ino Y, Betensky RA, Zlatescu MC, et al. Molecular subtypes of anaplastic oligodendroglioma: implications for patient management at diagnosis. Clin Cancer Res 2001;7:839–845.
25. Bauman GS, Ino Y, Yeki K, et al. Allelic loss of chromosome 1p and radiotherapy plus chemotherapy in patients with oligodendroglioma. Int J Radiat Oncol Biol Phys 2000;48:825–830.
26. Raff MC, Miller RH, Noble M. A glial progenitor cell that develops in vitro into an astrocyte or an oligodendrocyte depending on the culture medium. Nature 1983;303:390–396.
27. Bögler O, Wren D, Barnett SC, et al. Cooperation between two growth factors promotes extended self-renewal and inhibits differentiation of oligodendrocyte-type-2 astrocyte (O-2A) progenitor cells. Proc Natl Acad Sci USA 1990;87:6368–6372.
28. Shoshan Y, Nishiyama A, Chang A, et al. Expression of oligodendrocyte progenitor cell antigens by gliomas: implications for the histogenesis of brain tumors. Proc Natl Acad Sci USA 1999;96:10361–10366.
29. van Heyningen P, Calver AR, Richardson WD. Control of progenitor cell number by mitogen supply and demand. Curr Biol 2001;11:232–241.
30. Dai C, Celestino JC, Okada Y, et al. PDGF autocrine stimulation dedifferentiates cultured astrocytes and induces oligodendrogliomas and oligoastrocytomas from neural progenitors and astrocytes in vivo. Genes Dev 2001;15:1913–1925.
31. Di Rocco F, Carroll RS, Zhang J, Black PM. Platelet-derived growth factor and its receptor expression in human oligodendrogliomas. Neurosurgery 1998;42:341–346.
32. Robinson SW, Cohen M, Prayson R, et al. Constitutive expression of growth-related oncogene and it receptor in oligodendrogliomas. Neurosurgery 2001;48:864–874.
33. Smith JS, Wang XY, Qian J, et al. Amplification of the platelet-derived growth factor receptor-A (PDGFRA) gene occurs in oligodendrogliomas with grade IV anaplastic features. J Neuropathol Exp Neurol 2000;59:495–503.
34. Holland EC, Celestino JC, Dai C, et al. Astrocytes give rise to oligodendrogliomas and astrocytomas after gene transfer of polyoma virus middle T antigen in vivo. Am J Pathol 2004;157:1031–1037.
35. Nutt CL, Costello JF, Bambrick LL, et al. O^6 methylguanine-DNA methyltransferase in tumors and cells of the oligodendrocyte lineage. Can J Neurol Sci 1995;22:111–115.

36. Nutt CL, Noble M, Chambers AF, et al. Differential expression of drug resistance genes and chemosensitivity in glial cell lineages with differential response of oligodendrogliomas and astrocytomas to chemotherapy. Cancer Res 2000;60:4812–4818.
37. Rogers LR, Estes ML, Rosenbloom SA, et al. Primary leptomeningeal oligodendroglioma: case report. Neurosurgery 2000;36:166–169.
38. Chen R, Chir B, Macdonald DR, et al. Primary diffuse leptomeningeal oligodendroglioma. J Neurosurg 2000;83: 724–728.
39. Lee Y, van Tassel P. Intracranial oligodendrogliomas: imaging findings in 35 untreated cases. Am J Roentgenol 1989; 152:361–369.
40. Ginsberg LE, Fuller GN, Hashmi M, et al. The significance of lack of MR contrast enhancement of supratentorial brain tumors in adults: histopathological evaluation of a series. Surg Neurol 1998;49:436–440.
41. Kondziolka D, Lunsford LD, Martinez AJ. Unreliability of contemporary neurodiagnostic imaging in evaluating suspected adult supratentorial (low-grade) astrocytoma. J Neurosurg 1993;79:533–536.
42. Derlon JM, Chapon F, Noël MH, et al. Non-invasive grading of oligodendrogliomas: correlations between in vivo metabolic pattern and histopathology. Eur J Nucl Med 2000;27:778–787.
43. Vuori K, Kankaanranta L, Häkkinen A-M, et al. Low-grade gliomas and focal cortical developmental malformations: differentiation with proton MR spectroscopy. Radiology 2004;230:703–708.
44. Reifenberger G, Kros JM, Burger P, et al. Oligodendroglioma. In: Kleihues P, Cavenee WK, eds. World Health Organization classification of tumours. Pathology and genetics of tumours of the nervous system. Lyon, France: IARC Press, 2000: 55–70.
45. Smith MT, Ludwig CL, Godfrey AD, et al. Grading of oligodendrogliomas. Cancer 1983;52:2107–2114.
46. Shaw EG, Scheithauer BW, O'Fallon JR, et al. Oligodendrogliomas: the Mayo Clinic experience. J Neurosurg 1992;76:428–434.
47. Kros JM, de Jong AA, van der Kwast TH. Ultrastructural characterization of transitional cells in oligodendrogliomas. J Neuropathol Exp Neurol 1992;51:186–193.
48. Hart MN, Petito CK, Earle KM. Mixed gliomas. Cancer 1974;33:134–140.
49. Kim L, Hochberg FH, Thornton AF, et al. Procarbazine, lomustine, and vincristine (PCV) chemotherapy for grade III and grade IV oligoastrocytomas. J Neurosurg 1996; 85:602–607.
50. Krouwer HGJ, van Duinen SG, Kamphorst W, et al. Oligoastrocytomas: a clinicopathological study of 52 cases. J Neuro-Oncol 1997;33:223–238.
51. Mork SJ, Halvorsen TB, Lindegaard K-F, et al. Oligodendroglioma. Histologic evaluation and prognosis. J Neuropathol Exp Neurol 1986;45:65–78.
52. Tanaka J, Hokama Y, Nakamura H. Myelin basic protein as a possible marker for oligodendroglioma. Acta Pathol Jpn 1988;38:1297–1303.
53. Kennedy PG, Watkins BA, Thomas DG, et al. Antigenic expression by cells derived from human gliomas does not correlate with morphological classification. Neuropathol Appl Neurobiol 1987;13:327–347.
54. Perentes E, Rubinstein LJ. Recent applications of immunoperoxidase histochemistry in human neuro-oncology. An update. Arch Pathol Lab Med 1987;111: 796–812.
55. Lu QR, Park JK, Noll E, et al. Oligodendrocyte lineage genes (OLIG) as molecular markers for human glial brain tumors. Proc Natl Acad Sci USA 2001;98:10851–10856.
56. Marie Y, Sanson M, Mokhtari K, et al. Olig2 as a specific marker of oligodendroglial tumour cells. Lancet 2001; 358:298–300.
57. Bouvier C, Bartoli C, Aguirre-Cruz L, et al. Shared oligodendrocyte lineage gene expression in gliomas and oligodendrocyte progenitor cells. J Neurosurg 2003;99: 344–350.
58. Donahue B, Scott CB, Nelson JS, et al. Influence of an oligodendroglial component on the survival of patients with anaplastic astrocytomas: a report of radiation therapy oncology group 83–02. Int J Radiat Oncol Biol Phys 1997;38:911–914.
59. Pignatti F, van den Bent MJ, Curran D, et al. Prognostic factors for survival in adult patients with cerebral low-grade glioma. J Clin Oncol 2002;20:2076–2084.
60. Shaw EG, Scheithauer BW, O'Fallon JR, et al. Mixed oligoastrocytomas: a survival and prognostic factor analysis. Neurosurgery 1994;34:577–582.
61. Surma-aho O, Niemelä M, Vilkki J, et al. Adverse long-term effects of brain radiotherapy in adult low-grade glioma patients. Neurology 2001;56:1285–1290.
62. Leighton C, Fisher B, Bauman G, et al. Supratentorial low-grade glioma in adults: an analysis of prognostic factors and the timing of radiation. J Clin Oncol 1997;15:1294–1301.
63. Shaw EG, Scheithauer BW, O'Fallon JR. Supratentorial gliomas: a comparative study by grade and histologic type. J Neurooncol 1997;31:273–278.
64. Winger MJ, Macdonald DR, Cairncross JG. Supratentorial anaplastic gliomas in adults. J Neurosurg 1989;71:487–493.
65. Giannini C, Scheithauer BW, Weaver A, et al. Oligodendrogliomas: reproducibility and prognostic value of histologic diagnosis and grading. J Neuropathol Exp Neurol 2001;60:248–262.
66. Daumas-Duport C, Tucker ML, Kolles H, et al. Oligodendrogliomas: Part II. a new grading system based on morphological and imaging criteria. J Neurooncol 1997; 34:61–78.
67. Kros JM, Troost D, Van Eden CG, et al. Oligodendroglioma: a comparison of two grading systems. Cancer 1988;61: 2251–2259.
68. Ribom D, Eriksson A, Hartman M, et al. Positron emission tomography ^{11}C-methionine and survival in patients with low-grade gliomas. Cancer 2001;92:1541–1549.
69. Matthew J, Fuller G, Goodman JC, et al. The impact of histology and 1p/19q status on the outcome of patients with anaplastic oligodendroglioma [abstract]. Neuro-oncol 2002;4:344.
70. Nutt CL, Mani DR, Betensky RA, et al. Gene expression-based classification of malignant gliomas correlates better with survival than histological classification. Cancer Res 2003;63:1602–1607.

71. Watson MA, Perry A, Budhjara V, et al. Gene expression profiling with oligonucleotide microarrays distinguishes between world health organization grade of oligodendrogliomas. Cancer Res 2001;61:1825–1829.
72. Reijneveld JC, Sitskoorn MM, Klein M, et al. Cognitive status and quality of life in suspected versus proven low-grade gliomas. Neurology 2001;56:618–623.
73. Klein M, Heimans JJ, Aaronson NK, et al. Effect of radiotherapy and other treatment-related factors on mid-term to long-term cognitive sequelae in low grade gliomas: a comparative study. Lancet 2002;360:1361–1368.
74. Barker FG, Chang CH, Huhn SL, et al. Age and the risk of anaplasia in magnetic resonance-nonenhancing supratentorial cerebral tumors. Cancer 1997;80:936–941.
75. Berger MS, Deliganis AV, Dobbins J, et al. The effect of extent of resection on recurrence in patients with low grade cerebral hemisphere gliomas. Cancer 1994;74:1784–1791.
76. Schiffer D, Dutto A, Cavalla P, et al. Prognostic factors in oligodendroglioma. Can J Neurol Sci 1997;24:313–319.
77. Kros JM, Pieterman H, Van Eden CG, et al. Oligodendroglioma: the Rotterdam-Dijkzigt experience. Neurosurgery 1994;34:959–966.
78. Walker MD, Alexander E, Hunt WE, et al. Evaluation of BCNU and/or radiotherapy in the treatment of anaplastic gliomas. A cooperative clinical trial. J Neurosurg 1978; 49:333–343.
79. Karim ABMF, Afra D, Bleehen NM, et al. Randomized trial on the efficacy of radiotherapy for cerebral low-grade glioma in the adult: European Organization for Research and Treatment of Cancer study 22845 with the Medical Research Council study BRO4: an interim analysis. Int J Radiat Oncol Biol Phys 2002;52:316–324.
80. Gannett DE, Wisbeck WM, Silbergeld DL, et al. The role of postoperative irradiation in the treatment of oligodendroglioma. Int J Radiat Oncol Biol Phys 1994;30: 567–573.
81. Wallner KE, Gonzales M, Sheline GE. Treatment of oligodendrogliomas with or without postoperative irradiation. J Neurosurg 1988;68:684–688.
82. Bullard DE, Rawlings CE III, Philllips B, et al. Oligodendroglioma. An analysis of the value of radiation therapy. Cancer 1987;60:2179–2188.
83. Nijjar TS, Simpson WJ, Gadalla T, et al. Oligodendroglioma. The Princess Margaret Hospital experience (1958–1984). Cancer 1993;71:4002–4006.
84. Karim ABMF, Maat B, Hatlevoll R, et al. A randomized trial on dose-response in radiation therapy of low grade cerebral glioma: European Organization for Research and Treatment of Cancer (EORTC) study 22844. Int J Radiat Oncol Biol Phys 1996;36:549–556.
85. Shaw E, Arusell RM, Scheithauer B, et al. A prospective randomized trial of low versus high dose radiation in adults with a supratentorial low grade glioma: initial report of a NCCTG-RTOG-ECOG study. J Clin Oncol 2002;20:2267–2276.
86. Kiebert GM, Curran W, Aaronson NK, et al. Quality of life after radiation therapy of cerebral low-grade gliomas of the adult: results of a randomised phase III trial on dose–response (EORTC trial 22844). Eur J Cancer 1998;34:1902–1909.
87. Soffietti R, Ruda R, Bradac GB, et al. PCV chemotherapy for recurrent oligodendrogliomas and oligoastrocytomas. Neurosurgery 1998;43:1066–1073.
88. Mason WP, Krol GS, DeAngelis LM. Low-grade oligodendroglioma responds to chemotherapy. Neurology 1996;46: 203–207.
89. van den Bent MJ, Taphoorn MJ, Brandes AA, et al. Phase II study of first-line chemotherapy with temozolomide in recurrent oligodendroglioma: the European Organisation of Research and Treatment of Cancer Brain Tumor Group study 26971. J Clin Oncol 2003;21:2525–2528.
90. Yung WKA, Prados M, Yaya-Tur R, et al. Multicenter phase II trial of temozolomide in patients with anaplastic astrocytoma or anaplastic oligoastrocytoma at first relapse. J Clin Oncol 1999;17:2762–2771.
91. van den Bent MJ, Keime-Guibert F, Brandes AA, et al. Temozolomide chemotherapy in recurrent oligodendroglioma. Neurology 2001;57:340–342.
92. van den Bent MJ, Chinot O, Boogerd W, et al. Second-line chemotherapy with temozolomide in recurrent oligodendroglioma after PCV (procarbazine, lomustine and vincristine) chemotherapy: EORTC Brain Tumor Group phase II study 26972. Ann Oncol 2003;14:599–602.
93. Constanza A, Borgogne M, Nobile M, et al. Temozolomide in recurrent oligodendroglioma: a phase II study [abstract]. Neuro-oncol 2001;3:S66.
94. Chinot O, Honore S, Dufour H, et al. Safety and efficacy of temozolomide in patients with recurrent anaplastic oligodendrogliomas after standard radiotherapy and chemotherapy. J Clin Oncol 2001;19:2449–2455.
95. Triebels V, Taphoorn MJB, Brandes AA, et al. Second-line PCV chemotherapy in recurrent oligodendroglioma after first line temozolomide chemotherapy. Neurology 2004; 63:904–906.
96. Peterson K, Paleologos N, Forsyth P, et al. Salvage chemotherapy for oligodendroglioma. J Neurosurg 1996;85:597–601.
97. Chamberlain MC, Kormanik PA. Salvage chemotherapy with paclitaxel for recurrent oligodendrogliomas. J Clin Oncol 1997;15:3427–3432.
98. Chamberlain M. Salvage chemotherapy with CPT-11 for recurrent oligodendroglioma. J Neurooncol 2002;59: 157–163.
99. Soffietti R, Nobile M, Rudà R, et al. Second-line treatment with carboplatin for recurrent or progressive oligodendroglial tumors after PCV (procarbazine, lomustine and vincristine). Cancer 2004;100:807–813.
100. Belanger K, Macdonald DR, Cairncross G, et al. A phase II study of topotecan in patients with anaplastic oligodendroglioma or anaplastic oligoastrocytoma. J Neurooncol 2003;21:473–480.
101. Brandes AA, Basso U, Vastola F, et al. Carboplatin and teniposide as third-line chemotherapy in patients with recurrent oligodendroglioma or oligoastrocytoma: a phase II study. Ann Oncol 2003;14:1727–1731.
102. Cairncross JG, Swinnen LJ, Bayer R, et al. Myeloablative chemotherapy for recurrent aggressive oligodendroglioma. Neuro-oncol 2000;2:114–119.
103. Abrey LE, Childs BH, Paleologos N, et al. High-dose chemotherapy with stem cell rescue as initial therapy for

anaplastic oligodendroglioma. J Neurooncol 2003;65: 127–134.
104. Glioma Meta-Analysis Group. Chemotherapy in adult high-grade glioma: a systematic review and meta-analysis of individual patient data from 12 randomised trials. Lancet 2002;359:1011–1018.
105. DeAngelis LM, Burger PC, Green SB, et al. Adjuvant chemotherapy for malignant glioma: who benefits? Ann Neurol 1998;44:691–695.
106. Streffer J, Schabet M, Bamberg M, et al. A role for preirradiation PCV chemotherapy for oligodendroglial brain tumors. J Neurol 2000;247:297–302.
107. Brada M, Viviers L, Abson C, et al. Phase II study of primary temozolomide chemotherapy in patients with WHO grade II gliomas. Ann Oncol 2003;14:1715–1721.
108. Buckner JC, Gesme D, O'Fallon JR, et al. Phase II trial of procarbazine, lomustine, and vincristine as initial therapy for patients with low-grade oligodendroglioma or oligoastrocytoma: efficacy and and associations with chromosomal abnormalities. J Clin Oncol 2003;21: 251–255.
109. van den Bent MJ, van der Rijt CCD, Enting RE, et al. PCV: chemotherapy in newly diagnosed and recurrent low grade oligodendroglial tumors. Cancer 2005 (in press).

CHAPTER 16

Brainstem Gliomas

BRUCE H. COHEN / CAMERON L. NICHOLSON

The term brainstem glioma *refers to a number of pathologically and clinically distinct tumors that arise in brainstem tissue. Each subtype of tumor has a surprisingly well-defined clinical course. Although many of the subtypes have an indolent course that requires invasive treatment, they tend to have a favorable outcome with often minimal impact on the patient's ultimate quality of life. Other tumors tend to be resistant to therapy and are most often fatal. Brainstem tumors may occur in adults, but are far more common in the pediatric population. In children, they account for 10% to 20% of all brain tumors.*[1–4]

For this discussion, the brainstem includes brain structures located between the midbrain, including the tectal plate, and the cervicomedullary junction. Although the epicenter of the diffuse intrinsic pontine glioma is in the pons, there is often contiguous spread into the cerebellum and diencephalic regions. Because of their location and magnetic resonance imaging (MRI) that improves certainty of diagnosis, the vast majority of these tumors are not biopsied and therefore histologic diagnosis is assumed to represent glioma.

The majority of this discussion focuses on the most aggressive brainstem glioma, specifically the diffuse infiltrating pontine glioma. However, the other forms of brainstem gliomas are also discussed.

Before the advent of the MRI, the certainty of diagnosis was often in question. Because of technical limitations with CT technology, imaging the posterior fossa, especially those tumors in the pons and medulla that are often obscured by bone artifact, did not always lead to an exacting diagnosis. Detecting those tumors that had a more indolent course, such as those located in the tectal plate region or the cervicomedullary junction was often difficult. Differentiating the more malignant diffuse pontine glioma from the less aggressive focal pontine glioma was not certain. Finally, other diseases, such as acute disseminated encephalomyelitis (ADEM) (also known as brainstem encephalitis), that affect the brainstem often have a benign course, but could mimic the early course of the diffuse pontine glioma. Therefore, the natural history of many of these tumors could not be well defined until the late 1980s, and the validity of retrospective studies are questionable, because the current and more accurate methods of correct diagnosis could not be certain.[5–7]

▶ SYMPTOMS

The patient's symptoms depend on the exact location of the tumor within the brainstem, the tumor's rate of growth, and whether or not the flow of cerebral spinal fluid (CSF), typically through the aqueduct of Sylvius, is affected. Because of the varying nature of the neoplasms that occur within the brainstem, the speed of symptom onset and the character of the neurologic deficit will vary. In general, there is often involvement of cranial nerves, along with motor difficulties and disturbances of coordination. Bulbar symptoms, including swallowing and speech difficulties, are common. If CSF flow is disrupted, headache and vomiting may occur, along with limitation of upgaze and alteration of motor tone. Exophytic lesions and those involving the cervicomedullary junction may not cause cranial nerve dysfunction early in the course of the illness, but tend to present with unsteadiness, nausea, and vomiting. Symptoms may develop over the course of days, or may stretch out for months or years. In general, gliomas of the posterior midbrain and tectal plate present with macrocrania and symptoms of hydrocephalus. Depending on the extent of the lesion, impairment of upgaze and pupils that do not react to light (but will react to near accommodation) may also be present (Table 16-1).

Tumors of the medulla and upper cervical spinal cord will generally present with hypotonia in the infant, or varying combinations of long-track signs.[1,3,4]

▶ DIAGNOSIS

Neuroimaging

The availability of MRI allows for a rapid, and usually accurate, diagnosis. Although there is little role for the use of computerized tomography (CT) in the diagnosis or management of these diseases, some patients come to clinical presentation by way of CT. The CT appearance of the diffuse pontine glioma typically is a low-density lesion in the brainstem with associated compression and obliteration of the surrounding cisterns. The fourth ventricle is often distorted and displaced posteriorly. There is little, if any enhancement, even with high-grade gliomas. Less frequently, the lower-grade gliomas affecting the brainstem are isodense or hyperdense and contain cystic areas. Exophytic portions of the tumor are only moderately well delineated on CT. If the diagnosis of a brainstem glioma is suspected by CT, the diagnosis should be confirmed with an MRI.[5–7]

MRI demonstrates the presence and extent of infiltrating brain stem gliomas extremely well. The higher-grade infiltrating gliomas are usually seen as decreased signal intensities on T_1-weighted images and increased signal intensity lesions on T_2-weighted images. These tumors usually will expand the entire pons, and sometimes extend into the higher brainstem regions and beyond, as well as caudally into the medulla and upper cervical spinal cord. These tumors tend not to enhance, or do so only minimally. In some cases the tumor seems surprisingly demarcated and localized to one brainstem site, which is often associated with a less aggressive tumor.[5–7] Because the higher grade gliomas can disseminate early in the course of the disease, many centers are performing complete spinal cord MRIs with and without contrast at the time of diagnosis to investigate for leptomeningeal spread.[8–11]

▶ TABLE 16-1. FEATURES OF BRAINSTEM GLIOMAS

Tumor	Clinical Features	Predominant Pathology	MRI	Treatment
Intrinsic pontine glioma	Cranial nerve palsy, long tract signs, ataxia	High grade	Hypointense on T_1, hyperintense on T_2, patchy enhancement, hydrocephalus common	Radiotherapy, shunting for hydrocephalus
Exophytic brainstem glioma	Symptoms of increased intracranial pressure, occasional cranial nerve palsies	Variable grade	Hypointense on T_1, hyperintense on T_2, intense enhancement, sharp borders, hydrocepahlus common	Surgery; chemotherapy and/or radiotherapy are options for recurrent or high-grade tumors
Cervicomedullary glioma	Lower cranial nerve signs, mixed motor and sensory signs, nausea or vomiting	Low grade	Hypointense on T_1, hyperintense on T_2, variable enhancement pattern	Surgery or observation
Tectal glioma	Symptoms of increased intracranial pressure	Low grade	Hypointense on T_1, hyperintense on T_2, no enhancement, hydrocephalus almost universal	Observation or, rarely, surgery; shunting usually required

Source: Pollack I, Hoffman H, Humphreys R, et al. The long-term outcome after surgical treatment of dorsally exophytic brain-stem gliomas. J Neurosurg 1993;78:859–863.

Pathology, Pathophysiology, and Management of Brainstem Gliomas

Treatment decisions for the vast majority of brain tumors are deferred until after tissue has been obtained for pathologic examination. Several investigators have developed a proxy pathologic–pathophysiologic paradigm for brainstem gliomas based on the MRI appearance of the tumor. Although a biopsy can be safely performed on most brainstem tumors, a risk remains and it is questionable as to whether there is any benefit to the biopsy procedure given the excellent predictive value of the MRI. The principal prognostic factors found for patients with brainstem gliomas have been the location of the tumor and its histology; however, there is a good correlation between the location and appearance of the tumor on MRI and the clinical course. The diffuse infiltrating pontine glioma has an aggressive course, even when the histology may suggest the tumor is a low-grade glioma. There is no evidence to suggest improved survival with surgery for those with diffuse infiltrating tumors. In general, infiltrating tumors in the upper portion of the brainstem, particularly those of the diencephalon and upper midbrain, tend to be lower grade and have longer survival following radiotherapy, when compared with the survival in patients with intrinsic pontine gliomas, but like the intrinsic pontine gliomas, are not amenable to resection. Patients with cervicomedullary tumors, which may be intrinsic or exophytic, tend to have a benign histology, usually that of a pilocytic astrocytoma, and some can be cured with surgery alone, although the routine use of surgery has been recently questioned. The focal brainstem and exophytic pontine gliomas have a variable degree of aggressiveness and debulking surgery followed by radiotherapy may lead to a longer survival, although the risk of worsening the neurologic function should be considered.[11–15]

▶ SPECIFIC SUBTYPES

Diffuse Infiltrating Pontine Glioma

This tumor may occur at any age but is most common between the ages of 5 and 10 years, and is distinctly uncommon before the age of 2 years.[16] The typical presentation of this tumor is a triad of cranial nerve palsies, ataxia, and cerebrospinal tract dysfunction. Most often cranial nerves VI and VII are involved (sometimes unilaterally), and the motor signs and cerebellar signs often involve contralateral limbs. Symptoms may be present for several weeks but some patients come to medical attention within hours of their first complaint. On occasion, signs and symptoms of hydrocephalus (headache, irritability, and limited upgaze) may be the factor that brings the patient to medical attention. The MRI appearance and clinical course for these tumors is quite typical and there is seldom a question of diagnosis. These tumors are hypointense on T_1-weighted images and hyperintense on T_2-weighted images. They may involve the entire pons and appear to expand the entire body of the affected portion of the brainstem. There is patchy and variable enhancement of the mass. At times the tumor appears to wrap around the basilar artery. These tumors may have exophytic components, and may also invade through the cerebellar peduncles or extend up into the midbrain or down into the medulla (Fig. 16-1).[5–7,14] As part of the routine evaluation of patients with these tumors, a complete spinal MRI should be considered to evaluate for the leptomeningeal spread of tumor, which is not an uncommon finding.[10,11]

The initial neurologic symptoms often respond quickly with the use of dexamethasone or another corticosteroid, although this response is only temporary. The dose of steroids is variable and should be the minimal dose necessary to control symptoms. Many patients will ultimately require these steroids for weeks to months, and because of side effects, close monitoring of blood pressure and blood sugar is recommended. Although not routinely practiced, the use of prophylactic antibiotic therapy (usually trimethoprim-sulfamethoxazole or pentamidine) may be considered for prevention of *Pneumocystis carinii* pneumonia. Because of risk of gastric ulceration, the use of proton pump inhibitors, H_2-blockers, or buffering agents are commonly used, but it has not been shown that this practice will decrease the risk of ulceration. Approximately one-third of patients will present with symptomatic hydrocephalus, and either a shunting procedure or a third ventriculostomy should be considered. An occasional patient will have asymptomatic or presymptomatic hydrocephalus, which will need close monitoring during the initiation of therapy, as symptoms of progressive hydrocephalus will often mimic the side effects of treatment.[3,4,11] Because the MRI diagnosis is now an accepted part of management, most patients do not need to have a pathology-confirmed diagnosis.

The standard approach to treatment has been focal radiotherapy with 1- to 2-cm margins around the tumor, usually at a dose of 45 to 55 Gy delivered in daily fractions of 1800 to 2000 cGy. There does seem to be a survival advantage to those children treated with more than 5000 cGy.[17] Many patients show a clinical and radiographic response with this treatment, and both the examination and MRI improve and occasionally return to normal. However, the median time to progression is on the order of 6 months, with the overall duration of survival in the range of 9 to 13 months, with approximately only 10% of patients alive in a relapse-free state 18 months after diagnosis. In the 1980s there were a number of successive studies that treated patients with hyperfractionated radiotherapy, using twice-daily (or thrice-daily) smaller fractions (typically using 100

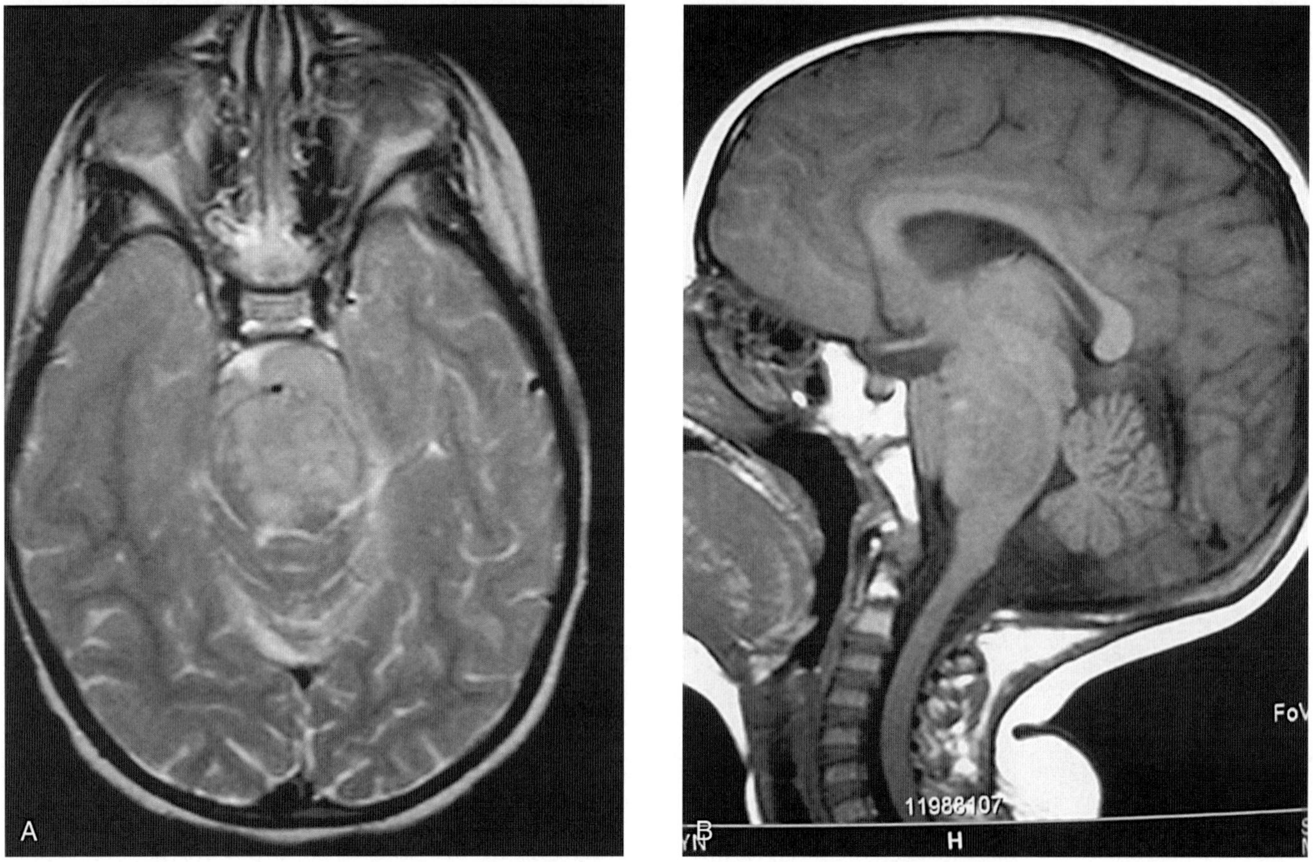

Figure 16-1. Intrinsic brainstem glioma. (A) This T_2-weighted image demonstrates the massive expansion of the pons by an infiltrating tumor, which extends around and in front of the basilar artery. (B) Sagittal T_1-weighted image of the same tumor. This patient presented with subacute ataxia and was treated with standard-dose radiotherapy (5400 cGy in 180-cGy fractions) and improved clinically. She had a radiographic progression 10 months after presentation and a clinical progression 11 months following the radiographic progression. She was then placed on low-dose oral etoposide and was free of any signs of progression for the last 12 months.

cGy doses in a BID regimen). The rationale was twofold: First, normal brain tissue is better able to tolerate higher total dosages of radiotherapy if the individual dose fractions are smaller. Second, the rapidly dividing tumor cells could not repair DNA breaks during the time between dose fractions, whereas the healthier (and relatively nonproliferating neurons and glial and endothelial cells of the brain) would be relatively spared. A trial conducted by The Children's Cancer Group used 7800 cGy of hyperfractionated radiotherapy in 100 cGy BID fractions to treat 66 children with this tumor. Treatment was well-tolerated but the 1-year survival rate of 35% and 3-year survival rate of 11% was no different than historical controls.[18] Similar findings were reported in a Pediatric Oncology Group study of 136 children treated with either 6600 cGy, 7020 cGy, or 7560 cGy in 110 cGy BID fractions. The 1-year survival was 47% and the 2-year survival was 6%, with a median time to progression of 6.5 months.[19] Another study investigated total treatment doses of 64.8, 66, 72, and 78 Gy. The response rate using hyperfractionated radiotherapy ranged from 62% to 77% but did not result in improvement in time-to-disease progression or impact on ultimate survival.[20,21] Therefore, at this time the standard radiotherapy treatment consists of standard daily (5 days a week) fractions of 180 to 200 cGy with a total treatment dose of about 5400 cGy. There does not seem to be a role for either stereotactic radiosurgery such as would be delivered by the Gamma Knife because of the increased risk for radiation necrosis and the diffuse nature of this tumor.

There have been numerous trials of chemotherapy in an adjuvant or neoadjuvant setting. Most of the earlier trials involved single agents in a phase II setting, although some involved multiple agents. More recent studies involved the use of neoadjuvant chemotherapy or concurrent chemotherapy and/or radiation sensitizers with irradiation. Although results from some of these trials were initially encouraging, the final results have been uniformly disappointing.[22–26]

Etoposide was used to treat tumors at relapse, demonstrating a 50% response rate that was durable for a median of 8 months in 12 patients. The dosing of etoposide was a conventional regimen (50 mg/m^2/d × 21 days with 14 days of rest between cycles). All patients had received prior radiotherapy at diagnosis.[27] Subsequent studies using various agents have failed to show consistent results and to date there is no standard relapse therapy given to patients with this tumor.

In a Children's Cancer Group study of intensive chemotherapy prior to hyperfractionated radiotherapy, 32 patients were randomly assigned to receive three courses of carboplatin, etoposide, and vincristine (arm A), and 31 patients were assigned to receive cisplatin, etoposide, cyclophosphamide, and vincristine (arm B). Granulocyte colony-stimulating factor was used in both arms. Following chemotherapy, both groups received 7200 cGy of radiation in 100 cGy BID fractions. The radiographic response rate to the chemotherapy was 10 ± 5% in arm A and 18 ± 9% in arm B. Event-free survival was 17 ± 5% at 1 year and 6 ± 3% at 2 years. Although those children that responded to the chemotherapy had a longer survival, the authors concluded that neither chemotherapy regimen meaningfully improved response rate, event-free survival, or overall survival.[28]

The most intensive chemotherapy regimen has employed high-dose chemotherapy with autologous bone marrow rescue, which failed to improve survival for children with this tumor.[29]

It is not uncommon for these tumors to develop a cystic component following radiotherapy. These cysts do have mass effect and often require intervention. The use of steroids will usually improve symptoms. However, in any individual patient, the differential diagnosis includes both tumor necrosis or tumor recurrence. If the patient does not respond to steroids, the question of surgical intervention in order to drain the cyst needs to be addressed in those patients that remain symptomatic and that might benefit in terms of quality of life, even if the ultimate prognosis is not favorable. The occurrence of tumor necrosis seems to be more common in the patients treated with higher dosages of radiotherapy, although most often viable tumor remains outside the necrotic cavity, without any outcome benefit in patients that develop this finding.

Most investigators conclude that the standard approach to treating these tumors begins with staging of the tumor and if contained to the pons, treating with standard dose radiotherapy delivered in a single daily fraction to the tumor plus a 1- to 2-cm margin. However, leptomeningeal dissemination can occur at diagnosis and about one-third of patients developed disseminated disease early in the course of illness. If disseminated disease is found at diagnosis, or at any time in the illness, radiotherapy can be used with a palliative attempt to treat the involved areas of disseminated disease. Although there is no evidence that neoadjunctive or adjunctive chemotherapy prolongs the time to relapse, the use of low-dose etoposide or experimental agents may be warranted at relapse. The survival in patients with this particular tumor has not improved in the last several decades despite escalating both radiation and cytotoxic chemotherapy dosing to the maximum tolerated levels. Further advances will likely require a unique chemotherapeutic agent or biologic agent.

Dorsal Exophytic Brainstem Tumors

Dorsal exophytic brainstem gliomas are a distinct subgroup of neoplasms that account for 20% of all brainstem tumors. They have a relatively benign histology and slow growth characteristics, and do not carry the near-universal dismal prognosis seen in the intrinsic pontine gliomas. These tumors may present in early infancy and generally appear before puberty.[30] They generally arise out of the floor of the fourth ventricle and grow into the ventricle as opposed to invading the brainstem itself. Because of their location, they may obstruct the flow of CSF. These tumors tend to be hypointense on T_1-weighted MRI and hyperintense on T_2-weighted MRI, but unlike the more malignant intrinsic pontine glioma, these tumors have sharp borders and enhance intensely with contrast. Unlike many other brainstem tumors, they are sometimes amenable to surgical excision with a positive outlook.

Symptoms are often insidious, a symptomatic period of months or years before diagnosis. Initial symptoms may be caused by the initial intermittent and eventual obstruction of CSF flow as the tumor grows into the fourth ventricle. Intermittent vomiting and failure to thrive without overt neurologic signs may result in prolonged evaluations by specialists without considering this diagnosis. These symptoms are not specific for increased intracranial pressure and patients often have only mild or intermittent cranial nerve paresis, and an absence of pyramidal tract findings. Symptoms will vary by age, with failure to thrive and chronic vomiting seen in infants, whereas older patients present with a combination of headache, vomiting, and ataxia.[6] Examination frequently reveals papilledema, ataxia, torticollis, nystagmus, and cranial nerve dysfunction. Because this tumor usually is not highly invasive, significant long-tract signs are absent.

These tumors most often have a low-grade glial histology. Tumor histology is typically grade I or grade II astrocytomas, frequently classic juvenile pilocytic astrocytomas, although higher-grade astrocytomas and gangliogliomas have been reported.

The treatment for these tumors is primarily surgical. A complete surgical excision is usually not feasible because there is not a plane between the tumor and brainstem, and often the invasion involves a large area of the brainstem surface, therefore only the exophytic component can be removed. Some of these tumors have cysts that cause local mass effect and are amenable to surgical drainage. CSF flow may be reestablished with successful debulking, but if this is not possible a ventriculoperitoneal shunt or third ventriculostomy will be necessary.

The small percentage of tumors that recur typically remain benign histologically and are amenable to repeat tumor excision (Fig. 16-2). Following a surgical excision, even if there is remaining tumor, it is reasonable to withhold radiotherapy or other treatments in favor of expectant observation with interval MRI and examinations.[30–32]

Radiation therapy has been generally reserved for patients with either high-grade gliomas or progression that is not amenable to repeat surgery. For those patients with high-grade neoplasms, it is recommended that surveillance MRI of the spine be performed to properly stage the patient's disease. Unless there is evidence of tumor spread, involved-field radiotherapy using standard dose and dose-fractions is recommended.

Cervicomedullary Tumors

Cervicomedullary region are predominantly low-grade neoplasms with a slowly progressive clinical course. Reported histology is predominately fibrillary astrocytomas, but ependymomas, gangliogliomas, pilocytic astrocytomas, and, rarely, high-grade astrocytomas are reported.[1] Patients present with lower cranial nerve signs and a variety of motor and sensory signs, depending on the exact location of the tumor. The presenting clinical syndromes reflect either cervical cord involvement, medullary dysfunction, or both. Symptoms associated with the cervical cord are predominantly motor deficits localized to the cervical cord, such as upper motor neuron hemiparesis or quadriparesis. Typical presenting symptoms associated with medullary involvement include protracted nausea and vomiting, which is not caused by increased intracranial pressure but by local effects on the area postrema, abnormal breathing patterns, dysphonia, dysarthria, and dysphagia. In infants, the syndrome may cause a failure-to-thrive presentation. The clinical course of these symptoms is often protracted; symptoms in one study had been present for a mean of more than 2 years. Children can also present with neck pain and torticollis. The largest study in children demonstrated a mean age at diagnosis of 6 years. The diagnosis is confirmed by MRI, which typically shows a hypointense mass on T_1-weighted images and a hyperintense mass on T_2-weighted images. The enhancement pattern is variable. Hydrocephalus does not typically occur, although rarely these tumors can invade the fourth ventricle and cause CSF flow obstruction (Fig. 16-3).

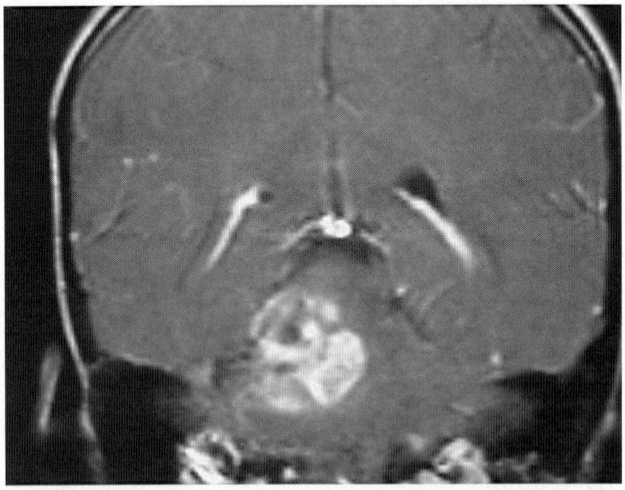

Figure 16-2. Low-grade brainstem glioma. This is a T_1-weighted contrast-enhanced MRI of a 16-year-old girl at the time of a second recurrence of a low-grade astrocytoma. She had been treated previously with chemotherapy following a partial resection and then radiotherapy following the first recurrence. The patient had a third resection of this tumor and was clinically stable 4 years later without signs of progressive disease.

As a general rule, these tumors are amenable to surgical resection, and because most are exophytic and low-grade tumors, surgery is the primary treatment.[33] The approach to these tumors has been an attempt at a gross total resection, although there is a continued debate as to the overall benefit of aggressive surgery. Five-year progression-free survival of 60% was reported in one series in which aggressive surgery was attempted. When the low-grade tumors were considered, 4 of 10 patients with gross total resections eventually progressed, compared with a 32% progression rate in 25 patients with incomplete resections.[34] Surgical morbidity is increased with more aggressive surgery, so the risk of neurologic worsening must be taken into account when attempting to remove all visible tumor. As a general rule, those patients with a slower clinical presentation tend to have a better chance at long-term progression-free survival. Following surgery, observation with interval examination and MRI is required, but there does not seem to be a role for either adjuvant radiotherapy or chemotherapy. At progression, additional surgery is usually warranted. These tumors are rare and there is little experience to suggest a definitive role for either radiotherapy or chemotherapy in the early management or at the time of first relapse in these low-grade tumors. If the pathology proves to be a high-grade neoplasm, the tumor should be treated as such, with either radiotherapy, chemotherapy or both.

Intrinsic Tectal Gliomas

Tumors intrinsic to the tectum tend to be low-grade astrocytomas. As with many tumors that occur in the brainstem, the exact histology is presumed, given that

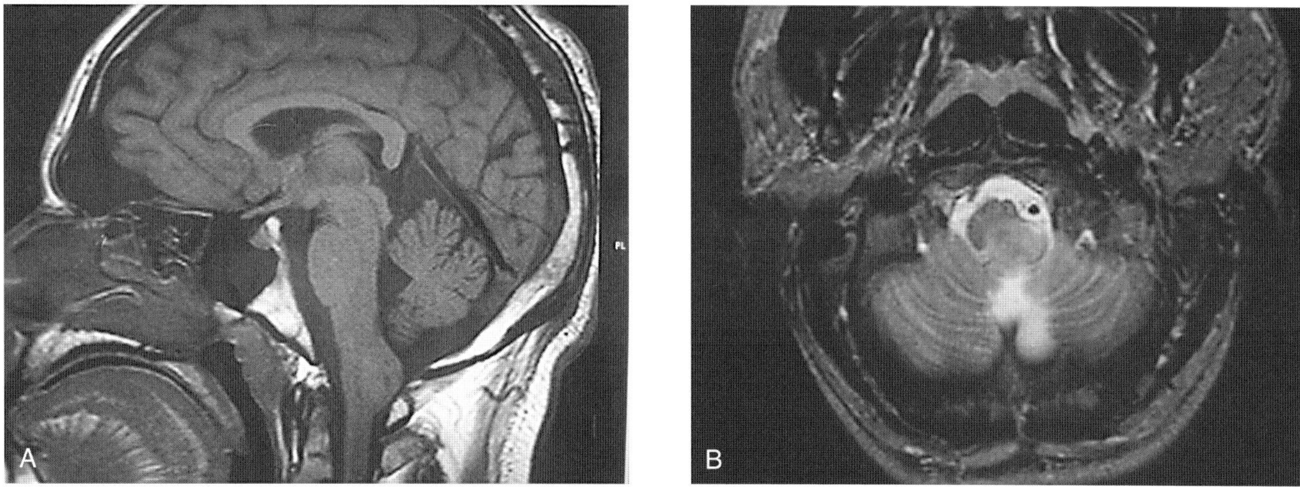

Figure 16–3. (A and B) Cervicomedullary glioma. These T_1-weighted sagittal and T_2-weighted axial images demonstrate an intrinsic focal mass in the lower medulla and upper cervical cord region. This patient presented with mild, long-standing, left arm weakness and was being observed pending progression.

most of these tumors are never biopsied. The low-grade tectal glioma is labeled based on the clinical presentation, classical MRI features, and subsequent favorable clinical course. By definition, because these tumors occur adjacent to the aqueduct of Sylvius, the clinical presentation is usually a result of hydrocephalus that results from obstruction of CSF flow. These tumors may be quite small; consequently, prior to MRI these tumors often went undetected during otherwise appropriate management for symptomatic hydrocephalus. Even with MRI, these tumors are often unnoticed at presentation and only become evident after correction of the hydrocephalus. The tumors may extend longitudinally along the nerve fibers without invading nearby structures; others grow exophytically.

Patients typically present with signs and symptoms of hydrocephalus, usually without cranial nerve palsies or long tract signs. In a patient with upgaze paresis or long-track signs following a CSF diversion procedure, one should consider an alternative diagnosis, such as a pineal astrocytomas, primitive neuroectodermal tumor (PNET), or germ cell neoplasm. In one study of 9 children with a mean age of 11.6 years at the time of initial operation and a mean duration of symptoms of 16 months, MRI revealed noncommunicating hydrocephalus and tectal distortion characterized by bulbous enhancement of the tectum with a clearly marginated intrinsic mass lesion with abnormal signal intensity. Lesions are hypointense on T_1-weighted images and hyperintense on T_2-weighted images. None of the lesions enhance with gadolinium. Good prognostic signs have been described, such as being in the pediatric age group, small tumor size, absence of contrast enhancement, intrinsic localization, and lack of tumor extension (Fig. 16-4).[35]

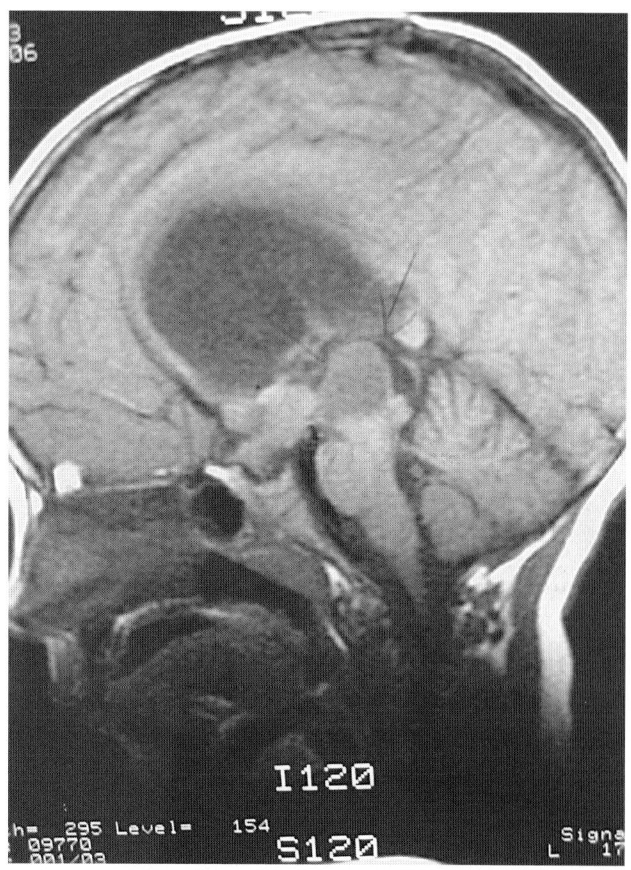

Figure 16–4. Tectal glioma. This is a T_1-weighted sagittal MRI showing the tectal mass and hydrocephalus. The patient presented with headaches and macrocrania, suggesting long-standing ventriculomegaly. This patient was treated with a third ventriculostomy and became free of symptoms. She remained under continued observation.

The literature is full of studies with small numbers of patients, so most studies indicate that tumors of the tectal region in children have an indolent clinical course.[35–37] In one study of 16 patients, the median interval from diagnosis and shunt insertion to progression of symptoms was almost 8 years, and more than 11 years from the first onset of initial symptoms.[37] As a general rule, the intrinsic tectal gliomas that measure less than 2 cm in diameter, without extension or contrast enhancement, represent the specific subgroup with an indolent course and should be managed conservatively, specifically with CSF diversion and observation. Larger tumor size and contrast enhancement have been cited as predictors of the need for eventual radiotherapy or chemotherapy. CSF diversion procedures, primarily third ventriculostomy and long-term interval physical examinations, and MRI are recommended.[38] By definition, the hydrocephalus would not have occurred if the tumor had not grown, but the observation that once the tumor is diagnosed, subsequent growth of the tumor occurs years later, and in one study patients did not progress in a time frame of up to 17 years.[39]

Brainstem Tumors and Neurofibromatosis Type I

Brain tumors, primarily gliomas, are more common in those with neurofibromatosis type 1 (NF1) than in the general population. Although most of these tumors occur along the visual pathway (optic nerves, optic chiasm with or without hypothalamic involvement, and extending into the optic tracks), some may occur in the brainstem.[40] It is critical during the evaluation to distinguish true neoplasm from the focal areas of signal intensity (although the more common jargon of "unidentified bright objects" appears in the literature this may be offensive to some) that are commonly found in children with NF1. These focal areas of signal intensity, which are bright on both fluid-attenuated inversion recovery and T_2-weighted images, are common in the deep gray masses, the brainstem, and the cerebellum, and may have some mass effect. These MRI abnormalities are often found on surveillance scanning or on scanning performed for clinical problems unrelated to brainstem function. In most instances, treatment with radiotherapy is not necessary and followup scanning alone is recommended unless the child has progressive neurologic findings related to brainstem function. Because many children with NF1 have long-standing fine and gross motor difficulties, these static problems should not be assumed to be caused by a neoplasm, unless they are clearly worsening. If however, there are progressive neurologic signs or clear-cut increases in the size of these MRI abnormalities, radiotherapy is recommended. Children with NF1 and intrinsic brainstem masses have a better prognosis than does the typical child with a pontine glioma.[40–43]

▶ CONCLUSION

Brainstem gliomas constitute approximately 10% to 20% of tumors in childhood. These tumors can be subtyped based on their MRI appearance into the diffuse infiltrating, focal intrinsic, exophytic, and the intrinsic medullary gliomas. The most common subtype, the diffuse pontine glioma, has a peak age of occurrence between 5 and 8 years of age and a bleak prognosis, even with intensive therapy. Surgical removal is not an option and, unfortunately, little advances in survival have been seen with this tumor. Although most children respond to radiotherapy, the duration of response is brief and most children with diffuse infiltrating lesions die within 18 to 24 months after diagnosis. The other tumor subtypes tend to have an indolent course. Surgical treatment, either resection of the tumor or diversion of CSF can result in a lengthy remission or symptom improvement in the majority of patients.

REFERENCES

1. Panitch ES, Berg BO. Brainstem tumors of childhood and adolescence. Am J Dis Child 1970;119:465–467.
2. Albright AL, Guthkelch AN, Packer RJ, et al. Prognostic factors in pediatric brain-stem Gliomas. J Neurosurg 1986;65: 751–755.
3. Cohen BH, Garvin J. Brain tumors. In: Rudolph, Hoffman, Rudolph, eds. Rudolph's Pediatrics, 21st ed. Stamford, CT: Appleton & Lange, 2002;2207–2231.
4. Walker DA, Punt JAG, Sokal M. Clinical management of brain stem glioma. Arch Dis Child 1999;80:558–564.
5. Fischbein NJ, Prados MD, Wara W, et al. Radiologic classification of brain stem tumors: correlation of magnetic resonance imaging appearance and clinical outcome. Pediatr Neurosurg 1996;24:9–23.
6. Zimmerman, RA. Neuroimaging of pediatric brain stem diseases other than brain stem glioma. Pediatr Neurosurg 1996;25:83–92.
7. Packer RJ, Zimmerman RA, Luerssen TG, et al. Brainstem gliomas of childhood: magnetic resonance imaging. Neurology 1985;35:397–401.
8. Donahue B, Allen J, Siffert J, et al. Patterns of recurrence in brain stem gliomas: evidence for craniospinal dissemination. Int J Radiat Oncol Biol Phys 1998;40(3):677–680.
9. Packer RJ, Allen J, Nielsen S, et al. Brainstem glioma: clinical manifestations of meningeal gliomatosis. Ann Neurol 1983;14:177–182.
10. Motoyama Y, Ogi S, Nabeshima S. Pontine glioblastoma multiforme initially presenting with leptomeningeal gliomatosis. Neurol Med Chir 2002;42(7):309–313.
11. Packer RJ. Brain tumors in children. Arch Neurol 1999; 56(4):1999;421–425.
12. Cartmill M, Punt J. Brain stem gliomas, the role of biopsy. Br J Neurosurg 1997;11:177.
13. Albright AL. Diffuse brainstem tumors. When is a biopsy necessary? Pediatric Neurosurg 1996;24:252–255.

14. Albright AL, Packer RJ, Zimmerman R, et al. Magnetic resonance scans should replace biopsies for the diagnosis of diffuse brain stem gliomas: a report from the Children's Cancer Group. Neurosurgery 1993;33:1026–1030.
15. Epstein F, McCleary EL. Intrinsic brain-stem tumors of childhood: surgical indications. J Neurosurg 1986;64:11–15.
16. Cohen BH, Packer RJ, Siegel KR, et al. Brain tumors in children under two years: treatment, survival and long-term prognosis. Pediatr Neurosurg 1993;19(4):171–179.
17. Packer RJ, Nicholson SH, Venzina FL, et al. Brainstem gliomas. Neurosurg Clini N Am 1992;3:863–880.
18. Packer RJ, Boyett JM, Zimmerman RA, et al. Outcome of children with brain stem gliomas after treatment with 7800 cGy of hyperfractionated radiotherapy. Cancer 1994;74: 1827–1834.
19. Freeman CR, Krischer J, Sanford RA, et al. Hyperfractionated radiotherapy in brainstem tumor: results of a Pediatric Oncology Group Study. Int J Radiat Oncol Biol Phys 1998; 15:311–318.
20. Packer RJ, Boyett JM, Zimmerman RA, et al. Hyperfractionated radiation therapy (72 Gy) for children with brain stem gliomas: a Children's Cancer Group phase I/II trial. Cancer 1993;72:1414–1421.
21. Jennings MT, Freeman ML, Murray MJ. Strategies in the treatment of diffuse pontine gliomas: the therapeutic role of hyperfractionated radiotherapy and chemotherapy. J Neurooncol 1996;28:207–222.
22. Lashford LS, Thiesse P, Jouvet A, et al. Temozolomide in malignant gliomas of childhood: A United Kingdom Children's Cancer Study Group and French Society for Pediatric Oncology Intergroup Study. J Clin Oncol 2002; 20(24):4684–4691.
23. Freeman CR, Kepner J, Kun LE, et al. A detrimental effect of a combined chemotherapy-radiotherapy approach in children with diffuse intrinsic brain stem gliomas?. Int J Radiat Oncol Biol Phys 2000;47(3):561–564.
24. Allen J, Siffert J, Donahue B, et al. A phase I/II study of carboplatin combined with hyperfractionated radiotherapy for brainstem gliomas. Cancer 1999;86(6):1064–1069.
25. Kaplan AM, Albright AL, Zimmerman RA, et al. Brainstem gliomas in children. A Children's Cancer Group review of 119 cases. Pediatr Neurosurg 1996;24(4):185–192.
26. Marcus K, Dutton S, Barnes P, et al. A phase I trial of etanidazole and hyperfractionated radiotherapy in children with diffuse brainstem glioma. Int J Radiat Oncol Biol Phys 2003;55:1182–1185.
27. Chamberlain MC. Recurrent brainstem gliomas treated with oral VP-16. J Neurooncol 1993;15(2):133–139.
28. Jennings MT, Sposto R, Boyett JM, et al. Preradiation chemotherapy in primary high-risk brainstem tumors: phase II study CCG-9941 of the Children's Cancer Group. J Clin Oncol 2002;20:3431–3437.
29. Dunkel IJ, Finlay JL. High-dose chemotherapy with autologous stem cell rescue for brain tumors. Crit Rev Oncol Hematol 2002;41(2):197–204.
30. Pollack IF, Hoffman HJ, Jumphreys RP. The long-term outcome after surgical treatment of dorsally exophytic brainstem gliomas. J Neurosurg 1993;78:859–863.
31. Pollack IF, Pang D, Albright AL. The long-term outcome in children with late onset aqueduct stenosis resulting from benign intrinsic tectal tumors. J Neurosurg 1994;80:681– 688.
32. Hoffman HJ. Dorsally exophytic brain stem tumors and midbrain tumors. Pediatr Neurosurg 1996;24:256–262.
33. Epstein F. Intra-axial tumors of the cervico-medullary junction in children. Concepts in Pediatr Neurosurg 1987;7:117.
34. Weiner HL, Freed D, Woo HH, et al. Intra-axial tumors of the cervicomedullary junction: surgical results and long-term outcome. Pediatr Neurosurg 1997;27:12–18.
35. Daglioglu E, Cataltepe O, Akalan N. Tectal gliomas in children: the implications for natural history and management strategy. Pediatr Neurosurg 2003;38:223–231.
36. Bowers DC, Georgiades C, Aronson LJ, et al. Tectal gliomas: natural history of an indolent lesion in pediatric patients. Pediatr Neurosurg 2000;32:24–29.
37. Pollack IF, Pang D, Albright AL. The long-term outcome in children with late onset aqueduct stenosis resulting from benign intrinsic tectal tumors. J Neurosurg 1994;80:681–688.
38. Javadpour M, Mallucci C. The role of neuroendoscopy in the management of tectal gliomas. Childs Nerv Syst 2004;20:852–857.
39. May PL, Blaser SI, Hoffman HJ, et al. Benign intrinsic tectal "tumors" in children. J Neurosurg 1991;74:867–871.
40. Hughes RAC. Neurological complications of neurofibromatosis 1. In: Huson SM, Hughes RAC, eds. The neurofibromatoses. A pathogenetic and clinical overview. London: Chapman & Hall Medical, 1994:204–222.
41. Bilaniuk LT, Molloy PT, Zimmerman RA, et al. Neurofibromatosis type 1: brain stem tumours. Neuroradiology 1997;39(9):642–53.
42. Pollack IF, Shultz B, Mulvihill JJ. The management of brainstem gliomas in patients with neurofibromatosis 1. Neurology 1996;46:1652–1660.
43. Rosser T, Packer RJ. Intracranial neoplasms in children with neurofibromatosis 1. J Child Neurol 2002;17:630–637.
44. Broniscer A, Gajjar A, Bhargava R, et al. Brain stem involvement in children with neurofibromatosis type 1: role of magnetic resonance imaging and spectroscopy in the distinction from diffuse pontine glioma. Neurosurgery 1997;40:331–337.

CHAPTER 17

Primary Central Nervous System Lymphoma

BRIAN PATRICK O'NEILL / DAVID SCHIFF

Primary central nervous system non-Hodgkin lymphoma (PCNSL) is invariably lethal, targets especially vulnerable populations, and is increasing in incidence. PCNSL, like any other brain tumor, may have a disproportionate effect on quality of life because of its disabling impact on cognition, memory, language, mobility, and adaptive skills. This morbidity is further amplified because of the advanced age of the average patient and the well-documented neurotoxicity of standard therapy. PCNSL is very responsive to treatment, and aggressive management may lead to prolonged remission. Nevertheless, current treatments do not increase cure rates and the quality of such survival is often poor. Clearly more effective and less toxic regimens are needed for this treatable and potentially curable tumor.

Bailey[1] *first recognized PCNSL as a distinct entity in 1929; he called the tumor "perithelial sarcoma" because of its perivascular localization. Nine years later Yuile*[2] *noted the resemblance of these tumors to those of lymph node origin that were at that time known as "reticulum cell sarcoma." However, it was not until the report of Henry and associates*[3] *that the unique nature of this tumor was first realized.* Primary central nervous system lymphoma, *or PCNSL, is now the accepted term and is defined as lymphoma confined to the brain, spinal cord, or leptomeninges without evidence of concurrent systemic lymphoma. It is considered a unique, extranodal non-Hodgkin lymphoma (NHL) ("extranodal lymphoma" refers to those NHL varieties that present in tissues other than lymph nodes) because (a) light and electron microscopic and immunohistochemical studies confirm that PCNSL cells are identical to malignant lymphocytes elsewhere in the body; (b) gene array studies demonstrate that most PCNSL lymphocytes are of germinal cell origin; (c) PCNSL responds to traditional NHL treatments; (d) occult systemic non-Hodgkin lymphoma (sNHL) is found at presentation; and (e) late systemic relapses occur, typically without recurrent PCNSL.*

PCNSL begins and develops in the nervous system and, in most cases, fails there. Systemic disease is identified in fewer than 5% of cases and, when present, is typically in retroperitoneal lymph nodes.[4] *The mechanisms of disease production and relapses are completely unknown. PCNSL occurs in two groups of patients: immunosuppressed patients, such as those infected with the human immunodeficiency virus (HIV), solid-organ transplant recipients, and patients with acquired or congenital immunodeficiencies; and older patients (median 60 years of age) with no known immunosuppression. Among the latter, PCNSL is an uncommon neoplasm, representing less than 1% of all NHLs and less than 5% of all primary brain tumors.[5] However, since 1995 the incidence of this tumor in this latter group has more than doubled.*

PCNSL may involve, simultaneously or sequentially, a number of sites in the central nervous system including the eyes.[6] The vast majority of "immunocompetent" patients present with the "solitary mass lesion" syndrome.[7] In fact, as an example of how modern imaging has informed classification, several PCNSL variants were hitherto unknown until magnetic resonance imaging (MRI) was introduced into standard clinical practice in the late 1980s.[6] Hochberg and Miller[6] are credited with defining four distinct clinical profiles; in descending order of frequency, they are: "single or multiple discrete intracranial nodules," "uveal or vitreous deposits," "diffuse meningeal or periventricular lesions," and "localized intradural spinal masses." Even rarer forms are lymphoma of peripheral nerves and roots ("neurolymphomatosis"[8]), primary dural lymphoma,[9] and intravascular lymphoma.[10]

▶ EPIDEMIOLOGY

Incidence

As recently as the mid-1990s PCNSL was projected to eventually become the most common primary brain tumor of adults.[11] This no doubt represented the impact of the acquired immunodeficiency syndrome (AIDS) epidemic as PCNSL is an AIDS-related malignancy. Highly active antiretroviral therapy (HAART) and the subsequent improved immune status of HIV-infected patients led to a rapid fall in HIV-associated PCNSL. The current estimated incidence of PCNSL (in all forms) is approximately 1:100,000 persons per year.[12] Among putative immunocompetent persons, the incidence of PCNSL is increasing beyond that which can be accounted for by improved diagnostic capabilities alone and exceeds the increasing incidence of systemic lymphoma. As the population ages, increasing numbers of older patients are expected as are proportionally increasing numbers of PCNSL patients.

Eby and associates[13] are credited with the first alert that PCNSL was increasing in incidence and that the increase could not be accounted for by HIV infection, referral patterns, or a change in nosology. They demonstrated that PCNSL incidence increased more than 10-fold between 1973 and 1984, from 2.7 to 30 cases per 10 million persons per year. Subsequent reports confirmed their findings.[14,15] These reports, however, did not address whether the observation of increasing incidence was an effect of ascertainment and referral biases. To address the effects on incidence of imaging, stereotactic neurosurgery, molecular neuropathology, and increasing age, and to revisit the issue of HIV infection, Olson and associates[16] reexamined the National Cancer Institute (NCI) Surveillance, Epidemiology, and End Results (SEER) resource (same one used by Eby and associates [v.s.]) to determine if those conclusions were still apt. They ascertained the age-adjusted incidence rates for PCNSL for all persons from 1975 through 1996 and demonstrated a significant increase in PCNSL for all populations studied and that the most significant increases were seen in patients 65 years of age and older (Fig. 17-1). As surrogates for new technology, SEER data were reviewed by dates of diagnosis (surrogate for imaging) and per glioma diagnosis (surrogates for stereotactic neurosurgery and improved diagnostic neuropathology). By convention, the rates were then calculated excluding the cases from the San Francisco SEER Registry and also by excluding never-married males and females and persons of unknown marital status. They also used SEER data (with exactly the same parameters) for Kaposi sarcoma as a surrogate for the effects of HIV infection. Greater incidence rates were seen for PCNSL than for sNHL, but the estimated annual percent change in incidence was less for both during the period 1985–1997 than during the period 1973–1984.

Etiology

A number of factors are implicated in the causation of systemic NHL, including genetic predisposition syndromes, medical treatments for cancer, phenytoin use, environmental accidents, farming, and certain chemical exposures (see reference 17 for a review). The most robust associations have been with infectious agents (Tables 17-1 and 17-2). Paradoxically, with rare exceptions, the Eby report[13] did not stimulate hypothesis-generating PCNSL epidemiologic studies. DeAngelis[18] reviewed the Memorial Sloan Kettering Cancer Center experience and noted a prior history of cancer in 13% of HIV-negative PCNSL patients, suggesting either a shared genetic predisposition to neoplastic transformation, a common environmental factor, or a causal role of the antineoplastic treatment in PCNSL development. Tomlinson's review[7] of the Mayo Clinic experience showed that autoimmune disease, a personal history of cancer, and a family history of malignancy were common in their HIV-negative PCNSL patients. The most definitive study was the case-control study (with both neurologic and cancer controls) by Schiff and colleagues.[19]

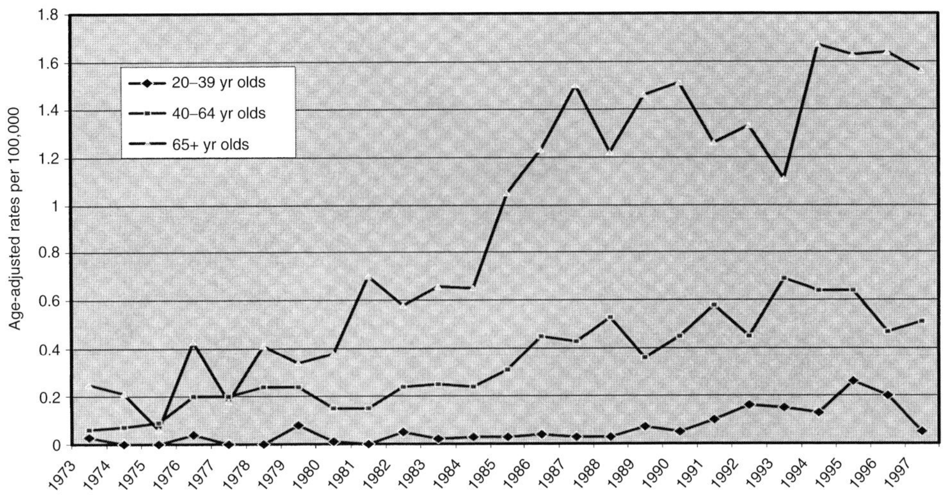

Figure 17-1. Age-adjusted incidence rates of primary central nervous system lymphoma by age groups in non–San Francisco SEER registries (excluding never married and unknown marital status cases). [*With permission from Olson JE, Janney CA, Rao RD, et al. The continuing increase in primary central nervous system (CNS) lymphoma: a surveillance, epidemiology, and end results (SEER) analysis. Cancer 2002;95:1504–1510.*]

"Host Factors"

The outcome of patients with PCNSL is very different from the outcome of patients presenting at other extranodal sites. For example, the clinical profile of stage I_E gastric lymphoma is similar to PCNSL but has a much different outcome. This has led to the proposition that host factors may play a role in outcome, for example, the association of some forms of gastric lymphoma with infection by *Helicobacter pylori* (see "Infectious Agents" below) where early-stage treatment with antibiotics alone may result in tumor regression. However, the immune system likely plays a significant role in the control/eradication of NHL at other extranodal sites, and the lack

▶ **TABLE 17-1.** INFECTIOUS AGENTS ASSOCIATED WITH THE DEVELOPMENT OF LYMPHOID MALIGNANCIES

Infectious Agent	Lymphoid Malignancy
Epstein-Barr virus	Burkitt lymphoma
	Postorgan transplant lymphoma
	Primary CNS diffuse large B-cell lymphoma
	Hodgkin disease
	Extranodal NK/T-cell lymphoma, nasal type
HTLV-1	Adult T-cell leukemia/lymphoma
HIV	Diffuse large B-cell lymphoma
	Burkitt lymphoma
Hepatitis C virus	Lymphoplasmacytic lymphoma
Helicobacter pylori	Gastric MALT lymphoma
Human herpesvirus 8	Primary effusion lymphoma
	Multicentric Castleman disease

CNS = central nervous system; HTLV = human T-cell lymphotropic virus; MALT = mucosa-associated lymphoid tissue; NK = natural killer.
Source: Reproduced with permssion from Kasper DL, Braunwald E, Fauci AS, et al. Harrison's online. URL=www3.accessmedicine.com.aspx?aID=65732.

▶ **TABLE 17-2.** DISEASES OR EXPOSURES ASSOCIATED WITH INCREASED RISK OF DEVELOPMENT OF MALIGNANT LYMPHOMA

Inherited immunodeficiency disease
Klinefelter syndrome
Chédiak-Higashi syndrome
Ataxia-telangiectasia syndrome
Wiskott-Aldrich syndrome
Common variable immunodeficiency disease
Acquired immunodeficiency diseases
Iatrogenic immunosuppression
HIV-1 infection
Acquired hypogammaglobulinemia
Autoimmune disease
Sjögren syndrome
Celiac sprue
Rheumatoid arthritis and systemic lupus erythematosus
Chemical or drug exposures
Phenytoin
Dioxin, phenoxyherbicides
Radiation
Prior chemotherapy and radiation therapy

Source: Reproduced with permission from Kasper DL, Braunwald E, Fauci AS, et al. Harrison's online. URL=www3.accessmedicine.com.aspx?aID=65732.

of an intrinsic immune system, all other things being equal, hinders the CNS from achieving the durable responses seen elsewhere.

As they seem to do in sNHL, age, performance status, and histology affect PCNSL outcome independent of treatment. Because immunocompetency declines steeply after age 50 years, these conclusions may simply reflect the vulnerability of older patients' nervous systems and/or the decline in immunocompetence over time. Noteworthy in one report's analysis was the sevenfold increase in survival among patients 45 years of age or younger.[20] However, within age groups, survival to identical therapies vary, especially between genders. These data suggest the interesting proposition that estrogen-based therapies, as in hormone-replacement therapies, may have a protective effect on oncogenesis.[21,22] However, even though PCNSL is a tumor that affects older males disproportionately, the female survival advantage persists among postmenopausal women who do *not* take hormone replacement therapy (HRT). Nevertheless, survival varies even within age and gender groups.[23]

Infectious Agents

Although rare in non-AIDS PCNSL, Epstein-Barr virus (EBV) genome expression in brain and cerebral spinal fluid (CSF) occurs in nearly all AIDS-associated and post-transplantation PCNSL.[24] EBV is a ubiquitous DNA herpesvirus; more than 90% of adults are seropositive. EBV binds to cells via the CD212 molecule, a B-cell surface molecule. Following B-cell infection, the virus becomes latent, maintaining its genome in episomes and retaining the potential for reactivation. Transcription of the viral protein LMP-1 immortalizes B cells, protecting against apoptosis. Cytotoxic T cells normally keep these immortalized B cells in check. Disruption of cell-mediated immunity, whether from HIV, immunosuppressive drugs in the posttransplantation state, or congenital immunodeficiency leads to the development of polyclonal or monoclonal B-cell lymphoproliferative disorders. Two problems remain with these studies. Firstly, double-labeling studies have not confirmed that the infectious agent was in tumor cells.[25] Secondly, immunosuppressed patients may have a number of infectious agents in tissues. Thus the infectious agents may be nothing more than "background noise." Furthermore, in the aforementioned gastric mucosa-associated lymphoid tissue (MALT) lymphomas, the bacterium does not transform lymphocytes to produce lymphoma; rather the vigorous immune response to the bacterium and the chronic antigenic stimulation leads to the neoplasia.[24] Nevertheless, viral oncogenesis remains a potent field of study and EBV is a major focus (see reference 26 for a review). However, other viruses have been investigated in brain tumors (Table 17-3). The best-documented studies have involved the detection of polyomavirus sequences in specimens of human brain tumors.

TABLE 17-3. JC VIRUS, BK VIRUS, AND SV40 SEQUENCES IN SELECTED NERVOUS SYSTEM TUMOR

	Virus (No. Positive/No. Tested)		
Tumor Type	**JCV**	**BKV**	**SV40**
Choroid plexus papilloma	1/16	0/16	6/16
			5/6
Ependymoma			10/11
	0/16	0/16	9/16
			0/10
			8/11
			4/13
Medulloblastoma	10/11		
	0/17	1/17	9/17
Other gliomas	0/75	0/75	
	1/1		
	0/52		
	3/150	5/150	51/150
			10/30
			3/20
Neuroblastoma		18/18	

Source: Adapted from Shah KV. Polyoma Viruses (JC virus, BK virus, and Simian virus 40) and Human Cancer. In Goedert JJ, ed. Infectious Causes of Cancer. Totowa, NJ: Humana Press, 2000:465.

Antigen Discovery

Antigen discovery is the term for the field devoted to identifying stimuli for the pathologic process that results in acute or chronic illnesses of epithelial, immune system, or neural origin (e.g., trigeminal neuralgia). These antigen discovery efforts so far have focused on diseases of the affluent world, that affect all ethnic groups after migration, and are increasing in incidence. A complementary, or perhaps necessary, second component, such as genetic susceptibilities, is not inconsistent with an antigen model. That within these regions its burden of disease falls disproportionally on highly vulnerable populations is supportive of an autoimmune, environmental, or infectious cause. PCNSL is predominantly a disease of Western Europe and the Americas, and does not appear to select any one ethnic group. Recent epidemiologic studies from the United States and Europe attest to this.[19,27,28] The aforementioned Schiff study identified a positive correlation with tonsillectomy (a similar observation was noted in the 1970s with Hodgkin disease[29]) and with educational level, the latter considered to be a surrogate for socioeconomic class.[19]

Given the robust association of EBV in brain lymphomas associated with intense immunosuppression, infectious particles are a major focus of investigation.

So far there has been no convincing demonstration of viral nucleic acid incorporation in tumor specimens from "immunocompetent" PCNSL patients. Furthermore, as a surrogate for such, the use of antiviral therapies have not been reported to impact the course of this group of PCNSL patients as they have been reported to do in AIDS-related PCNSL.[30] Unlike transplant recipients where one may be able to reduce or even eliminate the immunosuppression (and presumably interrupt the cascade toward neoplasm), PCNSL patients are ostensibly "immunocompetent" so there is no identifiable strategy to render them more so.

Immunocompetence

Lymphomas are disimmune disorders. Understanding normal lymphocyte function will likely yield clues into initiation and progression of lymphomas (see reference 28 for a review). Understanding normal lymphocyte differentiation is useful for an understanding of lymphoma classification and biology. Immunoglobulin or T-cell receptor gene rearrangement is an early event. B cells then become mature but naive small lymphocytes. Once exposed to antigen, lymphocytes begin to proliferate in germinal centers and are termed *immunoblasts*. The variable portion for the immunoglobulin gene undergoes further point mutations to improve antigen specificity; these are termed *somatic hypermutations*.

Some insights have already been provided by study of PCNSL occurring in the setting of profound immunosuppression. For example, PCNSL is the second most common intracranial mass lesion (after brain abscess) in persons infected with HIV and the risk is inversely proportional to CD4 counts.[31] Furthermore, some PCNSL cases are salvaged by reversal of immunosuppression, either by the use of HAART[32] in AIDS or discontinuation of organ-rejection suppression.[33] Furthermore, if immunocompetency is maintained, PCNSL does not recur. This reversal of immunosuppression likely exploits regulatory pathways inherent in germinal center–derived B lymphocytes; although the brain has no germinal centers, these tumors are derived from lymphocytes that have passed through a germinal center environment.[28]

The special situation of PCNSL occurring in the context of immunodeficiency such as in AIDS (HIV+ PCNSL) or following organ transplantation (central nervous system posttransplantation lymphoproliferative disease [CNS-PTLD]) has further epidemiologic implications. Prior to the introduction of HAART, patients developed PCNSL when they were in the advanced stages of AIDS. Survival was measured in months and the cause of death might be PCNSL, cerebral abscesses, organ failure, or overwhelming systemic infection. With HAART, incidence, age of onset, response to treatment, and overall survival are favorably influenced. It remains to be seen whether the form of HIV-PCNSL that will develop post-HAART are phenotypically different. The experience with CNS-PTLD suggests that they might be. Prior to 1998 there were fewer than 40 CNS-PTLD cases described in English-language scientific publications. Then a large series[33] from a single institution documented that although CNS-PTLD occurred in only 0.3% of organ transplantations and 12.4% of all posttransplantation non-Hodgkin lymphoma cases during the study period, CNS involvement accounted for 24% of all extranodal PTLD. CNS-PTLD cases predominated among patients with kidney or kidney and pancreas transplantations. None of the 134 patients who had a heart transplant developed CNS-PTLD.[33]

Until recently the standard immunosuppressive agents for organ transplantation were prednisone, azathioprine, and cyclosporine. Newer agents, such as tacrolimus and mycophenolate mofetil, are beginning to be used clinically (and being applied to other nontransplantation conditions). The mechanism of immunosuppression (and presumably the risk of immunosuppression-mediated disorders) varies among these new agents. In one study, nearly three-fourths of cases occurred in the late 1990s after the patients' long-term immunosuppression regimen was switched from azathioprine to mycophenolate mofetil.[34] An interesting co-association found in that study was the increased incidence of non–AIDS-defining cancers in HIV-infected patients before and after the use of HAART relative to that observed in the French general population of the same age and gender.[35]

▶ BASIC SCIENCE THAT INFORMS PATHOGENESIS

PCNSL tumor bulk comprises dividing cells, reactive cells, and accumulating cells. PCNSL likely develops from (and perhaps through) a progressive acquisition of "destabilizers," that is, cellular regulators of apoptosis, mismatch repair, and other intracellular regulators of cell division, that the lymphocyte acquires in its phenotypic evolution from "normal" to "reactive" to "cancer." This balance between apoptosis and cell survival in response to intra- or extracellular signaling is vital for maintaining tissue homeostasis. Aberrant control of cell-survival signaling can result in tumor generation and resistance to chemopreventive agents used in cancer treatment. This concept has already been formulated for systemic lymphoma with the discovery and elucidation of the function of the *bcl-2* oncogene. Follicular lymphoma patients with the *t(14q;18q)* translocation have modulation of the apoptotic cascade as a consequence of overexpression or inappropriately expressed function of *bcl-2*. In experimental lymphomas, *bcl-2* does not cause cancer directly but allows the cell to survive to undergo subsequent mutations involving rearrangements at other oncogenes, such as the *c-myc*, that result in accelerated progression of the lymphoma (see references 36 and 37 for reviews).

Until now most of what we know about PCNSL was derived by extrapolation from systemic NHL or by empiric information gained over the last two decades. For example, how PCNSL develops was informed by data obtained from gene expression profiling in systemic lymphoma. At least three groups of diffuse large B-cell lymphoma (the counterpart to the most common PCNSL histology [see "Pathology" below]) can be identified: a germinal center type; an activated B-cell type; and an ill-defined group. Additionally, NHL molecular "signatures" with both prognostic and predictive significance have been defined.[38] Most data suggest a germinal center origin for PCNSL based on sequence analysis of immunoglobulin genes or of other genes undergoing somatic hypermutations.[39] For example the *bcl-6* gene is strongly expressed in germinal center–derived B cells and *bcl-6* expression has been proposed as a marker of especially good PCNSL outcome.[40] Mutations are derived in the 5′ noncoding region correlate with the transition of B cells through its "phenotypic evolution" to cancer.[41] However, the basic question as to whether PCNSL is a unique lymphoma that *arises in* the nervous system or a lymphoma that *goes to* the nervous system is still unresolved.

Studies of alterations to tumor suppressor genes and protooncogenes in immunocompetent cases of PCNSL have been slowed by the uncommon nature of the disease and small amounts of tissue available. Nonetheless, several important observations have been made in recent years. The *p16/CDKN2A* (cyclin-dependent kinase N2A) tumor suppressor gene, which normally blocks cell-cycle progression through its effects on retinoblastoma protein (Rb) via CDK4 and CDK6, is usually inactivated either by homozygous deletion or a combination of hemizygous deletion and gene methylation.[42,43] The *p14* gene, which acts by inhibiting the effects of the *MDM2* gene on p53, is often inactivated.[44,45] *RB1* and *p53* are rarely mutated or lost, and *MDM2, CDK4*, and *MYC* are generally not amplified.

B-cell homeostasis is essential for normal immunity, and dysregulation of this homeostasis is an underlying aspect of lymphoid neoplasms. Signaling pathways control B-cell homeostasis and reflect the balance between proliferation and cell death. Many cytokines including members of the tissue necrosis factor (TNF) family function as potent survival factors for specific lymphoid populations. For example, B-lymphocyte stimulator (BLyS; also known as BAFF, TALL-1, THANK) is a recently defined member of the TNF family and is critical for survival of peripheral B lymphocytes.[46,47] Recent evidence implicates aberrant activation of the BLyS signaling network in some types of B-cell lymphoma.[48,49]

Even if disordered B-cell homeostasis is important in lymphoma genesis, one needs to explain how lymphoma cells get to the brain and from where they come. There are at least three mechanisms by which malignant white blood cells may access and enter the CNS. First, there may be direct extension from contiguous sites such as dura.[50] Second, cells may track along the Virchow-Robin spaces from the CSF as occurs in carcinomatous meningitis where infiltrating carcinoma cells produce parenchymal spinal cord disease.[51] Third, there may be lymphocyte "homing," whereby circulating malignant lymphocytes pass across the endothelium to enter perivascular spaces and eventually into the CNS. Convincing evidence for this type of CNS colonization exists from studies in experimental leukemia,[52] and myeloma cells have been tracked from the bone marrow to CSF. What is not known is how and why this "homing" occurs.

There is no resident lymphocyte population in the CNS. In the past, pluripotential cells intrinsic to the CNS were thought to have the capacity to differentiate into lymphocytes.[1] Supporting data for this concept were based on morphologic and a priori considerations only. The scant resident lymphocyte population of the CNS is now thought to arise by "trafficking" of normal T lymphocytes across capillary endothelia within the blood–brain barrier and epithelia at the choroid plexus. Human leukocyte antigen (HLA)-presenting cells are conspicuously lacking in normal brain, as are B lymphocytes. At the present time, these "trafficking" movements of T lymphocytes are thought to be random.[53] Further knowledge should lead to novel therapies such as dendritic cell therapy in sNHL.[54]

Lymphocytes enter the CNS in response to a signal provided within. This signal may be an infectious particle or may be some other antigen such as a "foreign body" (e.g., fragment of metal). The cascade that follows is consistent irrespective of the signal. Recent work derived from a mouse model of brain and eye lymphoma gives support to this concept.[55] Specific homing of these cells to the CNS followed intraperitoneal inoculation of S49 mouse lymphoma cells. These studies suggest that the first site of ingress was the choroid plexus and the ganglia of cranial nerves. Once in CNS cells, lymphocytes appear to spread within the brain and migrate along the optic nerve to the eyes.

No marker has yet been identified that can account for the CNS "homing." Chromosomal imbalances in PCNSL are similar to those of systemic diffuse large B-cell lymphomas, suggesting that genomic lesions alone do not explain the apparent neurotropism. However, malignant transformation *may* take place in lymphocyte subpopulations that already possess neurotropism for whatever reason. In other words, if "programmed" lymphocytes get into CNS they may evolve, depending on their molecular signature.[40] Recent work suggests that this may be the case. Early gene expression profile analysis of PCNSL specimens has defined approximately 100 genes with more than a twofold level of differential expression between PCNSL, nodal lymphomas, and nonneoplastic brain.[56] The signature appears to involve genes involved in B-cell differentiation, proliferation, apoptosis, and cytokine signaling. A major barrier to meaningful discovery in PCNSL has been the need to do such molecular biologic and gene microarray studies in fresh-frozen tumor specimens. Virtually all PCNSL patients have their diagnoses established by stereotactic biopsy.[57] Typically one to two 100-μm × 1-cm cores are removed and submitted for diagnostic workup. Standard and special stains often exhaust all or virtually all of this tissue. Newer techniques that permit messenger RNA (mRNA) retrieval from paraffin should obviate this problem and lead to exciting advances in knowledge of PCNSL.

▶ PATHOLOGY

PCNSL is typically a deep-seated, bulky tumor without corresponding mass effect (Fig. 17-2). The lesions are typically soft and granular and they often have contact with a CSF surface. Unlike metastatic tumors, PCNSL lesions are poorly defined because of infiltration into adjacent brain tissue. In presumed immunocompetent patients, PCNSL is typically a solitary mass lesion or, at most, two lesions. In contrast, immunocompromised patients (such as organ transplant recipients and patients infected with HIV) have multiple lesions in more than half of the instances. Associated necrosis, hemorrhage, and neovascularity are uncommon except in immunodeficiency-related cases. Microscopically, PCNSL (Fig. 17-3) is a diffuse lesion with an angiocentric growth pattern. Malignant lymphocytes freely invade normal surrounding brain, and autopsy studies demonstrate widespread infiltration of normal brain. Solid tumor bulk comprises sheets of fairly monotonous, atypical, mitotically active cells. Toward the edge of a lesion, tumor cells are preferentially arranged in small clumps around blood vessels. Within the tumor bulk is the perivascular layering of argyrophilic reticulum-rich basement membrane reduplications that produces an "onion ring"–like appearance. Hortega (and the silver stain that now bears his name) is credited with describing this phenomenon (which gave rise to its early name of "reticulum cell sarcoma"). Although still unexplained, this unique pathologic feature remains the morphologic hallmark of this disorder (see reference 58 for a review).

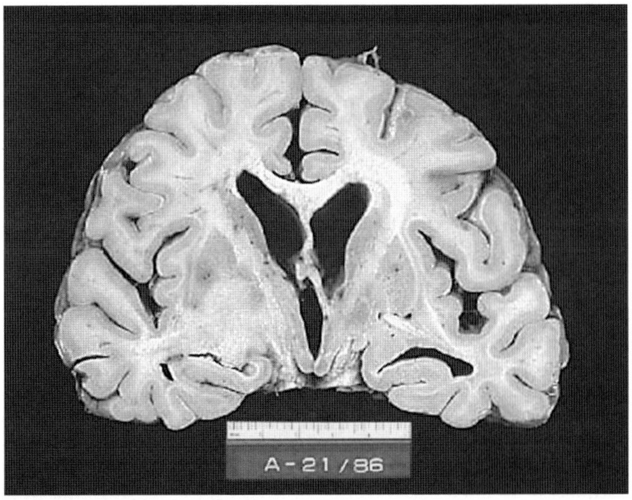

Figure 17-2. Cut section of brain with two PCNSL lesions—a large mass in right basal ganglia and a small lesion at apex of left lateral ventricle.

The most common PCNSL histologic subtype is diffuse large B-cell lymphoma, occurring in at least 80% of cases. Lower-grade B-cell and T-cell forms are rare, much less common than their frequency in systemic lymphomas. The reason for this difference in histologies between PCNSL and systemic lymphoma is unknown (Table 17-4). Tumor infiltrates are characterized by large centroblasts or immunoblasts expressing B-cell markers CD19, CD20, and CD79a. The cells are embedded within a matrix composed of CD3+ T cells, CD68+ macrophages, and small, mature, polyclonal CD20+ B cells. Typically PCNSL tumor cells demonstrate monoclonal surface or cytoplasmic immunoglobulin, most commonly IgM *kappa* (see reference 59 for a review). A study of gene sequences indicated tumor cell derivation from highly mutated germinal center B cells.[38]

PCNSL from immunocompromised patients tend to be exclusively B-cell tumors and are more likely to show lymphoplasmacytic differentiation, be more pleomorphic, and be interspersed with areas of necrosis or hemorrhage (or both). The brains of these patients may be swollen and there may be areas of hemorrhage visible over the surface or in CSF. Foci of necrosis are common—nearly 75% of the patients in one series.[55] Parenchymal hemorrhage, whether spontaneous or following biopsy, is not uncommon.[60] In fact, postbiopsy hemorrhage can be fatal, even if the procedure is done flawlessly and preoperative coagulation studies are normal[33] (see also "Clinical: All Forms" below).

The pathology of PCNSL associated with states of immunodeficiency such as HIV+ PCNSL and CNS-PTLD may be strikingly different from each other. HIV+ PCNSL is characterized by an increased frequency of high-grade tumors of either large cell or immunoblastic subtype. By immunohistochemistry, neoplastic cells are CD20+/CD3– B cells. In almost all instances the B-cell tumors are monoclonal.[61,62] Some forms are classified as "null"; in these instances, the extensive necrosis may have precluded the display of cell surface markers. The cellularity that comprises PTLD-CNS forms may vary from monomorphous

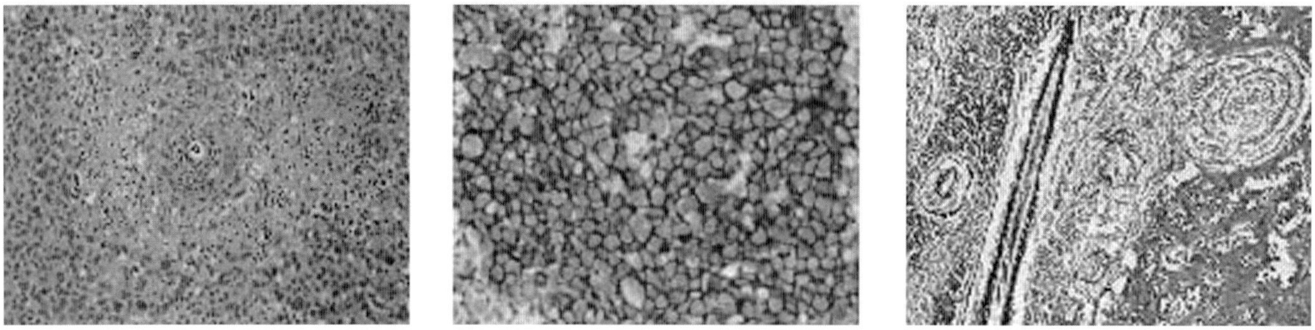

Figure 17-3 (PLATE 49). (Left) Typical light microscopic appearance: angiocentric infiltrate with, in this case, extensive PCNSL infiltration into parenchyma (hematoxylin and eosin [H&E], ×20). (Center) Most cases are large, CD20+ B-cell tumors (CD20, ×20). (Right) Characteristic "onion-ring" appearance with silver stains (Hortega, ×20).

small lymphocytes, to dense polymorphous lymphoplasmacytic infiltrates composed of small lymphocytes and plasma cells, to frank, large B-cell lymphoma cells indistinguishable from those of typical PCNSL. The polymorphous B-cell variety is approximately four times as common as the immunoblastic monomorphous variety.[63] Immunodeficiency-associated PCNSL T-cell forms have been described by Penn and Porat[64] but are very uncommon.

The association of immunodeficiency-related tumors with EBV is most easily shown by in situ hybridization (ISH). Cells are typically strongly positive in more than 95% of the cases. The specificity of the test is extremely high but the sensitivity is unknown. Traditional serology is useful in evaluating acute versus remote infection in healthy individuals, but titers are not dependable in immunocompromised hosts. EBV viral load testing by quantitative DNA amplification of blood samples has proven useful for early diagnosis and monitoring patients. Even more useful may be detection of EBV in CSF by polymerase chain reaction (PCR), which in one study was equivalent to brain biopsy (see references 65 and 66 for reviews). Recent studies also suggest a role for EBV viral load testing in nasopharyngeal carcinoma, Hodgkin disease, and AIDS patients with brain lymphoma.[67] Gene expression profiling, currently under development, may improve the subclassification of EBV-related diseases and help to predict response to therapy.

▶ **TABLE 17-4.** REPORTED INCIDENCE OF SUBTYPES OF PCNSL

Non-AIDS cases	
Diffuse follicle center cell lymphoma grade III	40%
Diffuse large B-cell lymphoma	20%
Diffuse follicle center cell lymphoma grades I–II	10%
Diffuse small lymphocytic and lymphoplasmacytoid lymphoma	10%
Peripheral T-cell lymphoma	<1%
AIDS cases	
Diffuse large B-cell lymphoma	65%
Diffuse follicle center cell lymphoma grade III	20%
Diffuse follicle center cell lymphoma grades I–II	5%
Diffuse small lymphocytic and lymphoplasmacytoid lymphoma	<5%
High-grade B-cell lymphoma, Burkitt-like	<5%
Peripheral T-cell lymphoma	<5%

The majority of all forms of PCNSL are diagnosed via stereotactic biopsy.[52] Careful coordination among clinician, surgeon, and pathologist is required. Patients should not be on corticosteroids, or should be withdrawn from them (if medically safe to do so), prior to biopsy, to avoid false-negative results.[68] Even under optimal circumstances the surgeon's first sample may reveal only reactive tissue. With a high clinical suspicion, more samples are obtained until the pathologist determines that there is diagnostic tissue within the specimen. Often a tumor smear will secure the diagnosis or make it highly likely. In that situation a portion of tumor containing tissue should be frozen at −70°C for additional diagnostic and/or research studies. Harris and colleagues recommend[59] that stereotactic core-needle biopsies be bisected longitudinally and the tips of each half smeared for histology.

Endothelial cells are often plump, and electron microscopy of PCNSL brain capillaries shows endothelial cell disruption with apoptotic changes.[69] These changes did not occur in a comparison group of gliomas of different cell type and grade. Unlike glioblastoma multiforme (GBM), a similarly lethal primary brain tumor, PCNSL lacks endothelial proliferation. Endothelial proliferation may be a result of stimulation by vascular endothelial growth factor (VEGF), which is expressed in high concentrations in GBM[70]; this has not been studied in PCNSL. However, there are data that angiogenesis

▶ **TABLE 17-5.** RECOMMENDED EVALUATION OF A SPECIMEN SUSPECTED TO BE PCNSL

Marker	Rationale
Leukocyte common antigen (CD45)	Confirms hematopoietic neoplasm
Cytokeratin	Excludes metastasis
B-cell antigen (CD20)	Distinction of B-cell from T-cell lymphoma
T-cell antigen (CD3)	Distinction of B-cell from T-cell lymphoma; marker of T-cell infiltration
BCL-6	Follicle center origin; may have prognostic importance
CD10 (optional)	Follicle center origin; may have prognostic importance
BCL-2 (optional)	May have prognostic importance
Ki-67 (optional)	Labels mitotic cells; may have prognostic significance

does occur in lymphoproliferative disorders,[71] and, by inference, in PCNSL.[66] Newer laboratory techniques promise to give more insights into pathogenesis and serve predictive and prognostic aims. Table 17-5 is an example of the application of newer immunohistochemical techniques to patient specimens.[59]

The blood–brain barrier is assumed to reside at the level of the endothelia of brain capillaries and postcapillary venules. The relative exclusion of intravascular contents is thought to be a result of fixed "tight junctions" between endothelial cells and a more dynamic active process that includes metabolic "pumps" (see reference 72 for a review). The blood–brain barrier is not intact in and around infiltrative primary brain tumors, which is likely the basis of imaging contrast enhancement. Little is known, however, about the mechanisms that lead to a "leaky" blood–brain barrier. The cellular disintegration and frank endothelial cell discontinuities shown in electron micrographs[69] have been proposed as the morphologic counterpart to the contrast enhancement seen on neuroimaging. However, this increased blood–brain barrier permeability may be secondary rather than primary and may be a consequence of a nonspecific (although distinctive) effect of cytokines on the endothelia, because similar imaging changes may be seen in inflammation and in infection. The PCNSL microenvironment includes T-cell infiltrates that are recognized as a source of cytotoxic cytokines.[68,73] There are rare cases of PCNSL *without* MRI contrast enhancement, basement membrane reduplication, or perivascular infiltrates.[74,75] This occurrence would argue for either an unusual pathologic phenotype, or PCNSL serendipitously captured prior to the development of the characteristic perivascular "fingerprint" and the corresponding contrast enhancement. Because pathologic specimens clearly show tumor cells in intact brain intermixed with normal-appearing blood vessels, this latter supposition is not unreasonable.

The true incidence of leptomeningeal tumor is unknown. Most of what we now know comes from postmortem specimens.[76] Stereotactic biopsies rarely include the pia-arachnoid. Analysis of CSF is now much more common; the fluid is normal or mildly abnormal with elevated total protein (including elevated immunoglobulins in some cases), a lymphocytic pleocytosis, and, in about a third of cases, "atypical cells."[77,78] However, criteria for calling a CSF cytology "positive" vary from merely the presence of atypical lymphocytes, to monoclonality of surface immunoglobulins, to frankly malignant cells, ideally with mitotic figures; in fact, spinal fluid contains tumor cells in only a minority of cases.[59] For example, one study attempted to correlate the CSF profile, MR images, and pathology slides for evidence of leptomeningeal tumor.[78] In that study the incidence of leptomeningeal tumor was 42% at diagnosis and 41% at recurrence, but the authors included patients with atypical lymphocytes, a nonspecific finding. Meningeal biopsy may be useful to demonstrate that a leptomeningeal process with abnormal but nondiagnostic spinal fluid is a result of PCNSL.[79] Because PCNSL comprises a polyclonal and polytypic lymphocytosis, it is not surprising that cells of any type may be shed into the CSF. Flow cytometry, CSF biomarker analyses, and proteomic profiles have the potential to be much more informative and useful.

▶ CLINICAL: ALL FORMS

All forms of PCNSL share common features of subacute onset and progression, distinctive (and nearly pathognomonic) imaging, potential for dramatic response in imaging *and* neurologic function to methotrexate (MTX)-based treatment (and corticosteroids), and lethality if untreated. What is also common is the influence of the host, the narrow "safety margin" of the CNS, the inherent neurotoxicity of the current menu of treatment options, and the vulnerability of the patients. This section has arbitrarily chosen to address the clinical issue as a whole. Nevertheless there are important distinctions between the categories of "immunocompetent" PCNSL, HIV-positive PCNSL, and those forms seen in posttransplantation

► **TABLE 17-6.** COMPARATIVE FEATURES OF PCNSL

	CNS-PTLD	HIV-positive PCNSL	PCNSL
Age	40 years	Any	60 years
Gender	M = F	Male > female	Male > female
Symptom duration	4–6 weeks	Variable; typically days to weeks	4–6 weeks
Imaging	"Abscessoid" (see text)	"Abscessoid"	"Snowball"
EBV status	Positive	Positive	Negative
Pathology	Polymorphic > monomorphic	Small cell, immunoblastic	Large, CD20+, B cell
Treatment	See text	Varies with patient's clinical stage	MTX-based drug
Median survival	See text	Varies with patient's clinical stage	30 months

CNS-PTLD = central nervous system posttransplantation lymphoproliferative disease; HIV = human immunodeficiency virus; PCNSL = primary central nervous system lymphoma.

patients (CNS-PTLD). Some of these were alluded to in prior sections of this chapter. Table 17-6 summarizes the features of these three forms, which are discussed where appropriate.

The typical PCNSL patient is between 55 and 70 years old and presents with the subacute mass lesion syndrome.[80] Men outnumber women by approximately a 3:2 ratio.[6] In patients with immunodeficiency, the male-to-female ratio is even greater (>7:1), likely reflecting the influence of infection with HIV. Children of HIV-positive mothers have been diagnosed as PCNSL as early as 2 years of age. The median duration of symptoms is 4 weeks, and some patients may have an explosive onset. At least a third of patients have prodromal symptoms that are flu-like and have been dubbed a "cytokine sickness." A prompt, although typically brief, clinical and imaging response to corticosteroids is considered a pathognomonic feature of PCNSL in all forms.[68,81] Rare reports of spontaneous remissions have been described.

There are four distinct anatomic distributions for PCNSL.[82] Similar profiles occur in immunocompetent and immunodeficient patients, but the proportions may vary. Those distributions inform the presenting clinical syndromes.[6] For example, cognitive and personality changes reflect the predilection of PCNSL to affect the frontal lobes, corpus callosum, and periventricular structures, whereas seizures are uncommon because these tumors usually reside in subcortical areas. In the largest single series reported, focal deficits occurred in 70% of patients, neuropsychiatric symptoms in 43%, symptoms of increased intracranial pressure in 33%, and seizures in 14%.[77] Approximately a quarter of immunocompetent patients have multifocal disease at presentation, whereas AIDS and postorgan transplant patients with PCNSL are just as likely to have multiple as solitary lesions. Several uncommon but characteristic PCNSL syndromes have been described, including intraocular lymphoma,[78] primary leptomeningeal lymphoma,[79] spinal cord PCNSL, and a fulminant syndrome with multiple lesions including brain, eye, spinal cord, and meninges.[6] Of these, intraocular lymphoma (IOL; also known as "lymphomatous uveitis") is the most common and has the broadest management implications.

Intraocular Lymphoma

IOL is an infrequent cause of uveitis in the general population.[83] However, its significance in the context of PCNSL is considerable (see reference 84 for a review). IOL typically presents as "floaters" or visual dimming in one eye. Careful ophthalmic evaluation shows subretinal infiltrates of large monoclonal lymphoid cells and vitreous cells arranged in clumps, both with morphologic and immunohistochemical features of NHL. Infiltrates are typically bilateral even in patients with monocular symptoms. Tumor typically involves the vitreous, subretinal pigment epithelial space, retina, or optic nerve in the absence of CNS or systemic disease (Fig. 17-4).[85] Figure 17-5 is an

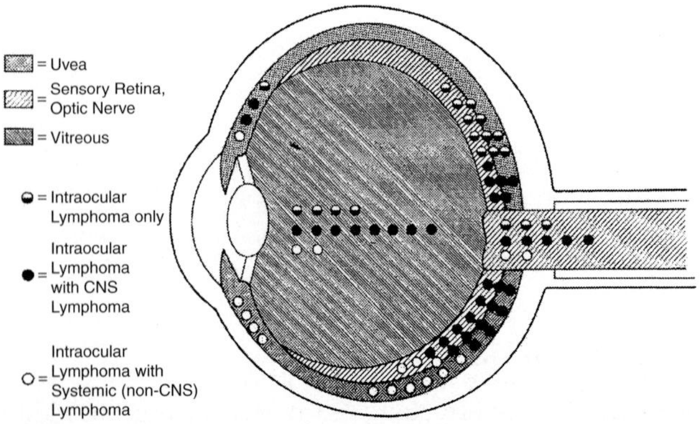

Figure 17-4. Distribution of loci of intraocular lymphoma and relationship to stage of disease. *(Reproduced with permission from Qualman SJ, Mendelsohn G, Mann RB, et al. Cancer 1983;52:878–886.)*

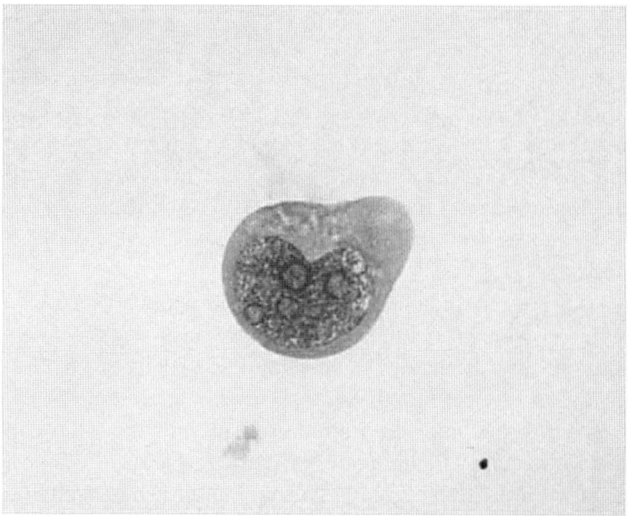

Figure 17-5 (PLATE 50). Vitrectomy specimen demonstrating single lymphoma cell. (*Courtesy of Dr. Karen Grogg, Department of Pathology, Mayo Clinic, Rochester, MN.*)

example of the usefulness of pars plana vitrectomy, which, if positive, may obviate the need for brain biopsy. Most clinical protocols allow enrollment of patients if there is a characteristic clinical syndrome and imaging, *and* diagnostic vitreal or CSF. The use of flow cytometry, immunohistochemistry, microbiologic, and cytokine analyses have all been used on vitreal fluid.

Age and gender distributions are the same as other forms of PCNSL, and IOL has been described in HIV+ PCNSL. Prognosis depends upon early diagnosis; those patients who are diagnosed before a cerebral lesion have more than a fivefold longer median survival.[86] However, subretinal infiltrates appear to correlate with permanent visual loss. More typically, the patient has months of symptoms until neurologic symptoms prompt brain imaging.[87] If IOL is diagnosed, other CNS lesions may be found on neurologic staging, usually a silent ipsilateral brain parenchymal mass.[85] If not initially found, parenchymal disease occurs in more than three-quarters of patients within months of diagnosis. Furthermore, IOL may be asymptomatic and detectable only by a careful eye examination by an experienced ophthalmologist; as many as 20% of newly diagnosed PCNSL patients will have concurrent IOL.

PCNSL Associated with Profound Immunodeficiency

Both AIDS-related PCNSL and CNS-PTLD are invariably EBV-driven expansions of oligo- or monoclonal populations of germinal center–derived B lymphocytes occurring in patients with profound immunodeficiency. This is most obvious in organ transplant recipients where the immunodeficiency is intentional (see reference 88 for a review). In other conditions where the immunodeficiency is congenital, inherited, or virally mediated, the effect (and the phenotype) is similar. In these latter conditions, the immunodeficiency is not so easily manipulated (although the recent use of HAART modulates this statement). We have had some patients who presumably did not cross the "point of no return" and were salvaged by HAART with clinical and imaging improvement coincident with a marked lowering of their viral load.

Delayed hemorrhage at the biopsy site and brain hemorrhage at other sites, is characteristic of these forms, rather than any fault of the biopsy technique.[33] There are reports of hemorrhage, before treatment, in PCNSL associated with acquired immunodeficiency syndrome and rare reports of hemorrhage as a late complication after treatment of childhood CNS lymphoma.[60] There are no identifiable predictive characteristics of the patient or of the neuroimaging features. Hemorrhage in other organs following transplant has led to the concept of "sick endothelia."[89]

AIDS-PCNSL formerly affected approximately 5% of patients infected with HIV and was an AIDS-defining illness in approximately 1% of patients.[90] Unlike typical PCNSL, seizures are more common, occurring in perhaps as many as 25% of patients. This may relate to the multiple and sometimes superficial location of the tumors. Seizures may also be a result of comorbid conditions such as infections, organ failure, or toxicity. The incidence of AIDS-PCNSL correlates with CD4 counts.[31] The use of HAART has decreased the incidence of AIDS-PCNSL and has redefined the phenotype.[91] AIDS-PCNSL patients are now older, of better performance status, and present later in the course of their HIV infection.[91] Table 17-6 lists the clinical features of AIDS-PCNSL and contrasts them with those of CNS-PTLD and typical PCNSL.

CNS-PTLD occurs in two forms of roughly equal frequency: a primary form where there is no evidence of other sites of involvement, and a secondary form where the CNS infection occurs in the context of recognized systemic disease.[65] These two forms are likely versions of the same disease. They are both EBV-driven. Both require the substrate of induced immunosuppression. In both forms the serologic status for EBV of donor and recipient correlates with outcome, as do peripheral blood CD4 counts. Unlike AIDS-PCNSL, the incidence of both forms is rising, probably because of more intense immunosuppressive regimens employed to prevent organ rejection.[34] Generalizations about the clinical and neuroimaging characteristics or treatment of CNS-PTLD cannot be made. The younger age of patients in earlier reports is probably because of selection bias and organ triage. As with AIDS-PCNSL, Table 17-6 represents the current state of knowledge about CNS-PTLD. The median time from transplantation to onset of CNS-PTLD is

12.6 months (range: 2–50 months). In approximately 20% of patients, tumor occurred more than 3 years after transplantation. These "late-form" patients are purported to be biologically distinct, although this may only represent different cohorts of patients or the effects of newer immunosuppressive regimens.[92] As in other forms of PCNSL, patients typically present with a subacute focal neurologic syndrome. Mean duration of symptoms before diagnosis is approximately 1 month, although an explosive onset (duration 0–5 days) is not uncommon. Rejection phenomena are not uncommon, occurring in more than half of the patients who developed CNS-PTLD.[88]

Secondary Forms

Brain parenchymal involvement is unusual in sNHL. An autopsy-based series found that 2 of 121 consecutive postmortem examinations of NHL patients harbored parenchymal lymphomatous deposits.[76] More recent studies have confirmed the rarity. A review of the Mayo Lymphoma Database for all patients who presented as PCNSL and had staging for the presence of occult systemic disease showed that 3.9% had systemic lymphoma, nearly all in intraabdominal or intrapelvic lymph nodes.[4] Because this population is a highly selected one, the actual incidence is probably much lower. When parenchymal lymphoma has been diagnosed it has usually been as a late complication, occurring at a time when there is widespread systemic disease and bone marrow involvement.[93,94] The widespread use of rituximab does not appear to have influenced the rate of secondary CNS involvement. A recent report of 20 elderly patients (median age of 69 years) correlated secondary involvement with the International Prognostic Index (IPI) only.[95] The authors opined that the poor rituximab diffusion into the CNS accounted for this.[96]

A special situation involves "Richter transformation," where CNS parenchymal lymphoma occurs some years after another hematologic malignancy, usually sNHL, and Hodgkin disease.[97,98] In some cases no treatment for the original tumor had been administered, thus excluding an induced second malignancy.[97] In other patients, the histology of the treated systemic lymphoma and the parenchymal disease have been discordant. These appear to be "second malignancies" rather than "recurrence," because there are distinct molecular genetic differences between the two tumors of similar histology (e.g., large-cell lymphoma[99]). The imaging features of these instances of Richter transformation are similar to those seen in "de novo" PCNSL, that is, intense and homogeneous contrast enhancement, less mass effect proportional to the tumor bulk, and contact with a CSF surface.

Spinal cord involvement has been demonstrated far less frequently than brain involvement. Except for the

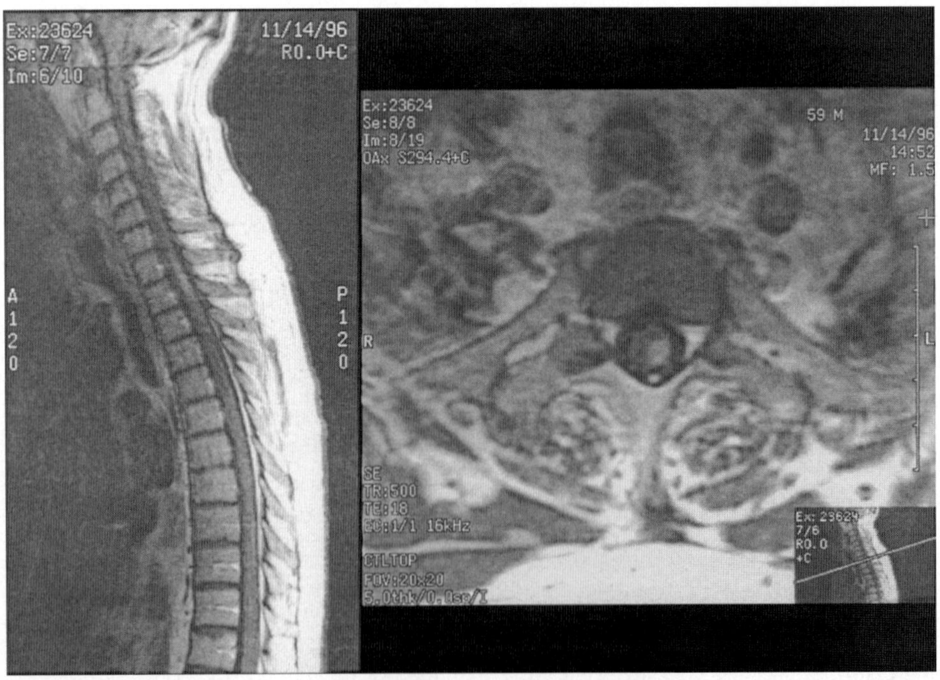

Figure 17-6. Spinal cord lymphoma. Gadolinium-enhanced sagittal (left) and axial (right) scans of cervical spine demonstrate homogeneously enhancing intramedullary mass.

special circumstance of cord involvement in the context of leptomeningeal lymphoma,[51] this is an underrecognized complication of systemic lymphoma. Because cord lymphoma rarely expands the cord, a myelogram would be unlikely to give diagnostic information.[100] The more recent widespread use of MRI scanning of the spine has contributed to the increased number of reports in the past decade compared with the two decades prior.[6] Furthermore, it is likely that a certain number of enhancing cord masses without significant mass effect occurring in the context of systemic non-Hodgkin lymphoma were assumed to be infectious, inflammatory, or postirradiation, as these often occurred as end-of-life illnesses and an aggressive workup may not have been considered (Fig. 17-6).

▶ IMAGING

Computerized tomography (CT) gave the first meaningful imaging representation of PCNSL. The use of CT contributed to the dramatic increase in reports of the condition because previously available imaging techniques, such as angiography and pneumoencephalography, were normal or nonspecifically abnormal. Furthermore, CT scans provided clinicians the first opportunity to define presentation, response to therapy, patterns of relapse, and complications of treatment. Although no CT appearance was absolutely diagnostic, a homogeneously enhancing lesion (or lesions) located in the corpus callosum or central gray matter was considered highly suspicious, the so-called cerebral "snowball" (Fig. 17-7).

In early clinical trial design, the appearance was felt to be so characteristic that a person could be enrolled in a study without a histologic diagnosis.[101] Similar images were later demonstrated in "tumefactive" multiple sclerosis, and sarcoid. Thus these "false-positives" may have contaminated early clinical trial reports and trial results. Several reports documented as much as a 20% discordance rate between the CT imaging diagnosis and the subsequent histologic diagnosis.[102,103] Another radiographic finding that almost attained pathognomonic status was the "ghost tumor," prompt partial to complete resolution to the administration of corticosteroids.[68] However, other lesions, including GBM and metastasis, may display identical imaging.[104] Nevertheless, the imaging characteristics in "immunocompetent" patients may be sufficient to define treatment decisions and even enter an otherwise eligible patient onto protocol, *provided that there is* positive cytology from cerebrospinal fluid or vitreous.

Because of its greater resolution and its ability to display the meninges and posterior fossa far better than CT, MRI greatly improved the imaging yield in PCNSL patients. MRI also proved superior to CT in monitoring

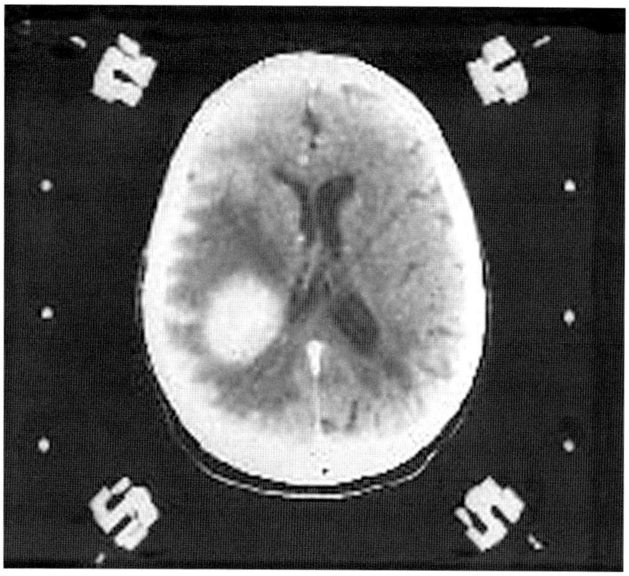

Figure 17-7. Characteristic "snowball" lesion of PCNSL; enhanced CT scan of head (in stereotaxic frame).

response to therapy, characterizing patterns of failure, and displaying the complications of therapy. In each of these domains, earlier and more accurate detection occurred with MR over CT (Fig. 17-8). The typical MRI features of PCNSL include (a) isointense to hyperintense parenchymal masses on T_1, T_1-T_2, and T_2 scans; (b) homogeneous and intense contrast enhancement; (c) characteristic locations such as basal ganglia and corpus callosum; (d) contact with the CSF, either at the ependymal or the pial surfaces; (e) less mass effect than correspondingly sized GBM; and (f) prompt response of the contrast enhancement to the administration of corticosteroids.

MRI also provided insights into the biology of PCNSL. These observations include the degree of leptomeningeal involvement and, by virtue of its superiority in the posterior fossa and the spinal canal, the multiplicity of lesions (see Fig. 17-8). MR also gave a much clearer view of neurotoxicity from PCNSL treatment; the onset, tempo, and extent of white matter disease and brain atrophy are displayed better on MR than CT.[105] MRI also provided a critical insight into the biology of PCNSL: when PCNSL recurs it usually does so in a different anatomic location *if* there has been a complete response at the primary site.[106] This is unprecedented for malignant gliomas and has led to research into mechanisms of recurrence and, by extrapolation, initial oncogenesis.

Modern imaging has also had a transforming effect on syndromic classification. In fact it is unlikely that some of these "orphan" types such as spinal cord parenchymal

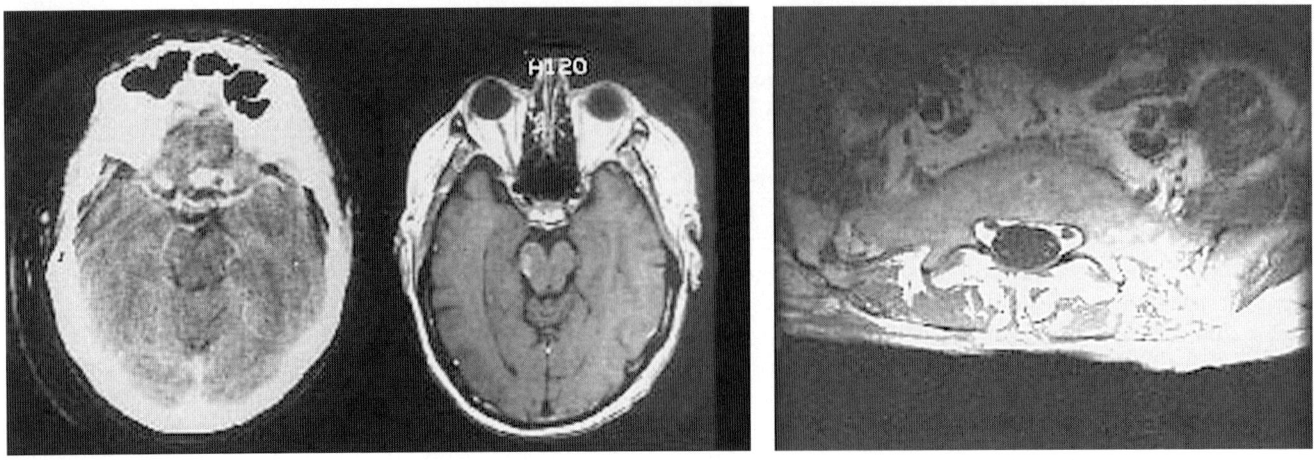

Figure 17-8. (Left) Contrast-enhanced CT and MR at same imaging level from same patient demonstrates the superiority of MR in identifying small lesions in the posterior fossa. (Right) Enlarged nerve roots of cauda equina in patient with leptomeningeal lymphoma.

lymphoma,[6] "lymphomatosis cerebri,"[74] and the primary leptomeningeal form[107] could have been recognized without contrast-enhanced MRI scanning. Our own experience does not indicate that this mix, described by Hochberg and Miller,[6] is substantially different now. Lastly, MRI and, to a lesser extent, CT have defined the approach toward the patient suspected of having PCNSL. In immunosuppressed patients, especially in the patient with AIDS, the choice of empiric therapy with antimicrobials versus radiation therapy is sometimes based on imaging characteristics if the clinical situation is consistent (see "Clinical: All Forms" above).

"Sentinel Lesions"

Approximately a third of patients will have premonitory symptoms and a presumably small number of patients will have a "sentinel lesion" syndrome. The former are not unlike the symptoms associated with the common cold—fatigue, sore throat, tender lymphadenopathy, mild fever—and has been called "cytokine sickness." The latter was first addressed by Alderson and colleagues[108] who described a specific episode of neurologic dysfunction, abnormal imaging, and brain biopsy evidence for inflammatory demyelination. Our experience indicates that

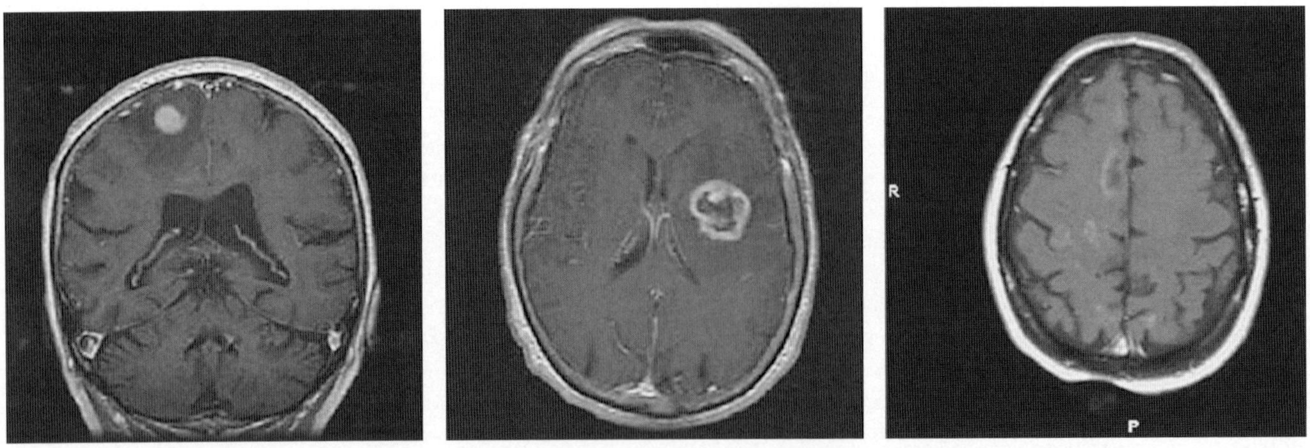

Figure 17-9. "Three faces of CNS lymphoma." (Left) Typical "snowball" lesion of PCNSL. (Center) Necrotic, ring-enhancing "abscessoid" lesion in EBV-positive CNS-PTLD. (Right) AIDS-related CNS lymphoma.

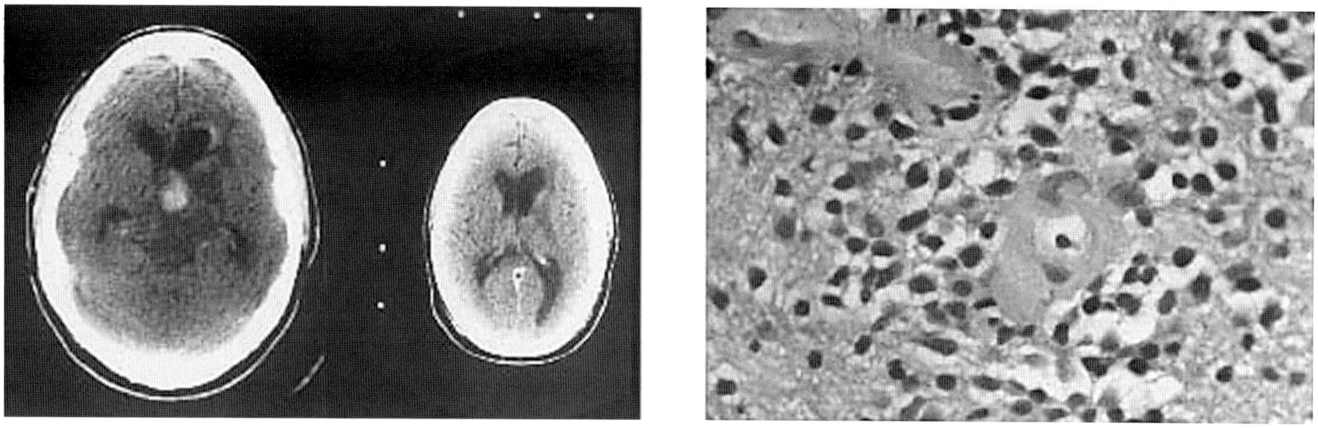

Figure 17-10 (PLATE 51). The "ghost tumor" effect of corticosteroids: (Left) A disappearance of a contrast-enhancing mass at the foramen of Munro following dexamethasone. (Right) Apoptotic nuclei in a biopsy specimen taken 6 hours later.

when the tumor appears it does so relatively soon after the "sentinel lesion," that the imaging abnormalities are often in different loci, and that the biopsy appearance is typical PCNSL.

HIV-PCNSL and CNS-PTLD

The imaging of CNS-PTLD is strikingly similar to that seen in AIDS-associated PCNSL (see Table 17-6). These patients present nonspecifically and progress rapidly on serial imaging studies. Admittedly, immunosuppressed patients may be tested more frequently than other patients. New symptoms with neurologic characteristics such as headache, fever, and confusion likely lead to early imaging and earlier detection. Contrast enhancement, often thought pathognomonic for PCNSL, may be a late phenomenon. There are reports of infiltrative PCNSL without contrast enhancement.[33] Thus, presence or absence of enhancement may indicate only the stage of tumor evolution. The features include variable T_2-signal and heterogeneous enhancement or rim enhancement with contrast; this is likely related to the necrosis seen on histologic examination.[88] The pattern of progressive heterogeneous contrast enhancement, multiplicity of the lesions, and ring-like features are similar to the imaging features of intracerebral abscesses (hence the "abscess-oid" description). In contrast, PCNSL imaging of immunocompetent patients is usually that of a solitary lesion with dense and homogeneous enhancement. Figure 17-9 displays representative scans from each of these three forms. A robust steroid response, the so-called ghost tumor,[68] can occur in all forms (Fig. 17-10). Because these patients are immunosuppressed there may be more than one diagnosis, such as concurrent vasculitis, infection, and neurotoxicity of treatment. In immunosuppressed patients, especially AIDS, the choice of empiric therapy with antimicrobials versus radiation therapy is sometimes based on the imaging characteristics of the particularly virulent form of PCNSL that occurs in these patients. However, widely disparate disorders may image similarly.[109] Figure 17-11 demonstrates the

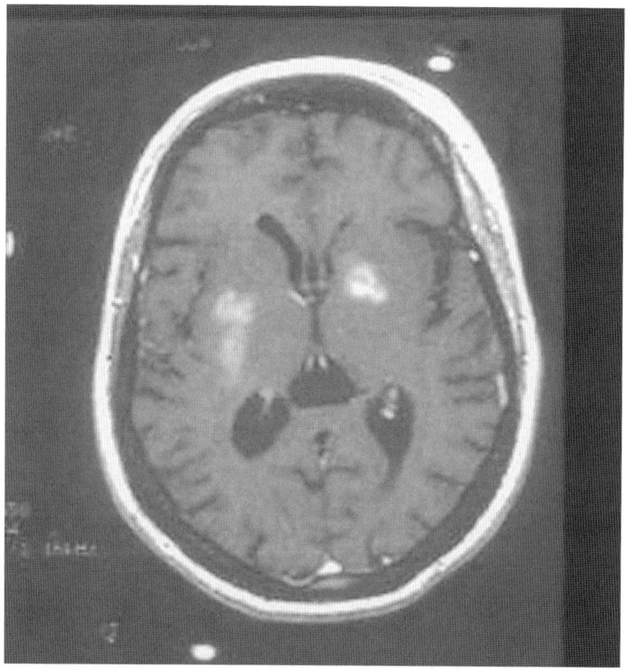

Figure 17-11. False-positive MRI. Multiple, deep-seated contrast-enhancing lesions with minimal mass effect consistent with CNS-PTLD. Pathologic diagnosis was toxoplasmosis. Prophylactic use of cotrimoxazole has now reduced the frequency of this in transplant recipients.

pitfalls of MRI in immunosuppressed patients. Because PCNSL may concurrently involve more than one site in the neuraxis, such as eyes, brain parenchyma, and leptomeninges, entire axis imaging is often performed. Imaging in secondary forms have not been reported to differ from the imaging characteristics of PCNSL.

▶ TREATMENT

Treatment principles applicable to sNHL should be applicable to PCNSL. However, the results of multiple, single, and combined modality treatment trials show that the fate of the PCNSL patient is very different than that of similar patients with large B-cell lymphomas at other extranodal sites. The prognosis for patients with PCNSL approaches that of glioblastoma multiforme; the median survival of untreated PCNSL patients is 2.2 months[3] and is 11.6 months following whole-brain radiation therapy (WBRT); the median survival for patients 60 years of age and older following WBRT is 7.6 months.[110]

Unlike GBM, however, considerable strides in PCNSL treatment have resulted in longer survival, less overall toxicity, and more options at disease recurrence. More specifically, median survival can be extended to the 30-month range if chemotherapy regimens include methotrexate. However, the number of cured patients does not appear to have been changed and neurotoxicity continues to be a major concern. Table 17-7 displays the evolution of PCNSL treatment over the past four decades. (Note that most experts rely upon reports that encompass the modern neuroimaging era; in the United States the CT era began in the mid-1970s and the MRI era in the mid-1980s.)

PCNSL is a treatable tumor and a responsive tumor. Whether chemotherapy, WBRT, or combined modality therapy is used, a response is seen in at least 80% of patients. Furthermore, a complete response (defined by a resolution of contrast enhancement) to initial therapy is seen in more than half of treated patients. Approximately 10% to 15% of patients do not respond to any treatment. Responding patients almost always recur, typically at the initial site if there is less than complete response, or elsewhere in the nervous system if there has been a complete response at the primary site. For a tumor whose demographics and clinical presentation are so similar to those of glioblastoma multiforme, the potential for clinical improvement is far greater. Most brain tumor clinical trials use imaging as a discriminator for response to therapy. Less attention is given to clinical improvement, especially because function may be altered by the therapy itself (e.g., a symptomatic neuropathy from spindle-inhibiting chemotherapy). For example, a person who is hemiparetic with a GBM will rarely improve to the level of full functionality, but a PCNSL patient with the same deficit may improve dramatically. This is in addition to the clear imaging improvement.

Because at least half the patients with PCNSL are 60 years of age or older, the possibility of long-term sequelae is important but poorly studied. No significant

▶ TABLE 17-7. EVOLUTION OF PCNSL TREATMENT

1960–1980s: Era of modern radiotherapy. WBRT effective in inducing a response but not curative. Dose response >40 Gy needed. Spinal irradiation ineffective. *RTOG 8310* was definitive. Surgical resection offered no advantage and several disadvantages (neurologic deterioration, delayed start of WBRT). See references 80, 110, and 114.
1980–1990s: Era of early chemo and CMT trials. Most were single-institution studies with small numbers composed of relatively young and healthy patients. Hint of improved outcome with CMT. See references 115, 148, and 149.
1996: Analysis of published series of 10 or more patients (total of 140 patients): median survival 9–44.5 mo; median age 54.1 y (approximately decade younger than the typical patient). Little mention of toxicity in survivors. See reference 105.
1996, 1997: Two Cooperative Groups (NCCTG/ECOG 86 72 52; RTOG 8806) published phase II data: median survival of 11.4 and 16.1 mo, respectively. Conclusion of limited effectiveness of typical NHL regimens because of poor CNS penetration. See references 111 and 147.
2000: RTOG review of 83-15 and 93-10 reported a clear advantage of methotrexate-based CMT over WBRT alone (30.4 vs. 11.6 mo). See reference 119.
2003: Comprehensive review by a working group of European and North American investigators. Patient- and disease-related predictors of response and survival defined from a pooled cohort of 378 immunocompent patients with PCNSL. A PCNSL IPI was proposed. See reference 117.

CMT = combined modality trial; IPI = International Prognostic Index; NCCTG/ECOG = North Central Cancer Treatment Group/Eastern Cooperative Oncology Group; RTOG = Radiation Therapy Oncology Group; WBRT = whole-brain radiotherapy.

differences in response rates have been reported between young (i.e., < 60 years of age) and old (60 years of age and older) patients on chemotherapy, and the older group of patients appeared to tolerate chemotherapy as well as the group as a whole.[23] Nevertheless, this older group of patients is at increased risk for long-term declines in both cognitive and physical function. Radiation in older patients has a clear risk of neurotoxicity.[111,112] Typically, this is a subcortical demyelination syndrome with varying degrees of dementia, gait apraxia, and urinary urgency and incontinence (Fig. 17-12).

Although all age groups incur the risk of this syndrome, careful fractionation schedules and a total dose below tolerance can minimize the effects on healthy brain. The older patient is less tolerant of the same schedule, at least in part from the presence of comorbid conditions such as stroke, alcoholism, and degenerative diseases of the CNS. A series of recent trials incorporated objective measures of cognitive function, performance, or both. Thus, the very patients who need effective treatment are the ones most at risk for disabling neurotoxicity from factors including age, comorbidity, the disease itself, and its treatment. Whether such declines in quality of life can be prevented by neuroprotective strategies such as delayed or lower-dose radiotherapy, blood–brain barrier disruption, or non-neurotoxic chemotherapy remains to be answered by appropriate clinical trials. Similarly, further studies are needed to determine if there are cohorts with inherent susceptibilities to neurotoxicity.[112] Because PCNSL patients are older, comorbid conditions confound the toxicity issue.[113] The following represent current approaches to treatment of PCNSL. Table 17-8 provides an approach to the patient.

Surgery

No benefit from surgical resection has been demonstrated.[3] The role of surgery is to establish a diagnosis, typically via stereotactic biopsy.[57]

Corticosteroids

Steroids are often used in primary brain tumors to reduce vasogenic edema caused by the intracranial mass. However, unless there is a strong medical reason for their use (clinical deterioration), their use should be withheld until after a histologic diagnosis has been established. As mentioned previously, corticosteroids may have a potent oncolytic effect on lymphomas.[68,81] The onset is visible clinically and by imaging within 24 hours.

Radiation Therapy

The diffuse nature of the tumor requires whole-brain irradiation. Results from different radiation regimens suggest that at least 40 Gy to the whole brain is necessary to achieve local control.[110,114] A boost to the tumor bed does not improve control.[110] Craniospinal radiation did not improve survival and considerably interferes with administration of subsequent chemotherapy. In patients

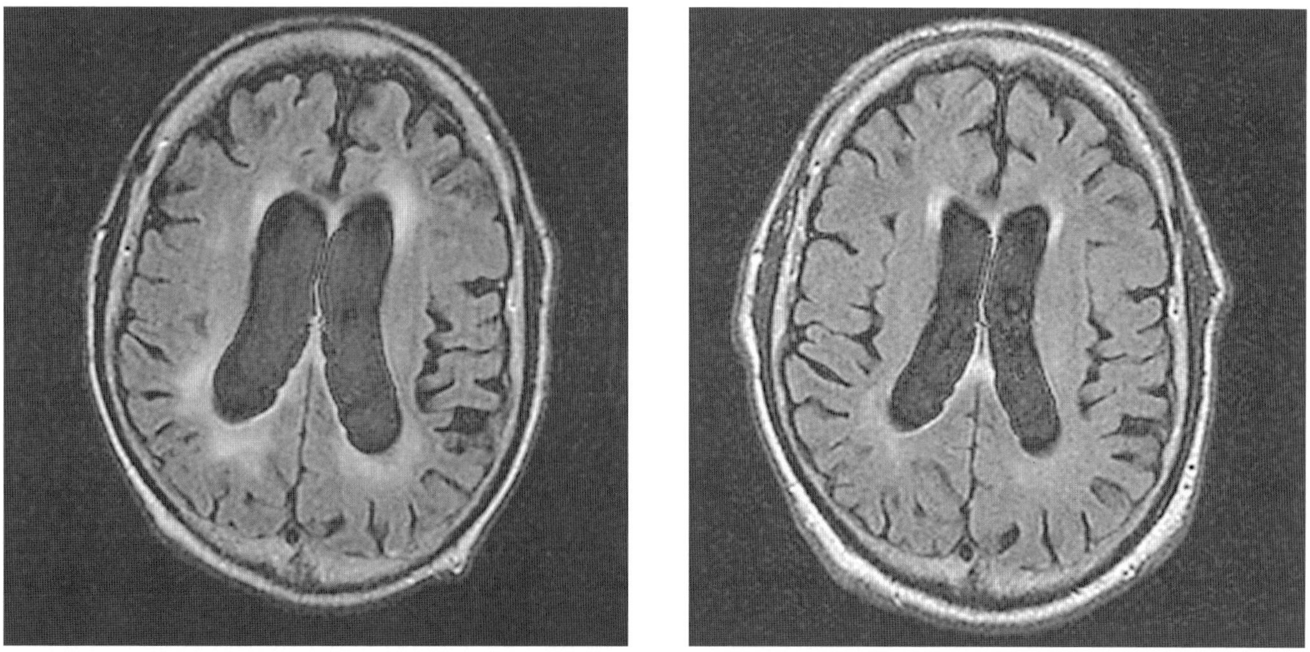

Figure 17-12. A 58-year-old man with PCNSL. Progressive ventricular dilatation, white matter hyperintensity, and cerebral atrophy 27 months after high-dose methotrexate and brain irradiation (FLAIR [fluid-attenuated inversion recovery] sequence).

▶ **TABLE 17-8.** APPROACH TO THE PATIENT

Patient with neurologic symptoms (or high-risk patient without symptoms)?
- Neuroimaging, preferably contrast-enhanced MRI

Imaging consistent with PCNSL?
- Withhold steroids (if medically safe to do so)
- Biopsy (if biopsy cannot be performed, obtain CSF and ophthalmology consult)
- Coordinate tissue management between neurosurgeon and pathologist; ideally, a component of fresh tissue should be available for special studies
- Alternative is to start with slit lamp examination and CSF and go to brain biopsy if these are negative

"Staging"
- Ophthalmology consult (if not already done)
- CSF examination (if safe to do so and if not already done)
- Contrast-enhanced MRI of remaining neuraxis
- HIV (HTLV-1 according to circumstances)
- Lactic acid dehydrogenase
- Bilateral iliac crest bone marrow aspiration and biopsy
- Chest/abdomen/pelvis contrast-enhanced CT

Treatment (all may be modified because of performance status, prior treatment, patient, and/or family interest)
- Eye only? Consider systemic methotrexate, bilateral ocular irradiation, intraocular chemotherapy
- Brain only? Systemic methotrexate with delayed irradiation is considered standard treatment (at the time of this writing)
- Brain and eye? See above. If irradiation is performed, posterior two-thirds of globes should be included in field
- Leptomeningeal only? Systemic methotrexate. No role for craniospinal radiation
- Immunosuppression? See above. In addition, if HIV+, consider HAART (or change in dose or drugs); if CNS-PTLD, consider reduction of immunosuppression
- Relapsed disease? No standard therapy

with intraocular lymphoma, the posterior two-thirds of both globes were also radiated. Nevertheless, most failures occurred within the treatment volume.[115]

Radiosurgery

Stereotactic radiosurgery either employing stereotactic LINAC or the Gamma Knife has not been systematically employed in PCNSL. Because PCNSL is considered a "whole-brain disease," its use has been limited to salvage situations. Given that it can be employed in patients who previously had received brain irradiation, it is not unreasonable to consider if there is a single lesion recurrence that meets treatment guidelines.[116]

Chemotherapy, Alone or in Combination with Radiation Therapy

Standard regimens employed in systemic non-Hodgkin lymphoma do not appear to be effective in PCNSL, presumably because of their inability to penetrate infiltrative tumor. A meta-analysis concluded that regimens that employed high-dose methotrexate (at least 3.5 g/m^2) were the most successful, and this has become the current standard of care.[117,118] The current approach of regimens containing at least 3.5 g/m^2 methotrexate (and more typically 8 g/m^2) followed by whole-brain irradiation results in response rates approaching 90% and median survivals between 30 and 60 months.[117,119–123] The current debate revolves around whether irradiation is necessary as consolidation therapy, whether methotrexate can be used as monotherapy (and, if not, what other agents should be employed), and whether there is a role for transplantation (as there seems to be in the treatment in systemic lymphoma).

Autologous Stem Cell Transplant

The initial evidence for the benefit of high-dose therapy and autologous stem cell transplant (ASCT) came initially from systemic non-Hodgkin lymphoma patients who had a history of CNS involvement. The European Bone Marrow Transplantation (EBMT) registry data showed that 42% of patients with NHL and a history of CNS involvement, in remission at the time of ASCT, had durable remissions.[124] Compared to a matched control group of patients without CNS involvement, there was no difference in survival. Similar results were shown in a U.S. study where 4 of 17 patients with active CNS lymphoma involvement at the time of ASCT were long-term survivors but not cures.[125] In these studies there was a high incidence of CNS complications in patients who previously had received cranial radiotherapy.

The first report in PCNSL demonstrated that 14 of 20 refractory or relapsed patients (70%) remained alive with a median followup of 41.5 months.[126] The event-free survival post-ASCT was 53%. The conditioning regimen used was a combination of thiotepa, busulfan, and cyclophosphamide. Given the costs, need for specialized centers and expertise, and the often poor status of patients at time of refractory or relapsed disease, focus then shifted to the role of ASCT as initial therapy. A multicenter study entered 24 PCNSL patients; 12 patients had response to induction chemotherapy that consisted of methotrexate and cytarabine and proceeded to ASCT. Conditioning was with BEAM (BCNU, cytarabine, etoposide, and melphalan). At a median followup of 4 months (range: 1–17 months), 58% remain in remission. Four patients relapsed before day 100 post-ASCT.[127] The transplant was well tolerated with no treatment-related mortality and no treatment-related neurotoxicity. The role of ASCT is thus not settled as of the time of writing.

Blood–Brain Barrier Disruption Therapy

A series of studies examined whether chemotherapy alone could be used for PCNSL, especially in vulnerable individuals such as patients older than age 70 years. One report claimed to achieve results comparable to combined treatment with less morbidity.[128] However, median survival of those patients who were biopsy-proven was no different than with brain irradiation.[110] Neuwelt demonstrated the safety, feasibility, and efficacy of intraarterial chemotherapy with osmotic opening of the blood–brain barrier for the treatment of PCNSL.[72] To date, more than 50 patients have been treated; 40 of 53 (75%) achieved complete response with a median survival of 44.5 months.[129] However, this technique requires highly specialized centers, is costly, and is accompanied by acute toxicities including seizures, cerebral ischemia, cerebral edema, and arterial trauma.[129,130] Furthermore, the long-term neurotoxicity risk has not yet been determined.[130]

Immunosuppressed Forms of Primary Central Nervous System Lymphoma

Immunosuppressed patients, such as organ transplant recipients and persons with AIDS, represent a particular treatment challenge because (a) PCNSL is only one of several causes of brain mass lesions in such patients; (b) the imaging of these lesions may be strikingly similar; (c) in the case of CNS-PTLD, a potentially effective treatment (reduction of immunosuppression) may lead to organ rejection; and (d) patients may develop the disease at a time when surgical diagnosis is not feasible and aggressive treatment problematic.

HIV+ Primary Central Nervous System Lymphoma

Although WBRT may produce complete response, the median survival for AIDS patients with PCNSL is 2 to 4 months, and is only weeks with supportive care alone.[131,132] Chemotherapy has been studied, but the results were no better than whole-brain irradiation and was accompanied by considerable toxicity.[133] Newer studies suggest that combined modality therapy could prolong survival for up to 16 months with acceptable toxicity.[134] The changing profile of AIDS-PCNSL since the introduction of HAART may mean that the results of treatment will be even better.

Central Nervous System Posttransplantation Lymphoproliferative Disease

There has been a disappointingly poor outcome in CNS-PTLD despite multimodal therapy. The experience reported in the literature indicates that fewer than 10% of reported cases were alive at the time of the reports; in one study, survival was 2.2 months following a variety of therapies.[33] Snanoudj and associates[34] described an outcome far better than previous literature. With a median followup time of 37 months, they reported an overall survival rate of 40%. They attributed this improvement to a number of features: earlier detection (prompt stereotactic biopsy), restitution of immunocompetence, induction of a complete response, routine use of cotrimoxazole prophylaxis against toxoplasmosis, and treatment regimens that included high-dose methotrexate.[34] Because all patients reported in the literature who survived had received the combination of antiviral therapy, reduced immunosuppressive therapy, and "antilymphoma" therapy (chemotherapy, radiotherapy, or both), perhaps all modalities should be combined at the outset of treatment. The "step-up" approach of adding one agent on top of another currently being tested in systemic PTLD is not appropriate for CNS-PTLD because of the rapid course.

"Secondary" and "Orphan" Forms

In these forms the decision making regarding treatment ultimately rests with the responsible clinician and is based on realistic goals and expectations. Treatment may be supportive care, palliative radiotherapy, or salvage attempts with "penetrating" chemotherapy, typically high-dose intravenous methotrexate or high-dose intravenous cytarabine. Only anecdotal reports support the use of one form of treatment over another. These conditions are far too seldom diagnosed for clinical trials to be available. A possible exception is intraocular lymphoma (see "Clinical: All Forms" above), where corticosteroids, ocular irradiation, systemic chemotherapy, and intravitreal chemotherapy[135] have all given impressive results.[86] However, relapse is common and, as mentioned earlier, may be in one eye or both eyes or the brain. If ocular irradiation was used, subsequent brain irradiation may be problematic because of overlapping fields.[85] Another exception is "neurolymphomatosis," where there are a series of recent reports and one review that summarizes the potential for effective treatment.[136,137]

Prophylaxis

Although standard in the treatment of children and adolescents with hematologic malignancies, the value of prophylactic treatment in adult patients is controversial. A high incidence of intradural "failure" has been described in NHL at certain sites, such as sinus and testicular lymphomas and Burkitt lymphoma.[138–140] Furthermore, this failure risk is bimodal, occurring early in their clinical course or even at presentation, or at a time later in their illness when they are well. Much literature has accumulated on the preventive treatment of the intradural nervous system, its type of treatment (or treatments), the timing, and indications.[141,142] The assumption is that prophylaxis is necessary to prevent CNS relapse and even systemic reseeding. Because many of the reports on which these recommendations are based preceded the modern neuroimaging era, it is not clear whether patients had been properly staged. Even with prophylaxis a substantial number of patients will still develop CNS disease, and, as was discussed earlier (see "Secondary Forms"), these late "recurrences" in fact may be second malignancies. Prophylactic therapy may be neurotoxic and has the potential of precluding the use of a potentially effective therapy later on.[142] Based on our experience with testicular lymphoma, we have taken a cautious view toward prophylaxis.[140]

Salvage Therapies

Recurrent Disease

There is no established salvage therapy for relapsed, recurrent, or progressive disease. Because of prior therapies, comorbidities, age, and, in the case of immunodeficiency states, reduced immunocompetence, patients at this stage may have no realistic options. The treatment decision ultimately rests with the patient, the patient's family, and the responsible clinician and is based on realistic goals and expectations.

Treatment may be supportive care, palliative radiotherapy, or salvage attempts with "penetrating" chemotherapy.[143] Occasionally, a biopsy or CSF examination is warranted, such as in an immunosuppressed patient with good performance status. Case reports and small series describe re-irradiation, radiosurgery, and various chemotherapy agents such as rituximab, temozolomide, topotecan, and blood–brain barrier disruption-based therapy.[144] Unlike in the primary setting, intensive therapies, such as transplantation, are rarely employed.[145,146]

A commonly asked question is whether the original chemotherapy could be tried. Each case is different, but one approach would at least consider a return to the original regimen *if* there had been a robust response when used initially, if there are no medical contraindications (allergic reaction, bone marrow failure, etc.), and there has been at least a year interval without evidence of disease. As mentioned previously (see "Secondary Forms"), two references suggest that true "recurrences" may be new malignancies.[98,99] Thus, high-dose methotrexate is often used. In approximately 10% of cases, the relapse is systemic with or without (but typically without) CNS involvement.[4] In these instances, treatments are often based on standard NHL regimens such as cyclophosphamide, adriamycin, vincristine, and prednisone (CHOP) plus rituximab.[147]

REFERENCES

1. Bailey P. Intracranial sarcomatous tumors of leptomeningeal origin. Arch Surg 1929;18:1359–1402.
2. Yuille CL. Case of primary reticulum cell sarcoma of the brain. Relationship of microglial cells to histiocytes. Arch Pathol 1938;26:1037–1044.
3. Henry JM, Heffner RR Jr, Dillard SH, et al. Primary malignant lymphomas of the central nervous system. Cancer. 1974;34:1293–302.
4. O'Neill BP, Dinapoli RP, Kurtin PJ, et al. Occult systemic non-Hodgkin's lymphoma (NHL) in patients initially diagnosed as primary central nervous system lymphoma (PCNSL): how much staging is enough? Med Oncol 1995;25:67–71.
5. CBTRUS. Statistical report: primary brain tumors in the United States, 1992–1997. Chicago: Central Brain Tumor Registry of the United States, 2000.
6. Hochberg FH, Miller DC. Review article: primary central nervous system lymphoma. J Neurosurg 1988;68:835–853.
7. Tomlinson FH, Kurtin PJ, Suman VJ, et al. Primary intracerebral malignant lymphoma: a clinicopathologic study of 89 patients. J Neurosurg 1995;82:36–44.
8. Diaz-Arrastia R, Younger DS, Hair L, et al. Neurolymphomatosis: a clinicopathologic syndrome re-emerges. Neurology 1992;42:1136–1141.
9. Lyons MK, O'Neill BP, Marsh WR, et al. Primary spinal epidural non-Hodgkin's lymphoma: report of eight CT era cases and review of the literature. Neurosurgery 1992;30: 675–680.

10. Glass J, Hochberg FH, Miller DC. Intravascular lymphomatosis. A systemic disease with neurologic manifestations. Cancer 1993;71:3156–3164.
11. Corn BW, Marcus SM, Topham A, et al. Will primary central nervous system lymphoma be the most frequent brain tumor diagnosed in the year 2000? Cancer 1997;79: 2409–2413.
12. Schabet M. Epidemiology of primary CNS lymphoma. J Neurooncol 1999;43(3):199–201.
13. Eby NL, Grufferman S, Flannelly CM, et al. Increasing incidence of primary brain lymphoma in the US. Cancer 1988;62:2461–2465.
14. Werner MH, Phuphanich S, Lyman GH. The increasing incidence of malignant gliomas and primary central nervous system lymphoma in the elderly. Cancer 1995;76: 1634–1642.
15. Lutz JM, Coleman MP. Trends in primary cerebral lymphoma. Br J Cancer 1994;70:716–718.
16. Olson JE, Janney CA, Rao RD, et al. The continuing increase in primary central nervous system (CNS) lymphoma: a surveillance, epidemiology and end results (SEER) analysis. Cancer 2002;95:1504–1510.
17. Pearce N, Bethwaite P. Increasing incidence of non-Hodgkin's lymphoma: occupational and environmental factors. Cancer Res 1992;52(Suppl 19):5496s–5500s.
18. DeAngelis LM. Primary central nervous system lymphoma as a second malignancy. Cancer 1991:67:1431–1435.
19. Schiff D, Suman VJ, Yang P, et al. Risk factors for primary central nervous system non-Hodgkin's lymphoma (PCNSL). Cancer 1998;82:975–982.
20. Schaller C, O'Fallon JR, Kelly PJ. Primary central nervous system lymphoma (PCNSL): does age and histology at presentation affect outcome? Zentralbl Neurochir 1996; 57:156–162.
21. Palackdharry CS. The epidemiology of non-Hodgkin's lymphoma: why the increased incidence? Oncology 1994;8:67–73.
22. Bernstein L, Ross RK, Henderson BE. Relationship of hormone use to cancer risk. J Natl Cancer Inst 1992;12: 137–147.
23. O'Neill BP, Wang C-H, O'Fallon JR, et al. Primary central nervous system non-Hodgkin's lymphoma (PCNSL): survival advantages with combined initial therapy update. Int J Radiat Oncol Biol Phys 1999;43:559–563.
24. Zucca E, Bertoni F, Roggero E, et al. Molecular analysis of the progression from *Helicobacter pylori*–associated chronic gastritis to mucosa-associated lymphoid-tissue lymphoma of the stomach. N Engl J Med 1998;338: 804–810.
25. Geddes JF, Bhattacharjee MB, Savage K, et al. Primary cerebral lymphoma: a study of 47 cases probed for Epstein-Barr virus genome. J Clin Pathol 1992;45:587–590.
26. de Thé G. Epstein-Barr virus and Burkitt's lymphoma. In: Goedert JJ, ed. Infectious causes of cancer. Totowa, NJ: Humana Press, 2000:77–92.
27. Krogh-Jensen M, D'Amore F, Jensen MK, et al. Clinicopathological features, survival and prognostic factors of primary central nervous system lymphomas: trends in incidence of primary central nervous system lymphomas and primary malignant brain tumors in a well-defined geographical area. Population-based data from the Danish Lymphoma Registry, LYPO, and the Danish Cancer Registry. Leuk Lymphoma 1995;19:223–233.
28. Hennessy BT, Hanrahan EO, Daly PA. Non-Hodgkin's lymphoma: an update. Lancet Oncol 2004;5:341–353.
29. Bonelli L, Vitale V, Bistolfi F, et al. Hodgkin's disease in adults: association with social factors and age at tonsillectomy: case-control study. Int J Cancer 1990;45: 423–427.
30. Raez L, Cabral L, Cai JP, et al. Treatment of AIDS-related primary central nervous system lymphoma with zidovudine, ganciclovir, and interleukin 2. AIDS Res Hum Retroviruses 1999;15:713–719.
31. Fine HA, Mayer RJ. Primary central nervous system lymphoma. Ann Intern Med 1993;119:1093–1104.
32. Skiest DJ, Crosby C. Survival is prolonged by highly active antiretroviral therapy in AIDS patients with primary central nervous system lymphoma. AIDS 2003;17: 1787–1793.
33. Phan T, O'Neill BP, Kurtin PJ. Post-transplant primary CNS lymphoma. Neuro-oncol 2000;2:229–238.
34. Snanoudj R, Durrbach A, Leblond V, et al. Primary brain lymphomas after kidney transplantation: presentation and outcome. Transplantation 2003;76:930–937.
35. Herida M, Mary-Krause M, Kaphan R, et al. Incidence of non-AIDS-defining cancer before and during the highly active antiretroviral therapy era in a cohort of human immunodeficiency virus-infected patients. J Clin Oncol 2003;21:3447–3453.
36. Armitage JO, Longo DL. Malignancies of lymphoid cells. In: Kasper DL, Braunwald E, Fauci AS, et al, eds. Harrison online. New York: McGrawHill.www3.accessmedicine.com/resourcetoc.aspx?resourceID24&part=5. For specific citation: www3.accessmedicine.com/content.aspx?aID=65651.
37. Alizadeh A, Eisen M, Botstein D, et al. Probing lymphocyte biology by genomic-scale gene expression analysis. J Clin Immunol 1998;18:373–379.
38. Alizadeh A, Eisen MB, Davis RE, et al. Distinct types of diffuse large B-cell lymphoma identified by gene expression profiling. Nature 2000;403:503–511.
39. Thompsett AR, Ellison DW, Stevenson FK, et al. V (H) gene sequences from primary central nervous system lymphomas indicate derivation from highly mutated germinal center B cells with ongoing mutational activity. Blood 1999;94:1738–1746.
40. Braaten KM, Betensky RA, de Leval L, et al. BCL-6 expression predicts improved survival in patients with primary central nervous system lymphoma. Clin Cancer Res 2003;9: 1063–1069.
41. Migliazza A, Martinotti S, Chen W, et al. Frequent somatic hypermutation of the 5N noncoding region of the BCL6 gene in B-cell lymphoma. Proc Natl Acad Sci USA 1995;92:12520–12524.
42. Zhang SJ, Endo S, Ichikawa T, et al. Frequent deletion and 5N CpG island methylation of the p16 gene in primary malignant lymphoma of the brain. Cancer Res 1998;58: 1231–1237.
43. Cobbers JM, Wolter M, Reifenberger J, et al. Frequent inactivation of DCKN2A and rare mutation of TP53 in PCNSL. Brain Pathol 1998;8:263–276.

44. Nakamura M, Sakkaki T, Hashimoto H, et al. Frequent alterations of the p14(ARF) and p16(INK4a) genes in primary central nervous system lymphomas. Cancer Res 2001;61: 6335–6339.
45. Larocca LM, Capello D, Rinelli A, et al. The molecular and phenotypic profile of primary central nervous system lymphoma identifies distinct categories of the disease and is consistent with histogenetic derivation from germinal center related B cells. Blood 1998;92:1011–1019.
46. Moore PA, Belvedere O, Orr A, et al. BLyS: member of the tumor necrosis factor family and B-lymphocyte stimulator. Science 1999;285:260–263.
47. Schiemann B, Gommersman JL, Vora K, et al. An essential role for BAFF in the normal development of B-cells through a BCMA-independent pathway. Science 2001;293: 2111–2114.
48. Briones J, Timmerman JM, Hilbert DM, et al. BLyS and BLyS receptor expression in non-Hodgkin's lymphoma. Exp Hematol 2002;30:135–141.
49. He B, Chadburn A, Jou E, et al. Lymphoma B cells evade apoptosis through the TNF family members BAFF/BLyS and APRIL. J Immunol 2004;172:3268–3279.
50. Herkes GK, Partington MD, O'Neill BP. Neurologic presentation of cranial vault lymphomas: report of two cases. Neurosurgery 1991;29:898–901.
51. Dunne JW, Harper CG, Pamphlett R. Intramedullary spinal cord metastases: a clinical and pathological study of nine cases. Q J Med 1986;61:1003–1020.
52. Azzarelli B, Easterling K, Norton JA. Leukemic cell-endothelial cell interaction in leukemic cell dissemination. Lab Invest 1989;60:45–64.
53. Ransohoff RM, Kivisakk P, Kidd G. Three or more routes for leukocyte migration into the central nervous system. Nat Rev Immunol 2003;3:569–581.
54. Whiteside TL, Odoux C. Dendritic cell biology and cancer therapy. Cancer Immunol Immunother 2004;53:240–248.
55. Hochman J, Assaf N, Deckert-Schluter M, et al. Entry routes of malignant lymphoma into the brain and eyes in a mouse model. Cancer Res 2001;61:5242–5247.
56. Rubenstein JL, Shen A, Fridlynad J, et al. Gene expression profile analysis of primary CNS lymphoma: class distinction and outcome prediction. Neuro-oncol 2003;5:314.
57. O'Neill BP, Kelly PJ, Earle JD, et al. Computer-assisted stereotactic biopsy for the diagnosis of primary central nervous system lymphoma. Neurology 1987;37:1160–1164.
58. Miller DC, Hochberg FH, Harris NL, et al. Pathology with clinical correlations of primary central nervous system non-Hodgkin's lymphoma. Cancer 1994;74:1383–1397.
59. Pfannl R, Ferry JA, Harris NL. Pathology of primary central nervous system lymphoma and related conditions. In: Batchelor T, ed. Lymphoma of the nervous system. Amsterdam: Butterworth-Heinemann, 2004:29–42.
60. Poussaint TY, Siffert J, Barnes PD, et al. Hemorrhagic vasculopathy after treatment of central nervous system neoplasia in childhood: diagnosis and follow-up. AJNR Am J Neuroradiol 1995;16:693–699.
61. Neuwelt EA, Frenkel EP, Gumerlock MK, et al. Developments in the diagnosis and treatment of primary CNS lymphoma: a prospective study. Cancer 1986;58: 1609–1620.
62. Grant JW, Isaacson PG. Primary central nervous system lymphoma. Brain Pathol 1999;2:97–109.
63. Nalesnik MA, Jaffe R, Starzl TE, et al. The pathology of posttransplant lymphoproliferative disorders occurring in the setting of cyclosporine A-prednisone immunosuppression. Am J Pathol 1988;133:173–192.
64. Penn I, Porat G. Central nervous system lymphomas in organ allograft recipients. Transplantation 1995;59:240–249.
65. Paya CV, Fung JJ, Nalesnik MA, et al. Epstein-Barr virus-induced posttransplant lymphoproliferative disorders. ASTS/ASTP EBV-PTLD Task Force and the Mayo Clinic Organized International Consensus Development meeting. Transplantation 1999;68:1517–1525.
66. Buteau B, Paya CV. Clinical usefulness of Epstein-Barr viral load in solid-organ transplantation. Liver Transpl 2001;7:157–159.
67. Piriou ER, van Dort K, Nanlohy NM, et al. Altered EBV viral load setpoint after HIV seroconversion is in accordance with lack of predictive value of EBV load for the occurrence of AIDS-related non-Hodgkin lymphoma. J Immunol 2004;172:6931–6937.
68. Vaquero J, Martinez R, Rossi E, et al. Primary cerebral lymphoma: the "ghost tumor." J Neurosurg 1984;60:174–176.
69. Molnar PP, O'Neill BP, Scheithauer BW, et al. The blood–brain barrier in primary CNS lymphomas: ultrastructural evidence of endothelial cell death. Neuro-oncology 1999;1:89–100.
70. Zhou YH, Tan F, Hess KR, et al. The expression of PAX6, PTEN, vascular endothelial growth factor, and epidermal growth factor receptor in gliomas: relationship to tumor grade and survival. Clin Cancer Res 2003;9:3369–3375.
71. Aref S, Mabed M, Zalata K, et al. The interplay between c-Myc oncogene expression and circulating vascular endothelial growth factor (sVEGF), its antagonist receptor, soluble Flt-1 in diffuse large B cell lymphoma (DLBCL): relationship to patient outcome. Leuk Lymphoma 2004;45(3): 499–506.
72. Neuwelt EA. Mechanism of disease: blood–brain barrier. Neurosurgery 2004;54:131–140.
73. Bashir R, Chamberlain M, Ruby E, et al. T-cell infiltration of primary CNS lymphoma. Neurology 1996;46:440–444.
74. Bakshi R, Mazziotta JC, Mischel PS, et al. Lymphomatosis cerebri presenting as a rapidly progressive dementia: clinical, neuroimaging and pathologic findings. Dement Geriatr Cogn Disord 1999;10:152–157.
75. Deangelis LM. Cerebral lymphoma presenting as a nonenhancing lesion on computed tomographic/magnetic resonance scan. Ann Neurol 1993;33:308–311.
76. Schaumburg HH, Plank CR, Adams RD. The reticulum cell sarcoma-microglioma group of brain tumours. Brain 1972; 95:199–212.
77. Chamberlain MC. Leptomeningeal metastases: a review of evaluation and treatment. J Neurooncol 1998;37:271–284.
78. Balmaceda C, Gaynor JJ, Sun M, et al. Leptomeningeal tumor in primary central nervous system lymphoma: recognition, significance, and implications. Ann Neurol 1995;38: 202–209.
79. Cheng TM, O'Neill BP, Scheithauer BW, et al. Chronic meningitis: the role of meningeal or cortical biopsy. Neurosurg 1994;34(4):590–596.

80. O'Neill BP, Illig JJ. Primary central nervous system lymphoma. Mayo Clin Proc 1989;64:1005–1020.
81. Gametchu B. Glucocorticoid receptor-like antigen in lymphoma cell membranes: correlation to cell lysis. Science 1987;236:456–461.
82. Bataille B, Delwail V, Menet E, et al. Primary intracerebral malignant lymphoma: report of 248 cases. J Neurosurg 2000;92:261–266.
83. Chan CC, Buggage RR, Nussenblatt RB. Intraocular lymphoma. Curr Opin Ophthalmol 2002;13:411–418.
84. McCannel CA, Holland GN, Helm CJ, et al. Causes of uveitis in the general practice of ophthalmology. UCLA Community-Based Uveitis Study Group. Am J Ophthalmol 1996;121:35–46.
85. Qualman SJ, Mendelsohn G, Mann RB, et al. Intraocular lymphomas. Natural history based on a clinicopathologic study of eight cases and review of the literature. Cancer 1983;52:878–886.
86. Hoffman PM, McKelvie P, Hall AJ, et al. Intraocular lymphoma: a series of 14 patients with clinicopathological features and treatment outcomes. Eye 2003;17:513–521.
87. Gill MK, Jampol LM. Variations in the presentation of primary intraocular lymphoma: case reports and a review. Surv Ophthalmol 2001;45:463–471.
88. O'Neill BP, Schiff D. Post-transplant lymphoproliferative disorders of the central nervous system. In: Roos K, ed. Neurologic complications of organ transplantation. Continuum, Philadelphia: Lippincott, 2004:48–60.
89. Wijdicks EFM. Abnormal conscious state and coma in transplant recipients. In: Roos K, ed. Neurologic complications of organ transplantation. Continuum, Philadelphia: Lippincott, 2004:9–18.
90. Blumenthal DT, Raizer JJ, Rosenblum MK, et al. Primary intracranial neoplasms in patients with HIV. Neurology 1999;52:1648–1651.
91. Newell ME, Hoy JF, Cooper SG, et al. Human immunodeficiency virus-related primary central nervous system lymphoma: factors influencing survival in 111 patients. Cancer 2004;100:2627–2636.
92. Leblond V, Dhedin N, Mamzer Bruneel MF, et al. Lymphoproliferative disorders after organ transplantation: a report of 24 cases observed in a single center. J Clin Oncol 1998;16:2052–2059.
93. Levitt LJ, Dawson DM, Rosenthal DS, et al. CNS involvement in the non-Hodgkin's lymphomas. Cancer 1980;45:545–552.
94. Macintosh FR, Colby TV, Podolsky WJ, et al. Central nervous system involvement in non-Hodgkin's lymphoma: an analysis of 105 cases. Cancer 1982;49:586–595.
95. Feugier P, Virion JM, Tilly H, et al. Incidence and risk factors for central nervous system occurrence in elderly patients with diffuse large-B-cell lymphoma: influence of rituximab. Ann Oncol 2004;15:129–133.
96. Rubenstein JL, Combs D, Rosenberg J, et al. Rituximab therapy for CNS lymphomas: targeting the leptomeningeal compartment. Blood 2003;101:466–468.
97. O'Neill BP, Banks PM, Habermann TM, et al. Primary central nervous system lymphoma as a variant of Richter's Syndrome in two patients with chronic lymphocytic leukemia. Cancer 1989;64:1296–1300.
98. DeAngelis LM. Primary central nervous system lymphoma as a secondary malignancy. Cancer 1991;67:1431–1435.
99. Lossos A, Ben-Yahuda D, Bokstein F, et al. Does late CNS relapse of systemic non-Hodgkin's lymphoma (NHL) represent a residual primary disease or a second novel lymphoma? Neurology 2000;54:A39–A40.
100. Winkelman MD, Adelstein DJ, Karlins NL. Intramedullary spinal cord metastasis. Diagnostic and therapeutic considerations. Arch Neurol 1987;44:526–531.
101. Deangelis LM, Yahalom J, Heinemann MH, et al. Primary CNS lymphoma: combined treatment with chemotherapy and radiotherapy. Neurology 1990;40:80–86.
102. Kondziolka D, Lunsford LD, Martinez AJ. Unreliability of contemporary neurodiagnostic imaging in evaluating suspected adult supratentorial (low-grade) astrocytoma. J Neurosurg 1993;79:533–536.
103. O'Neill BP, Kelly PJ, Earle JD, et al. The value of stereotactic biopsy in the diagnosis of primary brain tumors. Neurology 1986;36:187.
104. Watling CJ, Lee DH, Macdonald DR, et al. Corticosteroid-induced magnetic resonance imaging changes in patients with recurrent malignant glioma. J Clin Oncol 1994;12:1886–1889.
105. O'Neill BP, Wang C-H, O'Fallon JR, et al. The consequences of treatment and disease in patients with primary central nervous system non-Hodgkin's lymphoma (PCNSL): cognitive function and performance status. Neuro-oncol 1999;1:196–203.
106. Jack CR Jr, O'Neill BP, Banks PM, et al. Primary central nervous system lymphoma: histologic subtypes and CT appearance. Radiology 1988;167:211–215.
107. Lachance DH, O'Neill BP, Macdonald DR, et al. Primary leptomeningeal lymphoma: report of 9 cases, diagnosis with immunocytochemical analysis, and review of the literature. Neurology 1991;41:95–100.
108. Alderson L, Fetell MR, Sisti M, et al. Sentinel lesions of primary CNS lymphoma. J Neurol Neurosurg Psychiatry 1996;60:102–105.
109. Tefferi A, O'Neill BP, Inwards DJ. Late-onset cerebral toxoplasmosis after allogeneic bone marrow transplantation. Bone Marrow Transplant 1998;21:1285–1286.
110. Nelson DF, Martz KL, Bonner H, et al. Non-Hodgkin's lymphoma of the brain: can high dose, large volume radiation therapy improves survival? Report on a prospective trial by the Radiation Therapy Oncology Group (RTOG): RTOG 8315. Int J Radiat Oncol Biol Phys 1992;23:9–17.
111. O'Neill BP, Wang CH, O'Fallon JR, et al: Primary central nervous system non-Hodgkin's lymphoma (PCNSL): survival advantages with combined initial therapy? A final report of the North Central Cancer Treatment Group (NCCTG) Study 86–72–52. Int J Radiat Oncol Biol Phys 1999;43:559–563.
112. Blay JY, Ongolo-Zogo P, Sebban C, et al. Primary cerebral lymphomas: unsolved issues regarding first-line treatment, follow-up, late neurologic toxicity and treatment of relapses. The FNCLCC. French Federation Nationale des Centers de Lutte contre le Cancer. Ann Oncol 2000;11:39–44.
113. Harder H, Holtel HH, Bromberg JEC, et al. Cognitive status and quality of life after treatment for primary CNS lymphoma. Neurology 2004;62:544–547.

114. Murray K, Kun L, Cox J. Primary malignant lymphoma of the central nervous system: results of treatment of 11 cases and review of the literature. J Neurosurg 1986; 65:600–607.
115. Michalski JM, Garcia DM, Kase E, et al. Primary central nervous system lymphoma: analysis of prognostic variables and patterns of treatment failure. Radiology 1990;176: 855–860.
116. Dong Y, Pan L, Wang B, et al. Stereotactic radiosurgery in the treatment of primary central nervous system lymphoma. Chin Med J (Engl) 2003;116:1166–1170.
117. Ferreri AJ, Abrey LE, Blay JY, et al. Summary statement on primary central nervous system lymphomas from the Eighth International Conference on Malignant Lymphoma, Lugano, Switzerland, June 12 to 15,2002. J Clin Oncol 2003; 21:2407–2414.
118. Blay J-Y, Conroy T, Chevreau C, et al. High-dose methotrexate for the treatment of primary cerebral lymphomas: analysis of survival and late neurologic toxicity in a retrospective series. J Clin Oncol 1998;16:864–871.
119. DeAngelis LM, Seiferheld W, Schold SC, et al. Radiation Therapy Oncology Group Study 93–10. Combination chemotherapy and radiotherapy for primary central nervous system lymphoma: Radiation Therapy Oncology Group Study 93–10. J Clin Oncol 2002;20:4643–4638.
120. Gabbai AA, Hochberg FH, Linggood RM, et al. High-dose methotrexate for non-AIDS primary central nervous system lymphoma. J Neurosurg 1989;70:190–194.
121. Glass J, Gruber ML, Cher L, et al. Preirradiation methotrexate chemotherapy of primary central nervous system lymphoma: long-term outcome. J Neurosurg 1994;81:188–195.
122. Bessell EM, Graus F, Punt JAG, et al: Primary non-Hodgkin's lymphoma of the CNS treated with BVAM or CHOD/BVAM chemotherapy prior to radiotherapy. J Clin Oncol 1996;14:945–954.
123. Batchelor T, Carson K, O'Neill A, et al. Treatment of primary CNS lymphoma with methotrexate and deferred radiotherapy: a report of NABTT 96–07. J Clin Oncol 2003;21:1044–1049.
124. Goldman JM, Schmitz N, Niethammer D, et al. Allogenic and autologous transplantation for haematological diseases, solid tumors, and immune disorders: current practice in Europe in 1998. Bone Marrow Transplant 1997;20:745–752.
125. Popat U, Hosing C, Saliba RM, et al. Prognostic factors for disease progression after high-dose chemotherapy and autologous hematopoietic stem cell transplantation for recurrent or refractory Hodgkin's lymphoma. Bone Marrow Transplant 2004;33:1015–1023.
126. Soussain C, Suzan F, Hoang-Xuan K, et al. Results of intensive chemotherapy followed by hematopoietic stem-cell rescue in 22 patients with refractory or recurrent primary CNS lymphoma or intraocular lymphoma. J Clin Oncol 2001;19:742–749.
127. Abrey LE, Rosenblum MK, Papadopoulos E, et al. High-dose chemotherapy with autologous stem cell rescue in adults with malignant primary brain tumors. J Clin Oncol 1999;44:147–153.
128. Freilich RJ, Delattre JY, Monjour A, et al. Chemotherapy without radiation therapy as initial treatment of primary CNS lymphoma in elderly patients. Neurology 1996;46: 435–439.
129. Doolittle ND, Miner ME, Hall WA, et al. Safety and efficacy of a multicenter study using intraarterial chemotherapy in conjunction with osmotic opening of the blood-brain barrier for the treatment of patients with malignant brain tumors. Cancer 2000;88:637–647.
130. Dahlborg SA, Braziel R, Crossen JR, et al. Non-AIDS primary CNS lymphoma: first example of a durable response in a primary brain tumor using enhanced chemotherapy delivery without cognitive loss and without radiotherapy. Cancer J Sci Am 1996;2:166–174.
131. Formenti SC, Parkash SC, Lean E, et al. Primary central nervous system lymphoma in AIDS. Cancer 1989;63;1101–1107.
132. Baumgartner JE, Raichlin JR, Beckstead JH, et al. Primary central nervous system lymphoma with a natural history and response to radiotherapy in 55 patients with acquired immunodeficiency syndrome. J Neurosurg 1990;73; 206–211.
133. Forsyth P, DeAngelis LM. Biology and management of AIDS-associated primary CNS lymphoma. Hematol Oncol Clin North Am 1996;5:1125–1134.
134. Matthews GV, Bower M, Mandalia S, et al. Changes in acquired immunodeficiency syndrome-associated lymphoma since the introduction of highly active antiretroviral therapy. Blood 2000;96:273–2734.
135. Fisburne BC, Wilson DJ, Rosenbaum JT, et al. Intravitreal methotrexate as an adjunctive treatment of intraocular lymphoma. Arch Ophthalmol 1997;115:1152–1157.
136. Ghobrial IM, Buadi F, Spinner RJ, et al. High-dose intravenous methotrexate followed by autologous stem cell transplantation as a potentially effective therapy for neurolymphomatosis. Cancer 2004;100:2403–2407.
137. Baehring JM, Damek D, Martin EC, et al. Neurolymphomatosis. Neuro-oncol 2003;5:104–115.
138. Ratech H, Burke JS, Blayney DW, et al. A clinicopathologic study of malignant lymphomas of the nose, paranasal sinuses, and hard palate, including cases of lethal midline granuloma. Cancer 1989;64:2525–2531.
139. Todeschini G, Tecchio C, Degani D, et al. Eighty-one percent event-free survival in advanced Burkitt's lymphoma/ leukemia: no differences in outcome between pediatric and adult patients treated with the same intensive pediatric protocol. Ann Oncol 1997;8 (Suppl 1): 77–81.
140. Fonseca R, Inwards DJ, Habermann TM, et al. Testicular lymphoma is associated with a high incidence of extranodal relapse. Cancer 2000;88:154–161.
141. Young RC, Howser DM, Anderson T, et al. Central nervous system complications of non-Hodgkin's lymphoma. The potential role for prophylactic therapy. Am J Med 1979;66: 435–443.
142. Recht L, Straus DJ, Cirrincione C, et al. Central nervous system metastases from non-Hodgkin's lymphoma: treatment and prophylaxis. Am J Med 1988;84:425–435.
143. Reni M, Ferreri AJ. Therapeutic management of refractor or relapsed primary central nervous system lymphomas. Ann Hematol 2001;80(Suppl 3):B113–B117.

144. Tyson RM, Siegal T, Doolittle ND, et al. Current status and future of relapsed primary central nervous system lymphoma (PCNSL). Leuk Lymphoma 2003:44:627–633.
145. Cheng T, Forsyth P, Chaudhry A, et al. High-dose thiotepa, busulfan, cyclophosphamide and ASCT without whole-brain radiotherapy for poor prognosis primary CNS lymphoma. Bone Marrow Transplant 2003:31:679–685.
146. Arellano-Rodrigo E, Lopez-Guillermo A, Bessel EM, et al. Salvage treatment with etoposide (VP-16), ifosfamide and cytarabine (Ara-C) for patients with recurrent primary central nervous system lymphoma. Eur J Haematol 2003;70:219–224.
147. Schultz C, Scott C, Sherman W, et al. Preirradiation chemotherapy with cyclophosphamide, doxorubicin, vincristine, and dexamethasone for primary CNS lymphomas: initial report of Radiation Therapy Oncology Group protocol 88–06. J Clin Oncol 1996;14:556–564.
148. Abrey LE, Yahalom J, DeAngelis LM. Treatment for primary CNS lymphoma: the next step. J Clin Oncol 2000;18: 3144–3150.
149. Reni M, Ferreri AJ, Garancini MP, et al. Therapeutic management of primary central nervous system lymphoma in immunocompetent patients: results of a critical review of the literature. Ann Oncol 1997;8:227–234.

CHAPTER 18

Primary Meningeal Neoplasms

John K. Park / Peter McL. Black

Meningiomas are the second most common primary brain tumors and are usually histologically benign. They are thought to arise from the cap cells of the arachnoid villi that project into the venous sinuses of the dura (Fig. 18-1). Asymptomatic tumors are commonly left untreated and patients are given careful clinical and radiographic followup. Symptomatic and growing tumors are generally treated surgically, with good long-term results. Atypical and anaplastic meningiomas and those located near critical brain structures, however, are sometimes difficult to resect completely and may require adjuvant treatments such as radiation or chemotherapy.

▶ EPIDEMIOLOGY AND KNOWN INFLUENCES ON TUMOR

Meningiomas have an overall incidence of approximately 2 per 100,000 persons and account for one-fifth of all intracranial tumors.[1] In one study, 50% of tumors were first found at autopsy, particularly those occurring in people greater than 60 years of age.[2] In a separate study, 76 cases of meningiomas were found in 7345 autopsies performed over a 20-year period (1.03%).[3] Ninety percent of tumors are benign and most commonly occur between the ages of 40 and 70 years. Approximately 2% of meningiomas occur in patients younger than age 20 years,[4] and when they do occur, they are commonly associated with neurofibromatosis type 2 (NF2). In one series, 5 of 27 pediatric meningioma patients had NF2,[5] whereas 3 of 22 did in another series.[6] Meningiomas are two to three times more prevalent in women than men, and the peak decades of incidence are the seventh and sixth, respectively. Five percent to 15% of patients have multiple meningiomas, most commonly in association with NF2.

There is an increased incidence of tumors in patients who have had previous cranial irradiation. In one study, the cumulative actuarial risk of secondary meningioma in a cohort of 445 children age 16 years or younger treated with high-dose cranial irradiation (≥10 Gy) was 0.53%, 1.2%, and 8.18% at 10, 20, and 25 years, respectively.[7] This study reported that 4 of 9 of the histologically graded tumors were atypical, whereas a larger study of 19 tumors reported that 29% displayed anaplastic features.[8] In a cohort study of 10,000 children treated with 1.5 Gy of cranial radiation for tinea capitis, the relative risk ratio for meningioma development was 9.5 and tumors were more likely to be atypical or anaplastic than benign.[9]

Studies also cite an association between meningiomas and breast carcinomas in women. In a population-based, retrospective cohort analysis, the relative risk of subsequent breast carcinoma in women who were diagnosed with meningioma was 1.54 (95% confidence interval [CI], 0.77–2.75), whereas the relative risk of subsequent meningioma in women who were diagnosed with breast carcinoma was 1.64 (95% CI, 0.79–3.02). These results

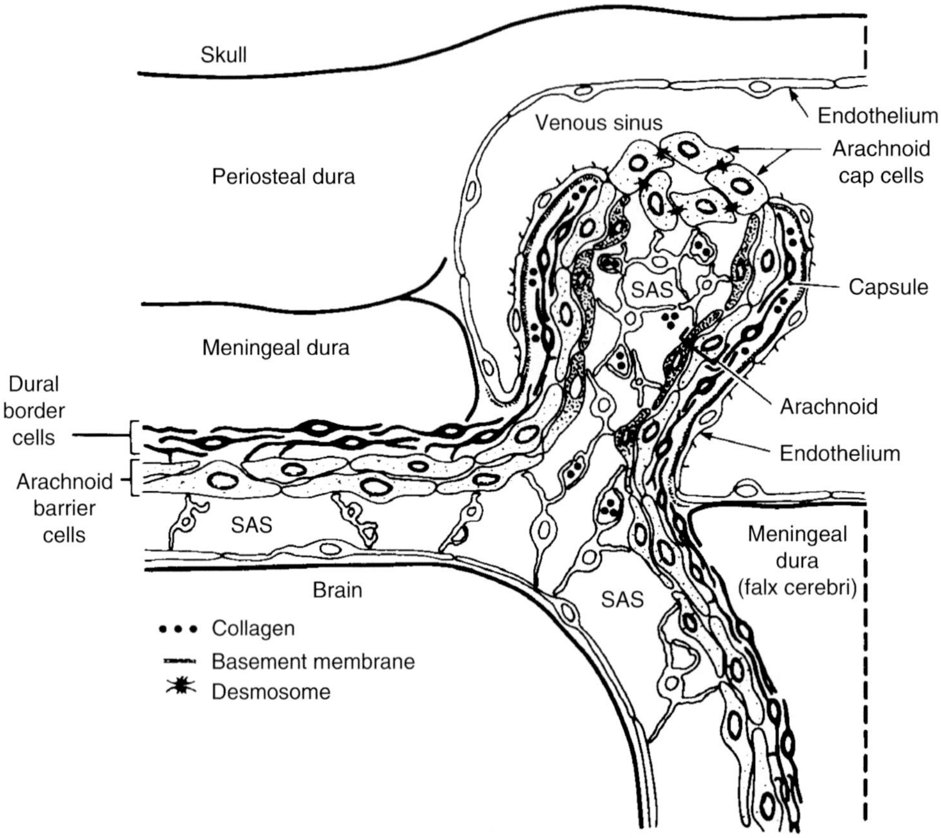

Figure 18-1. Semidiagrammatic representation of the arachnoid granulation showing its relation to the superior sagittal sinus (venous sinus) and the continuity of its layers and spaces with those of the meninges on the surface of the brain. The individual layers or cell clusters are not intended to be proportional but are drawn to emphasize the cytoarchitectural features of the granulation. SAS = subarachnoid space. (*Reproduced with permission from Haddad G, Al-Mefty O. Meningiomas: an overview. In: Wilkins R, Rengachary S, eds. Neurosurgery. New York: McGraw Hill, 1996:833–841.*)

are similar to those of other studies examining this relationship and the authors concluded that shared risk factors may account for the relatively weak bidirectional associations.[10]

The role of head trauma in tumor development is unclear. In a cohort study of 228,055 Danish head injury patients followed for an average of 8 years (maximum: 17 years), brain neoplasms were identified by linking the study roster with records of the Danish Cancer Registry for the corresponding years. This approach avoids the differential reporting of injuries by study participants as an explanation for any associations seen, the major weakness of many other studies. Intracranial tumors occurred more often than expected based on incidence rates for the Danish population; but most of the excess occurred during the first year after the injury and likely was due to the detection of tumors that were present before the injury occurred. Excluding the first year of followup, the standardized incidence ratio for meningioma was 95% CI = 0.8–1.7.[11]

▶ GENETICS AND MOLECULAR BIOLOGY

Genetics

The primary genetic defect underlying meningioma development is currently unknown. Loss of heterozygosity or deletions of the long arm of chromosome 22 have been reported in more than 40% of examined tumors.[12,13] The *NF2* gene, which encodes for the protein merlin, is found in this chromosomal region. Merlin is a membrane-associated cytoskeletal protein that plays a role in actin–cytoskeleton organization.[14] NF2 patients have an increased incidence of meningiomas, and mutations of merlin resulting in decreased protein expression are associated with many sporadic meningiomas. Approximately 40% of tumors, however, appear to have normal merlin expression and no deletions within chromosome 22.[15] Another chromosomal deletion that is associated with meningiomas is 18q, which contains the gene for DAL-1, a putative tumor suppressor protein absent in approximately 60% of non–small-cell lung carcinomas.[16]

Several different chromosomal abnormalities are associated with meningioma anaplasia (malignancy). Loss, as well as gain, of chromosome 22 has been demonstrated in anaplastic tumors. Anaplastic tumors have also been found to harbor loss of heterozygosity for chromosomes 1p, 2p, 6q, 9q, 10q, and/or 14q. The chromosomally deleted genes that are responsible for the anaplastic phenotype have yet to be identified.[17,18] However, a particular gene that has been implicated in the anaplastic progression of meningiomas is *p53*, which has been found at increased levels in anaplastic tumors.[19] Increased telomerase activity has also been reported in anaplastic, but not benign, meningiomas.[20]

Growth Factors and Receptors

As in many tumor types, the expression of growth factors and their receptors have been examined in meningioma specimens. Among the growth factors expressed by meningiomas, as determined by messenger RNA (mRNA) expression or immunocytochemistry, are epidermal growth factor (EGF), transforming growth factor-α (TGF-α), platelet-derived growth factor (PDGF), insulin-like growth factors (IGF)-I and -II, and vascular endothelial growth factor (VEGF). VEGF expression is of particular interest as it may be responsible for edema formation in the peritumoral brain white matter.[21] Receptors for the above mentioned growth factors are also expressed in meningioma specimens, allowing for the possibility of an autocrine loop mechanism of growth stimulation.[22]

Given the increased incidence of meningiomas in women, the slightly greater incidence in women with breast carcinoma, and the documented growth of some tumors during pregnancy, the role of steroid hormones in tumor pathogenesis has been investigated. Progesterone receptors are expressed in 70% to 80% of meningiomas and may be associated with a more benign phenotype. Estrogen and androgen receptors are also expressed by tumors, but in a smaller percentage.[23]

▶ SPECIFIC CLINICAL PRESENTATIONS

The most common findings in patients presenting with symptoms are seizures, headaches, and focal neurologic deficits. Seizures occur almost exclusively with supratentorial tumors, which comprise 90% of all intracranial tumors. Of patients with intracranial tumors 30% to 40% have seizures preoperatively and the median duration of seizures is 1 month.[24] Increased peritumoral edema is also associated with increased seizure likelihood.

Clinical syndromes associated with meningiomas usually correlate with anatomic location. The following describes site frequency of occurrence along with clinical syndrome:

- Falx and parasagittal meningiomas (25% of tumors) can lead to bilateral leg weakness or visual field deficits, depending on their location.
- Convexity meningiomas (20%) most commonly occur over the frontal lobes and frequently remain asymptomatic until they reach a large size. Seizures and mental status changes are common presenting symptoms.
- Medial sphenoid wing meningiomas (20%, which includes middle and lateral sphenoid wings) can result in cranial nerve palsies when there is spread to or pressure on the cavernous sinus and its contents (Fig. 18-2). Oculomotor palsies and facial numbness are not uncommon, and involvement of the carotid artery can lead to vascular occlusion symptoms. Middle and lateral sphenoid wing meningiomas are more akin to convexity meningiomas, both in terms of symptomatology and in surgical approach (Fig. 18-3).
- Olfactory groove meningiomas (10%) can also attain relatively large sizes prior to symptom development. The altered taste sensation and subtle mental status changes that can occur sometimes go unnoticed by patients and their families without specific questioning. Larger tumors can lead to optic nerve atrophy in the ipsilateral eye and papilledema in the contralateral eye (Foster-Kennedy syndrome) and result in visual symptoms.
- Sellar and parasellar meningiomas (10%) can lead to similar symptoms as olfactory groove meningiomas but visual symptoms are noticeable with relatively smaller-sized tumors.
- Posterior fossa meningiomas (10%) can present with facial numbness, facial weakness, hearing loss, swallowing difficulties, and/or shoulder weakness, depending on their proximity to and involvement of the cranial nerves. Tumors in the foramen magnum characteristically present with progressive weakness of the ipsilateral leg, followed by the contralateral leg, and the contralateral arm (Fig. 18-4).
- Intraventricular meningiomas (2%) often present with headaches as a consequence of the blockage of cerebrospinal fluid flow causing secondary hydrocephalus and increased intracranial pressure.
- Spinal meningiomas account for fewer than 10% of all meningiomas and commonly occur in the intradural thoracic spine as extramedullary tumors. They generally present with back and radicular pain that can progress to leg weakness and numbness, as well as bowel and bladder difficulties with further tumor growth.

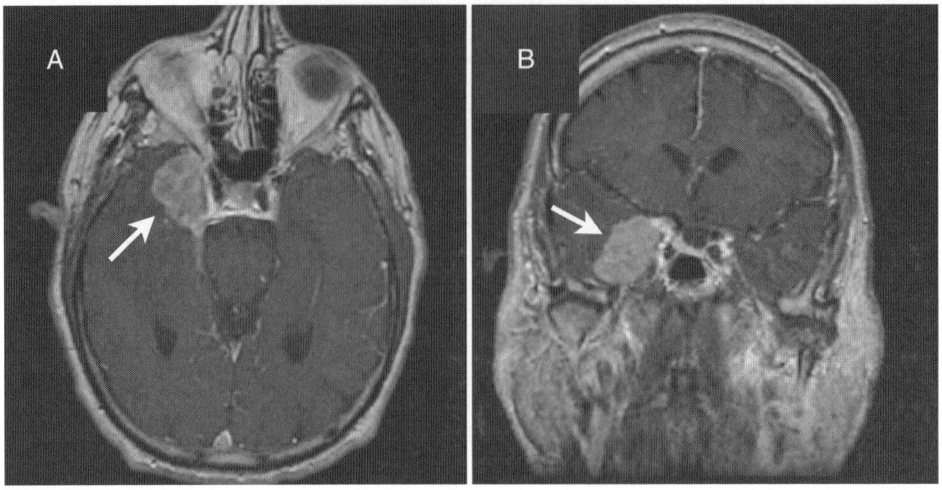

Figure 18-2. Cavernous sinus meningioma. A 60-year-old male presented with diplopia and mild right-sided facial numbness. (A) Axial T_1-weighted magnetic resonance imaging (MRI) following contrast administration. (B) Coronal T_1-weighted MRI following contrast administration.

▶ DIAGNOSTIC EVALUATION

Confirmation of a suspected meningioma can usually be made radiographically. On computerized tomography (CT) scan, tumors are usually isointense with normal surrounding brain. They are dural based, with the exception of intraventricular tumors, and frequently have a smooth contour, although some tumors can have irregular margins. There can be hyperostosis or erosion of the overlying skull, and some tumors themselves contain calcifications. Tumors can also contain hemorrhage, necrosis, and/or cysts, all of which can be seen on CT. Following the administration of intravenous contrast, tumors usually enhance brightly and are readily differentiated from the surrounding brain.

Magnetic resonance (MR) scanning is also very helpful in confirming a meningioma diagnosis. Tumors are usually isointense or hypointense to gray matter on T_1-weighted images and isointense or hyperintense on T_2-weighted and proton-density images. Tumors often brightly enhance following the administration of intravenous contrast, and frequently a "dural tail" of enhancement can be seen. Heterogeneous tumor enhancement, irregular tumor borders, and significant edema in the surrounding brain are suggestive of a more anaplastic phenotype but this cannot be predicted with a significant degree

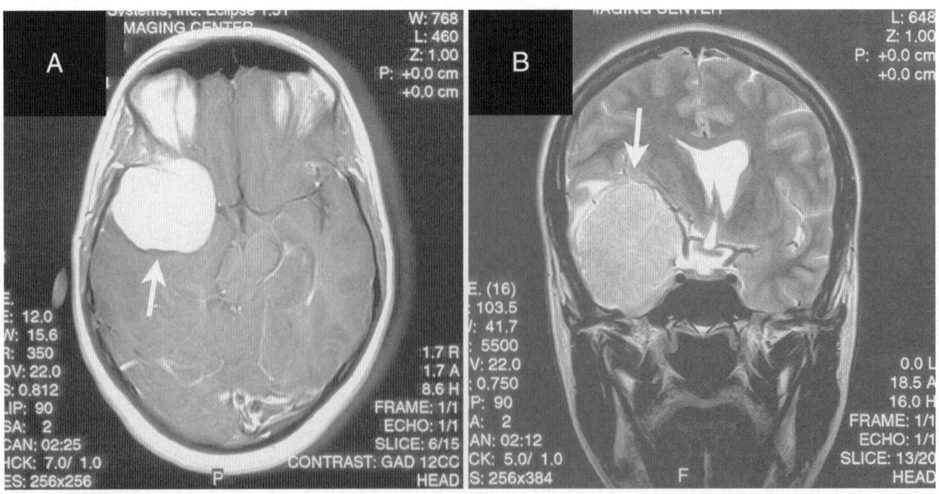

Figure 18-3. Sphenoid wing meningioma. A 29-year-old female presented with headaches. (A) Axial T_1-weighted MRI following contrast administration. (B) Coronal T_2-weighted MRI.

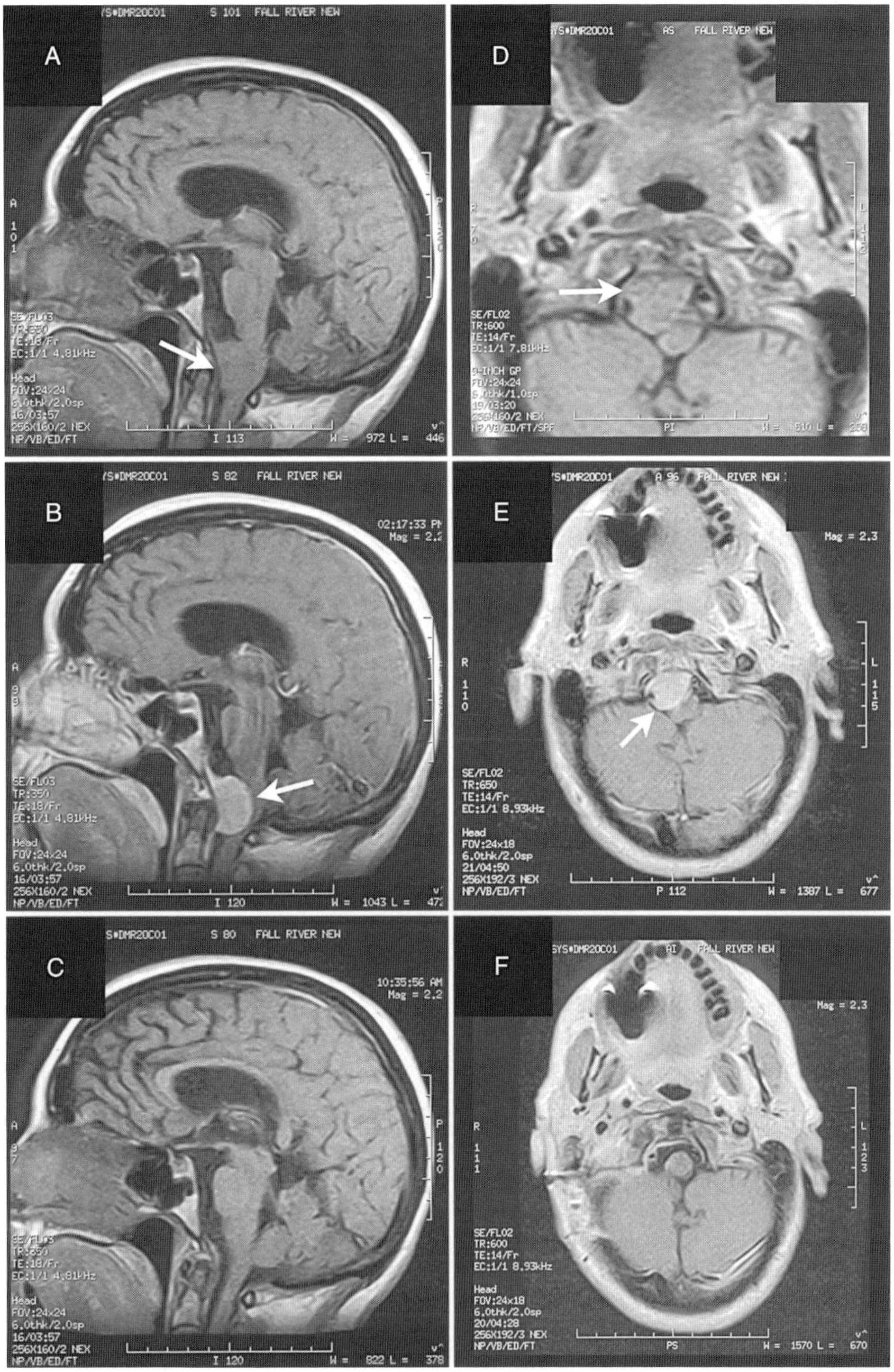

Figure 18-4. Foramen magnum meningioma. A 63-year-old female presented with a progressive history of right leg weakness followed by left leg weakness. A, B, D, and E are preoperative scans; C and F are postoperative scans. (A) Sagittal T_1-weighted MRI; (B) sagittal T_1-weighted MRI following contrast administration; (C) sagittal T_1-weighted MRI following contrast administration; (D) axial T_1-weighted MRI; (E) axial T_1-weighted MRI following contrast administration; (F) axial T_1-weighted MRI following contrast administration.

of specificity. While most dural-based enhancing lesions are meningiomas, the differential diagnosis also includes solitary fibrous tumors, gliosarcomas, leiomyosarcomas, hemangiopericytomas, melanocytomas, Hodgkin disease, plasmacytomas, inflammatory pseudotumors, neurosarcoidosis, plasma cell granulomas, Rosai-Dorfman disease, Castleman disease, xanthomas, rheumatoid nodules, and tuberculomas.[25]

MR scans, when combined with MR venography and MR arteriography, are useful if surgery is contemplated, as they can identify the course, and sometimes the patency, of associated vascular structures such as tumor-feeding vessels, the carotid arteries and their major branches, and the venous sinuses. A more detailed assessment of vascular structures requires the use of angiography. Tumors usually display a vascular blush which "arrives early and leaves late." Angiography has the added potential benefit of allowing for the embolization of larger tumor-feeding arteries.

Both [^{18}F]fluorodeoxyglucose positron emission tomography (FDG-PET) scanning and thallium-201 single-photon emission computed tomography (SPECT) scanning have been used to predict tumor malignancy prior to surgery and recurrence following surgery, but their utility in everyday clinical practice has yet to be demonstrated.[26,27]

▶ NEUROPATHOLOGY

Although meningiomas are classically described as consisting of whorls of tissue that form around a central region of hyaline material, the tumors, as a group, are somewhat heterogeneous in their histologic appearances. As can be seen radiographically, hemorrhage, calcifications, and cysts can be seen both grossly and microscopically. Many, but not all, tumors contain psammoma bodies, interlacing bundles of elongated fibroblasts. Although most tumors express vimentin and epithelial membrane antigen and are negative for glial fibrillary acidic protein and Leu-7, there is currently no single definitive marker for meningiomas.

The most commonly used classification scheme for meningiomas is that of the World Health Organization (WHO) (Table 18-1).[28] Tumors are grouped according to their predominant histologic appearance as well as degree of malignancy (Fig. 18-5). Grade I tumors are benign and have a low risk of recurrence or aggressive growth; grade II tumors are atypical and have an intermediate risk; and grade III tumors are anaplastic and have a high risk. Approximately 90% of tumors are grade I, of which the three most common subtypes are meningothelial, fibrous (fibroblastic), and transitional (mixed) meningioma. Tumors are considered atypical if they contain 4 mitoses per 10 high-power fields or 3 or more of the following: increased cellularity, small cells with a high nuclear-to-cytoplasmic ratio, uninterrupted patternless or sheet-like growth, or foci of spontaneous or geographic necrosis. Anaplastic tumors are those with abundant mitoses, nuclear pleomorphism, loss of the usual meningioma growth patterns, infiltration of the underlying brain, and multiple foci of microscopic necrosis. Many reports use the terms *anaplastic* and *malignant* interchangeably.

▶ TABLE 18-1. WHO CLASSIFICATION OF MENINGIOMAS

WHO grade I—Benign meningiomas
Meningothelial meningioma
Fibrous (fibroblastic) meningioma
Transitional (mixed) meningioma
Psammomatous meningioma
Angiomatous meningioma
Microcystic meningioma
Secretory meningioma
Lymphoplasmacyte-rich meningioma
Metaplastic meningioma
WHO grade II—Atypical meningiomas
Atypical meningioma
Clear cell meningioma (intracranial)
Chordoid meningioma
WHO grade III—Anaplastic meningioma
Rhabdoid meningioma
Papillary meningioma
Anaplastic (malignant) meningioma

Source: Reproduced with permission from Louis DN, Scheithauer BW, Budka H, et al. Meningiomas. In: Cavenee WK, ed. Pathology and genetics of tumours of the nervous system. Lyon, France: IARC Press, 2000:175–196.

▶ NATURAL HISTORY

The majority of meningiomas are benign, slow-growing tumors. Those that are asymptomatic and found incidentally can be followed clinically and radiographically until there is evidence of symptom development or tumor growth. In one study of 60 asymptomatic patients with a mean followup of 32 months, none of the patients developed new symptoms referable to the tumor. Forty-five of the patients had followup radiographic studies at 3 months, 9 months, and then every 1 to 2 years following initial evaluation. During this followup period, 10 patients had growth ranging from 0.2 cm to 1.0 cm and 35 patients exhibited no growth.[29] Another study followed 47 asymptomatic patients for a mean followup period of 43 months. Forty-one of the patients underwent conservative management for the duration of the study period and were found to have absolute tumor growth rates ranging from 0.03 to 2.62 cm^3/y, with a majority

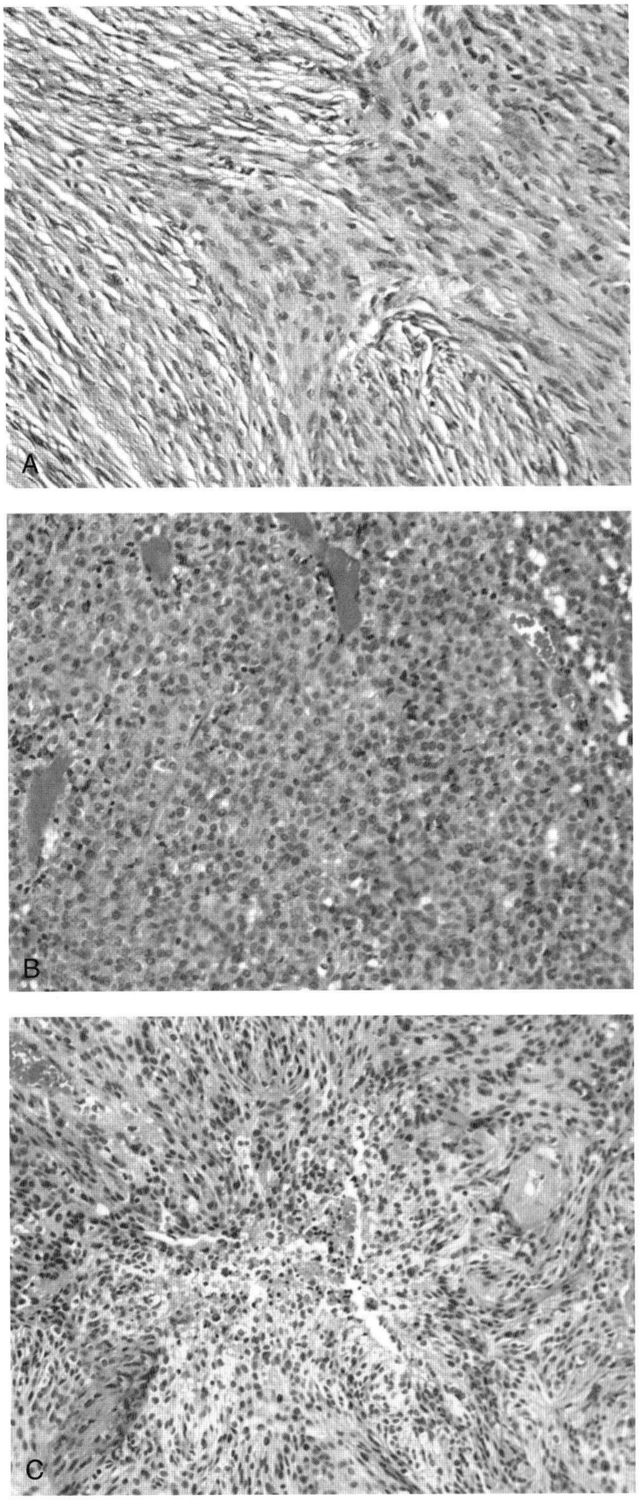

Figure 18-5 (PLATE 52). Hematoxylin and eosin-stained sections of meningiomas. (A) WHO grade I: benign meningioma of the transitional subtype; (B) WHO grade II: atypical meningioma showing "sheeting" of tumor cells; (C) WHO grade III: malignant meningioma with small cells with high nuclear cytoplasmic ratio, irregular growth, necrosis, and high mitotic index. (*Photomicrographs courtesy of Alexander Vortmeyer, MD, Surgical Neurology Branch, NINDS, NIH.*)

(66%) having tumor growth rates of less than 1 cm^3/y. Six of the patients, however, showed significant enough growth that resection was recommended and carried out.[30]

Tumors that are symptomatic, expanding, or have radiographic features suggestive of atypia or malignancy are typically resected. The natural history of such tumors is therefore not well studied.

▶ SURGICAL MANAGEMENT

When indicated and technically feasible, complete resection of a meningioma is the treatment goal. For tumors of the cerebral and cerebellar convexity, olfactory groove, lateral sphenoid wing, anterior falx, and anterior third of the superior sagittal sinus, this is usually possible. Tumors involving the medial sphenoid wing, posterior falx, posterior two thirds of the superior sagittal sinus, cavernous sinus, optic nerve sheath, and skull base are more difficult to remove completely; tumor residuum is usually preferable to permanent neurologic or vascular morbidity. Tumors that are incompletely resected can be treated with adjuvant radiation therapy with some success as discussed in "Role of Radiation."

Neurologic disability and mortality can result from direct injury to the brain, cranial nerves, or blood vessels. Leakage of cerebrospinal fluid and meningitis are potential concerns following the resection of large tumors or those located at the skull base. Deep venous thrombosis (DVT) is also a relatively common occurrence following meningioma resection. In one study, the incidence of postoperative DVTs in patients with meningiomas was 72%.[31] The etiology of this apparent hypercoagulable state is currently unknown. Operative mortality rates in large patient series are generally below 10%. In one study of 652 patients, the mortality rate was 7% and significant risk factors were poor preoperative clinical condition, absence of epilepsy, age greater than 65, incomplete tumor removal, pulmonary embolism, and an intracranial hematoma requiring evacuation.[32]

Tumor recurrence and life expectancy following surgery are dependent on the degree of resection and the histologic grade of the tumor. The completeness of tumor resection is frequently graded according to the Simpson scale, which, in turn, correlates with 10-year recurrence rates (Table 18-2).[33]

Two large patient series have also shown the benefits of a gross total resection. In one study of 581 patients, progression-free survival at 5 years for patients with gross total versus partial resections was 88% versus 61%. At 10 years, the corresponding percentages were 75% and 39%, respectively.[34] A separate study of 935 patients found a 4.2-fold relative excess risk of death for patients with incomplete tumor removals when compared with those with complete removals.[32]

▶ TABLE 18-2. SIMPSON GRADING SCALE

Grade	Extent of Removal	10-Year Recurrence Rate
1	Complete removal including resection of dura and bone	9%
2	Complete tumor removal with coagulation of dural attachment	19%
3	Complete tumor removal without resection or coagulation of dural attachment	29%
4	Subtotal removal	40%
5	Decompression	

Source: Reproduced with permission from Simpson D. Recurrence of intracranial meningiomas after surgical treatment. J Neurol Neurosurg Psychiatr 1957;20:22–39.

In addition to degree of tumor resection, histologic grade can also serve as a predictor of recurrence and survival. In a study of 936 patients, at 5 years after complete removal, the rate of recurrence was only 3% for benign meningiomas, but 38% for atypical ones, and 78% for anaplastic ones. The median recurrence times were 7.5, 2.4, and 3.5 years, respectively.[35] In a different study comparing 42 atypical and 29 anaplastic (malignant) meningiomas, the 5-year survival rates for patients were 95% and 64.3%, and the 10-year rates were 79% and 34.5%, respectively. As expected, recurrence-free survival and median time to recurrence were also significantly longer in patients with atypical meningiomas than in those with anaplastic meningiomas.[36]

▶ ROLE OF RADIATION

Radiation therapy for meningiomas is typically administered using one of two dosing regimens and one of three radiation sources. Stereotactic *radiosurgery* is a technique whereby multiple convergent beams of radiation are delivered to a discrete, radiographically determined volume with the goal of minimizing radiation to surrounding, nontumor structures. This is administered during a single treatment session using an electron source (linear accelerator), a gamma-emitting cobalt-60 source (gamma knife), or a proton source (proton beam). Stereotactic *radiotherapy* is based on the same principle of providing maximal radiation to tumor tissue while minimizing injury to surrounding tissues except that the radiation dose is fractionated and delivered over multiple treatment sessions. Theoretically, this decreases the risk of injury to radiosensitive structures such as the optic nerves and chiasm.

Some tumors, particularly those that involve cranial nerves or critical vascular structures, may not be completely resectable. Both stereotactic radiosurgery and radiotherapy have been used to treat these incompletely resected as well as recurrent tumors. In one retrospective study of 84 patients with subtotally resected tumors, the recurrence rate for patients who received radiation was 32% (17 of 54) versus 60% (18 of 30) for those who did not. Additionally, the median time to recurrence was significantly longer in the irradiated group than in the nonirradiated group (125 months vs. 66 months, $p < 0.05$).[37] A second retrospective study of 132 patients reported actuarial 10-year local control rates of 18% for subtotal excision alone and 82% for subtotal excision plus postoperative radiation therapy (and 77% for total excision alone). The actuarial 10-year survival rates were 49% and 81% (and 93%), respectively.[38]

More recently, patients with small- to medium-size meningiomas have been treated primarily with radiosurgery. In a retrospective series of adult meningioma patients with a mean followup of 64 months, 136 patients underwent surgical resection and 62 underwent radiosurgery. Tumor recurrence/progression was more common in the surgical group (12%) than the radiosurgical group (2%, $p = 0.04$) as were complications (22% and 10%, respectively, $p = 0.02$). Three- and 7-year actuarial progression-free survival rates were no different in the radiosurgical (100% and 95%, respectively) and Simpson grade 1 patients (100% and 96%, respectively), but were significantly higher in the Simpson grade 2 (91% and 82%, respectively; $p < 0.05$) and Simpson grades 3 to 4 (68% and 34%, respectively; $p < 0.001$). The authors of this study did not, however, recommend radiosurgery as the primary treatment for all patients with small- to moderate-size meningiomas. They cited the need for a minimal followup of 10 or more years to assess this treatment approach adequately. Also, unlike surgery, radiosurgery is ineffective at relieving the mass effect caused by some tumors.[39]

In the absence of any randomized trials comparing meningioma therapies, surgical resection remains the recommended primary treatment modality for most meningiomas that are symptomatic or enlarging. Radiation therapy is indicated for the treatment of atypical or anaplastic residual lesions and unresectable recurrent lesions of all histologic grades. Stereotactic radiosurgery is the preferred type of radiation therapy for radiographically discrete lesions away from radiosensitive structures such as the optic nerves and chiasm, whereas stereotactic radiotherapy is the preferred type for more diffuse lesions or discrete lesions close to radiosensitive structures.

▶ ROLE OF CHEMOTHERAPY

Studies of chemotherapies in the treatment of anaplastic meningiomas are few in number and report mixed results. Among the combination regimens tried with little significant benefit are cyclophosphamide, doxorubicin (Adriamycin), and vincristine (CAV)[40]; doxorubicin and dacarbazine[41]; and ifosfamide and mesna.[41] The initial report of hydroxyurea administration involved four patients who had undergone multiple resections for persistently growing tumor. One patient had stabilization of tumor size whereas the other patients had decreases in tumor volumes of 15%, 60%, and 74%.[42] Subsequent larger studies of hydroxyurea administration have reported good tolerability but less dramatic results. Delayed tumor progression has been much more common than actual tumor shrinkage.[43,44] Interferon-α2B, an immunomodulatory agent,[45] and mifepristone, a progesterone receptor antagonist,[46] have also been administered with some limited success.

▶ OTHER MENINGEAL NEOPLASMS

Hemangiopericytomas

Meningeal hemangiopericytomas, previously also referred to as angioblastic meningiomas, are radiographically indistinguishable from most meningiomas. They are, however, more akin to peripheral soft-tissue hemangiopericytomas than meningiomas and so the term *angioblastic meningioma* is no longer used.[47] Hemangiopericytomas arise from perivascular pericytes and comprise less than 1% of all brain tumors. In one of the largest series reported to date (44 patients), there was a slight preponderance of males (55%). The average age at diagnosis was 42 years, the average duration of preoperative symptoms was 11 months, and, as expected, symptomatology was related to tumor location. All patients were treated initially with surgical resection and the average time to first recurrence was 47 months, with recurrence rates of 15%, 65%, and 76% at 1, 5, and 10 years, respectively. Twenty-three percent of patients developed extraneural metastasis, a phenomenon that rarely occurs with meningiomas. The average survival period for the patients in the study was 7 years, with 5-, 10-, and 15-year survival rates following surgery of 67%, 40%, and 23%, respectively. As with meningiomas, gross total tumor resection favorably affected recurrence and survival, and metastasis adversely affected survival. Radiation therapy after the first operation improved the average time to first recurrence from 34 to 75 months, and extended survival from 62 to 92 months.[47]

Meningeal Sarcomas

Primary meningeal sarcomas are highly aggressive tumors that occur mostly in children and young adults and represent 0.1% to 5.5% of intracranial pediatric tumors.[48] They can arise from the dura mater, the leptomeninges, or the adventitial fibroblasts of the cerebral blood vessels. When they occur in adults, they sometimes develop following radiation therapy for other brain tumors. Meningeal sarcomas can grow sharply demarcated from the underlying brain, spread like a sheath over the cortex, or frankly infiltrate the brain parenchyma. In the WHO classification of tumors, they are referred to as meningeal sarcomatosis.[28] Among the tumor types that should be immunohistochemically excluded in the differential diagnosis are metastatic sarcoma, gliosarcoma, medulloblastoma with mesenchymal differentiation, malignant meningioma, and pleomorphic xanthoastrocytoma. Radiographically, tumors can resemble anaplastic meningiomas and typically have clear attachment to the dura, poorly defined margins with brain, and heterogeneous contrast enhancement.[48]

The clinical course for most patients is a rapid recurrence following surgery. The average 1-year survival is 50%,[49] and the average length of survival is 32 months.[48] Radical resection appears to provide a better chance for extended survival, but the number of patients reported in the literature has been too small to draw any firm conclusions. Likewise, the effectiveness of radiation and chemotherapy has not been determined.

Melanocytic Tumors

Melanocytic tumors are those arising from the melanocytes of the leptomeninges. The group is comprised of melanocytomas, diffuse melanocytosis (diffuse melanosis), and malignant melanomas.[50] The most common of these are melanocytomas, benign lesions that are themselves rare. They account for only 0.06% to 0.1% of brain tumors and have an annual incidence of approximately 1 per 10 million persons.[50] As of this writing, approximately 100 cases have been reported in the literature, with a roughly equal distribution between intracranial (47.5%) and spinal (52.5%) cases. Intracranial lesions tended to occur in slightly younger patients than spinal lesions (40 years and 49 years, respectively, $p = 0.016$), and 57.9% of patients were female. Melanocytes are found in higher densities in the infratentorial and cervical areas, but tumors occur more frequently in the supratentorial (26.3%) and thoracic (26.3%) regions. During a mean followup period of 46 months, patients who had complete resections fared slightly better than did those patients with subtotal resections, but this was not statistically significant.

The overall rates of tumor recurrence and tumor-related death were 26.3% and 10.5%, respectively.[51] Patients with melanocytoma can present with myelopathy, radiculopathy, cranial nerve deficits, chronic basilar meningitis, seizures, and hydrocephalus, depending on the tumor(s) location. Radiographically, lesions are typically hyperintense on T_1-weighted images and hypointense on T_2-weighted images as a consequence of their melanin content. They enhance with contrast and the differential diagnosis on gross examination includes pigmented meningioma, melanotic schwannoma, melanomatosis, and malignant melanoma. An accurate diagnosis requires immunohistochemistry and, rarely, electron microscopy.[52]

Diffuse melanocytosis can involve the supratentorial and/or infratentorial leptomeninges, and patients frequently present with seizures, psychiatric disturbances, or hydrocephalus.[53] Radiographically, there is diffuse thickening and enhancement of the meninges. Patients have a poor prognosis even in the absence of histologic malignancy because of the progressive extension of the tumor.[50]

Primary meningeal melanomas are similar to melanocytomas in many respects except they are histologically more malignant and carry a much poorer prognosis.[50]

▶ SUMMARY

Approximately 90% of meningiomas are benign, slow-growing tumors. Surgery is recommended for those that are symptomatic, enlarging, or have radiographic features suggestive of malignancy. Those that are found incidentally should be clinically and radiographically followed. When surgery is indicated, a gross total resection should be attempted as this provides the best opportunity for recurrence-free survival for all histologic subtypes. In cases where a complete removal is not feasible because of an unacceptable risk of neurologic injury, a subtotal resection should be undertaken followed by adjuvant radiation therapy if there is clinical or radiographic evidence of residual tumor growth. The role of chemotherapy in the treatment of anaplastic meningiomas is under active study at this time.

REFERENCES

1. Radhakrishnan K, Mokri B, Parisi JE, et al. The trends in incidence of primary brain tumors in the population of Rochester, Minnesota. Ann Neurol 1995;37(1):67–73.
2. Staneczek W, Janisch W. Epidemiologic data on meningiomas in East Germany 1961–1986: incidence, localization, age and sex distribution. Clin Neuropathol 1992;11(3):135–141.
3. Bellur SN, Chandra V. Meningioma size. Its relationship to other diseases. Arch Neurol 1981;38(7):458–459.
4. Zwerdling T, Dothage J. Meningiomas in children and adolescents. J Pediatr Hematol Oncol 2002;24(3):199–204.
5. Lund-Johansen M, Scheie D, Muller T, et al. Neurosurgical treatment of meningiomas in children and young adults. Childs Nerv Syst 2001;17(12):719–723.
6. Rochat P, Johannesen HH, Gjerris F. Long-term follow up of children with meningiomas in Denmark: 1935 to 1984. J Neurosurg 2004;100(2):179–182.
7. Strojan P, Popovic M, Jereb B. Secondary intracranial meningiomas after high-dose cranial irradiation: report of five cases and review of the literature. Int J Radiat Oncol Biol Phys 2000;48(1):65–73.
8. Pollak L, Walach N, Gur R, et al. Meningiomas after radiotherapy for tinea capitis—still no history. Tumori 1998;84(1):65–68.
9. Modan B, Baidatz D, Mart H, et al. Radiation-induced head and neck tumours. Lancet 1974;1(7852):277–279.
10. Custer BS, Koepsell TD, Mueller BA. The association between breast carcinoma and meningioma in women. Cancer 2002;94(6):1626–1635.
11. Inskip PD, Mellemkjaer L, Gridley G, et al. Incidence of intracranial tumors following hospitalization for head injuries (Denmark). Cancer Causes Control 1998;9(1):109–116.
12. Seizinger BR, de la Monte S, Atkins L, et al. Molecular genetic approach to human meningioma: loss of genes on chromosome 22. Proc Natl Acad Sci USA 1987;84(15):5419–5423.
13. Dumanski JP, Carlbom E, Collins VP, et al. Deletion mapping of a locus on human chromosome 22 involved in the oncogenesis of meningioma. Proc Natl Acad Sci USA 1987;84(24):9275–9279.
14. Rouleau GA, Merel P, Lutchman M, et al. Alteration in a new gene encoding a putative membrane-organizing protein causes neuro-fibromatosis type 2. Nature 1993;363(6429):515–521.
15. Ruttledge MH, Sarrazin J, Rangaratnam S, et al. Evidence for the complete inactivation of the NF2 gene in the majority of sporadic meningiomas. Nat Genet 1994;6(2):180–184.
16. Gutmann DH, Donahoe J, Perry A, et al. Loss of DAL-1, a protein 4.1-related tumor suppressor, is an important early event in the pathogenesis of meningiomas. Hum Mol Genet 2000;9(10):1495–1500.
17. Lamszus K, Kluwe L, Matschke J, et al. Allelic losses at 1p 9q 10q 14q, and 22q in the progression of aggressive meningiomas and undifferentiated meningeal sarcomas. Cancer Genet Cytogenet 1999;110(2):103–110.
18. Ozaki S, Nishizaki T, Ito H, et al. Comparative genomic hybridization analysis of genetic alterations associated with malignant progression of meningioma. J Neurooncol 1999;41(2):167–174.
19. Nagashima G, Aoyagi M, Yamamoto M, et al. P53 overexpression and proliferative potential in malignant meningiomas. Acta Neurochir (Wien) 1999;141(1):53–61; discussion 60–61.
20. Chen HJ, Liang CL, Lu K, et al. Implication of telomerase activity and alternations of telomere length in the histologic characteristics of intracranial meningiomas. Cancer 2000;89(10):2092–2098.
21. Kalkanis SN, Carroll RS, Zhang J, et al. Correlation of vascular endothelial growth factor messenger RNA expression with peritumoral vasogenic cerebral edema in meningiomas. J Neurosurg 1996;85(6):1095–1101.

22. Shamah SM, Alberta JA, Giannobile WV, et al. Detection of activated platelet-derived growth factor receptors in human meningioma. Cancer Res 1997;57(18):4141–4147.
23. Carroll RS, Zhang J, Dashner K, et al. Androgen receptor expression in meningiomas. J Neurosurg 1995;82(3):453–460.
24. Chozick BS, Reinert SE, Greenblatt SH. Incidence of seizures after surgery for supratentorial meningiomas: a modern analysis. J Neurosurg 1996;84(3):382–386.
25. Johnson MD, Powell SZ, Boyer PJ, et al. Dural lesions mimicking meningiomas. Hum Pathol 2002;33(12):1211–1226.
26. Cremerius U, Bares R, Weis J, et al. Fasting improves discrimination of grade 1 and atypical or malignant meningioma in FDG-PET. J Nucl Med 1997;38(1):26–30.
27. Jinnouchi S, Hoshi H, Ohnishi T, et al. Thallium-201 SPECT for predicting histological types of meningiomas. J Nucl Med 1993;34(12):2091–2094.
28. Kleihues P, Burger PC, Scheithauer BW. The new WHO classification of brain tumours. Brain Pathol 1993;3(3):255–268.
29. Olivero WC, Lister JR, Elwood PW. The natural history and growth rate of asymptomatic meningiomas: a review of 60 patients. J Neurosurg 1995;83(2):222–224.
30. Nakamura M, Roser F, Michel J, et al. The natural history of incidental meningiomas. Neurosurgery 2003;53(1):62–70; discussion 70–71.
31. Sawaya R, Zuccarello M, Elkalliny M, et al. Postoperative venous thromboembolism and brain tumors: Part I, Clinical profile. J Neurooncol 1992;14(2):119–125.
32. Kallio M, Sankila R, Hakulinen T, et al. Factors affecting operative and excess long-term mortality in 935 patients with intracranial meningioma. Neurosurgery 1992;31(1):2–12.
33. Simpson D. Recurrence of intracranial meningiomas after surgical treatment. J Neurol Neurosurg Psychiatr 1957; 20:22–39.
34. Stafford SL, Perry A, Suman VJ, et al. Primarily resected meningiomas: outcome and prognostic factors in 581 Mayo Clinic patients 1978 through 1988. Mayo Clin Proc 1998;73(10):936–942.
35. Jaaskelainen J, Haltia M, Servo A. Atypical and anaplastic meningiomas: radiology, surgery, radiotherapy, and outcome. Surg Neurol 1986;25(3):233–242.
36. Palma L, Celli P, Franco C, et al. Long-term prognosis for atypical and malignant meningiomas: a study of 71 surgical cases. J Neurosurg 1997;86(5):793–800.
37. Barbaro N, Gutin P, Wilson C, et al. Radiation therapy in the treatment of partially resected meningiomas. Neurosurgery 1987;20:525.
38. Taylor BJ, Marcus RJ, Friedman W, et al. The meningioma controversy: postoperative radiation therapy. Int J Radiat Oncol Biol Phys 1988;15:299.
39. Pollock BE, Stafford SL, Utter A, et al. Stereotactic radiosurgery provides equivalent tumor control to Simpson Grade 1 resection for patients with small- to medium-size meningiomas. Int J Radiat Oncol Biol Phys 2003;55(4):1000–1005.
40. Chamberlain MC. Adjuvant combined modality therapy for malignant meningiomas. J Neurosurg 1996;84(5):733–736.
41. Kyritsis AP. Chemotherapy for meningiomas. J Neurooncol 1996;29(3):269–272.
42. Schrell UM, Rittig MG, Anders M, et al. Hydroxyurea for treatment of unresectable and recurrent meningiomas. II. Decrease in the size of meningiomas in patients treated with hydroxyurea. J Neurosurg 1997;86(5):840–844.
43. Mason WP, Gentili F, Macdonald DR, et al. Stabilization of disease progression by hydroxyurea in patients with recurrent or unresectable meningioma. J Neurosurg 2002;97(2):341–346.
44. Rosenthal MA, Ashley DL, Cher L. Treatment of high risk or recurrent meningiomas with hydroxyurea. J Clin Neurosci 2002;9(2):156–158.
45. Kaba SE, DeMonte F, Bruner JM, et al. The treatment of recurrent unresectable and malignant meningiomas with interferon alpha-2B. Neurosurgery 1997;40(2):271–275.
46. Grunberg SM, Weiss MH, Spitz IM, et al. Treatment of unresectable meningiomas with the antiprogesterone agent mifepristone. J Neurosurg 1991;74(6):861–866.
47. Guthrie BL, Ebersold MJ, Scheithauer BW, et al. Meningeal hemangiopericytoma: histopathological features, treatment, and long-term follow-up of 44 cases. Neurosurgery 1989;25(4):514–522.
48. Buttner A, Pfluger T, Weis S. Primary meningeal sarcomas in two children. J Neurooncol 2001;52(2):181–188.
49. Rueda-Franco F, Lopez-Corella E. Sarcomas in the central nervous system of children 1982. Pediatr Neurosurg 1995;22(1):49–55; discussion 56.
50. Jellinger K, Chou P, Paulus W. Melanocytic lesions. In: Kleihues P, Cavenee WK, eds. Pathology and genetics of tumours of the nervous system. Lyon, France: IARC Press, 2000:193–195.
51. Rahimi-Movaghar V, Karimi M. Meningeal melanocytoma of the brain and oculodermal melanocytosis (nevus of Ota): case report and literature review. Surg Neurol 2003;59(3):200–210.
52. Bydon A, Gutierrez JA, Mahmood A. Meningeal melanocytoma: an aggressive course for a benign tumor. J Neurooncol 2003;64(3):259–263.
53. Allcutt D, Michowiz S, Weitzman S, et al. Primary leptomeningeal melanoma: an unusually aggressive tumor in childhood. Neurosurgery 1993;32(5):721–729; discussion 729.

CHAPTER 19

Pituitary Adenomas and Sellar Lesions: Multidisciplinary Management

John A. Jane, Jr. / Aaron S. Dumont / Mary Lee Vance / Edward R. Laws, Jr.

Pituitary adenomas account for 10% to 15% of primary brain tumors and are the third most frequently encountered primary intracranial neoplasm after gliomas and meningiomas.[1] These tumors present with an annual incidence of between 0.5 and 8.2 per 100,000 persons.[1–6] The prevalence may be much higher than these data indicate; autopsy series suggest that as many as 25% of the population harbor unrecognized adenomas.[7,8] However, most series estimate the prevalence to be approximately 10%, a figure supported by data from magnetic resonance imaging (MRI) series.[9–12] Although incidence varies according to tumor type, taken together, men and women appear equally affected.[2,6]

Depending on the tumor type and growth characteristics, patients present with a variety of endocrinologic and neurologic signs and symptoms. The hormonally active tumors cause characteristic syndromes and include Cushing disease (corticotropin [ACTH] adenomas), acromegaly (somatotroph/growth hormone [GH] adenomas), and amenorrhea-galactorrhea (lactotroph/prolactin [PRL] adenomas). Local intrasellar growth causes varying degrees of pituitary dysfunction. Extrasellar growth classically causes bitemporal hemianopsia, but an array of neurologic signs can be encountered. Although patients with nonfunctioning adenomas (NFAs) present exclusively with signs and symptoms of mass effect, the neurologic sequelae of mass effect may be experienced regardless of tumor type.

Although pituitary adenomas comprise the most common type of sellar tumor, other pathologic entities are encountered in this region and/or its contiguous surroundings. Pituitary apoplexy, which almost invariably occurs in the presence of an underlying adenoma,[13] represents a distinct pathologic syndrome with unique management challenges and is discussed separately. Additionally, other less common but important tumors, such as pituitary carcinomas, craniopharyngiomas and Rathke cleft cysts, possess their own characteristic biologic, pathoanatomic, radiologic, and clinical profiles and are also considered individually.

Significant advances occurred during the last three decades of the 20th century in the classification, pathogenesis, diagnosis, and treatment of pituitary adenomas and other lesions of the sellar region and its surroundings. This chapter focuses on current concepts in the understanding and management of these diverse pathologic entities.

▶ NORMAL ANATOMY AND NEUROIMAGING OF THE SELLAR REGION

The pituitary gland is situated in a cup-shaped depression, the sella turcica, in the body of the sphenoid bone in the central skull base (Fig. 19-1A). The sella turcica is demarcated anteriorly by the tuberculum sellae and posteriorly by the dorsum sellae. Its roof is formed by a dural covering called the diaphragma sellae, which has a central opening through which the pituitary stalk extends. The suprasellar subarachnoid space is located above the diaphragma sellae (containing the optic nerves, chiasm and upper part of the infundibular stalk). A carotid sulcus is found along the lateral surface of the body of the sphenoid bone along which the carotid artery courses. The sphenoid bone is also comprised of two lesser wings that extend from the superolateral part of the body, two greater wings that extend upward from the lower part of the body, and two pterygoid processes that course downward from the body. The anterior clinoid process, an important surgical landmark, is located at the medial termination of the lesser wing (one on either side). The posterior clinoid process may be found at the superolateral margin of the dorsum sellae (one on either side). The optic strut, which separates the optic canal (superior) from the superior orbital fissure (inferior), extends from the anterior clinoid process in an inferomedial direction to the body of the sphenoid (Fig. 19-1B) and is also an important surgical landmark. The cavernous sinus (lateral sellar compartment) is found on either side of the pituitary gland. Through it traverses the cavernous portion of the carotid artery along with cranial nerves III, IV, VI, and V1, which may be involved with lateral extension of sellar pathology producing cranial neuropathies (Fig. 19-2). The optic apparatus lies above the sella, explaining visual loss as sellar lesions grow superiorly to compress the optic chiasm, often producing bitemporal hemianopsia as a consequence of compression of the central chiasm through which fibers subserving the temporal visual fields run (Fig. 19-3). The internal carotid artery loops posteriorly as it passes the anterior clinoid and subsequently bifurcates into the anterior and middle cerebral arteries. The anterior cerebral arteries are found above the optic apparatus. They may, however, be encountered during transsphenoidal surgery during the approach to certain types of suprasellar pathology and this relationship

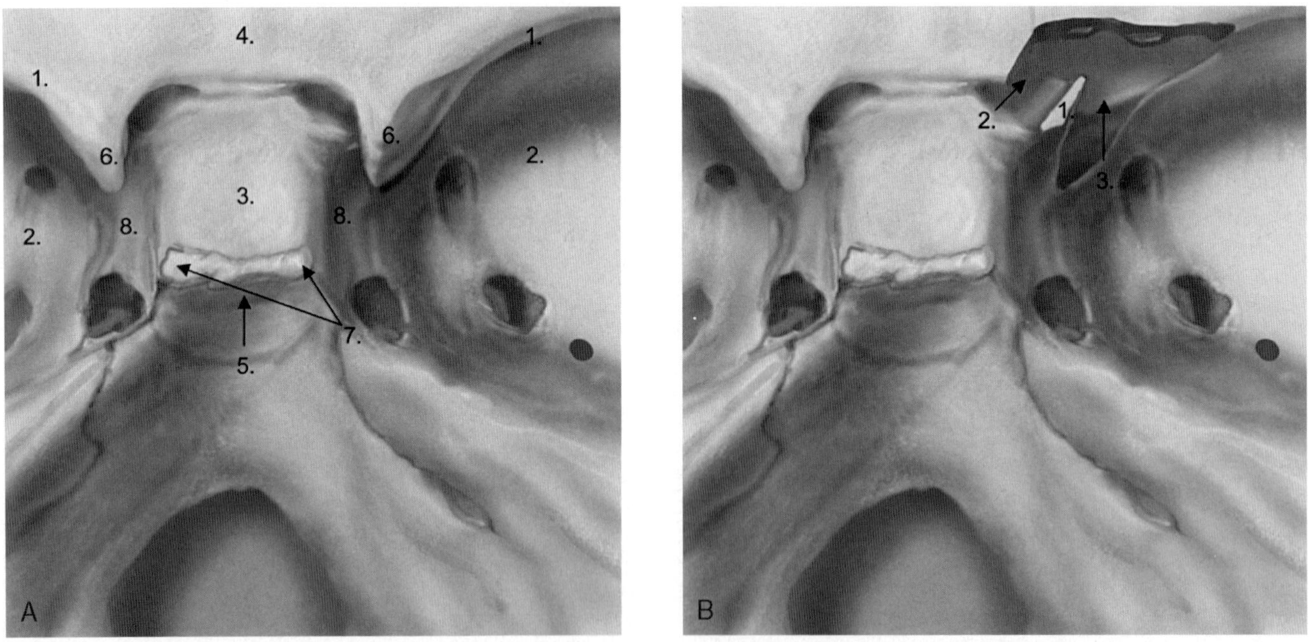

Figure 19-1. Central skull base: sphenoid bone viewed from above. (A) The sphenoid bone consists of two lesser wings (1), two greater wings (2) and two pterygoid processes (not shown). The sella turcica (3) is demarcated by the tuberculum sellae (4) anteriorly and by the dorsum sellae (5) posteriorly. The anterior (6) and posterior (7) clinoid processes are illustrated. The carotid sulcus (8), along which the carotid artery courses, is located on the lateral aspect of the sphenoid body. (B) The right anterior clinoid process has been removed and the right optic canal has been unroofed, exposing the optic strut (1), which runs from the anterior clinoid process in an inferomedial direction to the body of the sphenoid bone and separates the optic canal (2) (above) from the superior orbital fissure (3) (below).

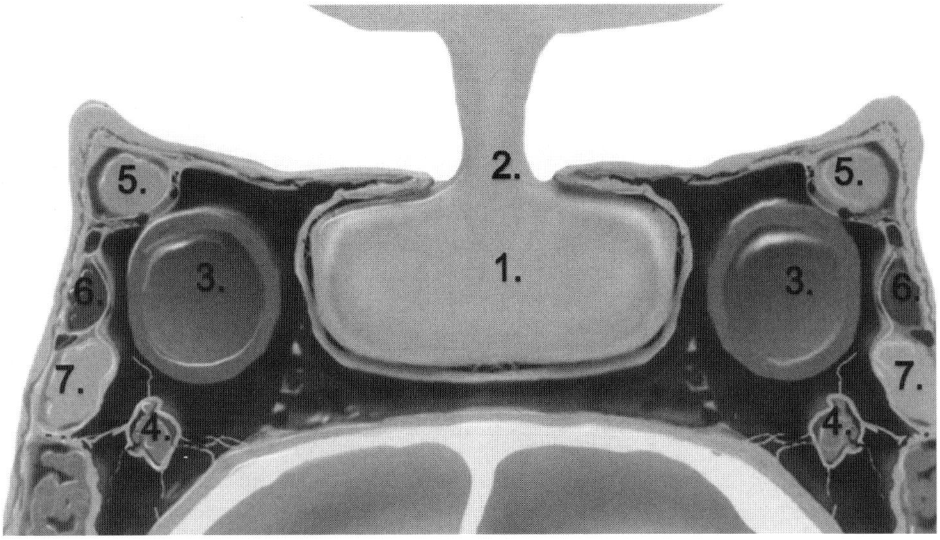

Figure 19-2. Coronal section: pituitary gland, cavernous sinus, sphenoid sinus. The pituitary gland (1) is illustrated within the sellar confines. Its stalk extends through an aperture in the diaphragma sellae (2). Within the cavernous sinus, the carotid artery (3) and cranial nerve VI (4) course through the venous network within the cavernous sinus, whereas cranial nerves III (5), IV (6), and V1 (7) are located within the wall of the cavernous sinus. The sphenoid sinus (8), located below the sella, is also illustrated and demonstrates the potential access to the pituitary gland afforded through a sphenoid sinus (transsphenoidal) approach.

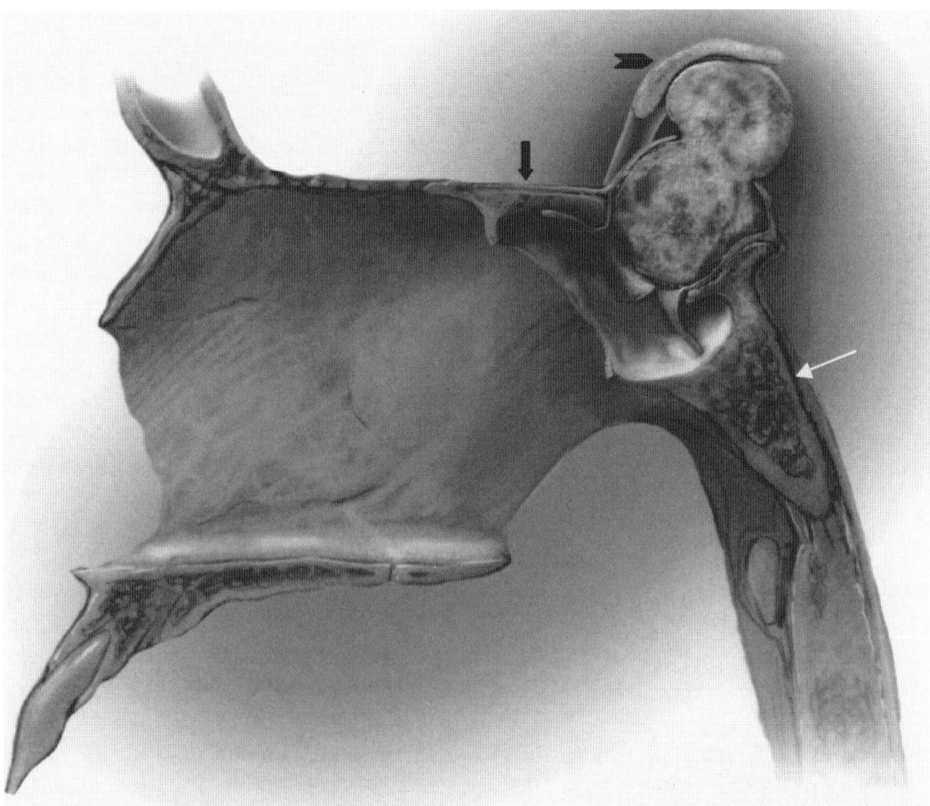

Figure 19-3. Optic chiasm compression from suprasellar extension of a macroadenoma. A sagittal view demonstrating the transsphenoidal trajectory to the sella and a macroadenoma compressing the optic chiasm. The face of the sphenoid sinus has been opened and the sellar floor and dura have also been opened. The tuberculum sellae/planum sphenoidale (black arrows) can also be seen. The pituitary tumor has extended into the suprasellar space and compresses the optic apparatus, which leads to visual disturbance, most commonly bitemporal hemianopsia (black arrowhead). The clivus is continuous inferiorly (white arrow).

must be respected to avoid inadvertent intraoperative injury.

The sphenoid sinus is a characteristically heterogeneous structure.[14] It is poorly developed at birth and the majority of maturation occurs after puberty. Its size, shape, aeration, and the presence and extent of septations are variable. The rostrum or face of the sphenoid sinus (as encountered during a transsphenoidal approach) can also vary in thickness, and may be absent, being covered only by a mucosal layer. Upon entering the sphenoid sinus, the normal convex bulging of the sellar floor is apparent. The clivus is situated below the sella and the tuberculum sellae and planum sphenoidale are located superiorly and anteriorly (see Fig. 19-3). The sellar floor may be particularly thin if eroded by a large sellar tumor.

The pituitary gland itself is comprised of two distinct lobes, anterior (adenohypophysis) and posterior (neurohypophysis) (Fig. 19-4). The anterior lobe is the larger lobe, traditionally thought to arise embryologically from the primitive oral cavity and its embryonic ectoderm, the stomodeum. It is composed of the pars tuberalis (consisting of part of the infundibular stalk and median hypothalamic eminence), pars intermedia (which is poorly developed in humans), and the pars distalis (most of the intrasellar anterior lobe). The anterior lobe does not have direct arterial supply, but rather is supplied by the hypophyseal portal system. Glandular epithelial cells produce endocrine hormones with ACTH- and thyrotropin-stimulating hormone (TSH)-secreting cells located in the central mucoid wedge, PRL- and GH-secreting cells located in the lateral wings, and leuteinizing hormone (LH)- and follicle-stimulating hormone (FSH)-producing cells located diffusely throughout the anterior lobe. These relationships help to explain the location of tumors (at least in the early stages before massive extension and loss of normal gross architecture) that arise from specific cell types. The posterior lobe, in contrast, is thought to arise from neuroectoderm of the diencephalon. The posterior lobe, stalk, and supraoptic and paraventricular nuclei collectively comprise the neurohypophysis. The posterior lobe is the caudal termination of the hypothalamohypophysial tract and stores oxytocin and vasopressin (antidiuretic hormone [ADH]) synthesized in the hypothalamus. This relationship is important to note, as disturbances of the pituitary stalk and hypothalamus (from a tumor or during surgery) can result in abnormalities of ADH, leading to clinical syndromes such as diabetes insipidus and the syndrome of inappropriate antidiuretic hormone (SIADH). These are commonly monitored for in the postoperative period after transsphenoidal surgery. The posterior lobe is supplied by the inferior hypophyseal arteries (from the cavernous carotid artery), whereas the stalk is supplied by the superior hypophyseal branches from the supraclinoid carotid artery (Fig. 19-5). Additionally, McConnell capsular artery, present in approximately 25% of people, may arise from the distal, medial cavernous carotid artery and supply the capsule of the gland or the sellar dura.

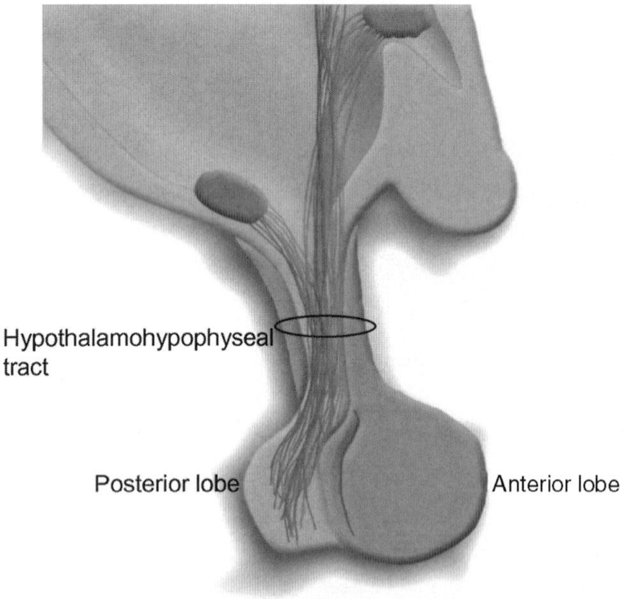

Figure 19-4. Anatomy of the pituitary gland. The relationship of the pituitary gland, situated within the sella, to the sphenoid sinus (inferiorly) and the optic chiasm (superiorly) is illustrated. The pituitary gland consists of an anterior (subdivided into the pars tuberalis, pars intermedia and pars distalis) and a posterior lobe. The supraoptic and paraventricular nuclei in the hypothalamus synthesize antidiuretic hormone (ADH) and oxytocin, which are transported to the posterior lobe for storage via the hypothalamohypophysial tract.

The sellar region is best visualized by magnetic resonance images dedicated to the region. Computerized tomography (CT) scans may provide complementary data, such as in delineation of acute hemorrhage in apoplexy, bony erosion from tumor growth, tumor calcification (with craniopharyngiomas, for example), and may also be useful in combination with frameless stereotaxy for intraoperative neuronavigation[15,16]; however, MR imaging is the current preferred study for delineating pathoanatomic features. The normal anterior pituitary lobe appears isointense to gray matter on T_1-weighted non-contrast enhanced and T_2-weighted MR images.[17] The posterior pituitary lobe is normally hyperintense on T_1-weighted images,[18] which is thought to be caused by the presence of neurosecretory vesicles.[19] This high-intensity signal often disappears with central diabetes insipidus.[20,21] Under normal circumstances, the pituitary parenchyma normally enhances rapidly and homogenously (Fig. 19-6). Indeed, this property is used in identifying a microadenoma within the parenchyma, as thin

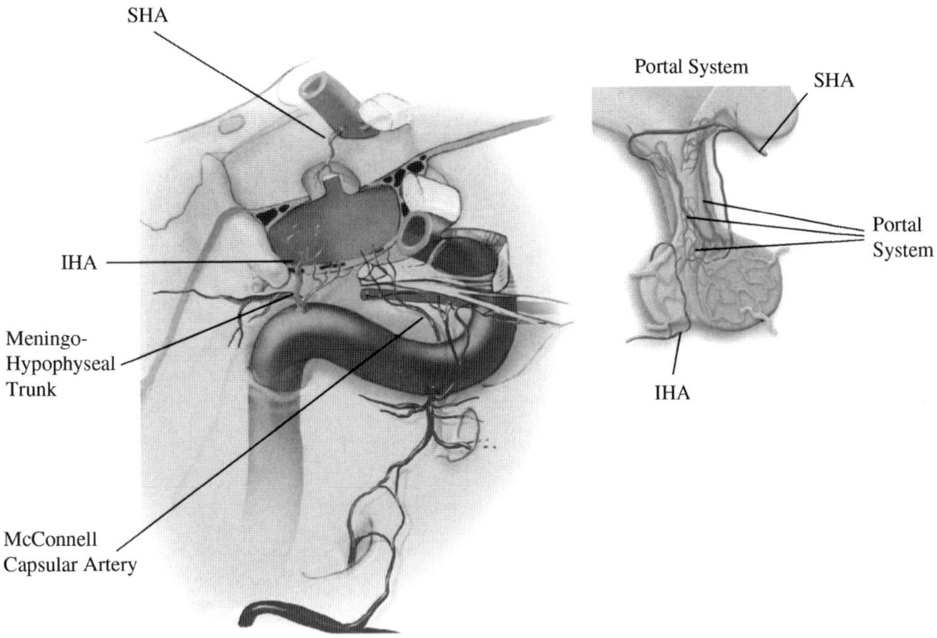

Figure 19-5 (PLATE 53). Vascular anatomy of the pituitary gland. Vascular supply of the pituitary gland is provided by the superior hypophyseal artery (SHA) and inferior hypophyseal artery (IHA) from the carotid arteries bilaterally, and their anastomoses. The SHA actually refers to a series of arteries that arise from the supraclinoid portion of the carotid artery bilaterally. These vessels largely supply the stalk and inferior surface of the optic apparatus and anastomose with their contralateral counterpart forming a vascular plexus. The IHA arise from the meningohypophyseal trunk of the cavernous segment of the carotid artery and supply the posterior lobe. These also anastomose with their contralateral counterpart and form a vascular plexus. The adenohypophysis is largely supplied by the hypophyseal portal venous system (inset) which arises as the anastomotic network between the vascular plexus formed from the SHA (superiorly) and IHA (inferiorly) and is also the means by which releasing hormones are transferred from the hypothalamus to adenohypophysis. McConnell capsular artery, present in approximately 25% of people, may arise from the distal, medial cavernous carotid artery and supply the capsule of the gland or the sellar dura.

coronal images are obtained rapidly during intravenous injection of contrast agent. The microadenoma enhances in delayed fashion relative to normal gland, and hence can be delineated as a hypointense lesion against a rapidly enhancing homogeneous background of normal pituitary gland.[22,23]

▶ PITUITARY ADENOMAS

Classification

Given the variety of tumor types and clinical presentations, an assortment of classification systems has been proposed to codify these tumors. Clinically, our approach primarily distinguishes tumors based on size and functional status (Table 19-1). Pituitary adenomas that are 10 mm or smaller are termed *microadenomas*; those larger than 10 mm are identified as *macroadenomas*. Clinically NFAs are actually a diverse group of tumors that include glycoprotein adenomas (α-subunit, LH, FSH), the null cell adenoma, and oncocytoma. Clinically hyperfunctioning tumors include the GH, prolactin, ACTH, and TSH adenomas.

This classification system has limitations. Confusing the picture somewhat are those tumors that secrete more than one clinically significant hormone. The most common plurihormonal tumors secrete both GH and PRL either in a mixed population of cells or by a single-cell population secreting both hormones.[24–26] Furthermore, although the clinical and biochemical functional status generally correlates with the immunohistochemical findings, exceptions do exist. For example, the silent corticotroph adenoma clinically behaves as a nonfunctioning adenoma but stains positively for ACTH. The most comprehensive classification schema that accounts for virtually all the exceptions is that of the World Health Organization, which codifies

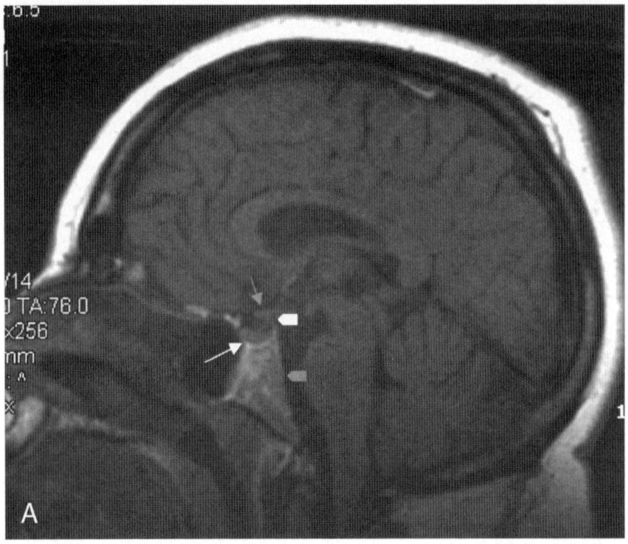

Figure 19-6. Normal MRI of the sellar region. (A) Precontrast T_1-weighted sagittal image. The white arrow, situated in the sphenoid sinus, points at the sellar surface and anterior pituitary lobe. The optic chiasm (gray arrow) and pituitary stalk (white arrowhead) are also depicted. The clivus extends caudally (gray arrowhead). (B) Pre- (left) and postcontrast (right) T_1-weighted sagittal images. The optic chiasm (white arrow), pituitary stalk (white arrowhead), pituitary gland (black arrow), and the flow voids of the cavernous carotid arteries (gray arrows) are illustrated. Note the marked enhancement of the normal pituitary gland following contrast administration.

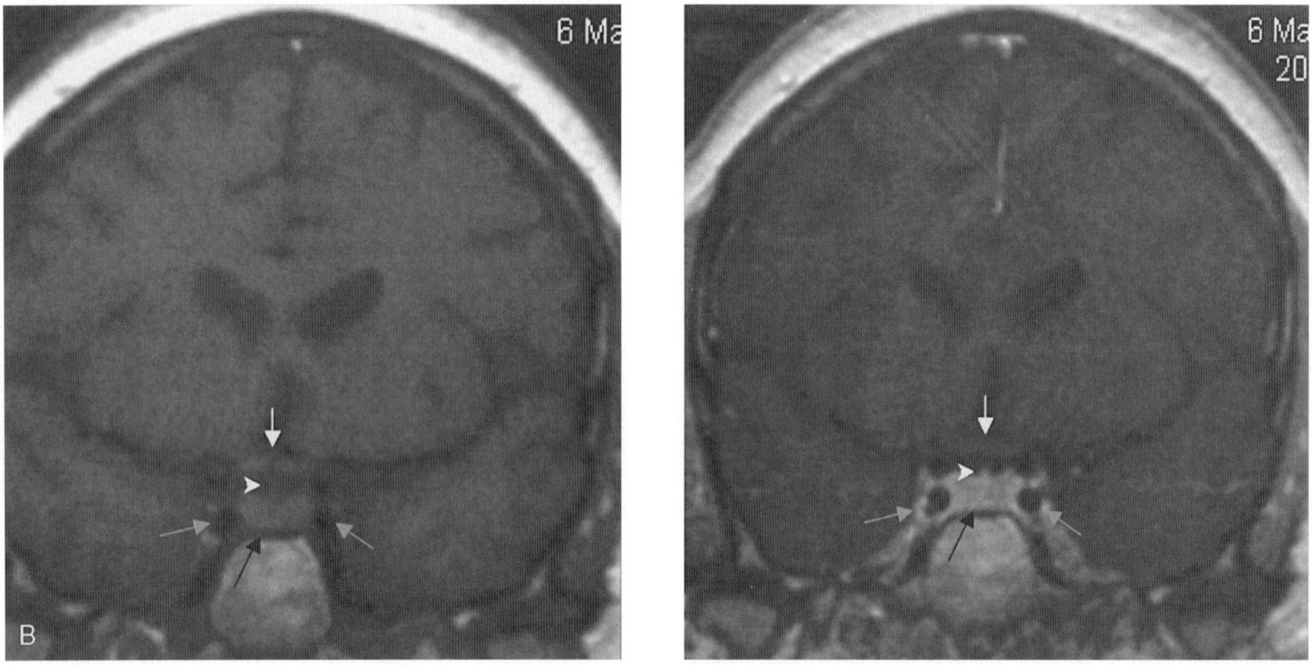

tumors based on (a) clinical presentation and biochemical secretory activity, (b) size and invasiveness (i.e., micro- vs. macroadenoma), (c) histologic features (adenoma vs. carcinoma), (d) immunohistochemical profile, and (e) ultrastructural features on electron microscopy.[27]

▶ PATHOGENESIS

Authors have generally argued that pituitary tumors result from either an abnormal response to hypothalamic stimulation or from intrinsic abnormalities within the pituitary gland itself. These theories are not mutually exclusive as extrinsic factors can provide a permissive environment for molecular events to occur within the gland. At the beginning of the previous decade, it was recognized that pituitary tumors are monoclonal in origin.[28,29] This phenomenon suggested that pituitary tumors result from genetic mutations in a single cell involving activation of oncogenes, inactivation of tumor suppressor genes, and alterations of transcription factors regulating cell growth and differentiation (Table 19-2). Although the precise mechanisms of tumorigenesis are yet to be fully elucidated, the previous decade has provided some clues as to the origin and progression of pituitary adenomas.

▶ **TABLE 19-1.** INCIDENCE AND CLINICAL PRESENTATION

Tumor Type	Incidence	Clinical Features
Nonfunctioning adenoma	25%–35%	Local mass effect causes hypopituitarism Extrasellar growth causes visual deficits, cavernous sinus syndrome, seizures, hydrocephalus
Prolactinoma	30%–45%	Female preponderance Women: amenorrhea and galactorrhea Men: impotence, decreased libido, mass effect
Growth hormone adenoma	15%–20%	Male preponderance Adults: acromegaly Children: gigantism 20%–30% have prolactin cosecretion
Corticotropin adenoma	10%–15%	Female preponderance Cushing disease
Thyrotrophin adenoma	1%	Hyperthyroidism in majority Mass effect

Oncogenes

Several oncogenes have been implicated in the development of pituitary adenomas. Located on chromosome 20, mutation of the α-subunit of the stimulatory guanine nucleotide-binding protein (gsp) gene produces an independently active adenyl cyclase signaling system that increases cyclic adenosine monophosphate (cAMP), leading to cell-cycle progression and GH hypersecretion.[30,31] Mutations of the gsp gene have been noted in approximately 40% of GH adenomas, 10% of NFAs, and 6% of ACTH adenomas.[32–39]

Cyclin D1 (CCND1), located on chromosome 11q13, is known to regulate progression through the cell cycle.

▶ **TABLE 19-2.** GENETIC CHANGES INVOLVED IN TUMORIGENESIS

Genetic Alteration	Features
Oncogenes	
gsp (stimulatory guanine nucleotide-binding protein)	Chromosome 20 40% growth hormone (GH) adenomas
CCND1 (cyclin D1)	Chromosome 11q13 Nonfunctioning adenomas (NFAs) Invasive adenomas
H-ras	Chromosome 5p13 Aggressive prolactinomas
c-myc	Chromosome 8q24 One-third of all adenomas
PTTG (pituitary tumor-transforming gene)	Prolactinomas, GH adenomas, corticotrophin (ACTH) adenomas, NFAs
Tumor suppressor genes	
MEN-1 (multiple endocrine neoplasia-1	Chromosome 11q13 25% of patients with inherited MEN-1 syndrome develop pituitary adenoma Some sporadic tumors
p53	Chromosome 17p13 Invasive NFAs ACTH adenomas
11q13 13q12-14 10q26	Case series; further confirmatory results pending

Reports indicate that CCND1 amplification may be more frequent in NFAs and invasive tumors.[40,41] The H-ras oncogene, located on chromosome 5p13, has been reported in pituitary carcinomas and aggressive prolactinomas.[42–44] The absence of this oncogene in clinically benign tumors indicates that the activation of this oncogene may be a late event, causing progression to a more aggressive type, and is evidence against it having a major role in initiating tumor formation.[34] The c-myc oncogene, located on chromosome 8q24, has been reported in nearly one-third of all pituitary adenomas, including prolactinomas, NFAs, and GH and ACTH adenomas.[45–47]

The pituitary tumor-transforming gene (*PTTG*) appears to induce basic fibroblast growth factor (bFGF) expression and secretion and may foster genetic instability.[48,49] Using sensitive assay methods, *PTTG* is expressed at very low levels in normal pituitary gland.[49] *PTTG* gene expression is increased in nearly all prolactinomas, GH and ACTH adenomas, and a majority of NFAs.[48,49] Relatively higher expression is also noted in functioning adenomas that have more aggressive growth characteristics.[50]

Tumor Suppressor Genes

Tumor suppressor gene inactivation has also been implicated in the development of pituitary adenomas. Among the earliest recognized tumor suppressor genes associated with pituitary adenomas is the multiple endocrine neoplasia-1 (MEN-1) gene located on chromosome 11q13.[51,52] Twenty-five percent of patients with the autosomal dominant inherited germ line mutation (MEN-1 syndrome) develop pituitary tumors. Although results are not fully accepted, MEN-1 mutations have been reported in sporadic tumors of all major subtypes, including ACTH and GH adenomas, prolactinomas, and NFAs.[29,31,32,52–54]

The mutated p53 gene, located on chromosome 17p13, has been reported in invasive NFAs and in the majority of both noninvasive and invasive ACTH adenomas.[55–57] Although discordant results have been demonstrated with regard to the retinoblastoma (Rb) gene, a yet uncharacterized deletion in a locus in propinquity to the Rb gene (on the long arm of chromosome 13) has been reported in invasive adenomas.[44,58,59] Several gene loci have been implicated in increased tumor invasiveness, including loss of heterozygosity (LOH) on chromosomes 11q13, 13q12–14, and 10q26.[58]

Other Transcription Factors

Transcription factors, which regulate cell proliferation and differentiation, have been implicated in determining the hormonal activity and proliferative potential of pituitary adenomas. In addition to PTTG and c-myc, several other transcription factors have been reported to be overexpressed in pituitary adenomas. These include Pit-1, estrogen receptor-α (ER-α), c-fos, and c-myc.[34] Overexpression of Pit-1, which is known to bind promoter regions for GH, PRL, and TSH, has been demonstrated in prolactinomas and GH and TSH adenomas, but is absent from ACTH and most NFAs.[60–64] ER-α, a nuclear receptor transcription factor, binds the PRL promoter and is overexpressed in prolactinomas.[65] It has also been detected in gonadotroph adenomas but rarely in GH adenomas.[65–67] c-fos binds the LH, FSH, ACTH, and TSH promoters and is overexpressed in GH, PRL, and NFAs.[47,68]

Autocrine/Paracrine Stimulation, Growth Factors, Cytokines

Although pituitary tumors arise from a clonal expansion of a single cell, this monoclonal expansion may occur within the context of a permissive hyperplastic milieu.[48] Abnormal response to target-organ feedback may play a role in creating this permissive milieu. It is recognized that prolactin cells become hyperplastic in response to estrogen stimulation during pregnancy and lactation. Loss of negative feedback is known to promote tumor growth in the setting of adrenalectomy (Nelson syndrome), thyroidectomy, and hypogonadism.[69] Exogenous estrogen is associated with the tumorigenesis of prolactinomas.[70] Part of this abnormal response may relate to hormone receptors. Higher estrogen receptor expression is also noted in macroprolactinomas than in microprolactinomas.[65,66] This estrogen responsivity may not be exclusive to prolactinomas. Indeed, increased estrogen receptor expression has been demonstrated in all tumor subtypes.[65]

In addition to abnormal feedback, the possible role of either abnormal pituitary responses to hypothalamic stimulation or abnormal feedforward signals from the hypothalamus has been investigated. GH adenomas do not appear to contain mature copies of somatostatin peptides.[71] Some GH adenomas express abnormal growth hormone-releasing hormone (GHRH) receptors, but these abnormal receptors are not constitutively active.[72] Similarly, abnormal gonadotropin-releasing hormone (GnRH) receptors have been reported in gonadotroph adenomas, but these also do not exhibit constitutive activity.[73] Abnormal corticotropin-releasing hormone (CRH) receptors have not been described in ACTH adenomas.[74] Taken together, convincing evidence for an abnormal pituitary response to hypothalamic stimulation remains elusive.

Among the possible growth factors involved in tumorigenesis is fibroblast growth factor (FGF)-4b, which is overexpressed in some prolactinomas.[75,76] The potent angiogenic growth factors bFGF and vascular endothelial growth factor (VEGF) are also implicated in providing a tumorigenic environment.[50] Because inhibitory signals reach the pituitary via its established vasculature, angiogenic factors that establish an independent blood supply may foster unrestricted growth and cell transformation.

In addition, investigators have shown overexpression of interleukin (IL)-6, IL-8, IL-11, and leukemia inhibitory factor (LIF) in some pituitary adenomas.[50,77,78]

▶ PATHOLOGY

Pituitary tumors are macroscopically yellow-gray to purple, and many have a soft consistency that is quite distinct from the firm normal pituitary parenchyma. The normal pituitary gland consists of a combination of different cell types arranged in a highly organized acinar pattern. In contradistinction, pituitary adenomas exhibit cellular monomorphism with disruption of the aforementioned highly organized acinar stromal pattern. The normal distribution of cell types within the anterior lobe of the pituitary gland was described earlier. Although somewhat variable, the location of small pituitary adenomas within the gland reflects the distribution of native cell types. For example, ACTH-secreting adenomas are generally found within the central mucoid wedge, whereas PRL- and GH-secreting adenomas may arise laterally within the anterior lobe. Of course, with continued growth these tumors extend beyond these typical confines. Additionally, because gonadotropin-positive cells are distributed throughout the anterior lobe and gonadotropin-secreting tumors are typically macroadenomas that disrupt local anatomy significantly, these tumors typically evade precise prediction of location.

Although adenomas were once histologically classified based on staining characteristics into acidophilic, basophilic, and chromophobic adenomas, this antiquated scheme (with limited specificity and applicability) has been supplanted by more sophisticated methods combining classical staining methods with immunohistochemistry for specific identification of secretory cell type(s) and ultrastructural analysis with electron microscopy to further delineate secretory granule size, type, and cellular synthetic activity.

To obtain an intraoperative diagnosis expeditiously, a smear preparation is often sufficient in identifying adenomatous tissue with high cell density (in contrast with less cellular tissue comprising normal gland in which the native acinar structure affords intercellular cohesiveness). Routine staining typically includes hematoxylin and eosin (H&E) along with periodic acid-Schiff (PAS) stain (because of positivity in ACTH-secreting and some glycoprotein-secreting adenomas). Immunohistochemistry routinely implements testing batteries surveying immunoreaction to LH, FSH, TSH, α-glycoprotein subunit, PRL, ACTH, and GH. Although this complement of tests is generally supportive of a given diagnosis, ultrastructural investigation with electron microscopy lends further credence. Electron microscopy can be used to characterize cell and nuclear morphology, secretory granule morphology and distribution, definition of endoplasmic reticulum and Golgi apparatuses, and microfilament aggregations. The following sections briefly review important pathologic features of selected types of pituitary adenomas.

Prolactin-Secreting Adenomas

Prolactin-secreting adenomas are commonly encountered. The diagnosis can occasionally be secured on the basis of H&E staining alone when characteristic psammomatous calcification is seen (approximately 10% of cases[79]). Calcification is rare across other tumor types. Deposition of amyloid may also be seen with prolactinomas and is rare in other tumor types.[80] Prolactinomas typically are sparsely granulated on routine staining, and may appear chromophobic or basophilic on H&E sections because of accumulation of rough endoplasmic reticulum (ER). Paranuclear immunoreactivity for PRL is also generally seen.[80] Ultrastructurally, abundant rough ER and "misplaced" exocytosis (direct exchange of granules between tumor cells rather than at their capillary interface)[80] may be seen.

Growth Hormone-Secreting Adenomas

Most GH-secreting adenomas are comprised of sheets of monomorphous cells and many GH-secreting adenomas also co-stain for other hormones (such as PRL or TSH).[81] With equal frequency, GH-secreting adenomas can either have densely or sparsely granulated (acidophilic or chromophobic, respectively) cell populations. In the densely granulated type, immunoreactivity for GH is strong and diffuse (Fig. 19-7). Additionally, this subtype most often coexpresses other hormones. On ultrastructural analysis, tumor cells contain large numbers of secretory granules and resemble normal GH-secreting cells.[81] In the sparsely granulated subtype, immunoreactivity for GH is often weak. Fibrous bodies (consisting predominantly of cytokeratin) may also be seen. Ultrastructurally, these fibrous bodies are comprised of whorled intermediate filaments found in a paranuclear distribution.[80] These sparsely granulated or chromophobic subtypes tend to be more aggressive.[80]

Adrenocorticotropic-Secreting Adenomas

Although there are three clinical subtypes of ACTH-producing adenomas (adenomas of Cushing disease, adenomas of Nelson syndrome [progression of ACTH-secreting tumors after adrenalectomy], and silent corticotroph cell adenomas [without elevation in ACTH or clinical evidence of Cushing disease]) only the most common adenoma of Cushing disease is discussed here. These tumors are classically basophilic and less than 10 mm in size (microadenomas). They are often PAS-positive and are immunoreactive to ACTH (and other derivatives of the precursor proopiomelanocortin such as melanocyte-stimulating hormone and β-endorphin)[80]

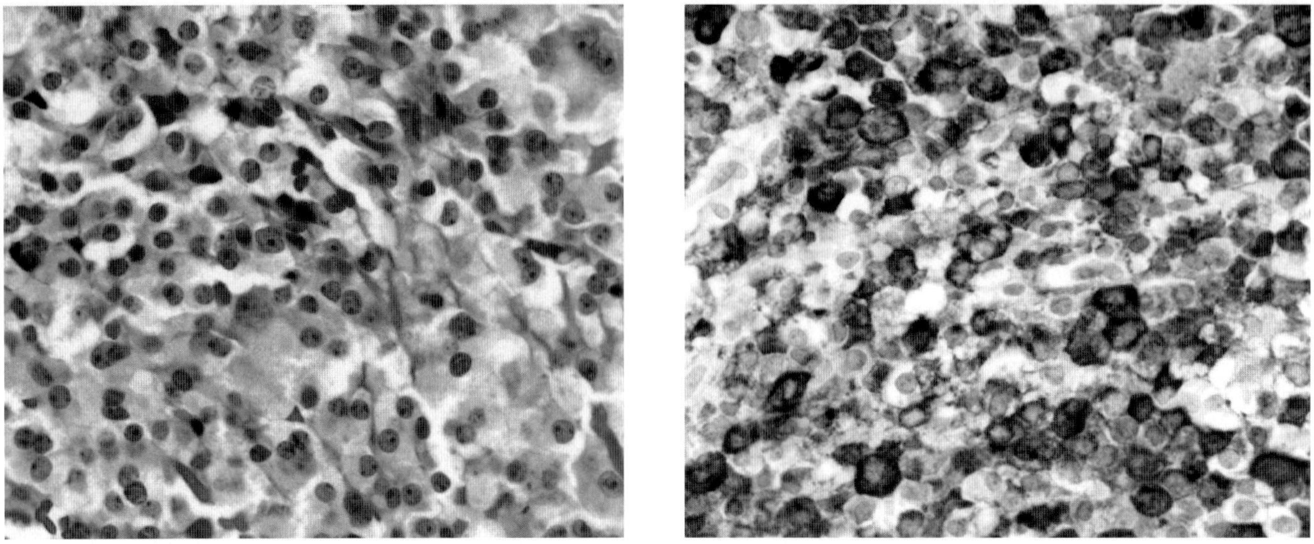

Figure 19-7 (PLATE 54). Growth hormone-secreting adenoma. H&E (left) preparation demonstrating a somatotroph cell adenoma that is strongly and diffusely immunoreactive for growth hormone (right).

(Fig. 19-8). Ultrastructurally, tumor cells appear densely granulated and have similar morphology to normal corticotrophs with teardrop-shaped secretory granules and perinuclear conglomerations of cytokeratin intermediate filaments.[81] Given the small size of some of these tumors (at times not delineated by neuroimaging), pathologic identification of tumor type within surgical specimens can be problematic. Another characteristic feature, often encountered in response to glucocorticoid excess in nonneoplastic tissue surrounding an adenoma, is Crooke hyaline change. Crooke hyaline change is characterized by robust accumulation of keratin microfilaments in nonneoplastic corticotrophs.[82] Rarely such changes may be found within neoplastic cells themselves (seen in so-called Crooke cell adenomas) and these tumors appear to have a more aggressive biology.[83]

Glycoprotein Adenomas

Glycoprotein-secreting adenomas include both gonadotropic (LH-FSH) and thyrotropic adenomas (TSH). This group of tumors is characterized by the production of

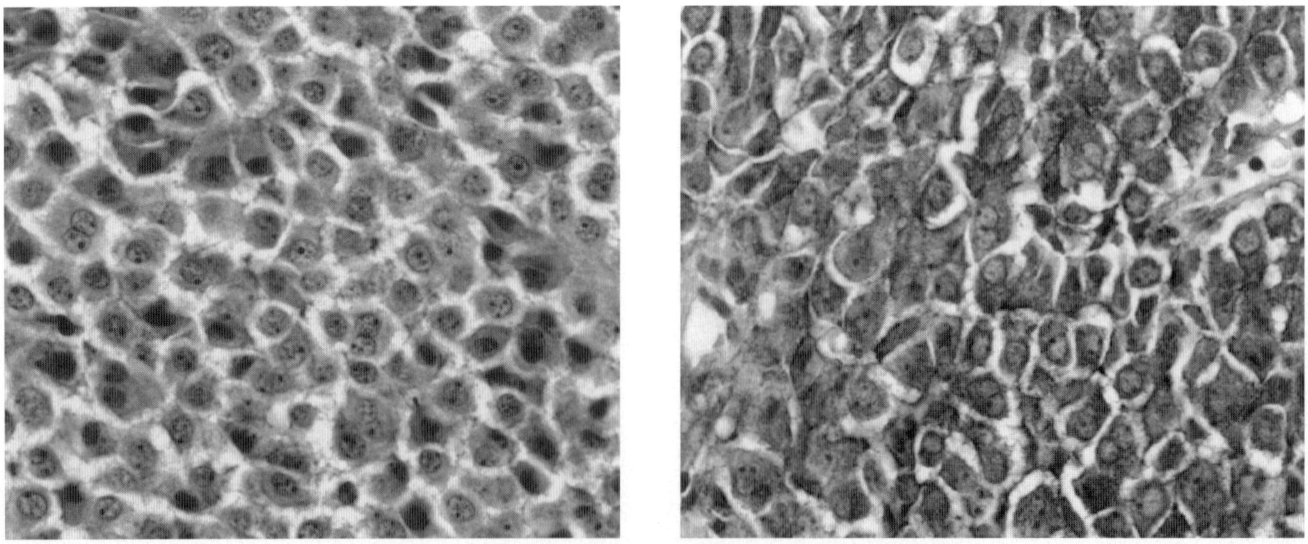

Figure 19-8 (PLATE 55). Adrenocorticotropic hormone-secreting adenoma. H&E (left) slide demonstrating a basophilic corticotroph that immunoreacts strongly for ACTH (right).

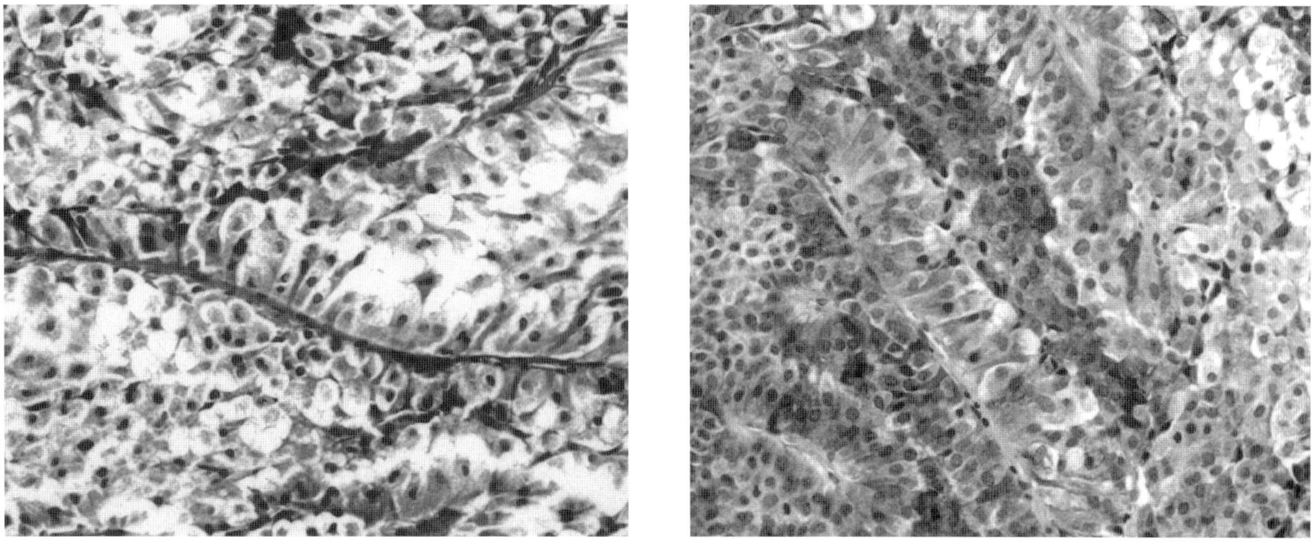

Figure 19-9 (PLATE 56). Gonadotrophic hormone-secreting adenoma. H&E (left) preparation demonstrating a sparsely granulated (chromophobic) gonadotroph cell adenoma that demonstrates patchy immunoreactivity with FSH (right).

hormones consisting of PAS-positive carbohydrate constituent in addition to two amino acid chains (an α-subunit common to all glycoprotein hormones and a β-subunit that differs among glycoprotein hormones, thereby conferring specificity).

Gonadotroph cell adenomas are typically sparsely granulated (and hence, chromophobic) and many demonstrate perivascular pseudorosette formation and/or oncocytic change (with abundance of intracellular mitochondria).[84,85] The pattern of granule distribution can be delineated by PAS positivity beneath the cell membrane. Furthermore, staining for LH, FSH and/or α-subunit can appear patchy and variable (Fig. 19-9). On ultrastructural analysis, gonadotroph adenomas are quite variable in terms of differentiation. Although the basis remains unclear, tumors from female patients often display a distinctive "honeycomb" appearance of the Golgi complex.[86]

Thyrotroph cell adenomas are rare lesions. These tumors are often comprised of elongated, weakly PAS-positive cells arranged in pseudorosette formation.[81] Immunoreactivity for TSH varies, and α-subunit staining is frequently encountered. Ultrastructurally, thyrotroph cell adenomas contain abundant synthetic organelles with few, small secretory granules.[80] Additionally, large lysosomes and cell processes containing microtubules can be observed.

Null Cell Adenomas

Null cell adenomas comprise approximately 15% to 25% of all pituitary tumors and the majority of nonfunctioning tumors.[80,87] They are typically immunonegative for pituitary hormones or may demonstrate very scant positivity for glycoprotein hormones or α-subunit.[88] Most null cell adenomas are chromophobic and similar to other sparsely granulated tumors. A few may be oncocytic.[80]

▶ IMAGING

Contemporary neuroimaging can accurately detect the presence of small lesions and can provide precise tumor localization and define relationships to adjacent structures (e.g., cavernous sinus, optic chiasm) in the case of larger tumors.

CT scanning with and without contrast enhancement can provide some important data concerning pituitary adenomas. Pituitary adenomas are typically isodense to brain parenchyma on unenhanced images and display marked contrast enhancement following contrast administration. Bone window images can accurately depict bony erosion and sellar expansion. In addition, acute hemorrhage and calcification, although rare, can be effectively illustrated. CT images can also be used with frameless intraoperative stereotaxy.[15]

Magnetic resonance imaging has become the imaging modality of choice because of its anatomic detail, lack of exposure to radiation, and sensitivity in detecting small adenomas. Microadenomas exhibit variable appearance on T_2-weighted images,[89] are typically hypointense to normal pituitary gland on T_1-weighted images, and usually exhibit less enhancement than normal gland with contrast administration (Fig. 19-10). With dynamic

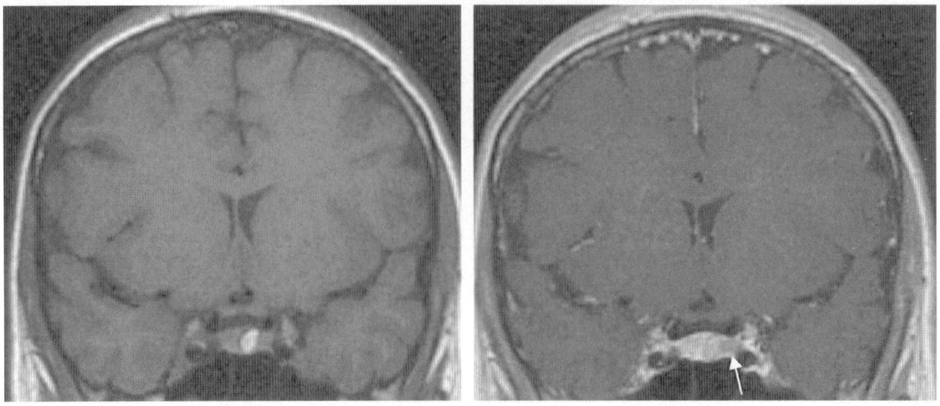

Figure 19-10. Microadenoma. Pre- (left) and postcontrast (right) coronal T_1-weighted MR images demonstrating an eccentrically placed microadenoma in the left wing of the gland. On the precontrast image, a hyperintense signal is apparent, which represents a small hemorrhage that was clinically silent (confirmed at surgery). The microadenoma exhibits delayed contrast enhancement relative to normal gland (arrow).

contrast-enhanced imaging studies, most pituitary adenomas exhibit early enhancement before the normal gland; however, this washes out while the pituitary gland shows intense enhancement, thereby ultimately leading to less enhancement in the pituitary tumor. Other imaging signs of pituitary tumors include deviation of the stalk and/or gland. Macroadenomas are typically well visualized as enhancing masses following contrast administration and may produce sellar expansion along with extension into adjoining spaces (cavernous sinus, suprasellar space, infrasellar space) (Fig. 19-11). Preoperatively, it is important to define the relationship of a macroadenoma with the visual apparatus and determine cavernous sinus invasion and potential carotid artery encasement. Hemorrhage can be detected as high signal intensity on T_1-weighted images even in the absence of clinical data suggesting apoplexy[90] (see Fig. 19-10).

Postoperative changes following transsphenoidal surgery are commonly encountered on imaging studies.[91–93] Packing of the operative site (sella and sphenoid sinus) with material such as fat is common. Fat is seen as hypodense material on CT scanning whereas it appears hyperintense on T_1-weighted MR imaging (nonfat suppressed). With time, this graft material is reabsorbed and there may be reexpansion of the normal gland and swelling of the optic chiasm.[94] Immediate or delayed (3 months or so following surgery) postoperative MRI can provide an accurate appraisal of tumor resection. Scans performed in an

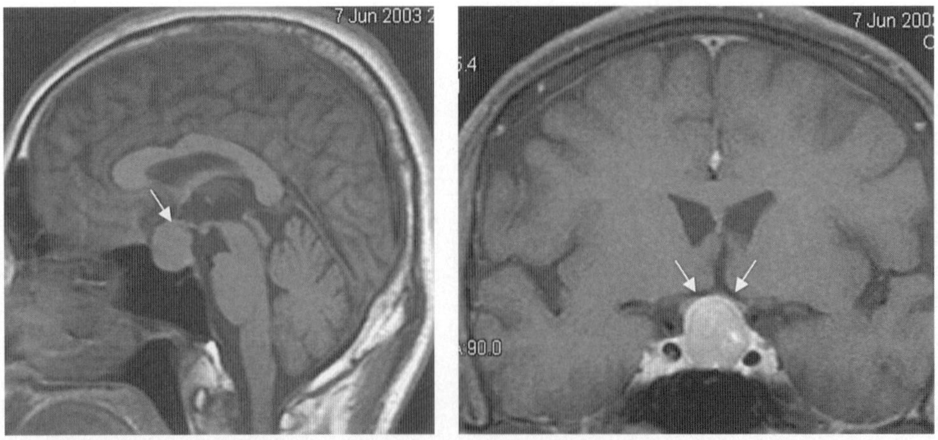

Figure 19-11. Macroadenoma. Precontrast sagittal (left) and postcontrast coronal (right) T_1-weighted MR images demonstrating a macroadenoma with superior extension compressing the optic chiasm (arrows).

intermediate time are difficult to interpret because of other postoperative changes during this period.

▶ CLINICAL DIAGNOSIS AND MANAGEMENT

Widespread availability of high-quality neuroimaging has resulted in the discovery of previously undetected asymptomatic tumors (*pituitary incidentalomas*). Incidentalomas are defined here as any tumor that is incidentally found in the absence of signs and symptoms related to the tumor (however, on careful evaluation, approximately 5% will have evidence of visual deficits and approximately 15% will have some degree of pituitary dysfunction[95]). The prevalence of such lesions in the general population has been well recognized from autopsy data[7,8] and is increasingly being corroborated with contemporary neuroimaging. For the most part, these lesions are nonfunctioning microadenomas (approximately two-thirds of cases at diagnosis); however, macroadenomas and hormone-secreting tumors can be found incidentally as well.[95] Considerable attention has been given to defining the natural history of incidentalomas.[95–101] Although the behavior of a given incidental tumor cannot be predicted with certainty, data have accrued to suggest that the natural history of many pituitary incidentalomas is benign.[95–101] Risks include enlargement with subsequent compression of the optic chiasm and/or invasion of the cavernous sinus, new onset of pituitary hormone deficiencies, and possibly apoplexy (particularly in patients on anticoagulation). Each patient presenting with an incidentally discovered tumor should be evaluated with endocrine screening and neuroophthalmologic examinations in addition to routine neurologic and general physical examination. In a prospective evaluation, macroadenomas and hormone-secreting tumors were not uncommon in an unselected series of patients with incidental lesions.[95] Practices regarding followup and treatment vary among institutions. At our institution, all data are presented to each patient and options, including risks, benefits, and alternatives, are discussed in detail. Our practice generally has been to observe patients with truly incidental, asymptomatic, and endocrinologically silent microadenomas. Patients with secreting tumors (e.g., prolactinomas) are managed as discussed for each type below. Patients with an otherwise normal evaluation (including vision and endocrine status) and an incidental macroadenoma may be carefully monitored with serial neuroimaging; however, when chiasmal compromise is observed radiologically, surgical resection may be recommended (although options are again discussed with each patient). Of note, more than one-third of incidental macroadenomas will show significant growth on serial imaging.[10,95,96,98,102] In our practice, most patients with large tumors in proximity to the optic apparatus generally opt for surgical management in lieu of the demonstrated safety and efficacy of transsphenoidal surgery in the contemporary neurosurgical era.

The ensuing discussion focuses on the diagnosis and management specific to each tumor subtype. Despite the individualized approach, certain protocols are universal. A careful neurologic and endocrinologic history is essential in all patients. The subsequent biochemical diagnosis should be followed by a careful screening of the pituitary axis to establish any preoperative endocrine insufficiency. Reasonable laboratory evaluation should include baseline PRL, GH, insulin-like growth factor type 1 (IGF-1), ACTH, cortisol, LH, FSH, TSH, thyroxine, testosterone, and estradiol. Of particular importance is the detection of cortisol and thyroid deficiency because failure to establish this preoperatively can have dire consequences. All patients will also need pretreatment high-resolution MRI using specific pituitary protocols. The gadolinium-enhanced sagittal and coronal planes are most helpful in surgical planning, but serial volumetric analysis also is essential in gauging the efficacy of therapy. Prior to medical or surgical therapy, patients should also have neuroophthalmologic testing including funduscopy, formal visual field testing (automated perimetry), and quantified visual acuity.

The goals of therapy are improved quality of life and survival, relief of mass effect and reversal of its associated signs and symptoms, normalization of hormonal hypersecretion, preservation or recovery of normal pituitary function, and prevention of recurrence. This effort requires a multidisciplinary team approach that includes endocrinologists, neurosurgeons, neuroophthalmologists, radiation therapists, and neuroradiologists.

Those patients undergoing surgery are administered perioperative hydrocortisone for the first 24 hours following surgery. Morning cortisol levels are measured on postoperative days 2 and 3. Patients with serum cortisol levels less than 8 μg/dL (225 nmol/L) are given steroid replacement. Those with preoperative cortisol deficiency are tapered postoperatively to their preoperative regimen. Patients with Cushing disease are not given perioperative steroid replacement and are monitored postoperatively for signs of adrenal insufficiency. Patients are also monitored closely for diabetes insipidus by monitoring daily weight, urine specific gravity every 4 hours, fluid intake and output, and serum sodium.

Nonfunctioning Adenomas

Clinical Presentation and Diagnosis

Clinically, NFAs account for approximately 25% to 35% of tumors resected surgically.[103,104] These lesions actually represent a diverse group of tumors, including gonadotroph adenomas and null-cell adenomas. Gonadotroph adenomas occur at approximately twice the frequency as the true nonsecreting adenomas.[105] Despite this diversity, the tumor subtypes appear to behave clinically in a uniform manner.[106,107] Patients generally present with signs and symptoms relating to local (sellar) and extrasellar mass effect. It bears repeating that the endocrinologic and neurological sequelae of tumor growth are not limited to patients with NFAs. Indeed, patients with any tumor subtype can experience the following sequelae.

Local intrasellar growth may cause varying degrees of pituitary dysfunction. The cell populations that appear most susceptible are the gonadotrophs (LH and FSH) and somatotrophs, followed by the thyrotrophs (TSH) and corticotrophs. Hypogonadism in men causes diminished libido and erectile dysfunction. Female hypogonadism causes amenorrhea and diminished libido. Growth hormone deficiency is characterized by decreased exercise tolerance, increased central adiposity, anxiety, and mood changes. Hypothyroidism can cause an array of symptoms including headache, weight gain, constipation, cold intolerance, depression, and diminished mental acuity. Relative adrenal insufficiency manifests with proximal weakness, fatigue, anorexia, myalgias, arthralgias, gastrointestinal symptoms, and orthostasis. Sudden pituitary insufficiency may occur in the setting of pituitary apoplexy. When acute, cortisol deficiency, or Addisonian crisis, may cause headache, visual disturbance, hyponatremia, mental status changes, and cardiovascular collapse.

As the tumor expands beyond the confines of the sella, neurologic signs begin to manifest. Headache, a common complaint, occurs as the expanding tumor stretches the sellar dura and diaphragma sellae. Suprasellar growth and resultant chiasmal compression commonly causes varying degrees of visual disturbance and bitemporal hemianopsia. Massive suprasellar growth may, less commonly, cause obstructive hydrocephalus. Lateral growth into the cavernous sinus may cause diplopia and facial pain or numbness. Further lateral growth into the mesial temporal lobe may also provoke seizures. An expanding tumor often compresses the pituitary stalk and disrupts the tonic hypothalamic inhibition of prolactin secretion. This "stalk effect" causes increased prolactin levels mimicking those seen in prolactinomas; however, elevation in prolactin levels secondary to stalk effect should be mild and absolute levels generally do not exceed 150 ng/mL.

Although two-thirds of the NFAs are glycoprotein adenomas, these tumors do not efficiently secrete α-subunit, FSH, or LH. Only about one-third of these have biochemical elevations in one of these markers.[107–109] For this reason, the preoperative diagnosis of NFA entails ruling out the secretory syndromes and confirming a pituitary mass on MRI.

Therapy

The primary treatment of NFAs is transsphenoidal surgery (Table 19-3). Visual field deficits improve in 70% to 87% of patients with preoperative deficits.[104,110,111] Normalization of vision is reported in approximately

▶ TABLE 19-3. DIAGNOSIS AND THERAPEUTIC RESULTS

Tumor Type	Diagnostic Features	Results of Primary Therapy
Nonfunctioning adenoma	PRL normal to moderate elevations	Transsphenoidal surgery 87% improve visual field deficit 27% improvement in preoperative endocrine deficits
Prolactin (PRL) secreting adenoma	PRL >200 ng/mL	Dopamine agonist 89% PRL normalized 90% visual improvement
Growth hormone (GH) adenoma	IGF-1 elevated Nadir GH >1 μg/L during oral glucose tolerance test	Transsphenoidal surgery Biochemical remission in 85% of microadenomas 50% of macroadenomas
Corticotropin (ACTH) adenoma	Elevated urinary free cortisol Failure to suppress with low-dose dexamethasone Suppression with high-dose dexamethasone Loss of diurnal variation	Transsphenoidal surgery Biochemical remission in 90% of microadenomas 60% of macroadenomas
Thyrotrophin (TSH) adenoma	Inappropriately elevated TSH for given thyroid hormone levels Elevated α-subunit (αSU) Molar ratio αSU/TSH >1	Transsphenoidal surgery 50% remission

25% of patients.[110] Improvement in pituitary deficiency is seen in up to 27% of patients and normalized endocrine function in nearly 15% of patients.[110–112] Normal pituitary function is preserved in approximately 70% of patients.[113] Nevertheless, 90% of premenopausal women with preoperative preserved menstruation retain normal menstruation postoperatively.[114] Regular menstruation is restored in 56% of those with preoperative amenorrhea.[114]

New endocrine deficits, seen more frequently in macroadenomas, have been reported in up to 40% of patients[110,111,113]; however, recent results indicate that only 3% of patients with microadenomas and 5% of patients with macroadenomas with preoperative normal pituitary function experience new hormonal deficits.[115] Immediate postoperative polyuria occurs in approximately 30% of patients, but in only 3% to 10% of patients does this polyuria persist beyond the first week of surgery.[115,116] Delayed hyponatremia, occurring most often 7 to 10 days after surgery, is evident in 1% to 2.4% of patients.[115,116] Worsening in preoperative vision can be seen in 1% to 4%.[112,117] Anatomic complications include nasal septal perforations in 7% and fat graft hematomas in 4% of patients.[113,117] Postoperative cerebrospinal fluid leaks and meningitis are reported in 0.5% to 3.9% of patients.[117,118]

Recurrence does develop over time and in our series, 16% of patients experience recurrent disease at 10 years.[104] However, recurrence requiring repeat surgery occurs in only 6% of patients. Completeness of resection as judged on postoperative MRI can predict recurrence. Although one-third of patients with residual tumor have recurrent tumor growth, fewer than 3% with complete resection experience recurrent disease (mean followup of 3.3 years).[119]

For tumors with incomplete resection, medical and radiation therapy can be considered; however, neither medical therapy nor radiation therapy is recommended as primary treatment. Although dopamine agonists, GnRH agonists, and octreotide therapy have been employed, their efficacy has not been proved. Postoperative adjuvant radiation therapy has been advocated for incompletely removed tumors and tumors with cavernous sinus invasion.[87,120] Our practice is to delay radiation therapy until there is evidence of progressive regrowth of the tumor. In many such cases, repeat transsphenoidal surgery for debulking is recommended prior to radiation therapy for cytoreduction and to ensure a margin of safety in targeting the tumor during radiation therapy (the tumor should be at least 3 mm away from the optic chiasm before administering radiation therapy). Radiation treatment to tumors involving the sellar region and its surroundings must consider the critical neighboring neural and vascular structures. Potential late complications of radiation therapy include optic neuropathy and other cranial nerve palsies, new endocrinologic deficits, hypothalamic injury and radiation necrosis, stroke, and development of secondary tumors. The risk of visual loss varies in reported series but adherence to strict criteria should minimize the risk to well below 1%.[121–129] The incidence of new hormone deficiencies varies (10% to more than 90%[121–129]), according to technique of radiation administration, as well as according to vigilance and length of followup in screening for deficits.

Prolactinomas

Clinical Presentation and Diagnosis

Although prolactinomas account for approximately 30% of the tumors treated in large surgical series, they actually comprise approximately 45% of all adenomas treated clinically.[3,104] These tumors have a female predominance with a ratio of about 4:1.[130,131] Women present in their second and third decades of life and nearly half present with microadenomas.[3,131] By contrast, men present most often in their fifth decade of life with macroadenomas.

Women present with amenorrhea and galactorrhea. Although men may experience galactorrhea, they more often come to clinical attention secondary to mass effect and often report headache, visual disturbance, diminished libido, and decreased energy. The biochemical diagnosis of prolactinoma is typically straightforward. Some pitfalls in the diagnosis must be avoided. Certain drugs (dopamine antagonists, estrogens), renal and liver failure, hypothyroidism, and "stalk effect" can produce moderate elevations in basal PRL levels. Nevertheless, serum PRL levels greater than 200 ng/mL are consistent with the diagnosis of a PRL-secreting adenoma. Another pitfall is the serum PRL "hook effect" that may misdiagnose a macroprolactinoma as a NFA.[132] The radioimmunoassay for PRL can provide falsely low values in the absence of serial dilutions. In fact, this may apply in any situation in which extremely high prolactin levels are encountered (micro- and macroadenomas, although most common with macroadenomas). Patients with macroadenomas and moderate elevations in PRL levels (or in any situation in which extremely high prolactin levels are suspected but not initially confirmed biochemically) should have repeated serum PRL testing with serial dilutions.

Therapy

Although some continue to advocate surgical treatment for microprolactinomas, our bias is to use medical therapy as the first-line therapy for all prolactinomas (see Table 19-3). Dopamine agonists, including bromocriptine, pergolide, and cabergoline, effectively normalize prolactin levels in as many as 89% of patients.[133–136] These medications are not only effective biochemically; tumor volume decreases by at least 50% in more than two-thirds of patients within the first few months of therapy, and, more importantly, visual field deficits improve in all but 10% of patients.[134] For women who wish to become pregnant, bromocriptine has been used in several thousand women who became pregnant while taking the medication.[137] There appeared to be no increased risk of birth defects in more than 2000 babies born to women taking bromocriptine.[138] More limited experience exists with cabergoline in women taking this medication during pregnancy, but the body of data at present suggests no increased risk above baseline in terms of birth defects in babies exposed to this medication during gestation.[139]

Although medical therapy can be highly effective, some patients are intolerant of the medications and some tumors are resistant to pharmacotherapy. Tumor resistance is characterized by either failure to normalize PRL levels or inadequate tumor volume reduction. In these situations, we advocate transsphenoidal surgery.

Transsphenoidal surgery is most successful in obtaining remission in the setting of microprolactinomas. In this population, prolactin levels can be normalized in 50% to 90% of patients, with experienced centers reporting results of approximately 85%.[102,104,105,140–142] Not unexpectedly, results with macroprolactinomas are less successful. Surgical remission may be expected in 28% to 56% of patients, with most experienced centers reporting remission in approximately 50% of patients.[104,140–143]

In the face of medical and surgical failure, radiation therapy is a reasonable adjunct. Conventional fractionated radiation therapy is reported to provide an additional 50% of patients normalized prolactin levels within a mean of 8.5 years.[144] We recently reported that gamma knife radiosurgery can achieve remission in 11% of patients within a mean of 1.7 years.[145] We expect that with continued followup the percentage of patients achieving remission will increase and then more meaningful conclusions can be made regarding the efficacy of stereotactic radiosurgery versus conventional radiation therapy. Regardless of what type of radiation therapy has been used, patients must have continued, long-term endocrinologic followup to monitor for late endocrinopathy. Hypopituitarism after radiation therapy is progressive. After conventional radiation therapy, at least partial hypopituitarism is evident in between 50% and 90% of patients by 10 years.[122,123,129,146]

If hyperprolactinemia persists in patients who desire fertility, medical therapy to facilitate ovulation or spermatogenesis may be implemented.[137] Clomiphene can be used to induce ovulation in women with mild, persistent hyperprolactinemia, whereas gonadotropin therapy (LH and FSH) can be used if the former is unsuccessful. Gonadotropin administration can be used in males to induce spermatogenesis; however, protracted therapy for more than 1 year may be necessary.[137]

Growth Hormone-Secreting Adenomas

Clinical Presentation and Diagnosis

GH adenomas account for 15% to 20% of all pituitary tumors.[104,147–149] Approximately 40 to 60 individuals per 1 million population have acromegaly.[150–153] Patients present in their third to fifth decades of life, often after many years of progressive and insidious symptoms.[152] Men present with twice the frequency of women, and most patients present with macroadenomas.[154,155] The densely granulated adenoma is more common in women, is frequently associated with plurihormonal adenomas, and is more frequently aggressive.[103] Approximately 20% to 30% of patients with acromegaly also have prolactin hypersecretion.[156]

GH adenomas present with the characteristic syndromes of acromegaly in adults and gigantism in children. Acromegalic patients experience cosmetic changes including frontal bossing, prognathism, macroglossia, and increased hand and foot size. This external hypertrophy is mirrored internally and patients have hypertension, congestive heart failure, colonic polyps, sleep apnea, lumbar stenosis, and carpal tunnel syndrome. Patients also have impaired glucose metabolism and can develop frank diabetes mellitus. Acromegalic patients also appear to have a higher incidence of cancers, although some reports have confirmed only an increased risk of colon cancer.[157–159] As a result of these complications, acromegalic patients have an increased risk of mortality compared with normal age-matched controls.[151,160]

The diagnosis of acromegaly is often apparent on physical examination. However, biochemical confirmation is imperative and easily obtained. Because GH secretion is pulsatile, random serum GH levels are of limited diagnostic value. Nevertheless, serum IGF-1 and GH levels following a standard glucose load (oral glucose tolerance test [OGTT]) may be used to diagnose acromegaly and to monitor for remission and recurrence.[161] Serum growth hormone levels are drawn in the fasting patient at –30, 0, 30, 60, 90, and 120 minutes around the time of an oral glucose load of 75 to 100 g. Failure to suppress GH levels to less than 1 μg/L (<2 mU/L) confirms the diagnosis.

Therapy

Although medical therapy is increasingly improving, transsphenoidal surgery remains the first-line therapy for GH adenomas (see Table 19-3). Surgery can achieve biochemical remission (normal IGF-1 levels, nadir GH <1 μg/L during OGTT) in approximately 85% of patients with microadenomas and in 50% of those with macroadenomas.[104,162–168] Once in remission, approximately 8% of patients have GH adenoma recurrence at 10 years.[169] Of these patients, 48% can achieve remission with repeated transsphenoidal surgery.[165,170,171]

In addition to relieving the symptoms of acromegaly, remission following surgery reduces the long-term mortality rates in patients with acromegaly.[168] Patients with persistent disease have a 3.5-fold relative increased risk of mortality compared with those in remission. Successful surgery also improves cardiac function and reduces hypertension.[172,173]

Somatostatin is a native factor that inhibits GH secretion. Somatostatin analogues (such as octreotide) may be more suppressive of GH than native somatostatin and more suppressive of GH secretion than insulin.[174] Debate lingers as to the possible beneficial effects of preoperative octreotide therapy. Although some investigators report reduced morbidity and improved biochemical results, definitive answers are lacking.[175–178] Preoperative GH levels greater than 50 μg/L predict failure of remission.[164,165,179] Early postoperative GH levels less than 2 μg/L are predictive of remission.[180] Patients with known cavernous sinus invasion and large incompletely removed tumors require adjuvant therapy.

Impressive advances have occurred with regard to the medical therapy of GH adenomas. Until recently, the two options for medical therapy were dopamine agonists and somatostatin analogues. Dopamine agonists provide symptomatic relief in the majority of patients, but normalize IGF-1 levels in only approximately 20% to 40% of patients.[181–185] Somatostatin analogues (octreotide [Sandostatin LAR], lanreotide, lanreotide-SR) can normalize IGF-1 levels in up to 60% of patients and have a more favorable side-effect profile than do dopamine agonists.[186–193] However, pegvisomant, the recently introduced GH receptor antagonist, has normalized IGF-1 levels in 90% to 100% of patients with refractory disease, although reported experience with administration for more than 2 years is limited.[194–197]

Radiation therapy can provide hormonal remission and is a reasonable choice for patients with refractory disease. Conventional fractionated radiation therapy can achieve remission in approximately 25% of patients by 5 years, and in approximately 60% of patients by 10 years.[122,198,199] Gamma knife radiosurgery can achieve remission in a shorter interval in 36% of patients.[145,200,201]

Corticotropin-Secreting Adenomas

Clinical Presentation and Diagnosis

ACTH adenomas account for 10% to 15% of pituitary adenomas and most are microadenomas.[103,104] Cushing disease occurs between five and eight times more frequently in women than in men and most women present in their third or fourth decades of life.[103,131,202–204] The prevalence is approximately 39 per 1 million population with an annual incidence of 0.24 per 100,000 population.[3] Cushing syndrome refers to a syndrome resulting from cortisol excess from any cause, whereas Cushing disease is used to describe a hypercortisolemic state resulting from an ACTH-secreting pituitary tumor.

Patients present with characteristic changes in body habitus. These changes include hirsutism, truncal obesity, purple striae, moon facies with plethora, easy bruisability, and fat deposition in the supraclavicular and postcervical region (buffalo hump). Patients report headache, fatigue, menstrual irregularities, proximal muscle weakness, labile affect, and depression. Excess cortisol is also associated with osteoporosis and hypokalemia. Patients with Cushing disease have a high incidence of hypertension and diabetes mellitus, which leads to cardiovascular disease and premature mortality.[204,205]

The initial workup in a patient suspected as having cortisol excess is the objective demonstration and establishment of the diagnosis of Cushing syndrome. The next step is to localize the source of cortisol excess (i.e., a pituitary adenoma in the context of Cushing disease). The diagnosis of Cushing disease can be problematic not only because these tumors are often not evident on MRI, but because pseudo-Cushing states can be difficult to distinguish definitively from true Cushing disease. Pseudo-Cushing syndrome results in a hypercortisolemic state and may also include physical features indistinguishable from those of Cushing disease. It results from an underlying disease process (such as alcohol use, depression, other psychiatric disorders, or other underlying illnesses) although the precise mechanism remains unclear. It appears to be centrally mediated and may involve excessive hypothalamic secretion of CRH.[206–208] However, this condition resolves with treatment of the underlying disease. Hence, the initial examination of a patient suspected of having Cushing disease should screen for disorders that may lead to pseudo-Cushing syndrome. Nonetheless, hypercortisolemia can be screened using a 24-hour urinary free cortisol (UFC) test or a low-dose dexamethasone suppression test (LDDST). UFC values greater than 220 to 330 nmol/24 h (80–120 μg/24 h) are sensitive, but relatively nonspecific, for the diagnosis of Cushing syndrome.[209,210] Failure to suppress morning (8 AM) serum cortisol levels to 100 to 200 nmol/L (3.6–7.2 μg/dL) the morning following a midnight dose of 0.5 to 2.0 mg of dexamethasone is also indicative of Cushing syndrome.[211,212] Suppression to less than 50 nmol/L or 1.8 μg/dL is highly specific for the exclusion of Cushing syndrome. When doubt remains as to the possibility of pseudo-Cushing syndrome, a combined CRH-LDDST may be used.[213] As described, patients are administered 0.5 mg of dexamethasone every 6 hours for 24 hours followed by a 1 μg/kg IV dose of CRH. In patients with Cushing syndrome, CRH should overcome the suppressive effects of dexamethasone and serum cortisol level at 15 minutes should be greater than 1.4 μg/dL.

Once the presence of Cushing syndrome is established, the source of cortisol excess must be determined. Although low ACTH levels (<5 pg/mL) exclude Cushing disease, higher levels require further testing to distinguish a pituitary from an ectopic source of ACTH secretion.[214] No single test provides an absolute distinction, but the combined results of several tests generally provide a preponderance of evidence.[215] These tests include the high-dose dexamethasone suppression test (HDDST), metyrapone (750 mg every 4 hours for 6 doses), CRH (1 μg/kg intravenously), and inferior petrosal sinus sampling (IPSS).

The HDDST compares steroid levels (either serum cortisol, 24-hour urinary 17-hydroxycorticosteriods [OHCSs], or 24-hour UFC) prior to and the morning after either 2 mg of dexamethasone every 6 hours for 48 hours or a single evening (11 PM) 8-mg dexamethasone dose. Patients with pituitary-dependent ACTH secretion should suppress serum cortisol levels greater than 50%, UFC levels greater than 90%, and 17-OHCS levels greater than 64% to 69%.[216,217]

In patients with Cushing disease, metyrapone, a potent inhibitor of cortisol synthesis, should raise baseline levels of serum 11-deoxycortisol (>400%) and also raise urinary 17-OHCS (>70%) and 11-deoxycortisol levels.[218,219] In CRH testing, serum ACTH and cortisol levels are drawn prior to and after (−15, 0, 15, 30, 60, 90, and 120 minutes) an intravenous dose of CRH. In patients with Cushing disease, cortisol, and ACTH levels should rise quantitatively more than those with ectopic ACTH syndromes (peak ACTH ≥50%; ACTH ≥35% at 15 or 30 minutes; peak cortisol ≥20%).[220,221]

IPSS is an invasive test that can be used not only to confirm the pituitary source of ACTH secretion but also to localize the tumor in preparation for planned adenomectomy. Bilateral inferior petrosal sinus measurements allow comparison between central and peripheral serum ACTH levels. This test is augmented using CRH.[222–226] Central to peripheral ratios greater than 2:1 are considered diagnostic of Cushing disease. CRH stimulation (100 μg IV) is reported to increase test sensitivity, and ratios greater than 3:1 are considered significant.[227–229] Furthermore, intersinus ratios greater than 1.4 correlate reasonably well (60%–70% accuracy) with lateralization of the adenoma.[222,230–232]

Therapy

The primary mode of therapy for Cushing disease is transsphenoidal surgery (see Table 19-3). Our tendency has been to withhold postoperative steroid replacement and to measure serum cortisol levels every 6 hours. When symptoms of adrenal insufficiency are noted or when the serum cortisol falls below 3μg/dL (85 nmol/L), we initiate steroid replacement.

Biochemical remission (normal 24-hour UFC) is obtained in 90% of patients with microadenomas and up to 60% of patients with macroadenomas.[104,230,233] Recurrence after biochemical remission occurs in just over 10% of patients.[104,234,235] Remission may be predicted if postoperative cortisol levels taken at 12 PM on the first postoperative day are less than the preoperative midnight cortisol.[236] In the typical Cushing ACTH microadenoma, neither negative preoperative MRI nor failure to obtain histologic confirmation of an adenoma has significant negative predictive value on outcome.[230,237]

Patients who fail selective adenomectomy are often offered early reoperation with the goal of total hypophysectomy. For patients with continued refractory disease, therapeutic choices include radiation therapy and/or adrenalectomy. Medical therapy in the form of ketoconazole, mitotane, aminoglutethimide, and metyrapone can reduce UFC levels but normalization is seen in less than half of those treated.[238–241] Medical therapy is not considered a definitive alternative to either radiation therapy or adrenalectomy.

Although mixed results have been reported, conventional fractionated radiation therapy has been reported to obtain remission in approximately 80% of patients after long-term followup.[129,233,242,243] Gamma knife radiosurgery is also effective and appears to achieve results more rapidly.[145,200,244–246] Our experience suggests that nearly 75% of patients achieve remission and do so within a mean of 16 months.[145]

Thyroid-Stimulating Hormone-Secreting Adenomas

Clinical Presentation and Diagnosis

Thyrotrophic adenomas account for approximately 1% of pituitary adenomas and most present as macroadenomas.[104,247,248] There does not appear to be a significant male or female predominance. Although the majority of patients with TSH adenomas present with severe clinical signs of hyperthyroidism, patients can present with either mild hyperthyroid symptoms or even hypopituitarism.[248] Patients may present with hypervigilance, palpitations, weight loss despite preserved appetite, heat intolerance, and excessive sweating.

TSH levels, although frequently normal, are inappropriately elevated for the given serum thyroid levels.[249] The serum α-subunit levels are increased and the molar ratio of α-subunit and TSH should be greater than 1.[248] Further confirmatory data can be obtained using thyroid-releasing hormone (TRH) stimulation which generally fails to increase TSH levels. The primary diagnostic dilemma is to distinguish TSH adenomas from patients whose pituitary gland is thyroid resistant but whose peripheral tissues are not.[105] Unlike the typical patient with a TSH adenoma who is clinically hyperthyroid,

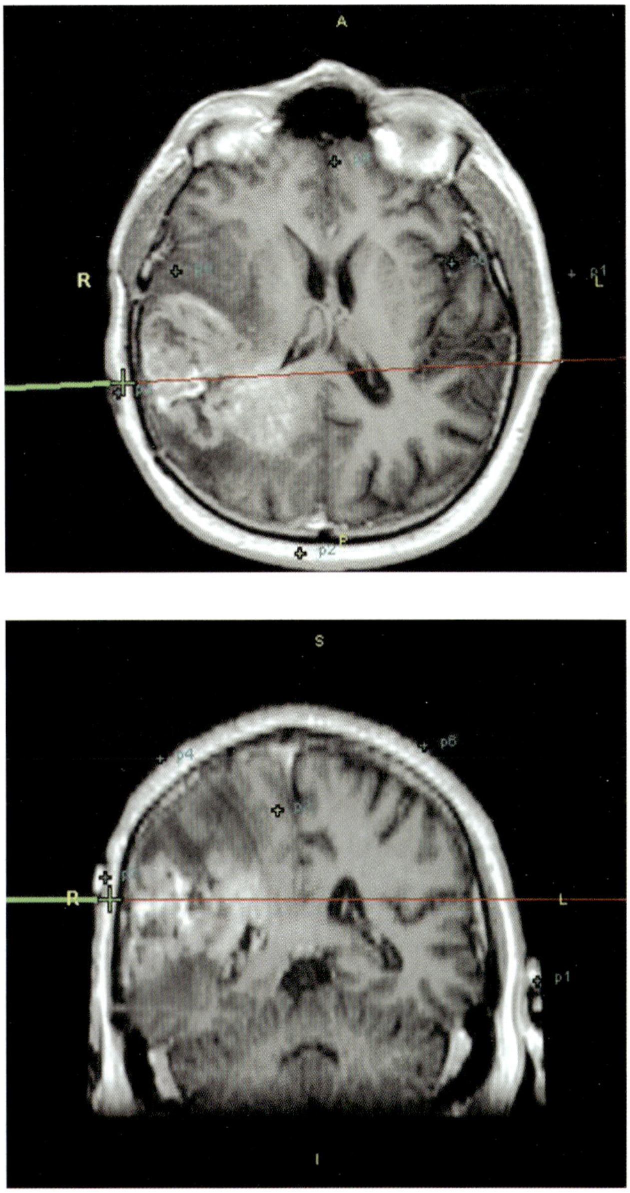

PLATE 35 (Figure 6-4). In-house (i.e., not commercially available) surgical navigation system (frameless stereotaxy) used to localize a recurrent tumor prior to the scalp incision. This was done to see if the previous scalp and/or bone flap would require revision to access the tumor. The navigation system was also used during the tumor resection. The end of the pointer tool in the surgeon's hand is demonstrated on the screen as the tip of the line.

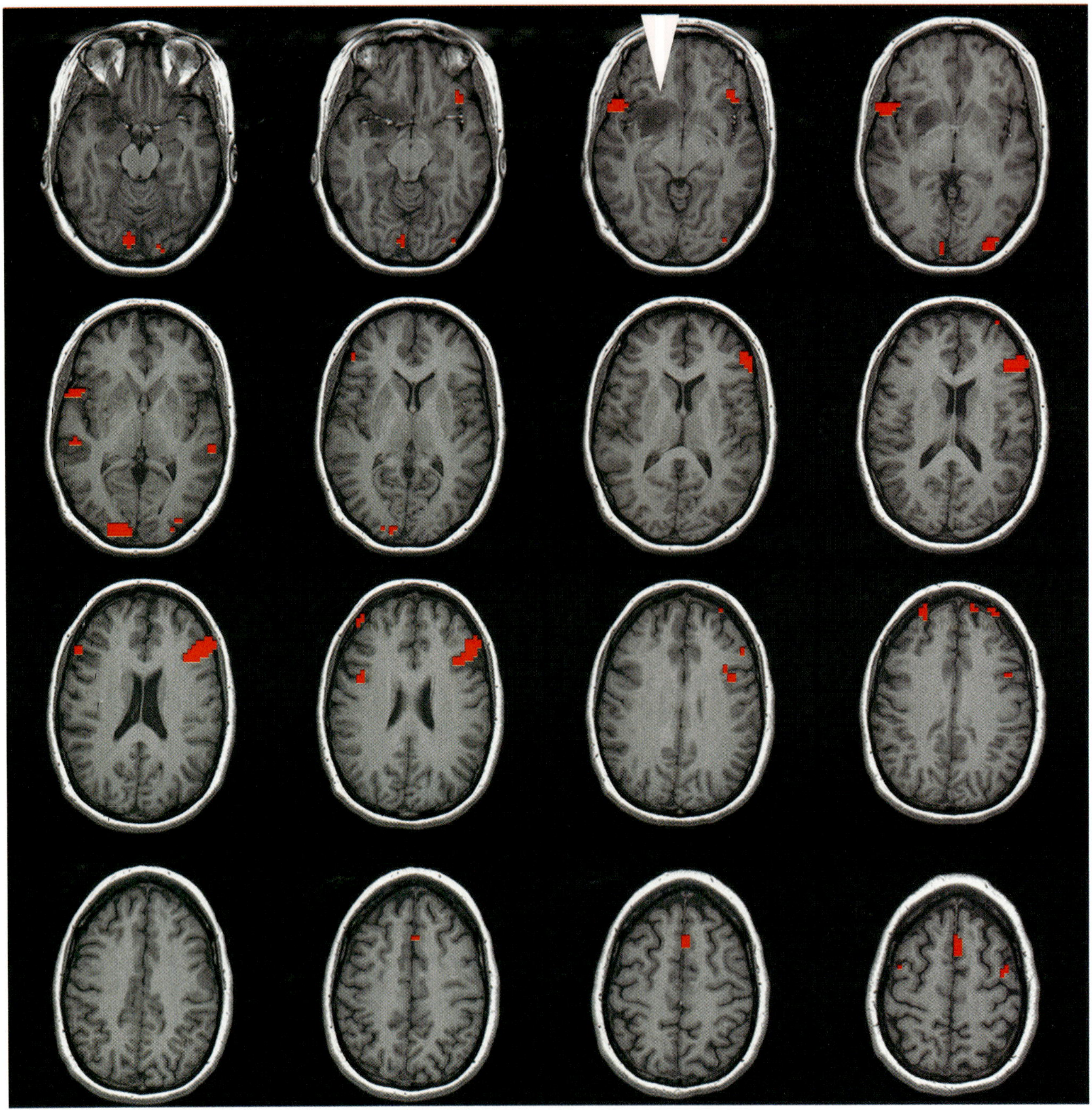

PLATE 36 (Figure 6-6). A 51-year-old left-handed lady presented with seizures and a right-sided perisylvian low-grade glioma (see arrowhead). Functional MRI in this left-handed patient revealed that her speech center was located in her left frontal lobe, thereby increasing the surgeon's confidence that this lesion could be safely resected without causing aphasia.

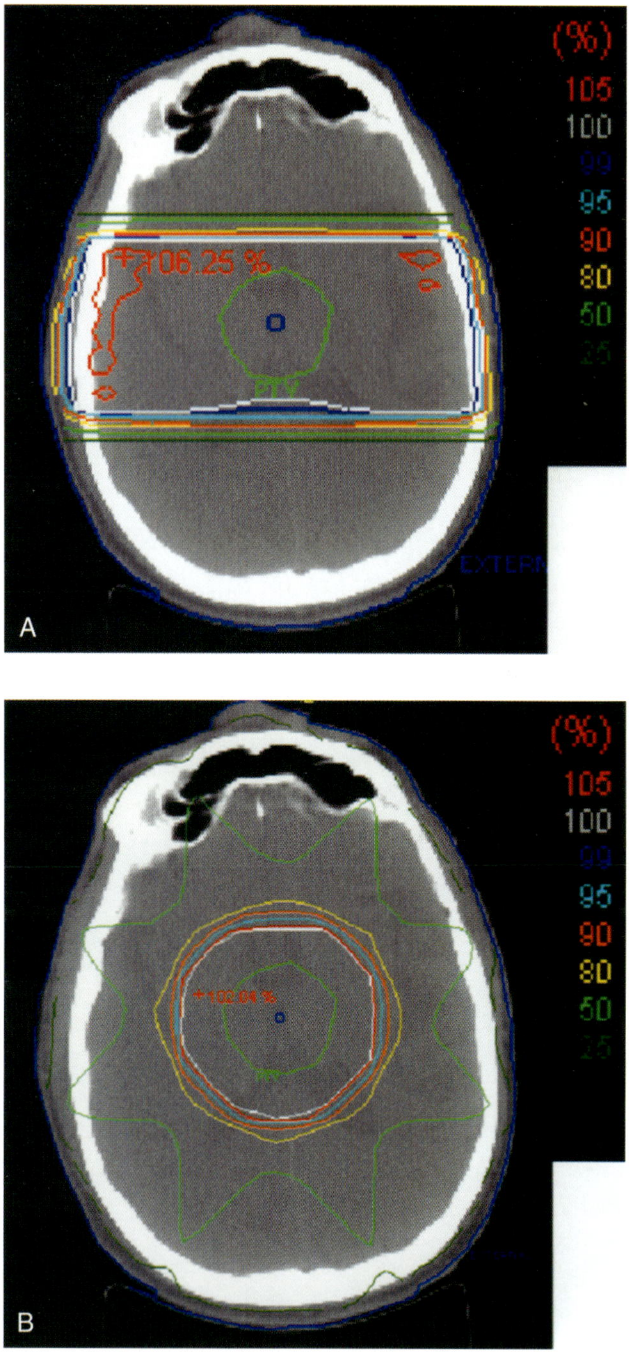

PLATES 37 and 38 (Figure 7-2). These two radiation plans illustrate one of the basic principles of three-dimensional conformal radiotherapy. For plan (A), a pair of equally weighted parallel opposed fields treat a centrally positioned lesion. In plan (B), four pairs of opposed fields treat the lesion. Both radiation plans encompass the target lesion with the 100% isodose curve. For plan (B) there is an approximately fourfold reduction in dose per field while maintaining the full dose at the intersection of all fields. This results in a significant reduction in the amount of brain receiving the full dose of radiation while increasing the amount of brain receiving lower doses of radiation.

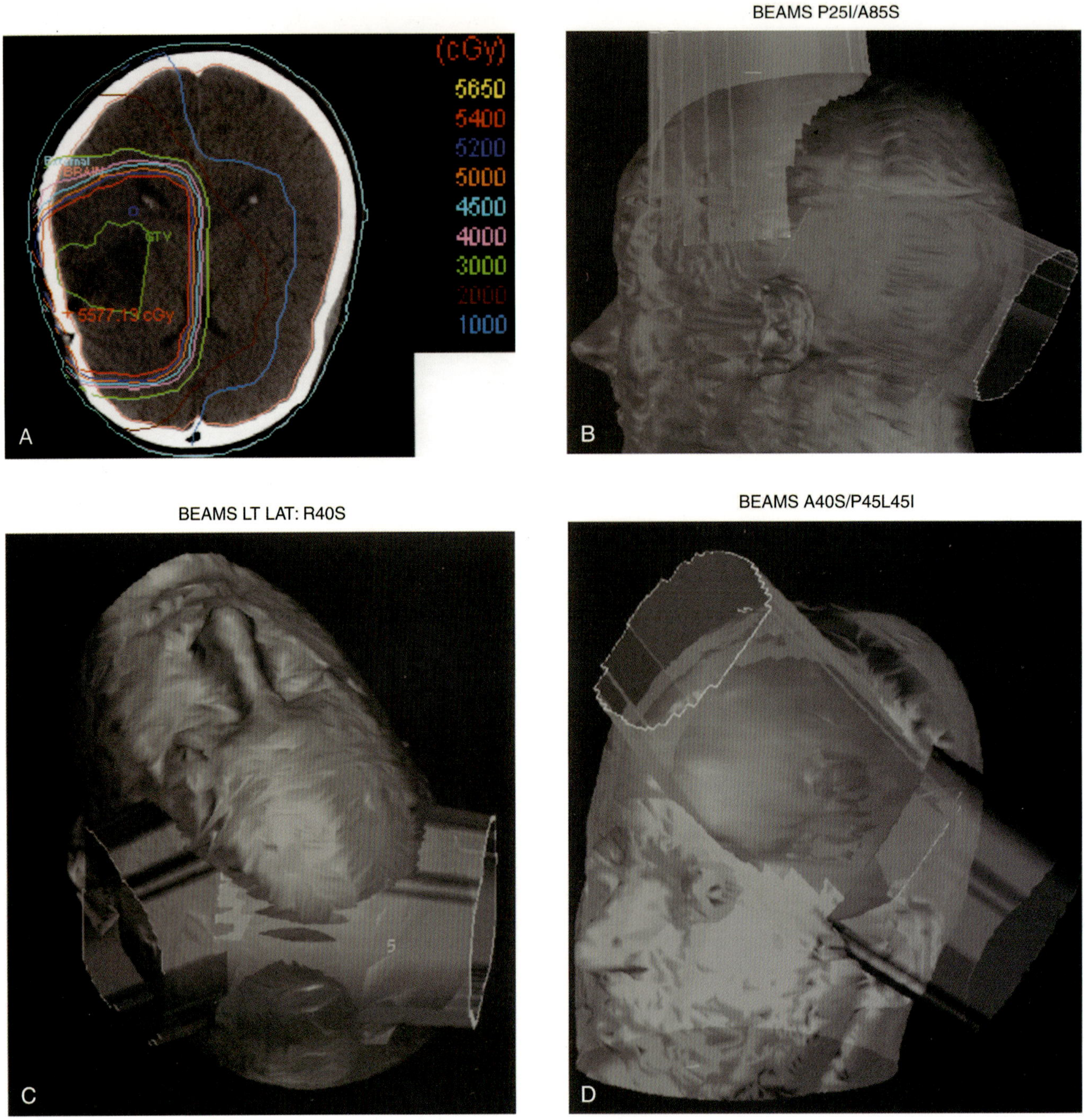

PLATES 39 (Figure 7-6). (A) Axial isodose distribution through the geometric center of a recurrent oligodendroglioma. The patient was placed in the prone position to obviate mechanical constraints of the linear accelerator, allowing a wider selection of beam angles. A thermoplastic mask was fabricated to immobilize the patient's head. Axial T2-weighted MRI images were fused with a planning CT scan to define the gross tumor volume (GTV). Two-centimeter margins were added to the tumor volume to account for patient setup variability and subclinical tumor infiltration. The margin was decreased medially because the tumor did not involve the corpus callosum and therefore contralateral hemispheric involvement was not a concern. This step was taken to decrease the dose to the contralateral hemisphere. The three-dimensional treatment plan called for six beams (B, posterior 25 degrees inferior and anterior 85 degrees superior; C, left lateral and right 40 degrees superior; D, anterior 40 degrees superior and posterior 45 degrees left 45 degrees inferior) employing various wedging (to improve dose homogeneity) to deliver a total dose of 5400 cGy in 30 fractions.

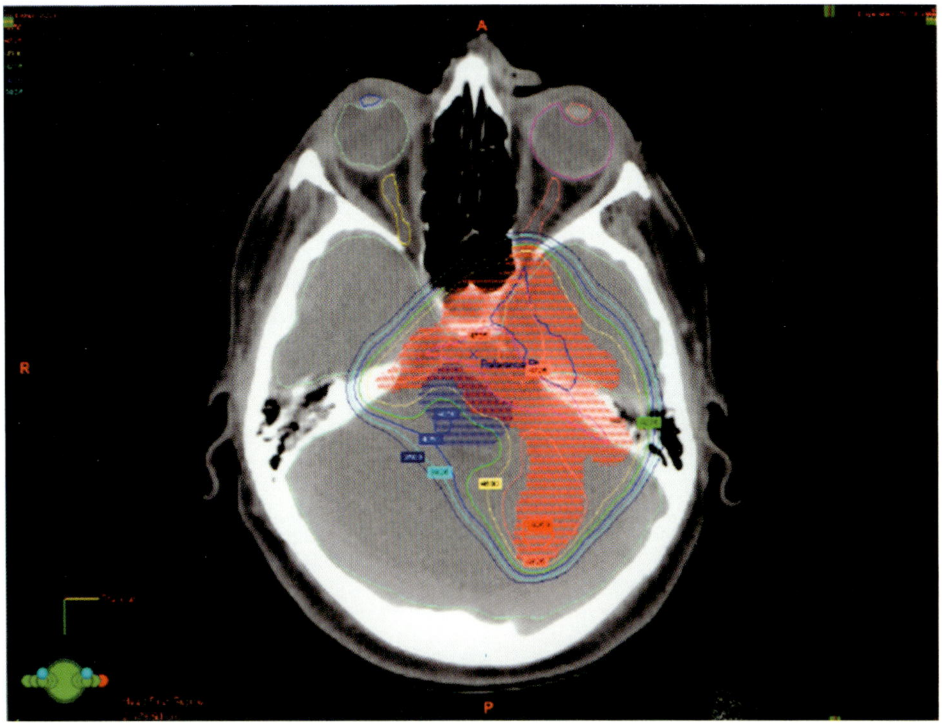

PLATE 40 (Figure 7-12). Dose distribution of an intensity-modulated radiation therapy plan for a 51-year-old female with an extensive skull-based meningioma (shaded) with involvement of clivus, left petrous apex, and left tentorium. The plan conforms the dose to the irregular tumor volume, allowing greater sparing of the brainstem and other critical structures.

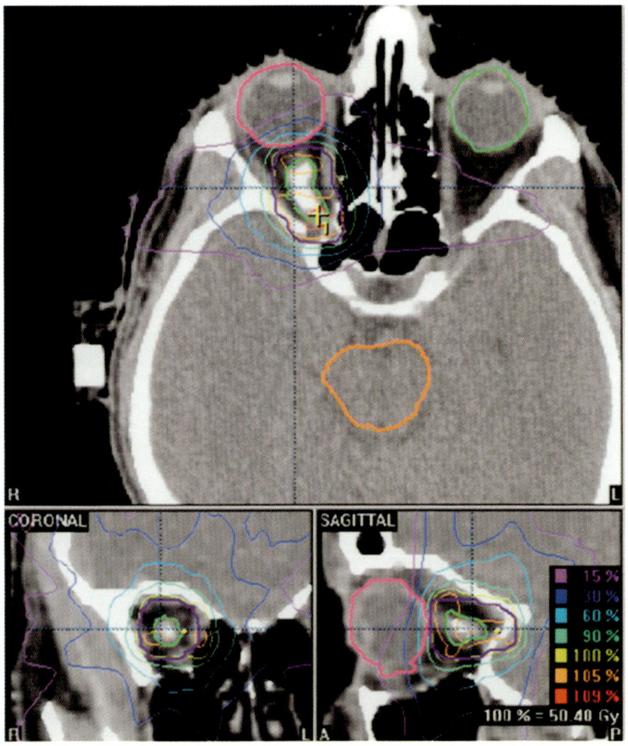

PLATE 41 (Figure 7-13). A patient with a right optic nerve sheath meningioma treated to 50.4 Gy with fractionated stereotactic radiotherapy system using a relocatable head frame stabilized by a mouth-guard bite block.

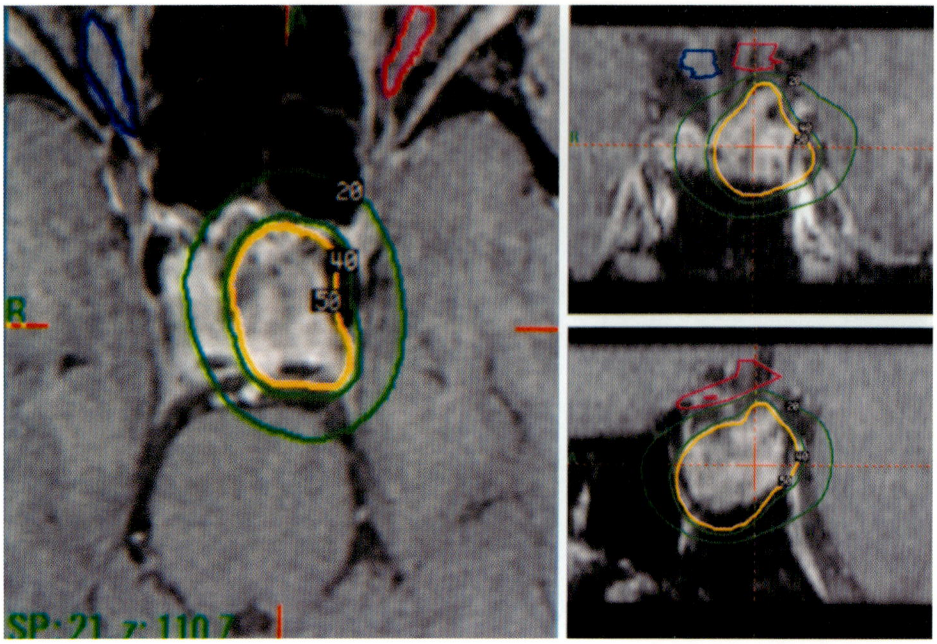

PLATE 42 (Figure 7-14). Dose plan of a patient with an enlarging nonfunctional pituitary adenoma after prior transsphenoidal resection. Six isocenters of radiation were used to cover a volume of 3.2 cm3. The tumor margin dose was 16 Gy; the maximum radiation dose to the adjacent left optic nerve was 6.1 Gy.

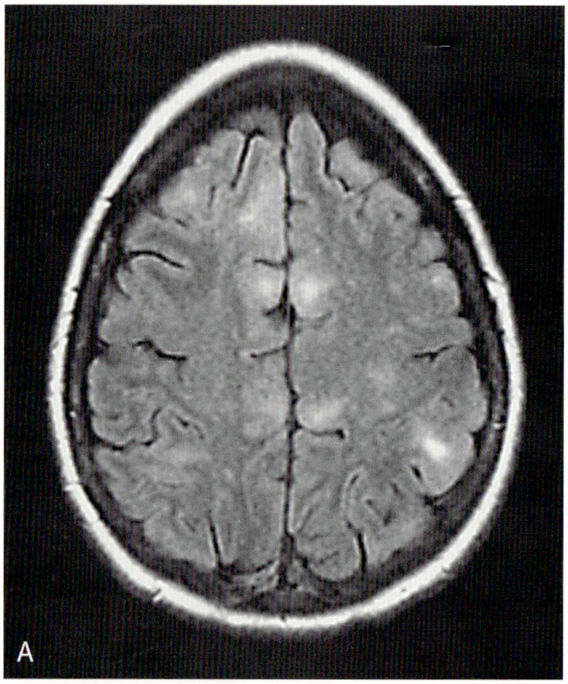

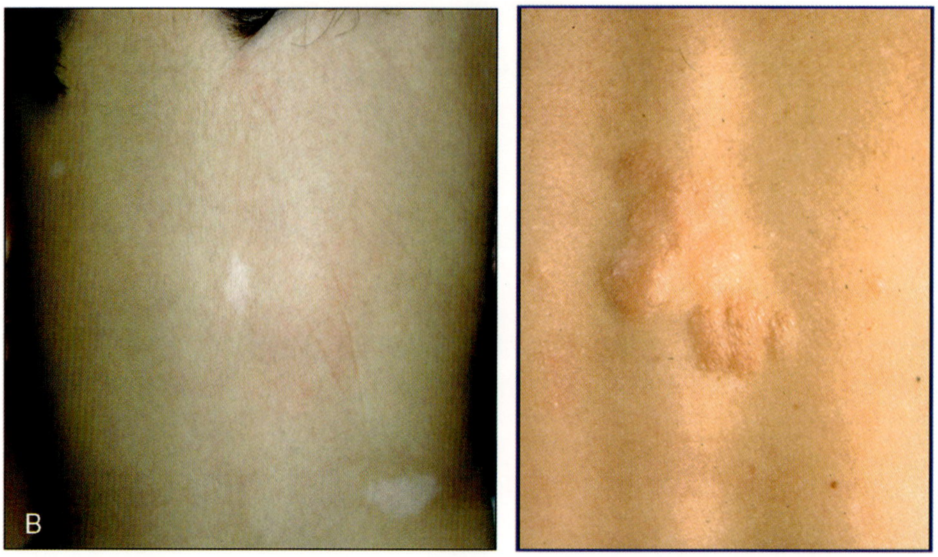

PLATE 43A and B (Figure 12-6A and B). (A) Multiple subcortical tubers. (B) "Ash leaf" depigmentation (left) and Shagreen patch (right) in TSC (courtesy of Dusica Babovic MD, DSc, Department of Human Genetics, Mayo Medical School, Rochester MN 55905).

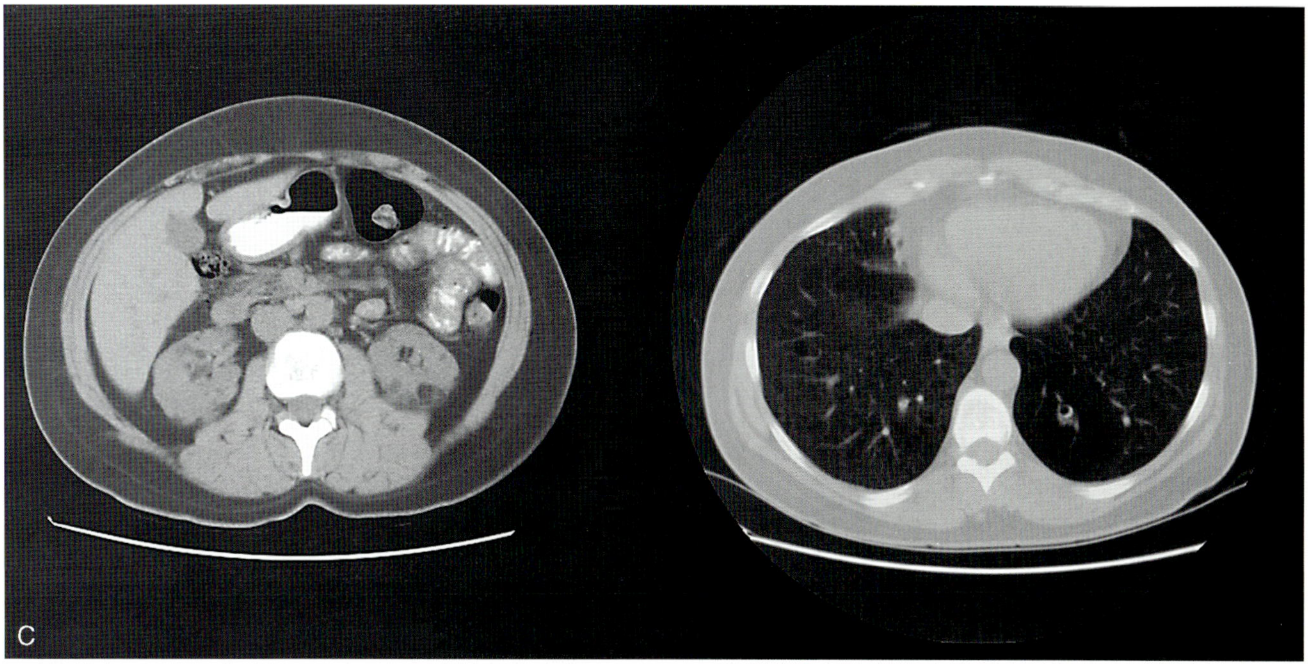

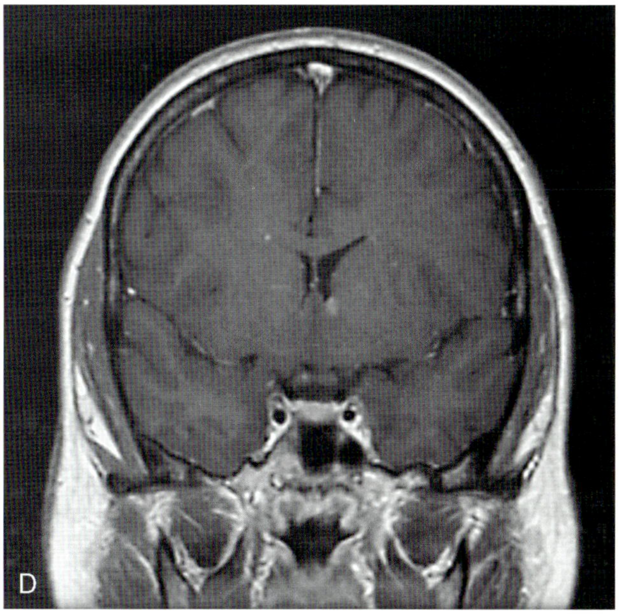

PLATE 43 C and D (Figure 12-6C and D). (C) Multiple angiomyolipomas and cysts in kidneys (left) and lungs (right) typical of TSC. (D) Subependymal giant cell astrocytoma (SEGA). Lesion (arrow) is small with no ventricular enlargement. Lesion found on routine screening and will serve as baseline for comparison to subsequent imaging.

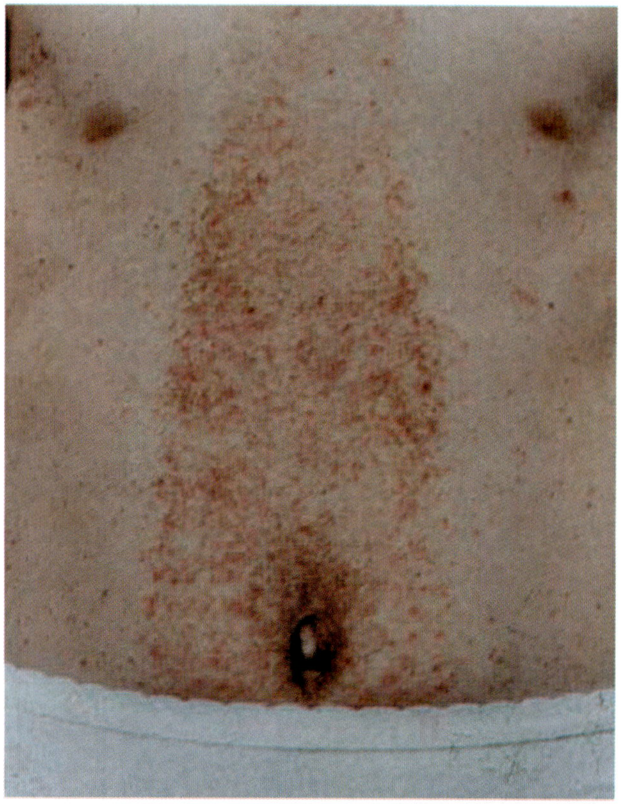

PLATE 44 (Figure 12-8). Subsequent development of nevoid basal cell carcinomas in treatment field of medulloblastoma patient who received neuraxis irradiation.

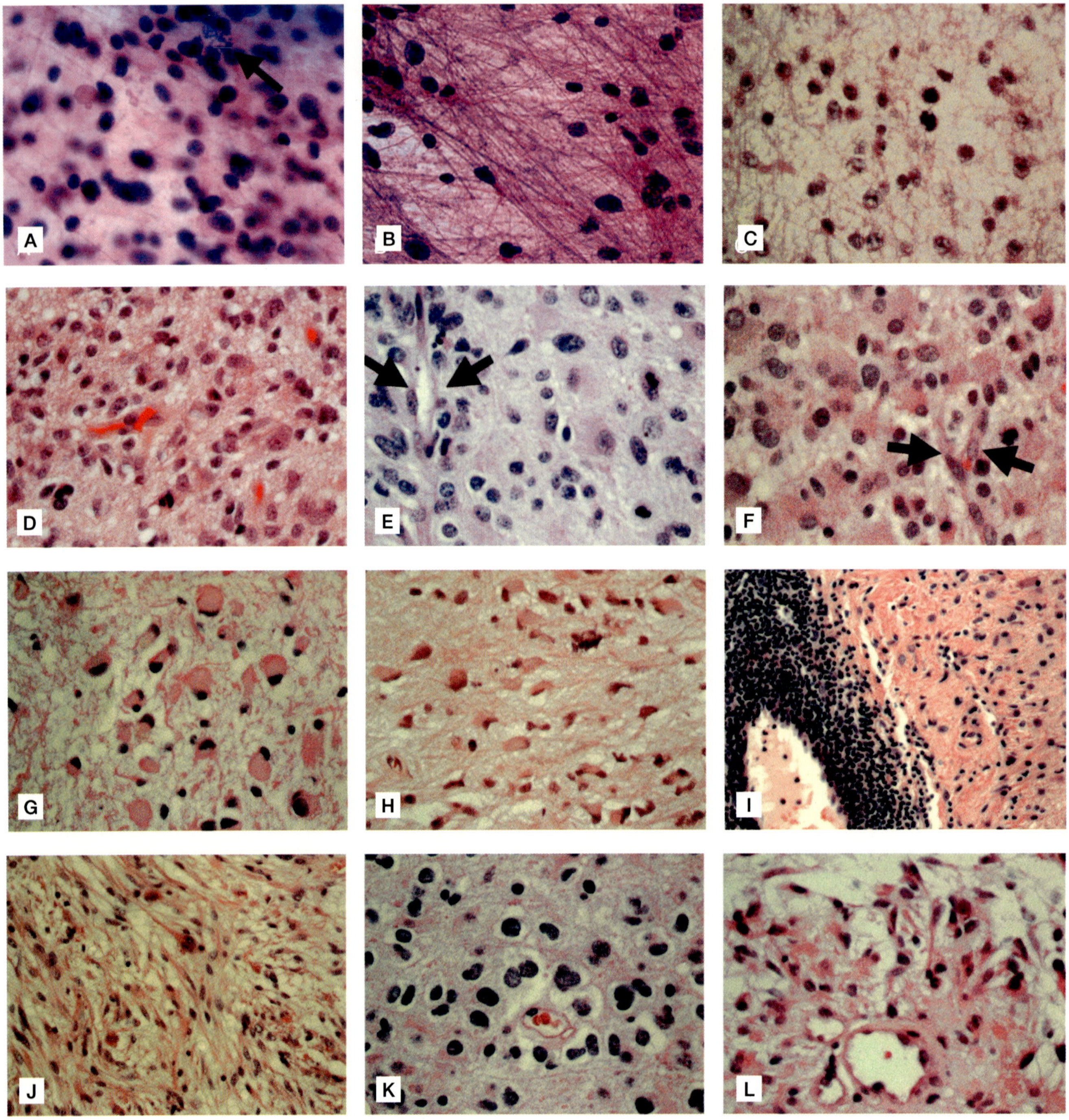

PLATE 45 (Figure 13-5). Histopathology of anaplastic astrocytoma. (A and B) Smear preparations. Smears are often useful for intraoperative consultation in conjunction with a frozen section. On this smear, note the mitotic activity (A, arrowhead) and the eosinophilic astrocytic processes (B). (C to F) Representative examples of AA. Each example shows mitoses, moderate to high cellularity, but with delicate, nonproliferative vasculature (E and F, arrows). (G to I) Gemistocytic astrocytoma. Tumor cells with defined eosinophilic cytoplasm. This is often accompanied by perivascular lymphocytic cuffing (I). An example of fibrillary anaplastic astrocytoma (J) is shown for comparison. (K and L) Diagnostic mimics. Occasional examples can show perinuclear haloes (K) or perivascular structuring (L). Although reminiscent of oligodendroglioma (K) or ependymoma (L), the cytologic features are more consistent with an astrocytic tumor.

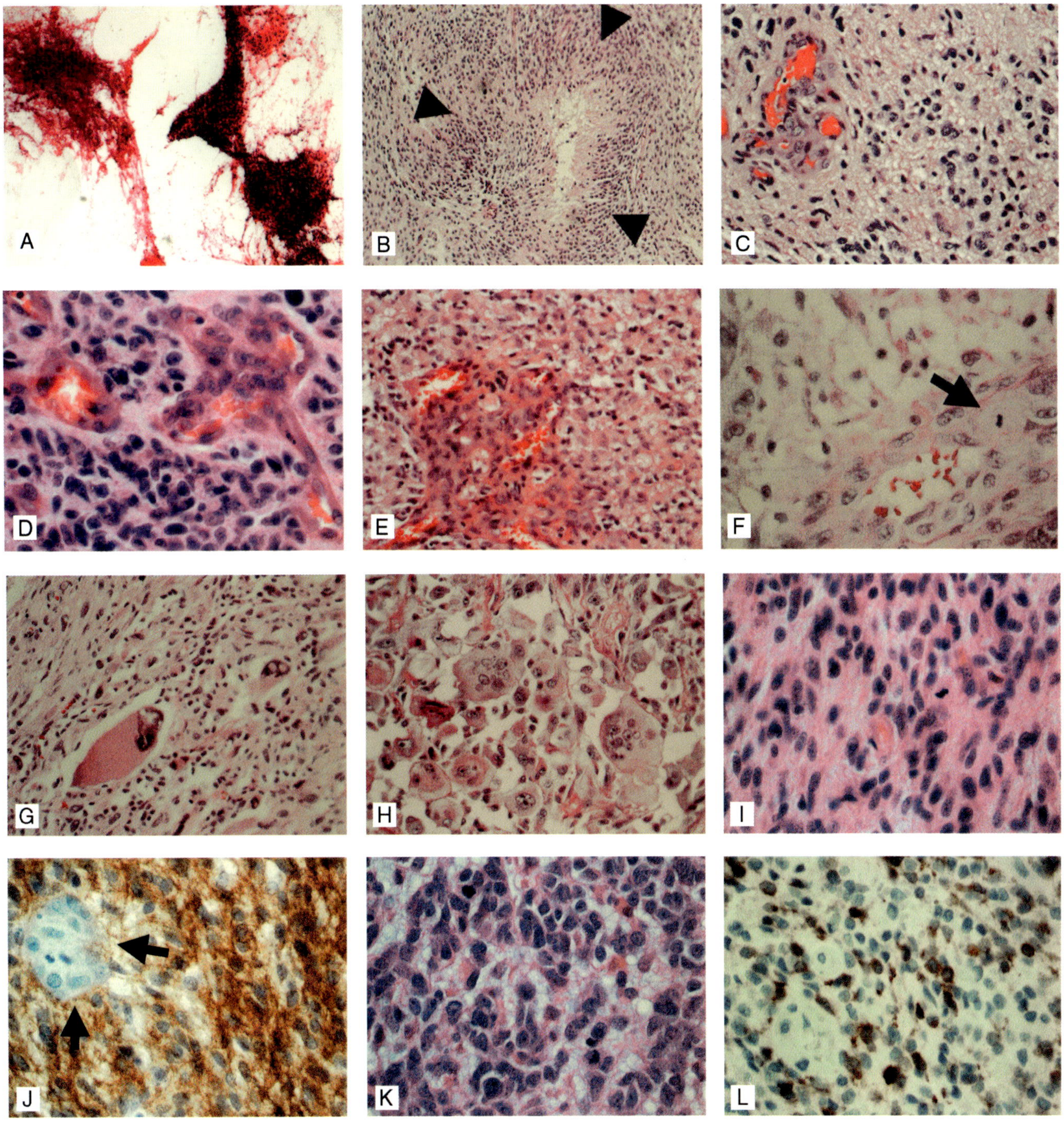

PLATE 46 (Figure 13-6). Histopathology of GBM. (A) A smear preparation of GBM typically shows viable tumor (right) in association with acellular necrotic material (left). (B) Pseudopalisading around necrotic areas is typical (arrowheads). (C to F) Microvascular proliferation. Piling-up of cells within vascular structures is another hallmark. The vascular structure in (E) resembles the glomerulus of the kidney, and is referred to as "glomeruloid" microvascular proliferation. Mitotic activity within the vessel is seen in (F, arrow), highlighting the proliferation of cells within vessels. Occasional large bizarre cells are seen (G), which when they compose the majority of the tumor, are called giant-cell GBM (H). (I and J) Small-cell GBM. Tumors with small minimally atypical nuclei which are also highly proliferative (note mitoses) are seen in approximately 10% of cases. Most of these tumors overexpress EGFR, as shown in the positive, predominately membrane, immunostaining using an anti-EGFR antibody (J). Note the lack of staining in the vessel (arrows), which serves as an internal negative control. (K and L) Use of tumor markers to supplement histology. Some specimens are highly cellular, but lack tumor necrosis or microvascular proliferation (K). By strict criteria, a glioblastoma diagnosis cannot be made. Staining for EGFR vIII (L) confirms that this tumor is best regarded as GBM.

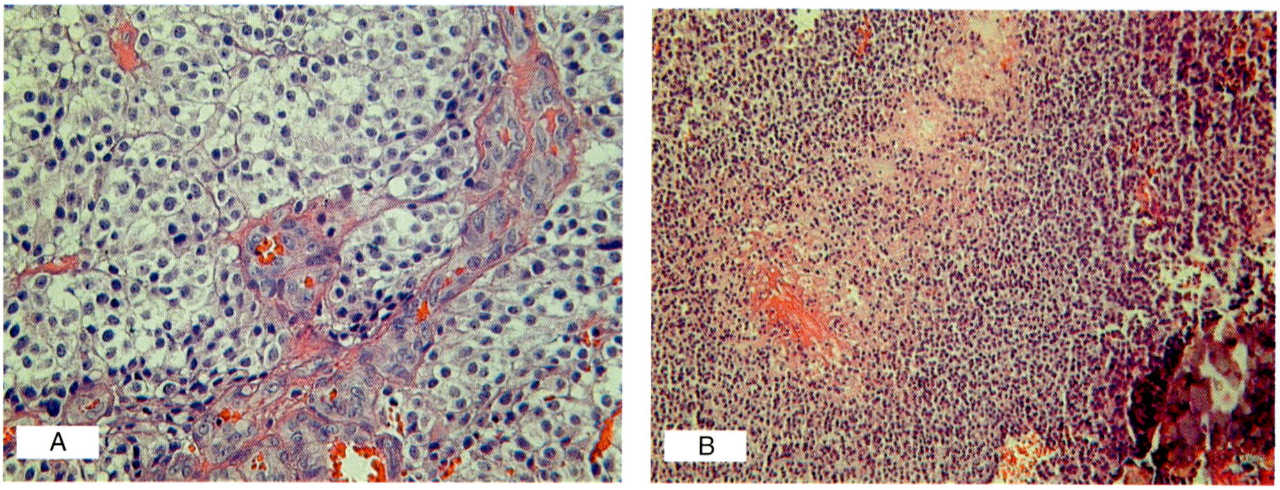

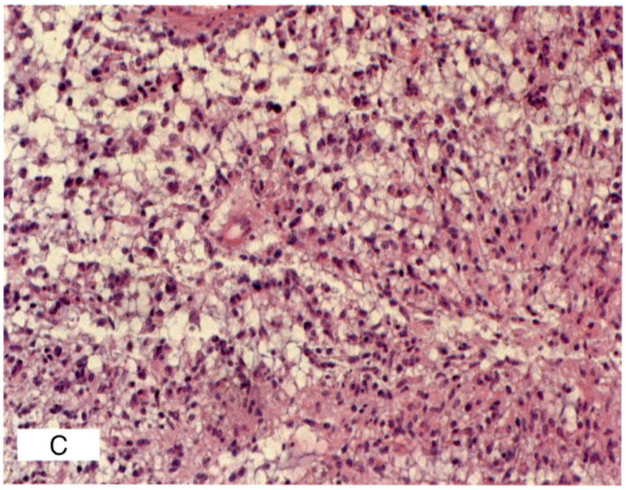

PLATE 47 (Figure 15-3). (A) High-grade (anaplastic) oligodendroglioma. The tumor cell nuclei are more pleomorphic as compared to the tumor in Fig. 15-1. There is pronounced microvascular (glomeruloid) proliferation (hematoxylin and eosin [H&E] stain, x200). (B) Glioblastoma ex oligodendroglioma. In this high-grade glioma, there are still unequivocal oligodendroglial hallmarks such as the perinuclear halos and the presence of calcifications. Overall, the tumor met the criteria for making the diagnosis of oligodendroglioma (H&E, x40). (C) Mixed oligoastrocytoma, showing tumor cells with oligodendroglial phenotypes and tumor cells with astrocytic phenotypes (H&E, x100).

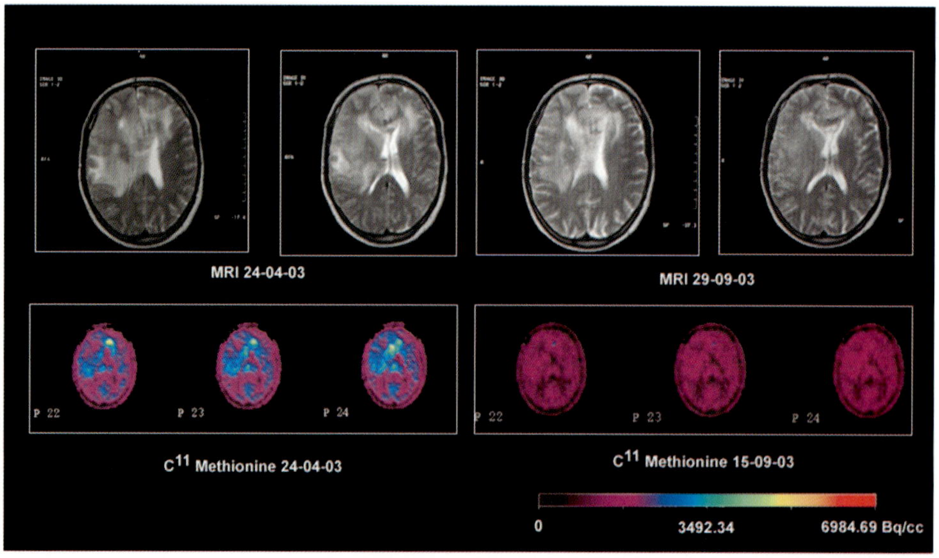

PLATE 48 (Figure 15-9). PCV chemotherapy in low-grade oligodendroglioma: T2-weighted MR images and 11C-methionine positron emission tomography scan before (left) and after (right) two cycles of PCV chemotherapy in a patient with gliomatosis cerebri with oligodendroglial morphology (1p/19q status unknown). Although there is some improvement of the MRI abnormalities, this does not qualify for a partial response according to Macdonald's criteria. In contrast, there is a marked reduction of the abnormal uptake of 11C-methionine. During treatment, behavioral abnormalities that had been present for 2 years normalized.

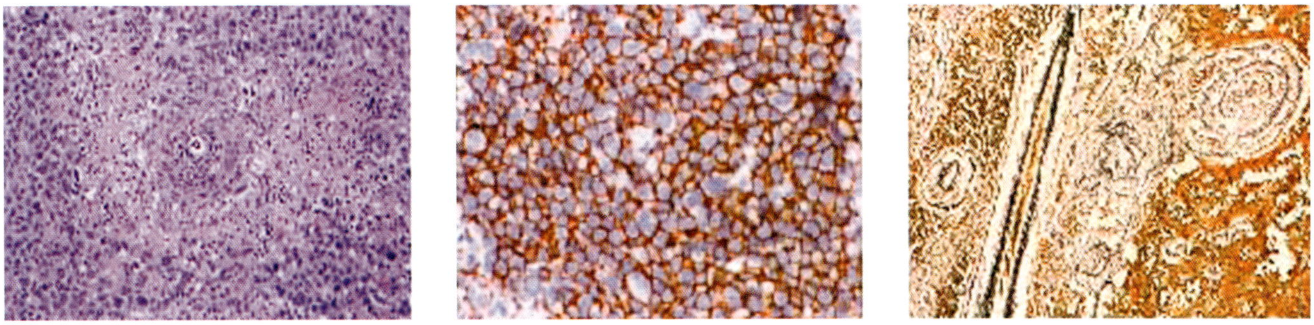

PLATE 49 (Figure 17-3). (Left) Typical light microscopic appearance: angiocentric infiltrate with, in this case, extensive PCNSL infiltration into parenchyma (hematoxylin and eosin [H&E], x20). (Center) Most cases are large, CD20_ B-cell tumors (CD20, x20). (Right) Characteristic "onion-ring" appearance with silver stains (Hortega, x20).

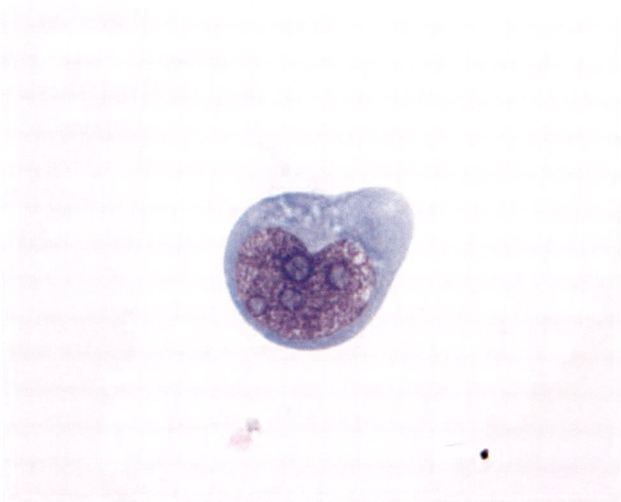

PLATE 50 (Figure 17-5). Vitrectomy specimen demonstrating single lymphoma cell. (Courtesy of Dr. Karen Grogg, Department of Pathology, Mayo Clinic, Rochester, MN.)

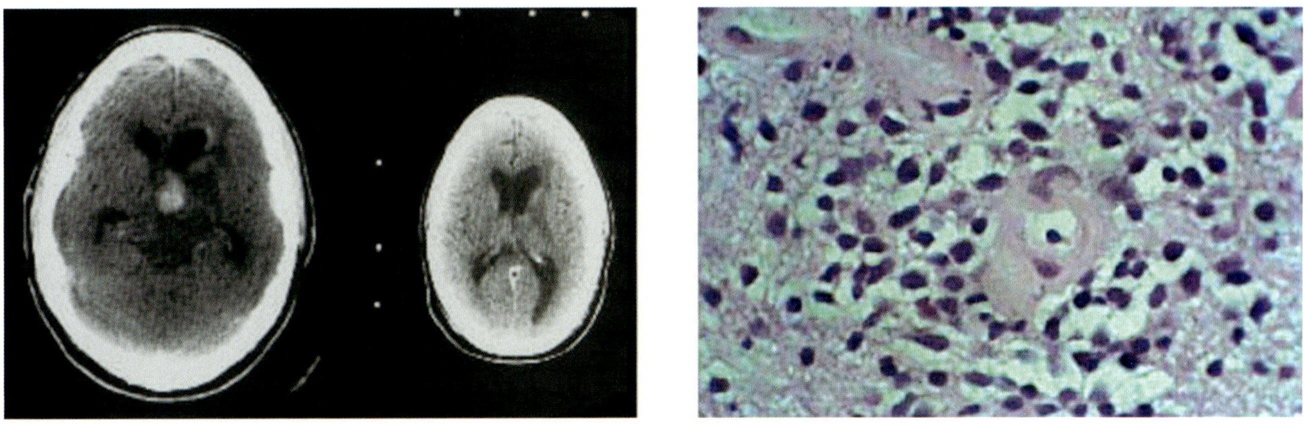

PLATE 51 (Figure 17-10). The "ghost tumor" effect of corticosteroids: (Left) A disappearance of a contrast-enhancing mass at the foramen of Munro following dexamethasone. (Right) Apoptotic nuclei in a biopsy specimen taken 6 hours later.

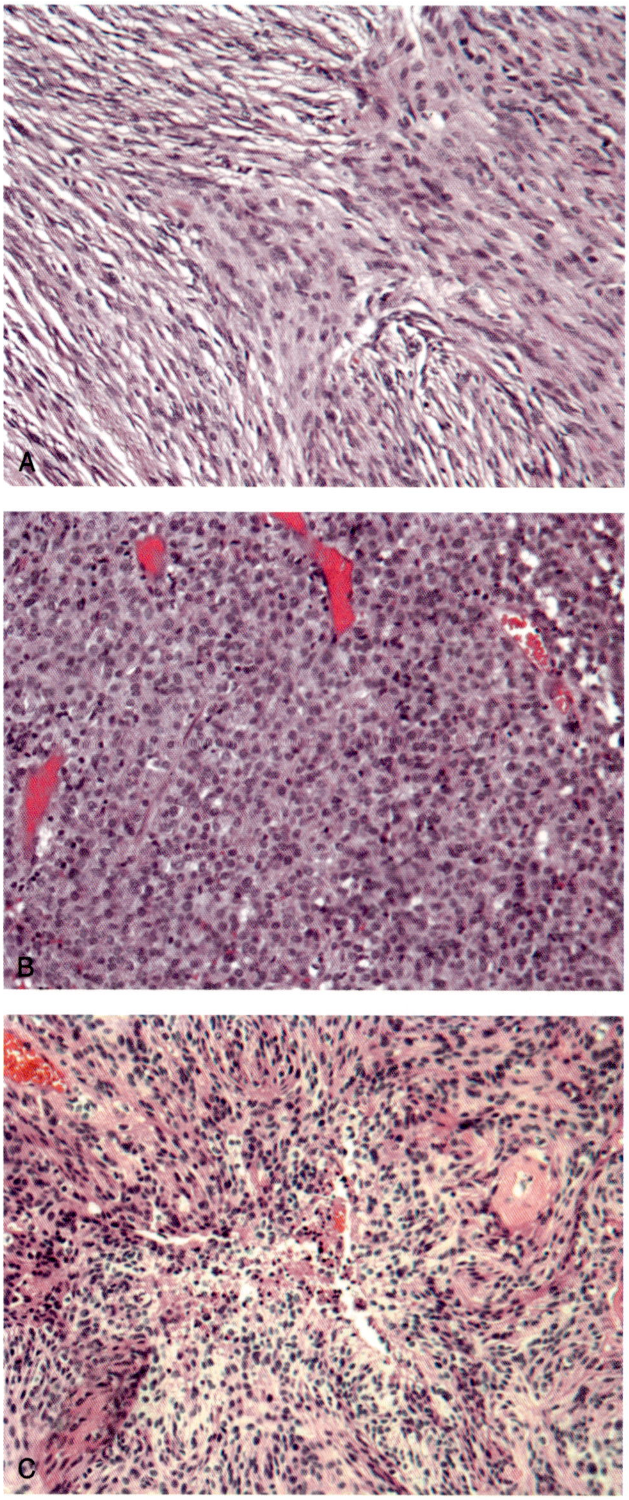

PLATE 52 (Figure 18-5). Hematoxylin and eosin-stained sections of meningiomas. (A) WHO grade I: benign meningioma of the transitional subtype; (B) WHO grade II: atypical meningioma showing "sheeting" of tumor cells; (C) WHO grade III: malignant meningioma with small cells with high nuclear cytoplasmic ratio, irregular growth, necrosis, and high mitotic index. (Photomicrographs courtesy of Alexander Vortmeyer, MD, Surgical Neurology Branch, NINDS, NIH.)

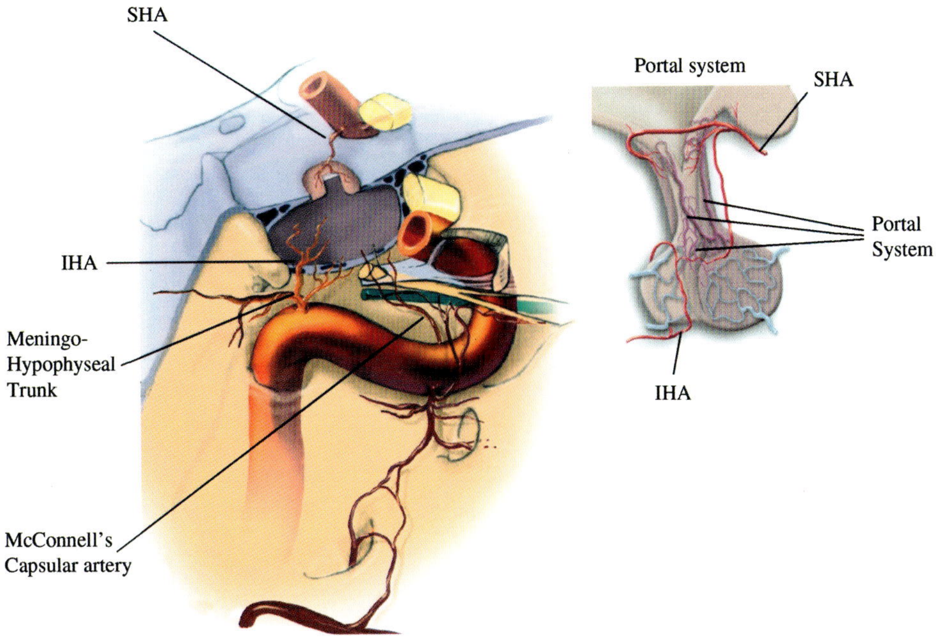

PLATE 53 (Figure 19-5). Vascular anatomy of the pituitary gland. Vascular supply of the pituitary gland is provided by the superior hypophyseal artery (SHA) and inferior hypophyseal artery (IHA) from the carotid arteries bilaterally, and their anastomoses. The SHA actually refers to a series of arteries that arise from the supraclinoid portion of the carotid artery bilaterally. These vessels largely supply the stalk and inferior surface of the optic apparatus and anastomose with their contralateral counterpart forming a vascular plexus. The IHA arise from the meningohypophyseal trunk of the cavernous segment of the carotid artery and supply the posterior lobe. These also anastomose with their contralateral counterpart and form a vascular plexus. The adenohypophysis is largely supplied by the hypophyseal portal venous system (inset) which arises as the anastomotic network between the vascular plexus formed from the SHA (superiorly) and IHA (inferiorly) and is also the means by which releasing hormones are transferred from the hypothalamus to adenohypophysis. McConnell capsular artery, present in approximately 25% of people, may arise from the distal, medial cavernous carotid artery and supply the capsule of the gland or the sellar dura.

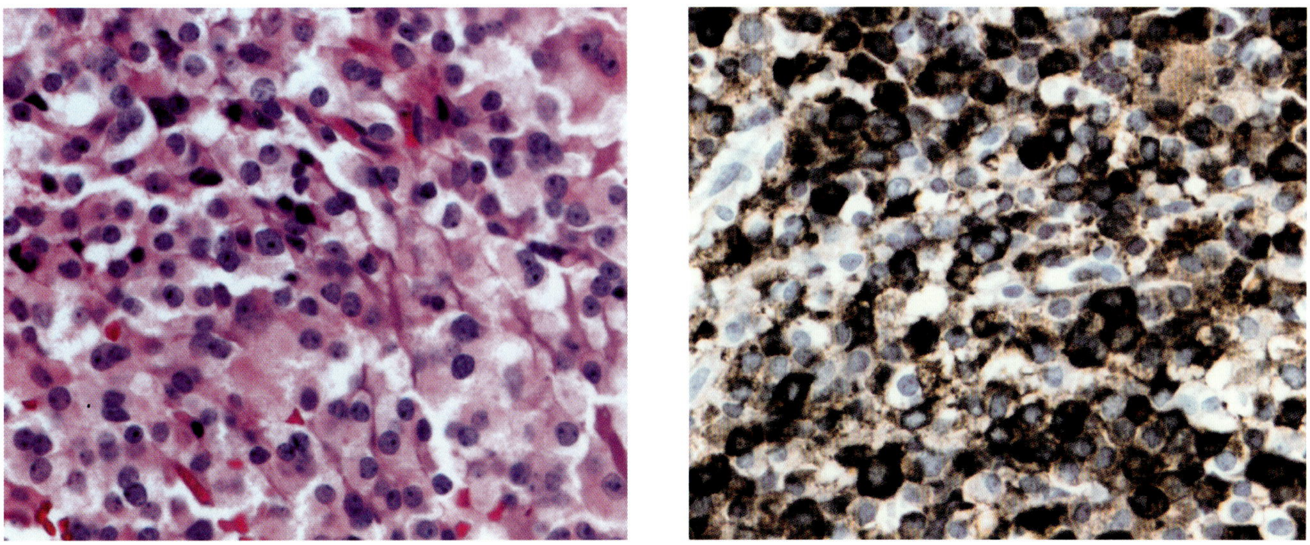

PLATE 54 (Figure 19-7). Growth hormone-secreting adenoma. H&E (left) preparation demonstrating a somatotroph cell adenoma that is strongly and diffusely immunoreactive for growth hormone (right).

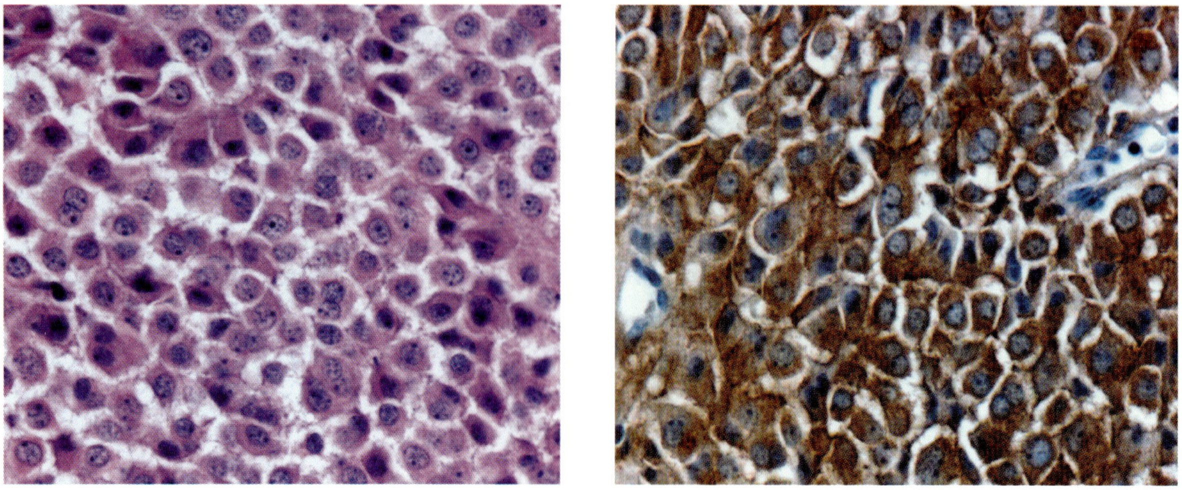

PLATE 55 (Figure 19-8). Adrenocorticotropic hormone-secreting adenoma. H&E (left) slide demonstrating a basophilic corticotroph that immunoreacts strongly for ACTH (right).

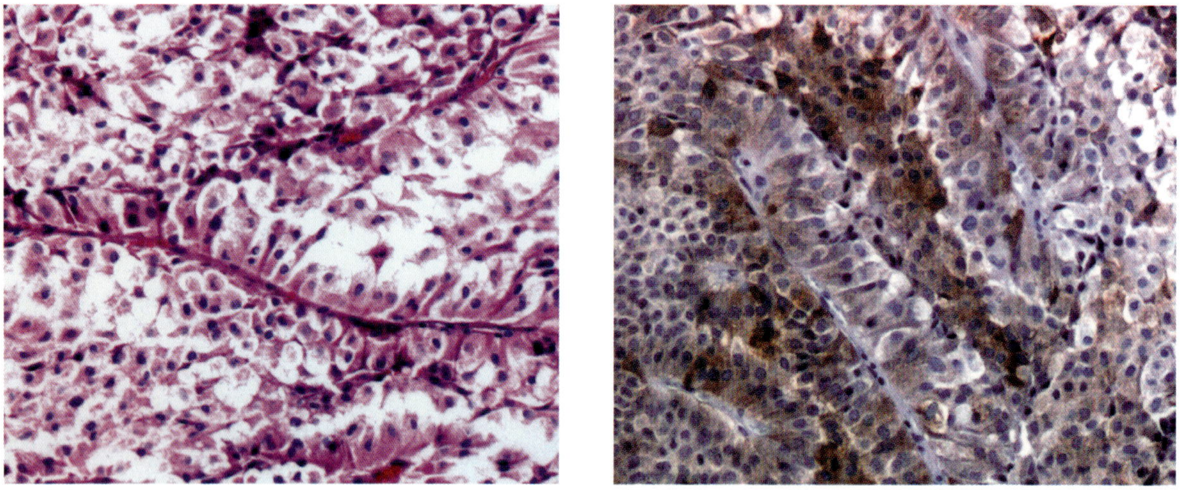

PLATE 56 (Figure 19-9). Gonadotrophic hormone-secreting adenoma. H&E (left) preparation demonstrating a sparsely granulated (chromophobic) gonadotroph cell adenoma that demonstrates patchy immunoreactivity with FSH (right).

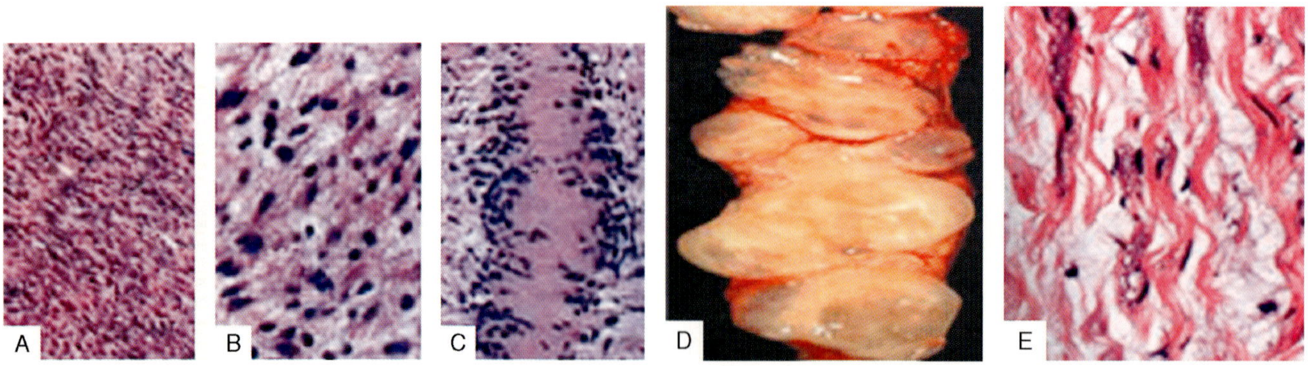

PLATE 57 (Figure 25-5). Histology of a typical schwannoma with (A) Antoni A hypercellular regions of transformed Schwann spindle-like cells. (B) Antoni B hypocellular loose myxoid regions. (C) Verocay bodies. (D) Gross picture of a neurofibroma with myxoid heterogeneous regions and intrafascicular growth. (E) Histopathology of a typical neurofibroma with loose myxoid architecture containing several cellular elements, including the transformed Schwann cells and axons, consistent with intrafascicular growth.

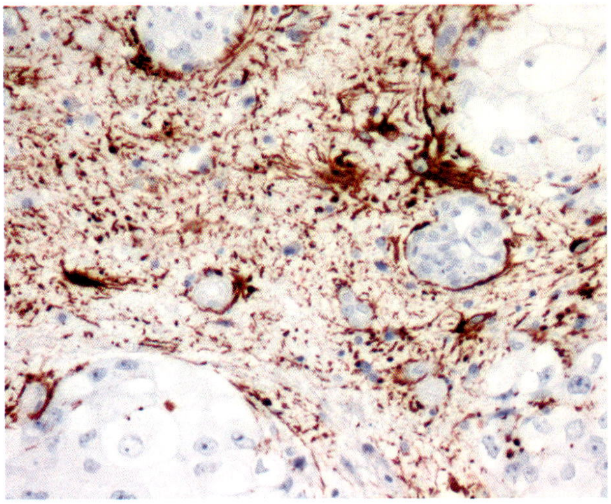

PLATE 58 (Figure 26-2). Histologic specimen with GFAP (glial fibrillary acidic protein) stain showing reactive astrocytosis adjacent to a metastasis (reactive astrocytes designated by arrow).

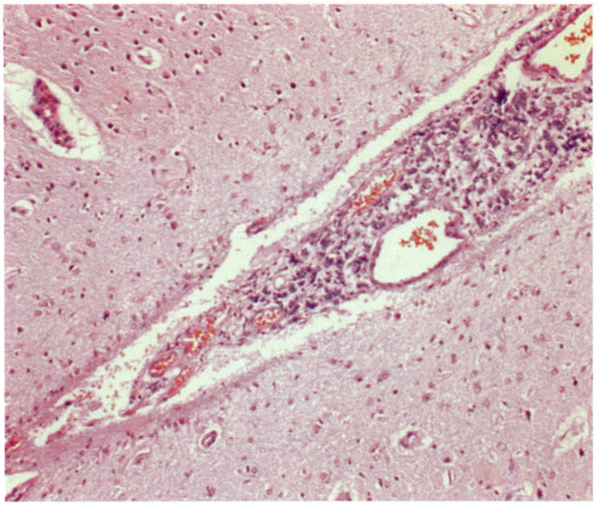

PLATE 59 (Figure 26-3). Microscopic view of leptomeningeal metastases. Note the invasion of the Virchow-Robin (perivascular) space (arrow) which is typical for this pathologic entity.

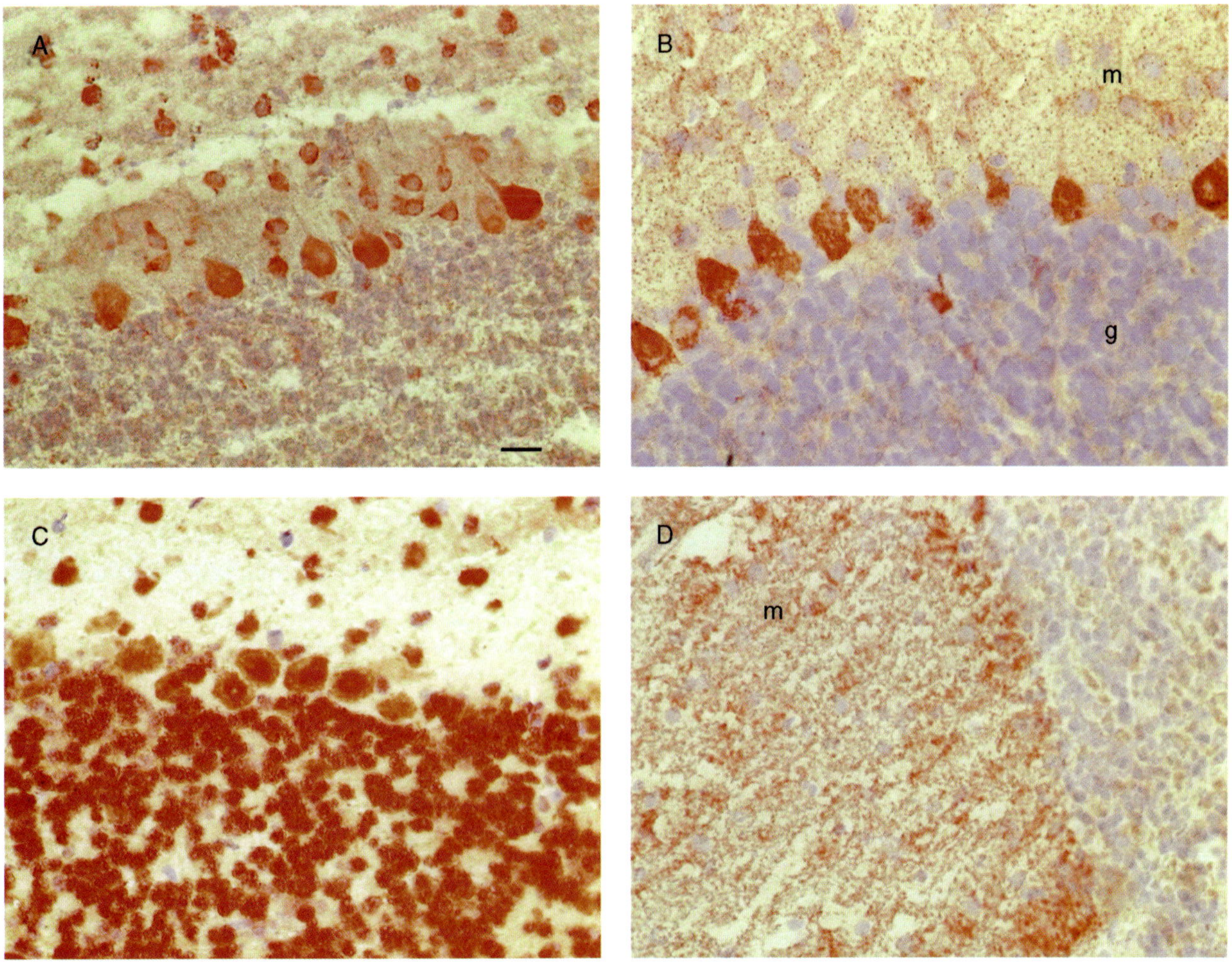

PLATE 60 (Figure 30-1). Paraneoplastic antibodies associated with "pure" PCD. (A) Anti-Yo antibodies label cytoplasm of Purkinje cells. (B) Incubation with anti-Tr antibodies results in strong immunoreactivity of Purkinje cell cytoplasm and dot-like labeling of the molecular layer. (C) Anti-Ri antibodies stain nuclei more than cytoplasm of all central neurons with sparing of the nucleolus. (D) Anti-mGluR1 strongly stains molecular layer and, to a lesser extent, the Purkinje cells. Frozen sections of rat cerebellum were incubated with the patients' sera after acetone fixation. The scale bar represents 20 mm; m = granular layer; g = molecular layer.

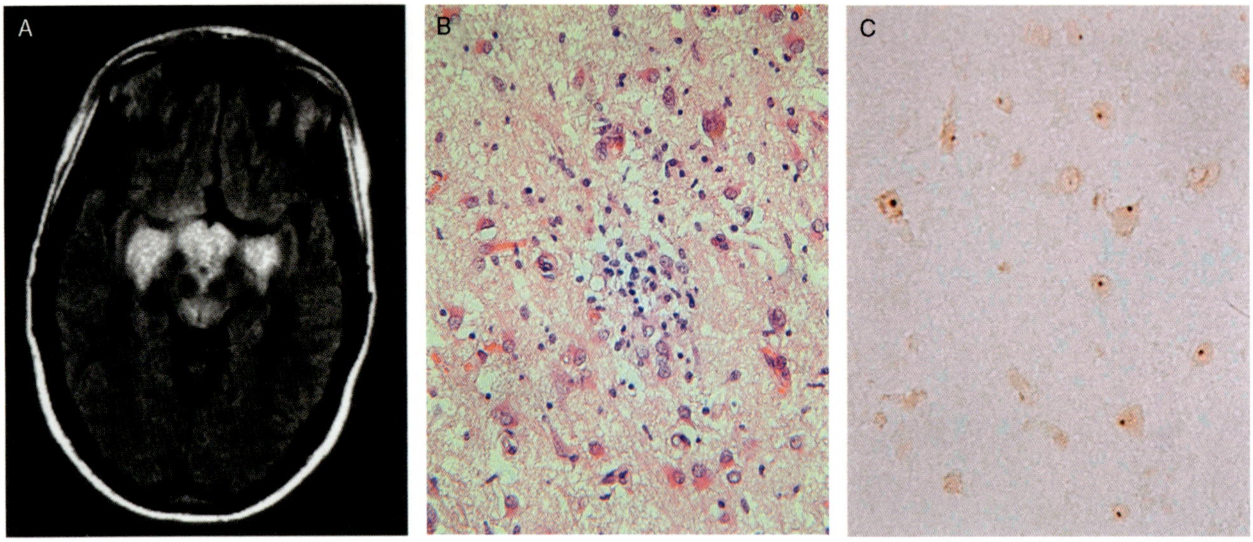

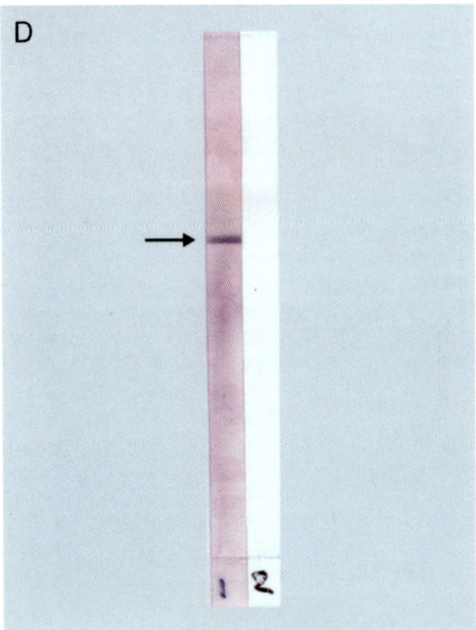

PLATE 61 (Figure 30-2). Paraneoplastic limbic encephalitis and anti-Ma2 antibodies. (A) MRI shows increased signal intensities in the medial temporal lobes, diencephalon and brainstem (FLAIR). (B) At autopsy, the medial temporal lobe showed parenchymal inflammatory infiltrates, consisting mostly of mononuclear cells. (C) The patient's serum, when reacted with human cortex, showed strong immunoreactivity against neuronal nucleoli. (D) The patient's serum (lane 1) contains immunoreactivity against purified Ma2 fusion protein (arrow). Control serum (lane 2) is negative.

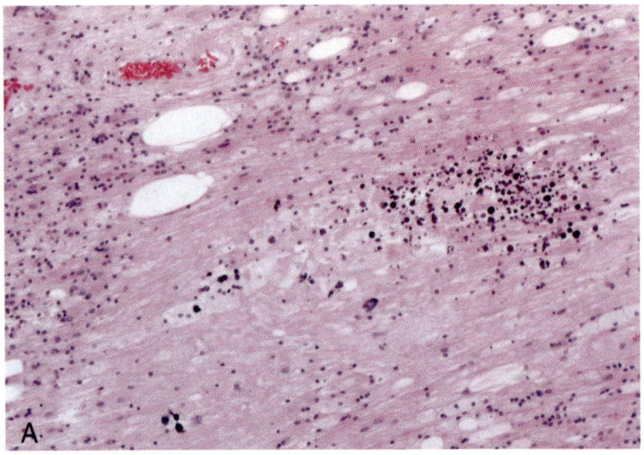

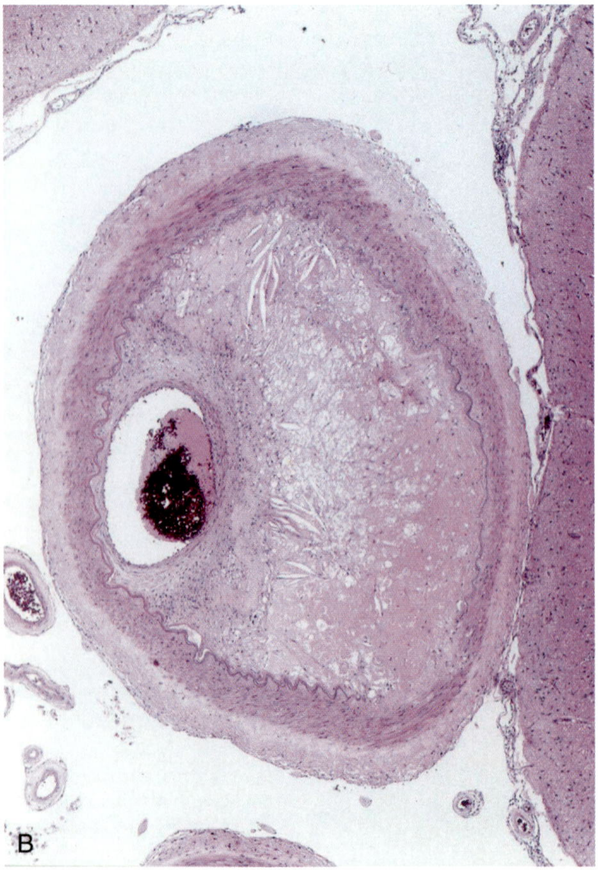

PLATE 62 (Figure 32-2). (A) Hematoxylin and eosin (H&E) stain of radiation-induced neurotoxicity demonstrating characteristic gliosis and spongiosis of the white matter with vacuolar change. (B) This panel demonstrates prominent atherosclerosis of the middle cerebral artery with thrombus in the vascular lumen.

these patients are more often clinically euthyroid despite elevated thyroid hormone and TSH levels. In addition, TRH stimulation causes increased TSH levels and serum α-subunit levels are not elevated.

Therapy

Surgery is the preferred therapy for these uncommon tumors (see Table 19-3). However, the rarity of this tumor has provided few centers the necessary clinical data to draw concrete conclusions. Transsphenoidal surgery appears to provide remission in approximately 50% of patients.[248,250,251] The addition of octreotide and radiation therapy appears to increase the rate of remission which has been achieved in 60% to 80% of patients.[248,250–254]

Overview of Surgical Approaches

There are two basic, common surgical approaches to the sellar region—transsphenoidal and transcranial—although modifications of these techniques or their derivatives are employed in specific instances. The transsphenoidal route is used to approach most pituitary adenomas. Through either a nasal or sublabial (gingival mucosa) incision, dissection is carried back to the front of the sphenoid sinus. We routinely use the nasal incision, which is more comfortable for the patient, except in instances where a wider exposure is necessary, such as with skull base extended transsphenoidal approaches, and where the nasal orifice is too narrow, such as in children. The front of the sphenoid sinus is opened and the sella and its junction with the clivus and tuberculum sellae is then identified. The sella can then be opened, thereby exposing the dura, which is subsequently coagulated and incised, exposing the normal gland and/or tumor. The approach is generally guided by intraoperative fluoroscopy although frameless stereotaxy may be used especially in cases of recurrent tumor and prior surgery where anatomic landmarks are obscured and/or absent. Knowledge of midline is imperative to ensure a safe approach. The carotid arteries lie lateral to the midline and are at risk with significant deviation from the midline.

The operating microscope with its inherent magnification and illumination facilitates careful tumor removal. Use of endoscopy, either as a primary means of visualization during the approach and tumor removal, or as an adjunct to the microscope, is becoming more common. The future of endoscopy appears promising, and may offer a less invasive approach with panoramic visualization to facilitate tumor removal. However, experience with this technique is considerably less than with standard microsurgery and current endoscopic optics that typically permit two-dimensional visualization remain limitations. We combine endoscopy with microsurgery at our institution. Both have advantages in certain circumstances and we have found endoscopy particularly useful during tumor resection in the suprasellar space and to explore the surgical site to ensure complete tumor removal.

Transsphenoidal approaches may not be ideal, for instance, in circumstances in which there is significant tumor extension into the anterior, middle, and posterior cranial fossae, with extreme suprasellar extension through a narrow diaphragmatic aperture or where the tumor is known or suspected to be tough and fibrous with suprasellar extension (thereby making resection from an inferior approach very difficult). Under these conditions a transcranial approach is superior. We generally perform a right-sided pterional craniotomy, usually with an orbital osteotomy to provide a basal trajectory of view with minimal brain retraction (Fig. 19-12). A lumbar drain may be placed preoperatively to facilitate cerebral relaxation in conjunction with other measures such as mild hyperventilation, osmotic diuresis with mannitol, and opening of the basal cisterns to minimize cerebral retraction. Under high magnification, the tumor is removed with microdissection. Patient, careful dissection around the optic apparatus and carotid arteries is imperative for tumor removal with minimal morbidity (Fig. 19-13). The optic apparatus can be decompressed under direct visualization and the anterior clinoid process can be removed along with unroofing of the optic canal if necessary.

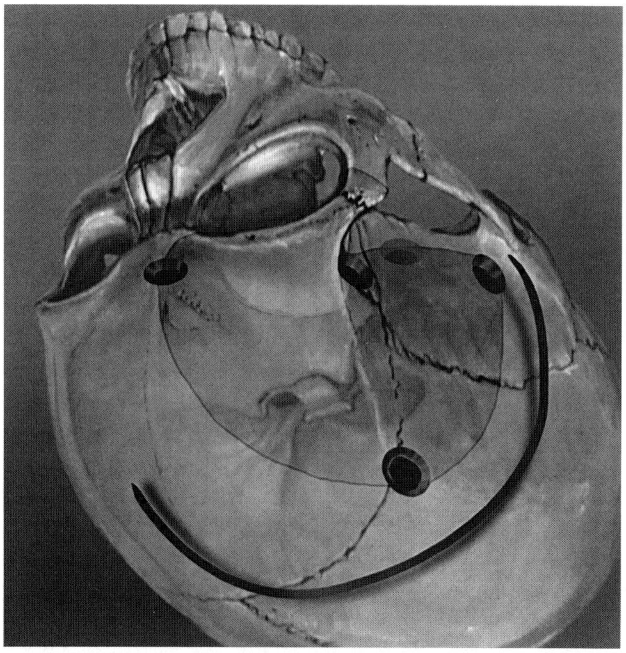

Figure 19-12. Transcranial approach to sellar tumors (cranio-orbital craniotomy). The skin incision and planned craniotomy (including osteotomy of the orbital roof) is depicted. The relationship of the sellar region is illustrated relative to the craniotomy.

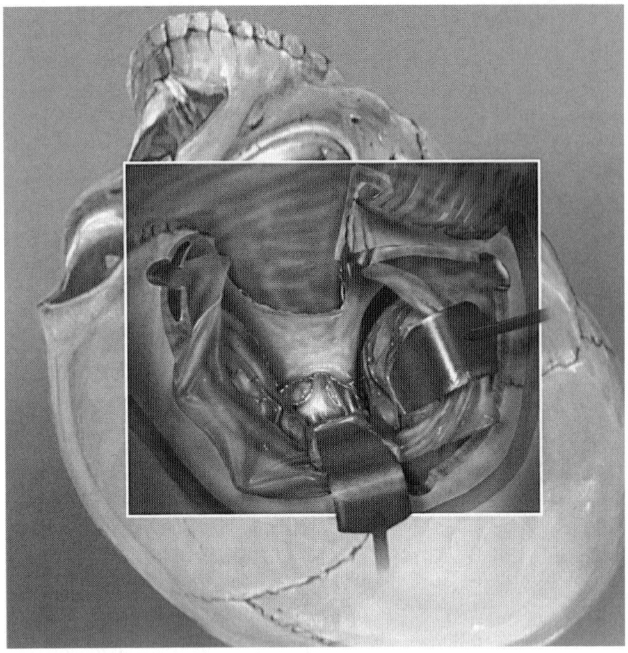

Figure 19-13. Intradural removal of a pituitary adenoma. The dura has been opened and the line of sight of the microscope is focused on the sellar region. The tumor is seen stretching the optic apparatus superiorly. The carotid artery is lateral to the optic apparatus and tumor dissection and removal is carried out through apertures between these vital structures.

▶ OTHER PATHOLOGIC ENTITIES

Pituitary Apoplexy

Pituitary apoplexy is used to describe an acute syndrome resulting from hemorrhage or infarction of the pituitary gland almost universally in the setting of a pituitary adenoma (Fig. 19-14). Although hemorrhage may occur without overt symptoms or in a subacute course, apoplexy is used to denote events in which there is an abrupt onset of characteristic signs and symptoms including headache, meningismus, nausea/vomiting, with visual or other neurologic impairment, with or without alterations in level of consciousness or hemodynamic instability related to abnormalities of hypothalamic–pituitary–end organ axes. Many patients presenting with pituitary apoplexy are unaware of a preexisting tumor (i.e., this is the initial manifestation). Apoplexy is a complication of 1% to 2% of all pituitary tumors and may be more common in males. There is considerable controversy concerning which tumor types are most prone to apoplexy. The reader is referred to several comprehensive reviews of the subject.[13,255–259]

The underlying pathophysiologic substrate(s) of pituitary apoplexy remain incompletely understood. Rapid tumor growth exceeding blood supply leading to ischemic necrosis, idiosyncratic vascular anomalies

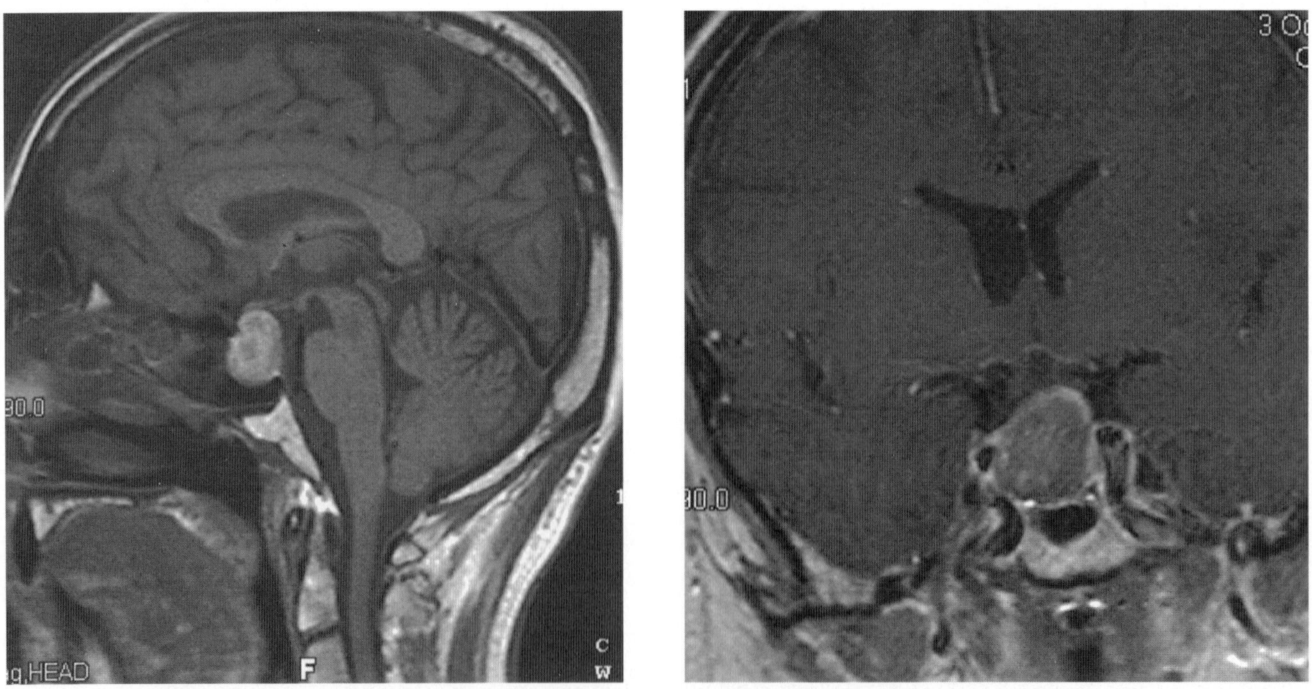

Figure 19-14. Pituitary apoplexy. Precontrast sagittal (left) and coronal (right) T_1-weighted MR images in a patient presenting with acute onset of headache, visual loss, and hypopituitarism. The hyperintense signal within the macroadenoma on T_1-weighted noncontrast images (indicating hemorrhage) coupled with the clinical scenario is consistent with pituitary apoplexy.

specific to pituitary tumors, and compression of the superior hypophyseal artery against the sellar diaphragm have been postulated as possible mechanisms. The posterior pituitary is generally spared as it has its own blood supply, and diabetes insipidus is relatively uncommon.[13]

Pituitary apoplexy represents a neurosurgical emergency. Initial management involves recognition of the syndrome and immediate corticosteroid replacement therapy. We have generally advocated prompt surgical decompression after medical stabilization, as delayed decompression appears to offer a lower chance of neurologic recovery (especially of vision).[13]

Pituitary Carcinoma

Pituitary carcinomas are rare lesions of the pituitary gland, and are defined as tumors of adenohypophyseal origin accompanied by demonstrated metastases (craniospinal or systemic).[81,260] Of note, typical criteria of malignancy in most human cancers (mitotic activity, necrosis, hemorrhage, nuclear atypical and polymorphism, invasiveness, etc.) are insufficient to qualify a pituitary tumor as a carcinoma as these features may be present in benign adenomas. Most pituitary carcinomas affect females. Three-quarters appear to be hormone-secreting (most commonly prolactin-secreting followed by corticotrophin-secreting) and one-quarter are nonfunctioning.[81] The initial clinical course of patients with pituitary carcinomas may resemble that of patients with benign pituitary adenomas. However, in patients with pituitary carcinomas, the clinical course is protracted with multiple local recurrences eventually being accompanied by metastatic dissemination. Metastases may occur via dissemination through cerebral spinal fluid (CSF), hematogenous spread, lymphatic spread, or a combination thereof. As the pituitary can be the site of metastatic spread of tumors from other sites, pituitary carcinoma must be distinguished from the more common occurrence of metastatic deposition of a non-adenohypophyseal tumor in the pituitary gland through careful clinical, radiologic, biochemical, and/or pathologic examination.[260,261] One of the interesting aspects of clinical history is that systemic metastases to the pituitary gland more frequently result in diabetes insipidus as a presenting manifestation. Indeed, Kimmel and O'Neill[261] found that of 100 consecutive cases of diabetes insipidus of any cause, 14 were a result of metastatic cancer. Moreover, diabetes insipidus was the initial presentation in 11 patients.

The management of pituitary carcinomas is based on anecdotal case series and clinical judgment because of their rarity. One or more surgical debulking procedures combined with radiation therapy and possibly pharmacologic therapy to provide local control, in conjunction with palliation of systemic disease, is reasonable, although long-term survival is uncommon.[260]

Craniopharyngioma

Craniopharyngiomas comprise a group of slow-growing, benign epithelial neoplasms of the sellar and suprasellar region. Although histologically benign, these lesions typically grow to involve vital surrounding structures, potentially producing endocrine deficits, visual loss, and mental disturbances with involvement of the hypothalamic–pituitary unit, optic apparatus, thalamus, and frontal and/or temporal lobes.

Craniopharyngiomas occur with an annual incidence of 0.5 to 2 cases per million population and occur with a bimodal age distribution with peaks between 5 and 10 years and between 50 and 60 years of age.[262–265] There appears to be no gender predilection.[262] Collectively, craniopharyngiomas account for 1% to 4% of intracranial tumors in the adult population and 6% to 10% of intracranial neoplasms in the pediatric population, respectively.[262,265] Craniopharyngiomas are generally sporadic and their molecular pathogenesis remains poorly defined.[266]

Embryologically, craniopharyngiomas arise from squamous epithelial remnants along the involuted craniopharyngeal duct.[267,268] During the fourth week of gestation, a diverticulum of embryonic stomodeum (oral cavity roof) gives rise to Rathke pouch, which subsequently migrates cranially to meet with the infundibulum (derived from diencephalic neuroectoderm). The path along which Rathke pouch migrates gives rise to the craniopharyngeal duct. Rathke pouch will eventually separate to form Rathke vesicle (surrounding the infundibulum) which gives rise to the constituents of the adenohypophysis, namely, the pars distalis, pars tuberalis, and the pars intermedia.[269] Craniopharyngiomas are postulated to originate from squamous cell rests deposited along the path of the primitive craniopharyngeal duct and adenohypophysis, either from remnants of the craniopharyngeal duct or from metaplasia of adenohypophyseal cells of the pituitary stalk.[80] To explain tumors contained solely within the third ventricle, aberrant growth of the pars tuberalis forward and backward with extension to the infundibulum and tuber cinereum of the floor of the third ventricle has been postulated.[270]

Grossly, craniopharyngiomas can be cystic, solid, or both. Histologically, there are two variants of craniopharyngioma—adamantinomatous and papillary—that have correspondingly unique clinical and radiologic features. Adamantinomatous craniopharyngiomas are epithelial neoplasms that arise in the suprasellar region and bear resemblance to odontogenic tumors.[80] These tumors typically affect a juvenile population (first two decades of life).[269] Internally, these tumors may contain a conglomeration of cysts, necrotic debris, fibrous tissue, calcification, and fluid filled with cholesterol particles.[80] This fluid, likened to machinery oil, may incite an intense sterile inflammatory reaction if spilled into the CSF space during surgery or through spontaneous rupture.[271–274]

Histologically, adamantinomatous craniopharyngiomas may be arranged in patterns of sheets, nodular whorls, trabeculae and "clover leaves," and cysts lined by attenuated epithelium.[80] The epithelial cells (all squamous in origin and immunoreactive for epithelial membrane antigen [EMA]) are arranged in a peripheral palisaded layer of columnar cells (stellate reticulum) and an intervening layer of polygonal cells.[80] Another characteristic feature of this variant is so-called wet keratin, formed by congregations of desquamated cells often undergoing calcification (which accounts for the calcification observed grossly and on imaging).[80] These lesions are also known to adhere to neurovascular structures and this can be observed histologically where intensive gliosis and Rosenthal formation is observed at tissue–tumor interface.[275] Papillary craniopharyngiomas are well-differentiated pseudopapillary tumors of squamous origin arising in the suprasellar region or third ventricle. The papillary craniopharyngioma variant, in contrast, occurs almost exclusively in adults.[276] Papillary craniopharyngiomas are mostly solid on gross inspection with papillations, but may exhibit a smaller cystic component and lack the cholesterol-rich machinery oil contents, calcification, and adherence to neurovascular structures as with adamantinomatous variants.[80] Microscopically, papillary craniopharyngiomas are comprised of well-differentiated squamous epithelium amidst a fibrovascular stroma. The epithelium appears to separate along fissures to form pseudopapillae.[80] Microscopic features of adamantinomatous tumors, including peripheral palisading of cells and nodules of wet keratin, are absent.

Imaging features reflect the pathology discussed above. Nonenhanced CT scans usually demonstrate a suprasellar mass that is cystic with a solid mural nodule. Calcification is present in the majority of pediatric craniopharyngiomas and in approximately half of adult cases.[94] The cyst content may be isodense to CSF but may also be hyperdense to CSF, reflecting protein content. Nodular or rim enhancement is also commonly seen. On MRI, the cystic component of craniopharyngiomas demonstrate considerable variability. Most commonly, the cyst is hypointense on T_1-weighted images and hyperintense on T_2-weighted images (Fig. 19-15). Increased signal intensity on T_1-weighted images is less common but may reflect high protein concentration or blood degradation products. Considerable contrast enhancement is usually demonstrated in the solid tumor component and cyst wall.

As mentioned, craniopharyngiomas are generally slow-growing neoplasms and the usual time interval between symptom onset and clinical presentation is 1 to 2 years.[269] Clinical presentation is dependent on the tumor's site of origin, vectors of growth, and involvement of surrounding structures. Headache, visual disturbances, and endocrine deficiencies are the most common presenting signs and symptoms.[264,277–279] Headaches may result from local mass effect or from CSF obstruction and hydrocephalus. Visual field loss, diminished acuity, diplopia and other visual deficits result from tumor involvement of the optic apparatus. Endocrine deficiencies result from disturbance of the hypothalamic–pituitary axis and up to 90% of patients may demonstrate deficiencies of one or more hormones at presentation.[262,280] Children commonly present with short stature and decreased growth velocity. Adolescents may report delayed or arrested puberty, whereas adult males may complain of decreased libido and adult females may report menstrual irregularities. Changes in mental status and behavior may also be encountered (although more common in adults) and seizures may also occur.[269]

As for pituitary adenomas, management of craniopharyngiomas requires a multidisciplinary approach. Thorough evaluation, including neurologic, endocrinologic, neuroophthalmologic, and neuropsychological evaluation, is imperative, in addition to oncologic consultation as indicated for adjuvant therapy. Hormonal deficiencies are corrected and hydrocephalus may be managed with either permanent ventriculoperitoneal shunting or temporary CSF diversion with ventriculostomy if surgical resection can correct the underlying obstruction. In general, surgical resection can be attempted through a transcranial or transsphenoidal approach (often an extended skull base transsphenoidal approach with opening of the tuberculum sellae and anterior cranial fossa floor with suprasellar exploration via the transsphenoidal corridor, which is most applicable with smaller, midline tumors). The pattern of tumor burden and extension determines the approach and its trajectory. Many of the principles discussed earlier apply here. A pterional craniotomy with orbital osteotomy is useful for many tumors. Occasionally, when the tumor is located predominantly within the third ventricle, an interhemispheric, transcallosal approach may be undertaken for tumor removal. General surgical principles include decompression of the optic apparatus and removal of CSF outflow obstruction. Experience with adjuvant radiation therapy in cases of subtotal resection is accumulating, and both conventional and stereotactic radiosurgery have demonstrated some efficacy.[281–289] Previously discussed considerations in radiation of the sellar region and its immediate vicinity apply here as well. Stereotactic radiosurgery appears promising for tumors that are less than 3 cm in size with ample distance from the optic chiasm (at least 3 mm or more). New radiation paradigms including fractionated radiosurgery are presently being evaluated. Intracavitary irradiation, involving implantation of beta-emitting isotopes (such as ^{32}P) after cyst aspiration, has also demonstrated some effectiveness in stabilizing or decreasing cyst size (in up to 96% of patients).[290–292] Local or systemic chemotherapy can also be used as adjuvant therapy for recurrent or residual

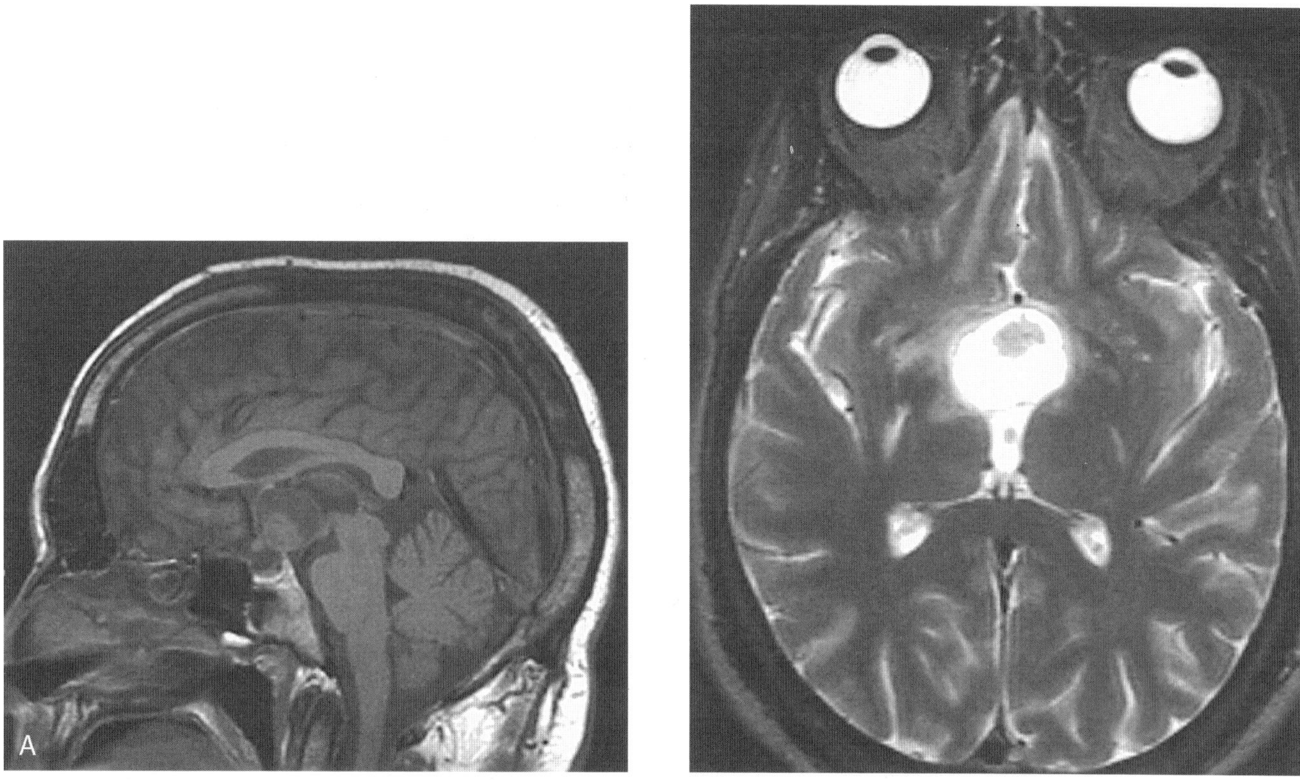

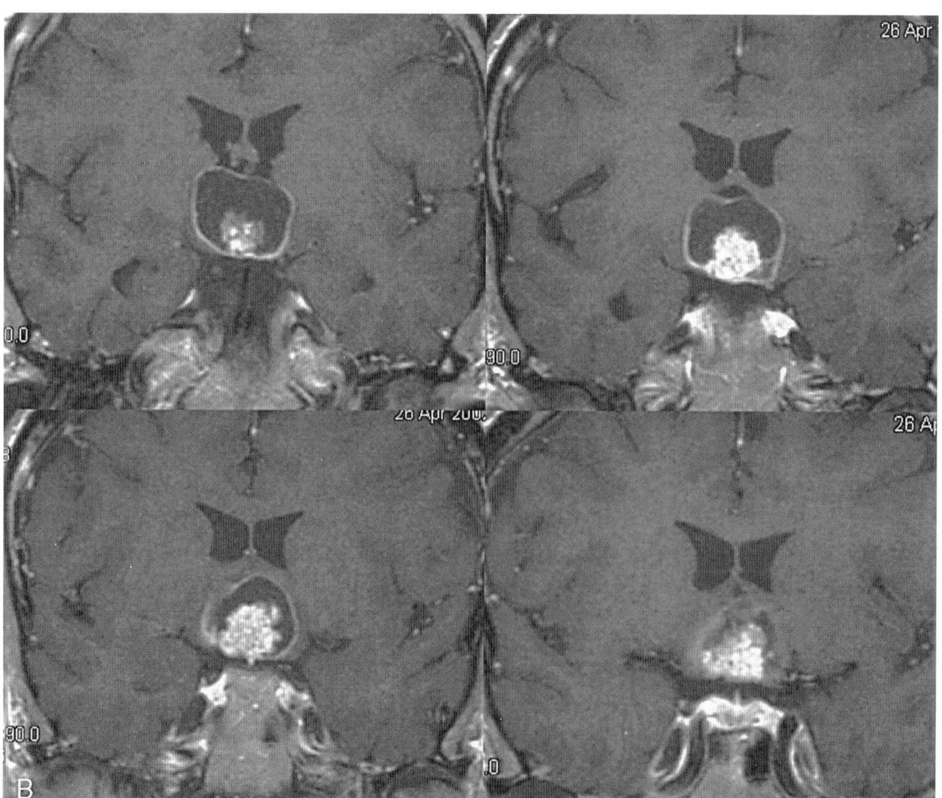

Figure 19-15. Craniopharyngioma. (A) Precontrast sagittal T_1-weighted and axial T_2-weighted MR images revealing a suprasellar mass with a solid and cystic component. The cystic component is hypointense on T_1 and hyperintense on T_2-weighted sequences. (B) Postcontrast coronal T_1-weighted images demonstrating the suprasellar lesion with its enhancing nodule and cyst wall.

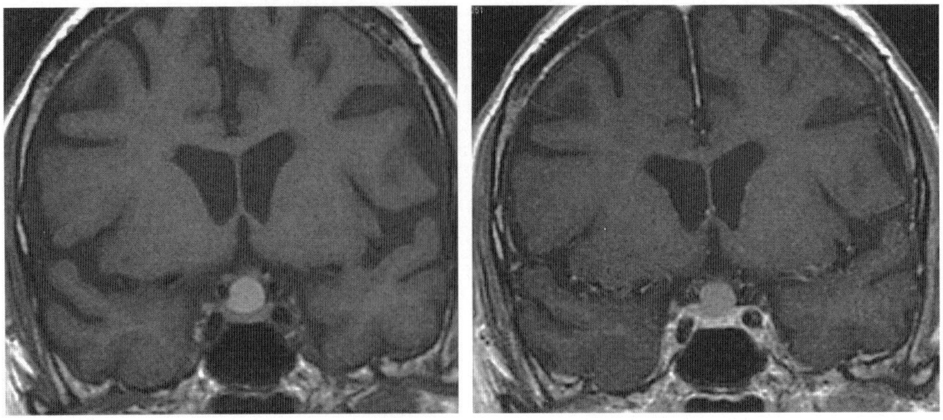

Figure 19-16. Rathke cleft cyst. Pre- (left) and postcontrast (right) T_1-weighted MR images demonstrating a cystic lesion that is hyperintense before contrast on T_1-weighted sequences. It appears to lie above the normal pituitary gland.

tumor; however, its definitive role is unclear and further data are needed. BCNU (1,3-bis (2-chloroethyl)-1-nitrosourea) and procarbazine have been used with some benefit.[293] Additionally, intracavitary chemotherapy (bleomycin[294–297] or carmustine[298]) has been used although the need for further experience is apparent and serious side effects of intracavitary bleomycin may occur.

Despite its benign histology, recurrence following treatment of craniopharyngioma remains relatively common (7%–19% after total resection with long-term followup[269,299]). Moreover, tumor growth is observed in more than 50% of subtotally removed tumors,[269] although this may be reduced to 30% when subtotal resection is combined with adjuvant radiotherapy.[300] Recurrence rates appear lower in adults than in children, perhaps attributable to differences in the histologic variants most common in the respective age groups.[269]

Our approach has generally been to resect as much tumor as safely possible (gross total resection whenever feasible) and to administer adjuvant radiation therapy on an individual case-by-case basis based upon discussion among a comprehensive neuro-oncology team. Repeat debulking is typically performed for recurrences, and other adjuvant therapy such as intracavitary therapy is reserved for recalcitrant cases.

Rathke Cleft Cysts

Rathke cleft cysts are nonneoplastic lesions derived from glandular rests of Rathke pouch (primitive stomodeum) in the region of the intermediate lobe. The rostral elongation of Rathke pouch gives rise to the craniopharyngeal duct whose proximal portion closes early during fetal development leaving a remnant between the pars distalis and pars nervosa.[301,302] This remnant may occasionally give rise to a Rathke cleft cyst. Symptomatic Rathke cleft cysts are uncommon (accounting for less than 1% of intracranial tumor-like masses), but autopsy series demonstrate small asymptomatic cysts in 2% to 26% of individuals.[303] Most lesions are found in adults and a female predilection exists.[302,303] These tumors are typically intra- and suprasellar,[303] whereas isolated suprasellar lesions are rare.[304] Patients harboring symptomatic Rathke cleft cysts may present with visual loss, pituitary dysfunction, or headaches.[303] Most lesions appear hypodense on CT, without calcification and may occasionally exhibit capsule enhancement.[302,303] Most lesions appear hyperintense on T_1-weighted MRI while T_2-weighted signal is more variable[302] (Fig. 19-16). Rathke cleft cysts may but usually do not enhance on MRI although an intensely enhancing rim of normal, compressed pituitary gland may be seen.[305] When symptomatic, Rathke cleft cysts can be treated effectively with transsphenoidal surgery. On pathologic examination, most cysts consist of a lining of pseudostratified or simple columnar epithelium with distinct cilia and scattered goblet cells.[303]

It is noteworthy that both Rathke cleft cysts and craniopharyngiomas are thought to arise from embryonic remnants of Rathke pouch suggesting a common origin. Histologically, these lesions appear to represent two ends of a continuum ranging from the simplest lesion (Rathke cleft cyst), through transitional states, to the most complex lesion (craniopharyngioma).[267]

▶ FUTURE PROSPECTS

Gene therapy may play a role in the future treatment of pituitary adenomas. Rats harboring estrogen-induced prolactinomas were treated with a tetracycline regulated adenovirus carrying the gene for tyrosine hydroxylase (the rate-limiting enzyme in dopamine synthesis). Researchers found a significant reduction in both tumor growth and plasma prolactin levels.[306]

Tissue specific promoters may also play a role in directing gene therapy. Researchers have shown that stereotactically injected recombinant adenoviruses containing the human growth hormone and the human glycoprotein hormone α-subunit promoter can selectively drive the expression of the β-galactosidase gene in cells expressing those hormones.[307,308] Tissue culture experiments have also indicated that these tissue-specific promoters can selectively drive the expression of toxic gene therapy with excellent cytotoxicity to specific pituitary cell lines. Future in vivo studies evaluating the efficacy of tissue-specific promoters that drive the expression of toxic gene therapy agents are anticipated.

▶ CONCLUSION

The management of pituitary adenomas and other sellar lesions must account for both the endocrine and neurologic sequelae of these tumors. Patients require thorough pre- and posttreatment evaluation by neuroendocrinologists, neurosurgeons, neurologists, neuroophthalmologists, and neuroradiologists. Medical therapy is the primary therapy for prolactinomas and recent advances also have brought forward the expectation of effective pharmacotherapy for GH adenomas. Transsphenoidal surgery offers effective relief of mass effect and not only restoration but the preservation of normal endocrine function in the majority of patients. Radiation therapy can offer remission for some patients with medically and surgically refractory tumors. With improved understanding of the molecular pathogenesis, future therapy should more effectively treat these tumors.

REFERENCES

1. Monson JP. The epidemiology of endocrine tumours. Endocr Relat Cancer 2000;7(1):29–36.
2. Annegers JF, Coulam CB, Abboud CF, et al. Pituitary adenoma in Olmsted County, Minnesota 1935–1977. A report of an increasing incidence of diagnosis in women of childbearing age. Mayo Clin Proc 1978;53(10):641–643.
3. Clayton RN. Sporadic pituitary tumours: from epidemiology to use of databases. Best Pract Res Clin Endocrinol Metab 1999;13(3):451–460.
4. Lovaste MG, Ferrari G, Rossi G. Epidemiology of primary intracranial neoplasms. Experiment in the Province of Trento, (Italy) 1977–1984. Neuroepidemiology 1986;5(4):220–232.
5. Percy AK, Elveback LR, Okazaki H, et al. Neoplasms of the central nervous system. Epidemiologic considerations. Neurology 1972;22(1):40–48.
6. Robinson N, Beral V, Ashley JS. Incidence of pituitary adenoma in women [letter]. Lancet 1979;2(8143):630.
7. Costello RT. Subclinical adenoma of the pituitary gland. Am J Pathol 1936;12:205–216.
8. Tomita T, Gates E. Pituitary adenomas and granular cell tumors. Incidence, cell type, and location of tumor in 100 pituitary glands at autopsy. Am J Clin Pathol 1999;111(6):817–825.
9. Burrow GN, Wortzman G, Rewcastle NB, et al. Microadenomas of the pituitary and abnormal sellar tomograms in an unselected autopsy series. N Engl J Med 1981;304(3):156–158.
10. Molitch ME, Russell EJ. The pituitary "incidentaloma." Ann Intern Med 1990;112(12):925–931.
11. Hall JE, Martin KA, Whitney HA, et al. Potential for fertility with replacement of hypothalamic gonadotropin-releasing hormone in long-term female survivors of cranial tumors. J Clin Endocrinol Metab 1994;79(4):1166–1172.
12. Aron DC, Howlett TA. Pituitary incidentalomas. Endocrinol Metab Clin N Am 2000;29(1):205–221.
13. Bills DC, Meyer FB, Laws ER Jr, et al. A retrospective analysis of pituitary apoplexy. Neurosurgery 1993;33(4):602–608; discussion 608–609.
14. Rhoton AL Jr. The sellar region. Neurosurgery 2002;51(Suppl 4):S335–S374.
15. Elias WJ, Chadduck JB, Alden TD, et al. Frameless stereotaxy for transsphenoidal surgery [see comments]. Neurosurgery 1999;45(2):271–275; discussion 275–277.
16. Kaptain GJ, Vincent DA, Sheehan JP, et al. Transsphenoidal approaches for the extracapsular resection of midline suprasellar and anterior cranial base lesions. Neurosurgery 2001;49(1):94–100; discussion 100–101.
17. Johnsen DE, Woodruff WW, Allen IS, et al. MR imaging of the sellar and juxtasellar regions. Radiographics 1991;11(5):727–758.
18. Kucharczyk W, Lenkinski RE, Kucharczyk J, et al. The effect of phospholipid vesicles on the NMR relaxation of water: an explanation for the MR appearance of the neurohypophysis? Am J Neuroradiol 1990;11(4):693–700.
19. Mark LP, Haughton VM, Hendrix LE, et al. High-intensity signals within the posterior pituitary fossa: a study with fat-suppression MR techniques. Am J Neuroradiol 1991;12(3):529–532.
20. Colombo N, Berry I, Kucharczyk J, et al. Posterior pituitary gland: appearance on MR images in normal and pathologic states. Radiology 1987;165(2):481–485.
21. Sato N, Ishizaka H, Yagi H, et al. Posterior lobe of the pituitary in diabetes insipidus: dynamic MR imaging. Radiology 1993;186(2):357–360.
22. Doppman JL, Frank JA, Dwyer AJ, et al. Gadolinium DTPA enhanced MR imaging of ACTH-secreting microadenomas of the pituitary gland. J Comput Assist Tomogr 1988;12(5):728–735.
23. Dwyer AJ, Frank JA, Doppman JL, et al. Pituitary adenomas in patients with Cushing disease: initial experience with Gd-DTPA-enhanced MR imaging. Radiology 1987;163(2):421–426.
24. Guyda H, Robert F, Colle E, et al. Histologic, ultrastructural and hormonal characterization of a pituitary tumor

secreting both HGH and prolactin. J Clin Endocrinol Metab 1973;36(3):531–547.
25. Horvath E, Kovacs K, Scheithauer BW, et al. Pituitary adenomas producing growth hormone, prolactin, and one or more glycoprotein hormones: a histologic, immunohistochemical, and ultrastructural study of four surgically removed tumors. Ultrastruct Pathol 1983;5(2–3):171–183.
26. Landolt AM, Rothenbuhler V. Extracellular growth hormone deposits in pituitary adenoma. Virchows Arch 1978; 378(1):55–65.
27. Kovacs K, Scheithauer BW, Horvath E, et al. The World Health Organization classification of adenohypophysial neoplasms. A proposed five-tier scheme. Cancer 1996; 78(3):502–510.
28. Alexander JM, Biller BM, Bikkal H, et al. Clinically nonfunctioning pituitary tumors are monoclonal in origin. J Clin Invest 1990;86(1):336–340.
29. Herman V, Fagin J, Gonsky R, et al. Clonal origin of pituitary adenomas. J Clin Endocrinol Metab 1990;71(6):1427–1433.
30. Blatt C, Eversole-Cire P, Cohn VH, et al. Chromosomal localization of genes encoding guanine nucleotide-binding protein subunits in mouse and human. Proc Natl Acad Sci U S A 1988;85(20):7642–7646.
31. Thakker RV, Pook MA, Wooding C, et al. Association of somatotrophinomas with loss of alleles on chromosome 11 and with gsp mutations. J Clin Invest 1993;91(6):2815–2821.
32. Boggild MD, Jenkinson S, Pistorello M, et al. Molecular genetic studies of sporadic pituitary tumors. J Clin Endocrinol Metab 1994;78(2):387–392.
33. Clementi E, Malgaretti N, Meldolesi J, et al. A new constitutively activating mutation of the Gs protein alpha subunit-gsp oncogene is found in human pituitary tumours. Oncogene 1990;5(7):1059–1061.
34. Suhardja AS, Kovacs KT, Rutka JT. Molecular pathogenesis of pituitary adenomas: a review. Acta Neurochir 1999; 141(7):729–736.
35. Vallar L, Spada A, Giannattasio G. Altered Gs and adenylate cyclase activity in human GH-secreting pituitary adenomas. Nature 1987;330(6148):566–568.
36. Landis CA, Masters SB, Spada A, et al. GTPase inhibiting mutations activate the alpha chain of Gs and stimulate adenylyl cyclase in human pituitary tumours. Nature 1989;340(6236):692–696.
37. Tordjman K, Stern N, Ouaknine G, et al. Activating mutations of the Gs alpha-gene in nonfunctioning pituitary tumors. J Clin Endocrinol Metab 1993;77(3):765–769.
38. Williamson EA, Daniels M, Foster S, et al. Gs alpha and Gi2 alpha mutations in clinically non-functioning pituitary tumours. Clin Endocrinol 1994;41(6):815–820.
39. Williamson EA, Ince PG, Harrison D, et al. G-protein mutations in human pituitary adrenocorticotropic hormone-secreting adenomas. Eur J Clin Invest 1995;25(2): 128–131.
40. Hibberts NA, Simpson DJ, Bicknell JE, et al. Analysis of cyclin D1 (CCND1) allelic imbalance and overexpression in sporadic human pituitary tumors. Clin Cancer Res 1999;5(8):2133–2139.
41. Jordan S, Lidhar K, Korbonits M, et al. Cyclin D and cyclin E expression in normal and adenomatous pituitary. Eur J Endocrinol 2000;143(1):R1-R6.
42. Cai WY, Alexander JM, Hedley-Whyte ET, et al. ras mutations in human prolactinomas and pituitary carcinomas. J Clin Endocrinol Metab 1994;78(1):89–93.
43. Karga HJ, Alexander JM, Hedley-Whyte ET, et al. Ras mutations in human pituitary tumors. J Clin Endocrinol Metab 1992;74(4):914–919.
44. Pei L, Melmed S, Scheithauer B, et al. H-ras mutations in human pituitary carcinoma metastases. J Clin Endocrinol Metab 1994;78(4):842–846.
45. Wang DG, Johnston CF, Atkinson AB, et al. Expression of bcl-2 oncoprotein in pituitary tumours: comparison with c-myc. J Clin Pathol 1996;49(10):795–797.
46. Woloschak M, Roberts JL, Post K. c-myc, c-fos, and c-myb gene expression in human pituitary adenomas. J Clin Endocrinol Metab 1994;79(1):253–257.
47. Raghavan R, Harrison D, Ince PG, et al. Oncoprotein immunoreactivity in human pituitary tumours. Clin Endocrinol 1994;40(1):117–126.
48. Heaney AP, Melmed S. New pituitary oncogenes. Endocr Relat Cancer 2000;7(1):3–15.
49. Zhang X, Horwitz GA, Heaney AP, et al. Pituitary tumor transforming gene (PTTG) expression in pituitary adenomas. J Clin Endocrinol Metab 1999;84(2):761–767.
50. Heaney AP, Melmed S. Pituitary tumour transforming gene: a novel factor in pituitary tumour formation. Best Pract Res Clin Endocrinol Metab 1999;13(3):367–380.
51. Weil RJ, Vortmeyer AO, Huang S, et al. 11q13 allelic loss in pituitary tumors in patients with multiple endocrine neoplasia syndrome type 1. Clin Cancer Res 1998;4(7): 1673–1678.
52. Bystrom C, Larsson C, Blomberg C, et al. Localization of the MEN1 gene to a small region within chromosome 11q13 by deletion mapping in tumors. Proc Natl Acad Sci U S A 1990;87(5):1968–1972.
53. Eubanks PJ, Sawicki MP, Samara GJ, et al. Putative tumor-suppressor gene on chromosome 11 is important in sporadic endocrine tumor formation. Am J Surg 1994;167(1): 180–185.
54. Bale AE, Norton JA, Wong EL, et al. Allelic loss on chromosome 11 in hereditary and sporadic tumors related to familial multiple endocrine neoplasia type 1. Cancer Res 1991;51(4):1154–1157.
55. Buckley N, Bates AS, Broome JC, et al. p53 Protein accumulates in Cushings adenomas and invasive non-functional adenomas [republished in J Clin Endocrinol Metab 1995;80(2):692–696]. J Clin Endocrinol Metab 1994;79(5):1513–1516.
56. Clayton RN, Boggild M, Bates AS, et al. Tumour suppressor genes in the pathogenesis of human pituitary tumours. Horm Res 1997;47(4–6):185–193.
57. Thapar K, Scheithauer BW, Kovacs K, et al. p53 expression in pituitary adenomas and carcinomas: correlation with invasiveness and tumor growth fractions. Neurosurgery 1996;38(4):763–770; discussion 770–761.
58. Bates AS, Farrell WE, Bicknell EJ, et al. Allelic deletion in pituitary adenomas reflects aggressive biological activity and has potential value as a prognostic marker. J Clin Endocrinol Metab 1997;82(3):818–824.
59. Simpson DJ, Magnay J, Bicknell JE, et al. Chromosome 13q deletion mapping in pituitary tumors: infrequent loss of the retinoblastoma susceptibility gene (RB1) locus

despite loss of RB1 protein product in somatotrophinomas. Cancer Res 1999;59(7):1562–1566.
60. Ingraham HA, Chen RP, Mangalam HJ, et al. A tissue-specific transcription factor containing a homeodomain specifies a pituitary phenotype. Cell 1988;55(3): 519–529.
61. Asa SL, Puy LA, Lew AM, et al. Cell type-specific expression of the pituitary transcription activator pit-1 in the human pituitary and pituitary adenomas. J Clin Endocrinol Metab 1993;77(5):1275–1280.
62. Friend KE, Chiou YK, Laws ER Jr, et al. Pit-1 messenger ribonucleic acid is differentially expressed in human pituitary adenomas. J Clin Endocrinol Metab 1993;77(5):1281–1286.
63. Delhase M, Vergani P, Malur A, et al. Pit-1/GHF-1 expression in pituitary adenomas: further analogy between human adenomas and rat SMtTW tumours. J Mol Endocrinol 1993; 11(2):129–139.
64. Hoggard N, Callaghan K, Levy A, et al. Expression of Pit-1 and related proteins in diverse human pituitary adenomas. J Mol Endocrinol 1993;11(3):283–290.
65. Stefaneanu L, Kovacs K, Horvath E, et al. In situ hybridization study of estrogen receptor messenger ribonucleic acid in human adenohypophysial cells and pituitary adenomas. J Clin Endocrinol Metab 1994;78(1):83–88.
66. Nakao H, Koga M, Arao M, et al. Enzyme-immunoassay for estrogen receptors in human pituitary adenomas. Acta Endocrinologica 1989;120(2):233–238.
67. Friend KE, Chiou YK, Lopes MB, et al. Estrogen receptor expression in human pituitary: correlation with immunohistochemistry in normal tissue, and immunohistochemistry and morphology in macroadenomas. J Clin Endocrinol Metab 1994;78(6):1497–1504.
68. Chernavsky AC, Chervin A, Vitale M, et al. Human pituitary tumours: studies on genes expression. Neurol Res 1993;15(1):2–6.
69. Snyder PJ. Gonadotroph cell adenomas of the pituitary. Endocr Rev 1985;6(4):552–563.
70. Kovacs K, Stefaneanu L, Ezzat S, et al. Prolactin-producing pituitary adenoma in a male-to-female transsexual patient with protracted estrogen administration. A morphologic study. Arch Pathol Lab Med 1994;118(5):562–565.
71. Levy L, Bourdais J, Mouhieddine B, et al. Presence and characterization of the somatostatin precursor in normal human pituitaries and in growth hormone secreting adenomas. J Clin Endocrinol Metab 1993;76(1):85–90.
72. Hashimoto K, Koga M, Motomura T, et al. Identification of alternatively spliced messenger ribonucleic acid encoding truncated growth hormone-releasing hormone receptor in human pituitary adenomas. J Clin Endocrinol Metab 1995;80(10):2933–2939.
73. Alexander JM, Klibanski A. Gonadotropin-releasing hormone receptor mRNA expression by human pituitary tumors in vitro. J Clin Invest 1994;93(6):2332–2339.
74. Suda T, Tozawa F, Dobashi I, et al. Corticotropin-releasing hormone, proopiomelanocortin, and glucocorticoid receptor gene expression in adrenocorticotropin-producing tumors in vitro. J Clin Invest 1993;92(6):2790–2795.
75. Shimon I, Huttner A, Said J, et al. Heparin-binding secretory transforming gene (hst) facilitates rat lactotrope cell tumorigenesis and induces prolactin gene transcription. J Clin Invest 1996;97(1):187–195.
76. Shimon I, Hinton DR, Weiss MH, et al. Prolactinomas express human heparin-binding secretory transforming gene (hst) protein product: marker of tumour invasiveness. Clin Endocrinol 1998;48(1):23–29.
77. Auernhammer CJ, Melmed S. Interleukin-11 stimulates proopiomelanocortin gene expression and adrenocorticotropin secretion in corticotroph cells: evidence for a redundant cytokine network in the hypothalamo-pituitary-adrenal axis. Endocrinology 1999;140(4):1559–1566.
78. Renner U, Gloddek J, Pereda MP, et al. Regulation and role of intrapituitary IL-6 production by folliculostellate cells. Domest Anim Endocrinol 1998;15(5):353–362.
79. Lipper S, Isenberg HD, Kahn LB. Calcospherites in pituitary prolactinomas. A hypothesis for their formation. Arch Pathol Lab Med 1984;108(1):31–34.
80. Burger PC, Scheithaver BW, Vogel FS. Region of the sella turcica. Surgical pathology of the nervous system and its coverings, 4th ed. New York: Churchill Livingstone, 2002: 437–497.
81. Sanno N, Teramoto A, Osamura RY, et al. Pathology of pituitary tumors. Neurosurg Clin N Am 2003;14(1):25–39, vi.
82. Kovacs K. The pathology of Cushing's disease. J Steroid Biochem Mol Biol 1993;45(1–3):179–182.
83. George DH, Scheithauer BW, Kovacs K, et al. Crooke's cell adenoma of the pituitary: an aggressive variant of corticotroph adenoma. Am J Surg Pathol 2003;27(10): 1330–1336.
84. Ho DM, Hsu CY, Ting LT, et al. The clinicopathological characteristics of gonadotroph cell adenoma: a study of 118 cases. Hum Pathol 1997;28(8):905–911.
85. Esiri MM, Adams CB, Burke C, et al. Pituitary adenomas: immunohistology and ultrastructural analysis of 118 tumors. Acta Neuropathol (Berl) 1983;62(1–2):1–14.
86. Horvath E, Kovacs K. Gonadotroph adenomas of the human pituitary: sex-related fine-structural dichotomy. A histologic, immunocytochemical, and electron-microscopic study of 30 tumors. Am J Pathol 1984;117(3):429–440.
87. Ebersold MJ, Quast LM, Laws ER Jr, et al. Long-term results in transsphenoidal removal of nonfunctioning pituitary adenomas. J Neurosurg 1986;64(5):713–719.
88. Holm R. Null cell adenomas and oncocytomas of the pituitary gland. Pathol Res Pract 1995;191(4):348–352.
89. Kucharczyk W, Davis DO, Kelly WM, et al. Pituitary adenomas: high-resolution MR imaging at 1.5 T. Radiology 1986;161(3):761–765.
90. Ostrov SG, Quencer RM, Hoffman JC, et al. Hemorrhage within pituitary adenomas: how often associated with pituitary apoplexy syndrome? Am J Roentgenol 1989;153(1): 153–160.
91. Dina TS, Feaster SH, Laws ER Jr, et al. MR of the pituitary gland postsurgery: serial MR studies following transsphenoidal resection. Am J Neuroradiol 1993;14(3):763–769.
92. Steiner E, Math G, Knosp E, et al. MR-appearance of the pituitary gland before and after resection of pituitary macroadenomas. Clin Radiol 1994;49(8):524–530.
93. Steiner E, Knosp E, Herold CJ, et al. Pituitary adenomas: findings of postoperative MR imaging. Radiology 1992;185(2): 521–527.

94. Zee CS, Go JL, Kim PE, et al. Imaging of the pituitary and parasellar region. Neurosurg Clin N Am 2003;14(1):55–80, vi.
95. Feldkamp J, Santen R, Harms E, et al. Incidentally discovered pituitary lesions: high frequency of macroadenomas and hormone-secreting adenomas—results of a prospective study. Clin Endocrinol 1999;51(1):109–113.
96. Nishizawa S, Ohta S, Yokoyama T, et al. Therapeutic strategy for incidentally found pituitary tumors ("pituitary incidentalomas"). Neurosurgery 1998;43(6):1344–1348; discussion 1348–1350.
97. Sanno N, Oyama K, Tahara S, et al. A survey of pituitary incidentaloma in Japan. Eur J Endocrinol 2003;149(2):123–127.
98. Donovan LE, Corenblum B. The natural history of the pituitary incidentaloma. Arch Intern Med 1995;155(2): 181–183.
99. Molitch ME. Clinical review 65. Evaluation and treatment of the patient with a pituitary incidentaloma. J Clin Endocrinol Metab 1995;80(1):3–6.
100. Molitch ME, Russell EJ. The pituitary "incidentaloma." Ann Intern Med 1990;112(12):925–931.
101. Reincke M, Allolio B, Saeger W, et al. The "incidentaloma" of the pituitary gland. Is neurosurgery required? JAMA 1990;263(20):2772–2776.
102. Molitch ME, Thorner MO, Wilson C. Management of prolactinomas. J Clin Endocrinol Metab 1997;82(4):996–1000.
103. Horvath E, Scheitauer BW, Kovacs K, et al. Regional neuropathology: hypothalamus and pituitary. In: Lantos PL, ed. Greenfield's neuropathology. New York: Oxford University Press, 1997:1027–1035.
104. Laws ER, Jane JA Jr. Pituitary tumors—long-term outcomes and expectations. Clin Neurosurg 2001;48:306–319.
105. Arafah BM, Nasrallah MP. Pituitary tumors: pathophysiology, clinical manifestations and management. Endocr Relat Cancer 2001;8(4):287–305.
106. Samuels MH, Ridgway EC. Glycoprotein-secreting pituitary adenomas. Baillieres Clin Endocrinol Metab 1995;9(2): 337–358.
107. Snyder PJ. Extensive personal experience: gonadotroph adenomas. J Clin Endocrinol Metab 1995;80(4):1059–1061.
108. Daneshdoost L, Gennarelli TA, Bashey HM, et al. Recognition of gonadotroph adenomas in women [comment]. N Engl J Med 1991;324(9):589–594.
109. Daneshdoost L, Gennarelli TA, Bashey HM, et al. Identification of gonadotroph adenomas in men with clinically nonfunctioning adenomas by the luteinizing hormone beta subunit response to thyrotropin-releasing hormone. J Clin Endocrinol Metab 1993;77(5):1352–1355.
110. Colao A, Cerbone G, Cappabianca P, et al. Effect of surgery and radiotherapy on visual and endocrine function in nonfunctioning pituitary adenomas. J Endocrinol Invest 1998;21(5):284–290.
111. Kurosaki M, Ludecke DK, Flitsch J, et al. Surgical treatment of clinically nonsecreting pituitary adenomas in elderly patients. Neurosurgery 2000;47(4):843–848; discussion 848–849.
112. Laws ER, Jane JA Jr. Pituitary tumors—long-term outcomes and expectations. Clin Neurosurg 2001;48:306–319.
113. Webb SM, Rigla M, Wagner A, et al. Recovery of hypopituitarism after neurosurgical treatment of pituitary adenomas. J Clin Endocrinol Metab 1999;84(10):3696–3700.
114. Arita K, Uozumi T, Yano T, et al. Effect of surgery on gonadal function of premenopausal women with pituitary adenomas other than prolactinomas. Endocr J 1996;43(2): 131–138.
115. Laws ER Jr, Thapar K. Pituitary surgery. Endocrinol Metab Clin N Am 1999;28(1):119–131.
116. Hensen J, Henig A, Fahlbusch R, et al. Prevalence, predictors and patterns of postoperative polyuria and hyponatraemia in the immediate course after transsphenoidal surgery for pituitary adenomas. Clin Endocrinol 1999;50(4): 431–439.
117. Woollons AC, Balakrishnan V, Hunn MK, et al. Complications of trans-sphenoidal surgery: the Wellington experience. Aust N Z J Surg 2000;70(6):405–408.
118. Ciric I, Ragin A, Baumgartner C, Pierce D. Complications of transsphenoidal surgery: results of a national survey, review of the literature, and personal experience. Neurosurgery 1997;40(2):225–236; discussion 236–227.
119. Losa M, Franzin A, Mangili F, et al. Proliferation index of nonfunctioning pituitary adenomas: correlations with clinical characteristics and long-term follow-up results. Neurosurgery 2000;47(6):1313–1318; discussion 1318–1319.
120. Turner HE, Stratton IM, Byrne JV, et al. Audit of selected patients with nonfunctioning pituitary adenomas treated without irradiation—a follow-up study. Clin Endocrinol 1999;51(3):281–284.
121. Babinski JFF. Tumeur du corps pituitaire sans acromegalie et avect arret de developpement des organes genitaux. Rev Neurol 1900;8:531.
122. Barrande G, Pittino-Lungo M, Coste J, et al. Hormonal and metabolic effects of radiotherapy in acromegaly: long-term results in 128 patients followed in a single center. J Clin Endocrinol Metab 2000;85(10):3779–3785.
123. Biermasz NR, van Dulken H, Roelfsema F. Long-term follow-up results of postoperative radiotherapy in 36 patients with acromegaly. J Clin Endocrinol Metab 2000;85(7): 2476–2482.
124. Levy RP, Fabrikant JI, Frankel KA, et al. Heavy-charged-particle radiosurgery of the pituitary gland: clinical results of 840 patients. Stereotact Funct Neurosurg 1991;57(1–2): 22–35.
125. Rocher FP, Sentenac I, Berger C, et al. Stereotactic radiosurgery: the Lyon experience. Acta Neurochir (Wien) 1995;63:109–114.
126. Lunsford LD, Witt TC, Kondziolka D, et al. Stereotactic radiosurgery of anterior skull base tumors. Clin Neurosurg 1995;42:99–118.
127. Voges J, Sturm V, Deuss U, et al. LINAC-radiosurgery (LINAC-RS) in pituitary adenomas: preliminary results. Acta Neurochir (Wien) 1996;65:41–43.
128. Tsang RW, Brierley JD, Panzarella T, et al. Radiation therapy for pituitary adenoma: treatment outcome and prognostic factors. Int J Radiat Oncol Biol Phys 1994;30(3): 557–565.
129. Tsang RW, Brierley JD, Panzarella T, et al. Role of radiation therapy in clinical hormonally active pituitary adenomas. Radiother Oncol 1996;41(1):45–53.
130. Peillon F, Racadot J, Moussy D, et al. Prolactin-secreting adenomas. A correlative study of morphological and

clinical data. In: von Werder K, ed. Treatment of pituitary adenomas. Stuttgart: Georg Thieme, 1978:114.
131. Mindermann T, Wilson CB. Age-related and gender-related occurrence of pituitary adenomas [erratum appears in Clin Endocrinol (Oxf) 1994;41(5):700]. Clin Endocrinol (Oxf) 1994;41(3):359–364.
132. St-Jean E, Blain F, Comtois R. High prolactin levels may be missed by immunoradiometric assay in patients with macroprolactinomas. Clin Endocrinol 1996;44(3):305–309.
133. Acquati S, Pizzocaro A, Tomei G, et al. A comparative evaluation of effectiveness of medical and surgical therapy in patients with macroprolactinoma. J Neurosurg Sci 2001;45(2):65–69.
134. Molitch ME, Elton RL, Blackwell RE, et al. Bromocriptine as primary therapy for prolactin-secreting macroadenomas: results of a prospective multicenter study. J Clin Endocrinol Metab 1985;60(4):698–705.
135. Liuzzi A, Dallabonzana D, Oppizzi G, et al. Low doses of dopamine agonists in the long-term treatment of macroprolactinomas. N Engl J Med 1985;313(11):656–659.
136. Webster J, Piscitelli G, Polli A, et al. A comparison of cabergoline and bromocriptine in the treatment of hyperprolactinemic amenorrhea. Cabergoline Comparative Study Group. N Engl J Med 1994;331(14):904–909.
137. Vance ML. Medical treatment of functional pituitary tumors. Neurosurg Clin N Am 2003;14(1):81–87.
138. Turkalj I, Braun P, Krupp P. Surveillance of bromocriptine in pregnancy. JAMA 1982;247(11):1589–1591.
139. Robert E, Musatti L, Piscitelli G, et al. Pregnancy outcome after treatment with the ergot derivative, cabergoline. Reprod Toxicol 1996;10(4):333–337.
140. Gokalp HZ, Deda H, Attar A, et al. The neurosurgical management of prolactinomas. J Neurosurg Sci 2000;44(3): 128–132.
141. Randall RV, Laws ER Jr, Abboud CF, et al. Transsphenoidal microsurgical treatment of prolactin-producing pituitary adenomas. Results in 100 patients. Best Pract Res Clin Endocrinol Metab 1983;58(2):108–121.
142. Molitch ME. Pathologic hyperprolactinemia. Endocrinol Metab Clin N Am 1992;21(4):877–901.
143. Feigenbaum SL, Downey DE, Wilson CB, et al. Transsphenoidal pituitary resection for preoperative diagnosis of prolactin-secreting pituitary adenoma in women: long-term follow-up. J Clin Endocrinol Metab 1996;81(5):1711–1719.
144. Tsagarakis S, Grossman A, Plowman PN, et al. Megavoltage pituitary irradiation in the management of prolactinomas: long-term follow-up. Clin Endocrinol 1991;34(5):399–406.
145. Jane JA Jr, Vance ML, Woodburn BS, et al. Stereotactic radiosurgery for hypersecreting pituitary tumors: part of a multimodality approach. Neurosurg Focus 2003;14(5): Article 12.
146. Plowman PN. Radiotherapy for pituitary tumours. Baillieres Clin Endocrinol Metab 1995;9(2):407–420.
147. Wilson CB. A decade of pituitary microsurgery. The Herbert Olivecrona lecture. J Neurosurg 1984;61(5):814–833.
148. Scheithauer BW. Surgical pathology of the pituitary: the adenomas. Part II. Pathol Ann 1984;19(Pt 2):269–329.
149. Scheithauer BW. Surgical pathology of the pituitary: the adenomas. Part I. Pathol Ann 1984;19(Pt 1):317–374.
150. Lissett CA, Peacey SR, Laing I, et al. The outcome of surgery for acromegaly: the need for a specialist pituitary surgeon for all types of growth hormone (GH) secreting adenoma. Clin Endocrinol 1998;49(5):653–657.
151. Alexander L, Appleton D, Hall R, et al. Epidemiology of acromegaly in the Newcastle region. Clin Endocrinol 1980; 12(1):71–79.
152. Etxabe J, Gaztambide S, Latorre P, et al. Acromegaly: an epidemiological study. J Endocrinol Invest 1993;16(3): 181–187.
153. Ritchie CM, Atkinson AB, Kennedy AL, et al. Ascertainment and natural history of treated acromegaly in Northern Ireland. Ulster Med J 1990;59(1):55–62.
154. Robert F. Pituitary adenoma in acromegaly-gigantism. Macroscopic, histological and ultrastructural study. Neurochirurgie 1973;19(2)(Suppl 2):117–162.
155. Trouillas J, Girod C, Lheritier M, et al. Morphological and biochemical relationships in 31 human pituitary adenomas with acromegaly. Virchows Archiv A 1980;389(2):127–142.
156. Scheithauer BW, Horvath E, Kovacs K, et al. Plurihormonal pituitary adenomas. Semin Diagn Pathol 1986;3(1):69–82.
157. Ituarte EM, Petrini J, Hershman JM. Acromegaly and colon cancer. Ann Intern Med 1984;101(5):627–628.
158. Orme SM, McNally RJ, Cartwright RA, et al. Mortality and cancer incidence in acromegaly: a retrospective cohort study. United Kingdom Acromegaly Study Group. J Neurosurg 1998;83(8):2730–2734.
159. Popovic V, Damjanovic S, Micic D, et al. Increased incidence of neoplasia in patients with pituitary adenomas. The Pituitary Study Group. Clin Endocrinol 1998;49(4): 441–445.
160. Bengtsson BA, Eden S, Ernest I, et al. Epidemiology and long-term survival in acromegaly. A study of 166 cases diagnosed between 1955 and 1984. Acta Med Scand 1988; 223(4):327–335.
161. Giustina A, Barkan A, Casanueva FF, et al. Criteria for cure of acromegaly: a consensus statement. J Neurosurg 2000; 85(2):526–529.
162. Freda PU, Wardlaw SL, Post KD. Long-term endocrinological follow-up evaluation in 115 patients who underwent transsphenoidal surgery for acromegaly. J Neurosurg 1998;89(3):353–358.
163. Laws ER, Vance ML, Thapar K. Pituitary surgery for the management of acromegaly. Horm Res 2000;53(Suppl 3): 71–75.
164. Shimon I, Cohen ZR, Ram Z, et al. Transsphenoidal surgery for acromegaly: endocrinological follow-up of 98 patients. Neurosurgery 2001;48(6):1239–1243.
165. Kreutzer J, Vance ML, Lopes MB, et al. Surgical management of GH-secreting pituitary adenomas: an outcome study using modern remission criteria. J Clin Endocrinol Metab 2001;86(9):4072–4077.
166. Melmed S, Jackson I, Kleinberg D, et al. Current treatment guidelines for acromegaly. J Neurosurg 1998;83(8): 2646–2652.
167. Gittoes NJ, Sheppard MC, Johnson AP, et al. Outcome of surgery for acromegaly—the experience of a dedicated pituitary surgeon. QJM 1999;92(12):741–745.
168. Swearingen B, Barker FG 2nd, Katznelson L, et al. Long-term mortality after transsphenoidal surgery and adjunctive therapy for acromegaly. J Neurosurg 1998;83(10): 3419–3426.

169. Laws ER Jr. Acromegaly and gigantism. In: Rengachary SS, ed. Neurosurgery, vol 1, 2nd ed. New York: McGraw-Hill, 1996:1317–1320.
170. Laws ER Jr. Craniopharyngioma: transsphenoidal surgery. Curr Ther Endocrinol Metab 1997;6:35–38.
171. Davis DH, Laws ER Jr, Ilstrup DM, et al. Results of surgical treatment for growth hormone-secreting pituitary adenomas. J Neurosurg 1993;79(1):70–75.
172. Minniti G, Moroni C, Jaffrain-Rea ML, et al. Marked improvement in cardiovascular function after successful transsphenoidal surgery in acromegalic patients. Clin Endocrinol 2001;55(3):307–313.
173. Colao A, Cuocolo A, Marzullo P, et al. Impact of patient's age and disease duration on cardiac performance in acromegaly: a radionuclide angiography study. J Neurosurg 1999;84(5):1518–1523.
174. Plewe G, Beyer J, Krause U, et al. Long-acting and selective suppression of growth hormone secretion by somatostatin analogue SMS 201–995 in acromegaly. Lancet 1984;2(8406):782–784.
175. Biermasz NR, van Dulken H, Roelfsema F. Direct postoperative and follow-up results of transsphenoidal surgery in 19 acromegalic patients pretreated with octreotide compared to those in untreated matched controls. J Clin Endocrinol Metab 1999;84(10):3551–3555.
176. Abe T, Ludecke DK. Effects of preoperative octreotide treatment on different subtypes of 90 GH-secreting pituitary adenomas and outcome in one surgical centre. Eur J Endocrinol 2001;145(2):137–145.
177. Kristof RA, Stoffel-Wagner B, Klingmuller D, et al. Does octreotide treatment improve the surgical results of macro-adenomas in acromegaly? A randomized study. Acta Neurochir 1999;141(4):399–405.
178. Colao A, Ferone D, Cappabianca P, et al. Effect of octreotide pretreatment on surgical outcome in acromegaly. J Neurosurg 1997;82(10):3308–3314.
179. Sheaves R, Jenkins P, Blackburn P, et al. Outcome of transsphenoidal surgery for acromegaly using strict criteria for surgical cure. Clin Endocrinol 1996;45(4):407–413.
180. Valdemarsson S, Ljunggren S, Bramnert M, et al. Early postoperative growth hormone levels: high predictive value for long-term outcome after surgery for acromegaly. J Intern Med 2000;247(6):640–650.
181. Colao A, Ferone D, Marzullo P, et al. Effect of different dopaminergic agents in the treatment of acromegaly. J Neurosurg 1997;82(2):518–523.
182. Abs R, Verhelst J, Maiter D, et al. Cabergoline in the treatment of acromegaly: a study in 64 patients. J Neurosurg 1998;83(2):374–378.
183. Jaffe CA, Barkan AL. Treatment of acromegaly with dopamine agonists. Endocrinol Metab Clin N Am 1992; 21(3):713–735.
184. Cozzi R, Attanasio R, Barausse M, et al. Cabergoline in acromegaly: a renewed role for dopamine agonist treatment? Eur J Endocrinol 1998;139(5):516–521.
185. Wass JA, Thorner MO, Morris DV, et al. Long-term treatment of acromegaly with bromocriptine. Br Med J 1977;1(6065): 875–878.
186. Newman CB. Medical therapy for acromegaly. Endocrinol Metab Clin N Am 1999;28(1):171–190.
187. Lamberts SW, van der Lely AJ, de Herder WW, et al. Octreotide. N Engl J Med 1996;334(4):246–254.
188. Colao A, Ferone D, Marzullo P, et al. Long-term effects of depot long-acting somatostatin analog octreotide on hormone levels and tumor mass in acromegaly. J Clin Endocrinol Metab 2001;86(6):2779–2786.
189. Caron P, Arlot S, Bauters C, et al. Efficacy of the long-acting octreotide formulation (octreotide-LAR) in patients with thyrotropin-secreting pituitary adenomas. J Clin Endocrinol Metab 2001;86(6):2849–2853.
190. Baldelli R, Colao A, Razzore P, et al. Two-year follow-up of acromegalic patients treated with slow release lanreotide (30 mg). J Clin Endocrinol Metab 2000;85(11): 4099–4103.
191. Cannavo S, Squadrito S, Curto L, et al. Results of a two-year treatment with slow release lanreotide in acromegaly. Horm Metab Res 2000;32(6):224–229.
192. Barkan AL. New options for diagnosing and treating acromegaly. Cleve Clin J Med 1998;65(7):343,347–349.
193. Melmed S. Acromegaly. N Engl J Med 1990;322(14): 966–977.
194. Trainer PJ, Drake WM, Katznelson L, et al. Treatment of acromegaly with the growth hormone-receptor antagonist pegvisomant. N Engl J Med 2000;342(16):1171–1177.
195. Parkinson C, Trainer PJ. Growth hormone receptor antagonists therapy for acromegaly. Best Pract Res Clin Endocrinol Metab 1999;13(3):419–430.
196. Drake WM, Parkinson C, Akker SA, et al. Successful treatment of resistant acromegaly with a growth hormone receptor antagonist. Eur J Endocrinol 2001;145(4):451–456.
197. Herman-Bonert VS, Zib K, Scarlett JA, et al. Growth hormone receptor antagonist therapy in acromegalic patients resistant to somatostatin analogs. J Clin Endocrinol Metab 2000;85(8):2958–2961.
198. Cozzi R, Barausse M, Asnaghi D, et al. Failure of radiotherapy in acromegaly. Eur J Endocrinol 2001;145(6):717–726.
199. Powell JS, Wardlaw SL, Post KD, et al. Outcome of radiotherapy for acromegaly using normalization of insulin-like growth factor I to define cure. J Neurosurg 2000;85(5): 2068–2071.
200. Morange-Ramos I, Regis J, Dufour H, et al. Gamma-knife surgery for secreting pituitary adenomas. Acta Neurochir 1998;140(5):437–443.
201. Landolt AM, Haller D, Lomax N, et al. Stereotactic radiosurgery for recurrent surgically treated acromegaly: comparison with fractionated radiotherapy. J Neurosurg 1998;88(6): 1002–1008.
202. Tsigos C, Papanicolaou DA, Chrousos GP. Advances in the diagnosis and treatment of Cushing's syndrome. Baillieres Clin Endocrinol Metab 1995;9(2):315–336.
203. Howlett TA, Drury PL, Perry L, et al. Diagnosis and management of ACTH-dependent Cushing's syndrome: comparison of the features in ectopic and pituitary ACTH production. Clin Endocrinol 1986;24(6):699–713.
204. Etxabe J, Vazquez JA. Morbidity and mortality in Cushing's disease: an epidemiological approach. Clin Endocrinol 1994;40(4):479–484.
205. Sandler LM, Richards NT, Carr DH, et al. Long term follow-up of patients with Cushing's disease treated by interstitial irradiation. J Neurosurg 1987;65(3):441–447.

206. Kirkman S, Nelson DH. Alcohol-induced pseudo-Cushing's disease: a study of prevalence with review of the literature. Metabolism 1988;37(4):390–394.
207. Newell-Price J, Trainer P, Besser M, et al. The diagnosis and differential diagnosis of Cushing's syndrome and pseudo-Cushing's states. Endocr Rev 1998;19(5):647–672.
208. Tsigos C, Chrousos GP. Differential diagnosis and management of Cushing's syndrome. Annu Rev Med 1996;47:443–461.
209. Cizza G, Nieman LK, Doppman JL, et al. Factitious Cushing syndrome. J Neurosurg 1996;81(10):3573–3577.
210. Mengden T, Hubmann P, Muller J, et al. Urinary free cortisol versus 17-hydroxycorticosteroids: a comparative study of their diagnostic value in Cushing's syndrome. Clin Invest 1992;70(7):545–548.
211. Wood PJ, Barth JH, Freedman DB, et al. Evidence for the low dose dexamethasone suppression test to screen for Cushing's syndrome—recommendations for a protocol for biochemistry laboratories. Ann Clin Biochem 1997;34(Pt 3):222–229.
212. Newell-Price J, Trainer P, Perry L, et al. A single sleeping midnight cortisol has 100% sensitivity for the diagnosis of Cushing's syndrome. Clin Endocrinol 1995;43(5):545–550.
213. Yanovski JA, Cutler GB Jr, Chrousos GP, et al. Corticotropin-releasing hormone stimulation following low-dose dexamethasone administration. A new test to distinguish Cushing's syndrome from pseudo-Cushing's states. JAMA 1993;269(17):2232–2238.
214. Raff H, Findling JW. A new immunoradiometric assay for corticotropin evaluated in normal subjects and patients with Cushing's syndrome. Clin Chem 1989;35(4):596–600.
215. Orth DN. Cushing's syndrome [erratum appears in N Engl J Med 1995;332(22):1527]. N Engl J Med 1995;332(12):791–803.
216. Dichek HL, Nieman LK, Oldfield EH, et al. A comparison of the standard high dose dexamethasone suppression test and the overnight 8-mg dexamethasone suppression test for the differential diagnosis of adrenocorticotropin-dependent Cushing's syndrome. J Neurosurg 1994;78(2):418–422.
217. Flack MR, Oldfield EH, Cutler GB Jr, et al. Urine free cortisol in the high-dose dexamethasone suppression test for the differential diagnosis of the Cushing syndrome. Ann Intern Med 1992;116(3):211–217.
218. Avgerinos PC, Nieman LK, Oldfield EH, et al. A comparison of the overnight and the standard metyrapone test for the differential diagnosis of adrenocorticotropin-dependent Cushing's syndrome. Clin Endocrinol 1996;45(4):483–491.
219. Avgerinos PC, Yanovski JA, Oldfield EH, et al. The metyrapone and dexamethasone suppression tests for the differential diagnosis of the adrenocorticotropin-dependent Cushing syndrome: a comparison. Ann Intern Med 1994;121(5):318–327.
220. Nieman LK, Oldfield EH, Wesley R, et al. A simplified morning ovine corticotropin-releasing hormone stimulation test for the differential diagnosis of adrenocorticotropin-dependent Cushing's syndrome. J Neurosurg 1993;77(5):1308–1312.
221. Kaye TB, Crapo L. The Cushing syndrome: an update on diagnostic tests. Ann Intern Med 1990;112(6):434–444.
222. Oldfield EH, Doppman JL, Nieman LK, et al. Petrosal sinus sampling with and without corticotropin-releasing hormone for the differential diagnosis of Cushing's syndrome. N Engl J Med 1991;325(13):897–905.
223. Oldfield EH, Girton ME, Doppman JL. Absence of intercavernous venous mixing: evidence supporting lateralization of pituitary microadenomas by venous sampling. J Neurosurg 1985;61(4):644–647.
224. Oldfield EH, Chrousos GP, Schulte HM, et al. Preoperative lateralization of ACTH-secreting pituitary microadenomas by bilateral and simultaneous inferior petrosal venous sinus sampling. N Engl J Med 1985;312(2):100–103.
225. Trainer PJ, Grossman A. The diagnosis and differential diagnosis of Cushing's syndrome. Clin Endocrinol 1991;34(4):317–330.
226. Corrigan DF, Schaaf M, Whaley RA, et al. Selective venous sampling to differentiate ectopic ACTH secretion from pituitary Cushing's syndrome. N Engl J Med 1977;296(15):861–862.
227. Colao A, Faggiano A, Pivonello R, et al. Inferior petrosal sinus sampling in the differential diagnosis of Cushing's syndrome: results of an Italian multicenter study. Eur J Endocrinol 2001;144(5):499–507.
228. Bonelli FS, Huston J 3rd, Carpenter PC, et al. Adrenocorticotropic hormone-dependent Cushing's syndrome: sensitivity and specificity of inferior petrosal sinus sampling. Am J Neuroradiol 2000;21(4):690–696.
229. Wiggam MI, Heaney AP, McIlrath EM, et al. Bilateral inferior petrosal sinus sampling in the differential diagnosis of adrenocorticotropin-dependent Cushing's syndrome: a comparison with other diagnostic tests. J Clin Endocrinol Metab 2000;85(4):1525–1532.
230. Semple PL, Vance ML, Findling J, et al. Transsphenoidal surgery for Cushing's disease: outcome in patients with a normal magnetic resonance imaging scan. Neurosurgery 2000;46(3):553–558; discussion 558–559.
231. Lopez J, Barcelo B, Lucas T, et al. Petrosal sinus sampling for diagnosis of Cushing's disease: evidence of false negative results. Clin Endocrinol 1996;45(2):147–156.
232. Lienhardt A, Grossman AB, Dacie JE, et al. Relative contributions of inferior petrosal sinus sampling and pituitary imaging in the investigation of children and adolescents with ACTH-dependent Cushing's syndrome. J Clin Endocrinol Metab 2001;86(12):5711–5714.
233. Blevins LS, Christy JH, Khajavi M, et al. Outcomes of therapy for Cushing's disease due to adrenocorticotropin-secreting pituitary macroadenomas. J Clin Endocrinol Metab 1998;83(1):63–67.
234. Yap LB, Turner HE, Adams CB, et al. Undetectable postoperative cortisol does not always predict long-term remission in Cushing's disease: a single centre audit. Clin Endocrinol 2002;56(1):25–31.
235. Chee GH, Mathias DB, James RA, et al. Transsphenoidal pituitary surgery in Cushing's disease: can we predict outcome? Clin Endocrinol 2001;54(5):617–626.
236. Simmons NE, Alden TD, Thorner MO, et al. Serum cortisol response to transsphenoidal surgery for Cushing disease. J Neurosurg 2001;95(1):1–8.
237. Sheehan JM, Lopes MB, Sheehan JP, et al. Results of transsphenoidal surgery for Cushing's disease in patients

with no histologically confirmed tumor. Neurosurgery 2000;47(1):33–36; discussion 37–39.
238. Invitti C, Giraldi FP, de Martin M, et al. Diagnosis and management of Cushing's syndrome: results of an Italian multicentre study. Study group of the Italian Society of Endocrinology on the Pathophysiology of the Hypothalamic-Pituitary-Adrenal Axis. J Neurosurg 1999;84(2):440–448.
239. Chou SC, Lin JD. Long-term effects of ketoconazole in the treatment of residual or recurrent Cushing's disease. Endocr J 2000;47(4):401–406.
240. Sonino N, Boscaro M. Medical therapy for Cushing's disease. Endocrinol Metab Clin N Am 1999;28(1):211–222.
241. Sonino N, Boscaro M, Paoletta A, et al. Ketoconazole treatment in Cushing's syndrome: experience in 34 patients. Clin Endocrinol 1991;35(4):347–352.
242. Savage MO, Lienhardt A, Lebrethon MC, et al. Cushing's disease in childhood: presentation, investigation, treatment and long-term outcome. Horm Res 2001;55(Suppl 1):24–30.
243. Estrada J, Boronat M, Mielgo M, et al. The long-term outcome of pituitary irradiation after unsuccessful transsphenoidal surgery in Cushing's disease. N Engl J Med 1997;336(3):172–177.
244. Degerblad M, Rahn T, Bergstrand G, et al. Long-term results of stereotactic radiosurgery to the pituitary gland in Cushing's disease. Acta Endocrinol 1986;112(3):310–314.
245. Sheehan JM, Vance ML, Sheehan JP, et al. Radiosurgery for Cushing's disease after failed transsphenoidal surgery. J Neurosurg 2000;93(5):738–742.
246. Shin M, Kurita H, Sasaki T, et al. Stereotactic radiosurgery for pituitary adenoma invading the cavernous sinus. J Neurosurg 2000;93(Suppl 3):2–5.
247. Saeger W, Ludecke DK. Pituitary adenomas with hyperfunction of TSH. Frequency, histological classification, immunocytochemistry and ultrastructure. Virchows Archiv A 1982;394(3):255–267.
248. Brucker-Davis F, Oldfield EH, Skarulis MC, et al. Thyrotropin-secreting pituitary tumors: diagnostic criteria, thyroid hormone sensitivity, and treatment outcome in 25 patients followed at the National Institutes of Health. J Clin Endocrinol Metab 1999;84(2):476–486.
249. Gesundheit N, Petrick PA, Nissim M, et al. Thyrotropin-secreting pituitary adenomas: clinical and biochemical heterogeneity. Case reports and follow-up of nine patients. Ann Intern Med 1989;111(10):827–835.
250. Losa M, Mortini P, Franzin A, et al. Surgical management of thyrotropin-secreting pituitary adenomas. Pituitary 1999;2(2):127–131.
251. Sanno N, Teramoto A, Osamura RY. Long-term surgical outcome in 16 patients with thyrotropin pituitary adenoma. J Neurosurg 2000;93(2):194–200.
252. Comi RJ, Gesundheit N, Murray L, et al. Response of thyrotropin-secreting pituitary adenomas to a long-acting somatostatin analogue. N Engl J Med 1987;317(1):12–17.
253. Chanson P, Weintraub BD, Harris AG. Octreotide therapy for thyroid-stimulating hormone-secreting pituitary adenomas. A follow-up of 52 patients. Ann Intern Med 1993;119(3):236–240.
254. Caron P, Morange-Ramos I, Cogne M, et al. Three year follow-up of acromegalic patients treated with intramuscular slow-release lanreotide. J Neurosurg 1997;82(1): 18–22.
255. Ebersold MJ, Laws ER, Jr, Scheithauer BW, et al. Pituitary apoplexy treated by transsphenoidal surgery. A clinicopathological and immunocytochemical study. J Neurosurg 1983;58(3):315–320.
256. Laws ER Jr. Vascular complications of transsphenoidal surgery. Pituitary 1999;2(2):163–170.
257. Cardoso ER, Peterson EW. Pituitary apoplexy: a review. Neurosurgery 1984;14(3):363–373.
258. Mohr G, Hardy J. Hemorrhage, necrosis, and apoplexy in pituitary adenomas. Surg Neurol 1982;18(3):181–189.
259. Bonicki W, Kasperlik-Zaluska A, Koszewski W, et al. Pituitary apoplexy: endocrine, surgical and oncological emergency. Incidence, clinical course and treatment with reference to 799 cases of pituitary adenomas. Acta Neurochir (Wien) 1993;120(3–4):118–122.
260. Pernicone PJ, Scheithauer BW, Sebo TJ, et al. Pituitary carcinoma: a clinicopathologic study of 15 cases. Cancer 1997;79(4):804–812.
261. Kimmel DW, O'Neill BP. Systemic cancer presenting as diabetes insipidus. Clinical and radiographic features of 11 patients with a review of metastatic-induced diabetes insipidus. Cancer 1983;52(12):2355–2358.
262. Thomsett MJ, Conte FA, Kaplan SL, et al. Endocrine and neurologic outcome in childhood craniopharyngioma: review of effect of treatment in 42 patients. J Pediatr 1980;97(5):728–735.
263. Adamson TE, Wiestler OD, Kleihues P, et al. Correlation of clinical and pathological features in surgically treated craniopharyngiomas. J Neurosurg 1990;73(1):12–17.
264. Van Effenterre R, Boch AL. Craniopharyngioma in adults and children: a study of 122 surgical cases. J Neurosurg 2002;97(1):3–11.
265. Weiner HL, Wisoff JH, Rosenberg ME, et al. Cranio-pharyngiomas: a clinicopathological analysis of factors predictive of recurrence and functional outcome. Neurosurgery 1994;35(6):1001–1010; discussion 1010–1001.
266. Rickert CH, Paulus W. Lack of chromosomal imbalances in adamantinomatous and papillary craniopharyngiomas. J Neurol Neurosurg Psychiatry 2003;74(2):260–261.
267. Harrison MJ, Morgello S, Post KD. Epithelial cystic lesions of the sellar and parasellar region: a continuum of ectodermal derivatives? J Neurosurg 1994;80(6):1018–1025.
268. FitzPatrick M, Tartaglino LM, Hollander MD, et al. Imaging of sellar and parasellar pathology. Radiol Clin North Am 1999;37(1):101–121, x.
269. Moore KD, Couldwell WT. Craniopharyngiomas. In: Berger MS, ed. Neuro-oncology. The essentials. New York: Thieme Medical, 2000:409–418.
270. Kunishio K, Yamamoto Y, Sunami N, et al. Craniopharyngioma in the third ventricle: necropsy findings and histogenesis. J Neurol Neurosurg Psychiatry 1987;50(8):1053–1056.
271. Maeda T, Kazumi T, Hotta K, et al. Aseptic localized peritonitis in a patient with chemical meningitis associated with craniopharyngioma cysts. Intern Med 1993;32(4):340–342.
272. Satoh H, Uozumi T, Arita K, et al. Spontaneous rupture of craniopharyngioma cysts. A report of five cases and review of the literature. Surg Neurol 1993;40(5):414–419.
273. Shida N, Nakasato N, Mizoi K, et al. Symptomatic vessel narrowing caused by spontaneous rupture of craniopharyngioma cyst—case report. Neurol Med Chir (Tokyo) 1998;38(10):666–668.

274. Kulkarni V, Daniel RT, Pranatartiharan R. Spontaneous intraventricular rupture of craniopharyngioma cyst. Surg Neurol 2000;54(3):249–253; discussion 253.
275. Miller DC. Pathology of craniopharyngiomas: clinical import of pathological findings. Pediatr Neurosurg 1994;21(Suppl 1): 11–17.
276. Kahn EA, Gosch HH, Seeger JF, et al. Forty-five years experience with the craniopharyngiomas. Surg Neurol 1973;1(1):5–12.
277. Hoffman HJ. Surgical management of craniopharyngioma. Pediatr Neurosurg 1994;21(Suppl 1):44–49.
278. Hoffman HJ, De Silva M, Humphreys RP, et al. Aggressive surgical management of craniopharyngiomas in children. J Neurosurg 1992;76(1):47–52.
279. de Vries L, Lazar L, Phillip M. Craniopharyngioma: presentation and endocrine sequelae in 36 children. J Pediatr Endocrinol Metab 2003;16(5):703–710.
280. Sklar CA. Craniopharyngioma: endocrine abnormalities at presentation. Pediatr Neurosurg 1994;21(Suppl 1):18–20.
281. Merchant TE, Kiehna EN, Sanford RA, et al. Craniopharyngioma: the St. Jude Children's Research Hospital experience 1984–2001. Int J Radiat Oncol Biol Phys 2002;53(3): 533–542.
282. Jackson AS, St. George EJ, Hayward RJ, et al. Stereotactic radiosurgery. XVII: recurrent intrasellar craniopharyngioma. Br J Neurosurg 2003;17(2):138–143.
283. Barajas MA, Ramirez-Guzman G, Rodriguez-Vazquez C, et al. Multimodal management of craniopharyngiomas: neuroendoscopy, microsurgery, and radiosurgery. J Neurosurg 2002;97(5 Suppl):607–609.
284. Ulfarsson E, Lindquist C, Roberts M, et al. Gamma knife radiosurgery for craniopharyngiomas: long-term results in the first Swedish patients. J Neurosurg 2002;97(5 Suppl): 613–622.
285. Pollock BE, Natt N, Schomberg PJ. Stereotactic management of craniopharyngiomas. Stereotact Funct Neurosurg 2002;79(1):25–32.
286. Amendola BE, Wolf A, Coy SR, et al. Role of radiosurgery in craniopharyngiomas: a preliminary report. Med Pediatr Oncol 2003;41(2):123–127.
287. Kondziolka D, Nathoo N, Flickinger JC, et al. Long-term results after radiosurgery for benign intracranial tumors. Neurosurgery 2003;53(4):815–821; discussion 821–812.
288. Varlotto JM, Flickinger JC, Kondziolka D, et al. External beam irradiation of craniopharyngiomas: long-term analysis of tumor control and morbidity. Int J Radiat Oncol Biol Phys 2002;54(2):492–499.
289. Chiou SM, Lunsford LD, Niranjan A, et al. Stereotactic radiosurgery of residual or recurrent craniopharyngioma, after surgery, with or without radiation therapy. Neurooncol 2001;3(3):159–166.
290. Pollock BE, Lunsford LD, Kondziolka D, et al. Phosphorus-32 intracavitary irradiation of cystic craniopharyngiomas: current technique and long-term results. Int J Radiat Oncol Biol Phys 1995;33(2):437–446.
291. Lunsford LD, Pollock BE, Kondziolka DS, et al. Stereotactic options in the management of craniopharyngioma. Pediatr Neurosurg 1994;21(Suppl 1):90–97.
292. Van den Berge JH, Blaauw G, Breeman WA, et al. Intracavitary brachytherapy of cystic craniopharyngiomas. J Neurosurg 1992;77(4):545–550.
293. Bremer AM, Nguyen TQ, Balsys R. Therapeutic benefits of combination chemotherapy with vincristine, BCNU, and procarbazine on recurrent cystic craniopharyngioma. A case report. J Neurooncol 1984;2(1):47–51.
294. Savas A, Erdem A, Tun K, et al. Fatal toxic effect of bleomycin on brain tissue after intracystic chemotherapy for a craniopharyngioma: case report. Neurosurgery 2000;46(1):213–216; discussion 216–217.
295. Savas A, Arasil E, Batay F, et al. Intracavitary chemotherapy of polycystic craniopharyngioma with bleomycin. Acta Neurochir (Wien) 1999;141(5):547–548; discussion 549.
296. Sagoh M, Murakami H, Hirose Y, et al. Occlusive cerebrovasculopathy after internal radiation and bleomycin therapy for craniopharyngioma—case report. Neurol Med Chir (Tokyo) 1997;37(12):920–923.
297. Broggi G, Giorgi C, Franzini A, et al. Preliminary results of intracavitary treatment of craniopharyngioma with bleomycin. J Neurosurg Sci 1989;33(1):145–148.
298. Laws ER Jr, Morris AM, Maartens N. Gliadel for pituitary adenomas and craniopharyngiomas. Neurosurgery 2003; 53(2):255–259; discussion 259–260.
299. Yasargil MG, Curcic M, Kis M, et al. Total removal of craniopharyngiomas. Approaches and long-term results in 144 patients. J Neurosurg 1990;73(1):3–11.
300. Wisoff JH. Surgical management of recurrent craniopharyngiomas. Pediatr Neurosurg 1994;21(Suppl 1):108–113.
301. Crenshaw WB, Chew FS. Rathke's cleft cyst. Am J Roentgenol 1992;158(6):1312.
302. Ross DA, Norman D, Wilson CB. Radiologic characteristics and results of surgical management of Rathke's cysts in 43 patients. Neurosurgery 1992;30(2):173–178; discussion 178–179.
303. Voelker JL, Campbell RL, Muller J. Clinical, radiographic, and pathological features of symptomatic Rathke's cleft cysts. J Neurosurg 1991;74(4):535–544.
304. Itoh J, Usui K. An entirely suprasellar symptomatic Rathke's cleft cyst: case report. Neurosurgery 1992;30(4): 581–584; discussion 584–585.
305. Hua F, Asato R, Miki Y, et al. Differentiation of suprasellar nonneoplastic cysts from cystic neoplasms by Gd-DTPA MRI. J Comput Assist Tomogr 1992;16(5):744–749.
306. Williams JC, Stone D, Smith-Arica JR, et al. Regulated, adenovirus-mediated delivery of tyrosine hydroxylase suppresses growth of estrogen-induced pituitary prolactinomas. Mol Ther 2001;4(6):593–602.
307. Lee EJ, Anderson LM, Thimmapaya B, et al. Targeted expression of toxic genes directed by pituitary hormone promoters: a potential strategy for adenovirus-mediated gene therapy of pituitary tumors. J Clin Endocrinol Metab 1999;84(2):786–794.
308. Lee EJ, Thimmapaya B, Jameson JL. Stereotactic injection of adenoviral vectors that target gene expression to specific pituitary cell types: implications for gene therapy. Neurosurgery 2000;46(6):1461–1468; discussion 1468–1469.

CHAPTER 20

Primitive Neuroectodermal Tumors

COREY RAFFEL / CORMAC O. MAHER

Medulloblastomas (MBs) are primitive neuroectodermal tumors (PNETs) of the posterior fossa. They are the most common primary brain tumor of children and adolescents. Despite typical circumferential growth, MBs have a marked propensity for neuraxis dissemination. Dissemination correlates with the tumor's lethality and mandates irradiation and chemotherapy. Refinements in imaging, surgical technique, and adjunctive therapies have led to longer survival and an improving quality of life in MB patients. Although these gains are encouraging, MBs are often not cured by current techniques. Furthermore, treatment of MB still carries an unacceptably high incidence of neuropsychologic sequelae in young children and infants. Hopefully, advances in molecular biology should lead to more efficacious therapies in the future.

Bailey and Cushing first described medulloblastomas in 1925.[1] Ever since the nomenclature for this tumor has been controversial. Based on histologic and embryologic investigations, medulloblastomas were originally included in a group of primitive brain tumors of childhood, thought to arise from a hypothesized embryonal precursor cell called a medulloblast. Such a cell has never been identified. Nevertheless, this classification scheme, later refined by Rubinstein, became widely accepted in the decades that followed.[2] More recently, the classification of these tumors was revised. Because medulloblastomas are composed of undifferentiated neuroepithelial cells and are histologically indistinguishable from retinoblastomas, neuroblastomas, and pineoblastomas, Rorke has suggested that the term primitive neuroectodermal tumor *(PNET) be applied to each of these tumors instead of the formerly accepted nomenclature.[3] The World Health Organization classification system (WHO-II) currently uses the term PNET in preference to medulloblastoma. Recently, medulloblastomas have been differentiated from other primitive neuroectodermal tumors of the central nervous system based on gene expression pattern, suggesting that the lumping together of these tumors may be inappropriate.[4] However, even within that classification there are strata. Eventually, gene expression patterns may prove to be more useful for informing tumor biology than classification.[5,6] This chapter emphasizes the diagnosis and treatment of medulloblastoma. Other varieties of PNET of the central nervous system, such as pinealoblastoma, central neuroblastoma, and ependymoblastoma, are considered briefly.*

▶ MEDULLOBLASTOMA

There are between 250 and 500 new cases of medulloblastoma diagnosed each year in the United States.[7] Furthermore, the number of diagnosed cases of medulloblastoma has increased significantly over the past several decades.[8] Although medulloblastomas may occur at any age, approximately 75% are diagnosed before age 15 years,[9,10] and the median age at diagnosis is between 5 and 7 years of age.[9] In children, medulloblastomas account for 15% to 30% of all brain tumors and 30% to 55% of posterior fossa tumors.[7] Furthermore, medulloblastoma is the second most common primary brain tumor in children younger than 2 years of age.[11–14] Medulloblastomas have a male predominance that varies from 1.3:1 to 2.7:1 in different series.[10,15–17]

Most medulloblastomas arise in the cerebellar vermis and extend into the fourth ventricle. The tumor usually fills the fourth ventricle, partially or entirely. In contrast to ependymomas, extension through the foramen of Luschka into the cerebellopontine angle, or through the cerebral aqueduct into the third ventricle, is unusual in medulloblastomas. Although medulloblastomas may extend from the vermis into one of the cerebellar hemispheres, isolated cerebellar hemispheric involvement is not common. Medulloblastomas are more likely to arise in the cerebellar hemisphere in adults than in children.[18] Finally, there are several reported cases of medulloblastomas arising within the cerebellopontine angle.

Clinical Diagnosis of Medulloblastoma

Patients with medulloblastoma may present with symptoms of tumor mass effect on the cerebellum and nearby structures, symptoms of spinal "drop" metastases, or symptoms of hydrocephalus. Often, patients present with some combination of these symptoms. The clinical history of medulloblastoma is typically brief. Symptom onset is less than 6 weeks prior to presentation in approximately half of patients, and less than 12 weeks in approximately 75% of patients.[10]

Regardless of histology, midline posterior fossa tumors in children characteristically present with symptoms of increased intracranial pressure (ICP) as a consequence of hydrocephalus. At least 90% of patients with medulloblastomas present with symptoms of hydrocephalus such as headache and recurrent vomiting. As a consequence, it is usually clinically impossible to differentiate patients with medulloblastoma from those with other processes that may cause obstructive hydrocephalus. Symptoms of obstructive hydrocephalus are typically worse in the morning and usually include headaches, nausea, and vomiting. Infants presenting with hydrocephalus may be irritable, lethargic, and occasionally demonstrate progressive macrocephaly and fullness of the anterior fontanelle.[10,15] Older children usually complain of headaches and consequently may be referred for imaging sooner than infants. Older patients with a medulloblastoma arising in the cerebellar hemisphere may complain only of the onset of progressive appendicular ataxia. Patients with or without hydrocephalus often present with truncal ataxia as a result of mass effect on the cerebellar vermis. Spinal drop metastases may present with back pain, urinary retention, or leg weakness.

In as many as 10% of cases, patients may present with acute decompensation secondary to hemorrhage into the tumor, causing acute hydrocephalus or brainstem compression. Subarachnoid hemorrhage from bleeding into the fourth ventricle can also occur, but is rare. Patients with medulloblastomas can occasionally present with acute symptoms of brainstem compression necessitating immediate intervention.

On physical examination, papilledema is frequently noted in those patients presenting with hydrocephalus. Nystagmus and diplopia are also frequent findings. Diplopia generally represents impairment of cranial nerves IV or VI. The level of alertness may be affected and should be continuously assessed. Infants usually present with some combination of macrocrania, bulging of the fontanelle, lethargy, and vomiting.[13] Imaging of the posterior fossa is indicated in any of these clinical settings (see "Imaging Diagnosis of Medulloblastoma," below). Preoperative lumbar cerebrospinal fluid (CSF) sampling is often contraindicated in the presence of a posterior fossa tumor. If a lumbar puncture is not medically appropriate, intraoperative or postoperative CSF cytology is useful for staging these tumors.

Between 1% and 2% of all cases of medulloblastoma occur in association with a tumor syndrome[19] and these syndromes have characteristic phenotypes (see also "Molecular Biology of Medulloblastoma"). For example, the nevoid basal cell carcinoma syndrome (Gorlin syndrome) is a rare autosomal dominant syndrome that is associated with basal cell carcinomas, keratocysts of the jaw, spine and rib anomalies, calcification of the falx cerebri, and, in approximately 4% of cases, medulloblastomas.[20,21] Most reported cases of medulloblastoma in the setting of Gorlin syndrome occur during the first 7 years of life, and annual screening with magnetic resonance imaging (MRI) has been advocated for patients with this syndrome.[20]

Imaging Diagnosis of Medulloblastoma

On diagnostic imaging, medulloblastomas classically appear as well-defined, midline, cerebellar mass lesions. Brainstem involvement is seen radiographically in a large minority of patients with medulloblastoma, and radiographic evidence of hydrocephalus is very common.[22,23]

Medulloblastomas typically appear hyperdense on noncontrast computerized tomography (CT) scan because of their dense cellularity (Fig. 20-1). This is an important means of differentiating medulloblastomas from cerebellar astrocytomas and ependymomas, which are generally hypodense and isodense, respectively, on noncontrast CT. Regions of mineralization are noted in approximately 20% of CT scans, and cystic or necrotic regions in 20% to 50% of CT scans.[24] A predominantly cystic cerebellar tumor, however, is more likely an astrocytoma in a child or a metastasis in an adult. Although intratumoral hemorrhage is a rare feature of medulloblastoma, it is more common in medulloblastomas than in cerebellar astrocytomas or ependymomas.

Most medulloblastomas have low to intermediate signal on T_1-weighted magnetic resonance (MR) images (Fig. 20-2). T_2 signal is characterized by heterogeneity secondary to intratumoral cysts, vessels, and mineralization. Medulloblastomas almost always enhance with gadolinium; the pattern of enhancement may be uniform or heterogeneous. Diffuse or patchy enhancement following contrast administration is seen in at least 90% of medulloblastomas.[22,23]

The entire neuraxis should be imaged for the presence of metastatic spread of the medulloblastoma to other sites, ideally before surgical resection of the posterior fossa mass. The preoperative diagnosis of dissemination is important to the surgeon; if disseminated a less aggressive operation can be planned. In addition, postoperative scans are difficult to interpret because of blood and protein artifacts. If spinal imaging cannot be obtained preoperatively, then scans should be delayed at least 2 weeks to allow for resolution of these artifacts.

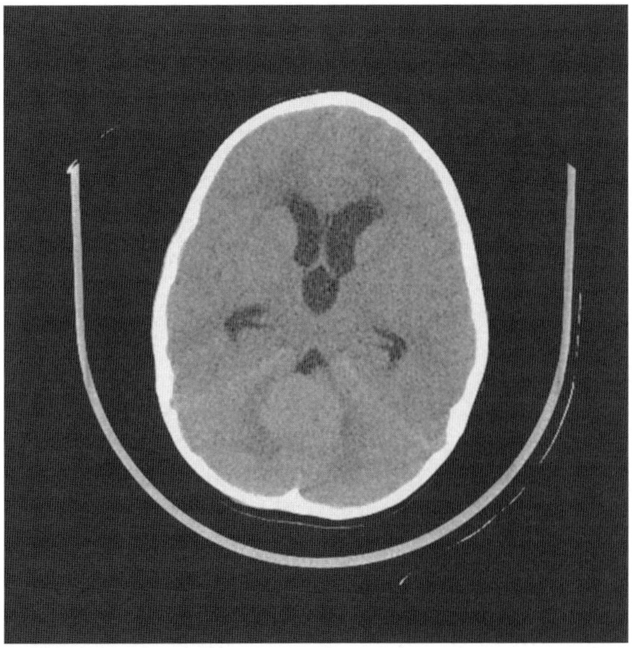

Figure 20-1. CT scan without contrast demonstrates a mildly hyperdense lesion in the posterior fossa with mass effect on the cerebellar hemispheres and the fourth ventricle, leading to obstructive hydrocephalus.

Medulloblastoma spreads along cerebrospinal fluid pathways. Drop metastases in the spinal canal are common, brightly enhance, and are almost always extramedullary, although intramedullary metastases have been reported. Less commonly, the tumor spreads to intracranial sites such as the basilar and suprasellar cisterns, sylvian fissures, infundibular recess, lateral ventricles, and subfrontal region. Metastatic disease is best evaluated with contrasted images (Fig. 20-3).

For a medulloblastoma arising from the cerebellar vermis, the major differential diagnostic consideration on imaging is ependymoma. Unlike ependymoma, medulloblastomas do not typically extend through the foramina of Luschka. Calcification is also more common in ependymomas than in medulloblastomas.

Medulloblastomas have been traditionally staged radiographically according to the Chang system, which assigns a stage based on tumor size (T stage) and metastatic spread (M stage).[25] The Chang stage has been criticized for including tumor size despite studies demonstrating no clear correlation between preoperative tumor size and outcome. In addition, the Chang stage does not include other factors, such as age, that are known to be predictive of outcome. For these reasons, the Chang staging system is no longer used. Although no other radiographic staging systems are widely accepted, patients are staged based on known prognostic factors (see "Non-Surgical Therapy for Medulloblastoma").

Postoperative MRI should be performed within 2 days of surgery to assess the extent of tumor resection. Postoperative enhancement is a common finding on imaging performed between 1 day and 1 year following surgery, and is most pronounced between postoperative days 3 and 21.[26,27] Nodular enhancement is characteristic of residual tumor as typical postoperative enhancement is thin and follows the outlines of the resection cavity without infiltration.

Pathologic Diagnosis of Medulloblastoma

Despite their uniform grade IV designation in the World Health Organization (WHO) classification of tumors,[28] medulloblastomas have several histologic subtypes that are of clinical relevance. The common cerebellar subtype is usually composed of small, densely packed, undifferentiated cells with hyperchromatic nuclei and scant cytoplasm. These cells may cluster into Homer-Wright rosettes.

The desmoplastic subtype is similar to the cerebellar subtype, but is further characterized by the presence of collagen bundles, and scattered, less cellular areas, or

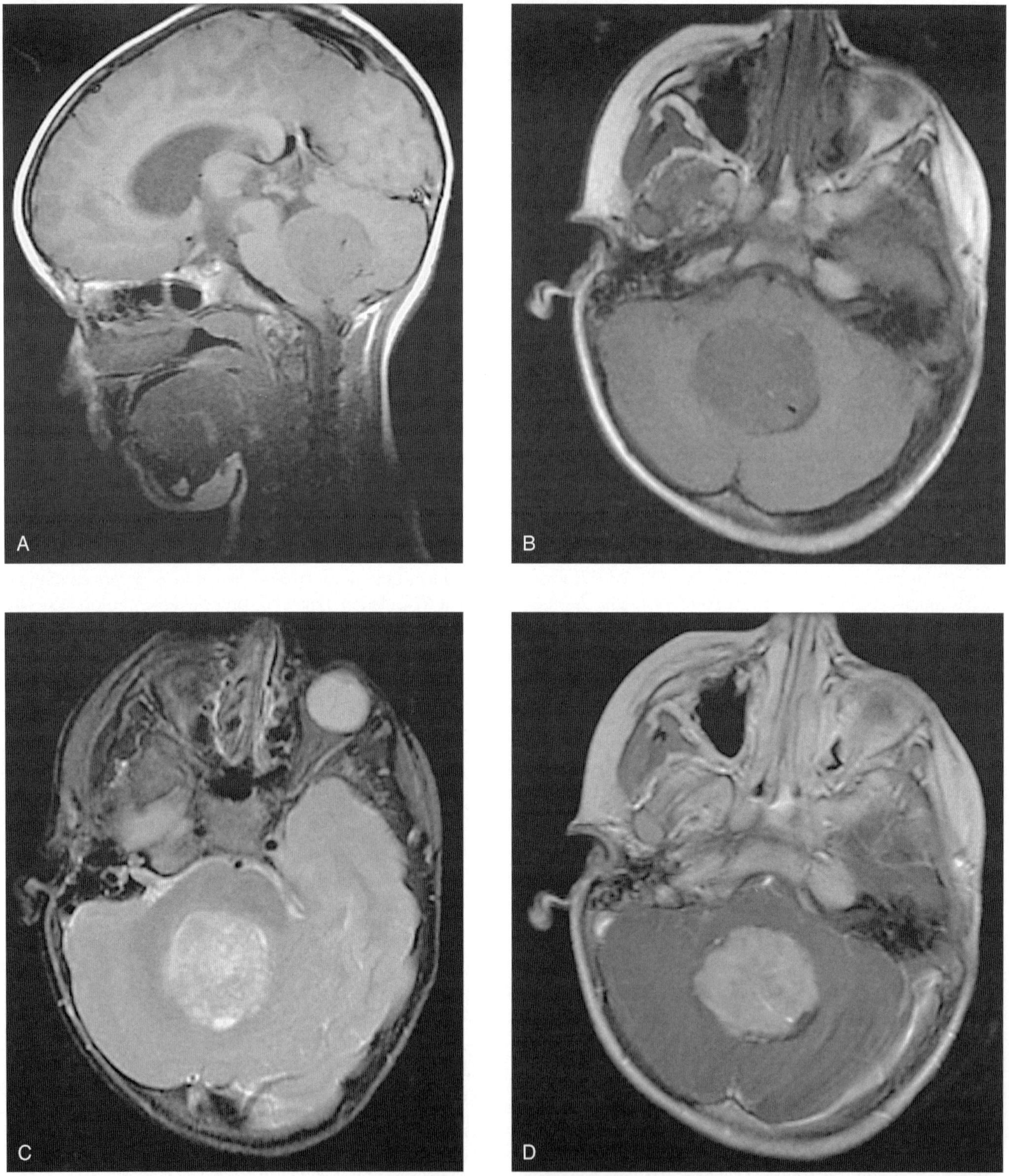

Figure 20-2. Typical appearance of medulloblastoma on MRI. (A) T_1 sagittal section showing a lesion filling the fourth ventricle. (B) Medulloblastoma is usually hypointense to isointense on T_1-weighted images, (C) hyperintense on T_2-weighted images, and (D) strongly enhancing.

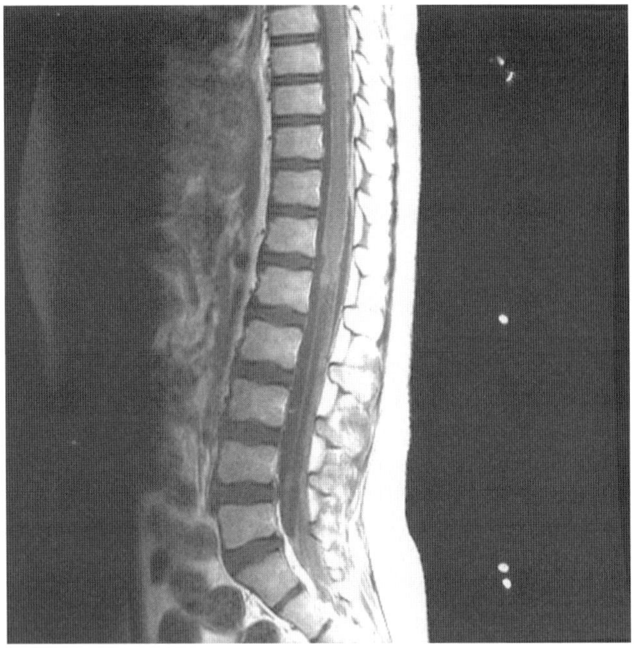

Figure 20-3. Gadolinium-enhanced sagittal MRI demonstrating the typical appearance of a spinal "drop metastasis" at the level of the conus medullaris and the cauda equina.

glomeruli, as well as prominent neuronal differentiation.[29] The desmoplastic subtype is found in approximately 6% of patients, is more common in adults, and may be associated with a more favorable prognosis, especially if extensive nodularity is noted.[18,30–32] Whereas most medulloblastomas are grossly friable and soft, desmoplastic variants are firmer. Both cerebellar and desmoplastic subtypes may occasionally calcify.

The large-cell subtype of medulloblastoma appears as sheets of large cells with round nuclei and prominent nucleoli.[29] Marked anaplasia is also characteristic of the large-cell subtype. This subtype is associated with a poorer prognosis.[29,33–35] Medulloblastomas with moderate to severe anaplastic features that lack other characteristics of the large-cell subtype may be classified simply as *anaplastic medulloblastomas*. This subtype is also associated with shorter survival.[29,30]

Cerebellar liponeurocytomas are low-grade neoplasms that have been referred to as "lipidized medulloblastomas"[33] in the past, but have been removed from the medulloblastoma category in the most recent WHO classification.[28] These indolent tumors are not further considered here.

Cell of Origin

Medulloblastomas are observed to differentiate along glial and neuronal pathways in situ, suggesting that these tumors are derived from primitive, pluripotent neuroepithelial stem cells. This conclusion is supported by studies of PNET cell lines that demonstrate expression of specific, developmentally regulated proteins in PNETs.[36] Medulloblastomas express *zic*, a gene normally expressed only in the external granular cell layer of the developing cerebellum and its derivatives, suggesting that medulloblastoma arises from external granular cell layer precursor cells.[37,38] Given the rapid proliferative capacity of external granular cell layer (EGL) precursors and the pattern of gene expression seen, EGL cells and their derivatives seem by far the most likely origin of medulloblastoma. Other cerebellar cells, such as Purkinje cells, basket neurons, or glial cells, are unlikely to be cells of origin for medulloblastoma.

Karyotypic Abnormalities

Only one karyotypic abnormality has been found to be typical of medulloblastoma, the presence of an isochromosome 17q, present in about 50% of tumors.[39] The breakpoint has been localized to 17p11.2,[40] but no tumor-specific gene rearrangement has been identified. Despite multiple studies, no tumor suppressor gene that can be implicated in the development of medulloblastoma has been found on chromosome 17p. Specifically, no alteration in p53 has been identified with more than 100 tumors investigated as of 2004. Other, less common karyotypic abnormalities, including loss of heterozygosity (LOH) on chromosome 9q, have been identified in approximately 20% of medulloblastomas. Interestingly, the loss of 9q in medulloblastoma correlates with the desmoplastic subtype.[32]

Analyses of Gene Expression in Medulloblastoma

Two reports of gene expression in medulloblastoma have added insights to the basic biology of these tumors. In the first, medulloblastoma samples were divided into two groups, depending on whether CSF dissemination of tumor was seen at the time the patient presented with the tumor.[41] Gene expression was analyzed on Affymetrix G110 cancer arrays, which are enriched for genes thought to be important in cancer biology. Fifty-nine genes were identified that had increased expression in the metastatic tumors compared with the nonmetastatic tumors. An additional 29 genes were identified that had decreased expression in the metastatic tumors. Two of theses genes, platelet-derived growth factor receptor [(PDGFR)-α] and secreted protein, acidic, cysteine-rich (SPARC), were shown by immunohistochemical staining to be expressed differentially between metastatic and nonmetastatic tumors. In addition, antibodies to PDGFR-α blocked tumor cell migration in in vitro assays. These investigators were able to use the pattern of gene expression to predict which tumors presented with CSF metastases in a blinded group of tumors. These results suggest that there may be genes important in the progression of medulloblastoma or that alterations in different pathways may be responsible for the differences in prognosis seen between tumors presenting without and with CSF dissemination.

The second study included a group of "embryonal tumors" of the central nervous system, including medulloblastomas, extracerebellar PNETs, atypical teratoid/rhabdoid tumors, and malignant gliomas.[4] Gene expression was analyzed on Affymetrix HuGene FL arrays, containing 5920 known genes and 897 expressed sequence tags. The first finding from this data set was that each tumor type could be easily distinguished from the others based on gene expression pattern. Especially interesting was the ability to distinguish medulloblastomas from other central nervous system (CNS) PNETs, suggesting that the lumping of these tumors together, as proposed by Rourke, may be inappropriate. The medulloblastomas often expressed genes normally expressed in the EGL, lending credence to the hypothesis that EGL precursors represent the cell of origin of medulloblastoma. Second, these investigators were able to distinguish "classical" medulloblastomas from desmoplastic medulloblastomas. The important genes with increased expression in the desmoplastic tumors were those involved in the sonic hedgehog/*PTCH* pathway (see below). Lastly, using an eight-gene model, these investigators were able to accurately predict outcome in their patients with medulloblastoma. Genes associated with favorable clinical outcome included *TRKC* and other genes characteristic of cerebellar differentiation. In contrast, these genes were underexpressed in tumors with poor prognosis, and genes involved in cell proliferation were overexpressed in a followup report from the same group.[5] In a cohort of 55 young patients, expression profiles were the only significant clinical prognostic factor in both univariate and multivariate analyses.

Molecular Biology of Medulloblastoma

Medulloblastomas may occur in association with two different inherited cancer syndromes: Gorlin syndrome and Turcot syndrome. Nevoid basal cell carcinoma syndrome (NBCCS), also called Gorlin syndrome or basal cell nevus syndrome, is an autosomal dominant disorder.[42] Affected individuals develop multiple basal cell carcinomas, multiple odontogenic keratocysts of the jaws, palmar and plantar dyskeratoses, and skeletal anomalies, especially rib malformations. In addition, at least 40 cases of medulloblastoma have been reported in patients with this syndrome, indicating that approximately 3% of Gorlin patients develop this tumor.[19,43] The gene for Gorlin syndrome is mapped to chromosome 9q22.3.[44,45] Two studies report loss of genetic markers mapped to 9q in medulloblastoma.[32,46] In these studies, 5 of 33 tumors demonstrated loss of genetic material in 9q, suggesting that a tumor suppressor gene important in medulloblastoma may be found in this region. Interestingly, all five of these tumors had the desmoplastic phenotype, suggesting that loss of genetic material in 9q is specific for this tumor subtype.

The gene at 9q22.3 responsible for NBCCS has been identified as the *PTCH* gene, the human homolog of the *Drosophila patched* gene.[47,48] The *Drosophila* gene encodes a protein with 12 putative transmembrane domains; it may function as a receptor or transporter.[49,50] The protein has an essential role in correct patterning of larval segments and imaginal discs during adult fruit fly development; a similar role in humans may explain the congenital anomalies associated with NBCCS.

PTCH mutations have been described in patients with NBCCS and in spontaneous basal cell carcinomas. A large number of such mutations has been reported, including single base substitutions, insertions ranging from a single base to 300 bases, and deletions ranging from a single base to 37 bases.[47,48,51–53] The described mutations are fairly evenly distributed throughout the *PTCH* gene; no "mutational hot spots" have been identified.

Based on these findings, sporadic medulloblastomas have been investigated for alterations of the *PTCH* gene. Inactivation of the *PTCH* locus by deletion and mutation has been found in approximately 10% of sporadic medulloblastomas, suggesting that *PTCH* functions as a classic tumor suppressor in this subset of tumors.[54–59] An analysis of the *SHH/PTCH* pathway reveals that other genes in the pathway might be altered to give a phenotype similar to that caused by *PTCH* inactivation. An investigation looking for these alterations in 15 other pathway genes has revealed only very rare mutations in v-smo and suppressor of fused (su[fu]).[55,60,61] This finding suggests that there is something unique about *PTCH* inactivation or that the *PTCH* locus is relatively easy to inactivate through mutation or deletion.

Turcot syndrome is a hereditary disorder in which affected individuals have multiple colonic polyps and a brain tumor, either glioblastoma multiforme or medulloblastoma.[62] In one study, mutations in the *APC* gene were identified in the group of patients with Turcot syndrome who developed medulloblastoma.[63] The relative risk for developing a medulloblastoma in patients with Turcot syndrome and an *APC* gene mutation is 92 times that in the general population.

APC functions as a key regulator in a complex developmental pathway. The control of the levels of free β-catenin in the cytoplasm by APC defines the role of APC as a tumor suppressor. Normally, free levels of β-catenin are low, as binding of β-catenin by APC sequesters β-catenin and targets the protein for degradation. APC only binds β-catenin when β-catenin is hyperphosphorylated. β-Catenin is phosphorylated by glycogen synthase kinase 3β (GSK-3β), a serine/threonine kinase. β-Catenin contains four phosphorylation sites for GSK-3β, three serines and one threonine, all encoded in exon 3 of the β-catenin gene. When APC is inactivated by mutation, for example, in colon carcinoma, levels of cytoplasmic β-catenin rise. Free β-catenin associates with members of the Tcf family.[64–66] When β-catenin associates with Tcf, the complex moves to the nucleus and upregulates the expression of genes that increase the rate of cell division, either by stimulating cell proliferation or by inhibiting apoptosis.

The *APC* gene has been investigated for inactivation in sporadic medulloblastoma. Surprisingly, in light of the association between germ line *APC* gene mutation and medulloblastoma seen in Turcot syndrome, *APC* gene mutations have rarely been identified in spontaneously occurring medulloblastomas. In one study, 47 sporadic medulloblastomas were examined for mutations in the *APC* mutation cluster region, comprising 10% of the gene, where more than two-thirds of the mutations seen in colorectal carcinoma occur.[67] No tumor had an *APC* mutation in this region. However, the entire gene was not investigated in this report. In a second study, DNA from 23 medulloblastomas was examined for deletions in the region of the *APC* gene.[68] No LOH was found in this region in any tumor. However, the four microsatellite markers used in this study, although the closest to *APC* available at the time, were at least 30 to 70 kilobases from the *APC* locus. In a third study, 2 tumors among 46 medulloblastomas were found to have *APC* mutations.[69] However, the mutations identified were very conservative, that is, alanine to valine and valine to isoleucine. The mutations did not occur in defined functional domains of the protein. The functional consequences of these mutations are not clear. Together these results indicate that APC mutations in sporadic medulloblastoma are quite rare and may have no functional consequence.

Because β-catenin/Tcf complexes are translocated to the nucleus, nuclear localization of β-catenin, demonstrated immunohistochemically, has been used as a marker for tumors with active β-catenin/Tcf transcription.[70–73] Nuclear localization of β-catenin occurs in tumors with inactivated APC or with oncogenic β-catenin mutations, suggesting that this finding identifies tumors with increased β-catenin/Tcf transcription, regardless of the mechanism responsible. Immunohistochemical staining for β-catenin has been performed in medulloblastoma.[74] Nine of 51 sporadic medulloblastomas were found to have nuclear localization of β-catenin. This result suggests that at least 20% of medulloblastomas have alteration in control of β-catenin levels other than APC inactivation.

In colon carcinoma, free β-catenin levels may be increased by two mechanisms. The first, inactivation of APC, was described above. The second mechanism involves mutation of the β-catenin gene (locus *CTNNB1*) itself.[66] Mutations of β-catenin that alter the GSK-3β phosphorylation sites in exon 3 have been described. These missense mutations change the serines or threonine that are GSK-3β phosphorylation sites to cysteine, and prevent β-catenin from being completely phosphorylated.

Given that germline APC mutations in Turcot syndrome give rise to an increased incidence of medulloblastoma, and given the rarity of APC mutations in sporadic medulloblastoma, sporadic medulloblastomas have been screened for oncogenic mutations in β-catenin, as these mutations result in the same phenotype as APC inactivation. Exon 3 of β-catenin, the location of all GSK-3β phosphorylation sites, was investigated by direct sequencing in 67 sporadic medulloblastomas.[75] Five tumors were found to have β-catenin mutations. In three cases, the alteration resulted in the substitution of a cysteine for a serine at a GSK-3β phosphorylation site. Sequencing of exon 3 in the constitutional DNA from these patients (available for two of the three patients) failed to show a mutation, indicating that the mutation identified is tumor specific. Two additional mutations were also found in exon 3, both of which altered an amino acid in the ubiquitin binding region. Thus, 5 of 67 (7.5%) tumors had oncogenic mutations in β-catenin. As expected, those tumors with β-catenin mutations also had nuclear localization of β-catenin. Similar results were reported from another group,[69] which reported that of 46 medulloblastomas, 4 (8.7%) were found to have oncogenic mutations in β-catenin. The finding that 25% of medulloblastomas have nuclear localization of β-catenin whereas only 7.5% contain oncogenic β-catenin mutations, suggests that alterations in this pathway other than β-catenin mutation that result in increased β-catenin/Tcf transcription may be occurring in a subset of medulloblastoma.

A third genetic alteration found in medulloblastoma is c-myc or N-myc amplification. Amplification of myc genes is rare, occurring in only 4% of medulloblastomas. Interestingly, c-myc amplification appears to correlate with the large-cell phenotype, which carries a particularly grim prognosis.

Other Growth Factor Pathways in Medulloblastoma

Gilbertson and coworkers investigated expression of erbB family members in medulloblastoma.[6,76–78] They showed that erbB2 and erbB4 are frequently expressed together in medulloblastoma. Interestingly, erbB4, but not erbB2, was expressed in the developing cerebellum. Expression of erbB2 and erbB4 was associated with simultaneous expression of neuregulin-1α, suggesting the possibility of an autocrine loop in tumors with expression of all three proteins. Indeed, erbB2/erbB4 dimerization was identified in tumors. This group also showed that novel splice variants of erbB4 are found frequently in medulloblastoma. Significantly, coexpression of erbB2 and erbB4 indicated a worse prognosis, and expression of these receptors with neuregulin-1α was associated with CSF dissemination at presentation. This preliminary finding was borne out in a study of 97 medulloblastoma patients. In that study, tumor erbB2 protein was an independent prognostic variable; children who met "average risk" clinical criteria and had no erbB2 detected had 100% 5-year survivals with conventional therapy, whereas only 54% of children who met "average risk" clinical criteria but had erbB2 detected were alive at 5 years.[6]

Activation of insulin-like growth factor receptor-1 (IGF-1R) has also been demonstrated in medulloblastoma cell lines.[79] Autophosphorylation of this receptor and induction of c-fos expression in the presence of exogenous IGF-1R have been shown, indicating a functional receptor. Tumor growth was inhibited by an anti-IGF-1R antibody that interferes with ligand binding. Similar results have been reported by others.[80]

Members of the neurotrophin family (nerve growth factor, brain-derived neurotrophic factor, NT-3, and NT-4/5) and their family of high-affinity receptors (trkA, trkB, and trkC) are important in the proliferation, differentiation, and survival of neuroepithelial cells. In addition to the trk receptors, a low-affinity receptor for neurotrophins ($p75^{LNGFR}$) has also been described in these cells. Because medulloblastoma is thought to arise from primitive neuroepithelial stem cells, neurotrophins and their receptors may be important in the development and growth of these tumors. Three studies have been performed examining the status of the low affinity nerve growth factor receptor in medulloblastoma.[81–83] About one-third of tumors studied had messenger RNA (mRNA) for this receptor. Expression of $p75^{LNGFR}$, however, may be restricted to the subset of PNET demonstrating neuronal differentiation. Addition of nerve growth factor had no effect on the growth characteristics or morphology of a PNET cell line expressing the receptor.

Trk expression has also been investigated. Interestingly, one study of a small number of tumors correlated good clinical outcome with high expression of full-length trkC mRNA.[84] This work has been corroborated in a larger study.[85] It has been suggested that expression of TrkC may lead to apoptosis of medulloblastoma cells when exposed to the TrkC ligand NT-3.[86]

▶ TREATMENT OF MEDULLOBLASTOMA

Surgical Treatment of Associated Hydrocephalus

Although hydrocephalus is noted preoperatively in the majority of patients presenting with medulloblastoma, routine placement of a ventricular shunt or external ventricular drain (EVD) prior to resection is no longer indicated in most cases.[87,88] In addition to the risk of infection, upward transtentorial herniation is a rare but significant complication of preoperative ventricular drainage in the setting of posterior fossa mass lesions. Furthermore, earlier tumor detection and the use of corticosteroids to control ICP has made preoperative drainage less necessary than in the past. In cases where symptoms of hydrocephalus are significant and refractory to maximal medical therapy, an external ventricular drain should be placed promptly. To decrease the risk of upward herniation, cerebrospinal fluid should be drained slowly and in a controlled manner.

When ventricular shunts were placed preoperatively, the overall rate of shunt dependency was substantially higher. Although the majority of patients will have resolution of the hydrocephalus following tumor resection, approximately 40% of medulloblastoma will require placement of a ventricular shunt within 4 weeks of the tumor resection. Patients with postoperative lethargy, especially if progressively worsening, and patients with a large pseudomeningocele should be screened for hydrocephalus. Three prognostic factors for permanent shunting have been identified: young age, extensive preoperative ventricular dilatation, and large tumors.[87] Importantly, patients with none of these characteristics rarely require permanent shunting. The theoretical risk of a ventriculoperitoneal shunt allowing seeding of the posterior fossa tumor into the peritoneum appears to be very small.[89]

Surgical Resection of Medulloblastoma

The goals of surgical resection include establishing a diagnosis, reestablishing normal CSF circulation, and removing all of the tumor. Although these goals may not be achieved in every case, surgical resection of posterior fossa medulloblastomas is almost always indicated as an initial therapy.[10] Furthermore, the extent of surgical resection is prognostically significant for these tumors.[90,91] For example, 2-year event-free survival and overall survival were significantly better for patients with nonmetastatic tumors that were completely removed at diagnosis than for those with metastases at diagnosis or those with less than total removal of tumor.[92] Any survival difference between a gross total resection and near-total resection (>90% of tumor removed), however, has not been proven prospectively.[90] Thus, aggressive resections that violate the plane of the floor of the fourth ventricle in pursuit of a gross total resection are not indicated.

Patient positioning for a posterior fossa tumor resection is dictated by the patient's age, the location of the tumor, and the individual preferences of the surgeon. Most surgeons favor the lateral decubitus or modified prone (concorde) positions. A midline suboccipital craniotomy or craniectomy followed by a vertical approach through the vermis is the standard technique for exposing a midline lesion of the posterior fossa. The tumor is usually carefully dissected off the floor of the fourth ventricle in a caudal-to-cranial direction. If extension of the tumor into the brainstem is anticipated preoperatively, intraoperative electromyogram (EMG) monitoring of the facial and abducens cranial nerves may be useful.[93] Medulloblastomas are usually soft and friable, and are resected piecemeal. Typically, the rostral extent of medulloblastomas may be dissected by following a plane between the tumor and the superior medullary velum. Most of these tumors have a cap of cerebrospinal fluid representing the superior fourth ventricle over the most rostral aspect of the tumor; this serves as a useful surgical landmark.

Complications of posterior fossa tumor resections include infection, cerebrospinal fluid leak, cranial nerve palsy, and cerebellar mutism. The syndrome of cerebellar mutism following a vermian tumor resection is now a well-known complication following the resection of any posterior fossa tumor, particularly medulloblastoma.[94] Cerebellar mutism usually develops during the first postoperative week, often after a period of normal postoperative recovery, and may persist for several months (mean: 6.8 weeks).[95] The mutism is followed in approximately 75% of cases with more slowly resolving dysarthric speech. Mutism may also be seen in association with a syndrome of pseudobulbar palsy.[96,97] Like isolated mutism, the syndrome of postoperative pseudobulbar palsy will usually abate after several weeks. Although various theories have been proposed, there is currently no consensus for either the etiology or the prevention of this syndrome. Minimizing midline cerebellar retraction or avoiding a midline vermian incision has been suggested to reduce the incidence.

Nonsurgical Therapy for Medulloblastoma

Patients with medulloblastoma are typically stratified into normal-risk and high-risk groups. Normal-risk patients are those older than 2 years of age at presentation who have had a near total resection of their tumor and who do not have disseminated disease. High-risk patients have one of the following characteristics: age younger than 2 years at presentation, less than near-total resection, or dissemination at presentation. This stratification has been devised after multiple prospective trials demonstrated the grave prognostic significance of any of the high-risk factors. The influence of molecular markers on the prognosis has been described, but these markers have yet to be used clinically (see "Molecular Biology of Medulloblastoma").

Medulloblastomas are both radiosensitive and chemoresponsive. Craniospinal radiation therapy in combination with surgery has improved survival and is indicated for most medulloblastomas. In support of this, the incidence of spinal metastasis following spinal radiation is 13%, compared to a 75% incidence without postoperative radiation to the neuraxis.[17] Furthermore, the incidence of supratentorial metastasis increases when the cranial volume is not radiated postoperatively.[98]

The optimal radiation dose remains a subject of debate. Neurotoxicity increases directly with the total dose of irradiation and inversely to the age of the patient at the start of treatment.[99] Local (i.e., tumor bed) control requires doses of at least 50 Gy, which has become the standard dose to the tumor bed.[100] What is not clear is what dose is required for the remainder of the posterior fossa and the spinal compartment. A typical plan included 40 to 45 Gy to the remainder of the intracranial compartment and 30 to 36 Gy to the spinal axis. To reduce neurocognitive, endocrine, hearing, and growth sequelae (see below), several studies used lower craniospinal doses (36 Gy reduced to 23.4 Gy) for children with standard-risk disease (younger than 3 years of age, localized disease at diagnosis, total or near-total resection). Use of the lower-dose radiation improved cognitive outcomes. However, when radiation was used without adjuvant chemotherapy, children who had received reduced-dose radiation had higher relapse rates, especially outside the primary site.[101]

The sequelae of radiation therapy in the developing nervous system can be profound and have become increasingly important as the survival of patients with medulloblastoma has improved. Cognitive impairment, growth retardation, endocrinopathies, and leukoencephalopathy are all associated with the use of radiotherapy in children.[102] The vast majority of children with medulloblastoma treated with adjuvant radiotherapy have a decrease in intelligence quotient.[103] Furthermore, the hypothalamic–pituitary axis is frequently depressed following posterior fossa radiation, as evidenced by the high incidence of growth hormone deficiency and an average patient height in the 25th percentile.[102,103]

Chemotherapy is now offered (alone or in combination with radiotherapy) to almost all patients after Packer and associates reported an 85% overall 5-year survival in high-risk patients receiving chemotherapy in addition to surgery and radiation.[104] Subsequent studies focused primarily on which regimen may deliver equivalent survival results while tempering the deleterious impact of craniospinal radiation on the developing nervous system. Children's Cancer Group (CCG) and Pediatric Oncology Group (POG) studies clearly demonstrated that modest reductions in the dose of craniospinal irradiation (to 23.4 Gy), if combined with adjuvant chemotherapy, preserved high rates of disease control with potential improvements in function.[105,106] Nevertheless, craniospinal radiation doses in excess of 20 Gy still posed a significant risk of neurocognitive decline, especially in children younger than age 8 years.

A series of contemporary treatment studies for young children and infants with MB (younger than 3 years of age at diagnosis) have relied on combination chemotherapy regimens intended to either eliminate or delay the need for irradiation. Unfortunately, these efforts have largely failed. For example, the largest study of primary chemotherapy for infant CNS tumors has been POG 8633/8634 where eligible patients received cyclophosphamide/vincristine and cisplatin/etoposide (VP16) in alternate cycles.[107] The progression-free survival (PFS) rate was only 41% at 1 year for children 24 to 36 months old at diagnosis and 39% at 2 years for those children younger than 24 months of age at diagnosis.[107] Progressive disease occurred early, with most failures occurring at the primary site and in the first 6 months. A CCG study employing the "eight-drugs-in-1-day" regimen yielded a 3-year PFS of 22% for medulloblastoma (it was employed for a series of pediatric brain malignancies).[108] A multicenter carboplatin/cyclophosphamide-based primary chemotherapy regimen resulted in a 3-year PFS of 22% for young children.[109] Studies from the United Kingdom[110] and Australasia[111] produced similar results. Replacement studies used dose-intensified chemotherapy. POG study 9233/34 compared standard-dose chemotherapy of 8633 to a dose-intensified regimen using the same agents with radiation delayed until completion of 72 weeks of chemotherapy or progression of disease on chemotherapy. However, young patients so treated failed to show an improvement in PFS or overall survival when compared to the standard regimen.[112] Most treatment failures occurred within the first year of diagnosis and at the primary site.[112]

Because the primary goal of using chemotherapy to delay or eliminate the need for radiation therapy had been achieved in only a minority of patients, newer studies have revisited the role of radiotherapy, albeit at a reduced dose. Single-institution series and pilot studies suggest that conformally directed radiation may control localized disease with acceptable toxicity. Two distinct cohorts have been reported. First, of ten patients with localized MB who received lower-than-conventional-dose craniospinal irradiation (<18 Gy) and standard dose boost in conjunction with conventional dose chemotherapy, seven were free of progression with near-normal neuropsychologic test results.[106] Second, instead of treatment of the entire posterior fossa after craniospinal irradiation, one study demonstrated comparable results using tumor bed irradiation in patients with a gross total resection at the primary site.[113] Studies testing whether a reduced dose of craniospinal radiation (to 18 Gy) in children 3 to 8 years of age compromises event-free survival and overall survival as compared to standard doses of 23.4 Gy, and whether reduction of the irradiated volume at the primary site from whole posterior fossa to the tumor bed only compromises event-free and overall survival, are under way.

Recurrent Medulloblastoma: Diagnosis and Treatment

Although a recent study failed to demonstrate a survival benefit, most groups continue to advocate regular surveillance scanning following surgical resection.[114,115] A majority of medulloblastoma recurrences are asymptomatic and could potentially benefit from early treatment. Protocols for surveillance imaging vary. Mendel and associates suggested obtaining a head MRI every 3 months for 2 years, then every 6 months for 2 years, then each year for 5 years.[115] Recurrences after the period of risk indicated by "Collins' rule" (a rule that suggests that a child with a malignant tumor should be cured if he or she survives for his or her age at presentation plus 9 months) have been noted in many cases of medulloblastoma.[13,116] Because late recurrences have been reported, the proper duration of surveillance scanning is not clear.

The majority of recurrences occur in the posterior fossa, usually in close proximity to the site of the primary tumor, although spinal and supratentorial recurrences are also common. The mean time to recurrence is approximately 15 months.[117] The average life expectancy for children with recurrent medulloblastomas varies from 8 months to greater than 27 months.[115] However, long-term survivors have been reported.[117] Local posterior fossa recurrences of medulloblastoma may be treated surgically or with stereotactic radiosurgery or conformal radiation.[118] Initial reports suggest that radiosurgery can prevent local progression in small recurrent (or residual) medulloblastomas.[119] Diffusely metastatic disease should be treated with chemotherapy.[120,121] Recurrent medulloblastoma will respond to "salvage" chemotherapy in approximately 50% of cases, achieving a second remission in approximately 25%.[121] For those patients who have not received radiation, studies indicate a clear superiority of control when radiation is added to the chemotherapy.[122]

Outcome of Medulloblastoma

Data from the Childhood Brain Tumor Consortium indicate that from 1930 to 1979, overall survival of patients with medulloblastoma did improve, although not significantly.[123] In recent years, however, with refinement of surgical and radiation therapy for these tumors and the introduction of chemotherapeutic measures, there is reason for greater optimism. Recent studies typically report 5-year survival rates exceeding 70%, and 5-year progression-free survival rates (survival with evidence of disease, but not of progression) of better than 50%.[90,104,105,117,124,125] Table 20-1 summarizes the five most frequently quoted series.

Clinical features that predict shorter survival include age younger than 3 years at the time of diagnosis, the presence of drop metastases, postoperative tumor volume, and possibly male gender.[30,90,91,126] Tumor histology is also of critical importance in predicting survival.

TABLE 20-1. SUMMARY OF STANDARD-RISK MB TREATMENTS

Author	CSRT (Gy)	CHEMO	5-Y EFS (%)	EPR
Evans[126]	35.0	CCNU/VCR/Pred	65	NA
		None	62	
Packer[104]	36.0	CDDP/CCNU/VCR	85	3/8
Thomas[101]	36.0	None	67	8/21
	23.4	None	52	14/25
Packer[105]	23.4	CDDP/CCNU/VCR	79	3/14
Goldwein[106]	18.0	CDDP/CCNU/VCR	69	2/3

CCNU = lomustine; CDDP = *cis*-diamminedichloroplatinum; Chemo = chemotherapy; CSRT = craniospinal radiotherapy; EFS = event-free survival; EPR = exoprimary relapse; Gy = Gray; NA = not applicable; Pred = prednisone; VCR = vincristine.

Fibrillary histology[127] and the desmoplastic subtype with extensive nodularity[30,31] are predictive of longer survival. Conversely, the large-cell subtype and anaplastic histology are associated with shorter survival.[34,35,128] Although there is no accepted tumor grading system for medulloblastomas, the degree of anaplasia is more closely associated with length of survival than tumor stage.[30] In the past several years, several molecular markers, such as TrkC and c-myc, have been found to have prognostic significance.[78,85,129,130] Further study of these markers may enhance our ability to predict the likely clinical course of a patient with medulloblastoma in the future.

Special attention should be devoted to distinguishing atypical teratoid/rhabdoid tumors (AT/RTs) from MB and PNET. Children with AT/RTs have lower progression-free and overall survival rates than do MB and PNET patients. In fact, the failure to cull these tumors from MB of infancy and early childhood may explain the overall poor outcome of patients less than two years of age as compared with the overall outcome of older children and adolescents. The gene for AT/RTs has been identified and mapped to chromosome band 22q11.2.[131] AT/RT patients may require more aggressive therapy than standard-risk medulloblastoma patients.

Long-term functional outcomes for children following treatment of a medulloblastoma are not well described. It is clear that many survivors experience significant neurocognitive, hearing, growth, and endocrine deficits as a result of radiation therapy,[102] particularly when this modality is used in younger patients. Radiation to the posterior fossa contributes a substantial dose to the parietal, occipital, and posterior temporal lobes bilaterally. The unique shape of the posterior fossa treatment volume necessitates inclusion of both posterior hippocampal formations, and the hypothalamic–pituitary axis (HPA). Conventional posterior fossa volumes also include both cochleae. Conformal techniques designed to spare the cochlea may increase dose to HPA (see Chapter 7). Furthermore, the additive effects of cisplatin chemotherapy and posterior fossa radiation likely contribute to high-frequency hearing loss of survivors. No study has yet been able to tease out what role cisplatin, vincristine, and nitrosourea chemotherapies may have had in producing neurocognitive decline. However, the amnestic dementia/apraxia of gait/urgent-type urinary incontinence syndrome well-described in adults likely occurs in these children as well, amplified by comorbidities caused by the tumor itself (hydrocephalus, papilledema, etc.).

Future directions for patients with MB and PNET will comprise (a) evaluation of local disease control, patterns of failure, progression-free and overall survival in patients treated with a radiation "boost" volume confined to the tumor bed rather than entire posterior fossa; (b) reduction of auditory, neurocognitive, and endocrinologic toxic effects of treatment of average-risk medulloblastoma by reducing the craniospinal radiation dose; and (c) determination of an optimal gene expression MB outcome predictor and tailoring treatment based on it.

▶ SUPRATENTORIAL PNETs

Recent clinical and molecular evidence has supported the distinction between medulloblastomas, pinealoblastoma (see Chapter 23 for details on this tumor), and other supratentorial PNETs.[132–134] Although supratentorial PNETs may be diagnosed at any age, most of these tumors occur during childhood.[135,136] The mean age at diagnosis in pediatric series varies between 3 and 7 years.[135,137] Furthermore, the median age of diagnosis even in adult series is 24 years, supporting a predilection for younger patients. Supratentorial PNET may occur as a congenital tumor and is occasionally diagnosed by ultrasonography in utero.[138] There appears to be a male predilection for this tumor,[135,139] although this is not a universal finding.[136,137]

Supratentorial PNETs are usually large (>5 cm) at the time of initial diagnosis, and symptoms most often are caused by the local tumor mass effect on the surrounding brain.[136] Symptoms of increased intracranial pressure such as headache, irritability, nausea, and vomiting are common.[140] Infants may present with a rapidly increasing head circumference.[140] Supratentorial PNETs arise within the cerebral hemispheres in most cases, although basal ganglia and pineal locations are frequently noted.[134,137,140,141] Tumor dissemination at the time of diagnosis is seen in approximately 20% of cases.[134,141,142]

On cranial imaging studies, supratentorial PNETs usually appear as large, relatively well circumscribed, heterogeneously enhancing lesions.[136,140] Intratumoral cysts and calcification are common findings.[136,140] Like medulloblastoma, supratentorial PNETs have a characteristic hyperdense appearance on CT.[140] In contrast to glial tumors, supratentorial PNETs usually exhibit a paucity of peritumoral edema.[140]

Supratentorial PNETs are usually treated with a combination of surgery, radiation, and chemotherapy.[134–137,139–141] The extent of surgical resection has been correlated with survival in several studies,[134,142] especially when a gross total resection can be achieved.[137] Craniospinal radiation is indicated for patients older than age 3 years.[137] Because of the high frequency of leptomeningeal dissemination, craniospinal irradiation confers a survival benefit over cranial radiation alone.[139]

The survival of patients with supratentorial PNETs is improving.[137] Recent series report 5-year progression-free survival rates between 27% and 37%,[134,141] and average survival between 5 and 7 years following diagnosis.[136,139] Positive prognostic predictors include extent of surgical resection and intratumoral calcification.[134–137] Negative prognostic factors include young age or tumor dissemination at the time of diagnosis.[134,137–139,143]

REFERENCES

1. Bailey P, Cushing H. Medulloblastoma cerebelli, a common type of midcerebellar glioma of childhood. Arch Neurol Psychiatry 1925;14:192–224.
2. Rubinstein L. Cytogenesis and differentiation of primitive central neuroepithelial tumors. J Neuropathol Exp Neurol 1972;31:7–26.
3. Rorke LB. The cerebellar medulloblastoma and its relationship to primitive neuroectodermal tumors. J Neuropathol Exp Neurol 1983;42(1):1–15.
4. Pomeroy SL, Tamayo P, Gaasenbeek M, et al. Prediction of central nervous system embryonal tumour outcome based on gene expression. Nature 2002;415:436–442.
5. Fernandez-Teijeiro A, Betensky RA, Sturla LM, et al. Combining gene expression profiles and clinical parameters for risk stratification in medulloblastomas. J Clin Oncol 2004;22:994–998.
6. Gajjar A, Hernan R, Kocak M, et al. Clinical, histopathologic, and molecular markers of prognosis: toward a new disease risk stratification system for medulloblastoma. J Clin Oncol 2004;22:984–993.
7. Schoenberg BS, Schoenberg DG, Christine BW, et al. The epidemiology of primary intracranial neoplasms of childhood: a population study. Mayo Clin Proc 1976;51:51–56.
8. Gilles FH, Sobel EL, Leviton A, et al. Temporal trends among childhood brain tumor biopsies. J Neurooncol 1992;13:137–149.
9. Roberts RO, Lynch CF, Jones MP, et al. Medulloblastoma: a population-based study of 532 cases. J Neuropathol Exp Neurol 1991;50:134–144.
10. Park T, Hoffman HJ, Hendrick EB, et al. Medulloblastoma: clinical presentation and management. J Neurosurg 1983; 58:543–552.
11. Farwell J, Dohrmann GJ, Flannery JT. Medulloblastoma in childhood: an epidemiological study. J Neurosurg 1984; 61:657–664.
12. DiRocco C, Iannelli A, Ceddia A. Intracranial tumors of the first year of life: a cooperative study of the 1986–1987 Education Committee of the ISPN. Childs Nerv Syst 1991;7: 150–153.
13. DiRocco C, Ceddia A, Iannelli A. Intracranial tumours in the first year of life: a report on 51 cases. Acta Neurochir (Wien) 1993;123:14–24.
14. Jooma R, Hayward RD, Grant DN. Intracranial neoplasms during the first year of life: analysis of one hundred consecutive cases. Neurosurgery 1984;14(1):31–41.
15. Albright AL. Posterior fossa tumors. Neurosurg Clin North Am 1992;3:8818–8891.
16. Chatty E, Earler KM. Medulloblastoma: a report of 201 cases with emphasis on the relationship of histologic variants to survival. Cancer 1971;28:977–983.
17. Hubbard J, Scheithauer BW, Kispert DB, et al. Adult cerebellar medulloblastomas: the pathological, radiographic, and clinical disease spectrum. J Neurosurg 1989;70:536–544.
18. Haie-Meder C, Song PY. Medulloblastoma: differences in adults and children. Int J Radiat Oncol Biol Phys 1995;32: 1255–1257.
19. Evans DG, Farndon PA, Burnell LD, et al. The incidence of Gorlin syndrome in 173 consecutive cases of medulloblastoma. Br J Cancer 1991;64(5):959–961.
20. Kimonis VE, Goldstein AM, Pastakia B, et al. Clinical manifestations in 105 persons with nevoid basal cell carcinoma syndrome. Am J Med Genet 1997;69:299–308.
21. Evans DGR, Ladusaris EJ, Rimmer S, et al. Complications of the naevoid basal cell carcinoma syndrome: results of a population based study. J Med Genet 1993;30:460–464.
22. Blaser S, Harwood-Nash DCF. Neuroradiology of pediatric posterior fossa medulloblastomas. J Neurooncol 1996; 29:23–34.
23. Barkovich AJ. Neuroimaging of pediatric brain tumors. Neurosurg Clin North Am 1992;3(4):739–769.
24. Sandhu A, Kendall B. Computed tomography in management of medulloblastomas. Neuroradiology 1987;29: 444–452.
25. Chang CH, Housepian EM, Herbert C. An operative staging system and a megavoltage radiotherapeutic technique for cerebellar medulloblastoma. Radiology 1969;93:1351–1359.
26. Sutton LN, Cnaan A, Klatt L, et al. Postoperative surveillance imaging in children with cerebellar astrocytomas. J Neurosurg 1996;84:721–725.

27. Schneider JH Jr, Raffel C, McComb JG. Benign cerebellar astrocytomas of childhood. Neurosurgery 1992;30:58–62.
28. Kleihues P, Louis DN, Scheithauer BW, et al. The WHO classification of tumors of the nervous system. J Neuropathol Exp Neurol 2002;61:215–225.
29. Perry A. Medulloblastomas with favorable versus unfavorable histology: how many small blue cell tumor types are there in the brain? Adv Anat Pathol 2002;9(6):345–350.
30. Eberhart CG, Kepner JL, Goldthwaite PT, et al. Histopathologic grading of medulloblastomas: a pediatric oncology group study. Cancer 2002;94:552–560.
31. Giangaspero F, Perilongo G, Fondelli MP, et al. Medulloblastoma with extensive nodularity: a variant with favorable prognosis. J Neurosurg 1999;91:971–977.
32. Schofield D, West DC, Anthony DC, et al. Correlation of loss of heterozygosity at chromosome 9q with histological subtype in medulloblastomas. Am J Pathol 1995;46:472– 478.
33. Giangaspero F, Cenacchi G, Roncaroli F, et al. Medullocytoma (lipidized medulloblastoma): a cerebellar neoplasm of adults with a favorable prognosis. Am J Surg Pathol 1996;20:656–664.
34. Brown HG, Kepner JL, Perlman EJ, et al. "Large cell/anaplastic" medulloblastomas: a Pediatric Oncology Group study. J Neuropathol Exp Neurol 2000;59:857–865.
35. Leonard JR, Cai DX, Rivet DJ, et al. Large cell/anaplastic medulloblastomas and medullomyoblastomas: clinicopathologic and genetic features. J Neurosurg 2001;95:82–88.
36. Trojanowski, JQ, Takashi T, Lee, VMY. Medulloblastomas and related primitive neuroectodermal brain tumors of childhood recapitulate molecular milestones in the maturation of neuroblasts. Mol Chem Neuropathol 1992;17: 121–135.
37. Aruga J, Yokota N, Hashimoto M, et al. A novel zinc finger protein, *zic*, is involved in neurogenesis, especially in the cell lineage of cerebellar granule cells. J Neurochem 1994; 63:1880–1890.
38. Yokota N, Aruga J, Takai S, et al. Predominant expression of human *zic* in cerebellar granule cell lineage and medulloblastoma. Cancer Res 1996;56:377–382.
39. Biegel JA, Rorke LB, Packer RJ, et al. Isochromosome 17q in primitive neuroectodermal tumors of the central nervous system. Genes Chromosomes Cancer 1989;1:139–147.
40. Scheurlen WG, Seranski P, Mincheva A, et al. High-resolution deletion mapping of chromosome arm 17p in childhood primitive neuroectodermal tumors reveals a common chromosomal disruption within the Smith-Magenis region, an unstable region in chromosome band 17p11.2. Genes Chromosomes Cancer 1997;18:50–58.
41. MacDonald TJ, Brown KM, LaFleur B, et al. Expression profiling of medulloblastoma: PDGFRA and the RAS/MAPK pathway as therapeutic targets for metastatic disease. Nat Genet 2001;29:143–152.
42. Gorlin R. Nevoid basal-cell carcinoma syndrome. Medicine 1987;66:98–113.
43. Lacombe D, Chateil JF, Fontan D, et al. Medulloblastoma in the nevoid basal-cell carcinoma syndrome: case reports and review of the literature. Genet Couns 1990;1:273–277.
44. Farndon P, Mastro RC, Evans D, et al. Location of gene for Gorlin syndrome. Lancet 1992;339:581–582.
45. Gailani MR, Bale SJ, Leffell DJ, et al. Developmental defects in Gorlin syndrome related to a putative tumor suppressor gene on chromosome 9. Cell 1992;69:111–117.
46. Albrecht S, von Deimling A, Pietsch T, et al. Microsatellite analysis of loss of heterozygosity on chromosomes 9q, 11p, and 17p in medulloblastomas. Neuropathol App Neurobiol 1994;20:74–81.
47. Johnson R, Rothman A, Xie J, et al. Human homologue of *Patched*, a candidate gene for the basal cell nevus syndrome. Science 1996;272:1668–1671.
48. Hahn H, Wicking C, Zaphiropoulos PG, et al. Mutations of the human homolog of Drosophila *patched* in the nevoid basal cell carcinoma syndrome. Cell 1996;85:841–851.
49. Hooper JE, Scott MP. The *Drosophila patched* gene encodes a putative membrane protein required for segmental patterning. Cell 1989;59:751–765.
50. Nakano Y, Guerrero I, Hidalgo A, et al. A protein with several possible membrane-spanning domains encoded by the drosophila segment polarity gene patched. Nature 1989;341:508–513.
51. Chidambaram A, Goldstein AM, Gailani MR, et al. Mutations in the human homologue of the *Drosophila patched* gene in Caucasian and African-American nevoid basal cell carcinoma syndrome patients. Cancer Res 1996;56:4599–4601.
52. Gailani MR, Stahle-Backdahl M, Leffell DJ, et al. The role of the human homolog of Drosophila patched in sporadic basal cell carcinomas. Nat Genet 1996;14:78–81.
53. Unden AB, Holmberg E, Lundh-Rozell B, et al. Mutations in the human homologue of Drosophila patched in basal cell carcinomas and the Gorlin syndrome: different in vivo mechanisms of PTCH inactivation. Cancer Res 1996;56: 4562–4565.
54. Raffel C, Jenkins RB, Fredrick L, et al. Sporadic medulloblastomas contain the PTCH mutations. Cancer Res 1997;57: 842–845.
55. Zurawel RH, Allen C, Chiappa S, et al. Analysis of PTCH/SMO/SHH pathway genes in medulloblastoma. Genes Chromosomes Cancer 2000;27:44–51.
56. Pietsch T, Waha A, Koch A, et al. Medulloblastomas of the desmoplastic variant carry mutations of the human homologue of *Drosophila patched*. Cancer Res 1997;57:2085–2088.
57. Vorechovsky I, Tingby O, Hartman M, et al. Somatic mutations in the human homologue of *Drosophila patched* in primitive neuroectodermal tumors. Oncogene 1997;15: 361–366.
58. Wolter M, Reifenberger J, Sommer C, et al. Mutations in the human homologue of the *Drosophila* segment polarity gene patched (PTCH) in sporadic basal cell carcinomas of the skin primitive neuroectodermal developmental abnormalities. Cancer Res 1997;57:2581–2585.
59. Xie J, Johnson RL, Zhang X, et al. Mutations of the PATCHED gene in several types of sporadic extracutaneous tumors. Cancer Res 1997;57:2369–2372.
60. Reifenberger J, Wolter M, Weber RG, et al. Missense mutations in SMOH in sporadic basal cell carcinomas of the skin and primitive neuroectodermal tumors of the central nervous system. Cancer Res 1998;58:1798–1803.
61. Taylor MD, Ling L, Raffel C, et al. Mutations in SUFU predispose to medulloblastoma. Nat Genet 2002;31:306–310.

62. Turcot J, Despres J-P, St Pierre F. Malignant tumors of the central nervous system associated with familial polyposis of the colon: report of two cases. Dis Colon Rectum 1959;2:465–468.
63. Hamilton SR, Liu B, Parsons RE, et al. The molecular basis of Turcot's syndrome. N Engl J Med 1995;332(13):839–847.
64. Korinek V, Barker N, Morin PJ, et al. Constitutive transcriptional activation by β-catenin-Tcf complex in $APC^{-/-}$ colon carcinoma. Science 1997;275:1784–1787.
65. Huber O, Korn R, McLaughlin J, et al. Nuclear localization of beta-catenin by interaction with transcription factor LEF-1. Mech Dev 1996;59(1):3–10.
66. Mori T, Nagase H, Horii A, et al. Germ-line and somatic mutations of the APC gene in patients with Turcot's syndrome and analysis of APC mutations in brain tumors. Genes Chromosomes Cancer 1994;9:168–172.
67. Morin PJ, Sparks AB, Korinek V, et al. Activation of β-catenin-Tcf signaling in colon cancer by mutations in β-catenin or APC. Science 1997;275:1787–1790.
68. Yong W, Raffel C, Deimling AV, et al. The APC gene in Turcot's syndrome. N Engl J Med 1995;333:524.
69. Huang H, Mahler-Araujo BM, Sankila A, et al. APC mutations in sporadic medulloblastomas. Am J Pathol 2000; 156:433–437.
70. Garcia-Rostan G, Tallini G, Herrero A, et al. Frequent mutation and nuclear localization of beta-catenin in anaplastic thyroid carcinoma. Cancer Res 1999;59:1811–1815.
71. Terris B, Pineau P, Bregeaud L, et al. Close correlation between beta-catenin gene alterations and nuclear accumulation of the protein in human hepatocellular carcinomas. Oncogene 1999;18:6583–6588.
72. Herter P, Kuhnen C, Muller KM, et al. Intracellular distribution of beta-catenin in colorectal adenomas, carcinomas and Peutz-Jeghers polyps. J Cancer Res Clin Oncol 1999;125:297–304.
73. Sparks AB, Morin PJ, Vogelstein B, et al. Mutational analysis of the APC/beta-catenin/Tcf pathway in colorectal cancer. Cancer Res 1998;58(6):1130–1134.
74. Eberhart CG, Tihan T, Burger PC. Nuclear localization and mutation of beta-catenin in medulloblastomas. J Neuropathol Exp Neurol 2000;59:333–337.
75. Zurawel R, Chiappa, SA, Allen C, et al. Sporadic medulloblastomas contain oncogenic beta-catenin mutations. Cancer Res 1998;58:896–899.
76. Gilbertson RJ, Perry RH, Kelly PJ, et al. Prognostic significance of HER2 and HER4 coexpression in childhood medulloblastoma. Cancer Res 1997;57:3272–3280.
77. Gilbertson RJ, Clifford SC, MacMeekin W, et al. Expression of the ErbB-neuregulin signaling network during human cerebellar development: implications for the biology of medulloblastoma. Cancer Res 1998;58:3932–3941.
78. Gilbertson R, Wickramasinghe C, Hernan R, et al. Clinical and molecular stratification of disease risk in medulloblastoma. Br J Cancer 2001;85:705–712.
79. Chin LS, Petersen DM, Raffel C. The insulin-like growth factor receptor activity is essential for growth of primitive neuroectodermal tumors in cell culture. Neurosurgery 1996;39:1183–1190.
80. Wang JY, Del Valle L, Gordon J, et al. Activation of the IGF-IR system contributes to malignant growth of human and mouse medulloblastomas. Oncogene 2001;20:3857–3868.
81. Pleasure S, Reddy R, Venkatakrishnan G, et al. Introduction of nerve growth factor (NGF) receptors into a medulloblastoma cell line results in expression of high- and low-affinity NGF receptors but not NGF-mediated differentiation. Proc Natl Acad Sci USA 1990;87:8496–8500.
82. Keles G, Berger M, Schofield D, et al. Nerve growth factor receptor expression in medulloblastomas and the potential role of nerve growth factor as a differentiating agent in medulloblastoma cell lines. Neurosurgery 1993;32:274–280.
83. Kokunai T, Sawa H, Tatsumi S, et al. Expression of nerve growth factor receptor by human primitive neuroectodermal tumors. Neurol Med Chir 1994;34:523–529.
84. Segal R, Goumnerova L, Kwon Y, et al. Expression of the neurotrophin receptor TrkC is linked to a favorable outcome in medulloblastoma. Proc Natl Acad Sci USA 1994; 91:12897–1287.
85. Grotzer MA, Janss AJ, Fung K-M, et al. TrkC expression predicts good clinical outcome in primitive neuroectodermal brain tumors. J Clin Oncol 2000;18:1027–1035.
86. Kim JY, Sutton ME, Lu DJ, et al. Activation of neurotrophin-3 receptor TrkC induces apoptosis in medulloblastomas. Cancer Res 1999;59:711–719.
87. Lee M, Wisoff JH, Abbott R, et al. Management of hydrocephalus in children with medulloblastoma: prognostic factors for shunting. Pediatr Neurosurg 1994;20:240–247.
88. Albright AL. The value of precraniotomy shunts in children with posterior fossa tumors. Clin Neurosurg 1983; 30:278–285.
89. Berger MS, Baumeister B, Geyer JR, et al. The risks of metastases from shunting in children with primary central nervous system tumors. J Neurosurg 1991;74:872–877.
90. Albright AL, Wisoff JH, Zeltzler PM, et al. Effects of medulloblastoma resections on outcome in children: a report from the Children's Cancer Group. Neurosurgery 1996;38: 265–270.
91. Jenkin D, Goddard K, Armstrong D, et al. Posterior fossa medulloblastoma in childhood: treatment results and a proposal for a new grading system. Int J Radiat Oncol Biol Phys 1990;19:265–274.
92. Tomita T, McLone DG. Medulloblastoma in childhood: results of radical resection and low-dose neuraxis radiation therapy. J Neurosurg 1986;64(2):238–242.
93. Grabb PA, Albright AL, Sclabassi RJ, et al. Continuous intraoperative electromyography of cranial nerves during resection of 4th ventricular tumors in children. J Neurosurg 1996;86:1–4.
94. Hirsch JF, Renier D, Czernichow P, et al. Medulloblastoma in childhood. Survival and functional results. Acta Neurochir 1979;48:1–15.
95. Erashin Y, Mutluer S, Cagli S, et al. Cerebellar mutism, Report of seven cases and review of the literature. Neurosurgery 1996;38:60–65.
96. Wisoff JH, Epstein FJ. Pseudobulbar palsy after posterior fossa operation in children. Neurosurgery 1984;15:707–709.
97. Pollack IF, Polinko P, Albright AL, et al. Mutism and pseudobulbar symptoms after resection of posterior fossa tumors in children: incidence and pathophysiology. Neurosurgery 1995;37:885–893.
98. Bouffet E, Bernard JL, Frappaz D, et al. M4 protocol for cerebellar medulloblastoma: supratentorial radiotherapy

may not be avoided. Int J Radiat Oncol Biol Phys 1992;24: 79–85.
99. Silber JH, Radcliffe J, Peckham V, et al. Whole-brain irradiation and decline in intelligence: the influence of dose and age on IQ score. J Clin Oncol 1992;10:1390–1396.
100. Hughes E, Shillito J, Sallan SE, et al. Medulloblastoma at the Joint Center for Radiation Therapy between 1968 and 1984: the influence of radiation dose on the patterns of failure and survival. Cancer 1988;61:1992–1998.
101. Thomas PRM, Deutsch M, Kepner JL, et al. Low stage medulloblastoma: final analysis of trial comparing standard-dose with reduced dose neuraxis irradiation. J Clin Oncol 2000;19:3004–3011.
102. Suc E, Kalifa C, Brauner R, et al. Brain tumors under the age of three: the price of survival. Acta Neurochir (Wien) 1990;106:93–98.
103. Johnson D, McCabe MA, Nicholson HS, et al. Quality of long-term survival in young children with medulloblastoma. J Neurosurg 1994;80:1004–1010.
104. Packer RJ, Sutton LN, Elterman R, et al. Outcome for children with medulloblastoma treated with radiation and cisplatin, CCNU, and vincristine chemotherapy. J Neurosurg 1994;81:690–698.
105. Packer RJ, Goldwein J, Nicholson HS, et al. Treatment of children with medulloblastomas with reduced-dose craniospinal radiation therapy and adjuvant chemotherapy: a Children's Cancer Group Study. J Clin Oncol 1999;17: 2127–2136.
106. Goldwein J, Radcliffe J, Johnson J, et al. Updated results of a pilot study of low doses craniospinal irradiation plus chemotherapy for children under five with cerebellar primitive neuroectodermal tumors (medulloblastoma). Int J Radiat Oncol Biol Phys 1996;34:899–904.
107. Duffner P, Horowitz M, Krisher J, et al. Postoperative chemotherapy and delayed radiation in children less than three years of age with malignant brain tumors. N Engl J Med 1993;24:1725–1731.
108. Geyer PM Jr, Zeltzer JM, Boyett LB, et al. Survival of infants with primitive neuroectodermal tumors or malignant ependymomas of the CNS treated with eight drugs in 1 day: a report from the Children's Cancer Group. J Clin Oncol 1994;12(8):1607–1615.
109. Heideman R, Phillips P, Li HJ. A cooperative study of of carboplatin (Carbo) based primary chemotherapy (Chemo) for infants and young children with embryonal CNS tumors. In: 7th International symposium on pediatric neuro-oncology. Washington, DC: 1996.
110. Lashford LSRH, Campbell H, Gattamaneni R, et al. An intensive multiagent chemotherapy regimen for brain tumours occurring in very young children. Arch Dis Child 1996;74(3):219–223.
111. White L, Kellie S, Gray E, et al. Postoperative chemotherapy in children less than 4 years of age with malignant brain tumors: promising initial response to a VATOPEC-based regimen. J Pediatr Hematol Oncol 1998;20:125–130.
112. Strother D, personal communication. 1999.
113. Merchant TEHL, Finlay JL, Leibel SA. Preliminary results of conformal radiation therapy for medulloblastoma. Neuro-oncol 1999;1:177–187.
114. Torres CF, Rebsamen S, Silber JH, et al. Surveillance scanning of children with medulloblastoma. N Engl J Med 1994;330:892–895.
115. Mendel E, Levy ML, Raffel C, et al. Surveillance imaging in children with primitive neuroectodermal tumors. Neurosurgery 1996;38:692–694.
116. Collins VP. Wilm's tumor: its behavior and prognosis. J La State Med Soc 1955;107:474–480.
117. David K, Casey ATH, Hayward RD, et al. Medulloblastoma: is the 5-year survival rate improving? J Neurosurg 1997; 86:13–21.
118. Elterman R, Bruce DA. The continued surveillance for recurrent medulloblastoma: primitive neuroectodermal tumors. Pediatr Neurosurg 1993;19:322.
119. Patrice S, Tarbell NJ, Goumnerova LC, et al. Results of radiosurgery in the management of recurrent and residual medulloblastoma. Pediatr Neurosurg 1995;22:197–203.
120. Finlay J, Garvin J, Allen J. High-dose chemotherapy with autologous marrow rescue in patients with recurrent medulloblastoma/primitive neuroectodermal tumors. Proc Am Soc Clin Oncol 1994;13:176.
121. Bouffet E, Doz F, Demaille MC, et al. Improving survival in recurrent medulloblastoma: earlier detection, better treatment or still an impasse? Br J Cancer 1998;77(8):1321–1326.
122. Kalifa C. Failure patterns and salvage therapy following post-operative chemotherapy for medulloblastoma in very young children for French Society of Pediatric Oncology (SFOP) In: 7th International symposium of pediatric neuro-oncology. Washington, DC: 1996.
123. Gilles FH, Sobel EL, Leviton A, et al. Age-related changes in diagnoses, histological features, and survival in children with brain tumors: 1930–1979. Neurosurgery 1995;37:1056–1067.
124. Merchant TE, Wang M-H, Haida T, et al. Medulloblastoma: long-term results for patients treated with definitive radiation therapy during the computed tomography era. Int J Radiat Oncol Biol Phys 1996;36:29–35.
125. Walter AW, Mulhern RK, Gajjar A, et al. Survival and neurodevelopmental outcome of young children with medulloblastoma at St. Jude Children's Research Hospital. J Clin Oncol 1999;17:3720–3728.
126. Evans A, Jenkin RDT, Sposto R, et al. The treatment of medulloblastoma: results of a prospective randomized trial of radiation therapy with and without CCNU, vincristine, and prednisone. J Neurosurg 1990;72:572–582.
127. Sobel EL, Gilles FH, Leviton A, et al. Survival of children with infratentorial neuroglial tumors. Neurosurgery 1996; 39(1):45–54.
128. Giangaspero F, Rigobello L, Badiali M, et al. Large-cell medulloblastomas: a distinct variant with highly aggressive behavior. Am J Surg Pathol 1992;16:687–693.
129. Scheurlen WG, Schwabe GC, Joos S, et al. Molecular analysis of childhood primitive neuroectodermal tumors defines markers associated with poor outcomes. J Clin Oncol 1998;16:2478–2485.
130. Herms J, Neidt I, Luscher B, et al. C-myc expression in medulloblastoma and its prognostic value. Int J Cancer 2000;89:395–402.
131. Biegel JA J-Y, Zhou LB, Rorke C, et al. Germline and acquired mutations of INI1 in atypical teratoid and rhaboid tumors. Cancer Res 1999;59:74–79.

132. Jakacki RI. Pineal and nonpineal supratentorial primitive neuroectodermal tumors. Childs Nerv Sys 1999;15:586–591.
133. Russo C, Pellarin M, Tingby O, et al. Comparative genomic hybridization in patients with supratentorial and infratentorial primitive neuroectodermal tumors. Cancer 1999;86:331–339.
134. Reddy AT, Janss AJ, Phillips PC, et al. Outcome for children with supratentorial primitive neuroectodermal tumors treated with surgery, radiation, and chemotherapy. Cancer 2000;88:2189–2193.
135. Yang HJ, Nam DH, Wang KC, et al. Supratentorial primitive neuroectodermal tumor in children: clinical features, treatment outcome and prognostic factors. Childs Nerv Sys 1999;15(8):377–383.
136. Kim DG, Lee DY, Paek SH, et al. Supratentorial primitive neuroectodermal tumors in adults. J Neurooncol 2002; 60(1):43–52.
137. Dirks PB, Harris L, Hoffman HJ, et al. Supratentorial primitive neuroectodermal tumors in children. J Neurooncol 1996;29(1):75–84.
138. Yamada T, Takeuchi K, Masuda Y, et al. Prenatal imaging of congenital cerebral primitive neuroectodermal tumor. Fetal Diagn Ther 2003;18(3):137–139.
139. Paulino AC, Cha DT, Barker JL Jr, et al. Patterns of failure in relation to radiotherapy fields in supratentorial primitive neuroectodermal tumor. Int J Radiat Oncol Biol Phys 2004;58(4):1171–1176.
140. Dai AI, Backstrom JW, Burger PC, et al. Supratentorial primitive neuroectodermal tumors of infancy: clinical and radiologic findings. Pediatr Neurol 2003;29(5):430–434.
141. Paulino AC, Melian E. Medulloblastoma and supratentorial primitive neuroectoderm tumors: an institutional experience. Cancer 1999;86(1):142–148.
142. Klisch J, Husstedt H, Hennings S, et al. Supratentorial primitive neuroectodermal tumors: diffusion-weighted MRI. Neuroradiology 2000;42(6):393–398.
143. Girschick HJ, Klein R, Scheurlen WG, et al. Cytogenetic and histologic studies of congenital supratentorial primitive neuroectodermal tumors: a case report. Pathol Oncol Res 2001;7(1):67–71.

CHAPTER 21

Ependymomas and Intraventricular Tumors

Joao Siffert / George Jallo

Tumors arising within or relating to the ventricular surface comprise a small but important proportion of all primary brain tumors. Intraventricular tumors are comprised of a unique spectrum of histological subtypes, the most common of which include ependymomas, central neurocytomas, subependymomas and subependymal giant cell astrocytomas. Other less common variants, including chordoid glioma, oligodendroglioma, choroid plexus papilloma and carcinoma, germ cell, and primary pineal tumors, have also been reported. Each type of intraventricular tumor has unique epidemiological, clinical, radiological, and pathological characteristics (Table 21-1). Furthermore, each type commands its own constellation of management considerations and is associated with distinct prognostic indicators and outcomes.

Considerable advances have been made in contemporary understanding and management of these tumors, particularly over the last several decades. The advent and widespread implementation of advanced microsurgical technique coupled with advancements and refinement in adjuvant therapies and their indications for use have helped to improve the care of patients harboring these lesions. Studies into the basic biology of these tumors utilizing modern molecular biological techniques are increasingly common. Despite this, however, the need for continued progress cannot be overemphasized, particularly in the management of ependymomas.

This chapter will address the individual types of intraventricular tumors, focusing on the unique characteristics and management considerations pertinent to each. Intracranial ependymomas, which occasionally have a parenchymal rather than an intraventricular location, are considered here as well. Spinal cord ependymomas are discussed in Chapter 24.

▶ EPENDYMOMAS

Ependymomas are relatively rare neuroepithelial tumors that account for 3% to 9% of all central nervous system (CNS) tumors. The incidence of ependymomas in children is approximately six times that in adults. In children, approximately two-thirds of ependymomas occur in the infratentorial compartment, whereas supratentorial ependymomas occur relatively more frequently in older children and adults.[1–10] In adults, approximately 75% of ependymomas arise within the spinal canal. Fewer than 5% of children present with metastatic disease, whereas in adults,

▶ **TABLE 21-1.** HISTOLOGY OF TUMOR BY LOCATION AND AGE GROUP

Site	Children	Adult
Lateral ventricle	PNET Choroid plexus tumor Teratoma Astrocytoma	Astrocytoma Subependymoma Neurocytoma Oligodendroglioma Metastasis Meningioma
Septum pellucidum	PNET JPA Subependymal giant cell astrocytoma	Astrocytoma Subependymoma Neurocytoma Lymphoma
Trigone	Choroid plexus tumor or cyst Ependymoma Meningioma	Choroid plexus tumor Oligodendroglioma Metastasis Meningioma
Third ventricle (anterior)	Colloid cyst JPA Germ cell tumors Craniopharyngioma Choroid plexus tumor	Colloid cyst Neurocytoma Subependymoma Meningioma Pituitary adenoma
Third ventricle (posterior)	Astrocytoma Pinealoma Teratoma	Colloid cyst Astrocytoma Pinealoma Metastasis Meningioma
Fourth ventricle	Ependymoma Medulloblastoma JPA	Ependymoma Subependymoma Choroid plexus

JPA = juvenile pilocytic astrocytoma; PNET = primitive neuroectodermal tumor.

neuraxis dissemination is exceedingly rare. Surgical resection with or without radiation therapy confers long-term remission in approximately half of patients newly diagnosed with ependymoma. A complete surgical resection is widely considered the single most important prognostic factor. Postoperative radiotherapy (RT) is believed to improve the prognosis in patients with ependymoma and remains the adjuvant treatment of choice, in particular for those patients with postoperative residual disease. However, the value of adjuvant therapy for patients with no postoperative residual disease remains unclear.[11,12] Chemotherapy has a limited role in the management of ependymoma; it is used in an attempt to defer radiation in newly diagnosed infants and for patients with recurrent disease under experimental protocols.[8,13–19] Although advances in diagnosis and management have improved the outcome of intraventricular tumors in general, the prognosis for intracranial ependymomas, particularly those arising in the posterior fossa, remains unsatisfactory. Surgical and radiation techniques have advanced substantially over the past decades, but future breakthroughs are likely to stem from a greater understanding of tumor biology.

Epidemiology

Ependymomas account for 3% to 9% of all CNS tumors.[20] In the United States, fewer than 200 patients younger than age 25 years are diagnosed with ependymomas each year. The incidence of ependymomas appears equally distributed between the two sexes. In children, the mean age at clinical manifestation is 6.4 years, with approximately 30% occurring in children younger than age 3 years. In adults, a second age peak at 30 to 40 years has been reported for spinal cord tumors.[1–10,20] Among pediatric CNS tumors, ependymomas are the third most common intracranial tumor (6%–12%); juvenile pilocytic astrocytomas and primitive neuroectodermal tumors being the most common.

The etiology of ependymomas is unknown. However, the virus SV40 is implicated in the pathogenesis of several tumors, including ependymomas. SV40 was discovered as a contaminant of poliovirus vaccines that were inadvertently administered to millions of people in Europe and the United States between 1955 and 1963. Shortly afterwards, SV40 was proven to be oncogenic in rodents and capable of transforming human and animal cells in vitro. Despite a lack of significant epidemiologic evidence, there are recent reports about the presence of SV40-like DNA in a high proportion of human mesotheliomas, ependymomas, and osteosarcoma (the three main types of tumors caused by virus in hamsters), renewing the question whether SV40 might be a human tumor virus.[21,22]

Pathology

Ependymomas are thought to be derived from the primitive neuroepithelial cells that line the ventricles and the central canal of the spinal cord and therefore can develop throughout the central nervous system. There are several different histologic variants of ependymomas that have been characterized according to degree of anaplasia or cellular derivatives. The World Health Organization (WHO) grading system has recognized four basic ependymoma groups as follows: the classic ependymoma (with cellular, papillary, clear cell, and fibrillary or tanycytic variants), WHO grade II; subependymoma, WHO grade I; myxopapillary ependymomas, WHO grade I; and anaplastic ependymoma, WHO grade III.[23]

Classic ependymomas are solid, well-demarcated dark gray-red tumors. In the posterior fossa, ependymomas generally originate either from the floor or the roof of the fourth ventricle and develop into the ventricular lumen. Tumor tissue may extend into the cerebellopontine angle through the foramina of Luschka, protrude into the cisterna magna through the foramen of Magendie, and extend along the surface of the brainstem and through the foramen magnum. Despite the insidious growth pattern along cerebral spinal fluid (CSF) pathways, these tumors are generally well demarcated, especially those arising in the supratentorial compartment, and only occasionally do they invade adjacent brain parenchyma. Rare intraparenchymal and extraneural metastases are described. Infrequently, there is spread via the CSF (less than 5%), particularly from infratentorial lesions.[8] Histologically, they are composed of uniform columnar and astrocyte-like fibrillary cells arranged in "true" ependymal rosettes around a central lumen resembling the ependymal epithelia, or in the form of perivascular pseudorosettes, more common but less specific. Ependymal rosettes are generally viewed as diagnostic findings. Intratumoral hemorrhage, calcifications, or myxoid degeneration are occasionally seen, but mitoses are rare or absent. Occasional nonpalisading foci of necrosis are compatible with this diagnosis. Variant forms of ependymomas have been characterized by the presence of increased cellularity, papillary growth pattern, and clear-cell morphology or fibrillary/tanycytic formation. Ependymomas will generally stain positive for glial fibrillary acidic protein (GFAP) and typically express S100 protein and vimentin. Electron microscope analysis may be necessary because of the significant variability in the histologic subtypes, especially because ependymomas maintain characteristic ultrastructural properties of ependymal cells. The presence of either cilia or basal cell blepharoplasts confirms the diagnosis of ependymoma.

Subependymomas and myxopapillary ependymomas are slow-growing ependymomas classified as WHO grade I. Subependymomas are nodular and arise from within the ventricular wall, primarily from the fourth ventricle in about half the reported cases. They appear as tufts of cells within a fibrillary matrix and are thought to be derived from the subependymal glial cells. In contrast, myxopapillary ependymomas are almost exclusively found in the lower spinal canal around the conus, cauda equina, and filum terminale area. Although generally localized at diagnosis, these low-grade tumors can be locally invasive, and residual or recurrent tumor can spread via the CSF pathways along the spinal axis and intracranially.[24] Histologically, this variant appears papillary with mucocystic cells around vascular networks. Myxopapillary ependymomas characteristically express GFAP, S100, and vimentin, but not cytokeratin.

Malignant or anaplastic ependymomas are given WHO grade III classification because of such histologic features as pleomorphism (giant-cell formation), endothelial hyperplasia, mitotic figures, vascular proliferation, and necrosis. This high-grade variant is locally invasive, and subarachnoid dissemination may be found, portending a poorer prognosis.

Molecular Biology and Cytogenetics

The molecular and cytogenetic studies of ependymomas are limited and much of the data are based on case reports and small series. Cytogenetic characterization of ependymomas has revealed significant heterogeneity. Several genetic alterations have been characterized, the most common of which are aberrations involving chromosome 22. The 22q region is of special interest because it contains the neurofibromatosis type 2 tumor suppressor gene, and spinal cord ependymomas are a major manifestation of this genetic disorder.[25] Despite this association, ependymomas are not otherwise hereditary. Other chromosomes implicated with ependymomas include chromosomes 6, 9, 10, 13, and 17 (no association with p53 has been demonstrated).[26,27] Despite the lack of a consistent cytogenetic pattern in ependymomas, recent progress has been made in its molecular understanding. An analysis of a large cohort of pediatric ependymomas (n = 121) compared immunohistochemistry, Western blotting, and reverse transcriptase polymerase chain reaction analysis with histologic markers of anaplasia (necrosis, microvascular proliferation, and Ki-67 proliferative index). Coexpression of erbB2 and erbB4 was identified in more than 75% of tumors. High-level coexpression of these receptors was significantly related to tumor proliferative activity [$p < 0.05$; Ki-67 labeling index (LI)], and a combined survival analysis of clinical (degree of surgical resection) and molecular (erbB2/erbB4 expression status and Ki-67 LI) factors enabled a greater resolution of patient prognosis than any individual variable alone.[28] This study suggests that erbB receptor signaling results in aggressive disease behavior in ependymoma by promoting tumor cell proliferation. Further genetic exploration of certain chromosomal regions may provide future direction for investigations of both diagnostic and therapeutic importance.

Clinical Manifestations

The clinical signs and symptoms of intracranial ependymomas depend on the location, size of the tumor, and the age of the patient (Table 21-2).[29] Ependymomas are typically large at time of presentation. Posterior fossa ependymomas usually present with signs and symptoms of increased intracranial pressure, a result of hydrocephalus caused by obstruction of CSF flow in the fourth ventricle. The most prominent presenting symptoms are vomiting (generally not accompanied by nausea or anorexia), headache, and occasionally diplopia as a consequence of pseudoabducens palsy. Arterial hypertension, bradycardia, and decreased level of consciousness are uncommon findings (possibly because of improved medical care and diagnostic capabilities), but when present they should prompt immediate attention as they indicate possible brainstem dysfunction and consequent risk of respiratory arrest. Frank ataxia, hemiparesis, and cranial nerve deficits are less common and are generally associated with other signs and symptoms of intracranial hypertension. The neurologic exam typically reveals bilateral papilledema, bilateral or unilateral esotropia, and subtle gait ataxia and dysmetria. The extension of the tumor into the cervical subarachnoid space, a rather common growth pattern for ependymomas, may result in neck pain, nuchal rigidity, and torticollis. Diagnosis of a brain tumor in children under the age of 2 years can be challenging, not only because of a communication barrier but also because of nonspecific clinical manifestations such as neck pain/nuchal rigidity, vomiting, lethargy, irritability, and failure to thrive.[1,3,15] Even in older children, it is important to keep in mind that ependymomas occasionally present with isolated symptoms such as recurrent daily vomiting (generally not associated with nausea or anorexia) or neck pain/torticollis, often without the more common signs and symptoms of increased intracranial pressure. Therefore, one should keep in mind the less common clinical manifestations of ependymomas in order to increase diagnostic acumen.

The signs and symptoms of supratentorial ependymomas, which occur more frequently in older children and adults, are primarily related to mass effect from the tumor. They typically present with headaches, focal neurologic deficits such as limb weakness, visual field defects, and less frequently with seizures.[1,7,10,19]

Diagnostic Evaluation and Imaging Characteristics

Ependymomas appear isodense or hyperdense to brain on precontrast computerized tomography (CT) (Table 21-2). They have mild to moderate heterogenous enhancement with intravenous contrast. Calcification occurs in nearly 50% of all cases. In the posterior fossa, ependymomas typically present as solid masses in the fourth ventricle with extension through the foramina of Luschka into the cerebellopontine angle or through the foramen magnum into the cervical spinal canal (Figs. 21-1 and 21-2). Supratentorial intraventricular ependymomas have a more variable appearance with heterogenous enhancement after contrast administration (Fig. 21-3). They tend to be cystic, calcified, and well-demarcated tumors.[30]

On magnetic resonance imaging (MRI), ependymomas may also have a variable appearance caused by small cysts or calcifications. On T_1-weighted imaging, ependymomas

▶ TABLE 21-2. TYPICAL CLINICAL AND RADIOLOGIC FEATURES OF EPENDYMOMA

Ependymoma	Clinical Manifestations	CT Findings	MRI Findings
Fourth ventricle/posterior fossa	• Vomiting • Headache • Esotropia secondary to increased intracranial pressure • Neck tilt/torticollis/neck pain • Ataxia • Lower cranial nerve deficits	• Iso-hyperdense precontrast • Heterogeneous enhancement • Presence of calcification • Extension into foramen magnum	• T_1: hypointense • T_2: isointense consistent with gray matter • Downward extension through foramen of Magendie into cervical canal and lateral extension through Lushka into cerebellar–pontine angle
Supratentorial	• Motor deficits • Visual field defects • Seizures • Sensory deficits • Headache • Vomiting	• Heterogeneous enhancement • Cystic • Well demarcated	• Well demarcated • Heterogeneous signal characteristics and enhancement pattern • No typical features

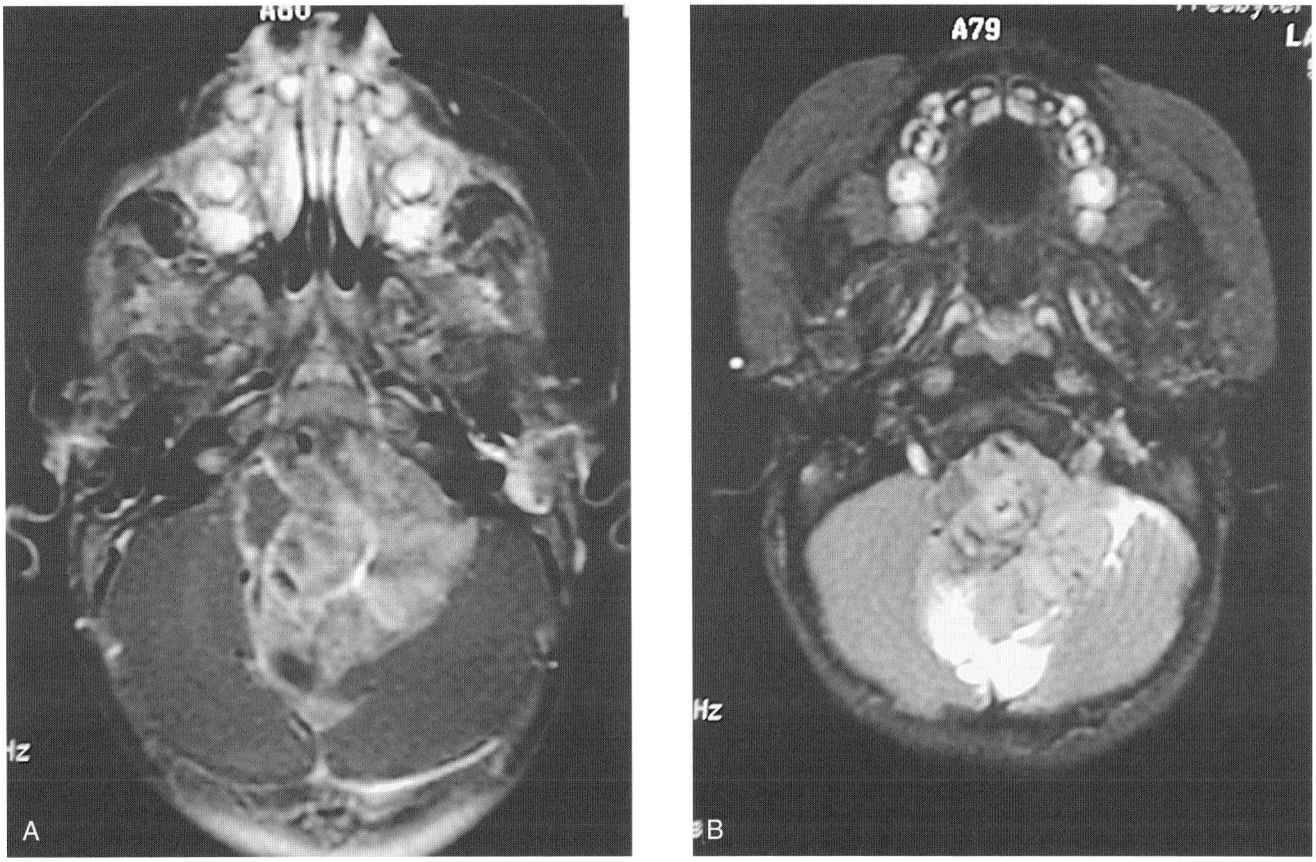

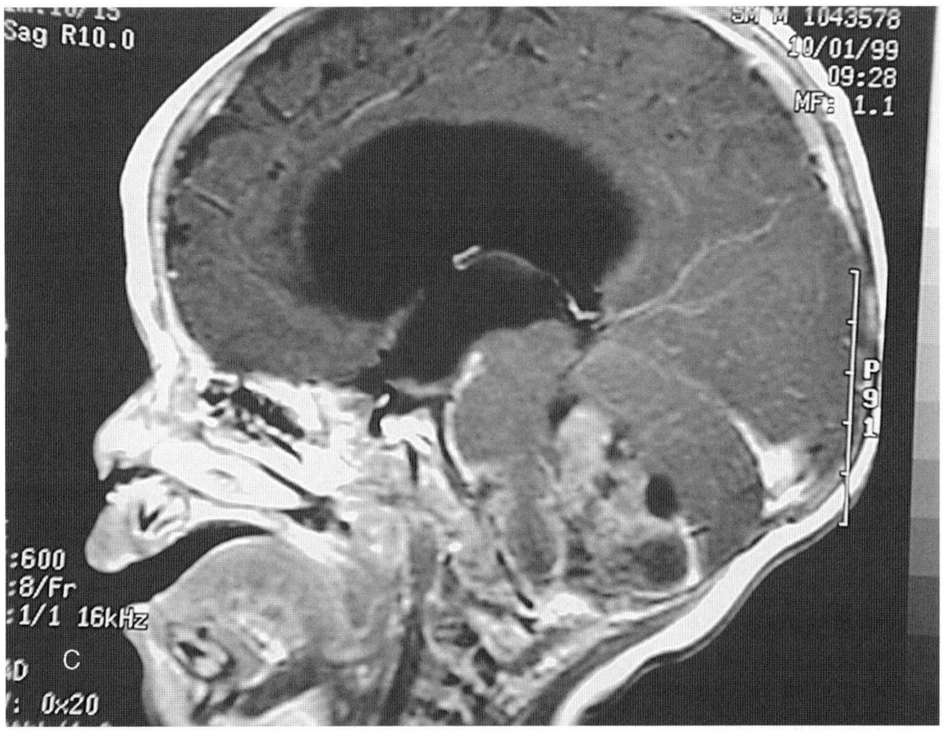

Figure 21-1. Imaging characteristics for a fourth ventricle ependymoma that extends out to the cerebellar–pontine angle. (A) T_1-weighted axial image with gadolinium demonstrates the location of the tumor within the fourth ventricle and extension out the left foramen of Luschka. (B) T_2-weighted axial image demonstrates the hyperintense signal characteristics. (C) T_1-weighted sagittal image.

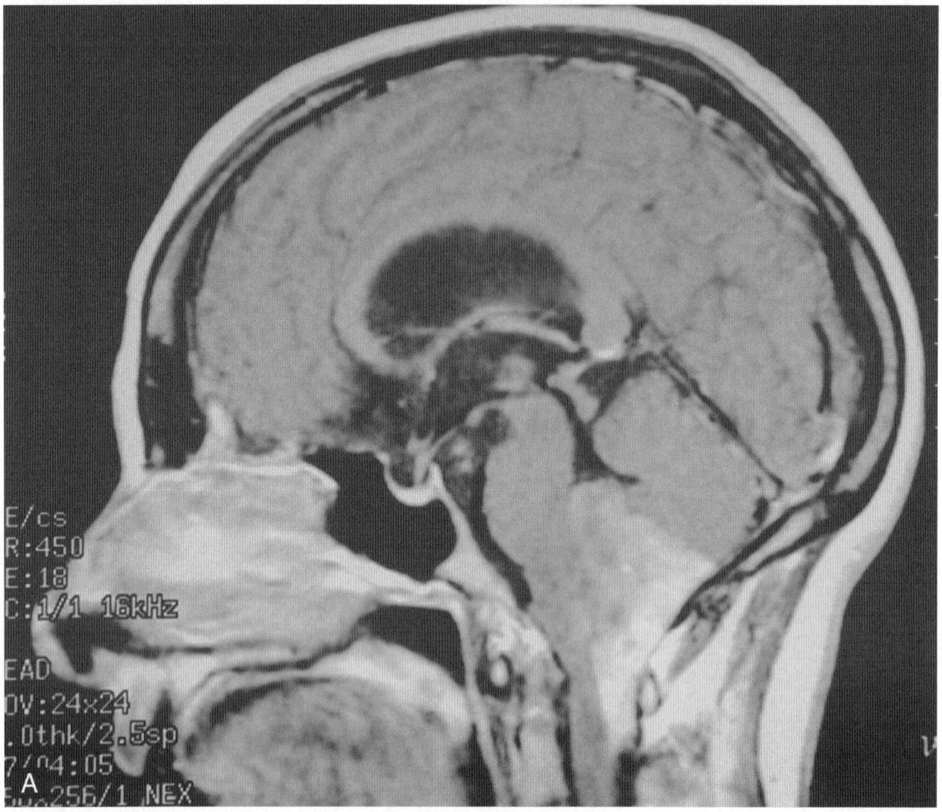

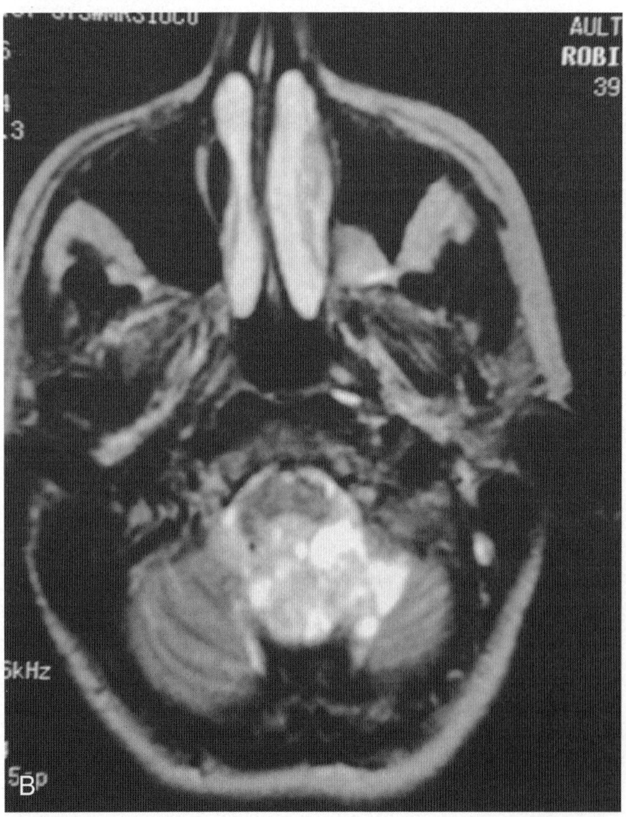

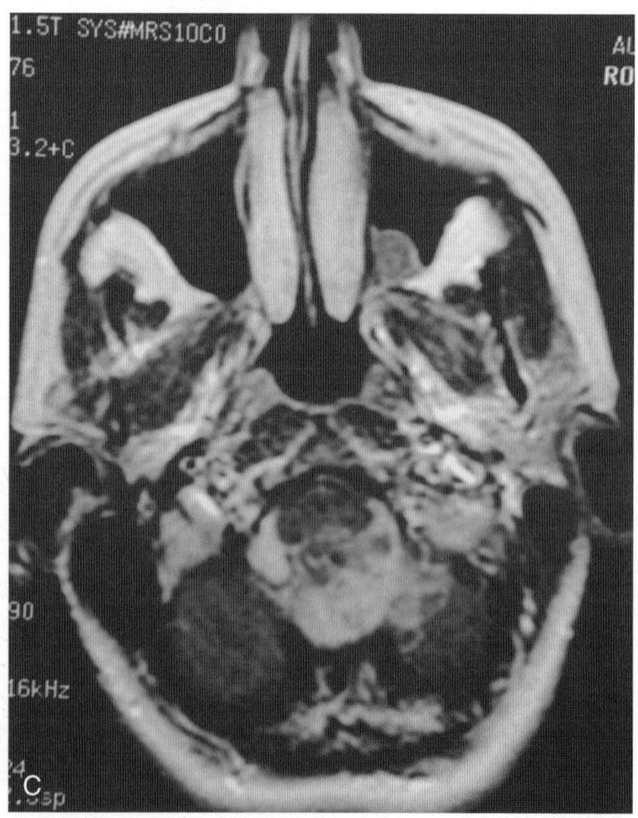

Figure 21-2. Imaging characteristics for a fourth ventricle ependymoma that extends down the cervical spinal cord. (A) T_1-weighted sagittal image with gadolinium demonstrates the location of the tumor within the fourth ventricle and extension. (B) T_2-weighted axial image demonstrates the hyperintense signal characteristics. (C) T_1-weighted axial image.

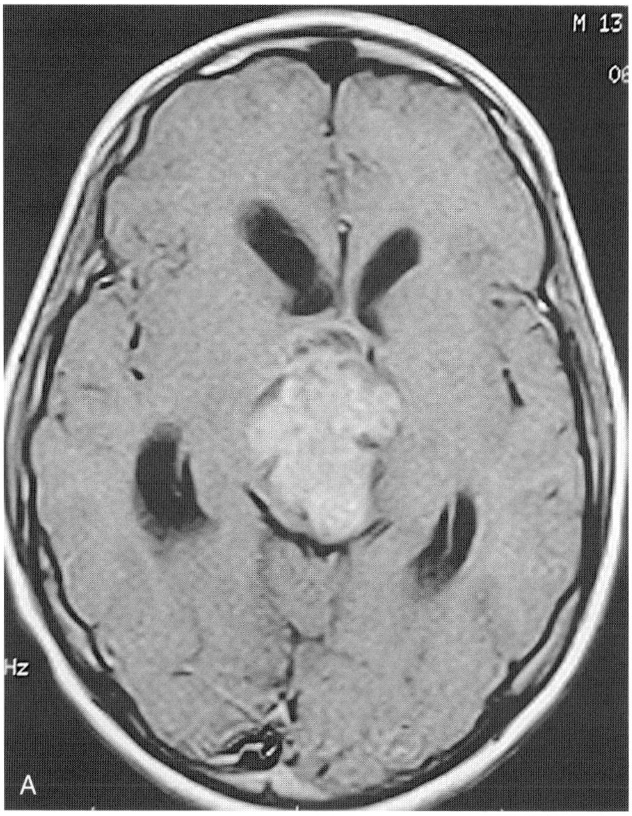

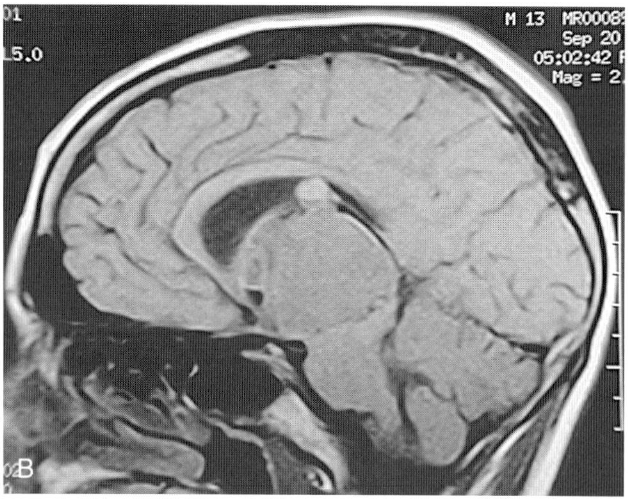

Figure 21-3. A supratentorial ependymoma located in the left frontal horn. (A) T_1-weighted axial image demonstrates a heterogenously enhancing tumor within the left lateral ventricle and hydrocephalus. (B) T_1-weighted sagittal image.

are hypointense as compared to brain parenchyma. On T_2-weighted imaging, these tumors are isointense with gray matter. However, the diverse signal characteristics may make the diagnosis of ependymoma difficult on MRI (see Table 21-2). The most characteristic finding to support a diagnosis for infratentorial ependymomas is downward extension of the tumor through the foramen of Magendie into the cervical subarachnoid space or through the foramina of Luschka into the cerebellopontine cistern (see Figs. 21-1 to 21-3).[3,15,30,31] This rather characteristic growth pattern helps preoperative differentiation of ependymomas from other posterior fossa tumors such as medulloblastoma and astrocytoma.

Preoperative survey of the entire neuraxis is recommended because the presence of metastases may impact the overall management strategy. Postoperative changes such as blood accumulation in the thecal sac may hinder optimal radiologic detection of the tumor in the spinal canal.

Treatment

Surgery

Surgery is the mainstay and the initial treatment for ependymomas.[8,15,17,32,33] Because of its prognostic importance for improved long-term survival, a total or near-total tumor resection should be attempted at initial surgery. Technological advances, such as image-guided surgery, intraoperative MRI, ultrasonic aspirator, and neurophysiologic monitoring, have increased the chances of a total or near-total resection of tumor with minimal morbidity.[8,15] According to recent literature, the rate of total resection for supratentorial ependymomas ranges from 53% to 72%, and for infratentorial ependymoma, from 27% to 55%.[2,6–8,17,19,24,33–36]

Infratentorial Ependymomas

The most common location for infratentorial ependymoma is within the fourth ventricle. The surgical approach, therefore, is a suboccipital craniotomy with or without C1 laminectomy, depending on the extent of the tumor in the cervical region. Tumoral extension through the foramen of Magendie, into the cisterna magna, and downward to the cervical spinal canal, can be removed without difficulty as there is no infiltration of the pia. The tumor in the fourth ventricle can be exposed by elevation of cerebellar tonsils and the inferior vermis and occasionally by opening the sulcus between the tonsil and vermis. Splitting of the inferior cerebellar vermis should be avoided as it is implicated as a potential cause for posterior fossa/cerebellar mutism syndrome (see discussion below).[37] The majority of the tumor bulk is resected in piecemeal fashion using the bipolar cautery-suction and the Cavitron Ultrasonic Surgical Aspirator (CUSA). However, attempts to resect tumor attachments to the floor of the fourth ventricle may result in significant postoperative morbidity as a consequence of injury of the nuclei of the sixth ventricle, the facial colliculi, the mesiolingual fossa, and of other lower cranial nerve nuclei. Thus, facial palsy, extraocular movement abnormalities, and swallowing dysfunction are relatively common postoperative complications.[15] Careful consideration is needed during the surgery to maximize the degree of resection while preserving neurologic function. Neurophysiologic mapping of the floor of the fourth ventricle can be helpful in the intraoperative decision-making process.[15]

In addition to direct surgical injury to brainstem and cranial nerves, postoperative complications include "posterior fossa syndrome" (also known as cerebellar mutism syndrome) and aseptic meningitis. The posterior fossa syndrome affects approximately 10% to 25% of patients following posterior fossa tumor (medulloblastomas, astrocytomas, and ependymoma) resections. Clinical manifestations develop several hours to a couple of days after surgery and generally last for several weeks. Typical neurologic deficits include reduced speech output (mutism in more severe cases), global cerebellar dysfunction, severe irritability, motor apraxia, hypotonia, dysphagia, and bowel and bladder incontinence. Patients remain alert throughout the clinical course, but they tend not to remember the periods during which symptoms were most severe. A complete recovery occurs in most patients, but long-term cerebellar dysfunction may persist in the more severely affected individuals despite intensive rehabilitation.[3,37–39]

Aseptic meningitis is also occasionally observed in patients undergoing posterior fossa tumor resection. Subarachnoid blood products are believed to cause chemical irritation of the meninges. Nuchal rigidity, fever, and irritability arise 24 to 48 hours postoperatively and may be indistinguishable from clinical manifestation of infectious meningitis. CSF analysis usually shows increased protein and mild to moderate pleocytosis consisting of mononuclear and polymorphonuclear leukocytes, as well as red blood cells. CSF culture is negative. Clinical management with steroids is effective, and symptoms generally subside within 24 to 48 hours.

Determining the extent of resection is best done by both a postoperative MRI and the surgeon's intraoperative assessment. The postoperative MRI should ideally be performed before development of postoperative contrast enhancement, that is, within 24 to 48 hours after surgery. As discussed in greater detail later (see "Prognosis"), the extent of resection is relevant both for prognosis and for postoperative management, including the decision of a second-look surgery.

Several authors recommend that a second-look surgery be considered in order to maximize the extent of resection in cases of postoperative residual tumor.[40] The optimal timing for a second-look surgery, however, is a subject of debate. If the postoperative MRI shows residual tumor that appears readily resectable, immediate reoperation should be considered. In cases of more extensive postoperative tumor burden, or residual tumor that is deemed difficult to resect, a second-look surgery may be deferred several weeks. There is preliminary evidence that adjunctive chemotherapy or radiotherapy may facilitate a second surgery by either altering tumor characteristics or reducing the volume of residual tumor.[8,40] Whether chemotherapy, radiotherapy, or just time for healing is accountable for a potential improvement of the tumor resectability remains to be determined. The important fact is that an attempt at gross total resection is imperative in the management of ependymomas.

Supratentorial Ependymomas

Supratentorial ependymomas occur in either the ventricular system or a hemisphere and are usually large at time of diagnosis. Frameless image guidance, intraoperative MRI, and intraoperative ultrasonography provide good localization of the tumor and facilitate a complete resection of the tumor. Intraoperative neurophysiologic monitoring of motor and somatosensory-evoked potentials also help to minimize the risk of morbidity associated with surgery. The surgical corridors for intraventricular ependymomas include a transcallosal approach to avoid cortical injury and seizures, and a targeted transcortical approach for patients with large ventricles. Postoperative complications mainly relate to tumor location and may include seizures, language or visual field dysfunction, and motor or sensory deficits.

Management of Hydrocephalus

Obstructive hydrocephalus can be caused by obstruction of CSF pathways as a consequence of posterior third ventricle or fourth ventricle/posterior fossa tumors. In most patients, resection of the primary tumor suffices to manage obstructive hydrocephalus. However, patients who present acutely with severe signs of raised intracranial hypertension require immediate treatment. The treatment of choice in such patients is endoscopic third ventriculostomy. If there is effacement of the interpeduncular cistern because of anterior displacement of the brainstem or cisternal tumor seeding, this procedure is contraindicated because of risk of injury to the brainstem or basilar artery. External ventricular drainage or ventriculoperitoneal shunting are reasonable alternatives, but carry a risk of infection, overdrainage producing subdural hematoma formation, and, in rare cases, peritoneal tumor seeding, upward transtentorial herniation, and intratumoral hemorrhage.[3,15,18,19] Only approximately 20% of patients with fourth ventricular ependymoma will require shunt placement after resection.[19] There is evidence that infants are more likely to require some form of shunting procedure.[41]

Adjuvant Therapy

Radiotherapy

Postoperative RT has long been considered the standard adjuvant treatment for patients with intracranial ependymomas. Concerns about long-term neurologic and endocrine effects,[42] especially for infants and children less than 5 years, have led to attempts to defer or completely avoid radiation therapy in select subsets of patients. Although no randomized trial has been conducted to definitively evaluate the benefit of RT, several retrospective studies have reported a better prognosis for patients treated with postoperative RT as compared with those treated with surgery alone.[17,34,43–45] However, questions remain regarding the need of postoperative RT for children who have both intraoperative and radiographic confirmation of a complete resection, particularly those with supratentorial ependymomas.[1,11,12,19,32,46,47]

The optimal volume (local field vs. whole brain vs. craniospinal axis) and dose of radiation are still matters of some debate. Most experts recommend local field RT, unless there is evidence of subarachnoid tumor dissemination. Several factors support this recommendation for local radiation: tumor relapse occurs mainly at the primary site, the risk of dissemination is low, and there is no evidence that CNS dissemination can be prevented by whole-brain or craniospinal irradiation.[2,6,18,19,24,34,48–51] Most national study protocols in the United States and abroad recommend focal radiotherapy of at least 5400 cGy in 30 fractions over 6 weeks for low-grade ependymomas and 5940 cGy in 33 fractions over 6.5 weeks for high-grade ependymomas.[2,52,53] Conformal or stereotactic techniques for fractionated radiation treatment planning and delivery have been quickly adopted by most specialized centers with the aim of reducing radiation-related side effects and potentially increasing the dose of radiation delivered to the volume considered at risk. Even though recent data suggest that increased accuracy may not come at an increased risk of local failure, the possibility that a reduction in the size of the targeted volume will result in a higher rate of local failure needs to be kept in mind during radiation planning.[33,48,52] Most radiation therapists currently agree that the appropriate and safe volume for nondisseminated and low-grade infratentorial ependymomas should encompass the tumor bed with a <2-cm safety margin.[35,52] In fact, results of a cohort of 64 pediatric patients (median age at diagnosis: 3 years) with localized ependymoma treated with conformal radiotherapy (5940 cGy) at St. Jude Children's Research Hospital showed that the most common pattern of failure is within the primary radiation target. After a median followup of 17 months (range: 3–43 months), only 1 of 6 failures occurred outside the prescribed volume.[35] Pending a longer-term followup of this cohort, use of highly conformal radiotherapy may be more readily considered, especially in younger patients.

Stereotactic radiosurgery (SRS) has been applied to manage recurrent or residual intracranial tumor in some institutions. Sanford and Gajjar reported that in-field local control was achieved for 14 of 17 recurrent intracranial ependymomas and the 3-year local control rate was 68%.[9] However, Hodgson and associates found that SRS provided a 3-year local control in children with recurrent or residual intracranial ependymomas of only 29%.[54]

Chemotherapy

The role of chemotherapy in the adjunctive care of ependymoma is not fully established. In young children with newly diagnosed ependymoma, chemotherapy has been used in an attempt to defer radiation, but there is no conclusive benefit from use of chemotherapy in older children or adults.[13,18,32,55] The largest chemotherapy studies in ependymoma have been in children with recurrent disease, and active agents identified in such studies are candidates for prospective trials in newly diagnosed patients. More recently, chemotherapy has been considered as an adjunct treatment when a second-look surgery is being planned (see "Infratentorial Ependymomas" above).[8,14–19,55,56]

The only well-controlled study that prospectively compared postoperative radiotherapy with or without chemotherapy was conducted by the Children's Cancer Group (CCG).[16] The CCG conducted a protocol in patients with infratentorial medulloblastomas and ependymomas, all of whom received postoperative craniospinal irradiation, were randomized to receive either adjuvant chemotherapy with lomustine (CCNU), vincristine, and prednisone for 1 year or no chemotherapy. Thirty-six of the 42 patients with ependymoma entered in the study were suitable for analysis; 22 received combined modality therapy and 14 received RT alone. The failure-free survival for the entire sample at 10 years was 36% and overall survival was 39%, with no difference in outcomes between the two regimens. Thus, adding chemotherapy to surgery and RT was not shown to confer an increase survival in patients with infratentorial ependymoma.

Several studies have assessed the use of chemotherapy and deferral of radiation in young children with newly diagnosed ependymoma.[13] The largest prospective trial was conducted by the French Society of Pediatric Oncology (SFOP) and reported in 2001.[57] Seventy-three children younger than 5 years of age with ependymoma (82% with high-grade tumors) were administered 16 months of adjuvant multiagent chemotherapy (alternating procarbazine and carboplatin, etoposide and cisplatin, vincristine and cyclophosphamide) after surgery. Radiotherapy was not planned as part of the protocol. Chemotherapy was generally well tolerated, but no radiologically documented response (>50% tumor reduction) was observed. With a median followup of 4.7 years (range: 5 months to 8 years), the 2- and 4-year survival rates of patients who never received radiotherapy were 40% (95% confidence interval [CI], 29% to 51%) and 23% (95% CI, 14% to 35%), respectively. In the multivariate analysis, the two factors associated with a favorable outcome were a supratentorial tumor location ($p = 0.0004$) and complete surgical resection

($p = 0.0009$). The relatively short median followup period, the lack of randomization, and unknown relative risk of long-term toxicity as a consequence of chemotherapy (including second malignancy) versus radiotherapy (CNS and endocrine, as well as neoplastic) limit the ability to determine if this strategy should be widely adopted.[57] A German prospective trial with 55 newly diagnosed anaplastic ependymomas in children showed that adjuvant chemotherapy did not influence survival.[45]

The role of chemotherapy in adults with ependymoma has not been prospectively studied. Thus, most newly diagnosed adult patients are managed conventionally with maximum surgical resection followed by radiotherapy. Those with recurrent disease are generally considered for additional surgery and radiotherapy/radiosurgery prior to enrollment in phase I or II chemotherapy trials.

In summary, there is no convincing evidence that chemotherapy improves survival in patients with intracranial ependymomas.

Prognosis

The outcome of patients with ependymoma remains poor when compared with the outcome for other pediatric brain tumors. Recently published reports demonstrate a 5-year overall survival rate of 40% to 65% for children with intracranial ependymomas.[2,8,16,17,44,55,57]

Prognostic factors have been a matter of discussion because much of the information is derived from retrospective series; prospective studies have generally included small cohorts of patients (Table 21-3). The one consistently identified favorable prognostic factor is a complete surgical resection for both patients with intracranial and spinal cord tumor ependymomas.[6,7,19,33,57,58] The reported overall 5-year survival rate for the patients with complete surgical resection ranges from 60% to 80%, compared to 22% to 41% for patients with incomplete surgical resection.[6,8,16,18,33,35,46,56,57,59,60] Several investigators have reported a long survival and progression-free survival for patients with completely resected ependymoma without adjuvant therapy (Table 21-4).[7,11,12,33]

The patient's age at diagnosis is also an important prognostic factor, even though treatment differences (deferral of radiotherapy), tumor location (predominantly in the posterior fossa), and histology (higher proportion of higher-grade tumors) may influence the outcome. Overall, children younger than 3 years with intracranial ependymomas have a worse prognosis than older children. Healey and associates reported that the overall actuarial survival rate at 12 years for children younger than 24 months at diagnosis was 0% as compared to 62% for older children.[61] Pollack and associates reported a 5-year overall survival rate of 22% in children younger than 3 years of age and 75% in children older than 3 years at diagnosis.[46,60] Lyons and associates found the 5-year survival rates for patients with posterior fossa tumors was 14% for children and 76% for adults.[6] It is not clear why children younger than 3 years have a worse prognosis than older children and adults. Some investigators report a higher incidence of high-grade ependymomas in the young children age group.[33,62] Also, these children typically have infratentorial tumors, which have a higher incidence of incomplete resection.[6,63] Young children, especially younger than 3 years of age, have a disadvantage regarding adjuvant therapy. They are frequently treated with chemotherapy and deferred radiotherapy.[55,57]

It is controversial whether histopathology affects survival. Ernestus and associates, using a multivariate analysis of 125 patients with intracranial ependymomas, found a statistically significant relevance of WHO grading for the long-term prognosis of intracranial ependymomas. They reported a median progression-free survival (PFS) time of 7.5 years for grade II, but 1.5 years for grade III tumors.[62] In other series, however, the histopathologic grade did not appear to significantly influence survival. A possible explanation for this lack of histopathologic correlation to the outcome in intracranial ependymomas is the difficulty in accurately diagnosing the anaplastic variant.[4,19,34,44]

Several retrospective studies indicated that supratentorial ependymomas have a better prognosis than infratentorial ones. The effect of the tumor location on the clinical outcome may result from the greater difficulty in obtaining a complete resection in the patients with infratentorial ependymomas.[6,63]

Advances in molecular biology are likely to provide a better understanding of the clinical behavior of ependymoma and cancer in general. One such example (discussed in

▶ TABLE 21-3. PROGNOSTIC FACTORS FOR EPENDYMOMA

Prognostic factor	Gross total resection*	High-grade histology	Young age at diagnosis	Infratentorial location	Radiotherapy	Chemotherapy
Relative contribution to overall survival	⇑⇑	⇓	⇓	⇓	⇑	⇐⇒

*Only independent prognostic factor.
⇑ = increase overall survival; ⇓ = decrease overall survival.

▶ **TABLE 21-4.** SURVIVAL OF PATIENTS WITH EPENDYMOMA BASED ON EXTENT OF RESECTION

Series, Year (Reference)	Number of Patients	Complete Resection (5-Year Survival in %)	Subtotal Resection (5-Year Survival in %)
Sutton et al., 1990[18]	45	60	21
Nazar et al., 1990[33]	35	87	30
Duffner et al., 1993[32]	48	61	30
Pollack et al., 1995[38]	40	80	22
Perilongo et al., 1997[59]	92	70	33
Grill et al., 2001[57]	73	74	35

"Molecular Biology and Cytogenetics" above) is a recent analysis of a large cohort of pediatric ependymomas (n = 121), which suggests that erbB receptor signaling results in aggressive disease behavior in ependymoma by promoting tumor cell proliferation.[28]

▶ OTHER INTRAVENTRICULAR TUMORS

There are several additional tumor types that may arise within the ventricles. These include gliomas, subependymomas, neurocytomas, choroid plexus tumors, germ cell tumors, and tumors arising in the pineal region (see Table 21-1).

Imaging

Intraventricular tumors are readily seen on neuroimaging, but a differential diagnosis may be elusive. Subependymomas and central neurocytomas have an affinity for the anterior portion of the lateral ventricle, and both commonly demonstrate a heterogeneous cystic appearance on cross-sectional images. Subependymomas are more common in adults older than age 40 years, whereas central neurocytomas are more common in adults younger than 40 years of age. Subependymal giant cell astrocytomas lie near the foramen of Monro and are characterized by frequent calcification, intense enhancement on contrast-enhanced studies, and the presence of other stigmata seen in tuberous sclerosis. When a mass is centered on the choroid plexus, a highly vascular tumor—either choroid plexus papilloma, choroid plexus carcinoma, meningioma, or metastasis—should be suspected. The characteristic heavily lobulated appearance of a choroid plexus tumor favors this diagnosis over other possibilities, although it is not always possible to distinguish between the more common benign form, the choroid plexus papilloma, and the less common malignant counterpart, the choroid plexus carcinoma.[64] The majority of germ cell tumors arise either on the pituitary/hypothalamic region (60%–70%) or in the pineal region (30%–40%).[65]

Clinical Manifestations

The clinical presentation of these intraventricular tumors depends more on location than on histology. The majority of intraventricular tumors (85%) grow slowly, and as a result may present insidiously until symptoms of raised intracranial hypertension become evident.

Pathology

The tumors found in the lateral ventricles (see Table 21-1) are varied in their pathology and arise from cellular elements found within and around the ventricle walls. There is an age- and location-dependent presentation of most tumor types. Slow-growing tumors include low-grade gliomas, which make up 50% of lateral ventricular tumors, and choroid plexus papillomas and meningiomas, which together account for an additional 35%. Neurocytomas, congenital tumors, ependymomas, and metastasis each account for 5% of these tumors. Most of the tumors arise in the trigone area, and the most common tumor of this location in an adult is meningioma followed by choroid plexus papillomas. The body of the lateral ventricle accounts for 35% of all ventricular tumors. In this location, gliomas and neurocytomas are most common.

Gliomas

This group comprises 50% of lateral ventricle tumors. These lesions arise from surrounding ependymal and subependymal tissues and expand into the ventricle. Astrocytomas are discussed in Chapter 14.

The subependymal giant cell astrocytoma (SEGA) is a variant of astrocytomas found in patients with tuberous sclerosis. SEGAs arise from the brain tissue surrounding the lateral ventricles and protrude into the ventricular lumen. In most cases, these generally asymptomatic lesions are multiple, but tumors arising in the region of the foramen of Monro can produce symptoms when they obstruct the flow of cerebrospinal fluid. Signs or symptoms of increased intracranial pressure along with the clinical stigmata of this phakomatosis make the diagnosis, although incidental findings are increasingly more common with widespread use of neuroimaging.

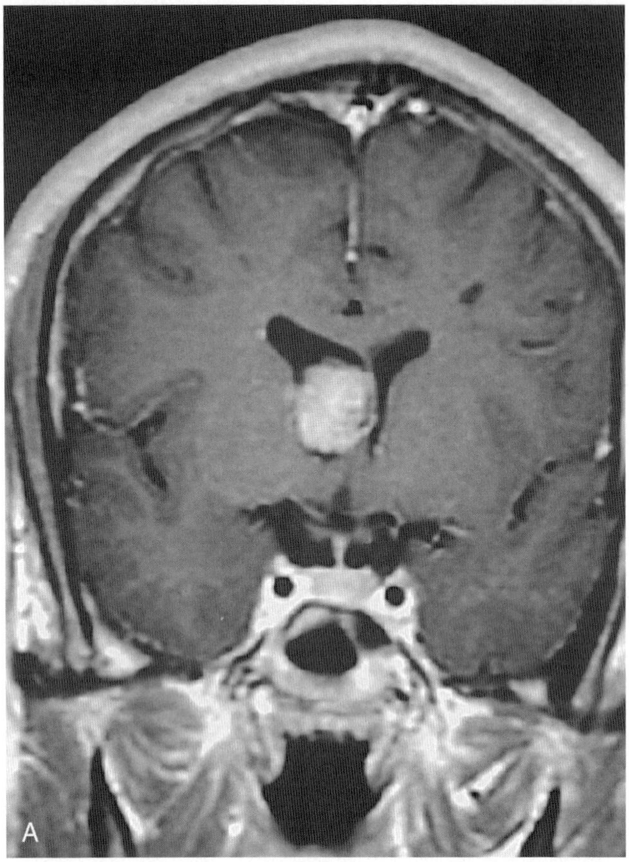

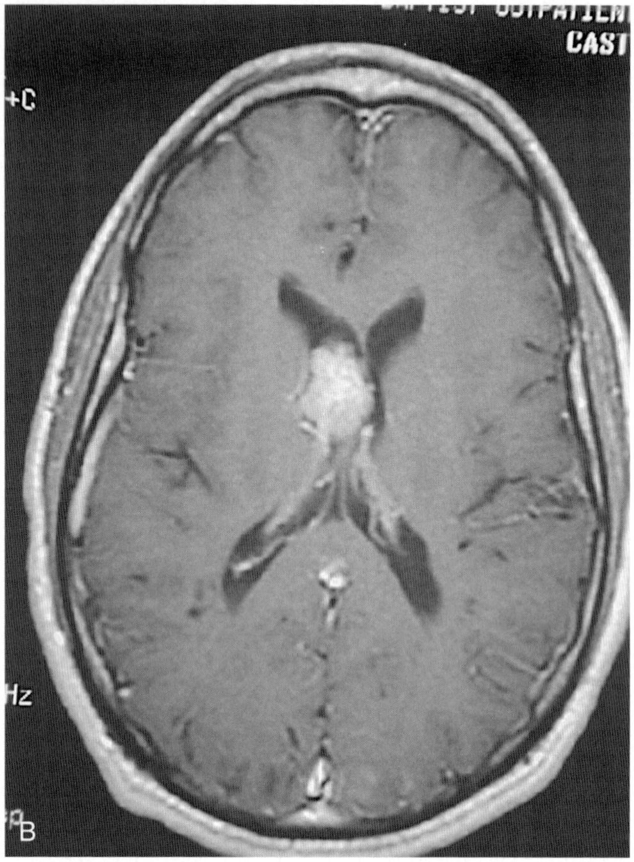

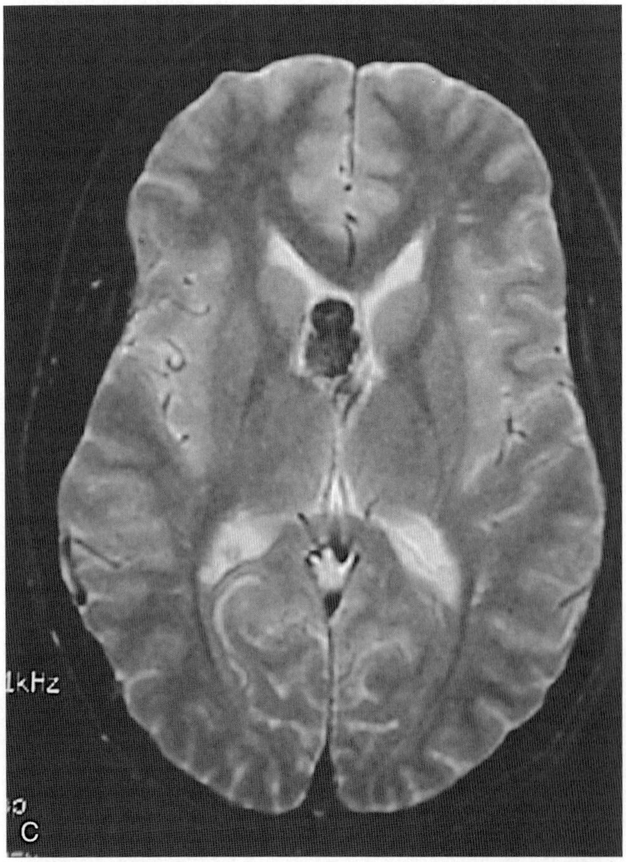

Figure 21-4. Imaging characteristics for an intraventricular neurocytoma. (A) Coronal T_1-weighted image with contrast demonstrates the location within the lateral ventricles. (B) T_1-weighted axial image with contrast. (C) T_2-weighted axial image demonstrates the hypointense signal.

Oligodendrogliomas

Intraventricular oligodendrogliomas are uncommon. Chapter 15 is specifically dedicated to oligodendrogliomas.

Subependymomas

These are rare tumors with a nodular appearance that may arise anywhere within the ventricular system, but typically are found in the fourth ventricle. They are very-slow-growing tumors that frequently remain asymptomatic and are occasionally found incidentally at autopsy. Surgical resection becomes necessary when obstructive hydrocephalus develops, but adjunctive therapy is usually not required.

Neurocytomas

CNS neurocytomas are rare neoplasms, with fewer than 240 cases reported in the literature. The majority of neurocytomas are found in the ventricular system at the septum pellucidum near the foramen of Monro (Fig. 21-4). They tend to occur in the second to fourth decade of life. These tumors, which typically present with obstructive hydrocephalus, are very slow growing, histologically low grade, and often well demarcated. Because of the low incidence of this tumor type, information on management and prognosis are based on case series. Gross total surgical resection generally confers an excellent prognosis. Radiotherapy may be considered for recurrent or inoperable tumors, and radiosurgery is sometimes employed for residual or recurrent tumors.[66]

Choroid Plexus Tumors

Choroid plexus tumors are rare epithelial brain tumors most commonly seen in children. There is limited information available regarding their biology and the best treatment. A review of the medical literature (1966–1998) revealed 566 well-documented cases of choroid plexus tumors. Most patients with a supratentorial tumor were children, with a median age of younger than 2 years, while the most common sites in adults were the fourth ventricle and the cerebellopontine angle. Histology was the most important prognostic factor, as 1-, 5-, and 10-year projected survival rates were 90%, 81%, and 77%, respectively, in choroid plexus papilloma ($n = 353$), compared to only 71%, 41%, and 35%, respectively, in choroid plexus carcinoma ($p < 0.0005$). Surgery was prognostically relevant for both choroid plexus papilloma ($p = 0.0005$) and choroid plexus carcinoma ($p = 0.0001$). Radiotherapy was associated with significantly better survival in choroid plexus carcinomas, although its role in infants with supratentorial tumors is limited. Eight of 22 documented choroid plexus carcinomas responded to chemotherapy. Relapse after primary treatment was a poor prognostic factor in choroid plexus carcinoma patients but not in choroid plexus papilloma patients.[67,68]

Germ Cell Tumors

Germ cell tumors comprise approximately 2% of all intracranial tumors. They tend to arise in the midline, either in the pineal or suprasellar region. The presenting symptoms depend on the site of growth and the dissemination pattern. For practical purposes, germ cell tumors are usually grouped as either pure germinoma or nongerminoma germ cell tumors. The most common tumor histology is pure germinoma, which typically presents in the second and third decades of life with diabetes insipidus with or without additional endocrine deficiencies. Germinomas are more common in males (60%). In general, surgery is performed for histologic diagnosis only, because these tumors are highly responsive to both chemotherapy and radiation. The overall survival of patients with pure germinoma exceeds 80% to 90% in most modern series.[69] Nongerminoma germ cell tumors, such as choriocarcinoma, endodermal sinus tumor, and teratocarcinoma, are also rare malignant tumors, but the overall prognosis is less favorable. These tumors are more frequently diagnosed in the pineal region. Typical signs and symptoms include intracranial hypertension due to obstructive hydrocephalus and Parinaud's syndrome caused by compression of the quadrigeminal plate. Their treatment includes radical surgery and adjuvant therapy consisting of chemotherapy and radiotherapy.[70] Mature teratomas, which also arise in the pineal region, are generally curable with complete removal without adjunctive therapy. Germ cell tumors are discussed more fully in Chapter 23.

Pineal Region Tumors

Tumors typically classified as pineal region tumors are quite rare, with pineoblastoma (a primitive neuroectodermal tumor [PNET]) being five times as common as pineocytoma. These tumors typically present with signs and symptoms of hydrocephalus and Parinaud syndrome. Pineocytomas and PNETs can share some imaging characteristics, but the benign tumors are typically well circumscribed, whereas the malignant tumors may demonstrate invasion into the thalamus or midbrain. Pineocytomas are generally managed with surgery alone. Pineoblastomas (PNET) require surgery and craniospinal radiotherapy with or without chemotherapy. A comprehensive discussion of the management of PNETs is presented in Chapter 20.

REFERENCES

1. Applegate GL, Marymont MH. Intracranial ependymomas: a review. Cancer Invest 1998;16(8):588–593.
2. Bouffet E, Perilongo G, Canete A, et al. Intracranial ependymomas in children: a critical review of prognostic factors and a plea for cooperation. Med Pediatr Oncol 1998;30: 319–331.

3. Duncan JA, Hoffman HJ. Intracranial ependymomas. In: Kaye AH, Laws ER, eds. Brain tumors. Edinburgh: Churchill Livingstone, 1995:493–504.
4. Gerszten PC, Pollack IF, Martinez AJ, et al. Intracranial ependymomas of childhood. Lack of correlation of histopathology and clinical outcome. Pathol Res Pract 1996; 192(6):515–522.
5. Hamilton RL, Pollack IF. The molecular biology of ependymomas. Brain Pathol 1997;7:807–822.
6. Lyons MK, Kelly PJ. Posterior fossa ependymomas: report of 30 cases and review of the literature. Neurosurgery 1991;28: 659–665.
7. Palma L, Celli P, Cantore G. Supratentorial ependymomas of the first two decades of life: long-term follow-up of 20 cases (including two subependymomas). Neurosurgery 1993;32: 169–175.
8. Robertson PL, Zeltzer PM, Boyett JM, et al. Survival and prognostic factors following radiation therapy and chemotherapy for ependymomas in children: a report of the Children's Cancer Group. J Neurosurg 1998;88(4): 695–703.
9. Sanford RA, Gajjar A. Ependymomas. Clin Neurosurg 1997; 44:559–570.
10. Wiestler OD, Schiffer D, Coons SW, et al. Ependymomas. In: Kleihues P, Cavenee WK, eds. World Health Organigation classification of tumors. Pathology and genetics of tumors of the nervous system. Lyon: IARC Press, 2000:71–80.
11. Hukin J, Epstein F, Lefton D, et al. Treatment of intracranial ependymoma by surgery alone. Pediatr Neurosurg 1998; 29:40–45.
12. Awaad Y, Allen J, Miller D, et al. Deferring adjuvant therapy for totally resected ependymoma. Pediatr Neurol 1996;14: 216–219.
13. Siffert J, Allen JC. Chemotherapy in recurrent ependymoma. Pediatr Neurosurg 1998;28(6):314–319.
14. Bouffet E, Foreman N. Chemotherapy for intracranial ependymomas. Childs Nerv Syst 1999;15:563–570.
15. Epstein FJ, Goh KYC. Ependymomas of the posterior fossa. In: Kaye AH, Black PM, eds. Operative neurosurgery. London: Churchill Livingstone, 2000:429–436.
16. Evans AE, Anderson JR, Lefkowitz-Boudreaux IB, et al. Adjuvant chemotherapy of childhood posterior fossa ependymoma: cranio-spinal irradiation with or without adjuvant CCNU, vincristine, and prednisone: a Children's Cancer Group study. Med Pediatr Oncol 1996;27(1):8–14.
17. Rousseau P, Habrand JL, Sarrazin D, et al. Treatment of intracranial ependymomas of children: review of a 15-year experience. Int J Radiat Oncol Biol Phys 1994;28(2):381–386.
18. Sutton L, Goldwein J, Perilongo G, et al. Prognostic factors in childhood ependymomas. Pediatr Neurosurg 1990;16:57–65.
19. Tomita T. Ependymomas. In: McLone DG, ed. Pediatric neurosurgery, 4th ed. Philadelphia: WB Saunders, 2001: 822–834.
20. Yates A, Becker L, Sachs L. Brain tumors in childhood. Childs Brain 1979;5:31–39.
21. Jasani B, Cristaudo A, Emri SA, et al. Association of SV40 with human tumours. Semin Cancer Biol 2001;11(1):49–61.
22. Klein G, Powers A, Croce C. Association of SV40 with human tumors. Oncogene 2002;21(8):1141–1149.
23. Wiestler OD, Schiffer D, Coons SW, et al. Ependymomas. In: Kleihues P, Cavenee WK, eds. World Health Organization classification of tumors. Pathology and genetics of tumors of the nervous system. Lyon: IARC Press, 2000:71–80.
24. Rezai AR, Woo HH, Lee M, et al. Disseminated ependymoma of the central nervous system. J Neurosurg 1996;85:618–624.
25. Parry DM, Eldridge R, Kaiser-Kupfer MI, et al. Neurofibromatosis 2 (NF2): clinical characteristics of 63 affected individuals and clinical evidence for heterogeneity. Am J Med Genet 1994;52(4):450–461.
26. Mazewski C, Soukup S, Ballard E, et al. Karyotype studies in 18 ependymomas with literature review of 107 cases. Cancer Genet Cytogenet 1999;113(1):1–8.
27. Biegel JA. Cytogenetics and molecular genetics of childhood brain tumors. Neuro-oncol 1999;1(2):139–151.
28. Gilbertson RJ, Bentley L, Hernan R, et al. ERBB receptor signaling promotes ependymoma cell proliferation and represents a potential novel therapeutic target for this disease. Clin Cancer Res 2002;8(10):3054–3064.
29. Allen J, Hukin J, Siffert J. Clinical manifestations of childhood ependymoma: a multitude of syndromes. Pediatr Neurosurg 1998;28:48–55.
30. Barkovich AJ. Pediatric neuroimaging. Philadelphia: Lippincott Williams & Wilkins, 2000.
31. Lefton DR, Pinto RS, Martin SW. MRI features of intracranial and spinal ependymomas. Pediatr Neurosurg 1998;28: 97–105.
32. Duffner P, Horowitz M, Krischer J, et al. Postoperative chemotherapy and delayed radiation in children less than three years of age with malignant brain tumors. N Engl J Med 1993;328:1725–1731.
33. Nazar G, Hoffman H, Becker L, et al. Infratentorial ependymomas in childhood: prognostic factors and treatment. J Neurosurg 1990;72:408–417.
34. McLaughlin MP, Marcus RB, Buatti JM, et al. Ependymoma: results, prognostic factors and treatment recommendations. Int J Radiat Oncol Biol Phys 1998;40(4):845–850.
35. Merchant TE. Current management of childhood ependymoma. Oncology (Huntingt) 2002;16(5):629–642, 644; discussion 645–646, 648.
36. Vinchon M, Soto-Ares G, Riffaud L, et al. Supratentorial ependymoma in children. Pediatr Neurosurg 2000;34:77–87.
37. Dailey AT, McKhann GM 2d, Berger MS. The pathophysiology of oral pharyngeal apraxia and mutism following posterior fossa tumor resection in children. J Neurosurg 1995; 83(3):467–475.
38. Pollack I, Polinko P, Albright A, et al. Mutism and pseudobulbar symptoms after resection of posterior fossa tumors in children: incidence and pathophysiology. Neurosurgery 1995;37(5):885–893.
39. Siffert J, Allen J, Epstein F. The posterior fossa syndrome following tumor resection: incidence, clinical features and long-term outcome [abstract]. Ann Neurol 1995;38(3):187.
40. Foreman NK, Love S, Gill SS, et al. Second-look surgery for incompletely resected fourth ventricle ependymomas: technical case report. Neurosurgery 1997;40(4):856–860.
41. Lee M, Wisoff J, Abbott I, et al. Management of hydrocephalus in children with medulloblastoma: prognostic factors for shunting. Pediatr Neurosurg 1994;20:240–247.
42. Dowell RE Jr, Copeland DR. Cerebral pathology and neuropsychological effects. Differential effects of cranial radiation as a function of age. Am J Pediatr Hematol Oncol 1987;9(1):68–72.

43. Donahue B, Steinfeld A. Intracranial ependymoma in the adult patient: successful treatment with surgery and radiotherapy. J Neurooncol 1998;37:131–133.
44. Schiffer D, Giordana MT. Prognosis of ependymoma. Childs Nerv Syst 1998;14:357–361.
45. Timmermann B, Hortmann RD, Huhl J, et al. Combined postoperative irradiation and chemotherapy for anaplastic ependymomas in childhood: results of the German prospective trials HIT 88/89 and HIT 91. Int J Radiat Oncol Biol Phys 2000;46(2):287–295.
46. Duffner PK, Krischer JP, Sanford RA, et al. Prognostic factors in infants and very young children with intracranial ependymomas. Pediatr Neurosurg 1998;28:215–222.
47. Palma L, Celli P, Mariottini A, et al. The importance of surgery in supratentorial ependymomas. Childs Nerv Syst 2000; 16:170–175.
48. Grill J, Pascal C, Chantal K. Childhood ependymoma: a systematic review of treatment options and strategies. Paediatr Drugs 2003;5(8):533–543.
49. Horn B, Heideman R, Geyer R, et al. A multiple-institutional retrospective study of intracranial ependymomas in children: identification of risk factors. J Pediatr Hematol Oncol 2000;21(3):203–211.
50. Merchant TE, Zhu Y, Thompson SJ, et al. Preliminary results from a phase II trial of conformal radiation therapy for pediatric patients with localised low-grade astrocytoma and ependymoma. Int J Radiat Oncol Biol Phys 2002;52(2): 325–332.
51. Vanuytsel L, Brada M. The role of prophylactic spinal irradiation in localized intracranial ependymoma. Int J Radiat Oncol Biol Phys 1991;21:825–830.
52. Paulino AC. The local field in infratentorial ependymoma: does the entire posterior fossa need to be treated? Int J Radiat Oncol Biol Phys 2001;49:757–761.
53. Paulino AC, Wen BC. The significance of radiotherapy treatment duration in intracranial ependymoma. Int J Radiat Oncol Biol Phys 2000;47(3):585–589.
54. Hodgson DC, Goumnerova LC, Loeffler JS, et al. Radiosurgery in the management of pediatric brain tumors. Int J Radiat Oncol Biol Phys 2001;50(4):929–935.
55. Souweidane MM, Bouffet E, Finlay J. The role of chemotherapy in newly diagnosed ependymoma of childhood. Pediatr Neurosurg 1998;28(5):273–278.
56. Needle M, Goldwein J, Grass J, et al. Improved relapse-free survival in incompletely excised childhood ependymoma with hyperfractionated radiotherapy (HFRT) followed by carboplatin (CBDCA), vincristine (VCR), ifosfamide (IFOS) and etoposide (ETP) chemotherapy. In: Sixth International Symposium on Pediatric Neuro-Oncology 1994:79.
57. Grill J, Le Deley MC, Gambarelli D, et al. Postoperative chemotherapy without irradiation for ependymoma in children under 5 years of age: a multicenter trial of the French Society of Pediatric Oncology. J Clin Oncol 2001;19(5): 1288–1296.
58. Constantini S, Allen J, Epstein F. Pediatric and adult primary spinal cord tumors. In: Black P, Loeffler J, eds. Cancer of the nervous system. Cambridge, MA: Blackwell Science, 1997:658–669.
59. Perilongo G, Massimino M, Sotti G, et al. Analyses of prognostic factors in a retrospective review of 92 children with ependymoma: Italian Pediatric Neuro-Oncology Group. Med Pediatr Oncol 1997;29:79–85.
60. Pollack IF, Gerszten PC, Martinez AJ, et al. Intracranial ependymomas of childhood: long-term outcome and prognostic factors. Neurosurgery 1995;37(4):655–666; discussion 666–657.
61. Healey E, Barnes P, Kupsky W, et al. The prognostic significance of postoperative residual tumors in ependymoma. Neurosurgery 1991;28:666–672.
62. Ernestus RI, Schroder R, Stutzer H, et al. The clinical and prognostic relevant grading in intracranial ependymomas. Br J Neurosurg 1997;11(5):421–428.
63. Sala F, Talacchi A, Mazza C, et al. Prognostic factors in childhood intracranial ependymomas: the role of age and tumor location. Pediatr Neurosurg 1998;28:135–142.
64. Koeller KK, Sandberg GD. From the archives of the AFIP. Cerebral intraventricular neoplasms: radiologic-pathologic correlation. Radiographics 2002;22(6):1473–1505.
65. Allen J. Management of primary intracranial germ cell tumors of childhood. Pediatr Neurosci 1987;13:152–157.
66. Brown DM, Karlovits S, Lee LH, et al. Management of neurocytomas: case report and review of the literature. Am J Clin Oncol 2001;24(3):272–278.
67. Packer RJ, Perilongo G, Johnson D, et al. Choroid plexus carcinoma of childhood. Cancer 1992;69(2):580–585.
68. Wolff JE, Sajedi M, Brant R, et al. Choroid plexus tumours. Br J Cancer 2002;87(10):1086–1091.
69. Allen J, DaRosso R, Donahue B, et al. A phase II trial of preirradiation carboplatin in newly diagnosed germinoma of the central nervous system. Cancer 1994;74: 940–944.
70. Robertson PL, DaRosso RC, Allen JC. Improved prognosis of intracranial non-germinoma germ cell tumors with multimodality therapy. J Neurooncol 1997;32(1):71–80.

CHAPTER 22

Primary Tumors of the Cranial Nerves and Skull Base

L. Gerard Toussaint III / Michael J. Link

The evaluation and management of tumors involving the cranial nerves and the skull base have evolved in parallel with advances in diagnostic imaging, intraoperative electrophysiologic monitoring, and microsurgical techniques. Tumors once deemed surgically inaccessible and without other treatment options can now be treated using a variety of modalities with good clinical outcome. The guiding principles underlying the care of patients with these lesions include prompt diagnosis, preservation of function, and prolongation of a meaningful quality of life. This chapter reviews the presentation, imaging, and management options for these lesions, with an emphasis on possible surgical interventions.

The history of surgical intervention for skull base lesions dates to the late 1800s and early 1900s. Pecchioli of Siena reported the successful removal of an olfactory groove meningioma in 1835.[1] Balance and Beevor reported surgical extirpation of an acoustic neuroma via a posterior fossa craniotomy in 1894.[2] In 1909, Harvey Cushing described the transnasal approach to the pituitary.[3] This approach was then abandoned until the development of antibiotics in the second half of the 20th century and has since become the standard route for removing pituitary tumors. Walter Dandy, in the first half of the 20th century, published what was to become the operative standard for acoustic tumor resection, until the advent of the operative microscope.[4] Donald credits Fisch and Yasargil with development of the infratemporal approach to the middle cranial fossa.[5] Approaches through the face and upper pharynx to the central skull base along with the transoral approach to the clivus and upper cervical spine are recent additions to the surgical armamentarium.[6–12]

The past 110 years of skull base surgery have seen a remarkable evolution of diagnostic and treatment options. Surgical planning has greatly benefited from the advent of computerized tomography (CT) and magnetic resonance imaging (MRI). Instruments for rigid facial and cranial fixation without significant infection rates have added numerous facial mobilization and reconstruction procedures to the surgical repertoire. Few contraindications to surgical extirpation of skull base lesions remain. Those that persist include carotid artery involvement without contralateral perfusion, bilateral optic nerve involvement, extensive brain invasion, and severe medical comorbidity.

The diversity of skull base tumors encompasses tissue origins as distinct as nerve sheaths, meninges, cartilage, bone, nasopharyngeal mucosa, and remote organs via metastasis. Their biology and growth patterns are heterogeneous, and, although they may present with similar signs owing to the dysfunction of local nervous and vascular structures, their outcomes are varied. The classification of clinical skull base syndromes—orbital, parasellar, middle fossa, jugular foramen, and occipital condyle—began with Greenberg and colleagues.[13] *Although their classifications were based on symptoms of metastatic lesions, they are applicable to the primary lesions discussed here. Tumors described in this chapter are grouped according to the area of the skull base from which they arise: anterior fossa/anterior skull base, sellar and parasellar, middle fossa/central skull base, posterior fossa, and extracranial cranial nerves. Yet, this categorization is manufactured, as many skull base lesions involve more than one of the aforementioned spaces. The tumors described herein represent those conditions that a neurologist and/or neurosurgeon might be asked to evaluate. A comprehensive discussion of all skull base tumors and their treatment is beyond the scope of this review and the reader can be directed to volumes dedicated to this topic alone. We focus here on lesion presentation, evaluation, and management, with an emphasis on surgical options. Adjunctive treatment of these lesions is expanding as the role of surgery grows and the outlook for survival is more positive.*[14]

▶ ANTERIOR SKULL BASE/ANTERIOR FOSSA LESIONS: THE CRISTA GALLI, CRIBRIFORM PLATE, ORBITAL ROOF, AND PLANUM SPHENOIDALE

Clinical Presentation

The presentation of anterior skull base lesions is quite varied. Nonspecific symptoms such as headache, lightheadedness, imbalance, and mild cognitive or memory impairment are difficult to localize and often attributed to stress or aging. Nasal congestion, rhinorrhea, purulent drainage, and epistaxis help to localize the tumor to the sinuses. Trismus can result from pterygoid or temporalis involvement by irritation of the muscles of mastication or branches of the trigeminal motor root. Even more specifically, cerebral spinal fluid (CSF) rhinorrhea can point to penetration of the dura. Paresthesias or hypesthesia in the distribution of the first or second divisions of the trigeminal nerve can herald the diagnosis of lesions along the course of these nerves. Orbital involvement can produce diplopia, ophthalmoplegia, proptosis, or pain with or without changes in visual acuity.[13] Personality changes, especially development of abulia or disinhibition, along with incontinence, point to significant encroachment of the frontal lobes. Anosmia, which may present as a change in taste, can precede these frontal lobe symptoms. Palpable cheek or forehead masses or cervical adenopathy are rarer presentations.[15]

Evaluation

The initial evaluation of a patient with an anterior skull base lesion has specific caveats. Historical information regarding occupational exposures may be valuable. Occupational exposure may occur in 44% of paranasal malignancies, with the highest-risk professions considered to be smelting, hydrocarbon refining, meat-curing, hardwood woodworking, cotton weaving, and leather tanning.[15] Physical examination should include a careful head, neck, and sinus examination. Transnasal endoscopic examination can visualize nearly all paranasal malignancies abutting the skull base.[15] Ten percent to 15% of patients will present with regional lymph node involvement, mostly secondary to lymphoma, melanoma, sarcoma, and squamous cell carcinoma.[15] The neurologic examination should include testing of the cranial nerves: especially olfaction, visual acuity, and extraocular movements. Additionally, visual fields, concentration, attention, memory, along with the motor, sensory, speech, and cerebellar examinations should be completed. A physical examination directed at finding a primary malignancy is important, as skull base lesions are frequently metastatic. The converse is not true. Skull base malignancies rarely present with distant metastases, but 5% to 10% of patients may expire from systemic disease, so liver function tests and a chest radiograph are important.[15] Lesions of the posterior portion of the anterior cranial fossa and skull base may affect pituitary function, and testing of the pituitary axes can be helpful.

Bony erosion of the skull base, orbits, and paranasal sinuses can be seen well with CT. Magnetic resonance (MR) scanning is required in nearly all skull base lesions. This imaging is particularly helpful to document dural invasion, perineurial spread, and soft-tissue planes.[15] Nonneoplastic entities can often be ruled out, as inflamed mucosa, polyps, and inspissated mucous all have abnormally high T_2 signal, whereas most tumors have isointense T_2 signal. Exceptions include salivary gland tumors, hemangiomas, and schwannomas of the paranasal sinuses.[15] On postcontrast T_1 images, nearly all tumors will enhance, with some angioinductive lesions enhancing heterogeneously. Dural and periorbital thickening and brain or periorbital edema usually indicate invasion.[16] Perineurial spread is often best seen on fat-suppressed images, but frequently does not predict the true extent of spread, as it is often microscopic and has to be assessed as a surgical margin at the time of operation. MR is also useful in detecting large, enhancing, high retropharyngeal lymph nodes suggestive of local lymphatic invasion. Radiographic staging of skull base tumors is variable between authors. Paranasal sinus tumors are often staged using the Kadish system.[17]

Skull base lesions encroaching on or encasing the carotid arteries deserve special evaluation. A conventional cerebral angiogram with external and internal carotid selective injections can document any vessel narrowing by the lesion, identify major feeding vessels to the tumor, and, in specific cases, can be used to embolize the lesion preoperatively. When there is a risk of vessel injury, a trial balloon occlusion of the internal carotid artery can help stratify risk of carotid sacrifice or temporary intraoperative occlusion. Clinical deterioration with occlusion, poor ipsilateral hemispheric perfusion, and delayed venous outflow are indicators of high risk. Formal metabolic and functional perfusion studies can augment this information.[18,19]

Because many of the tumors involving the anterior skull base are readily visible in the nasopharynx, preoperative biopsy can often be easily performed. Massive epistaxis, massive CSF leak, or tumor swelling are possible rare complications. The preoperative evaluation should also pay special attention to physical reconstruction and the need for possible speech, physical, or occupational therapy after surgery. The midface is the most scrutinized portion of the human in social interaction.[15] For this reason, consultation with ophthalmology, oral and maxillofacial surgery, and plastic or reconstructive surgery is useful. An anesthesia evaluation is helpful to address operative medical risks, any airway issues, and to allow planning for blood loss, hypotension, and possible carotid sacrifice. Consultation with a physiatrist is helpful in planning postoperative therapies.

Diagnoses and Management

Esthesioneuroblastoma

Esthesioneuroblastoma is a neoplasm of the olfactory neuroepithelium in the nasal cavity. There is a bimodal distribution of presentation with peaks in the second and sixth decades.[20] These tumors commonly invade the cribriform plate, orbits, dura, and frontal lobes (Fig. 22-1A). Symptoms can include nasal obstruction, epistaxis, nasal mass, anosmia or hyposmia, headache, rhinorrhea, proptosis, visual loss, diplopia, face pain, facial mass, and tooth pain. Family members may report the patient has abulia, personality change, and incontinence to which the patient may be indifferent. Presentation signs depend on extent of invasion. CT scanning defines the sinus anatomy, cribriform plate involvement, and orbital destruction, most notably the lamina papyracea. Coronal-enhanced MR images offer the best picture of tumor anatomy (Fig. 22-1B). Pial enhancement and parenchymal edema may be present. Often, the tumor has a cystic component on the edge leading the brain invasion (Fig. 22-1A).

The multimodality management of these lesions varies by institution. Surgery is the mainstay of therapy, and usually involves a bifrontal craniotomy and lateral rhinotomy for cranial and nasal exposure of the tumor. Recently, endoscopic approaches have been applied to esthesioneuroblastoma, with similar results among patients with small, less invasive tumors, and with adequate local control for aggressive lesions in patients with comorbidity limiting the extent of possible surgical intervention.[21] Endoscopic surgery can afford removal of the cribriform plate, olfactory bulbs, dura, and crista galli, but reconstruction of the skull base may prove problematic through a purely endoscopic approach. Reconstruction of the anterior skull base comprises a major portion of the operation after removal of all gross tumor and establishing negative margins.

The adjuvant therapy of esthesioneuroblastoma includes fractionated radiation and chemotherapy.[21] Preoperative therapy is common, but the decision to use radiation, chemotherapy, or both prior to surgery is unclear. Preoperative radiotherapy (50–60 Gy) is reported to decrease the recurrence rate from 50% to 20%. Those patients responding to preoperative radiation or chemotherapy have better outcome.[22] Typical chemotherapeutic agents used are cyclophosphamide, vincristine or cisplatin, doxorubicin, and infusional 5-fluorouracil (5-FU).

Survival in esthesioneuroblastoma patients is related either to tumor stage or grade. There are reports of a correlation of survival with histologic grade only, and other reports of correlation with tumor stage only.[17] In general, the overall survival at 5 and 10 years is 80% to 88% and 50%, respectively.[21,23] Tumors of Kadish stage A have a 57% to 88% 5-year survival rate, stage B tumors have a 58% to 60% 5-year survival rate, and stage C or D tumors have a 0% to 50% 5-year survival rate.[17] Distant metastases are present in 20% to 25% of patients.[22] Recurrence is possible in up to 18% to 20% of patients with gross total resection. Reoperation seems effective in disease control.

Complications of treatment include wound infection or breakdown from radiation or chemotherapeutic effects, cerebral infarction, contusion, CSF leak, pneumocephalus with lumbar CSF drainage, blindness, exophthalmus, visual acuity loss, and diplopia.

Chondrosarcoma and Chordoma

Both chondrosarcomas and chordomas are discussed in the section "Posterior Fossa/Clival: Posterior Temporal Bone, Occipital Bone, Clivus" below. Although chordomas involve the anterior skull base by extension from notochord remnants in the clivus and spheno-occipital

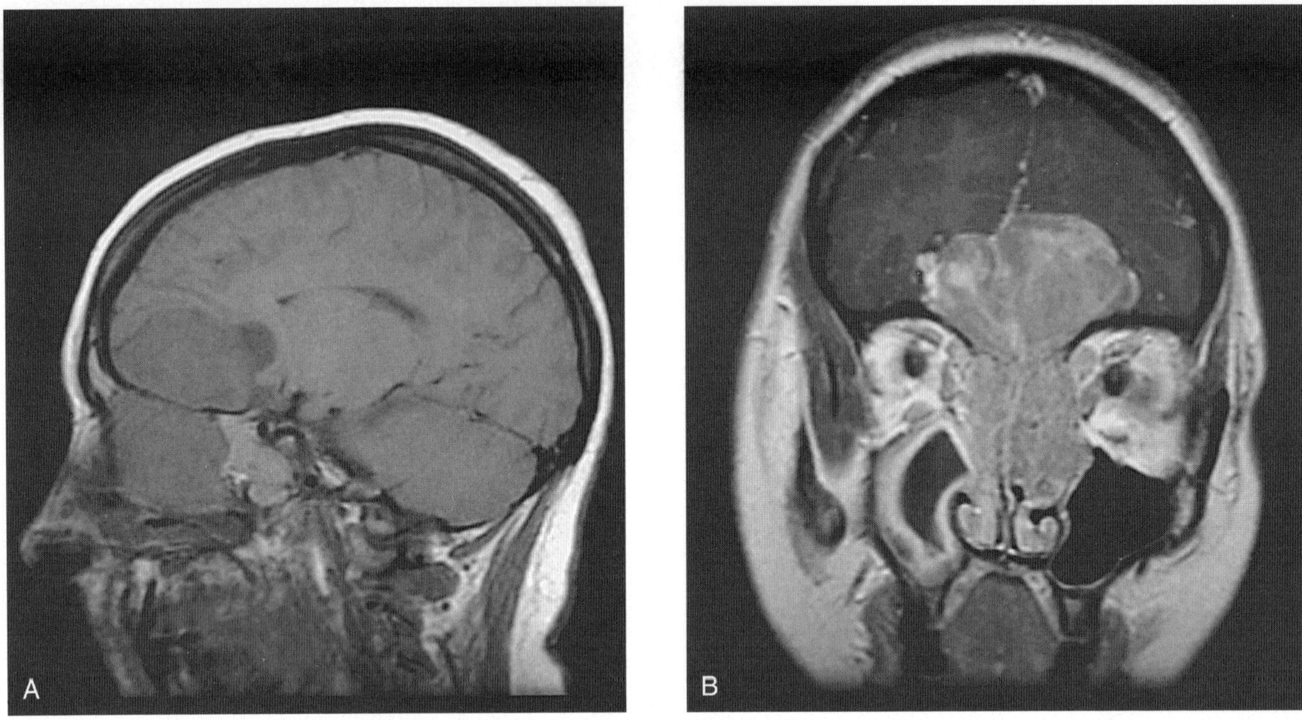

Figure 22-1. (A) Sagittal unenhanced T_1-weighted MRI scan of a patient with a large esthesioneuroblastoma. The tumor fills the nasal cavity and extends through the cribriform plate to markedly compress the frontal lobes. Note the sphenoid sinus is filled with trapped secretions and there is a cyst adjacent to the posterior margin of the tumor at the tumor–brain interface. (B) Coronal enhanced T_1-weighted MRI scan of the same patient in (A) shows an intensely enhancing mass filling the nasal cavity down to the inferior turbinates and extending through the destroyed anterior skull base to compress both frontal lobes. The tumor is easily biopsied through the nasal cavity to establish the diagnosis.

synchondrosis, chondrosarcomas can often originate from the frontonasal or sphenoethmoidal synchondroses. Surgical resection followed by proton beam radiotherapy is reported to maximize tumor control. Typically, low-grade chondrosarcoma has a slightly better prognosis than does chordoma. More information is offered in the section noted.

Rhabdomyosarcoma

Rhabdomyosarcoma is a soft-tissue sarcoma of childhood that can present as a primary lesion in the skull base. It represents 4% to 8% of tumors in patients younger than age 15 years.[24] The lesions show T_1 isointense signal, T_2 hyperintensity,[24] and avid enhancement with gadolinium, along with soft tissue as well as bony erosion on imaging.[20] The treatment is surgical with attempted en bloc resection. Chemotherapy and radiation therapy are used, with hyperfractionated radiation dosing showing similar results to conventionally fractionated doses.[25–27] The tumor histology does alter outcome, with alveolar and pleomorphic subtypes offering decreased rates of survival.[28] The embryonal subtype has intermediate survival. Parameningeal rhabdomyosarcoma carries a poor prognosis, and warrants more aggressive adjuvant therapies. Overall, more than two-thirds of patients are alive at 5-year followup.

Fibrous Histiocytoma

These lesions are common mesenchymal tumors in the sixth to eighth decades of life, with a male prevalence. Their skull base localization is typically in the orbit, causing exophthalmus. Although most tumors are benign, with nearly 100% long-term survival, 10% of these lesions may have a malignant phenotype resulting in a 10-year survival rate in the 25% range.[29] Surgical resection is the treatment of choice, with reports of chemotherapy and, especially, radiation therapy as adjuncts for the more aggressive variants. The histology of these lesions often determines radiosensitivity; more sensitive lesions have a small fibrous component in a histiocyte-rich lesion.[30] The malignant subset of these tumors requires orbital exenteration for complete resection. However, in tumors with negative margins in the periorbita, the orbit can be preserved, and when postoperative irradiation is added, the prognosis is favorable.[30] Preoperative arterial embolization has been described as a surgical adjuvant in these highly vascular lesions.[31]

Other Tumors of Bone, Cartilage, or Mesenchymal Origin: Osteogenic Sarcoma, Osteoclastoma/Giant Cell Tumor, Osteoma, Osteochondroma, Fibrosarcoma

The most useful distinction to make among these bony lesions is biologic behavior. Whereas fibrosarcoma and osteogenic sarcoma are rapidly growing, painful, expansile lesions, giant cell tumors and osteochondromas are more benign. Osteomas are benign bone lesions that, in the skull base, present in the ethmoid, maxillary, and sphenoid sinuses. CT is often sufficient for diagnosis of these well-circumscribed lesions. Treatment is curettage of the entire lesion. Multiple osteomas should prompt evaluation for Gardner syndrome.[16] Osteoblastomas share imaging features with osteomas, but are typically larger and present in the sphenoid region. Excision is again the treatment of choice.

Chondroma, or osteochondroma, is a benign neoplasm of bone formed by enchondral ossification. In the skull, these tumors are limited to the skull base, most often sphenoid, ethmoid, or occipital. Multiple chondromas are seen in Maffucci syndrome and Ollier disease. Symptoms are typically cranial neuropathy from direct compression.[16] Surgical intervention may have to be limited to nerve decompression, depending on access. There is no role for radiation or chemotherapy. Degeneration into chondrosarcoma is possible but extremely rare.

Giant cell tumor of the skull base is typically limited to the temporal or sphenoid bones.[16] The pathologic differential diagnosis includes Paget disease, brown tumor of hyperparathyroidism, and giant cell granuloma. The imaging differential includes lytic metastases, myeloma, and invasion of local carcinoma. Radiation may induce malignant dedifferentiation[16,32] and is usually reserved for multiple recurrences or particularly aggressive tumors in which only a subtotal resection can be performed. Treatment is wide excision if possible.

Fibrous dysplasia is a bone lesion that can also present with multiple cranial neuropathies from compression and/or exophthalmus and visual disturbance. McCune-Albright syndrome involves multiple areas of fibrous dysplasia. On CT imaging, the involved bone is expanded and has a ground-glass appearance. A lytic form can present with hypodense regions in the affected bones, and there is also a pagetoid variant with alternating sclerotic and lytic areas. Surgical excision is effective treatment, but in some patients, complex craniofacial reconstruction is necessary because of the extent of disease. The efficacy of bisphosphonates in slowing disease progression is a topic of debate.[33,34]

Skull base sarcomas are mainly of osteogenic and fibrous varieties. Paget disease and fibrous dysplasia can rarely degenerate into sarcoma. Osteogenic sarcoma is the most common bone malignancy. Although it affects primarily the mandible and maxilla in the head, its fast growth can lead rapidly to skull base encroachment. Fibrosarcoma can arise in the marrow space of the skull or in the sinus cavities, face, scalp, periosteum, or dura.[16] Both lesions are lytic on CT imaging with variable amounts of calcification. The fibrosarcomas enhance less than the osteogenic sarcomas, and have a bland bulky soft tissue component making up the lytic substrate. Osteoblastic osteosarcoma, a subset of osteogenic sarcoma, rarely presents with its typical long bone radiographic sunburst appearance when located in the skull. These lesions, because of anatomic constraints, are rarely amenable to en bloc resection. Therefore, adjuvant therapy is recommended. Metastases are predominantly to the lungs.

As with most sarcomas of the head and neck, radiation therapy is an adjuvant, and when combined with surgery, patients do better than with surgery alone.[35] Charged particle irradiation (Ne, He, and proton) is one possible therapy, with a reported 58% 5-year local control.[36,37] Sarcomas in young adults and children typically respond better to chemotherapy.[38] Osteogenic sarcoma, rhabdomyosarcoma, and Ewing sarcoma respond well. Advanced soft tissue sarcoma of the adult is typically not treated with chemotherapy. Doxorubicin and iphosphamide are the most frequently used drugs for palliative efforts, with concurrent chemoradiotherapy used to limit locoregional disease.[38] The Memorial Sloan-Kettering 5-year survival rate for sarcomas of the skull base is approximately 80% for low-grade sarcoma, and 47% for high-grade sarcoma.[23]

Plasmacytoma

Plasmacytoma of the skull base has been reported as a solitary lesion, as the presentation of occult multiple myeloma, and as secondary lesions in confirmed myeloma cases. This entity is rare, and can have protean manifestations. The orbit, sphenoid bone, clivus, and occipital skull base can be affected. Most patients present with cranial neuropathy—visual symptoms, diplopia, facial numbness, swallowing trouble, and even hearing loss. Radiation and surgery have been used alone or in combination for the management of these lesions, in addition to systemic therapy for widespread disease. Plasmacytoma is so radioresponsive that surgical treatment is usually limited to biopsy to establish the diagnosis (Fig. 22-2).

Neurofibroma

Comments on the management of facial and extracranial neurofibromas are offered in later sections of this chapter

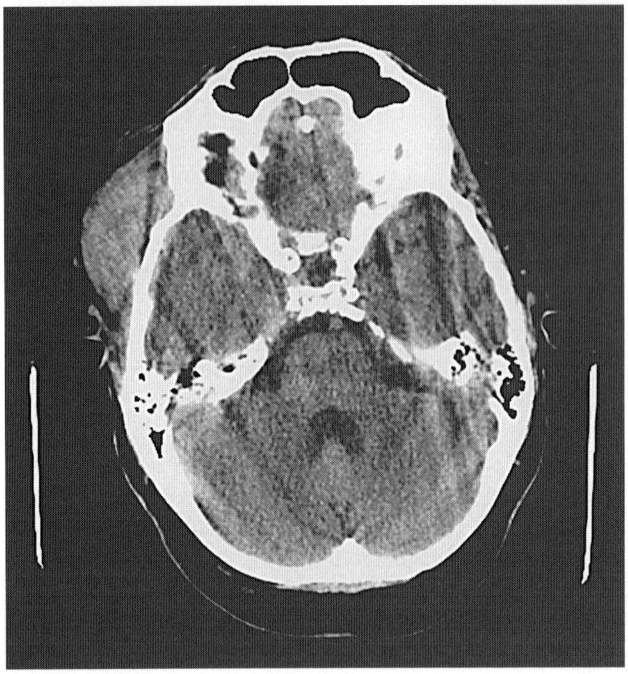

Figure 22-2. Axial unenhanced CT scan of the head reveals a right soft-tissue mass that extended from the anterior skull base through the lateral sphenoid wing beneath the temporalis muscle. A needle biopsy under local anesthesia was easily performed and revealed a plasmacytoma.

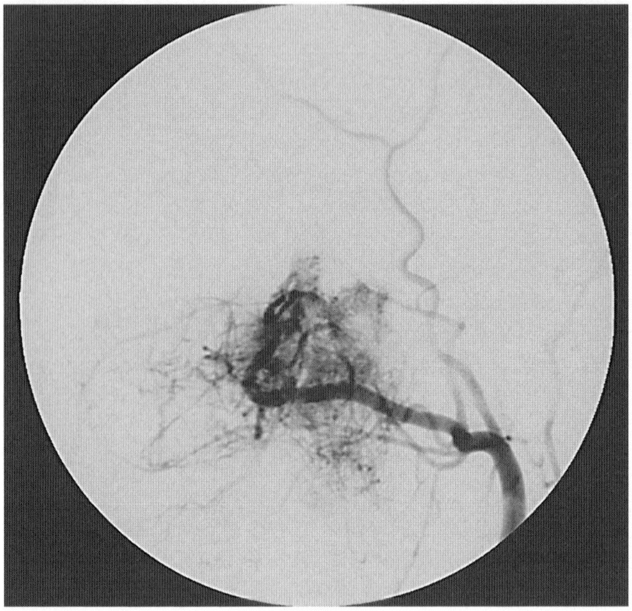

Figure 22-3. Lateral subtracted left external carotid artery injection in a 16-year-old male reveals an intense tumor blush in the infratemporal fossa. The angiofibroma is fed primarily from branches of the internal maxillary artery. This vessel was embolized preoperatively, which markedly reduces surgical blood loss.

such as "Cavernous Sinus/Middle Fossa Lesions" and "Extracranial Lesions." The typical course of management is one of treatment of symptomatic lesions by surgical resection. Solitary neurofibromas can be removed completely, whereas plexiform neurofibromas and diffuse facial/skull base neurofibromas evade total resection. Chemotherapy and radiation therapy are reserved for malignant peripheral nerve sheath tumors.

Juvenile Neuroangiofibroma

The juvenile neuroangiofibroma or nasopharyngeal angiofibroma is a lesion of young adolescent males. The presenting symptoms are epistaxis and nasal obstruction foremost, with rarer complaints of proptosis, hearing loss, sinusitis, and meningitis. Although benign in histology, these tumors are locally invasive. This highly vascular lesion originates in the nasopharynx, with extension through the sphenopalatine foramen into the pterygopalatine fossa and, occasionally, behind the maxillary sinus into the infratemporal fossa.[39,40] Extension through the vidian canal and foramen rotundum has been reported in lesions reaching the cavernous sinus. CT scanning demonstrates an enlarged sphenopalatine foramen with anterior skull base bony remodeling. Angiography demonstrates an extremely vascular mass supplied principally by ascending pharyngeal and internal maxillary arteries (Fig. 22-3), along with internal carotid supply in larger lesions.[31] Surgical resection after preoperative embolization offers good results, owing to the indolent nature of residual tumor and the reported spontaneous remission of small residual lesions. Radiographic residual/recurrent tumor is not considered an indication for further therapy until symptomatic or growing.

Meningioma

The presentation and management of cranial vault meningiomas is discussed in Chapter 18. Here we review the specific considerations for these lesions at the skull base.

In the anterior fossa, meningiomas are split somewhat evenly between sphenoid wing lesions and lesions of the olfactory groove or tuberculum sella. For the purposes of this review, we define tuberculum sella lesions as those midline or near-midline meningiomas arising from the tuberculum sella or diaphragma sella. Olfactory groove meningioma refers to those lesions arising from the floor of the anterior cranial fossa along the cribriform plate and frontosphenoidal suture. Lesions off the midline in the anterior fossa are sphenoid wing meningiomas. Medial sphenoid wing lesions arising around the anterior clinoid are considered anterior clinoid meningiomas.

Tuberculum sella meningiomas commonly present with visual findings—loss of acuity or unilateral blindness, or, more rarely, junctional scotoma and possibly Foster-Kennedy syndrome. Hemiparesis and anosmia are rare, 15% and 11% respectively.[41] In addition to examination and imaging, the evaluation of these patients includes neuroophthalmologic exam and pituitary function studies. Angiography with trial balloon occlusion is considered when the carotid arteries are endangered by resection efforts. The blood supply to these lesions is most often from the ethmoidal branches of the ophthalmic artery, whereas parasitization of pial vessels may result in anterior cerebral artery and anterior communicating artery supply.[41] Surgical intervention for these lesions includes the opening of both optic canals to allow for optic nerve decompression. Cerebrospinal fluid leak is a frequent concern following aggressive resection, and vascularized pericranial flaps can help provide a water-tight barrier.[41] The particular risk of surgery in this region is worsening of vision, reported to occur in 5% to 38% of cases.[41] Prognostic factors in favor of good visual outcome include tumor size less than 3 cm in diameter, normal optic discs, less than 50% loss of acuity, and symptoms for less than 2 years. Surgical mortality of tuberculum sella meningioma resection is related to large artery injury, with rates reported from 0 to 7% and higher for larger lesions.[41]

Olfactory groove meningiomas typically present with indolent changes in personality, headaches, visual symptoms in 50%, cognitive change in 33%, anosmia, or seizures.[41,42] Preoperative imaging may reveal growth of these lesions into the ethmoid sinuses, seen in 15% of these tumors.[41] These lesions have an arterial supply similar to tuberculum sella lesions, with the exception of an increased role of middle meningeal branches. Their growth displaces the olfactory bulbs and tracts superiorly, the optic nerves inferiorly and laterally, and the anterior cerebral/anterior communicating arteries posteriorly. The resection of olfactory groove meningiomas carries less risk to vision than do their tuberculum sella counterparts, and a greater chance of visual improvement.[42] Still, visual complications are a risk, along with CSF leak, seizures, and infection. Operative mortality from pooled data is estimated at 4.8%.[41]

Meningiomas arising from the anterior clinoid are a subset of sphenoid wing meningioma (Fig. 22-4A). They

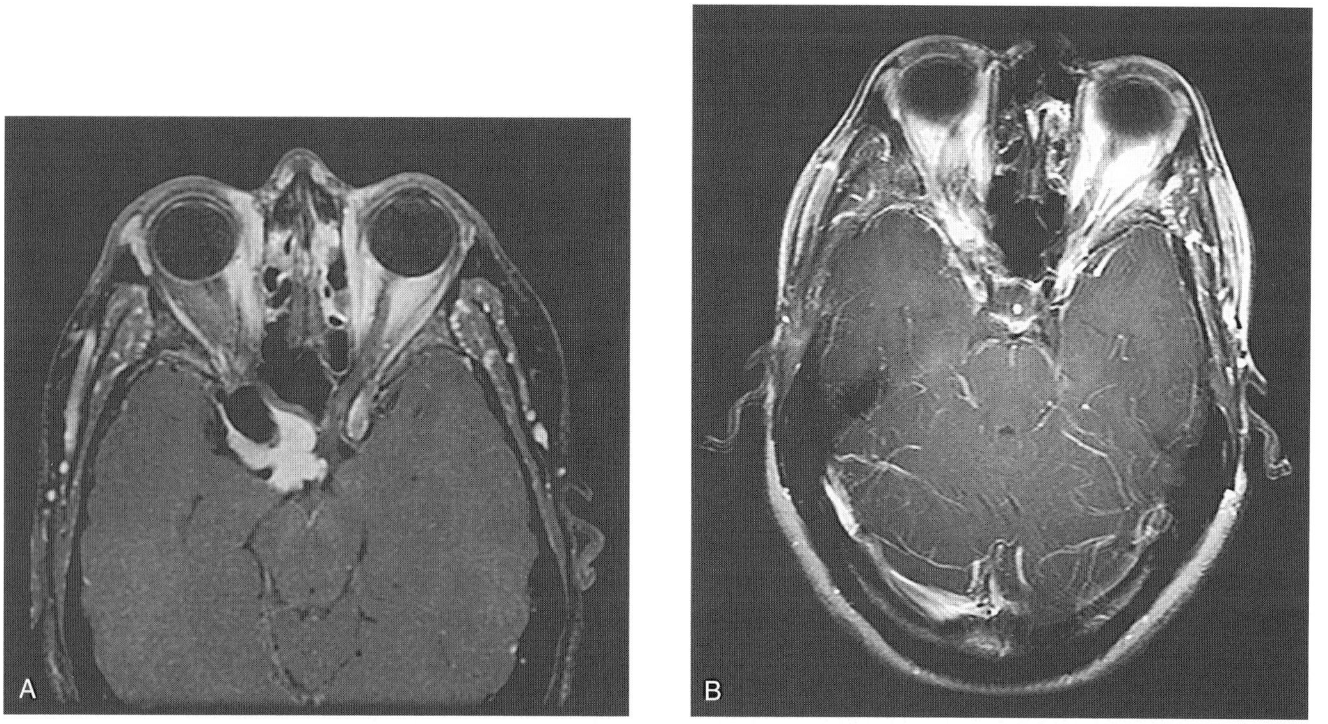

Figure 22-4. (A) Preoperative axial, enhanced, T_1-weighted MRI scan reveals a tumor arising from the right anterior clinoid displacing the right optic nerve medially. The anterior clinoid in this patient is markedly hypertrophied and pneumatized and appears as the black signal void in the center of the tumor. Great care must be taken to pack off the communication of the pneumatized clinoid to the sphenoid and ethmoid sinuses after the clinoid and tumor are removed to prevent postoperative CSF leak. (B) Postoperative axial, enhanced, T_1-weighted MRI scan reveals the tumor has been completely resected. The patient's vision is normal.

present with unilateral visual symptoms, occasionally progressing to unilateral blindness without contralateral eye findings.[41] Lesions extending into the cavernous sinus or superior orbital fissure can cause palsies of cranial nerves III through VI. The preoperative evaluation includes neuroophthalmologic exam, pituitary function studies, and consideration of cerebral angiography with some measurement of available cerebral collaterals in the event of carotid injury/occlusion. Surgery for these lesions, depending on the extent of tumor, may involve removal of the lateral and superior orbit, drilling of the sphenoid wing including removal of the anterior clinoid, cervical carotid exposure for control, orbital and zygomatic osteotomies for exposure, and carotid bypass if sacrificed. Al-Mefty described three types of clinoidal meningiomas depending on planes of arachnoid protecting the carotid or optic nerve.[43] The recovery of cranial nerve function after clinoidal meningioma resection is low.[41] Operative complications include worsened cranial nerve palsies, stroke, life-threatening vasospasm, diabetes insipidus, CSF leak, and visual loss. The mortality of surgery has been reported to be as high as 42%, although modern series have shown improvement (Fig. 22-4B).

Because of the complication rates for skull base meningioma resection, and a long-standing history of local control using radiation, both stereotactic radiosurgery and fractionated external beam radiotherapy have been used in treatment of skull base meningiomas.[42] The current dosage of radiation for skull base meningioma is typically 50 to 54 Gy in 28 to 30 fractions over 6 weeks using a 1-cm margin in typical meningiomas, and 5940 to 6000 cGy in 30 to 32 fractions using a 2-cm margin for atypical or malignant lesions.[35] Radiosurgical dosages generally should not exceed 8 to 10 Gy to the optic apparatus[42] or 12 Gy to the brainstem. In general, the drawbacks of radiosurgery include risk of damage to the visual apparatus, continued and occasionally worsened mass effect from the tumor, and, without biopsy, unknown histology. Advantages are avoidance of operative complications and good control of local growth. Of 190 patients treated with Gamma Knife radiosurgery at the Mayo Clinic and followed for a median of 47 months, patients with benign histology had a 93% 5-year local control rate. Patients with atypical histology had a 68% 5-year local control rate and patients with frankly malignant meningiomas had a 0% 5-year local control rate; 13% of patients experienced some treatment-related complications but only 3% exhibited a decrease in functional status related to the radiosurgical procedure.[44] Indications for radiation as primary treatment may include necessary anticoagulation, inaccessibility, patient preference, and comorbidity preventing surgery. In general, fractionated external beam radiation has offered comparable results to stereotactic radiosurgery in controlling tumor growth, whereas charged particle irradiation with protons, helium ions, or neon ions has shown little improvement over standard techniques.[36]

As adjuvant therapy, radiation has reduced recurrence of skull base meningiomas dramatically, from greater than 50% to less than 20%.[42] Indications for postoperative radiation in skull base meningioma management include residual tumor in a young patient, tumor growth, and atypical/malignant histology.[45] Combination therapy involving subtotal resection and postoperative radiation therapy has been reported to offer up to 98% 5-year progression-free survival to these patients.[35] The identified risk factors for subtotal resection include prior irradiation, vessel encasement, multiple cranial fossa involvement, and cranial nerve palsies (namely, cranial nerves III, V, and VI).[46] When two or more factors are present, there is a 60% chance of subtotal resection, and adjuvant therapy is warranted.[46]

The role of other adjuvant therapies is undergoing investigation. Hormone receptors on meningiomas are attractive sites for chemotherapeutic targeting. Preoperative embolization may reduce blood loss.[31] Finally, the use of three-dimensional virtual reality in training skull base surgeons in meningioma resection has been espoused, but its efficacy remains unproven.[45]

Hemangiopericytoma

Once considered angioblastic meningioma, the hemangiopericytoma is now classified as a sarcomatous lesion of the pericytes,[42] which accounts for 1% of blood vessel neoplasms and 3% of sarcomas.[47] The sites of origin in the head include the meninges, and extracranially, in order of frequency, the ethmoid sinuses, nasal cavity, maxillary sinus, cribriform plate, sphenoid sinus, nasal vestibule, and frontal sinus.[47] The signs at presentation parallel those of skull base meningiomas, with headaches, seizures, and focal cranial nerve deficits. These symptoms are typically more rapid in onset than in meningiomas, because hemangiopericytomas typically have a faster growth rate. Imaging features that distinguish this lesion from meningioma are a lack of hyperostosis, more frequent bony destruction and invasion, less frequent calcification, heterogeneous enhancement, and prominent vascular flow voids. The "dural tail" sign may or may not be present. On angiogram, these tumors have an impressive vascular blush of corkscrew vessels from the distal maxillary arteries, meningeal branches, and some internal carotid artery branches. They occasionally display early venous filling.[31] Embolization can help with operative blood loss.[47]

Surgical resection is similar to that of skull base meningiomas or sinus tumors. Metastases are unlikely with tumors smaller than 6.5 cm in diameter.[47] The propensity for larger tumors to metastasize, especially to the lung, has led some to recommend routine chest radiographs for surveillance.[48] Radiation and chemotherapy have had equivocal results. Although Coffey reported good results and dramatic tumor shrinkage with Gamma Knife radiosurgery for these lesions, he stressed tissue diagnosis prior to this treatment.[49] Radiosurgery may have a considerable role as adjuvant therapy (with surgery) in primary lesions and as treatment for recurrent disease.

Paranasal Sinus Lesions: Squamous Cell Carcinoma and Adenocarcinoma

Half of the tumors of the paranasal sinus have benign histology, the vast majority of which are inverted papillomas.[15] The malignant lesions include squamous cell carcinoma (80%), adenocarcinoma or adenoid cystic carcinoma (10%–15%), and others (melanoma, sarcoma, sinonasal undifferentiated carcinoma, mucoepidermoid carcinoma).[20] The management of inverted papilloma is discussed later in this section. Malignant lesions of the paranasal sinuses have been associated with both tobacco and occupational exposures. Nickel refining, hardwood furniture making, and rubbing alcohol manufacturing are linked to malignancy in the paranasal sinuses. These malignancies originate in any of the paranasal sinuses, with 60% from the maxillary sinus, 30% from the nasal walls, 10% to 15% in the ethmoid sinuses, and the remainder from the sphenoid sinus.[15] Staging criteria vary widely.[15,50]

The initial management of these lesions, even with extensive disease, is surgical. Preoperative radiation has been espoused, with an increase in the rate of preservation of orbital contents, as has been seen in esthesioneuroblastoma.[50–52] Intraarterial embolization of these lesions—removing external carotid feeders between 24 hours and 2 weeks in advance of surgery—is an adjunct that has some popularity. This is intended to limit blood loss without allowing time for growth of collaterals. Typically, when these lesions enter the intracranial space, their blood supply is from the anterior or posterior ethmoidal branches of the ophthalmic artery, or from the orbitofrontal branch of the anterior cerebral artery. These vessels are not considered for embolization because of the risk of stroke or visual loss.

The operative considerations are multiple. Placement of a catheter in the lumbar subarachnoid space preoperatively offers the surgical team a means of achieving brain relaxation. Lesions invading the palate and lower pharynx may necessitate tracheostomy placement prior to resection. The patient draping and positioning on the operating table must allow access not only to the face and cranium, but to all sites of donor tissue to be used in dural and facial repair. Antibiotics must be broad enough in spectrum to prevent sinus organisms from causing meningitis or abscess. The use of prophylactic anticonvulsants prior to tumor resection, although not studied in a randomized trial, is warranted when a postoperative seizure could have devastating consequences. Tumors that encase the carotid arteries as they pass lateral to the sphenoid sinuses may make hypothermia, barbiturate brain protection, electroencephalography (EEG) monitoring[18] intraoperative cardiac arrest, and high-flow vein graft carotid bypass,[53] tools to be considered.

The operative approaches are dictated by tumor anatomy. Lesions primarily of the anterior fossa are approached transfrontally, whereas extension into the nasopharynx or clivus extends the approach to include nasal or orbital opening. Nasopharyngeal lesions extending anteriorly, posteriorly, and inferiorly can be approached through a transnasomaxillary route with midfacial degloving or via a lateral rhinotomy. Large clival lesions with small nasopharyngeal components can be resected through transmaxillary routes, with Le Fort osteotomies. Lower clival lesions may necessitate palatal splitting.[54] Endoscopic approaches attempt to limit the extent of facial incisions. The extensive sampling of tissues at the tumor margins is practiced by the majority of skull base surgeons in treatment of these lesions. The reconstruction of large facial cavities and dural openings necessary in resection is often painstaking. Primary dural closure is frequently impossible. Pericranial flaps and free fascia lata reinforcement are readily available and should be planned preoperatively. The emphasis on dural closure and facial reconstruction is necessary in an area likely to be irradiated and certain to be scrutinized in social interaction.

Surgical complications are possible. Pulmonary embolism and pneumonia are the most common medical morbidities of these operations. Cerebrospinal fluid leak is present in 3% to 20% of patients,[15] and meningitis is present in 1% to 5% of patients. The rate of wound infection, including abscess, osteomyelitis, and meningitis, increases with preoperative radiation.[55] Intracranial hemorrhage occurs in 1% to 5% of patients, with a higher rate in patients who underwent resection of these lesions via craniotomy alone. This is likely related to the increased retraction needed to see the entire tumor from above only.[56] Stroke (1%–3% of patients), cranial nerve injury, and chronic seizures (1%–2% of patients) are the most common neurologic sequelae. Ocular complications are epiphora (36% of patients), partial visual loss (5% of irradiated patients), complete visual loss (5% of patients), permanent diplopia (3.5% of patients), temporary diplopia (10% of patients), ectropion (5% of patients), eye pain (3.5% of patients), and enophthalmos (3.5% of patients).[57] Pneumocephalus requiring intervention because of mass effect is rare, but can be related to aggressive postoperative CSF drainage. Flap necrosis of any vascularized flap is possible and usually requires return to the operating room for further wound reconstruction.

The use of adjuvant therapy in aggressive, extensive, and incompletely resected lesions is encouraged. In fact, some authors espouse induction chemotherapy or chemoradiotherapy prior to surgical resection,[22] with reported partial response in 90% to 95% of squamous cell lesions and complete response in 50%.[38] However, phase II and III trials of these regimens have failed to prove the survival advantage of preoperative chemotherapy.[38] Concurrent chemoradiotherapy prior to operating is showing some promise, but likely increases the risk of wound complications. Many of the agents used in the treatment of squamous cell carcinoma in other anatomic locations have been used to treat lesions of the paranasal sinuses, including methotrexate, bleomycin, cisplatin, 5-FU,[38] and hydroxyurea. Cisplatin and 5-FU are the most popular. Intraarterial chemotherapy with cisplatin, along with systemic sodium thiosulfate for tissue protection, is promising.[31,38] Neurotoxicity of intraarterial cisplatin precludes its use in the internal carotid distribution.[31] Patients responding to these chemotherapeutic regimens have increased rates of local control with the addition of radiation. Surveillance MR imaging in these patients should be done every 3 months in the first year to 18 months of followup, every 6 months for 2 to 3 years, and yearly thereafter.

The outcomes for treatment of paranasal sinus malignancy depend on histology, age, extent of resection, and preoperative functional capacity. The 5-year cancer-free survival in paranasal sinus squamous cell carcinoma is 50% and only 25% to 30% for advanced stages.[22] Of those tumors that invade the skull base from the paranasal sinuses, lesions affecting the skull anterior to the sphenoid sinus carry a better prognosis compared with centrally and posteriorly invasive lesions.[15] The most common cause of death in these patients is local recurrence (64%–91%). Distant recurrence was noted in 39 of 166 patients in the Sloan-Kettering series,[23] confirming the 25% rate of distant disease reported elsewhere.[55] Use of chemotherapy and radiation therapy without surgery has offered a poor success rate in the treatment of paranasal sinus malignancy. In fact, visual loss as a side effect of radiation is seen in up to 33% of patients.[52] Together, these data underscore the importance of attempting en bloc resection of these lesions when possible. Adjuvant postoperative radiation therapy is justified in partially resected lesions, lesions with positive surgical margins, and malignant histology regardless of extent of resection. The dose is typically 55 to 65 Gy of fractionated radiation starting 4 to 8 weeks after surgery to allow complete wound healing.[51,52] Indications for adjuvant therapy or newer novel therapies include dural or aggressive local invasion, aggressive pathologic grade, and positive surgical margins,[55] all of which have been reported to predict poor outcome.[23] The 5-year survival rates are nearly 70% for adenocarcinoma and 50% for squamous cell carcinoma.[23]

Management of recurrent paranasal sinus lesions is variable. Isolated recurrences with defined margins and pathology suggesting a low to moderate grade lesion could be amenable to repeat operations. Most centers base their management of recurrences on the histologic characteristics of the tumors.[55] Radiosurgery is another option for management of recurrent lesions not favorable for operative resection.[58] The role of Gamma Knife radiosurgery for primary lesions is undefined, although patients who are not candidates for aggressive surgical resection may be considered for this form of radiation.

Nasopharyngeal Carcinoma

The epidemiology of nasopharyngeal carcinoma is of interest. Southern Chinese ancestry is a significant risk factor. In this population, there is a 90% positivity rate for IgA anti-Epstein-Barr virus (EBV) antibodies.[39] In the United States, the risk is highest in the young black population, ages 10 to 19 years.[17] Epistaxis and nasal obstruction can herald presentation. MR images suggest a nasopharyngeal mass with intermediate T_1 signal and hyperintense T_2 signal with diffuse mild contrast enhancement.[39] Perineurial spread is common. Regional metastases typically travel to the lymph nodes of the posterior cervical triangle.[17]

This tumor is one of few skull base neoplasms often treated with radiation and chemotherapy prior to surgical intervention. Radiation with 65 to 70 Gy in 180 to 200 cGy fractions can afford a cure in stage I and stage II disease.[35] Cisplatin, anthracycline, and 5-FU regimens show promise as chemotherapeutic options.[38] Up to 80% of tumors respond to chemotherapy, with a complete response in 19%. Even metastatic disease can be controlled, with a 13% rate of remission with chemotherapy.[38] Combination chemoradiotherapy is most frequently advocated and has become the American treatment paradigm. Surgery is reserved for recurrent or unresponsive lesions. The survival rates at 5, 10, and 15 years in stage III tumors are 46%, 29%, and 17%, respectively. Patients with stage IV disease fare worse, with survival rates of 29%, 21%, and 8%, respectively.[35]

Mucosal Melanoma

Mucosal melanomas represent 2.5% of all melanomas and arise in the nasal cavity and paranasal sinuses more frequently than the oral cavity (Fig. 22-5). MRI reveals high T_1 signal, which is consistent with paramagnetic melanin or intratumoral hemorrhage.[20] The prognosis is often grave, in spite of surgery. Radiation therapy has been used to treat mucosal melanomas, reserving chemotherapy for systemic disease. Novel therapies, immunologic or genetic, may play a role in management of these lesions in the future.

Inverted Papilloma

A benign lesion of the paranasal sinuses, the inverted papilloma has the potential for malignant transformation. There is conflicting literature on the association of these lesions with EBV or human papillomavirus (HPV) infections. Surgical resection is the treatment of choice, and can be accomplished endoscopically when there is not extensive tumor spread. Cribriform plate and ethmoid sinus involvement allow for the very rare penetration of the intracranial space. There is a 7% rate of malignant dedifferentiation, usually into squamous cell carcinoma.[59]

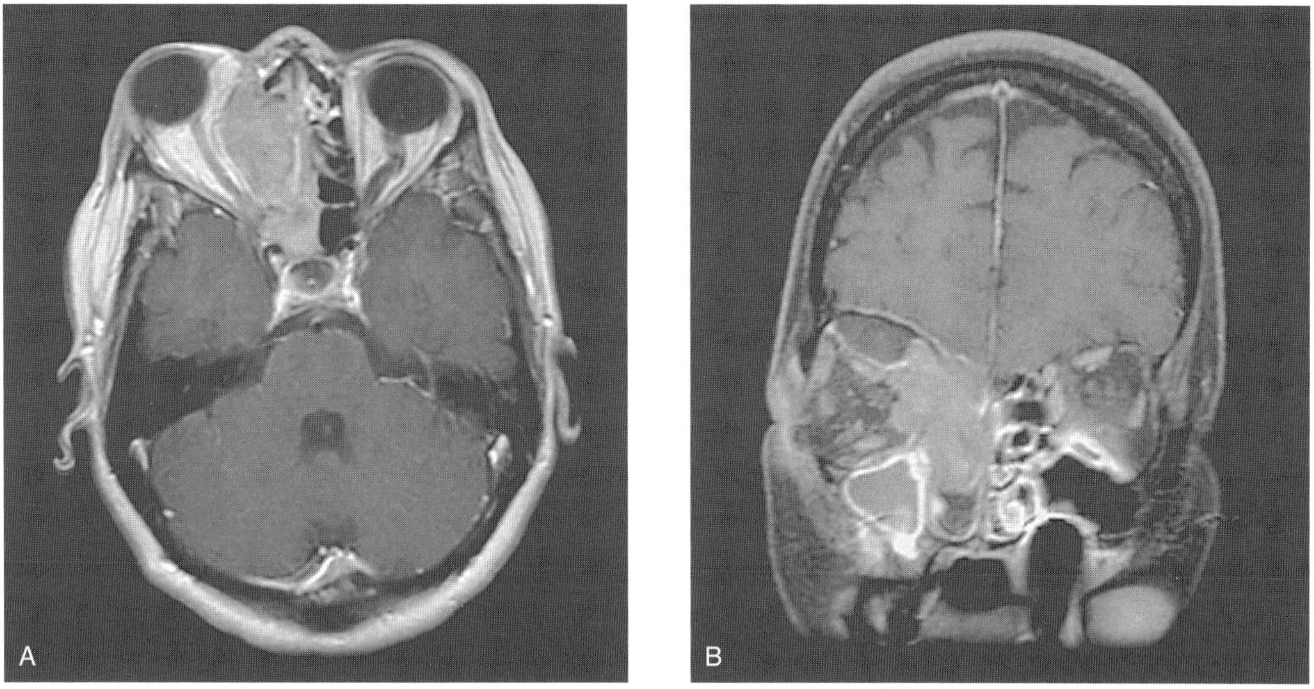

Figure 22-5. Axial (A) and coronal (B), enhanced, T_1-weighted MRI scans revealed an enhancing mass destroying the right ethmoid sinuses and invading the right orbit. Surgical treatment consisted of craniofacial resection, including exenteration of the right orbit and right cavernous sinus to achieve negative margins.

Surgical resection is the treatment of choice. Recurrence rates are around 10% to 20% with either endoscopic or open surgical techniques. Irradiation is controversial, with some concern for induction of malignant transformation.

Sinonasal Undifferentiated Carcinoma

The sinonasal undifferentiated carcinomas present a formidable challenge to surgeons and oncologists (Fig. 22-6). Even multimodality treatment has resulted in mean survival times of around 11.5 months.[35] Reports of some reduction in tumor volume by induction chemotherapy (carboplatin and paclitaxel) prior to surgery[22] have influenced care at our institution. Although some advocate preoperative radiation therapy as well, the task of achieving a healed, watertight dural closure is made more daunting in an irradiated field. The most practiced strategy for this tumor at our institution is aggressive resection followed by adjuvant chemotherapy and radiation.

Malignant Salivary and Lacrimal Gland Lesions

Tumors of the salivary and lacrimal glands vary in histology. Surgical resection followed by irradiation is the primary therapy for these lesions. Adenoid cystic carcinoma is the one most commonly seen by neurologists and neurosurgeons. It affects the skull base, typically originating from the lacrimal or parotid glands. This tumor is notorious for perineural spread from its origin through cranial foramina to the cavernous sinus and posterior fossa.[40] Surgery is the mainstay of therapy, and when used in combination with radiation offers a 3- to 5-year survival rate from 17% to 53%.[35] Chemotherapy is largely investigational in this setting.[22]

The survival rates generally depend on histologic tumor type and extension from their gland of origin. A report using the Swedish Population Registry to track survival in parotid and submandibular gland lesions demonstrated a 10-year survival rate of 74% for adenoid cystic carcinoma.[60] This study likely overestimates survival for lesions involving the skull base that, by implication, have grown farther from their gland of origin and are likely more aggressive. Furthermore, the accumulating neurologic morbidity from progressive cranial nerve involvement influences the quality of these periods of survival.

Neuroendocrine Carcinoma

Neuroendocrine carcinoma is treated in a fashion similar to esthesioneuroblastoma. Gross total resection is followed by adjuvant radiotherapy in high-grade lesions or if negative margins are not obtained at the time of surgery. There is some evidence in the literature, however, that surgical management may be delayed until after a

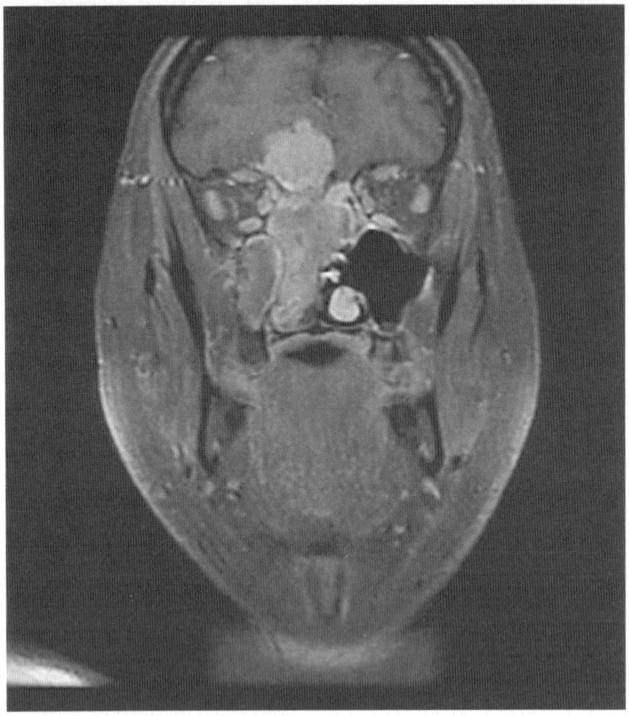

Figure 22-6. Coronal enhanced, T_1-weighted MRI scan reveals a mass involving the right nasal cavity, bilateral ethmoid sinuses, right orbit, and right anterior cranial fossa. Transnasal biopsy revealed sinonasal undifferentiated carcinoma. Following craniofacial resection the patient is receiving concurrent cisplatin chemotherapy and 5940-cGy radiotherapy in 33 fractions.

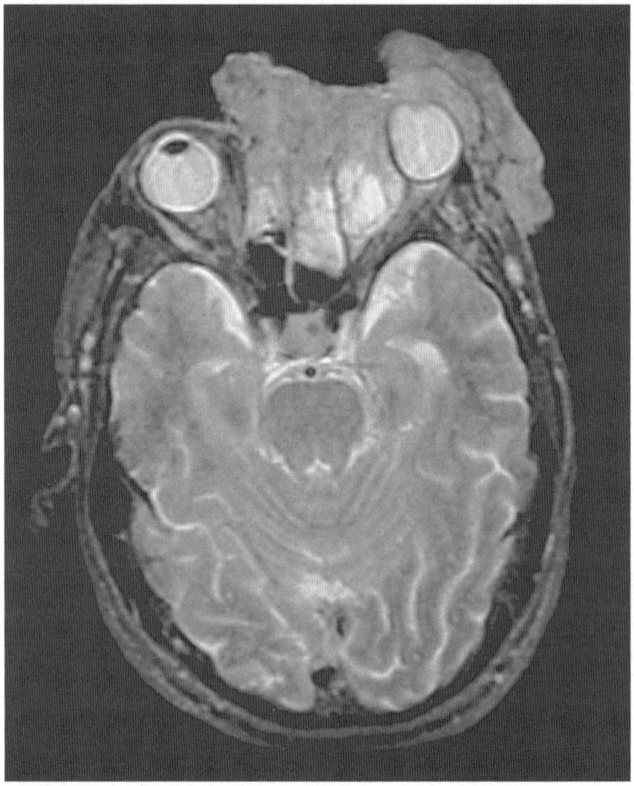

Figure 22-7. Axial, unenhanced, T_2-weighted MRI scan reveals a large mass completely engulfing the left orbit and globe, ethmoid sinuses, and skin of the forehead, nose, left cheek, and temporal region. Surgical resection required a combined effort with neurosurgery, otolaryngology, ophthalmology, and plastic surgery. Pathology was basal cell carcinoma.

trial of chemotherapy. Induction with a platinum-based regimen including etoposide may be an initial step.[22] At M. D. Anderson, responders go on to definitive radiation therapy, whereas nonresponders undergo resection. This regimen is used for small cell carcinomas as well.

Orbital Lesions

Lesions of the orbit are clearly not of uniform histology. A separate section is created here for the main purpose of drawing a differential diagnosis for lesions affecting the orbital cavity. The interested reader is referred to several excellent ophthalmology sources for these lesions. In general, the periorbita limits invasion, especially at sites of strong orbital attachment along the superior and inferior medial orbit.[40] When lesions extend into (and through) the skull base, surgery is a coordinated effort with ophthalmology (Fig. 22-7).

Mucocele

Mucoceles are nonneoplastic collections of sinus mucous formed when the ostium of a paranasal sinus is blocked, or normal sinus drainage is disrupted. Occasionally, these cysts can erode the posterior sinus walls and project into the intracranial space. Dural involvement is very rare, and may be limited to cases of previous craniotomy when the dura is not closed tightly. Surgical excision of the mucocele, drilling to remove any remaining mucosa, and packing of the sinus should be curative.

Encephalocele

Idiopathic encephaloceles, like nasal gliomas with which they may be confused,[16] present in children with nasal obstruction or glabellar deformity. Recurrent meningitis or chronic rhinorrhea is possible. Meningoceles and encephaloceles can emerge between sphenoid and ethmoid bone or through the sphenoid bone into nasal cavity.[40] In adults, they may occur after remote history of trauma with basilar skull fracture, or following prior surgical procedures in which the bony skull base and/or dura are breached. In neurofibromatosis, sphenoid dysplasia can result in large encephaloceles, especially into the orbit.[40] Treatment of these nonneoplastic lesions includes resection and dural repair.

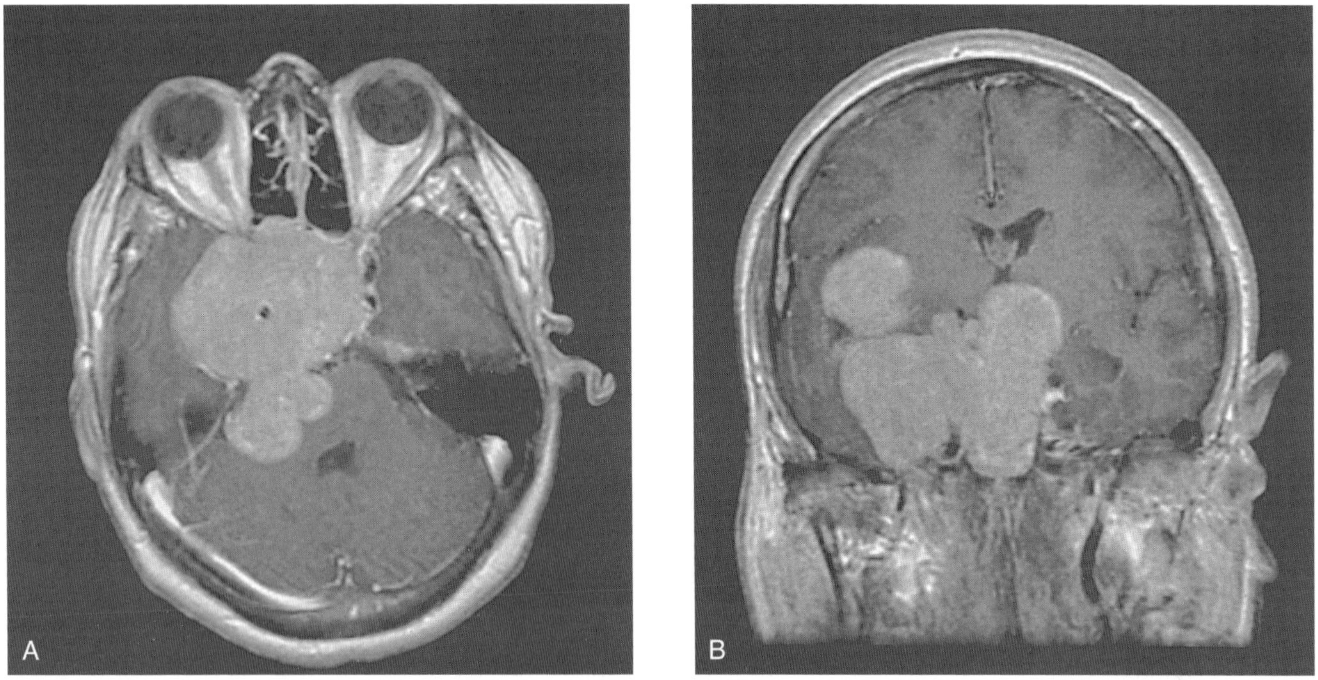

Figure 22-8. Axial (A) and coronal (B), enhanced, T_1-weighted MRI scans reveal a very large pituitary tumor involving the anterior, middle and posterior cranial fossas. It completely destroys the central skull base and encases the left carotid artery.

Brown Tumor of the Skull Base

Hyperparathyroidism can be complicated by lytic lesions of the skull or skull base without a sclerotic edge. These brown tumors are described as giant cell granuloma with osteitis fibrosa cystica. In the skull base, they present in the paranasal area, especially the ethmoid sinuses.[61] Whereas patients with primary hyperparathyroidism from parathyroid adenomas have a 3% to 7% risk of developing these lesions, patients with secondary hyperparathyroidism from renal failure have a 1% to 2% risk.[61] An evaluation for other tumors of the multiple endocrine neoplasia family is worthwhile. Imaging reveals soft tissue attenuation on CT, and low signal on T_1 and T_2 MR sequences with homogeneous gadolinium enhancement. High MR signal is suspicious for hemorrhage. Bone scan images show bright signal. The differential diagnosis includes plasmacytoma, giant cell reparative granuloma, giant cell tumor, aneurysmal bone cyst, and metastases, especially prostate.[61] The management typically includes biopsy and subsequent treatment of the hyperparathyroidism. The histologic differentiation from giant cell tumors may require multiple samples. Elimination of the hyperparathyroidism results in tumor shrinkage. If there is a progressive neurologic deficit, resection would be advisable.

Nasal Glioma

Nasal glioma, a developmental lesion in children, presents with nasal obstruction and glabellar deformity. It is often difficult to distinguish from encephalocele. Its treatment is surgical, and the approach depends on the presence of intracranial extension.[20] There is no adjuvant therapy.

▶ SELLAR/PARASELLAR

The evaluation and management of pituitary lesions are presented in Chapter 19 (Fig. 22-8).

▶ CAVERNOUS SINUS/MIDDLE FOSSA LESIONS: SQUAMOUS TEMPORAL BONE, GREATER SPHENOID WING, LOWER PARIETAL BONE, TEGMEN, AND PETROUS TEMPORAL BONE

Presentation

Cavernous sinus lesions often present with cranial nerve involvement, starting with the abducens, and proceeding to the oculomotor with pupillary involvement, trochlear, and first division of the trigeminal nerve. Posterior cavernous sinus lesions are more likely to involve the second and, occasionally, third divisions of the trigeminal nerve than more anterior cavernous or superior orbital fissure lesions. Proptosis, ocular hypertension, and disc edema can reflect mass effect in the cavernous sinus. The presentation of anterior middle fossa lesions outside the cavernous sinus is less specific than those involving the cavernous and parasellar region. Headache, V2 or V3 division trigeminal pain, and seizures are possible. Rarely, mass effect can lead to ipsilateral third nerve palsy from lesions outside the cavernous sinus. Large lesions can affect the optic radiations, cortical receptive language function, and visual associations. Lesions of the petrous ridge may manifest with otorrhea, pain, hearing loss (conductive or sensorineural), tinnitus, vertigo, facial weakness, or diplopia.[62,63] Cranial nerve VI is commonly affected in anterior petrous ridge lesions, whereas more posterior lesions can result in facial and vestibulocochlear nerve lesions. Involvement of the greater superficial petrosal nerve may be associated with dry eye.

Evaluation

Occasionally, vestibular testing or, more commonly, audiogrphy, offers further information for petrous ridge lesions, as some patients have asymptomatic hearing loss. CT evaluation of the temporal bone is extremely helpful for bony lesions or bone invasion, whereas MR scanning is essential for these lesions. MRI is also valuable in defining the anatomy and possible involvement of the infratemporal fossa. This space extends from the greater wing of sphenoid and temporalis muscle superiorly, to the pharyngeal space posterior and inferiorly, to the posterior wall of maxillary sinus anteriorly, and to the lateral pterygoid plate medially.[64] This is a challenging place to access surgically, and sound preoperative planning is required if a gross total resection of a lesion extending into the infratemporal fossa is going to be achieved.

Some differential diagnoses can be narrowed based on location. Lesions of the cavernous sinus arising above the foramen ovale are typically meningiomas, nerve sheath tumors, or aneurysms. Of these, meningiomas develop along the wall of the cavernous sinus or in Meckel's cave. Schwannomas and, rarely, neurofibromas grow within the cavernous sinus, and these nerve sheath tumors can follow their parent nerves through foramina.[40] Malignant or invasive skull base lesions can grow intracranially by extension into the cavernous sinus. The stage of invasion progresses as the lesion enters the cavernous sinus, then Meckel's cave, the intracranial/intradural space, followed by the posterior fossa along the cranial nerves.[40] Adenoid cystic tumors are notorious for this aggressive perineurial spread. Squamous cell carcinoma, melanoma, lymphoma, and basal cell carcinoma can also follow this pattern of invasion. Fat loss in the pterygopalatine fossa on CT scanning can indicate tumor compression. Juvenile nasopharyngeal angiofibroma, lymphoma, and nerve sheath tumors are common here.[40]

The anatomy of the tumor as it relates to the vertical, petrous, and cavernous carotid should be noted. Cerebral angiography with internal and external injections can be valuable in evaluation of lesions involving this area of the skull base. If the surgical approach will involve extensive temporal bone drilling and dissection, there is potential for loss of the facial nerve and the vestibulocochlear nerve, as well as violation of the middle and/or inner ear structures. Reanimation options when sacrifice of cranial nerve VII is possible need to be considered in surgical planning. Likewise, the hearing status of the contralateral ear must be known preoperatively if ipsilateral hearing may be lost during tumor resection.

Diagnoses and Management

General Management Considerations

The benign neoplasms of the cavernous sinus are generally meningioma and trigeminal schwannoma. Pituitary adenoma may extend into the cavernous sinus, and management of this tumor is well described in Chapter 19. Epidermoid and dermoid cysts are found here on occasion, with dermoid cysts arising more frequently in the midline and extending to the cavernous sinus after growth. Their management is surgical when symptomatic, and their natural history is of slow indolent growth.

The presence of the carotid arteries within the cavernous sinuses makes surgical approaches to the lesions tedious. Preoperative blood flow studies with trial balloon occlusion, along with intraoperative somatosensory-evoked potential or electroencephalographic recording, help to determine the tolerance of the brain to temporary occlusion. Radiation therapy for benign lesions of the cavernous sinus is not contraindicated. In fact, subtotal resection of these lesions is frequently followed by postoperative irradiation, with good rates of progression-free survival.[18] Lesions remote from the optic apparatus may be candidates for radiosurgery.

There are no randomized trial data guiding management decisions for cavernous sinus lesions. Considerations in the management of these lesions include likely pathology, growth rate, size less than or greater than 3 cm, extension through foramina or posteriorly, prior radiation, prior surgery, brainstem compression, carotid involvement (touching, partially encasing, encasing, encasing and narrowing, bilateral internal carotid artery involvement), and brain or pial invasion. Risks of surgery and radiation should be weighed. The cranial nerves at most risk in surgical resection tend to be the trigeminal and abducens, whereas the oculomotor and trochlear are less frequently injured.[65]

There are three main surgical approaches to the middle fossa and cavernous sinus for resection of skull base neoplasms. The intracranial approaches provide access to middle fossa lesions by entry through the temporal bone. Removal of the zygoma, orbital rim, and clinoid processes can permit greater exposure. Transpetrous exposure requires a good understanding of temporal bone anatomy. Extensive extradural mobilization may permit exposure of the sellar or suprasellar spaces, the middle fossa, or the basilar artery with minimal intradural work via an anterolateral temporopolar exposure.[66] Petrous apex meningiomas, schwannomas, superior chordomas, and epidermoid cysts can be reached extradurally on occasion in an anterior transpetrosal pathway.[66]

Schwannoma

True cavernous sinus schwannoma are very rare; the very few reports of schwannomas of cranial nerves III, IV, VI, XI, and XII are in stark contrast to the volumes of data on trigeminal and vestibulocochlear lesions.[67] Trigeminal schwannomas, the second most common type of intracranial schwannoma, typically involve the cavernous sinus via extension from the posterior fossa (Fig. 22-9) or from the Gasserian ganglion in Meckel's cave. The most common presenting symptom is facial hypesthesia, with fewer patients also reporting face pain.[68] A small, but significant proportion of patients will have neurofibromatosis type 2.[68] These schwannomas are often dumbbell-shaped tumors extending from mid-pons superiorly along the clivus medial to the petrous ridge, into Meckel's cave, the cavernous sinus, and, occasionally, to the extracranial space.[39] MRI of these lesions reveals T_1 hypointensity to isointensity, as compared to T_2 hyperintensity. Hemorrhage and calcification can cause heterogeneous signal. Computed tomograms show the tumors to be hypodense to brain. Heterogeneous signal on contrasted images may illustrate fatty or cystic change,[39] whereas neurofibromas have a target-shaped appearance based on a central collagenous core. In distinction from cavernous sinus hemangioma, they tend to originate more posteriorly.[69]

The extension of trigeminal schwannomas from the posterior fossa, through the middle fossa, and occasionally into the extracranial space, poses a formidable challenge to surgical resection. Two-step operations attacking the posterior and middle fossa components separately are one option, whereas anterior petrosectomy often can allow complete tumor removal in one stage. A tumor confined to the middle fossa may be approached via a frontotemporal epidural–interdural pathway.[68] Posterior fossa lesions can be addressed through a lateral suboccipital opening, and extracranial lesions through infratemporal dissection. Malignant schwannomas warrant adjuvant therapy with radiation, using chemotherapy only in the pediatric population.[68]

Neurofibroma

Patients with neurofibromatosis type 1 can present with intracranial, facial, and neck pathology. Sphenoid wing dysplasia, optic glioma, brainstem glioma, arachnoid cysts,[70]

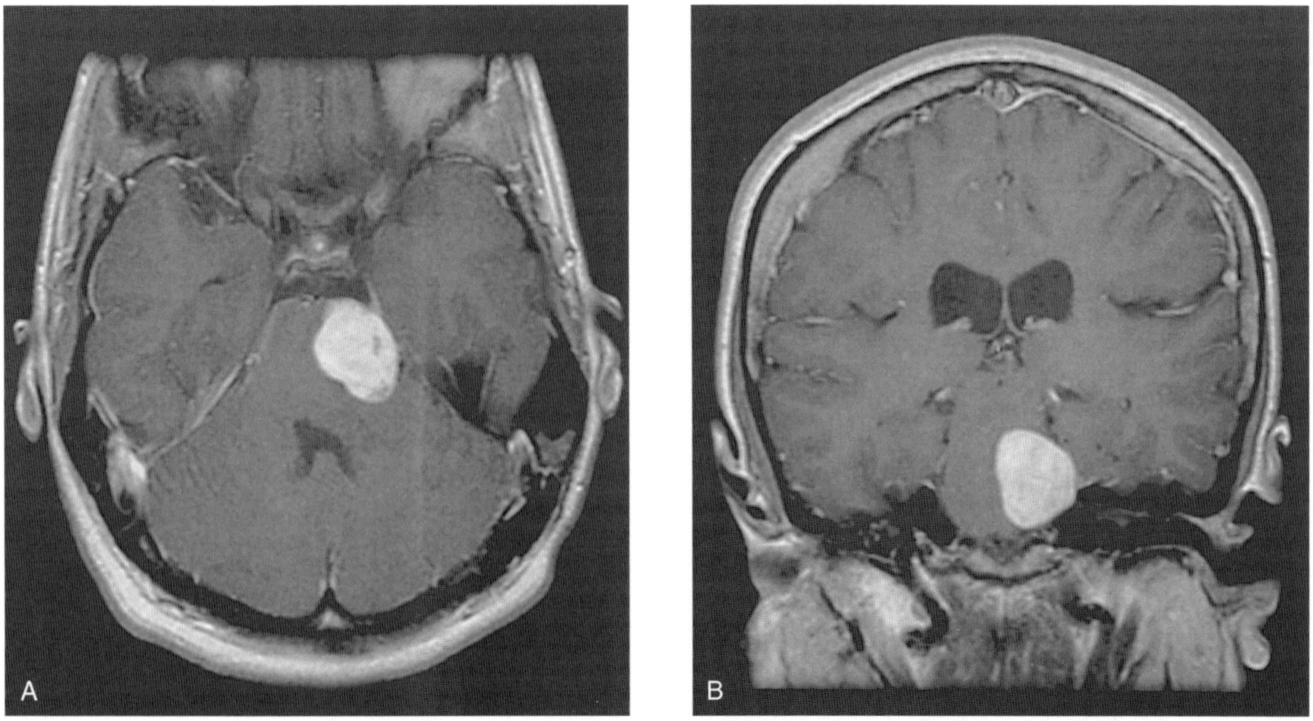

Figure 22-9. Axial (A) and coronal (B), enhanced T_1-weighted MRI scans reveal a homogeneously enhancing mass at the upper pontocerebellar junction at the expected site of the left trigeminal nerve. The tumor was completely removed via a presigmoid, retrolabyrinthine approach and was a trigeminal schwannoma.

large facial neurofibromas, orbital neurofibromas or malignant peripheral nerve sheath tumors, and intracranial/extracranial neurofibromas are seen. Neurofibromas of the cavernous sinus have been reported in patients without neurofibromatosis and not in connection with a cranial nerve.[71] Surgical excision of neurofibromas typically involves sacrifice of the affected nerve, or at least the affected fascicles. The histopathology explains this: axons are seen within the body of the tumor. Radiation of benign neurofibromas is rarely used, as reports implicate radiation in malignant transformation. The lesions are typically insensitive to chemotherapy.

Epidermoid Cyst/Dermoid Cyst

Epidermoid cysts and dermoid cysts are intracranial, and occasionally intraosseus, epidermal inclusions. Their bland epithelial histology describes their behavior: slow indolent growth. Dermoid cysts are typically in the midline, have epidermal appendages—hair, teeth, nails—and can cause aggressive chemical meningitis with rupture of lipid-containing cysts. Recurrent bacterial meningitis is possible when a dermal sinus tract connects the cyst to the skin. Epidermoid cysts are lines with squamous epithelium continuously sloughing off in the cyst. The dry keratin causes expansion of the cyst, and highly restricted diffusion on appropriate MR images. Both of these inclusion cysts should be surgically removed if their growth results in mass effect symptoms. They are very rarely found in the cavernous sinus, whereas epidermoids of the middle cranial fossa are more common. If curative resection is intended, all of the cyst wall must be meticulously removed. If the cyst wall is adherent to surrounding critical neurovascular structures, subtotal resection may be preferable.

Hemangioma

Cavernous sinus hemangiomas, if expanding and causing symptoms, may require resection. Intraoperative hemorrhage can be life-threatening. Unfortunately, preoperative differentiation of these lesions from meningioma is difficult.[69] Preoperative embolization is a new and promising adjunct to surgery.[72] At least one author reports response of cavernous sinus hemangioma to radiation therapy.[73] Radiosurgery has not been systematically evaluated in the treatment of these lesions, but could be considered in lesions with favorable morphology.

Meningioma

Although many of the considerations in the management of skull base meningiomas are presented in the "Anterior Skull Base/Anterior Fossa Lesions" section, meningiomas of the cavernous sinus, Meckel's cave, and petrous apex are separately described here. Forty percent of cavernous sinus lesions are meningioma.[42] Cavernous sinus lesions present with headache most commonly, followed by visual loss, ocular paresis, other visual disturbance, and facial sensory dysfunction (Fig. 22-10).[74] Meckel's cave lesions often present with weakness in mastication, face pain, or face numbness.[75] The natural history of these lesions is not benign, with a stroke rate nearing 25% and disease progression in the 25% to 75% range.[65] Growth from inside the cavernous sinus outward may be difficult to differentiate from extrinsic compression of the sinus on MR images, but this difference may greatly affect the risk of surgical intervention.[65]

The operative intervention for these lesions may include orbital and zygomatic osteotomies with extradural removal of the sphenoid wing, although outcome-oriented data regarding the efficacy on tumor control and complication avoidance are not available.[74] Larger middle fossa lesions may require removal of the mandibular condyle, drilling of the temporal bone, and mobilization of the petrous carotid.[42] Occasionally, the goal of operative intervention is to make room for stereotactic radiosurgery.[65] Although some authors advocate attempting gross total resection of cavernous sinus meningiomas in young patients,[65] other benign lesions of the cavernous sinus are more likely to be removed safely from the sinus, sparing the carotid artery.[54,76] Sacrifice of the cavernous internal carotid artery to obtain negative margins for cavernous sinus

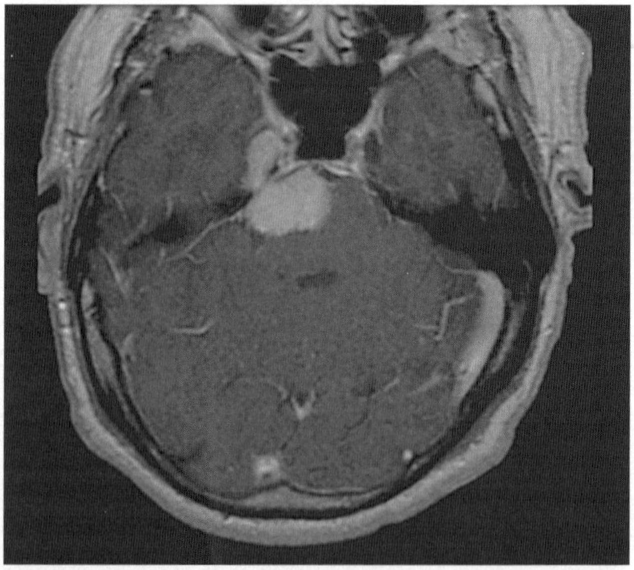

Figure 22-10. Axial, enhanced, T_1-weighted MRI scan shows a homogeneously enhancing tumor at the right petroclival junction extending into the right cavernous sinus. The patient presented with headache, diplopia, and mild left hemiparesis. The petroclival component was resected and the portion extending into the cavernous sinus was left. The patient had improvement in all his symptoms postoperatively. Pathology was meningothelial meningioma. Note imaging similarity to Fig. 22-9A.

meningioma had surprisingly little effect on recurrence when comparing two previously reported series.[54] With the risk of stroke from carotid sacrifice near 10%,[77] the practice is not advised. For older patients with cavernous sinus meningiomas encasing the carotid artery, subtotal resection and adjuvant radiation are advisable.

The surgical results for cavernous sinus meningioma resection are comparable to clinoidal meningioma resection. Complete cranial neuropathies very rarely improve, whereas incomplete palsies have some potential for recovery.[74] Total resection is possible in half to three-quarters of cases.[78,79] Worsening cranial nerve function is seen in 50% and any new deficit in 67% of patients.[74] Cranial nerve III palsies render the eye nonfunctional, whether they occur pre- or postoperatively. Palsies of cranial nerves IV and VI are not as devastating. Intraoperative monitoring of the cranial nerves is a possible, but unproven tool.[42] Other possible surgical complications include aphasia, hemiparesis, and seizures.

Focused external beam radiotherapy can offer local tumor control. In fact, one-third of tumors can actually decrease in size, and cranial nerve deficits have been reported to improve in 60% of patients.[74] Again, the treatment of skull base lesions based on imaging characteristics can be problematic. Sekhar reported that of 17 cases of cavernous sinus meningioma, 2 were labeled schwannoma and malignancy preoperatively and another 2 were misdiagnosed as meningioma with subsequent histology of plasmacytoma and hemangioma.[78]

The management of petroclival meningiomas is similar to cavernous sinus and Meckel's cave lesions. Presenting symptoms can include temporal lobe, cranial nerve, or brainstem dysfunction. Preoperative angiography reveals internal carotid, middle meningeal, and ascending pharyngeal blood supply,[42] and can define the venous anatomy, including dural sinuses. Surgery may be attempted through a low middle fossa subtemporal approach, a posterior fossa approach, or a combined approach. Wider exposure is needed for tumors approaching or crossing the midline. In all, there is a 75% to 84% rate of gross total resection with skull base approaches, and a 50% to 60% rate of good outcome.[42]

Temporal Bone Adenomatous Lesions

Adenomatous lesions of the temporal bone are either glandular, festooning, or aggressive papillary on histology.[80] The first two are soft tissue masses that enhance with contrast, but do not cause extensive bony destruction.[81] Resection through partial petrosectomy or partial mastoidectomy has been helpful.

Some authors call the aggressive papillary adenomas of the temporal bone endolymphatic sac tumors. This pathologic entity, if singular, is associated with the von Hippel–Lindau syndrome. The tumors arise in the vestibular aqueduct and have imaging characteristics of glomus tumors, including a vascular blush on angiogram. They almost always present with profound sensorineural hearing loss. These tumors can invade the middle and posterior fossa from the temporal bone, causing cranial neuropathies and, eventually, brainstem signs. Gross total resection is the treatment, but often is impossible. There is no current consensus on the use of radiation for treatment of these lesions.

Chordoma/Chondrosarcoma

Skull base chordoma and chondrosarcoma are discussed in the "Posterior Fossa/Clival" section. Extension of these tumors into the middle cranial fossa can be seen. Lesions of the superior clivus may require both middle and posterior fossa exposure for resection.

Cholesteatoma

The middle ear cholesteatoma is a lesion histologically identical to the intracranial epidermoid inclusion cyst. With continued desquamation into the epithelial lined cyst, the lesion expands. Hearing loss and recurrent otitis media can be the presenting findings. CT imaging shows some rim enhancement with bony erosion around the lesion, and MR images reveal an isointense T_1 and hyperintense T_2 lesion. Erosion into the middle fossa is possible and may contribute to meningitis if secondary rupture of the cholesteatoma occurs. The lesions are removed surgically, with no role for adjuvant medical or radiation therapy.

Cholesterol Granuloma

The exact etiology of cholesterol granuloma formation is unclear, but most agree that the process is started by hemorrhage into a petrous air cell. Inflammation induced by the blood products can block the normal egress pathways connecting the air cells. An abnormal granulomatous inflammatory reaction results and the lesion expands. Eventually, the most common presenting symptom is hearing loss, but cholesterol granulomas are thought to occasionally result in pain or trigeminal dysfunction. On CT images, the lesion expands the bony cortex around it, but does not have rim enhancement. They are usually seen at the petrous apex. MR images reveal a hyperintense lesion on T_1 and T_2 sequences.[40] The carotid artery, in its petrous portion, may be located at the periphery of the cyst. Surgical drainage of the cyst usually prevents further expansion and preserves cranial nerve function.

Nonneoplastic Lesions of the Temporal Bone and Middle Fossa

The differential diagnosis of a middle fossa or temporal bone mass includes important, nonneoplastic processes. Mucoceles are seen with low T_1 signal and bright T_2 signal on MR images.[40] Abscess is rarely a diagnostic dilemma, but indolent fungal or mycobacterial infections may mimic tumors. Large and giant aneurysms can erode bone when present for years, and often resemble ovoid tumors on contrasted images. Arachnoid cysts are most common in the middle fossa, can remodel overlying bone, and occasionally show enough of a difference from CSF on MR images to resemble a mass. Sarcoidosis has the potential to present with massive areas of non-caseating granulomas at the skull base. Fibrous dysplasia and Paget's disease of the bone have been discussed in connection with sarcomatous dedifferentiation. These latter two lesions can mimic frank bony neoplasia, and occasionally require surgery for symptomatic relief.

▶ POSTERIOR FOSSA/CLIVAL: POSTERIOR TEMPORAL BONE, OCCIPITAL BONE, CLIVUS

Presentation

The multiple vital functions of the brainstem, cerebellum, and cranial nerves make the presentation of posterior fossa skull base lesions potentially ominous and extremely varied. Headache and hydrocephalus from mass effect are common. Ataxic speech, gait, and posture are seen. Dysphagia, tongue weakness, shoulder droop, hearing loss, tinnitus, vertigo, diplopia, facial palsy, hemifacial spasm, and facial hypesthesia are possible. Long tract signs, including spasticity, Babinski responses, hemi- or quadriparesis, Horner syndrome, and spinothalamic or posterior column dysfunction, can prompt evaluation. Altered consciousness and coma are very rare without acute change in the tumor, hemorrhage, or acute occlusion of vascular supply to the brainstem. Clustering of signs and symptoms can hint at specific diagnoses. Sequential involvement of multiple cranial nerves, occasionally starting unilaterally and spreading, points to a growing clival lesion. The clival syndrome may involve a vertex headache worsening with neck flexion, or pain in the posterior neck or mastoid tip, with neck stiffness. Dysfunction of cranial nerves IX through XI can be manifest in jugular foramen lesions. A jugular foramen syndrome typically manifests with hoarseness, dysphagia, palatal weakness, atrophy of the sternocleidomastoid and upper trapezius, and either posterior auricular or vertex pain. An occipital condyle lesion can cause unilateral hypoglossal palsy with pain on neck flexion. Tinnitus, high tone hearing loss, early preservation of facial motor function with late facial weakness, and occasional loss of corneal reflexes are seen in patients with vestibular schwannomas. Cruciate paralysis is the classical presentation of foramen magnum meningiomas.

Evaluation

The evaluation of posterior skull base and posterior fossa lesions should adhere to caveats noted in earlier sections. Papilledema and a history of sudden loss of consciousness with Valsalva maneuver may prompt urgent hospitalization. In this region, it is again useful to ask about a history of recurrent bacterial or aseptic meningitis because dermoid and epidermoid inclusion cysts can predispose both to infection and leakage of irritating proteolipids into the cerebrospinal fluid. Careful evaluation of the cranial nerves is essential. Adjunctive evaluation with electromyography showing fasciculations can demonstrate subclinical irritation of the motor nerves VII, XI, and XII. Any cerebellopontine angle mass warrants an audiogram, and brainstem auditory-evoked potentials can further verify retrocochlear pathology as the cause of a subtle hearing loss. It is also important to document the status of hearing in the contralateral ear. Serviceable hearing is described as a speech discrimination of at least 50% and a threshold of 50 dB on a pure tone audiogram.

By far the most important testing modality is the MR scan, although CT scan of the temporal bone is critical to discern the pathology in relation to the middle and inner ear as well as the descending portion of the facial nerve. MR diffusion imaging makes epidermoid cyst conspicuous, while gadolinium enhancement of a dural tail can suggest meningioma rather than schwannoma. For small lesions, MRI can help to locate the center of the tumor, thus narrowing the differential. For example, lesions from the medial jugular fossa should be nerve sheath rather than glomus tumor.[40] CT scanning with bone windows can play a substantive role in evaluation of clival and posterior skull base neoplasms. Viewing the lateral jugular plate separating the jugular bulb from the middle ear establishes the difference between glomus tympanicum (present) and glomus jugulare (absent) tumors.[40] Fibrous dysplasia, chordoma, and chondrosarcoma are a few of the clival lesions requiring bony evaluation.

Diagnoses and Management

The diagnoses of posterior fossa masses in various ages reflect disparate differential diagnoses. The posterior fossa mass in children is rarely extraaxial, with only 2.4% of lesions being dermoid inclusion cysts, 1.4% sarcomas, 0.2% germ cell tumors, and 0.2% acoustic neuromas.[82] However, the cerebellopontine angle lesion in an adult is acoustic neuroma in 80%, with the rest a mix of meningioma, epidermoid, arachnoid cyst, lipoma, facial nerve schwannoma, metastasis, choroid plexus papilloma, and others.[83]

The surgical approaches to the posterior fossa and internal auditory canal are multiple. The retrosigmoid suboccipital craniectomy allows dissection in the cerebellopontine angle and lateral posterior fossa from the tentorium to the foramen magnum. The extreme lateral approach opens the foramen magnum and C1 and C2 if needed. Transpetrous approaches include the retrolabyrinthine presigmoid route to the cerebellopontine angle and opening of the internal auditory canal. A partial labyrinthectomy also exposes the porus acousticus. A translabyrinthine opening gives a wide avenue to the cerebellopontine angle and lateral middle clivus from the porus acousticus of the internal auditory canal to the fundus. The transcochlear approach offers further exposure to the ventral pons and middle clivus. Intraoperative monitoring via electromyogram (EMG) is possible for cranial nerves XII, XI, X, VII, VI, V, IV (more difficult), and III.[84] Complications of posterior fossa skull base surgery can include injury to the superior petrosal sinus, the transverse or sigmoid sinuses, the cranial nerves (especially cranial nerve IV where it is hidden in the tentorial folds), and venous air embolism in the sitting position.[85]

Acoustic Neuroma

Acoustic neuromas, or, more appropriately, vestibular schwannomas, make up 80% of cerebellopontine angle tumors.[83] They typically present with high-frequency hearing loss, and occasionally with vertigo. The hearing loss can occasionally be abrupt in onset, with a presumed vascular etiology in 26% of patients.[86] Most patients have gradual progressive hearing difficulty. Facial weakness is extraordinarily rare, even with very large tumors. Facial hypesthesia related to compression of the trigeminal nerve by the tumor may be found in up to 20% of patients in some series. Lower cranial nerve dysfunction is rare, but can occur in larger tumors. Given the wide availability of intracranial MRI, more tumors are being discovered incidentally during evaluation for nonspecific neurologic symptoms or headache, likely unrelated to the tumor (Fig. 22-11). A smaller number are found on screening for neurofibromatosis. These patients, surprisingly, can have large tumors. In one series, patients without hearing loss had an average tumor size of 19 mm with five tumors larger than 3 cm.[86]

Evaluation of the patient with acoustic neuroma should include a physical directed at locating any stigmata of neurofibromatosis, formal audiogram, brainstem auditory-evoked response testing as baseline, and, rarely, vestibular function testing. The diagnosis of acoustic neuroma is fairly reliable with high-quality MRI. Typically, acoustic neuromas appear hypo- to isointense on T_1 images, with contrast enhancement and variable T_2 signal.[83] The pathology most resembling acoustic neuroma in the cerebellopontine angle is meningioma. For that reason, the dural "pseudotail" from T_1 brightness in the bone marrow around the internal auditory canal (IAC) can cause confusion.[83] Consequently, it is helpful to look closely at MR images for IAC enlargement, and to determine whether the tumor's long axis is parallel to the canal (Fig. 22-12). CT imaging can help illustrate IAC enlargement, and CT contrast material is more avidly incorporated into meningioma than schwannoma. When there is fatty or cystic degeneration of the lesion on MR scans, the pathology is much more frequently schwannoma.[87]

Historically, the treatment of acoustic neuroma has been surgical. Data from many large radiosurgical series

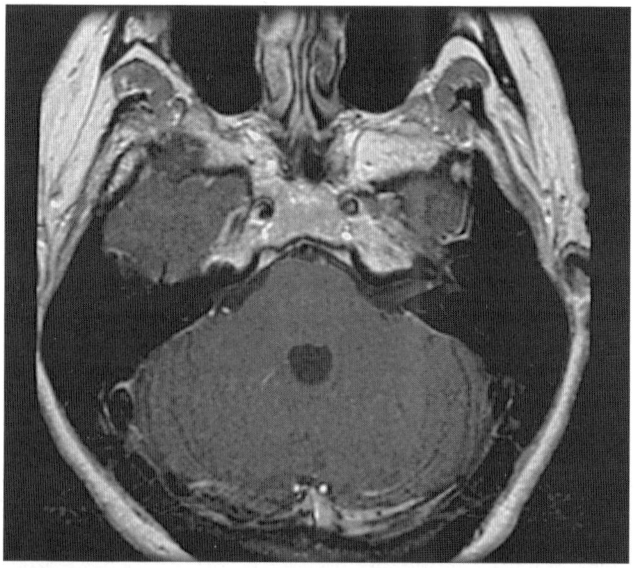

Figure 22-11. Axial, enhanced, T_1-weighted MRI scan reveals an incidental tiny vestibular schwannoma in the distal left internal auditory canal.

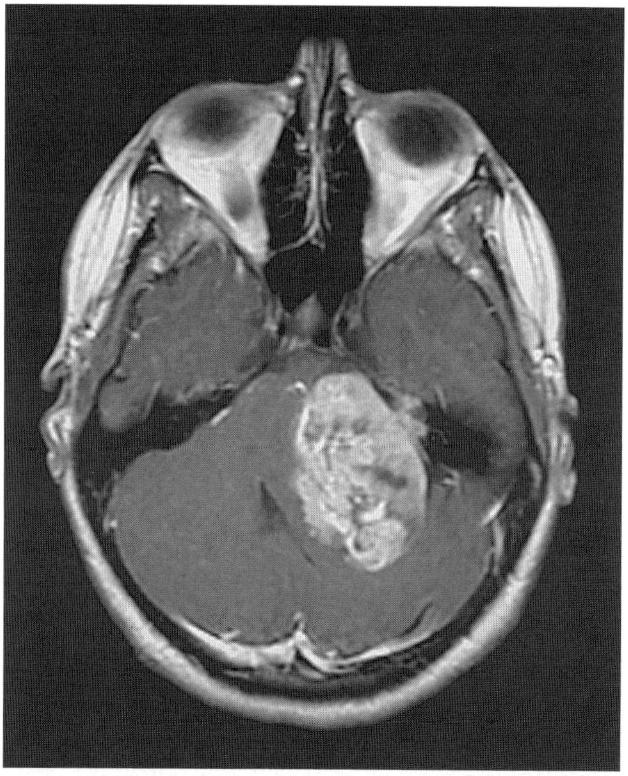

Figure 22-12. Axial, enhanced, T_1-weighted MRI scan reveals a giant left vestibular schwannoma markedly compressing the posterior fossa contents and enlarging the internal auditory canal.

now suggest that radiosurgery offers long-term tumor control with less morbidity when compared with microsurgical removal of the tumor. The choice of surgical approach is guided by the patient's ipsi- and contralateral hearing function, the patient's age, the location of the tumor within the IAC, and somewhat by surgeon preference. The middle fossa approach offers the best chance at hearing preservation for lesions that are intracanalicular. Superior vestibular tumors are more easily resected by this approach than are inferior vestibular lesions. A translabyrinthine approach is used when there is loss of functional hearing preoperatively, or there is very little likelihood that serviceable hearing could be preserved with tumor removal. This approach allows for the best exposure of the distal IAC and some authors report it provides better facial nerve preservation. The retrosigmoid, suboccipital posterior fossa approach offers excellent exposure of the entire cerebellopontine angle cistern, and the porus acousticus. Intraoperative monitoring of the facial nerve to reduce the risk of postoperative facial weakness is now a standard of care. Additionally, intraoperative monitoring of cranial nerves V and XI may be helpful in larger tumors. For patients with serviceable hearing preoperatively intraoperative monitoring of the brainstem auditory-evoked response waveforms is also a helpful adjunct. When operating on large tumors, the fascicles of the facial nerve can be difficult to distinguish, and may lie anterior, superior, or inferior to the acoustic neuroma. Facial nerve injury rate is proportional to the size of the lesion resected. Normal facial function is achieved in 75% of patients with small acoustic tumors at 1-year.[84] The surgical maneuvers important in hearing preservation include, foremost, the identification of anterior inferior cerebellar artery branches entering the IAC. Early identification of the vestibular nerve from which the tumor arises is helpful, and sacrifice of that branch is necessary. At 6-month followup there is no difference in subjective or objective vestibular function when the vestibular portion of one cranial nerve VIII is sacrificed.[84] Predictors of good hearing outcome include tumor size less than 2 cm, good preoperative hearing, short IAC penetration, low degree of IAC erosion, and reduced caloric responses ipsilaterally. The latter would indicate vestibular dysfunction greater than cochlear.[84] Brainstem auditory-evoked response monitoring can alert the surgeon when the wave V latency is prolonged more than 0.9 ms, and eventually 1.5 ms, the cutoff beyond which hearing is at high risk. A change of latency of more than 0.07 ms/min is also worrisome, and should prompt retractor removal or repositioning.[88]

Although fractionated radiation therapy was effective in the past for tumor control,[35] stereotactic radiosurgery is becoming an increasingly popular first-line radiotherapy treatment for acoustic neuromas less than 25 mm in diameter. Larger lesions can be treated in patients with contraindications to surgery. Typical doses are 12 to 14 Gy at the 50% isodose line. Relative contraindications to radiosurgery include large tumors, brainstem compression, long tracts signs, and, especially, T_2 signal change in the brainstem or cerebellum indicating vasogenic edema. The outcome of surgery and radiosurgery in the treatment of acoustic neuroma is excellent. Microsurgical techniques have heralded a new age in the treatment of these lesions, with very acceptable morbidity rates. For lesions with a mean diameter of 22 mm, the control rate of radiosurgery is nearly 94% at 5 years.[89] Risks included facial weakness in 23%, altered trigeminal sensation in 25%, with hearing loss in 49% of patients. In comparison, 5-year results in a series of resected tumors showed 100% local control, 1.3% facial weakness, and hearing loss in 43% of patients.[90]

In a direct comparison of Gamma Knife radiosurgery with microsurgical resection, patients who underwent radiosurgery had a better functional outcome.[91]

Meningioma

The cerebellopontine angle and foramen magnum are the most common sites of posterior fossa meningiomas. Between 5% and 8% of all meningiomas present in the cerebellopontine angle, and approximately 10% to 15% of cerebellopontine angle lesions are meningioma.[83] The presenting symptoms are similar to those of acoustic neuromas and include hearing loss, tinnitus, dysequilibrium, and facial numbness.[83] The characteristic "dural tail" (enhancing hypervascularity of the surrounding dura rather than tumor involvement) used to differentiate these lesions from acoustic neuromas is present in 56% of patients (Fig. 22-13).[83] These lesions are typically eccentric to the internal auditory canal and do not typically invade or expand the IAC. The T_1 hypointensity with brisk enhancement and T_2 variability in signal do not help in differentiating these tumors. A cystic degeneration making the enhancement more ring-like in appearance typically favors schwannoma. CT images can help in the diagnosis. Hyperostosis, although rare, is very suggestive of meningioma. Calcification within the tumor and hyperdensity of the lesion on CT points toward meningioma. Bony erosion of the petrous pyramid is also more common in meningioma.[83] Patients are more likely to have preserved hearing with large lesions (>2 cm) when they are meningiomas. Typically, these lesions are approached through a retrosigmoid route, although depending on the size and dural base of the tumor, the approaches mentioned above for acoustic neuroma may also be considered. Typically the tumor receives its vascular supply from the ascending pharyngeal, vertebral, or middle meningeal arteries, the meningohypophyseal trunk, or the petrous carotid.[42] There is an excellent rate of gross total resection and subsequent good neurologic outcome.[42]

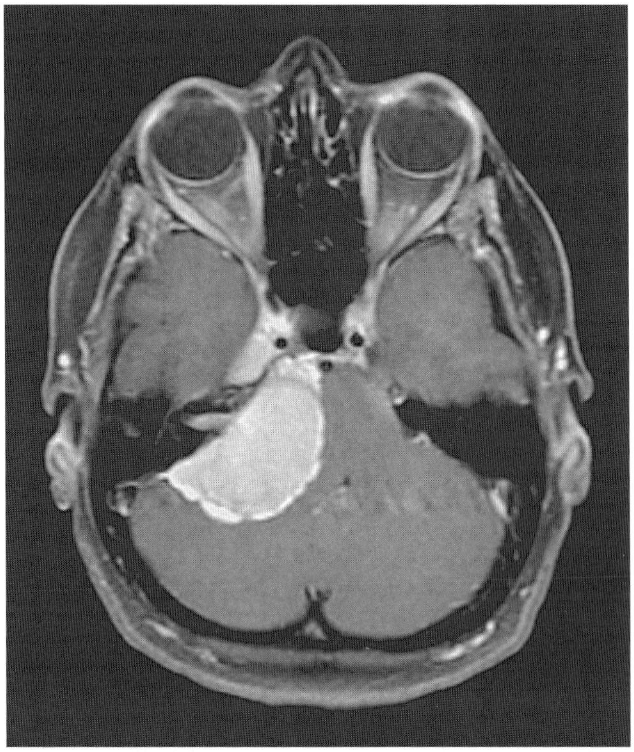

Figure 22-13. Axial, enhanced, T_1-weighted MRI scan reveals a large homogeneously enhancing right cerebellopontine angle meningioma. Even though the tumor extends out of the internal auditory canal, it does not significantly widen the canal. Additionally, the tumor has a broad dural base with some extension into the right cavernous sinus, making it easy to distinguish radiographically from a vestibular schwannoma.

Meningiomas of the foramen magnum classically present with cruciate paralysis—starting in one arm, progressing to the ipsilateral leg, then to the contralateral leg, and eventually the contralateral arm—owing to the somatotopic decussations of the pyramidal tracts. This classical presentation, unfortunately, is not the rule. Additional symptoms include headache, neck pain, weakness, lower cranial nerve dysfunction, and clumsy/atrophic hands. These lesions typically (if arising from the clivus and not the spinal canal) present anteriorly or anterolaterally. The vertebral artery is commonly encased by tumor, often along with the posterior inferior cerebellar artery. Approaches include far lateral transcondylar, transoral, and transcervical.[42] Mobilization of the upper dentate ligament and sacrifice of the first cervical nerve root often are necessary for tumor resection.[92] If preoperative imaging suggests pial invasion with T_2 signal change in the brainstem, a thin rim of tumor may need to be left.[92] Postoperative radiation therapy can be considered. There are reports of 60% to 77% good outcome.[42] Tumor size is predictive of postoperative deficits, most of which improve.[92]

Petroclival meningiomas were discussed in the "Cavernous Sinus/Middle Fossa Lesions" section but can be considered posterior fossa lesions. They involve the upper clivus and petrous ridge, occasionally extending into Meckel's cave or the cavernous sinus.[92] The posterior petrosectomy approach is most commonly used for these difficult lesions. This involves a retrolabyrinthine, presigmoid, subtemporal exposure with ligation of the superior petrosal sinus and dividing the tentorium. Mobilization of the trigeminal nerve may require opening of Meckel's cave. Frequently, surgeons prefer monitoring somatosensory-evoked potentials, brainstem auditory-evoked potentials, and EMG of cranial nerves V, VI, and VII during resection.[92] Total petrosectomy sacrifices ipsilateral hearing for further tumor resection. The most frequent cranial nerve palsies seen postoperatively are III, VII, and X.[92]

Radiation therapy as single therapy or adjuvant to surgery can be considered. The data supporting its use were presented earlier. The posterior fossa, in general, allows for less radiation-induced parenchymal swelling than the supratentorial space. The proximity of the brainstem may limit the possible radiosurgical dose. Careful treatment planning is necessary so that "fall-off" of radiation does not affect nearby structures. The use of preoperative embolization has been considered in the past, although tumor swelling and hemorrhage from alcohol embolization has resulted in one fatality in a patient with a posterior fossa meningioma.[92]

Facial Nerve Schwannomas

Facial nerve schwannomas are rare; by 1999, only 300 had been reported.[93] The presentation of facial nerve schwannomas is one of facial weakness or hemifacial spasm prior to hearing loss or vestibular dysfunction.[83] Although the majority of facial nerve schwannomas arise at the geniculate ganglion (Fig. 22-14), they can occur along the entire course of the nerve. Lesions contained within the temporal bone have been reported. More frequently, a soft tissue mass in the cerebellopontine angle extending into the internal auditory canal suggests a possible acoustic lesion.[83] Middle ear tumors are possible as well. When patients present with complete facial palsy, the decision to operate is straightforward. Patients with good facial nerve function, however, present a management dilemma. The risk of surgery to the facial nerve is significant, even with intraoperative cable grafts and anastomoses. Delaying surgery and following serial imaging is an acceptable mode of management. Radiosurgery can be used for control of growth of these lesions with reports of success.[94]

Chondrosarcoma

Chondrosarcomas arise from remnants of the skull base cartilaginous synchondroses: sphenooccipital, frontonasal, sphenoethmoidal, and petroclival.[95,96] In fact, chondrosarcoma leads the differential of petrooccipital fissure

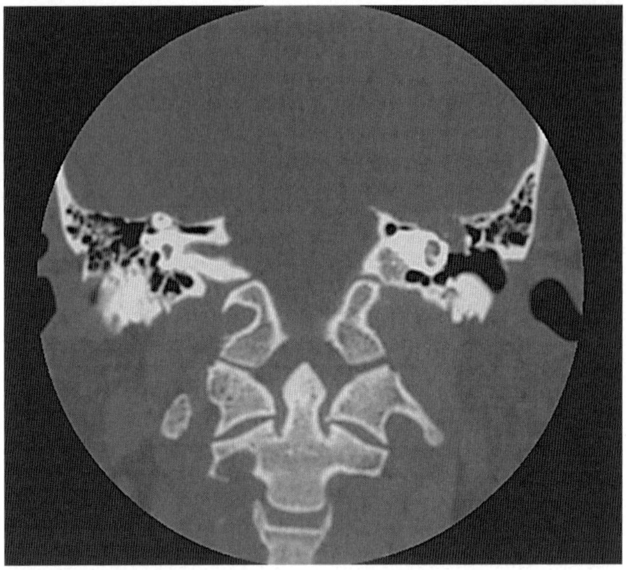

Figure 22-14. Axial CT scan of the temporal bones distinguishes a soft tissue mass in the region of the left genticulate ganglion destroying the surrounding bone and extending into the attic of the middle ear consistent with a facial nerve schwannoma. There remains only a thin rim of bone between the tumor and the cochlea.

lesions.[40] Occasionally, they arise from dedifferentiation of a chondroma. Patients with Maffucci syndrome or Ollier disease are at particular risk for degeneration of one or more of their multiple enchondromas into chondrosarcoma.[96] The histology of chondromyxoid fibroma is occasionally confused with that of chondrosarcoma and chordoma.[97] The fibrous component of the tumor separates it from these other two lesions.

Typically, chondrosarcomas are slow growing and discovered at sizes greater than 2 cm. The peak incidence is in the second through fourth decades of life. Of all chondrosarcomas, 5% to 7% occur in the skull base,[95] comprising 0.16% of intracranial tumors (Fig. 22-15).[98] Presentation symptoms and signs include headache and cranial nerve VI dysfunction in clival lesions affecting Dorello's canal, cranial nerves II through VI dysfunction with diffuse anterior skull base lesions, and lower cranial nerve palsies when tumor invades the jugular foramen and posterior fossa. The most common palsies are of cranial nerves X, VI, and IX.[99] Complete jugular foramen syndromes are not uncommon. Extracranial lesions can present with hoarseness, dysphagia, unilateral headache, and diplopia.[99] Occasionally, the occipitocervical junction is destabilized by tumor erosion. A rare and

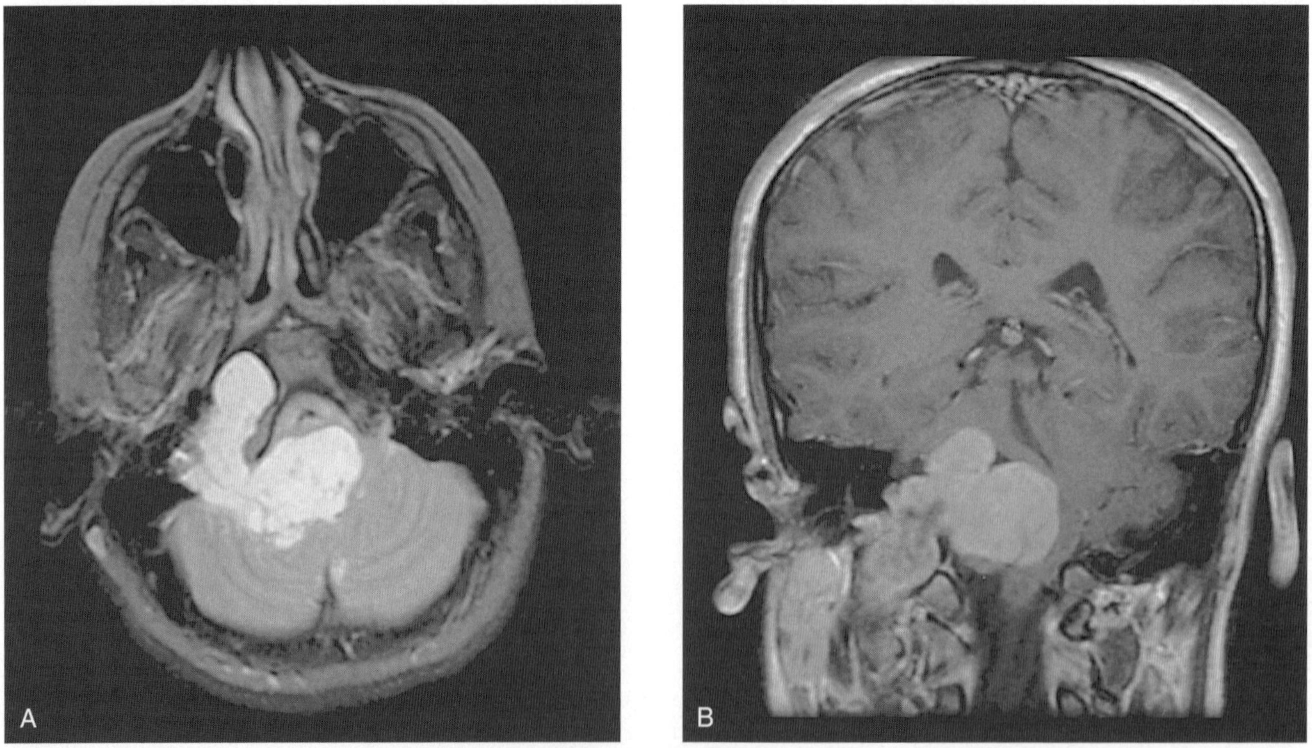

Figure 22-15. (A) Axial, unenhanced, first-echo, T_2-weighted MRI scan shows a large chondrosarcoma extending from the petroclival junction, destroying the right temporal bone and extending intracranially through the widely expanded jugular foramen to markedly compress the medulla. (B) Coronal, enhanced, T_1-weighted MRI scan (same case as [A]), shows the chondrosarcoma extends into the soft tissues of the right neck.

late complication is hydrocephalus from ventricular outflow obstruction. CT, MRI, and, occasionally, angiography where there is concern for vascular compromise, are the imaging modalities of choice. Plain radiographs show only a radiolucent lesion with punctate calcifications. CT can reveal overlying bony hyperostosis[98] and lesional calcification.[40] The MR signal is often heterogeneous with variable T_1 intensity and bright T_2 signal, except in calcified areas.[40] Bone and blood products can alter the MR signal of these lesions.[39] There is peripheral enhancement, occasionally with a dural tail. The angiogram reveals mass effect from a hypovascular lesion.

The management of these lesions is largely surgical. There is some controversy over the role of adjuvant radiotherapy in the form of charged particles, conventional photons, or brachytherapy. Some suggest partial resection and postoperative radiation therapy as a palliative mode of treatment. Proton beam and Gamma Knife radiosurgery hold more promise at the skull base than does conventional radiation.[35] Chemotherapy has poor results,[95] and its use is limited to higher-grade lesions only. In these cases, cisplatin, cyclophosphamide, vincristine, doxorubicin, and dacarbazine therapy have been attempted. There is some evidence of a response in these tumors to removal of growth hormone through hypophysectomy.[100]

The outcome of treatment in chondrosarcoma is typically better than that of chordoma. However, certain subtypes, such as mesenchymal, dedifferentiated, and clear-cell lesions, have a worse prognosis with higher rates of recurrence and more difficult operative resections.[97] Distant metastases are rare and usually limited to higher-grade lesions. Tumor grade, based on mitoses, naked nuclei, spindle nuclei, myxoid change, and loss of lacunar spaces, shows inverse correlation to survival.[99] Five- and 10-year survival rates for grades I, II, and III lesions are 90%/83%, 81%/64%, and 43%/29%, respectively. Excellent local control rates of 98% at 5 years and 94% at 10 years have been reported from Massachusetts General Hospital for proton beam therapy.[101] Possible side effects of proton beam therapy include myelopathy, temporal lobe injury, cranial nerve dysfunction, and endocrinopathy.[102] Larger lesions, greater than 25 cm^3, have a poorer outcome, even with use of proton beam radiotherapy.[101]

Chordoma

Chordoma represents 1% of the cranial tumors and 4% of the bone tumors.[103] Its comparison to chondrosarcoma is important, because the histopathology often overlaps. Chordomas are typically midline lesions (Fig. 22-16) derived from notochord remnants, often at the sphenooccipital synchondrosis,[39] presenting in the third or fourth decade of life (age range: 2–80 years old) with cranial nerve dysfunction (especially cranial nerve VI). White males are most frequently affected.[103] Their presentation can include headache, face pain, neck pain, torticollis, neuroendocrine changes, nasal obstruction, hearing loss, dizziness, hoarseness, swallowing dysfunction, tongue/palate paresis, craniofacial pain, visual loss, ptosis, diplopia, papilledema, and ataxia.[104,105] The lesions, although originating in the clivus, can extend into the suprasellar cistern, interpeduncular cistern, cerebellopontine angle, sphenoid sinus, cervical spinal canal, pharynx, petrous bone, jugular fossa, and atlas.[104] Chondroid chordomas are similar to chondrosarcomas histologically and in behavior.[17] They can have more frequent tumor calcification and less frequent bony sequestra on CT than their typical chordoma counterparts.[103]

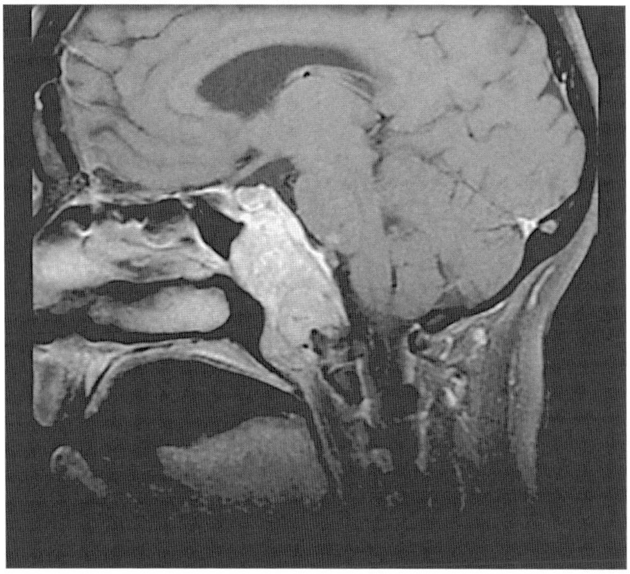

Figure 22-16. Sagittal, enhanced, T_1-weighted MRI scan reveals a chordoma expanding and destroying the clivus from the bottom of the sella to the opisthion. The tumor bulges into the nasopharynx but does not yet appear to extend through the dura.

Chordomas enhance minimally on imaging studies, and their characteristic pathologic hallmark is physaliferous ("bubbly") cells. They appear similar to chondrosarcomas on MR scans, with iso- to hypointense T_1 signal and high T_2 signal.[39] The T_1 signal may be high in areas of hemorrhage or proteinaceous fluid collection.[40] Fat-suppression MR sequences can outline these tumors well because these tumors are known to respect the dura and vasculature.[103] Their degree of enhancement is usually, but not reliably, more than that of chondrosarcoma. CT imaging of chordomas reveals a hypodense lesion in the clivus.[105]

The management of chordoma is surgical resection if possible, or debulking followed by proton beam radiotherapy or fractionated radiation. Craniotomy with orbitozygomatic extension is used to access the upper clivus, while transcondylar approaches can allow access to the lower clivus. Transfacial approaches (transnasal/transsphenoidal, lateral retropharyngeal, transmandibular with tongue splitting) gain access to lesions extending anteriorly into the nasopharynx.[103,105] With extensive clival and cervical spine involvement, patients may need upper cervical decompression, bone grafting, and occipitocervical fusion.[105] The surgical complication characteristic of this lesion is seeding of the path of exposure, especially in the nasal cavity for transfacial exposures.[104] General risks include pneumocephalus, CSF leak, syndrome of inappropriate antidiuretic hormone secretion, and pituitary or cranial nerve injury.[105]

Radiotherapy for this lesion parallels that of chondrosarcoma. Conventional radiotherapy is reportedly not as effective as proton beam radiotherapy, which has shown improvement in outcomes with each subsequent publication. Charged particle therapy with He/Ne/protons was reported to have a control rate of 63% at 5 years in 1994.[36] Later, proton beam alone was described as offering 73% local control at 5 years.[102] Most recently, local control with proton beam was reported to be 94% and 64% at 5 and 10 years, respectively.[35]

At a mean followup of 41 months, in patients with chordoma or low-grade chondrosarcoma, local control nears 82% with 76% disease-free survival.[106] When chordoma is separated, it usually fares worse than low-grade chondrosarcoma. In fact, the typical natural history is one of early local control, slow local invasive growth, very late metastases (7%–14%) to the liver, lungs, skeleton, and lymph nodes, and eventual death.[103,104] The 5-year local control rate in one series was 55% compared to 95% for chondrosarcoma.[104] Others have reported a 60% to 70% disease-free survival rate at 5 years following aggressive resections.[103] Predictors of poor outcome include female sex, tumor necrosis on microscopy, and tumor volume greater than 70 cm^3 [103] or 25 cm^3.[101]

Lipoma

Lipomas account for 0.1% of all intracranial tumors and for 0.14% of cerebellopontine angle lesions.[83] They are considered congenital malformations of the meninx primitiva rather than neoplasms. Other locations for intracranial lipoma include the corpus callosum, the cisterns (ambient, quadrigeminal, chiasmatic, sylvian, lateral pontine, interpeduncular), and the tela choroidea of the choroid plexus. More than half of patients with intracranial lipoma have other brain malformations, but this association is not seen with the cerebellopontine angle lesions.[83]

The clinical presentation usually involves males with tinnitus, vertigo, or hearing loss, while many more present incidentally or on autopsy. The lipoma may be present in the cerebellopontine angle, internal auditory canal, or both.[83] On CT scans, lipomas are very hypodense, resembling intracranial air. MRI reveals a lesion that is hyperintense on T_1-weighted images and isointense to hypointense on T_2-weighted images. Gadolinium does brighten these tumors above their baseline T_1 signal.

Surgical resection is the treatment of choice for progressively symptomatic lesions, whereas small incidental lesions can be observed. The conservative management can involve a weight-loss program, which may result in shrinkage of the intracranial lipoma. The resection of these lipomas puts the eighth and, less frequently, the seventh cranial nerves at high risk for injury. Complications could also include injury to cranial nerves IX, X, XI, XII, and V, along with meningitis and long-tract dysfunction. Sparing vital nerves and vasculature may require leaving some lipoma behind after resection. This alternative is clearly favored over injuring a patient for gross total resection.

Teratoma

In the past, teratomas have been described as congenital lesions containing tissue from three germ cell layers: ectoderm, mesoderm, and endoderm. Their histology is better characterized as primitive neoplastic lesions displaying divergent differentiation. They are more common in the supratentorial space, especially the pineal gland and parasellar area.[83] The cerebellar vermis and lateral ventricles are still more frequent locations than the cerebellopontine angle. Imaging studies show very heterogeneous signal. Immature teratoma can be treated with a trial of radiation or chemotherapy, especially when germ cell markers are positive. The remaining teratoma mass is usually the mature teratoma component, which can be observed or resected. Sarcomatous or carcinomatous dedifferentiation is possible.

Cavernoma

A cavernous hemangioma of the internal auditory canal can arise at the geniculate ganglion and spread medially to the cerebellopontine angle. The presentation involves facial spasm or weakness. Most of these are resected without losing facial function, but occasionally, a nerve graft is needed.[83] The middle fossa or translabyrinthine approaches are options, with the latter used when hearing is lost.

Epithelial Cyst

Benign epithelial cysts of the posterior fossa are developmental inclusions referred to as neurenteric cysts, neuroepithelial cysts, enterogeneous cysts, endodermal cysts, gastrocytomas, and foregut cysts.[83] Although neurenteric cysts have classically been described as arising from nondisjunction of the transient ectoderm-to-endoderm connection through the notochord called the neurenteric canal, some contend that these lesions are ectodermal in origin.[107] In the spine, neurenteric cysts are associated with split-cord malformations, and an abnormal vertebral column. In the skull, these cysts are seen in the posterior fossa, primarily in the cerebellopontine angle, and, occasionally, in the fourth ventricle. Recurrent meningitis is possible as are symptoms from cranial nerve dysfunction. The MRI of neurenteric cysts parallels CSF—high T_2 signal and low T_1 signal—with the exception of possible enhancement of the cyst wall. The treatment is generally surgical, and when the cyst is adherent to nerves and the brainstem, may consist of fenestration or shunting alone. Rare reports of malignancies arising from the epithelial lining of these cysts[108] have not altered the management of this lesion.

Arachnoid cysts are typically bounded by a bilayer of arachnoid that has filled with CSF via a ball valve mechanism. These cysts are rounded and can exhibit significant mass effect. They are not neoplastic, and their treatment is wide fenestration, complete excision, or CSF diversion.

Epidermoid Cyst

Whereas neurenteric cysts can be thought of as endodermal central nervous system (CNS) inclusions, epidermoid cysts and dermoid cysts are ectodermal inclusions. Epidermoid cysts are the most common embryonal intracranial lesion, accounting for 2% of all intracranial tumors and 4.6% to 9% of cerebellopontine angle lesions.[83] The cerebellopontine angle is a more common presenting location than the other sites of intracranial epidermoids—parasellar, chiasmatic, skull base, hemispheric, brainstem, and ventricular. The cyst lining is constantly desquamating keratinized epithelium, resulting in inexorable slow growth. The cysts spread along planes of least resistance until further progress is halted, and mass effect begins to cause symptoms. MRI is hypointense on T_1 (between brain and CSF) and hyperintense on T_2, with some matrix substance that distinguishes them from arachnoid cysts (Fig. 22-17A and B).[109] The MR sequence of choice is diffusion-weighted images, showing

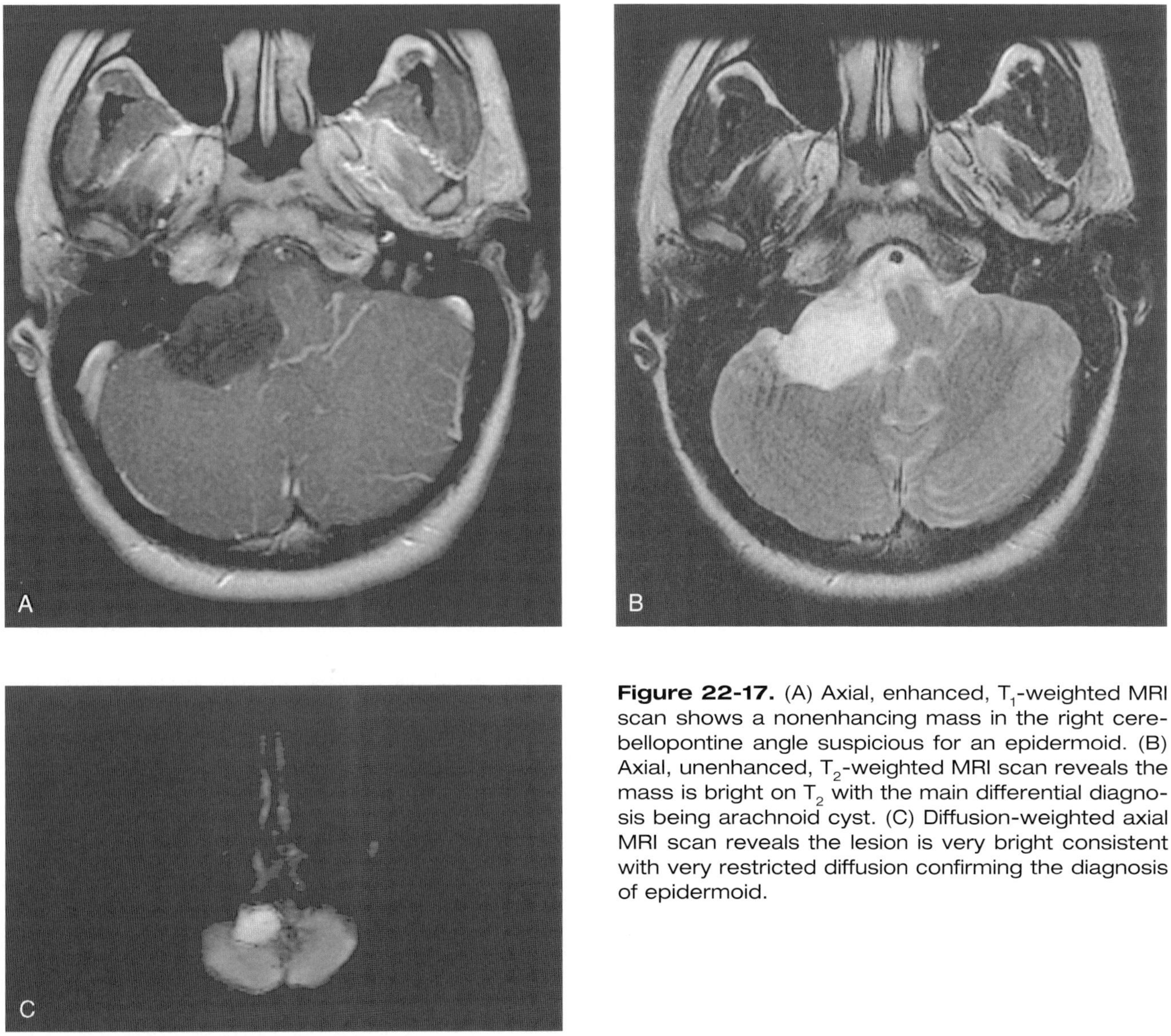

Figure 22-17. (A) Axial, enhanced, T_1-weighted MRI scan shows a nonenhancing mass in the right cerebellopontine angle suspicious for an epidermoid. (B) Axial, unenhanced, T_2-weighted MRI scan reveals the mass is bright on T_2 with the main differential diagnosis being arachnoid cyst. (C) Diffusion-weighted axial MRI scan reveals the lesion is very bright consistent with very restricted diffusion confirming the diagnosis of epidermoid.

very restricted diffusion of water in the dry keratin of these cysts (Fig. 22-17C). On CT scans, these are hypodense, with irregular borders, exhibiting almost no bony remodeling or mass effect. The treatment of epidermoid cysts is resection. Preoperative steroids are used to prevent aseptic meningitis associated with spillage of dry keratin.

Dermoid Cyst

Dermoid cysts are also ectodermal inclusions in the CNS. Their histology differs from epidermoids by the presence of dermal appendages—sebaceous glands, hair, nails, and teeth—in the lining of the cyst. These lesions are about one-tenth as common as epidermoid tumors. They are typically midline, and rarely present in the skull base of the posterior fossa. Dermoids present at an earlier age than do epidermoids, likely because they are less able to insinuate themselves into tight spaces, as they are firmer and cause earlier mass effect. Rupture of a dermoid cyst can result in debilitating chemical meningitis from sebaceous secretions. The therapy for these lesions is resection.

Choroid Plexus Papilloma

Although intraaxial lesions are not typically considered skull base neoplasms, some exophytic ones can enter the differential of cerebellopontine angle and posterior fossa skull base masses. The most typical are choroid plexus papillomas, which can extend through the foramina of Magendie and Luschka into the subarachnoid space. Cranial neuropathies can occur when enough tumor is growing in the cerebellopontine angle. Resection of these "cauliflower"-appearing lesions is the therapy of choice with adjuvant chemotherapy or radiation for malignant histology, or recurrence.[83]

Nerve Sheath Tumor of Jugular Foramen

Peripheral nerve sheath tumors can be found along cranial nerves throughout their course. The jugular foramen is no exception, with cranial nerves IX, X, and XI passing through. Typically, CT imaging of the area shows smooth enlargement of the foramen, while MR images reveal a mass that is hypointense on T_1, hyperintense on T_2, and enhances well.[81] As expected, the tumors center on the pars nervosa of the jugular foramen.[40] The constriction of the jugular foramen often results in dumbbell-shaped tumors. Angiography to assess patency of the sigmoid sinus–jugular vein system also shows the lesions to be hypovascular. Because of the morbidity of injury to multiple lower cranial nerves, some authors advocate radiosurgery as the first-line therapy for these lesions.[110] Although some authors espouse careful dissection of these lesions free of the lower cranial nerves,[111] others accept that tedious dissection of multiple lower cranial nerves carries high risk and decide that subtotal resection is sufficient with either serial scanning or immediate postoperative radiosurgery.[112]

Paragangliomas

The paragangliomas or chemodectomas of the posterior fossa and neck comprise a specific niche in the realm of skull base tumors. These lesions are of extraadrenal neuroendocrine origin, and are named by the location or structures from which they arise: glomus vagale, glomus tympanicum, glomus jugulare, and carotid body tumors.[81] Glomus vagale lesions are the least common, with carotid body tumors and jugulotympanic lesions seen nearly equally. Paragangliomas are the most common middle ear tumor, the most common cause of mass-producing pulsatile tinnitus, and the second most common temporal bone neoplasm after acoustic neuroma.[81] Other than carotid body tumors, paragangliomas outside the posterior skull base are rare. There is a female predominance in paraganglioma patients, with a female-to-male ratio of 2.7:1 for glomus vagale lesions, and 6 to 7:1 for jugulotympanic lesions. Interestingly, oxygen deprivation from high-altitude living or chronic obstructive pulmonary disease tends to increase the incidence of this lesion.[81]

Presenting symptoms of glomus tumors are hearing loss, swallowing difficulty, neck/ear pain or neck mass, pulsatile tinnitus, tongue weakness, shoulder weakness, or ear discharge.[81] The lesions are not typically painful. Physical examination may document palsies of cranial nerves IX to XII, with an occasional Horner syndrome. Very commonly, a red mass is seen behind the ear drum on otoscopic examination. Rarely, these tumors produce and can secrete catecholamines. A history of difficult-to-control hypertension or hypertensive crises should be noted. Also, all patients with paragangliomas should have pretreatment 24-hour urine catecholamine screen to investigate for a possible endocrinologically active tumor. If catecholamine production is documented, preoperative beta and alpha blockade is necessary to avoid intraoperative hypertensive crisis. Synchronous or metasynchronous paragangliomas are seen in 10% of patients.[20] This necessitates a careful search for another lesion when a paraganglioma is discovered. The glomus vagale lesions can arise anywhere along the vagus nerve.[81] Temporal bone paragangliomas arise from the tympanic branch of cranial nerve IX (Jacobsen nerve), the auricular branch of cranial nerve X (Arnold nerve), or the jugular bulb. The glomus tympanicum may be confined to the middle ear or extend to the mastoid air cells. Glomus jugulare tumors affect the mastoid air cells, vascular tracts, eustachian tube, and neural foramina. Erosion of the temporal bone takes place, with tympanic dehiscences, ossicular involvement, and bony labyrinth destruction.[81]

CT reveals isodense lesions and clear boundaries, with occasional tumor calcification and some bony erosion.[113,114] Jugular foramen erosion followed by middle ear involvement suggests glomus tumor. Preservation of the ossicles favors glomus tympanicum rather than jugulare.[81]

Erosion through the IAC into the cerebellopontine angle is possible. MR scans show isointense lesions on T_1 sequences with an occasional "salt and pepper"[81] appearance from the hypervascularity of the lesion. T_2 images show hyperintense lesions with flow voids possible.[113,114] Contrast enhancement is brisk, and angiography shows a hypervascular tumor blush (Fig. 22-18).[81] The most common feeding arteries to head and neck paragangliomas are ascending pharyngeal and ascending cervical, whereas jugulotympanic tumors receive additional blood from meningeal branches of the internal carotid, vertebral, and middle meningeal arteries.[81] Angiography allows for evaluation of the internal jugular vein. Indium-111 octreotide scans are often positive when lesions approach 1.5 cm in diameter.[81]

The differential diagnosis of these lesions in the jugular foramen includes nerve sheath tumor, meningioma, metastasis, bone tumors, histiocytosis X, lymphoma, multiple myeloma, jugular dehiscence, and jugular thrombosis.[81] In the middle ear, glomus tumors can mimic adenoma, endolymphatic sac tumor, choristoma, cholesteatoma, cholesterol granuloma, small cell carcinoma, adenocarcinoma, and sarcoma.[81] Before a middle ear lesion is biopsied, one should recall that an aberrant petrous internal carotid artery may infrequently pass through the middle ear and mimic a glomus tympanicum.

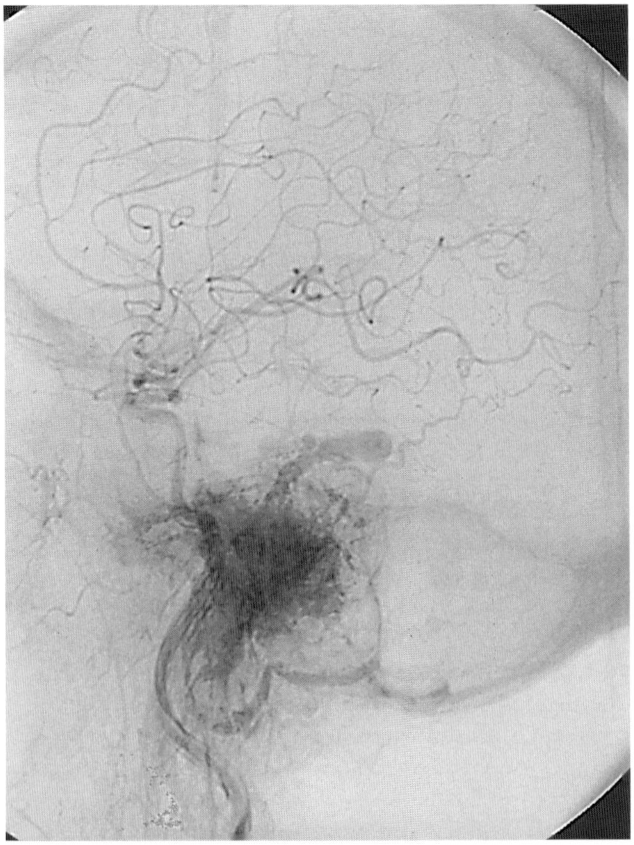

Figure 22-18. Lateral left common carotid angiogram reveals a very large vascular mass in the region of the jugular foramen consistent with a large glomus jugulare tumor. The left internal carotid artery is displaced forward by the mass.

The histology of these lesions is specific: chromogranin- and synaptophysin-positive cells in clusters, or "Zellballen" configuration. They are epithelial membrane antigen positive, whereas the sustentacular cells are S100 positive. There is variable cytokeratin staining. Vimentin is negative.[113,114] Malignant paragangliomas are rare, but have high mitotic rate, local invasiveness, invasion of vascular structures, necrosis of cell clusters, and local or distant metastases.[115]

The surgical resection of glomus tumors involves infratemporal fossa dissection to the jugular foramen. When there is intracranial extension, a suboccipital craniectomy is added to secure the intracranial component. Preoperative embolization 2 to 14 days in advance helps to reduce operative blood loss and allows for better visualization.[31,84,116] This requires complete embolization in tumors that are often fed by multiple feeding arteries to different tumor compartments.[81] Complications of angiographic embolization include passage of embolic agents through vascular channels to the systemic circulation, catecholamine release from the tumor, and cranial nerve infarction and palsy. Complications from surgery include transient or permanent facial nerve palsy, dysphagia or vocal cord paralysis, stroke, or death.[84] Raquet reported mostly transient cranial nerve deficits in 31 patients who underwent resection of jugular foramen lesions.[117]

The adjuvant therapy of these lesions with medications or radiation is unproven.[114] However, the reports of radiation insensitivity in carotid body tumors are contradicted by reports of glomus tumors responding to radiation. In fact, Suh reports an 80% to 90% response of these tumors to fractionated radiotherapy, using 1.8 to 2.0 Gy fractions for a total of 45 to 50 Gy.[35] When surgery for bilateral glomus vagale tumors would result in complete vocal cord paralysis, one side is often radiated.[81] In general, postoperative radiation is withheld after the original resection, but used if recurrence prompts another surgical intervention or if the tumor histology suggests the malignant variant.[113] Mortality from jugulotympanic lesions is 15%, while the recurrence rate for glomus jugulare ranges from 40% to 50%.[81]

Craniopharyngioma

The presence of craniopharyngioma in the posterior fossa has been reported both primarily[118] and by extension of large suprasellar lesions. Connolly reported on three patients presenting with hearing loss preceding other cranial nerve findings in suprasellar craniopharyngioma extended to the posterior fossa.[119] The three children underwent staged operations to address the suprasellar tumor and posterior fossa tumors separately. There was one new visual field cut, one trigeminal motor paresis, and endocrinopathy in all patients. Hearing did not improve.

There is controversy regarding the optimum initial treatment of these lesions with some authors espousing radiation, while others advocate surgery. When gross total resection is feasible, a surgical attempt can be made, even in giant lesions extending to the posterior fossa. If achieved, observation with serial MR scans is adequate management. Residual or recurrent disease can be treated with radiation. The role of stereotactic radiosurgery in management of children with these lesions is undefined.

▶ EXTRACRANIAL LESIONS

Extracranial tumors of the cranial nerves include nerve sheath and carotid body tumors.

Presentation

Extracranial lesions of the cranial nerves present typically either incidentally on examination, or with local mass effect or nerve dysfunction. Mass effect may include obstructive dysphagia, conductive hearing loss, stridor, and soft tissue fullness. Ear pain and otorrhea can be seen. The lower cranial nerves are more commonly affected. Highly vascular lesions can present with pulsatile tinnitus. Horner syndrome is occasionally seen, with irritation of the cervical sympathetic plexus around the carotid artery. Rarely, paragangliomas can present with symptoms of excess catecholamine synthesis—headache, palpitations, hypertension, and tachycardia.

Evaluation

The evaluation of the patient with cranial nerve lesions outside the skull base should include a thorough evaluation of the family history. Nerve sheath tumors are associated with neurofibromatosis, whereas carotid body tumors can have familial inheritance. The physical examination should focus on stigmata of neurocutaneous syndromes and auscultation of any cervical bruits. Patients with carotid body paragangliomas often have masses that can be moved horizontally with careful palpation, but not vertically. In general, regional lymph node enlargement is freely mobile.[120] Lymph node pathology (infection or tumor), carotid artery aneurysm or pseudoaneurysm, salivary tumor, branchial cleft cyst, or thyroid tumor are also possible in the neck.[120] For patients with transient or chronic hypertension, a screen for urine and serum catecholamines is reasonable. CT scanning is valuable for documenting skull or cervical spine erosion, whereas MRI delineates tissue planes. Special investigations in patients with these tumors should include color flow Doppler ultrasonography and angiography.[120] During angiography, embolization can be used to lessen operative blood loss.[121]

Diagnoses and Management

Carotid Body Tumor and Malignant Carotid Body Tumor

Paragangliomas and malignant paragangliomas of the carotid body share histologic features with the previously mentioned glomus tumors. This group of tumors arises from neural crest and third brachial arch mesoderm present in the jugular venous system, vagus nerve, aortic arch, visceral autonomic system, or carotid body.[122] The pathology of carotid body tumors parallels other paragangliomas, "Zellballen" clusters of chief cells in a fibrous unencapsulated tumor with peripheral sustentacular cells.[122] The chief cells have neurosecretory granules, and the sustentacular cells are S100 positive.

Carotid body tumors are often incidental findings on exam,[120] but can present with hoarseness, mechanical dysphagia, stridor, mobile palpable neck mass (most common), pulsatile tinnitus, discomfort, vertigo, and tongue weakness. Late in disease progression, tonsillar displacement by intraoral mass and paresis of cranial nerves X, XII, XI, IX, can occur.[81] Horner syndrome is seen in 25% of carotid body tumors, while hoarseness and vocal cord difficulty are rare. These lesions are familial in 7% to 10% of cases (mostly through paternal inheritance of a tumor suppressor gene mutation) of which 30% present bilaterally.[81,120] The general rate of bilaterality on presentation is 5% in all patients.[81] The relationship between some blood-clotting-factor deficiencies and carotid body tumors is surprising. Rarely, these tumors are part of a more syndromic neuroendocrine tumor disorder. Between 1% and 3% of these lesions are functionally active, secreting catecholamines.[81]

Ultrasonography is used as a screening tool for ruling out carotid body tumors, whereas angiography makes the diagnosis and offers possible embolization.[122] While glomus vagale lesions displace the internal and external carotid arteries away from the internal jugular vein, carotid body tumors typically splay the external and internal carotid arteries apart, rarely narrowing their lumens.[81] They grow at a rate of approximately 5 mm per year and can cause lower cranial nerve dysfunction.[81] The peak age of onset is 45 to 50 years, with no gender preference. Based on imaging findings, the differential includes nerve sheath tumor, nodal mets, abscess, and venous thrombosis.

Surgical treatment is preferred, with the aid of preoperative embolization when it is safe. Preoperative angiography offers the advantage of estimating the risks of carotid sacrifice—from cerebral blood flow and neurologic examination during trial occlusion. Biopsy of these lesions has been reported to carry significant risk of life-threatening hemorrhage.[120] Preparations for saphenous vein harvest or synthetic patching can be made if needed. Surgical dissection should include consideration of intraoperative EEG, with carotid shunting for EEG changes, observation of carotid back-flow if opened, and possible vein reconstruction or patch grafting. Periadventitial dissection offers the chance of carotid preservation where possible.[123] Regional lymphadenectomy is accomplished when feasible. Bone invasion may require mandibular resection, and significant carotid involvement has resulted in carotid sacrifice in the past.[120] Complications of surgery include a 67% rate of cranial nerve palsy when resectioning vagale lesions.[81] Cranial nerve XI injury can result in shoulder droop, pain, and internal rotation.

The response of these lesions to adjuvant radiotherapy is poor; paragangliomas of the skull base tend to respond more favorably.[81] For this reason, radiation of carotid body lesions is reserved for salvage therapy or in treatment of one side of bilateral lesions. Chemotherapy has also been used as a salvage procedure. Cyclophosphamide, dacarbazine, and vincristine are used in recurrent or metastatic disease.[38]

Malignant carotid body tumors represent 2% to 13% of all carotid body tumors.[81] They are defined by local, regional, or distant metastases. Although some authors report differences in malignant carotid body tumor histology, such as necrosis of cell clusters, high mitotic rate, local invasion (into vagus), vascular invasion,[115] and fewer sustentacular S100-positive cells,[81] there is no steadfast correlation of histology with metastasis.[122] In one series, 3 of 87 lesions were malignant, of which one resulted in death, one was cured at longest followup, and one was lost to followup.[115] All were treated with postoperative radiation therapy. Metastases, mostly to the lungs and bone, can be treated with surgical excision and local radiation. These metastases can be seen from 20 months to 20 years after resection.[115] The chemoresponsiveness of the tumors is poor.[115]

Benign and Malignant Nerve Sheath Tumors of the Head and Neck

Schwannomas and neurofibromas of the face and neck are managed by local excision of the tumors, along with nerve or fascicle sacrifice in the case of neurofibromas. Of 52 patients with extracranial head and neck schwannoma reported by Leu, 1 had malignant pathology.[124] Of these 52 patients, tumors were found most often in the scalp, face, and external ear canals. Schwannomas of major extracranial cranial nerves were most often found in the poststyloid compartment of the parapharyngeal space. Schwannomas have been reported in the orbit, oral and nasal cavities, ear canal, maxillary sinus, subcutaneous face, infratemporal fossa, scalp, and neck. Because of their less invasive nature, complete resection is common.

Neurofibromas are commonly seen in neurofibromatosis type I, and when affecting the head and neck, often involve the face and facial bones. Plexiform neurofibromas are often found expanding the maxillary sinuses, with cutaneous neurofibromas of the face.[125] Surgery often requires extensive facial dissection and can result in facial disfigurement, necessitating cosmetic repair. The rate of malignancy in neurofibromatosis type 1 is nearly 30%,[126] reflecting an additive risk with multiple lesions.

Malignant peripheral nerve sheath tumors (MPNSTs) of the cranial nerves are seen in the head and neck. Of all soft tissue sarcomas, MPNSTs comprise 5%, of which 8% to 15% are found in the head and neck.[127] They are associated with neurofibromatosis type 1 in 26% to 70% of cases. Therapy is primarily surgical with or without irradiation.

Outcome

The results of treatment for carotid body lesions are generally good. However, dural invasion, aggressive pathologic grade, and positive margins are predictive of poor outcome and should prompt consideration of adjuvant therapy or new novel interventions.[23] Operative complications could include cranial nerve palsies VII, IX, X, XII. Preoperative embolization does not affect these risks.[120] Of 19 patients treated by Muhm, 3 had tumor recurrence.[120] When there is question of whether MR changes reflect recurrent tumor or postoperative change, positron emission tomography scanning is helpful.[20] Mortality figures are approximately 9% for carotid body lesions with a recurrence rate of 10% (17% for vagale lesions).[81]

The outcome of head and neck schwannoma resection is most frequently complete cure. Neurofibromas requiring extensive dissection are difficult to remove completely, and multiple operations may be needed to treat symptomatic recurrence. Unfortunately, these facial incisions along with tumor regrowth are quite disfiguring. MPNST treatment has an even less favorable outcome.

▶ CONCLUSION

Cranial base tumors are a heterogeneous compilation of lesions that share a complex anatomic space. Their shared location leads to similar patterns of presentation, while their biologic diversity determines the chronicity of presentation, the extent of pretreatment neurologic deficits, and the success of therapy. Adjuvant therapies improve survival and quality of life in some settings, but surgical intervention remains the mainstay of treatment, when feasible, for many of these pathologies. Gamma Knife and linear accelerator–based radiosurgery, intravascular embolization, and vascularized flap closures of complex defects are part of the armamentarium used against these lesions. Future directions could include gene therapy.[128] The principle of treating these typically benign lesions continues to be tumor control—to prevent or alleviate mass effect without inducing new neurologic deficits.

REFERENCES

1. Giuffre R. Successful radical removal of an intracranial meningioma in 1835 by Professor Pecchioli of Siena. J Neurosurg 1984;60:47–51.
2. Stone JL. Sir Charles Ballance: pioneer British neurological surgeon. Neurosurgery 1999;44:610–631; discussion 631–632.
3. Cushing H. Partial hypophysectomy for acromegaly: with remarks on the function of the hypophysis. Ann Surg 1909;50:1002.
4. Dandy WE. Results of removal of acoustic tumors by the unilateral approach. AMA Arch of Surg 1942;42:1026–1033.
5. Donald PJ. History of skull base surgery. In: Donald PJ, ed. Surgery of the skull base. Philadelphia: Lippincott-Raven, 1998:3–13.
6. Smith RR, Klopp CT, Williams JM. Surgical treatment of cancer of the frontal sinus and adjacent areas. Cancer 1954;7:991–994.
7. Ketcham AS, Wilkins RH, Van Buren JM, et al. A combined intracranial facial approach to the paranasal sinuses. Am J Surg 1963;106:698–703.
8. Ketcham AS, Hoyle RC, Van Buren JM, et al. Complications of intracranial facial resections for tumors of the paranasal sinuses. Am J Surg 1966;112:591–596.
9. Millar HS, Petty PG, Wilson WF, et al. A combined intracranial and facial approach for excision and repair of cancer of the ethmoid sinuses. Aust N Z J Surg 1973;43:179–183.
10. Sisson GA, Bytell DE, Becker SP, et al. Carcinoma of the paranasal sinuses and cranial-facial resection. J Laryngol Otol 1976;90:59–68.
11. Bridger GP. Radical surgery for ethmoid cancer. Arch Otolaryngol 1980;106:630–634.
12. Cheesman AD, Lund VJ, Howard DJ. Craniofacial resection for tumors of the nasal cavity and paranasal sinuses. Head Neck Surg 1986;8:429–435.
13. Greenberg HS, Deck MD, Vikram B, et al. Metastasis to the base of the skull: clinical findings in 43 patients. Neurology 1981;31:530–537.
14. Schuller DE, Goodman JH, Mountain RE, et al. Adjunctive treatment of cranial base malignancies. J Craniofac Surg 1995;6:69–74.
15. Osguthorpe JD, Patel S. Craniofacial approaches to tumors of the anterior skull base. Otolaryngol Clin North Am 2001; 34:1123–1142.
16. Fewel ME, Gebarski SS, Hoff JT. Skull tumors. In: Winn HR, ed. Youmans neurological surgery. Philadelphia: WB Saunders, 2003:1383–1408.
17. Richardson MS. Pathology of skull base tumors. Otolaryngol Clin North Am 2001;34:1025–1042.
18. Chang CY, O'Rourke DK, Cass SP. Update on skull base surgery. Otolaryngol Clin North Am 1996;29:467–501.
19. Link MJ, Tomsick TA, Tew JM Jr. Honored guest presentation: therapeutic carotid occlusion. Clin Neurosurg 2000;46: 326–338.
20. Durden DD, Williams DW 3rd. Radiology of skull base neoplasms. Otolaryngol Clin North Am 2001;34:1043–1064.
21. Casiano RR, Numa WA, Falquez AM. Endoscopic resection of esthesioneuroblastoma. Am J Rhinol 2001;15:271–279.
22. Diaz EM Jr, Kies MS. Chemotherapy for skull base cancers. Otolaryngol Clin North Am 2001;34:1079–1085.
23. Bentz BG, Bilsky MH, Shah JP, et al. Anterior skull base surgery for malignant tumors: a multivariate analysis of 27 years of experience. Head Neck 2003;25:515–520.
24. Ginsberg LE. Neoplastic diseases affecting the central skull base: CT and MR imaging. Am J Roentgenol 1992; 159:581–589.
25. Donaldson SS, Meza J, Breneman JC, et al. Results from the IRS-IV randomized trial of hyperfractionated radiotherapy in children with rhabdomyosarcoma—a report from the IRSG [see comment]. Int J Radiat Oncol Biol Phys 2001;51:718–728.
26. Paulino AC. Role of radiation therapy in parameningeal rhabdomyosarcoma. Cancer Invest 1999;17:223–230.
27. Timmerman RD, Mendonca M. In regard to Donaldson et al: results from the IRS-IV randomized trial of hyperfractionated radiotherapy in children with rhabdomyosarcoma—a report from the IRSG. IJROBP 2001;51:718–728 [comment]. Int J Radiat Oncol Biol Phys 2002;54:1579–1580; author reply 1580.
28. Radner H, Katenkamp D, Reifenberger G, et al. New developments in the pathology of skull base tumors. Virchows Archiv 2001;438:321–335.
29. Dalley RW. Fibrous histiocytoma and fibrous tissue tumors of the orbit. Radiol Clin North Am 1999;37:185–194.
30. Ueda R, Hayashi T, Kameyama K, et al. Orbital malignant fibrous histiocytoma with extension to the base of the skull—case report. Neurol Med Chir (Tokyo) 2003;43: 263–266.
31. Turowski B, Zanella FE. Interventional neuroradiology of the head and neck. Neuroimaging Clin North Am 2003;13: 619–645.
32. Rock MG, Sim FH, Unni KK, et al. Secondary malignant giant-cell tumor of bone. Clinicopathological assessment of nineteen patients. J Bone Jt Surg Am 1986;68:1073–1079.
33. Kos M, Luczak K, Godzinski J, et al. Treatment of monostotic fibrous dysplasia with pamidronate. J Craniomaxillofac Surg 2004;32:10–15.
34. Plotkin H, Rauch F, Zeitlin L, et al. Effect of pamidronate treatment in children with polyostotic fibrous dysplasia of bone. J Clin Endocrinol Metab 2003;88:4569–4575.
35. Suh JH, Saxton JP. Conventional radiation therapy for skull base tumors: an overview. Neurosurg Clin North Am 2000;11:575–586.
36. Castro JR, Linstadt DE, Bahary JP, et al. Experience in charged particle irradiation of tumors of the skull base: 1977–1992 [see comment]. Int J Radiat Oncol Biol Phys 1994;29:647–655.
37. Nahum AE, Dearnaley DP, Steel GG. Prospects for proton-beam radiotherapy. Eur J Cancer 1994;30A:1577–1583.
38. Adelstein DJ. The role of chemotherapy for skull base carcinomas and sarcomas. Neurosurg Clin North Am 2000;11: 681–691.
39. Fischbein NJ, Kaplan MJ. Magnetic resonance imaging of the central skull base. Top Magn Reson Imaging 1999;10: 325–346.
40. Curtin HD, Chavali R. Imaging of the skull base. Radiol Clin North Am 1998;36:801–817.
41. DeMonte F. Surgical treatment of anterior basal meningiomas. J Neurooncol 1996;29:239–248.
42. Desai R, Bruce J. Meningiomas of the cranial base. J Neurooncol 1994;20:255–279.

43. Al-Mefty O. Clinoidal meningiomas. J Neurosurg 1990;73: 840–849.
44. Stafford SL, Pollock BE, Foote RL, et al. Meningioma radiosurgery: tumor control, outcomes, and complications among 190 consecutive patients. Neurosurgery 2001;49: 1029–1037; discussion 1037–1028.
45. Black PM. Hormones, radiosurgery and virtual reality: new aspects of meningioma management. Can J Neurol Sci 1997;24:302–306.
46. Goldsmith BJ, Larson DA. Conventional radiation therapy for skull base meningiomas. Neurosurg Clin North Am 2000;11:605–615.
47. Abdel-Fattah HM, Adams GL, Wick MR. Hemangiopericytoma of the maxillary sinus and skull base. Head Neck 1990;12:77–83.
48. Bastin KT, Mehta MP. Meningeal hemangiopericytoma: defining the role for radiation therapy. J Neurooncol 1992;14:277–287.
49. Coffey RJ, Cascino TL, Shaw EG. Radiosurgical treatment of recurrent hemangiopericytomas of the meninges: preliminary results. J Neurosurg 1993;78:903–908.
50. Osguthorpe JD. Sinus neoplasia. Arch Otolaryngol Head Neck Surg 1994;120:19–25.
51. Paulino AC, Marks JE, Leonetti JP. Postoperative irradiation of patients with malignant tumors of skull base. Laryngoscope 1996;106:880–883.
52. Parsons JT, Kimsey FC, Mendenhall WM, et al. Radiation therapy for sinus malignancies. Otolaryngol Clin North Am 1995;28:1259–1268.
53. Sen C, Sekhar LN. Direct vein graft reconstruction of the cavernous, petrous, and upper cervical internal carotid artery: lessons learned from 30 cases. Neurosurgery 1992;30:732–742; discussion 742–743.
54. Lawton MT, Hamilton MG, Beals SP, et al. Radical resection of anterior skull base tumors. Clin Neurosurg 1995;42: 43–70.
55. Boyle JO, Shah KC, Shah JP. Craniofacial resection for malignant neoplasms of the skull base: an overview. J Surg Oncol 1998;69:275–284.
56. McCutcheon IE, Blacklock JB, Weber RS, et al. Anterior transcranial (craniofacial) resection of tumors of the paranasal sinuses: surgical technique and results [see comment]. Neurosurgery 1996;38:471–479; discussion 479–480.
57. Andersen PE, Kraus DH, Arbit E, et al. Management of the orbit during anterior fossa craniofacial resection. Arch Otolaryngol Head Neck Surg 1996;122: 1305–1307.
58. Firlik KS, Kondziolka D, Lunsford LD, et al. Radiosurgery for recurrent cranial base cancer arising from the head and neck. Head Neck 1996;18:160–165; discussion 166.
59. Lawson W, Kaufman MR, Biller HF. Treatment outcomes in the management of inverted papilloma: an analysis of 160 cases. Laryngoscope 2003;113:1548–1556.
60. Wahlberg P, Anderson H, Biorklund A, et al. Carcinoma of the parotid and submandibular glands—a study of survival in 2465 patients. Oral Oncol 2002;38:706–713.
61. Al-Gahtany M, Cusimano M, Singer W, et al. Brown tumors of the skull base. Case report and review of the literature. J Neurosurg 2003;98:417–420.
62. Arena S, Keen M. Carcinoma of the middle ear and temporal bone. Am J Otol 1988;9:351–356.
63. Manolidis S, Pappas D Jr, Von Doersten P, et al. Temporal bone and lateral skull base malignancy: experience and results with 81 patients. Am J Otol 1998;19:S1–S15.
64. Branovan DI, Schaefer SD. Lateral craniofacial approaches to the skull base and infratemporal fossa. Otolaryngol Clin North Am 2001;34:1175–1195.
65. Sekhar LN, Buchanan RI, Wright DC, et al. The case for aggressive resection. Clin Neurosurg 1999;45:263–278.
66. Day JD, Fukushima T, Giannotta SL. Innovations in surgical approach: lateral cranial base approaches. Clin Neurosurg 1996;43:72–90.
67. Lanotte M, Giordana MT, Forni C, et al. Schwannoma of the cavernous sinus. Case report and review of the literature. J Neurol Sci 1992;36:233–238.
68. Yoshida K, Kawase T. Trigeminal neurinomas extending into multiple fossae: surgical methods and review of the literature. J Neurosurg 1999;91:202–211.
69. Eisenberg MB, Al-Mefty O, DeMonte F, et al. Benign nonmeningeal tumors of the cavernous sinus. Neurosurgery 1999;44:949–954; discussion 954–955.
70. Boltshauser E, Stocker H, Sailer H, et al. Intracranial abnormalities associated with facial plexiform neurofibromas in neurofibromatosis type 1. Neurofibromatosis 1989;2:274–277.
71. Ng HK, South JR. Supratentorial neurofibroma unassociated with cranial nerves. Aust N Z J Surg 1988;58:594–597.
72. Hashimoto M, Yokota A, Ohta H, et al. Intratumoral injection of plastic adhesive material for removal of cavernous sinus hemangioma. Technical note. J Neurosurg 2000;93: 1078–1081.
73. Jamjoom AB. Response of cavernous sinus hemangioma to radiotherapy: a case report. Neurosurg Rev 1996;19:261–264.
74. Long DM. The treatment of meningiomas in the region of the cavernous sinus. Childs Nerv Syst 2001;17:168–172.
75. Strang RD, al-Mefty O. Small skull base meningiomas. Surgical management. Clin Neurosurg 2001;48:320–339.
76. Lanzino G, Hirsch WL, Pomonis S, et al. Cavernous sinus tumors: neuroradiologic and neurosurgical considerations on 150 operated cases. J Neurol Sci 1992;36:183–196.
77. Lawton MT, Spetzler RF. Surgical management of giant intracranial aneurysms: experience with 171 patients. Clin Neurosurg 1995;42:245–266.
78. Sekhar LN, Sen CN, Jho HD, et al. Surgical treatment of intracavernous neoplasms: a four-year experience. Neurosurgery 1989;24:18–30.
79. Dolenc VV, ed. The cavernous sinus: a multidisciplinary approach to vascular and tumorous lesions. Wien, Germany: Springer-Verlag, 1987.
80. Bold EL, Wanamaker JR, Hughes GB, et al. Adenomatous lesions of the temporal bone immunohistochemical analysis and theories of histogenesis. Am J Otol 1995;16:146–152.
81. Rao AB, Koeller KK, Adair CF. From the archives of the AFIP. Paragangliomas of the head and neck: radiologic-pathologic correlation. Armed Forces Institute of Pathology. Radiographics 1999;19:1605–1632.
82. Matson DD. Surgery of posterior fossa tumors in childhood. Clin Neurosurg 1968;15:247–264.
83. Lalwani AK. Meningiomas, epidermoids, and other nonacoustic tumors of the cerebellopontine angle. Otolaryngol Clin North Am 1992;25:707–728.

84. Mann WJ, Maurer J, Marangos N. Neural conservation in skull base surgery. Otolaryngol Clin North Am 2002;35: 411–424.
85. Porter JM, Pidgeon C, Cunningham AJ. The sitting position in neurosurgery: a critical appraisal. Br J Anaesth 1999;82: 117–128.
86. Lustig LR, Rifkin S, Jackler RK, et al. Acoustic neuromas presenting with normal or symmetrical hearing: factors associated with diagnosis and outcome. Am J Otol 1998; 19:212–218.
87. Loevner LA. Imaging features of posterior fossa neoplasms in children and adults. Semin Roentgenol 1999;34:84–101.
88. Kileny PR, Niparko JK, Shepard NT, et al. Neurophysiologic intraoperative monitoring: I. Auditory function. Am J Otol 1988;9(Suppl):17–24.
89. Kondziolka D, Lunsford LD, McLaughlin MR, et al. Long-term outcomes after radiosurgery for acoustic neuromas [see comment]. N Engl J Med 1998;339:1426–1433.
90. Sampath P, Long DM. Acoustic neuroma. In: Winn HR, ed. Youmans neurological surgery. Philadelphia: WB Saunders, 2003:1147–1168.
91. Regis J, Pellet W, Delsanti C, et al. Functional outcome after gamma knife surgery or microsurgery for vestibular schwannomas. J Neurosurg 2002;97:1091–1100.
92. Sekhar LN, Wright DC, Richardson R, et al. Petroclival and foramen magnum meningiomas: surgical approaches and pitfalls. J Neurooncol 1996;29:249–259.
93. Yokota N, Yokoyama T, Nishizawa S. Facial nerve schwannoma in the cerebellopontine cistern. Findings on high resolution CT and MR cisternography. Br J Neurosurg 1999;13:512–515.
94. Mabanta SR, Buatti JM, Friedman WA, et al. Linear accelerator radiosurgery for nonacoustic schwannomas. Int J Radiat Oncol Biol Phys 1999;43:545–548.
95. Rapidis AD, Archondakis G, Anteriotis D, et al. Chondrosarcomas of the skull base: review of the literature and report of two cases. J Craniomaxillofac Surg 1997;25:322–327.
96. Ramina R, Coelho Neto M, Meneses MS, et al. Maffucci's syndrome associated with a cranial base chondrosarcoma: case report and literature review [see comment]. Neurosurgery 1997;41:269–272.
97. Keel SB, Bhan AK, Liebsch NJ, et al. Chondromyxoid fibroma of the skull base: a tumor which may be confused with chordoma and chondrosarcoma. A report of three cases and review of the literature. Am J Surg Pathol 1997;21:577–582.
98. Oikawa H, Satoh T, Masuda T, et al. Intracranial low-grade chondrosarcoma with hyperostosis of the skull: a case report. J Neurooncol 2000;49:249–254.
99. Seidman MD, Nichols RD, Raju UB, et al. Extracranial skull base chondrosarcoma. Ear Nose Throat J 1989;68:626–632.
100. Arlen M, Tollefsen HR, Huvos AG, et al. Chondrosarcoma of the head and neck. Am J Surg 1970;120:456–460.
101. Hug EB, Slater JD. Proton radiation therapy for chordomas and chondrosarcomas of the skull base. Neurosurg Clin North Am 2000;11:627–638.
102. Munzenrider JE, Liebsch NJ. Proton therapy for tumors of the skull base. Strahlenther Onkol 1999;175(Suppl 2):57– 63.
103. Erdem E, Angtuaco EC, Van Hemert R, et al Comprehensive review of intracranial chordoma. Radiographics 2003;23: 995–1009.
104. Weber AL, Liebsch NJ, Sanchez R, et al. Chordomas of the skull base. Radiologic and clinical evaluation. Neuroimaging Clin North Am 1994;4:515–527.
105. Mizerny BR, Kost KM. Chordoma of the cranial base: the McGill experience. J Otolaryngol 1995;24:14–19.
106. Austin-Seymour M, Munzenrider J, Goitein M, et al. Fractionated proton radiation therapy of chordoma and low-grade chondrosarcoma of the base of the skull. J Neurosurg 1989; 70:13–17.
107. Fleming H, Murayama S, Dacey RG Jr. Posterior fossa epithelial cyst of ectodermal origin. Neurosurgery 1991;29: 459–463; discussion 463.
108. Monaco R, Boscaino A, Di Blasi A, et al. Intraepithelial carcinoma arising in an endodermal cyst of the posterior fossa. Neuropathology 2003;23:219–224.
109. Wiot JG. Radiographic evaluation of the skull base. Ear Nose Throat J 1991;70:563–564.
110. Pollock BE, Foote RL, Stafford SL. Stereotactic radiosurgery: the preferred management for patients with nonvestibular schwannomas? Int J Radiat Oncol Biol Phys 2002;52:1002–1007.
111. Carvalho GA, Tatagiba M, Samii M. Cystic schwannomas of the jugular foramen: clinical and surgical remarks [see comment]. Neurosurgery 2000;46:560–566.
112. Goel A, Desai K. Cystic schwannomas of the jugular foramen: clinical and surgical remarks [comment]. Neurosurgery 2000;47:1470–1471.
113. Hertel F, Bettag M, Morsdorf M, et al. Paragangliomas of the parasellar region. Neurosurg Rev 2003;26:210–214.
114. Yamauchi T, Kubota M, Saeki N, et al. Paraganglioma in the frontal skull base—case report. Neurol Med Chir (Tokyo) 1999;39:308–312.
115. Pacheco-Ojeda L. Malignant carotid body tumors: report of three cases. Ann Otol Rhinol Laryngol 2001;110: 36–40.
116. Thornton J, Bashir Q, Aletich VA, et al. Role of magnetic resonance imaging and diagnostic and interventional angiography in vascular and neoplastic diseases of the skull base associated with vestibulocochlear symptoms. Top Magn Reson Imaging 2000;11:123–137.
117. Raquet F, Mann W, Maurer J, et al. Funktionseinschrankungen der kaudalen Hirnnerven nach Operationen von Tumoren im Foramen jugulare. Eine Langzeitkontrolle. Laryngorhinootologie 1991;70:284–288.
118. Link MJ, Driscoll CL, Giannini C. Isolated, giant cerebellopontine angle craniopharyngioma in a patient with Gardner syndrome: case report. Neurosurgery 2002;51:221–225; discussion 225–226.
119. Connolly ES Jr, Winfree CJ, Carmel PW. Giant posterior fossa cystic craniopharyngiomas presenting with hearing loss. Report of three cases and review of the literature. Surg Neurol 1997;47:291–299.
120. Muhm M, Polterauer P, Gstottner W, et al. Diagnostic and therapeutic approaches to carotid body tumors. Review of 24 patients. Arch Surg 1997;132:279–284.
121. Murphy TP, Brackmann DE. Effects of preoperative embolization on glomus jugulare tumors. Laryngoscope 1989;99:1244–1247.
122. Warshawski SJ, de Souza FM. The carotid body tumor. J Otolaryngol 1989;18:306–310.

123. Meyer FB, Sundt TM Jr, Pearson BW. Carotid body tumors: a subject review and suggested surgical approach. J Neurosurg 1986;64:377–385.
124. Leu YS, Chang KC. Extracranial head and neck schwannomas: a review of 8 years experience. Acta Otolaryngol 2002;122:435–437.
125. Friedrich RE, Giese M, Mautner VF, et al. Fehlbildungen der Kieferhohle bei Neurofibromatose Typ 1. Mund Kiefer Gesichtschir 2002;6:363–367.
126. Holt GR. E.N.T. manifestations of Von Recklinghausen's disease. Laryngoscope 1978;88:1617–1632.
127. Hoffmann DF, Everts EC, Smith JD, et al. Malignant nerve sheath tumors of the head and neck. Otolaryngol Head Neck Surg 1988;99:309–314.
128. Jane JA Jr, Helm GA. Gene therapy for skull base tumors. Neurosurg Clin North Am 2000;11:703–716.

CHAPTER 23

Intracranial Germ Cell Tumors

PATRICIA L. ROBERTSON

Primary intracranial germ cell tumors (GCTs) are rare neoplasms in Western countries, comprising only 1% and 3% of adult and pediatric brain tumor diagnoses.[1] *They are more frequent in Japan, where they constitute 4% of brain tumors overall and 16% of brain tumors in children.*[2] *They typically arise in midline central nervous system (CNS) locations, predominantly in pineal or suprasellar regions, and are virtually indistinguishable, histologically, from their systemic gonadal, mediastinal, or retroperitoneal counterparts.*[3]

Intracranial GCTs are classified by their cell of origin, into two main histopathologic groups: (a) the undifferentiated GCT, or germinoma (called seminoma or dysgerminoma in the testis or ovary, respectively), which is the most primitive histologically but the most readily cured by radiation therapy, and (b) the nongerminoma GCT (NGGCT), comprised of several histopathologic variants that are classified together as a separate entity because of their relative radioresistance and historically poorer prognosis, albeit improved with the use of combination chemotherapy and radiation therapy. The malignant NGGCT variants include immature or malignant teratoma, embryonal carcinoma, endodermal sinus tumor (yolk sac tumor), and choriocarcinoma, or may be a mixture of any of these elements (including germinoma). Mature or benign teratomas are also classified as GCTs, but behave much differently, with a good prognosis after total surgical resection. From a retrospective analysis in 1985 of all intracranial GCTs in the literature, 65% were germinomas and 35% NGGCTs,[1] *although a higher percentage of NGGCTs have been reported in Japanese series.*[4] *NGGCTs also predominate in younger children between birth and 9 years of age. It has also become apparent, as more extensive surgery has been attempted for these tumors, that the most common subtype is a mixed GCT, containing various combinations of the GCT variants.*[5]

The therapeutic approach and prognosis are very different between the germinoma and NGGCT subtypes of intracranial GCT, and have changed considerably over the last two decades as a result of several factors. First, there is a greater ability and willingness on the part of surgeons to biopsy or even resect these tumors, which in the past were considered inaccessible. This has led to more accurate diagnosis and ability to employ more appropriate treatment for each of the two subtypes of GCT, as well as for the broader spectrum of other non-GCTs diagnosed in the common GCT locations, the suprasellar or pineal regions, such as low-grade glioma, pinealoma, or pineoblastoma. Second, we have learned that chemotherapy useful against systemic GCTs is effective in the treatment of intracranial GCTs. This has permitted a significant reduction in the dosage of radiation therapy for germinomas without sacrificing survival, and has led to an improvement in the long-term outcome of NGGCTs when given along with radiation therapy.

▶ EPIDEMIOLOGY AND KNOWN INFLUENCES ON TUMOR

Intracranial GCTs can occur at any age, but their incidence peaks in the second and third decade, in adolescence and early adulthood. Overall, there is a male predominance for intracranial GCTs of 2 to 3:1, but this may prevail only with pineal location tumors, while those in the suprasellar region have no gender predominance.[1] Likewise, GCTs in younger children occur with equal frequency in boys and girls.[6]

Intracranial GCTs arise predominantly in midline CNS locations, the vast majority in pineal or suprasellar regions. A review of the reported cases of all types of intracranial GCTs in the literature found that 85% originated near the third ventricle along an axis between the suprasellar cistern (37%) and the pineal gland (48%), with 6% occurring sequentially or simultaneously in both sites, and the remaining 8% in other sites.[1] Intracranial GCTs also have a tendency to spread along cerebral spinal fluid (CSF) pathways, with a 10% to 42% incidence of metastatic seeding at diagnosis, making careful tumor staging critical in the initial evaluation of these tumors.[1,7] These may well be an underestimate of metastatic seeding, having been done largely in the premagnetic resonance imaging era.

▶ GENETICS AND MOLECULAR BIOLOGY

Tumor Pathogenesis

Because gonadal GCTs appear to arise from primordial germ cells in the developing embryo, the formation of intracranial GCTs is believed to arise from these primordial cells that somehow made their way into brain and subsequently transformed. Primordial germ cells normally migrate from the yolk sac endoderm along the dorsal mesentery, laterally to the genital ridges during the fourth week of embryogenesis, for eventual incorporation into the developing gonads.[8] This pathway of migration is probably orchestrated by complex molecular events that involve extracellular matrix glycoproteins such as fibronectin and laminin, probably through interaction with cell surface receptors such as integrins, and the involvement of other chemotropic factors.[9] Intracranial GCTs may arise because of defects in this intricate process that cause aberrant migration rostrally rather than laterally, with incorporation into midline diencephalic structures. Specific chemotrophic factors secreted in the hypothalamus, which undergoes maturation at the same time as the migration of primordial germ cells, may play a role in attracting the germ cells to the diencephalon.[10]

Extragonadal primordial germ cells have been demonstrated in otherwise normal embryos, but few actually develop tumors. The mechanism by which these cells become neoplastic and develop into tumors is not clear. Derangement of the normal biologic systems of programmed cell death or apoptosis, which is part of normal embryonic and postnatal development, is known to be involved in the development of some tumors, and could play a role in the pathogenesis of intracranial GCTs.[11] There may also be a connection between the pathogenesis of intracranial GCTs and the neuroendocrinologic mechanisms that regulate the complex physiologic functions of reproduction. This is suggested by both the predominance of the location of GCTs in the diencephalon where this regulation is centered and by the frequent temporal association of intracranial GCTs with puberty. It is possible that the hormonal surges of puberty may sometimes induce malignant changes in the normally quiescent primordial germ cells in the diencephalon.[1,12]

Tumor Cytogenetics

The cytogenetic abnormalities of GCTs and their role in pathogenesis have been studied most extensively in testicular GCTs. Isochromosome 12p is the most characteristic chromosomal anomaly, found in 80% of all histologic types of testicular GCT.[13] The isochromosome 12p may have from one to four or more copies; more than three copies is a prognostic indicator associated with progressive tumors that fail treatment. This suggests that gene amplification of a proto-oncogene somewhere in the 12p segment is involved in tumor pathogenesis.[14] Cytogenetic analysis of intracranial GCT has been reported for only five patients, of which only one pineal mixed NGGCT had an isochromosome 12p.[15]

However, mutations of the *p53* oncogene on chromosome 17 were found in approximately 5 (26%) of 19 intracranial GCTs.[16] Recently, gene amplification of the *mdm2* gene, which has important interaction with the p53 protein, was found in some types of intracranial GCTs, suggesting that the disruption of the balance of *p53–mdm2* interaction is involved in the tumorigenesis of intracranial GCTs.[17] Moreover, genetic alterations in a tumor suppresser gene at the inhibitor of kinase 4a (INK4a)–adenosine diphosphate-ribosylation factor (ARF) locus, whose gene product has a major influence on *p53–mdm2* interactions, were found in 15 (71%) of 21 intracranial GCTs, further supporting a role for *p53–mdm2* gene interactions in the tumorigenesis of intracranial GCTs.[18]

More recently, an increased number of X chromosomes, typically one extra copy, was observed in 23 (92%) of 25 intracranial GCTs (both germinoma and NGGCT), with the demonstration of hypomethylation of the additional X chromosome in 21 (84%). Taken together with the observed male predominance of some intracranial GCTs, the data argue that sex chromosome aberrations are integral in tumorigenesis.[19]

▶ SPECIFIC CLINICAL PRESENTATIONS

The clinical manifestations of intracranial GCTs of any histologic subtype—germinoma or NGGCT—depend on both the age at presentation and the tumor location. Intracranial GCTs develop predominantly in midline locations, most commonly in the suprasellar region or the pineal region, or in both regions simultaneously.

Congenital Teratomas

The teratoma subtype of NGGCT is frequently diagnosed by antenatal ultrasonography or soon after birth, and presents differently from GCTs of older children and adults, regardless of the tumor site.[20] A congenital teratoma is suggested by a history of polyhydramnios and hydrocephalus and by a heterogeneous echogenic mass with cystic and solid components; it is associated with an almost uniformly fatal prognosis.

Germ Cell Tumors in Young Infants

Young infants presenting with a GCT (most often teratoma or choriocarcinoma subtypes of NGGCT) most often have protean manifestations including irritability, listlessness, failure to thrive, macrocephaly, and a bulging fontanelle, all nonspecific signs of increased intracranial pressure.

Suprasellar Germ Cell Tumors in Older Children and Adults

After infancy, in older children and adults, GCTs in a suprasellar location (any subtype), because of proximity to the hypothalamic/pituitary axis, often present with hypopituitary endocrine deficits when they are diagnosed earlier in their course. Because signs and symptoms of these deficits can be relatively subtle, the prodrome before diagnosis, especially for germinomas, can be long, from many months to years. There may be deficits of anterior pituitary dysfunction with signs and symptoms of thyroid or cortisol deficiency, or both. Children may also have growth failure from growth hormone deficiency and delayed puberty from gonadotrophin deficiency. Children with such acquired hypopituitarism can harbor GCTs that are not yet visible on imaging and need to be followed closely with serial surveillance scans at regular intervals. Deficits of pituitary gonadotrophins also cause signs and symptoms of regression of sexual development or sexual dysfunction in adults.[1,21] A high proportion of GCT patients also present with posterior pituitary dysfunction (vasopressin deficiency) that causes the polyuria/polydipsia of diabetes insipidus. In Jennings' series of intracranial GCTs, 33% of patients with suprasellar tumors presented with some type of anterior pituitary dysfunction and 41% presented with diabetes insipidus.[1] Occasionally, precocious puberty may develop in a prepubertal child with a suprasellar GCT or even pineal tumor, either as a consequence of tumor-induced hypothalamic injury or from the human chorionic gonadotrophin secreted by the tumor.[1,22]

The symptoms of endocrine dysfunction from a suprasellar GCT may go undiagnosed for months or even years until visual symptoms, hydrocephalus, and signs of increased intracranial pressure call attention to it.[1] The visual signs and symptoms are typically deficits of visual acuity or fields, classically a bitemporal hemianopia caused by optic chiasm involvement. Suprasellar tumors can sometimes grow larger, invading the thalamus or basal ganglia and producing hemiparesis or movement disorder.

Pineal Region Germ Cell Tumors in Older Children and Adults

Pineal region GCTs tend to present more acutely than suprasellar tumors because they more frequently cause hydrocephalus and signs of increased intracranial pressure (headache, nausea, vomiting, lethargy, papilledema) as a consequence of obstruction of the ventricular system at the third ventricle and cerebral aqueduct. Situated at the posterior aspect of the third ventricle, pineal GCTs also compress the dorsal midbrain (tectum), interfering with cortical input to oculomotor nuclei and gaze centers and producing Parinaud syndrome (Fig. 23-1). This syndrome consists of (a) vertical upward-gaze paralysis, (b) decreased pupillary response to light, and (c) retractory or convergence nystagmus. Sometimes more extensive growth of pineal tumors into the cerebellum or cerebellar peduncles can cause ataxia and tremor, and growth into the brainstem may produce other cranial nerve deficits or long tract signs.[1,23] Diabetes insipidus and anterior hypopituitarism is also sometimes found in association with GCTs that appear to be isolated to the pineal region, suggesting that microscopic disease involving the pituitary axis is involved.

Patients with simultaneous pineal and suprasellar GCT masses can have the above-noted signs of either or both, depending on the size and sequence of development of the lesions (Fig. 23-2).

▶ DIAGNOSTIC EVALUATION

Table 23-1 illustrates an approach to the patient with a tumor of the pineal or suprasellar region.

▶ TABLE 23-1. APPROACH TO THE PATIENT WITH A PINEAL OR SUPRASELLAR TUMOR

Initial Diagnostic Evaluations

1. **Brain MRI + gadolinium**
2. **Spine MRI + gadolinium**
   preoperative if possible
3. **Tumor Markers—AFP and β = hCG**
   serum & CSF preoperative if possible
4. **Pituitary Function Tests**
   for suprasellar tumor or if any symptoms of pituitary dysfunction
5. **Visual Field Testing**
   suprasellar tumor

↓

Hydrocephalus

→ **Hydrocephalus** / → **No Hydrocephalus**

Hydrocephalus ↓

Hydrocephalus Management Options

1. **Preoperative External Ventricular Drainage**
   better control of increased ICP than shunt
2. **Pre- or postoperative VP Shunt**
   may not be necessary if tumor can be resected
3. **Endoscopically Guided Third Ventriculostomy**
   often optimal for pineal region tumors;
   avoids permanent shunt

↓

Tumor Markers
serum and/or CSF

Markers Positive
AFP + or hCG >50 IU/L confirms NGGCT; tissue not required for diagnosis

Markers Negative
Normal AFP or hCG ≤50 IU/L; tissue required for histologic diagnosis

↓

Surgical Approaches for Tissue Diagnosis

1. **Stereotactic Biopsy**
   avoids open craniotomy
2. **Open Craniotomy with Biopsy/Resection**
   allows for resection if indicated for treatment;
   resection may avoid shunt
3. **Endoscopic Biopsy**
   pineal tumors

(*Continued on page 485*)

Tumor Staging

1. **Postoperative Brain MRI + gadolinium**
2. **Total Spine MRI (postoperative if not done preoperative)**
3. **Serum and CSF Tumor Markers (if positive preoperative)**
4. **CSF cytology**

Adjuvant Therapy After Diagnosis

Germ Cell Tumors		Pineal Parenchymal Tumors		Gliomas	
Germinoma	**NGGCT** **EST, CC, EC, malignant TT**	**Pineocytoma**	**Pineoblastoma**	**Low-grade**	**High-grade**
Chemotherapy may permit RT dose-reduction + Radiation Therapy volume per staging disseminated: craniospinal + boost localized: whole ventricular + boost	+/– Surgery + Chemotherapy + Radiation Therapy craniospinal + primary site boost	Maximal Surgery +/– Radiation Therapy	Maximal Surgery + Radiation Therapy + Chemotherapy	Variable Therapy +/– Surgery +/– Chemotherapy +/– Radiation Therapy	

CC = choriocarcinoma; EC = embryonal catcinoma; EST = endodermal sinus tumor; TT = teratoma.

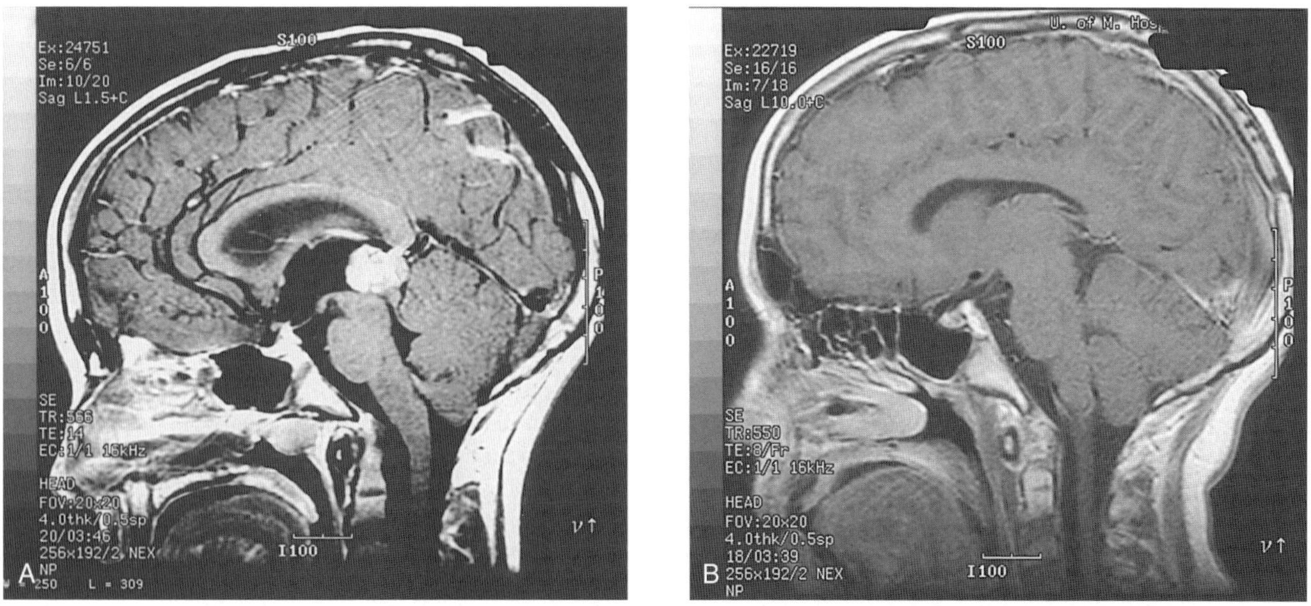

Figure 23-1. (A) Sagittal T_1 brain magnetic resonance imaging (MRI) with gadolinium of a 16-year-old boy who presented with symptoms of increased intracranial pressure and Parinaud syndrome, showing a homogeneously enhancing pineal region mass with hydrocephalus from obstruction of the cerebral aqueduct. The tumor proved to be a germinoma at histologic diagnosis. (B) Sagittal T_1 MRI with gadolinium of the same patient after treatment with carboplatin chemotherapy and radiotherapy, showing disappearance of the pathologically enhancing pineal region mass.

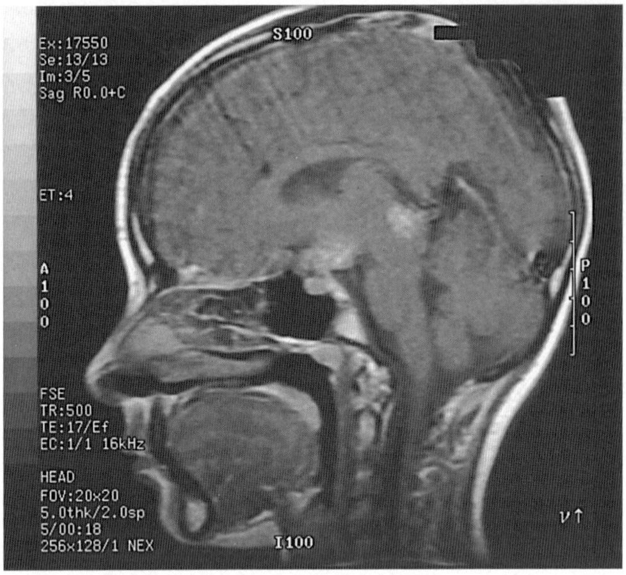

Figure 23-2. Sagittal T_1 brain magnetic resonance imaging (MRI) with gadolinium of an 8-year-old girl who presented with progressive changes in her visual acuity, bitemporal visual field deficits, and decreased upgaze with convergence nystagmus (Parinaud syndrome). The MRI shows homogeneously enhancing masses in both the suprasellar and pineal regions, which proved to be a mixed NGGCT on histopathologic diagnosis.

Neuroimaging

Neuroradiologic imaging is the first step in identifying a tumor of the pineal or suprasellar region that may prove to be a GCT. Computerized tomography (CT) will demonstrate a suspected tumor, although magnetic resonance imaging (MRI) with and without gadolinium is best for delineation of tumor anatomy, and may suggest specific histopathology, but does not substitute for a tissue diagnosis.[6]

Among NGGCT, benign teratomas tend to have mixed densities on MRI and CT, often with large cysts and areas of calcification or bone, and occasionally even teeth and hair, and the tumor has distinct margins.[24,25] Malignant teratomas are also heterogeneous, but they have fewer and smaller cystic areas, more irregular tumor margins (sometimes with peritumoral edema), and are less likely to be calcified than mature teratomas.[25] However, pineal parenchymal tumors and pineocytomas are also commonly calcified on CT. On MRI, germinomas tend to be of mixed T_1 signal with increased T_2 signal, but these characteristics do not distinguish them from NGGCT or from pineocytomas or even pineoblastoma/primitive neuroectodermal tumors (PNETs). Germinomas and nonteratoma NGGCTs are less likely to have calcifications on CT, suggesting that they are less likely to be teratomas, but neuroimaging does not differentiate them from one another. Thus, it is apparent that although these imaging modalities are good for defining tumor anatomy, neither CT nor MRI can predict specific tumor histology with a sufficient degree of certainty to be used alone when making a diagnosis.[24]

Histologic Diagnosis

Suprasellar Tumors

For suprasellar tumors, surgery to obtain tissue for histologic confirmation is usually the best approach to diagnosis. Suprasellar tumors are surgically accessible, and other diagnostic considerations for tumors in this location are not readily ruled out radiographically or by other means.[6] The possible exception to this, as with pineal region tumors, is the situation in which serum or CSF tumor markers human chorionic gonadotropin (hCG) or α-fetoprotein (AFP) are elevated, which unequivocally establishes the diagnosis of a secreting NGGCT. Histologic considerations other than GCTs in the differential diagnosis of suprasellar tumors include low-grade optic pathway/hypothalamic glioma, which can be difficult to differentiate radiographically if they do not distinctly involve the optic apparatus, craniopharyngioma, parasellar meningioma, and pituitary adenoma.

Pineal Region Tumors

Prior to the 1980s, a standard diagnostic approach for pineal region tumors was to observe their radiographic response to a small dose of irradiation.[4,7,26] This approach was justified by the relatively high incidence of germinomas in this location (especially in Japan), the known radiosensitivity of germinomas, and the morbidity of biopsy or resection of these deep tumors in the pineal region, encircled by major important veins. A prompt and marked reduction in tumor volume after a trial of 20 Gy of irradiation was taken as evidence that the tumor was a radiosensitive germinoma, and a full course of radiation therapy was then completed. This method of managing pineal tumors is still used in Japan and England.[7,27]

The diagnosis of pineal GCTs has changed since the 1990s, with a general consensus among most neurosurgeons, radiation oncologists, and neuro-oncologists that a tissue diagnosis is nearly always necessary for optimal management of both pineal and suprasellar lesions. The one exception to this is in the setting of elevated CSF or serum tumor markers, which are considered to be diagnostic of a malignant NGGCT and may obviate histologic confirmation. The change in approach to pineal tumors has come about mainly because of improvements in neurosurgical techniques that facilitate surgery in a location previously considered inaccessible, with resultant decreased morbidity and mortality. Operative morbidity for pineal region tumors is currently considered to be less than 2% to 5%.[28,29] Moreover, there is greater appreciation of the limitations of empiric diagnostic irradiation, especially in pediatric and Western populations where the incidence of radioresponsive germinomas is lower.[28,30]

Tumors in several categories other than GCTs also arise in the pineal region. These include (a) pineal parenchymal tumors such as low-grade differentiated pineocytomas and malignant pineoblastomas; (b) other neoplasms, including intraaxial glial tumors such as ependymomas, astrocytomas or mixed gliomas, and extraaxial tumors that derive from tissues surrounding the pineal gland such as meningiomas, dermoid and epidermoid tumors, and, rarely, systemic metastases; (c) nonneoplastic lesions such as simple pineal cysts and vein of Galen malformations. As more histopathologic confirmation of pineal tumors is obtained, these other tumor types are increasingly identified. Some may also respond promptly to radiation therapy like germinomas, but subsequently progress without additional therapy, underscoring the critical importance of histologic diagnosis.[30,31] Indeed, the improved prognosis of NGGCTs and pineoblastomas treated with current multimodality therapy regimens is absolutely dependent on making a correct initial histologic diagnosis. Furthermore, irradiation of the more benign tumors occurring in the pineal region could be inappropriate therapy, because curative surgical resection may be possible with less morbidity, and some of these lesions require no adjuvant therapy.[28,32]

Pineal Parenchymal Tumors

Neoplasms arising from the pineal parenchyma are relatively rare. They are traditionally categorized as pineocytomas (lower grade) and pineoblastomas (malignant), which are tumors resembling medulloblastomas and categorized as a type of PNET.[33] Russell and Rubenstein also described a classification of both pineocytomas and pineoblastomas into subgroups with various types differentiation.[34] In a Canadian population-based study of patients of all ages, these tumors comprised only 3 (1%) of 315 cases,[35] although 8 (32%) of 25 pediatric pineal region tumors in a series from Children's Hospital of Philadelphia were pineal parenchymal tumors.[30] They present very similarly to pineal region GCTs with the predominant symptoms of increased intracranial pressure from aqueductal stenosis or Parinaud syndrome from midbrain compression.

Pineocytomas consist of small cells that form rosettes but are more spread out than in pineoblastomas, and have large hypocellular areas that contain fibrillary stroma.[36] They differ from the normal pineal gland in having less uniform cells and no astroglial stroma. In midadulthood, when pineocytomas occur most often, they are generally thought to be only locally invasive and can be managed with radical surgical resection and local irradiation for any residual tumor.[37] However, they have been reported to have greater metastatic potential and a poorer prognosis when they occur in children and may require craniospinal irradiation and/or chemotherapy.[38]

Pineoblastomas are always high-grade tumors with a propensity to subarachnoid metastasis and resemble medulloblastoma/PNET tumors elsewhere in the CNS. They are similar both in their histology, consisting of dense populations of small round blue cells with little cytoplasm that form rosettes, and in their clinical behavior. These tumors occur predominantly in children or adolescents, and occasionally in young adults. Pineoblastomas are classified as high-risk PNET, and are optimally treated with multimodal therapy that includes maximal resection, craniospinal irradiation, and adjuvant chemotherapy. Extensive outcome data for this relatively rare tumor are lacking, but a 3-year progression-free survival of 61% was achieved among 15 pediatric patients treated in this way on a Children's Oncology Group protocol.[39]

Other Non–germ Cell Pineal Region Tumors

Glial neoplasms are the second most frequently occurring pineal region tumors in children and adults.[28,30,40] They arise from adjacent regions of the thalamus or midbrain and may be low-grade or high-grade neoplasms. They have no pathologic characteristics to distinguish them from glial neoplasms found elsewhere in the CNS, and are managed similarly, based on histologic grade. However, the prognosis, especially for high-grade tumors, is even poorer than for their counterparts elsewhere in brain because they are more surgically inaccessible, and radical resections are often not possible. Low-grade gliomas have a more variable prognosis. Fibrillary astrocytomas often do poorly, but pilocytic astrocytomas can have a more favorable outcome even without resection, after radiation or chemotherapy.[41] The tectal midbrain or pencil glioma appears to have a particularly benign course, often manageable only with CSF diversion.[42]

The pineal region is one of the most uncommon sites for metastatic involvement of systemic malignant tumors, and have been most frequently reported to be diagnosed at autopsy. Rarely metastasis to the pineal parenchyma can occur and mimic a primary pineal gland mass.[43] Bronchogenic carcinoma is reported to be the most frequent source of the primary lesion.[44] Imaging characteristics are often nonspecific, and in the absence of additional lesions to suggest metastatic disease, such lesions must be managed in the same way as other pineal region tumors.[45]

Benign cysts of the pineal gland are being incidentally diagnosed at a higher rate because of the increased performance of brain MRI scans for evaluation of symptoms unrelated to any pineal pathology. These are cystic lesions often with peripheral calcification and rim contrast enhancement. They usually require no therapy unless they increase in size and become symptomatic, an uncommon occurrence.[46] Occasionally, a cystic pilocytic astrocytoma can look similar radiographically, and serial imaging may be needed to verify the absence of growth.

Tumor Staging

See Table 23-1 for an approach to tumor staging.

Tumor Markers

The tumor markers AFP and hCG are produced and secreted by some NGGCTs and can be measured at elevated levels in the serum and CSF of these patients (Table 23-2). They can provide a sensitive means of following tumor response to therapy, and in some cases, the markers are sufficient to confirm tumor histology without obtaining biopsy tissue. Thus, the measurement of serum and CSF levels of AFP and hCG should be done preoperatively whenever possible, because the finding of any elevation of AFP or of a sufficiently high hCG (>50 IU/L) could make surgery unnecessary. Postoperative levels should also be measured as a baseline for following response to therapy.

AFP is the normal main serum protein of the fetus, first produced by the fetal yolk sac and later by liver cells of the fetus. An elevated AFP level in the serum or CSF of a patient with an intracranial tumor means that the tumor has elements of either pure endodermal sinus tumor (yolk sac), embryonal carcinoma, or malignant teratoma.[6,47] Endodermal sinus tumors appear to secrete only AFP, the levels of which may be very high, whereas embryonal carcinoma and malignant teratoma can produce less elevated levels of AFP (<700 IU/L), hCG, or both. Human chorionic gonadotrophin is a placental glycoprotein, of which the beta chain is present in fetal serum and in pregnant women.[6] Among GCTs where only hCG is elevated, the tumor may contain choriocarcinoma or germinoma elements, but the degree of the elevation of this marker distinguishes between them. High levels of hCG (>50 IU/L) suggest the presence of choriocarcinoma within the tumor, whereas lower values can occur with germinoma in the absence of any NGGCT elements.[47,48]

In summary, any elevation of AFP is confirmation that the tumor contains nongerminoma elements, either endodermal sinus tumor, or if hCG is also elevated, embryonal carcinoma or malignant teratoma. Likewise, levels of hCG greater than 50 IU/L predict the presence of a choriocarcinoma NGGCT.[47,48] These associations are sufficiently strong that presurgical detection of any elevation of AFP, or a high level (>50 IU/L) of hCG in serum or CSF of a patient with a pineal or suprasellar tumor means that a tissue diagnosis may not be absolutely necessary for diagnosis. If only a limited biopsy of a secreting tumor is possible, treating it as a presumed NGGCT, without histologic confirmation, is reasonable. However, if the patient might benefit therapeutically from a more radical resection of the tumor, surgery is not contraindicated. CSF marker levels usually exceed those of serum, and lumbar fluid levels frequently exceed ventricular levels.[47] Therefore, when serum levels are higher than those of the CSF, the possibility of metastases from a systemic GCT should be considered, although exceptions to this rule have occurred. Moreover, when tumor markers are measured simultaneously in serum and CSF, marker elevation may sometimes be found only in the CSF.[49] Thus, staging evaluations should include marker levels obtained from both locations to prevent missing the diagnosis of a secreting tumor.

▶ TABLE 23-2. SERUM/CSF TUMOR MARKER PROFILE FOR GERM CELL TUMORS

	AFP	hCG
Germinoma	–	+/– (≤50 IU/L)
Nongerminoma germ cell tumor (NGGCT)		
Endodermal sinus tumor (yolk sac tumor)	++	–
Choriocarcinoma	–	++
Embryonal carcinoma	+	+/–
Malignant teratoma	+/–	+/–

Radiologic Staging and Cerebrospinal Fluid Cytology

Staging evaluation to determine the amount of residual tumor at the primary site after surgery and the extent of metastatic disease is critical in the treatment planning for GCT. This is best accomplished by postoperative gadolinium-enhanced MRI of the brain and an MRI of the entire spine, preferably done before surgery if this is feasible. This type of staging is particularly important for GCTs because the incidence of CNS tumor spread via ventricular and subarachnoid pathways to third ventricles and the spinal cord is high.[1] Information about extent of the disease is needed to determine the total volume of radiotherapy required, as well as to determine where a boost of irradiation may be needed for any bulky disseminated metastatic deposits. As well, the knowledge of tumor spread could help determine whether an intracranial GCT could possibly represent metastasis from a primary systemic GCT. An isolated suprasellar or pineal mass virtually excludes this possibility, whereas the presence of leptomeningeal metastases could indicate the need for further evaluation.

After histologic confirmation of an intracranial GCT, postoperative staging should include CSF cytologic examination for malignant cells. Evaluation for spread of the disease outside the CNS is usually unnecessary unless the patient's symptoms suggest it, given the rarity of systemic metastases from primary intracranial GCTs. Fewer than 9 (4%) of 233 patients with pineal tumors had pulmonary or abdominal metastases, and these were all at relapse and in association with a ventriculoperitoneal shunt.[32]

▶ NEUROPATHOLOGY

As noted in the introduction, GCTs are histologically classified into two main groups based on their cell(s) of origin. The first group is the germinoma (called seminoma or dysgerminoma in the testis or ovary, respectively), which has the most undifferentiated histopathology, although it is the most readily cured by radiation therapy. The second group is the NGGCT, or differentiated GCT, made up of four different subtypes based on their specific differentiated cell type(s), but grouped together because of their historically poorer response to radiation therapy. The NGGCT include the teratoma (benign and malignant), embryonal carcinoma, endodermal sinus tumor (yolk sac tumor), and choriocarcinoma, listed in increasing order of malignant potential except for the mature teratoma, which is considered a benign tumor.[50] Mixed GCTs, containing components in various combinations of any of these cell types, are increasingly recognized.[5]

Each of the histologic GCT variants is derived from cells of a normal stage of embryonic development. Germinoma is the malignant correlate of the primordial germ cell itself. Teratomas are made up of a mixture of tissues derived from all three germinal cell layers, and mature (benign) teratomas are composed of fully differentiated ectodermal, mesodermal, and endodermal elements, and most frequently arise in the pineal region. Immature (malignant) teratomas have embryonal or fetal primitive elements with malignant potential. Pure mature teratomas are benign and can be cured surgically, but these tumors often have a mixture of mature and immature elements, making their behavior difficult to predict. Embryonal carcinoma arises from the pluripotential stem cell of the embryo; endodermal sinus tumor (yolk sac tumor) and choriocarcinoma are extraembryonic derivatives of the yolk sac and trophoblast, respectively.[51]

Germ cell tumors most commonly arise in gonadal tissue (testis or ovary), and the central nervous system is only one of several extragonadal sites of origin that also include the retroperitoneum, the sacrococcygeal region, the mediastinum, and, rarely, the nasopharynx, neck, thorax, abdomen, bladder, or prostate.[52] Each of the various subtypes of GCT are virtually indistinguishable histologically, by light and electron microscopy, no matter what its site of origin.[3]

By light microscopy, the undifferentiated germinoma consists of two cell types: large, polyhedral tumor cells that are intermixed with small lymphocytes. The large primitive-looking cells have round nuclei with prominent nucleoli and clear cytoplasm that contains abundant glycogen. Very frequently, these cells are reactive for the immunocytochemical marker placental alkaline phosphatase (PLAP), a diagnostically definitive marker for these tumors (Fig. 23-3).[53] Some germinomas also contain syncytiotrophoblastic cells that are immunopositive for the tumor marker hCa.

Endodermal sinus tumors (yolk sac tumors), derived from endoderm with differentiation along extraembryonic yolk sac lines, contain glomeruloid structures consisting of a vascular pedicle lined by a single layer of tumor cells.[34,54] Globules of periodic acid–Schiff (PAS)-positive proteins seen within the cells at higher magnification correlate with the presence of AFP, the tumor marker that appears in serum and CSF with these tumors. Choriocarcinomas also differentiate along extraembryonic trophoblastic lines and are composed of cytotrophoblastic or syncytiotrophoblastic cells without actual villous formation. The syncytiotrophoblastic cells are immunoreactive with antibodies for hCG, the tumor marker they secrete.[3,34] Embryonal carcinomas are thought to be derived from stem cells of the embryo itself, and are the least differentiated of the NGGCT, consisting of sheets or cords of anaplastic cuboidal or columnar epithelium with large nuclei. Pure teratomas, the most uncommon type of NGGCT, are composed of tissues derived from all three germ cell layers. Mature teratomas contain fully differentiated ectodermal, mesodermal, and endodermal tissues, whereas immature teratomas contain more variable and primitive elements that look more like embryonic or fetal tissues and can be more difficult to identify as specific germ cell layers.[3]

In most series, all subtypes of malignant NGGCTs, including mixed tumors with any malignant NGGCT component and all of the pure subtypes of NGGCT (choriocarcinoma, embryonal carcinoma, endodermal sinus,

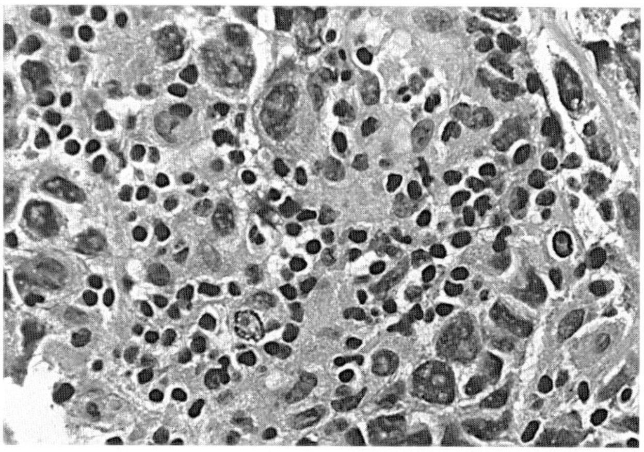

Figure 23-3. Histopathology of an intracranial germinoma containing large cells with clear cytoplasm intermixed with small lymphocytes (hematoxylin and eosin [H&E] stain).

malignant teratoma), are considered together for prognosis. However, in three Japanese series of GCTs in which malignant teratomas were evaluated separately from other malignant NGGCTs, their long-term survival (treated mainly with multimodality therapy), although not as good as germinoma or benign teratoma, was significantly better (70%) than any other pure or mixed tumors containing NGGCT elements (10%–25%).[5,55,56] Conversely, the 1985 review by Jennings of 398 intracranial GCTs found only 32% long-term survival among teratomas, even with benign and malignant teratomas grouped together.[1] Likewise, a small British series of malignant teratomas treated with radiation therapy between 1962 and 1987 determined a 5-year survival of only 18%.[7] The reason for this discrepancy is not clear, but it may lie in variances of specific therapy, as well as inherent differences between populations.

For discussion of the histopathology of NGGCT of the pineal region, see "Diagnostic Evaluation: Histologic Diagnosis: Pineal Region Tumors" above.

▶ SURGICAL MANAGEMENT

See Table 23-1 for an approach to surgical management of GCTs.

General Surgical Considerations for Germ Cell Tumors

There is general agreement that a tissue confirmation of histologic diagnosis is nearly always necessary in the management of patients with intracranial pineal and suprasellar tumors. However, the best method for obtaining tissue for histologic diagnosis of pineal and suprasellar tumors, whether by stereotactic biopsy or at open craniotomy, is debated among neurosurgeons. Stereotactic biopsy for both suprasellar and pineal tumors has been endorsed by some because of its low morbidity.[7] However, an open procedure is advocated by most, for two main reasons.[29] The first concerns the sampling error that can occur with small-needle biopsies, especially with GCTs that are frequently heterogeneous. The misdiagnosis of a NGGCT as a germinoma because of such an error would result in significant undertreatment of the tumor, with a high likelihood of a poor outcome. The second reason for an open surgical approach is that it allows for the possibility of more radical surgery for a tumor type that might benefit from a more extensive resection. This would be the case for patients with benign tumors in either the suprasellar or pineal location, such as mature teratomas, some low-grade gliomas, dermoids, or arachnoid cysts. In a suprasellar location, a craniopharyngioma could benefit from surgical resection, as could a pinealoma or pineal cyst in the pineal region. There is also a therapeutic role for resection of some non–germ cell malignant tumors in these locations, such as anaplastic gliomas or pineoblastoma/PNETs, prior to other adjuvant therapy.

The majority of patients with pineal region tumors, as well as some with suprasellar tumors, have symptomatic hydrocephalus that requires treatment at the time of presentation. The placement of an external ventricular drain prior to surgery is a way of temporarily managing preoperative increased intracranial pressure that affords a more gradual and controlled decompression of ventricles. This approach is more likely to avoid the upward brainstem herniation that can occur with the placement of a ventriculoperitoneal (VP) shunt in this setting. It also facilitates preoperative removal of CSF for marker analysis and cytologic examination. Moreover, if a more extensive tumor resection is feasible at the time of surgery, the hydrocephalus might be relieved without the need for a permanent indwelling shunt, thereby avoiding future problems of shunt malfunction, and, rarely, peritoneal tumor seeding. In the case of hydrocephalus caused by aqueductal obstruction by a pineal region tumor, an endoscopically guided third ventriculostomy is a reliable method of CSF diversion that also avoids the drawback of shunts. A small endoscope is passed through a burr hole into a lateral ventricle, and then through the floor of the anterior third ventricle into the prepontine subarachnoid cistern, providing an alternate route for CSF flow and absorption.[57,58] This approach has the possible added advantage of permitting an endoscopically guided biopsy of the tumor during the same procedure. If a germinoma GCT with negative markers is diagnosed in this way, a craniotomy can be avoided for this medically curable disease.

Surgical Management of Germinomas

Once a tissue diagnosis of germinoma is made at frozen section after biopsy of a tumor in either suprasellar or pineal location, it is generally agreed that a more extensive resection is not indicated, given the high degree of curability of this tumor with radiation or combination radiation–chemotherapy.

Surgical Management of Nongerminoma Germ Cell Tumors

More controversial is the therapeutic role for more radical surgery with histologically confirmed NGGCT. These tumors are much less responsive to radiotherapy than their germinoma counterparts, and with conventional radiotherapy alone, usually after a small biopsy, long-term survival has been poor with virtually no chance for survival with some of the histologic subtypes.[1] For such marginally responsive tumors, the prevailing wisdom in oncology is that decreasing tumor burden by surgical means should increase the curative potential of subsequent radiotherapy and chemotherapy.[21] Some data support this hypothesis for malignant pineal region tumors, in general (except for germinomas), although not specifically for NGGCTs.[59] A few studies suggest that an extensive resection improves survival. From a recent Japanese series of histologically confirmed intracranial GCTs treated between 1963 and 1994, among the 30 pineal malignant NGGCTs treated with surgery and radiotherapy alone (60%), surgery and radiation therapy plus chemotherapy (22%), or surgery and chemotherapy alone (18%), there was significantly better 5-year survival among 14 patients whose tumors were extensively resected (47%) than among 16 patients who had only partial removal or biopsy (53%).[5]

Conversely, the combined data from several European studies contradict a benefit for radical surgery for NGGCTs, demonstrating no positive correlation between extent of resection and event-free survival of 48 patients with intracranial NGGCTs.[60] Moreover, among more than 250 patients recruited (mainly from the United Kingdom, Germany, France, and Italy) to a recent international intracranial GCT study (SIOP CNS GCT 96), 48 tumor resections of secreting NGGCTs were considered unjustified, according to protocol, because the marker secretion was sufficient for diagnosis of NGGCT. The toxicity from surgery, considered likely to have been underreported because there is no specific protocol form for the purpose, nevertheless was severe in 10 patients, 3 of whom died from their complications.[61]

Second-Look Surgery

Another surgical consideration is that of so-called second-look surgery. Because NGGCTs have shown moderately high response rates to chemotherapy, it was proposed that more radical resection might better be reserved for those tumors that require second-look surgery after an incomplete response to initial chemotherapy.[49] This approach may be useful not only as a therapeutic measure after incomplete response to initial chemotherapy, but also as a diagnostic approach, to verify the histology of any residual tissue in this setting. In an increasing number of cases where this was done, remaining tissue was determined to be nonmalignant. In the context of a French Society of Pediatric Oncology study of 27 patients with intracranial NGGCTs, all 14 patients who underwent second-look surgery for residual radiographic abnormalities after chemotherapy were found to have only fibrosis, mature teratoma, or, in a few cases, immature teratoma.[62] Similar findings at second-look surgery for intracranial GCTs have been confirmed by others.[63,64] Clearly, most of such patients would not likely benefit from or require further chemotherapy, which could not have been determined without the second surgery. On the other hand, residual malignant tumor was found at planned surgery in 9 of 11 NGGCT patients after they received platinum-based chemotherapy and irradiation, with a resulting 8-year progression-free survival of 91%.[65] Why there is such a discrepancy between the fraction of patients found to have residual malignant tumor and those with nonmalignant tissue in these different studies employing similar presurgical therapy is unclear, but in both cases, the second-look surgery served a useful purpose.

The Growing Teratoma Syndrome

The so-called growing teratoma syndrome is another complication of intracranial pineal region mixed GCTs with surgical implications. This occurs in the setting of a mixed GCT with a secreting portion that responds to chemotherapy, and a nonsecreting portion, most often a mature teratoma, that continues to grow during or after chemotherapy. First observed among systemic gonadal or extragonadal mixed GCTs, usually with metastases, this syndrome has now been reported in four cases of pineal region NGGCT. The treatment of this type of tumor should include chemotherapy and radiation therapy for the secreting portion and surgery for the mature teratoma.[66–68]

▶ ROLE OF RADIATION THERAPY

See Table 23-1 for an approach to radiation therapy.

Radiation Therapy for Germinomas

For patients with pure germinoma, treatment issues surrounding the role of radiation therapy concern the dose and volume of irradiation. These, in turn, hinge on the respective role given to chemotherapy, which is being considered in modern treatment planning because of concerns about late effects of irradiation, especially in young children, as well as in adults.

Radiation therapy had been standard treatment for pure intracranial germinoma in the past. Conventionally, the radiation dose given to the primary tumor was 50 to 55 Gy, with whole-brain and spinal irradiation given at doses of 30 to 40 Gy, resulting in disease-free survival of germinomas in the range of 80% to 90%.[69] Some have proposed that an intracranial germinoma, similar to its gonadal counterpart, the seminoma, could be cured with lower doses of local radiotherapy, although this approach has not been adopted without the addition of other therapy.[70] However, the reduction or deletion of the craniospinal dose has been successfully used in cases where there is no evidence of metastatic spread of tumor at diagnosis.[71–73] Some have advocated whole-ventricular or whole-brain volume, rather than craniospinal volume, in patients with localized disease at diagnosis, because of the pattern of intracranial or intraventricular relapse seen in some series.[71,74] Others favor continuing to give craniospinal irradiation volumes, after finding a high likelihood of recurrence outside the focal field, including the spine, when craniospinal treatment was deleted.[7,75] Moreover, the outstanding results at a single institution over 25 years, where there were absolutely no relapses among 39 germinoma patients, all treated with craniospinal irradiation and followed for a median of 7 years, also bear careful consideration when evaluating approaches that reduce the radiation volume.[76]

With long-term survival rates of germinoma patients exceeding 80%, the potential for late effects of therapy is of greater concern. The radiotherapy used for these tumors has resulted in neuroendocrine deficits, including thyroid, cortisol, and/or growth hormone deficiencies in more than two-thirds of treated children.[77] Even more worrisome are the potential neurocognitive effects of cranial irradiation. In a prospective study of cognitive function in children after cranial radiotherapy, a mean decline in IQ of 15 points was seen 2 years after treatment, but was not seen in children with tumors in similar sites who had not received radiation therapy.[78] Cognitive dysfunction following cranial irradiation was found in more than 30% of adults treated for various types of brain tumors, the degree of which related to total dose of irradiation.[79]

More recent studies successfully reduced the dose and, in some cases, the volume, of irradiation by employing chemotherapy. Trials employing single-agent chemotherapy (cyclophosphamide or carboplatin) before irradiation have produced complete responses that permitted the reduction of radiation dosage to the primary site and craniospinal volume to 30 Gy and 20 Gy, respectively, in a significant fraction of patients. The long-term survival is comparable to standard-dose radiation treatment alone.[80–82]

Patients treated in several different European studies that employed multiagent chemotherapy regimens and various degrees of radiation dose/volume reductions, also had comparable outcomes compared with standard radiation therapy alone.[60,83,84]

In summary, although radiation therapy is very effective treatment for pure germinomas, resulting in long-term survival rates of 80% to 90% or higher, there *are* sufficient data to support an approach to treatment with adjuvant chemotherapy to permit the reduction of radiation dosage, and possibly volume, in the hope of mitigating potential deleterious neuroendocrine and neurocognitive effects of this therapy, especially in younger children. The minimum required dosage and volume of irradiation needed to preserve the high rate of survival already achieved with these tumors using radiation therapy alone needs to be studied in a large cooperative group setting. Whether this approach will reduce neurologic sequelae awaits confirmation as well.

Radiation Therapy for Nongerminoma Germ Cell Tumors

Malignant intracranial NGGCTs are much less sensitive to irradiation than are germinomas. In a review of patients treated before 1985, NGGCTs had disease-free survival rates of less than 25% after conventional radiation therapy (50–55 Gy primary site and 36–40 Gy craniospinal), with similar results echoed in later reports.[1,32] This left considerable, room for improvement, and it is now generally agreed that chemotherapy, along with irradiation, is an important part of the treatment of an intracranial NGGCT.[49,69,85,86]

The optimal volume of irradiation for NGGCTs is still somewhat controversial. It is generally agreed that craniospinal therapy should be given when there is evidence of CNS dissemination at diagnosis, including cases with positive CSF cytology, with MRI evidence of cranial or spinal metastases, and with multiple midline tumors such as simultaneous pineal and suprasellar sites of visible tumor.[21,69]

An adequate irradiation volume in cases of NGGCT with localized disease is still debated, and data pertaining to this issue are sparse. A British experience of 21 NGGCT patients (excluding malignant teratomas) reported that only 1 of 10 relapses was from outside the irradiated field. As well, the abstracted data of 27 secreting NGGCTs treated with chemotherapy and focal radiotherapy in a French Society of Pediatric Oncology study (except for patients with metastatic disease at diagnosis) had 4-year event-free survival of 70%, although the pattern of relapse was not reported.[62]

Conversely, several studies show a trend supporting the need for craniospinal volume for these tumors. From a recent study of 18 NGGCT patients treated with multimodality therapy, 4 of 6 relapses were isolated tumor recurrences outside the primary site, and all 4 were in patients who had not received craniospinal irradiation. There were no relapses among the five patients who received craniospinal irradiation.[86] In a recent retrospective analysis of 13 malignant NGGCT patients (excluding immature teratomas), there were no spinal relapses in any of the 5 patients who received craniospinal irradiation, but spinal relapses occurred in 3 of 8 patients who did not.[56] Yoshida and associates concluded from their study of 30 newly diagnosed GCTs that craniospinal axis irradiation was necessary in the treatment of NGGCT.[87] Moreover, the high rate of ventricular relapses among the 13 of 26 relapsed NGGCT patients after chemotherapy without initial radiotherapy (even among those with complete responses to chemotherapy) argues for, at least, whole-ventricular radiation volumes in this group.[49] Moreover, to date, the best 5-year progression-free survival rate of NGGCT (80%) was reported in 14 patients treated on a German protocol with chemotherapy and irradiation that included craniospinal fields.[60] Together, all of these findings certainly support a role for, at least, whole-ventricular irradiation, and probably for craniospinal volume in NGGCT patients, even with localized disease at diagnosis.

With regard to the optimal dosage of radiation therapy for NGGCT, extensive radiation dose–response data are lacking. Most patients treated with radiation therapy have received involved field doses between 40 and 60 Gy, and the majority, 50 to 54 Gy, but with broad variability of volume and other adjuvant therapy.[7,55,56,60,69,86] Among 13 NGGCT patients who received involved-field radiotherapy at a median dose of 43 Gy (± chemotherapy, ± craniospinal volume), local failure was seen in 3 of 10 patients who received less than 54 Gy, but in none of the 3 who received greater than or equal to 54 Gy (maximum 60 Gy).[56] Among 17 NGGCT patients treated with multimodality "sandwich" therapy, there were no local relapses among the 7 patients who received 54 to 55 Gy to the involved field, but locally progressive disease occurred in 1 of 9 patients who received 50 Gy to the involved field.[86] The best survival reported for NGGCT was 80% progression-free survival at a median of 53 months followup among 14 patients treated on a German protocol in which they received 50 Gy involved-field irradiation (plus craniospinal volume and cisplatin-based chemotherapy).[60]

Gamma Knife or radiosurgery has also been used as adjuvant local therapy to moderate success in the multimodal management of intracranial NGGCT in several small series, and could be considered as a treatment option for locally recurrent NGGCT.[88,89]

▶ ROLE OF CHEMOTHERAPY

See Table 23-1 for an approach to chemotherapy.

Basis of Chemotherapy for Intracranial Germ Cell Tumors

Systemic GCTs are highly chemosensitive, and cisplatin-based regimens containing vinblastine, bleomycin, or etoposide have greatly improved the survival of high-risk, disseminated gonadal GCTs.[90] Moreover, brain metastases from systemic GCT are responsive to chemotherapy. Speculation that this therapy might be effective for primary CNS GCT led to the demonstration of responses of recurrent CNS tumors (germinoma and NGGCT) to salvage chemotherapy.[23,54] The feasibility of using neoadjuvant chemotherapy to allow radiation therapy dose reduction for newly diagnosed CNS germinomas, as well as to improve the survival of NGGCT patients, was also demonstrated, and that earlier experience has been expanded.[80–82]

Chemotherapy for Germinomas

Some of the trials aimed at reducing the dose of radiotherapy for germinomas employed single-drug chemotherapy (cyclophosphamide or carboplatin), with radiation dose reduction for those with a complete response to chemotherapy.[81,82] Cyclophosphamide alone has produced objective responses in intracranial germinomas and was responsible for complete responses in 7 of 8 germinomas in a study in which patients with a complete response (CR) received reduced-dose irradiation.[80,81] This resulted in a long-term survival equivalent to that after full-dose radiation therapy.[81] Carboplatin, which avoided the fertility-reducing effects of cyclophosphamide, permitted radiation dose reduction to involved field and craniospinal volume, from 50 Gy to 30 Gy, and from 36 Gy to 21 Gy, respectively, with long-term survival comparable to standard radiotherapy alone.[82] Thirty patients were treated on several different European regimens employing various multidrug chemotherapy regimens (cisplatin- or carboplatin-based) combined with varying degrees of radiation dose reduction and experienced comparable progression-free survival.[60,83,84] There has been no direct comparison between the efficacy of cisplatin and of carboplatin for intracranial germinomas. However, in a trial for good-risk systemic GCTs, a regimen of cisplatin and etoposide was slightly superior to that of carboplatin and etoposide with respect to progression-free survival.[91] Most recently, in a trial of multiagent neoadjuvant chemotherapy for intracranial germinoma, in which response-driven radiation dose reduction was prescribed, 21 (68%) of 31 intracranial germinoma patients had a CR to 2 cycles of carboplatin and etoposide, and 7 (22%) had a subsequent CR to 2 additional cycles of cisplatin and cyclophosphamide, for a total of 90% who received reduced-dose irradiation. Ninety-six percent of these patients remain in continuous remission at a median followup of 19 months.[92]

Moreover, because of concern about potential late effects of irradiation, even at reduced dosage, on cognition and growth, attempts have been made to treat germinomas with chemotherapy alone and eliminate radiation therapy altogether. In an international study of intracranial GCTs, 45 germinoma patients were treated with multiagent chemotherapy that employed 6 cycles of carboplatin, etoposide, and bleomycin ± cyclophosphamide, and did not receive radiation therapy unless they had progressive disease.[49] A complete response to the chemotherapy was achieved in 37 (82%) of these patients, but nearly half (22 patients) subsequently relapsed. Most of them were salvaged with full-dose radiation therapy at relapse (19 patients; 86%) but with only 18 months median followup. However, the toxicity of the regimen was considerable, with a 10% toxic death rate from the chemotherapy. In view of these statistics, the advisability of treating pure germinomas with chemotherapy alone, especially with such an intensive regimen and attendant toxicity, is certainly controversial. Whether a less toxic chemotherapy regimen could obviate radiation therapy completely, and still produce the same outcome, has yet to be demonstrated. Moreover, the proven benefit, with regard to neurotoxicity, of eliminating versus reducing radiotherapy is also uncertain.

Chemotherapy for Nongerminoma Germ Cell Tumors

Multidrug chemotherapeutic regimens effective in the treatment of systemic GCTs have also proven useful in the treatment of the relatively radiotherapy-resistant intracranial NGGCT for which the prognosis is poor with radiation therapy alone. Responses of both recurrent and newly diagnosed NGGCTs to various combinations of these agents are well documented.[23,49,54,81,86,87,93,94]

In a number of small series, a trend toward improved survival rates was also seen among newly diagnosed intracranial NGGCT patients treated with multimodality therapy, with 2- to 4-year progression-free survival rates ranging from 40% to 100% reported with the use of various cisplatin-based chemotherapy regimens ± bleomycin, vinblastine, and etoposide.[94] Robertson and colleagues reported 5-year actuarial event-free survival of 67% (±9%) at a median followup of 4 years, among 18 newly diagnosed intracranial NGGCT patients treated in a multicenter study with a "sandwich" multimodality therapy regimen.[86] Preliminary data from a later study that employed neoadjuvant chemotherapy consisting of four cycles of cisplatin, etoposide, and ifosfamide, and for patients with less than a CR, two cycles of dose-intensified stem-cell-supported chemotherapy using carboplatin and cyclophosphamide, has a 66% progression-free survival rate at 3 years median followup.[95] The best outcome for intracranial NGGCT is reported among a small cohort of 14 patients treated according to a German protocol consisting of 4 cycles of cisplatin-based chemotherapy and craniospinal radiation therapy with a local tumor boost. The event-free survival for these patients is 80% with a median followup of 52 months.[60]

A critical effect of the platinum dosage on the outcome of intracranial NGGCT was seen in the combined data from several European studies. Seventeen patients who received 400 mg/m^2 or greater cumulative platinum dose in a multiagent regimen (plus irradiation) had an 86% event-free survival, compared with only a 56% event-free survival in the 15 who received 200 mg/m^2 cumulative platinum dose, when followed for 4 or more years.[60] Cisplatin has been used in the majority of platinum-based regimens for NGGCT, although a French group that reported 70% 4-year event-free survival among 27 intracranial NGGCTs employed carboplatin rather than cisplatin in its multiagent regimen, along with etoposide and ifosfamide.[62]

An approach using neoadjuvant platinum-based chemotherapy and radiation therapy, followed by complete excision of residual tumor was employed in 11 NGGCTs. Nine of 11 patients underwent surgery for residual tumor after the initial regimen, with an 8-year progression-free survival of 91%.[65]

As noted above, the possibility of withholding radiation therapy altogether in favor of chemotherapy alone, so far, has been a less successful strategy for intracranial NGGCTs. The approach was explored in an international trial in which both germinomas and NGGCTs were treated with intensive chemotherapy. The chemotherapy consisted of six cycles of carboplatin, etoposide, and bleomycin if there was a CR after four cycles, or four cycles followed by two cycles intensified by cyclophosphamide if there was less than a CR after four cycles.[49] Although there was a nearly 80% eventual CR rate of 26 NGGCT patients treated in this manner, 13 of 26 relapsed, of whom only half could be salvaged with irradiation or other therapy. The toxic death rate from the protocol was 10%, and the overall survival was 60%, at a median followup of only 18 months.

Chemotherapy may be effective in the particular setting of the relatively rare intracranial malignant teratoma type of NGGCT, which is most common in infants. Optimal therapy is not certain, but complete resection, where possible, is generally thought to be most beneficial. However, in a single case of an infant with a large intracranial malignant teratoma that recurred after a gross total resection, the tumor was completely responsive to eight cycles of platinum-based chemotherapy, and the child remained progression-free at least 2 years off therapy.[96]

From these observations taken together, a general consensus is that the most effective treatment for patients with intracranial NGGCTs includes some type of combination platinum-based chemotherapy that includes a minimum dose of platinum (cisplatin 400 mg/m^2 total dose or equivalent of carboplatin) as the cornerstone agent plus radiation therapy of at least whole-ventricular, and probably craniospinal, volume, even in patients with localized disease. It remains unclear why various patients with NGGCTs have different event-free survival rates after receiving similar therapy regimens, even those that included high-dose platinum-based chemotherapy and comparable radiotherapy doses and volumes. Possible explanations include the relatively small number of patients treated on the various protocols, differences in efficacy between cisplatin and carboplatin, unrecognized synergistic effects of the various combinations of drugs, the influence of time intervals between courses of chemotherapy, and the specific order in which the components of the multimodality therapy are given. How survival may be further improved is uncertain, but the question is best posed in a cooperative group setting where the number of patients treated for this rare tumor could be sufficient to answer it. Such a study was recently initiated within the Children's Oncology Group for these tumors in patients up to age 25 years.

In view of the chemosensitivity of systemic GCTs, it is possible that some of the poor outcomes of intracranial NGGCTs treated with prior chemotherapy regimens may have resulted from a failure to achieve adequate drug levels at tumor sites in the brain. Dose-intensification of chemotherapy may be a way to address this issue. Bone marrow ablative chemotherapy supported by autologous bone marrow or peripheral blood stem cell transplantation has curative potential for some relapsed systemic GCTs and may have promise as a consolidation of first-line therapy for some high-risk gonadal GCTs.[97] In an international pilot study of high-dose chemotherapy, 13 relapsed GCTs (9 NGGCTs, 4 germinomas) were treated with etoposide (1.5 g/m^2) and thiotepa (900 mg/m^2) followed by peripheral blood stem cell support plus focal radiation or further resection.[98] With a median follow-up of 16 months, 11 patients were still alive, 8 with no evidence of disease and 3 with stable disease. The optimal regimen for patients with relapsed intracranial GCTs is also best determined in a cooperative group setting.

▶ PROGNOSIS

Long-Term Survival of Germinomas

It is clear that a very high fraction of intracranial germinomas, approaching 100%, can be cured using craniospinal irradiation with a boost to the primary tumor site as sole therapy. This is true even for patients with disseminated CNS disease at diagnosis. As noted above in the discussions of the role of radiation and chemotherapy for these tumors, the controversial question is whether standard dosage and volumes of radiation therapy known to cure a high percentage of germinomas can safely be reduced or eliminated by substituting chemotherapy. This is being tried in the hope of reducing the potential neuroendocrine and neurocognitive sequelae resulting from nervous system irradiation, with promising results to date. However, the optimal chemotherapy regimen, the amount of reduction of radiation therapy, and the real benefit to be gained from such an approach is still being debated. Small single- and multiinstitution studies have suggested answers to these questions, which will be best addressed in future larger cooperative group trials for these relatively rare CNS tumors.

Long-Term Survival of Nongerminoma Germ Cell Tumors

Conversely, the outcome for intracranial NGGCTs treated with radiation therapy alone (at various dosages and volumes) has been poor, resulting in only 7% to 30% long-term survival rates.[1,26,32,72] The inferior outcome of patients with NGGCT treated solely with radiation therapy has led to other approaches, including treatment with the addition of chemotherapy to radiotherapy and with chemotherapy alone. The latter approach was not as successful as hoped, with a high percentage of relapses that could not be salvaged with irradiation.[49,99] The best outcomes for NGGCTs have been achieved with multimodality therapy that included chemotherapy and irradiation, with long-term progression-free survival in approximately two-thirds of patients.[60,62,86,100] A 5-year progression-free survival of 80% occurred among 14 NGGCT patients who were treated with 4 cycles of multiagent platinum-based chemotherapy and craniospinal irradiation.[60] A very good outcome was also recently reported after an approach using platinum-based neoadjuvant chemotherapy and radiation therapy, followed by resection of residual tumor in 9 of 11 NGGCT patients, resulting in a 91% 8-year progression-free survival.[65]

The optimal chemotherapy regimen, radiation dosage and volume, and the role and timing of surgery remain to be determined and should be evaluated in a large cooperative group setting, as is being done in the Children's Oncology Group study.

Tumor-Related Morbidity and Therapy-Related Sequelae

General

Patients with intracranial GCT tumors can have persistence of the neurologic or endocrinologic symptoms and signs with which they presented, even after successful treatment of the tumor. Abnormalities of visual acuity or visual fields from tumor compression of optic pathways or by prolonged elevation of increased intracranial pressure may not return to normal even after the tumor is gone. Endocrinologic deficits associated with suprasellar GCT almost always persist after the tumor is treated.[93]

Neurocognitive Sequelae

Successful treatment of intracranial GCT with radiation therapy, as with other primary CNS tumors, raises concerns about neurocognitive sequelae in survivors, particularly in those treated as young children. The deleterious effects on intelligence are related to radiation dose and volume and are inversely proportional to age at the time of therapy.[77] However, radiation therapy is also not totally without cognitive "cost" among older children and adults, with significant cognitive deficits reported in nearly 20% of patients with GCTs treated with cranial irradiation at mean ages of 15 to 16 years, and milder learning disabilities in 60%.[101,102] A Karnofsky score of less than 80 and some degree of cognitive dysfunction were found in 26 (31%) of 84 survivors of intracranial GCTs treated with radiation therapy. Radiologic evidence of possible radiation-induced brain injury was seen on MRI in 25 (30%) survivors, and 7 (8%) survivors had borderline to moderate mental retardation on psychometric testing.[55]

Neuroendocrine Sequelae

Generally, impaired pituitary functions present before treatment of intracranial GCTs persist or worsen after tumor remission.[93] These include posterior pituitary dysfunction with diabetes insipidus, anterior pituitary deficits with hypothyroidism, adrenal insufficiency, gonadotrophin deficiency causing delayed puberty or sexual dysfunction, and growth failure from growth hormone deficiency. Pituitary hormone replacement was required in 76 (68%) of Sawamura's 111 intracranial GCT patients. Five of 31 patients (16%) with no deficits before irradiation developed late-onset pituitary dysfunction, considered an effect of therapy.[55] Fourteen (82%) of 17 GCT patients in another series required some pituitary hormone replacement, and more than half had panhypopituitarism.[101]

Secondary Neoplasms

Both radiation therapy and chemotherapy of intracranial GCTs, like other CNS tumors, have the potential to produce secondary neoplasms.[103] Chemotherapy-related leukemias, most frequently of a myeloid type, are among the most common second malignancies in both adult and pediatric populations.[104] However, the incidence of such leukemias was low (only 0.37%) in a large series of 538 systemic GCT patients treated on clinical trials with etoposide and platinum-based regimens similar to that used for intracranial GCTs.[103] Radiation-induced secondary brain neoplasms occurred in 4 (4.8%) of 84 intracranial GCT survivors (2 glioblastomas, 2 meningiomas) in Sawamura's series.[55]

REFERENCES

1. Jennings MT, Gelman R, Hochberg F. Intracranial germ-cell tumors: natural history and pathogenesis. J Neurosurg 1985;63:155–167.
2. Kuratsu J, Takeshima H, Ushio Y. Trends in the incidence of primary intracranial tumors in Kumamoto, Japan. Int J Clin Oncol 2001;6:183–191.
3. Bjornsson J, Scheithauer BW, Okazaki H, et al. Intracranial germ cell tumors: pathobiological and immunohistochemical aspects of 70 cases. J Neuropathol Exp Neurol 1985;44:32–46.
4. Oi S, Matsumoto S. Controversy pertaining to therapeutic modalities for tumors of the pineal region: a worldwide survey of different patient populations. Childs Nerv Syst 1992;8:332–336.
5. Matsutani M, Sano K, Takakura K, et al. Primary intracranial germ cell tumors: a clinical analysis of 153 histologically verified cases. J Neurosurg 1997;86:446–455.
6. Heideman R, Packer RJ, Albright LA, et al. Principles and practice of pediatric oncology, 2nd ed. Philadelphia: Lippincott, 1993.
7. Dearnaley DP, A'Hern RP, Whittaker S, et al. Pineal and CNS germ cell tumors: Royal Marsden Hospital experience 1962–1987. Int J Radiat Oncol Biol Phys 1990;18:773–781.
8. Mc Kay DG, Hertig AT, Adams EC, et al. Histochemical observations on the germ cells of human embryos. Anat Rec 1953;117:201–219.
9. Hynes RO, Lander AD. Contact and adhesive specificities in the associations, migrations, and targeting of cells and axons. Cell 1992;68:303–322.
10. Horowitz MB, Hall WA. Central nervous system germinomas. A review. Arch Neurol 1991;48:652–657.
11. Marx J. Cell death studies yield cancer clues. Science 1993;259:760–761.
12. Styne D, Grumbach M. Reproductive endocrinology: physiology, pathophysiology and clinical management, 2nd ed. Philadelphia: WB Saunders, 1986.
13. Sandberg AA, Meloni AM, Suijkerbuijk RF. Reviews of chromosome studies in urological tumors: III. Cytogenetics and genes in testicular tumors. J Urol 1996;155:1531–1556.
14. Brison O. Gene amplification and tumor progression. Biochim Biophys Acta 1993;1155:25–41.
15. de Bruin TW, Slater RM, Defferrari R, et al. Isochromosome 12p-positive pineal germ cell tumor. Cancer Res 1994;54: 1542–1544.
16. Kim SK, Cho BK, Paek SH, et al. The detection of p53 gene mutation using a microdissection technique in primary intracranial germ cell tumors. Int J Oncol 2001;18:111–116.
17. Iwato M, Tachibana O, Tohma Y, et al. Alterations of the INK4a/ARF locus in human intracranial germ cell tumors. Cancer Res 2000;60:2113–2115.
18. Iwato M, Tachibana O, Tohma Y, et al. Molecular analysis for p53 and mdm2 in intracranial germ cell tumors. Acta Neuropathol (Berl) 2000;99:21–25.
19. Okada Y, Nishikawa R, Matsutani M, et al. Hypomethylated X chromosome gain and rare isochromosome 12p in diverse intracranial germ cell tumors. J Neuropathol Exp Neurol 2002;61:531–538.
20. DiGiovanni LM, Sheikh Z: Prenatal diagnosis, clinical significance and management of fetal intracranial teratoma: a case report and literature review. Am J Perinatol 11:420–422, 1994.
21. Allen JC. Controversies in the management of intracranial germ cell tumors. Neurol Clin 1991;9:441–452.
22. Rivarola MA, Mendilaharzu H, Warman M, et al. Endocrine disorders in 66 suprasellar and pineal tumors of patients with prepubertal and pubertal ages. Horm Res 37:1–6, 1992.
23. Allen JC, Bosl G, Walker R. Chemotherapy trials in recurrent primary intracranial germ cell tumors. J Neurooncol 1985;3:147–152.
24. Zee CS, Segall H, Apuzzo M, et al. MR imaging of pineal region neoplasms. J Comput Assist Tomogr 1991;15:56–63.
25. Fujimaki T, Matsutani M, Funada N, et al. CT and MRI features of intracranial germ cell tumors. J Neurooncol 1994; 19:217–226.
26. Nakagawa K, Aoki Y, Akanuma A, et al. Radiation therapy of intracranial germ cell tumors with radiosensitivity assessment. Radiat Med 1992;10:55–61.
27. Yamashita J, Handa H. Diagnosis and treatment of pineal tumours. Kyoto University experience (1941–1984). Acta Neurochir Suppl (Wien) 1988;42:137–141.
28. Bruce JN, Stein BM. Surgical management of pineal region tumors. Acta Neurochir (Wien) 1995;134:130–135.
29. Baumgartner JE, Edwards MS. Pineal tumors. Neurosurg Clin N Am 1992;3:853–862.
30. Packer RJ, Sutton LN, Rosenstock JG, et al. Pineal region tumors of childhood. Pediatrics 1984;74:97–102.
31. Linggood RM, Chapman PH. Pineal tumors. J Neurooncol 1992;12:85–91.

32. Fuller BG, Kapp DS, Cox R. Radiation therapy of pineal region tumors: 25 new cases and a review of 208 previously reported cases. Int J Radiat Oncol Biol Phys 1994; 28:229–245.
33. Rorke LB. The cerebellar medulloblastoma and its relationship to primitive neuroectodermal tumors. J Neuropathol Exp Neurol 1983;42:1–15.
34. Russell D, Rubenstein LJ. Tumors of specialized tissues of central neuroepithelial origin. Baltimore, MD: Williams & Williams, 1989.
35. Sutherland GR, Florell R, Louw D, et al. Epidemiology of primary intracranial neoplasms in Manitoba, Canada. Can J Neurol Sci 1987;14:586–592.
36. Schild SE, Scheithauer BW, Schomberg PJ, et al. Pineal parenchymal tumors. Clinical, pathologic, and therapeutic aspects. Cancer 1993;72:870–880.
37. Borit A, Blackwood W, Mair WG. The separation of pineocytoma from pineoblastoma. Cancer 1980;45:1408–1418.
38. D'Andrea AD, Packer RJ, Rorke LB, et al. Pineocytomas of childhood. A reappraisal of natural history and response to therapy. Cancer 1987;59:1353–1357.
39. Jakacki RI, Zeltzer PM, Boyett JM, et al. Survival and prognostic factors following radiation and/or chemotherapy for primitive neuroectodermal tumors of the pineal region in infants and children: a report of the Children's Cancer Group. J Clin Oncol 1995;13:1377–1383.
40. Regis J, Bouillot P, Rouby-Volot F, et al. Pineal region tumors and the role of stereotactic biopsy: review of the mortality, morbidity, and diagnostic rates in 370 cases. Neurosurgery 1996;39:907–912; discussion 912–904.
41. Petronio J, Edwards MS, Prados M, et al. Management of chiasmal and hypothalamic gliomas of infancy and childhood with chemotherapy. J Neurosurg 1991;74:701–708.
42. Robertson PL, Muraszko KM, Brunberg JA, et al. Pediatric midbrain tumors: a benign subgroup of brainstem gliomas. Pediatr Neurosurg 1995;22:65–73.
43. Vaquero J, Martinez R, Magallon R, et al. Intracranial metastases to the pineal region. Report of three cases. J Neurosurg Sci 1991;35:55–57.
44. Weber P, Shepard KV, Vijayakumar S: Metastases to pineal gland. Cancer 1989;63:164–165.
45. Korogi Y, Takahashi M, Ushio Y. MRI of pineal region tumors. J Neurooncol 2001;54:251–261.
46. Bodensteiner JB, Schaefer GB, Keller GM, et al. Incidental pineal cysts in a prospectively ascertained normal cohort. Clin Pediatr (Phila) 1996;35:277–279.
47. Allen JC, Nisselbaum J, Epstein F, et al. Alpha-fetoprotein and human chorionic gonadotropin determination in cerebrospinal fluid. An aid to the diagnosis and management of intracranial germ-cell tumors. J Neurosurg 1979;51: 368–374.
48. Inoue HK, Naganuma H, Ono N. Pathobiology of intracranial germ-cell tumors: immunochemical, immunohistochemical, and electron microscopic investigations. J Neurooncol 1987;5:105–115.
49. Balmaceda C, Heller G, Rosenblum M, et al. Chemotherapy without irradiation—a novel approach for newly diagnosed CNS germ cell tumors: results of an international cooperative trial. The First International Central Nervous System Germ Cell Tumor Study. J Clin Oncol 1996;14:2908–2915.
50. Brodeur GM, Howarth CB, Pratt CB, et al. Malignant germ cell tumors in 57 children and adolescents. Cancer 1981;48:1890–1898.
51. Takei Y, Pearl GS. Ultrastructural study of intracranial yolk sac tumor: with special reference to the oncologic phylogeny of germ cell tumors. Cancer 1981;48:2038–2046.
52. Gonzalez-Crussi R. Extragonadal teratomas: atlas of tumor pathology. Washington, DC: Armed Forces Institute of Pathology, 1982:Fascicle 18.
53. Cotran RS. Germinomas. In: Cotran RS, Kumar V, Collins T, eds. Robbins pathologic basis of disease, 6th ed. Philadelphia: WB Saunders, 1999:1350.
54. Kobayashi T, Yoshida J, Ishiyama J, et al. Combination chemotherapy with cisplatin and etoposide for malignant intracranial germ-cell tumors. An experimental and clinical study. J Neurosurg 1989;70:676–681.
55. Sawamura Y, Ikeda J, Shirato H, et al. Germ cell tumours of the central nervous system: treatment consideration based on 111 cases and their long-term clinical outcomes. Eur J Cancer 1998;34:104–110.
56. Aoyama H, Shirato H, Yoshida H, et al. Retrospective multi-institutional study of radiotherapy for intracranial non-germinomatous germ cell tumors. Radiother Oncol 1998;49:55–59.
57. Goodman RR. Magnetic resonance imaging-directed stereotactic endoscopic third ventriculostomy. Neurosurgery 1993; 32:1043–1047; discussion 1047.
58. Ferrer E, Santamarta D, Garcia-Fructuoso G, et al. Neuroendoscopic management of pineal region tumours. Acta Neurochir (Wien) 1997;139:12–20; discussion 20–21.
59. Stein BM, Bruce JN. Surgical management of pineal region tumors (honored guest lecture). Clin Neurosurg 1992;39: 509–532.
60. Calaminus G, Bamberg M, Baranzelli MC, et al. Intracranial germ cell tumors: a comprehensive update of the European data. Neuropediatrics 1994;25:26–32.
61. Nicholson JC, Punt J, Hale J, et al. Neurosurgical management of paediatric germ cell tumours of the central nervous system—a multi-disciplinary team approach for the new millennium. Br J Neurosurg 2002;16:93–95.
62. Baranzelli MC, Patte C, Bouffet E, et al. Carboplatin-based chemotherapy (CT) and focal irradiation (RT) in primary cerebral germ cell tumors (GCT): a French society of pediatric oncology (SFOP). Proc Annu Meet Am Soc Clinic Oncol, 1999;18:S538.
63. Brandes AA, Pasetto LM, Monfardini S. The treatment of cranial germ cell tumours. Cancer Treat Rev 2000;26:233–242.
64. Friedman JA, Lynch JJ, Buckner JC, et al. Management of malignant pineal germ cell tumors with residual mature teratoma. Neurosurgery 2001;48:518–522; discussion 522–523.
65. Kochi M, Itoyama Y, Shiraishi S, et al. Successful treatment of intracranial nongerminomatous malignant germ cell tumors by administering neoadjuvant chemotherapy and radiotherapy before excision of residual tumors. J Neurosurg 2003;99: 106–114.
66. Hanna A, Edan C, Heresbach N, et al. [Expanding mature pineal teratoma syndrome. Case report]. Neurochirurgie 2000;46:568–572.
67. O'Callaghan AM, Katapodis O, Ellison DW, et al. The growing teratoma syndrome in a nongerminomatous germ

cell tumor of the pineal gland: a case report and review. Cancer 1997;80:942–947.
68. Lee AC, Chan GC, Fung CF, et al. Paradoxical response of a pineal immature teratoma to combination chemotherapy. Med Pediatr Oncol 1995;24:53–57.
69. Wolden SL, Wara WM, Larson DA, et al. Radiation therapy for primary intracranial germ-cell tumors. Int J Radiat Oncol Biol Phys 1995;32:943–949.
70. Thomas GM: Controversies in the management of testicular seminoma. Cancer 1985;55:2296–2302.
71. Haas-Kogan DA, Missett BT, Wara WM, et al. Radiation therapy for intracranial germ cell tumors. Int J Radiat Oncol Biol Phys 2003;56:511–518.
72. Chao CK, Lee ST, Lin FJ, et al. A multivariate analysis of prognostic factors in management of pineal tumor. Int J Radiat Oncol Biol Phys 1993;27:1185–1191.
73. Dattoli MJ, Newall J: Radiation therapy for intracranial germinoma: the case for limited volume treatment. Int J Radiat Oncol Biol Phys 1990;19:429–433.
74. Tseng CK, Tsang NM, Wei KC, et al. Radiotherapy to primary CNS germinoma: how large an irradiated volume is justified for tumor control? J Neurooncol 2003;62:343–348.
75. Kersh CR, Constable WC, Eisert DR, et al. Primary central nervous system germ cell tumors. Effect of histologic confirmation on radiotherapy. Cancer 1988;61:2148–2152.
76. Maity A, Shu HK, Janss A, et al. Craniospinal radiation in the treatment of biopsy-proven intracranial germinomas: twenty-five years' experience in a single center. Int J Radiat Oncol Biol Phys 2004;58:1165–1170.
77. Duffner PK, Cohen ME: The long-term effects of central nervous system therapy on children with brain tumors. Neurol Clin 1991;9:479–495.
78. Packer RJ, Sutton LN, Atkins TE, et al. A prospective study of cognitive function in children receiving whole-brain radiotherapy and chemotherapy: 2-year results. J Neurosurg 1989;70:707–713.
79. Crossen JR, Garwood D, Glatstein E, et al. Neurobehavioral sequelae of cranial irradiation in adults: a review of radiation-induced encephalopathy. J Clin Oncol 1994;12:627–642.
80. Jereb B, Zupancic N, Petric J: Intracranial germinoma: report of seven cases. Pediatr Hematol Oncol 1990;7:183–188.
81. Allen JC, Kim JH, Packer RJ. Neoadjuvant chemotherapy for newly diagnosed germ-cell tumors of the central nervous system. J Neurosurg 1987;67:65–70.
82. Allen JC, DaRosso RC, Donahue B, et al. A phase II trial of preirradiation carboplatin in newly diagnosed germinoma of the central nervous system. Cancer 1994;74:940–944.
83. Gobel U, Bamberg M, Haas RJ, et al. [Non-testicular germ cell tumors: analysis of the therapy study MAKEI 83/86 and changes in the protocol for the follow-up study]. Klin Padiatr 1989;201:247–260.
84. Plantaz D, Kalifa C, Flamant F, et al. Primary germinal tumors of the nervous system in children and adolescents. A retrospective study of 35 cases from 1975 to 1987. Arch Fr Pediatr 1992;49:87–92.
85. Calaminus G, Andreussi L, Garre ML, et al. Secreting germ cell tumors of the central nervous system (CNS). First results of the cooperative German/Italian pilot study (CNS sGCT). Klin Padiatr 1997;209:222–227.
86. Robertson PL, DaRosso RC, Allen JC. Improved prognosis of intracranial non-germinoma germ cell tumors with multimodality therapy. J Neurooncol 1997;32:71–80.
87. Yoshida J, Sugita K, Kobayashi T, et al. Prognosis of intracranial germ cell tumours: effectiveness of chemotherapy with cisplatin and etoposide (CDDP and VP-16). Acta Neurochir (Wien) 1993;120:111–117.
88. Hasegawa T, Kondziolka D, Hadjipanayis CG, et al. Stereotactic radiosurgery for CNS nongerminomatous germ cell tumors. Report of four cases. Pediatr Neurosurg 2003;38:329–333.
89. Kobayashi T, Kida Y, Mori Y. Stereotactic gamma radiosurgery for pineal and related tumors. J Neurooncol 2001;54:301–309.
90. Einhorn LH. General Motors Cancer Research Prizewinners Laureates Lectures. Charles F. Kettering Prize. Clinical trials in testicular cancer. Cancer 1993;71:3182–3184.
91. Bajorin DF, Sarosdy MF, Pfister DG, et al. Randomized trial of etoposide and cisplatin versus etoposide and carboplatin in patients with good-risk germ cell tumors: a multiinstitutional study. J Clin Oncol 1993;11:598–606.
92. Allen J, Robertson P, Sieffert J, et al. Intensive chemotherapy followed by response-based radiotherapy: preliminary results of the Beth Israel Germinoma Consortium. In: abstracts of the 32nd annual meeting of the Child Neurology Society. Ann Neurol 2003;54(Suppl 7):S109.
93. Herrmann HD, Westphal M, Winkler K, et al. Treatment of nongerminomatous germ-cell tumors of the pineal region. Neurosurgery 1994;34:524–529; discussion 529.
94. Itoyama Y, Kochi M, Kuratsu J, et al. Treatment of intracranial nongerminomatous malignant germ cell tumors producing alpha-fetoprotein. Neurosurgery 1995;36:459–464; discussion 464–456.
95. Robertson PL, Siffert J, Jakacki R, et al. Multimodality therapy for CNS–non-germinoma germ cell tumors (NGGCT): results of a phase II consortium. Eleventh International Symposium on Pediatric Neuro-oncology. Boston: 2004.
96. Garre ML, El-Hossainy MO, Fondelli P, et al. Is chemotherapy effective therapy for intracranial immature teratoma? A case report. Cancer 1996;77:977–982.
97. Motzer RJ, Mazumdar M, Bajorin DF, et al. High-dose carboplatin, etoposide, and cyclophosphamide with autologous bone marrow transplantation in first-line therapy for patients with poor-risk germ cell tumors. J Clin Oncol 1997;15:2546–2552.
98. Baranzelli MC, Pichon F, Pattte C, et al. High dose etoposide and thiotepa for recurrent intracranial malignant germ cell tumors (CGT). Eighth International Symposium on Pediatric Neuro-Oncology. Rome, Italy: 1998:62A.
99. Baranzelli MC, Patte C, Bouffet E, et al. An attempt to treat pediatric intracranial alphaFP and betaHCG secreting germ cell tumors with chemotherapy alone. SFOP experience with 18 cases. Societe Francaise d'Oncologie Pediatrique. J Neurooncol 1998;37:229–239.
100. Nam DH, Cho BK, Shin HJ, et al. Treatment of intracranial nongerminomatous malignant germ cell tumor in children: the role of each treatment modality. Childs Nerv Syst 1999;15:185–191.

101. Kiltie AE, Gattamaneni HR. Survival and quality of life of paediatric intracranial germ cell tumour patients treated at the Christie Hospital, 1972–1993. Med Pediatr Oncol 1995; 25:450–456.
102. Shirato H, Nishio M, Sawamura Y, et al. Analysis of long-term treatment of intracranial germinoma. Int J Radiat Oncol Biol Phys 1997;37:511–515.
103. Nichols CR, Breeden ES, Loehrer PJ, et al. Secondary leukemia associated with a conventional dose of etoposide: review of serial germ cell tumor protocols. J Natl Cancer Inst 1993;85:36–40.
104. Aguiar RC. Therapy-related chronic myeloid leukemia: an epidemiological, clinical and pathogenetic appraisal. Leuk Lymphoma 1998;29:17–26.

CHAPTER 24
Primary Spinal Tumors

VOLKER W. STIEBER / STEPHEN B. TATTER / MARK E. SHAFFREY / EDWARD G. SHAW

Primary tumors of the spinal cord and canal are uncommon. Primary treatment for most spinal cord tumors involves surgical resection using advanced microsurgical techniques. Patients unable to undergo complete resection and those at high risk of recurrence are typically treated with radiation therapy. The role of chemotherapy in the management of spinal cord tumors remains to be elucidated.

▶ EPIDEMIOLOGY

Recent United States registry data show that the combined incidence of all primary neural axis tumors is 14.0 in 100,000 person-years.[1,2] Table 24-1 shows the distribution by benign versus malignant, male versus female, and by racial group. Incidence rates for all primary neural axis tumors are lowest in the pediatric population younger than 20 years of age (3.9), rises notably in the age 55 years and older population (17.2), and again in the age 65 years and older population (39.7).[2]

The overall incidence of primary spinal cord tumors is approximately 10% to 19% of all primary central nervous system (CNS) tumors[3] and, like that of primary neural axis tumors overall, appears to increase with age. The incidence of primary spinal cord tumors is 0.7, 1.0, 2.8, and 3.6 per 100,000 person-years in the age groups of 0 to 24, 25 to 44, 45 to 64, and 65 years and older, respectively.[4] The incidence ratio of intracranial to intraspinal tumors is up to four times higher in pediatric patients than in adults.

As Table 24-2 shows, the frequency of specific spinal cord tumors is quite different from that of their counterpart brain tumors. The incidence ratios of intracranial to intraspinal astrocytomas, ependymomas, and meningiomas are approximately 10:1, 3:1, and 18:1, respectively.[4] The age-adjusted incidence for spinal glioma is 0.11% to 0.14%; for meningioma it is 0.08% to 0.28%, depending on sex (female higher than male subjects); and for nerve sheath tumors it is 0.07% to 0.13%.[5] Schwannoma and meningioma account for approximately 60% of primary spinal tumors, with schwannoma being slightly more frequent; both types occur primarily in adults. Regional differences are also noted. Gliomas constitute 46% of primary intracranial tumors but only 23% of spinal tumors. Most primary spinal gliomas are ependymomas with a predilection for the cauda equina. Other less common spinal tumors are lipomas, dermoids, central neurocytomas, and hemangioblastomas.

Spinal tumors can also be classified according to location: extradural or intradural. Intradural tumors either arise within the spinal cord (intramedullary), or outside of it (extramedullary) (Fig. 24-1).[6] Approximately 70% of intradural tumors are extramedullary and 30% are intramedullary. Of the intradural tumors, intradural extramedullary schwannoma (neurilemmoma) and meningioma are the most common and are attached to sensory nerve roots and to dura, respectively. Occasionally they may present as extradural tumors. Other intradural extramedullary tumors include chordomas, epidermoids, and intradural drop metastases of intracranial primary tumors such as medulloblastomas. Of intramedullary tumors, 40% are

▶ **TABLE 24-1.** INCIDENCES OF PRIMARY NEURAL AXIS TUMORS

Category	Incidence*
Benign	6.3
Malignant	7.7
Male	14.2
Female	13.9
White	14.3
Black	9.9
Hispanic	10.8

*All numbers are per 100,000 person-years.

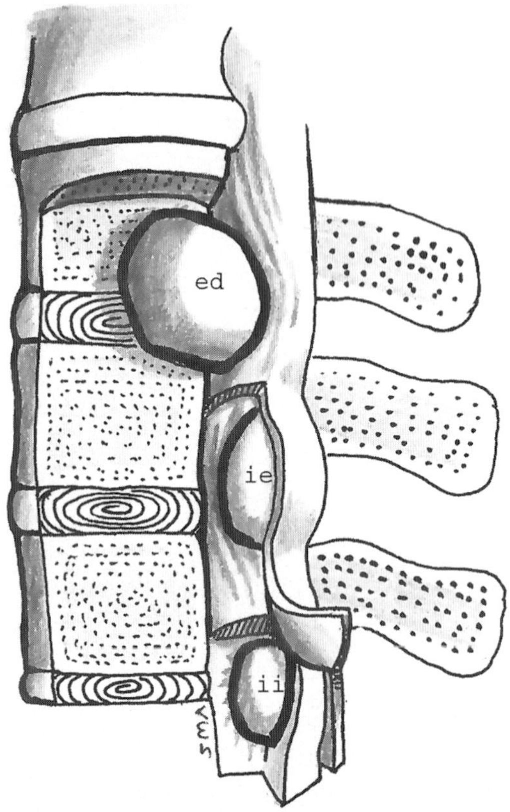

Figure 24-1. Location within the spinal column. ed = extradural; ie = intradural extramedullary; ii = intradural intramedullary.

▶ **TABLE 24-2.** DISTRIBUTION OF PRIMARY SPINAL CORD TUMORS BY HISTOLOGY

Histology	Incidence
Tumors of glial origin	23%
• Ependymoma	• 13%–15%
• Astrocytoma	• 7%–11%
Schwannoma	22%–30%
Meningioma	25%–46%
Vascular lesions	6%
Chordoma/chondrosarcoma	4%
Other miscellaneous tumors	3%–4%

Source: *From Preston MS*[5] *and Sloof JL.*[253]

▶ **TABLE 24-3.** ANATOMIC DISTRIBUTION OF SPINAL TUMORS BY HISTOLOGIC DIAGNOSIS

Extradural	Intradural Extramedullary	Intradural Intramedullary
Chondroblastoma	Ependymoma, myxopapillary type	Astrocytoma
Chordoma	Epidermoid	Ependymoma
Chondrosarcoma	Lipoma	Ganglioglioma
Hemangioma	Meningioma	Hemangioblastoma
Lipoma	Neurofibroma	Hemangioma
Lymphoma	Paraganglioma	Lipoma
Meningioma	Schwannoma	Medulloblastoma
Metastasis		Neuroblastoma
Neuroblastoma		Neurofibroma
Neurofibroma		Oligodendroglioma
Osteoblastoma		Teratoma (mature)
Osteochondroma		
Osteosarcoma		
Sarcoma		
Vertebral hemangioma		

ependymomas; next most common are the astrocytomas of low to intermediate grade. These are followed in frequency by less common histologies, such as oligodendroglioma, ganglioglioma, medulloblastoma, central neurocytoma, and hemangioblastoma. Table 24-3 classifies spinal axis tumors by location.

Approximately 50% to 55% of spinal tumors involve the thoracic spinal canal, 25% to 30% involve the lumbosacral spine, and the remaining 15% to 25% involve the cervical spine, including the foramen magnum. Meningiomas are dural based and arise preferentially at the foramen magnum and in the thoracic spine. Astrocytomas are distributed throughout the spinal cord, and most ependymomas involve the conus medullaris and the cauda equina. Spinal chordomas are characteristically sacral but may also occur in the mobile spine.

The predominant mode of spread of primary tumors is by direct extension. Spread along the subarachnoid space with spinal or cranial involvement of the meninges may also occur. Upward spread is seen with some spinal cord tumors and is discussed in the sections grouped by histologic diagnosis, when applicable.[7]

Finally, depending on histology, one should not always assume that the spinal cord tumor found on imaging is the primary lesion. Supratentorial tumors that show a tendency toward leptomeningeal metastases include 1.2% of glioblastomas and 1.5% of anaplastic gliomas.[8] Thus, imaging of the entire craniospinal axis is often necessary.

▶ PATHOLOGY

The diversity of primary spinal axis tumors results partly from the diversity of phenotypically distinct cells capable of transformation into tumors.[9] Because of changes in classification and reporting of these tumors, tumor registry data are not completely accurate. Table 24-2 shows the relative frequency of distribution of spinal tumors by histology.[5] The most common intramedullary tumors are those derived from glial precursors (astrocytes, ependymocytes, and oligodendrocytes).

▶ ANATOMY, CLINICAL PRESENTATION, AND NEUROLOGIC DIAGNOSIS

The clinical presentation of tumors of the spinal axis is a function of the local anatomy.[6] Within the spinal canal there exists a well-defined extradural space containing epidural fat and blood vessels. The extradural space communicates with adjacent extraspinal compartments via the intervertebral foramina. A spinal cord tumor produces local and distal symptoms and signs; the latter reflect involvement of motor and sensory long tracts within the spinal cord. These allow localization of the level of the lesion based on clinical findings.[6] However, the clinical presentation of a spinal tumor rarely indicates if it is extradural or intradural.

By Location[6]

Intramedullary

Tumors in this location can cause a characteristic neurologic syndrome. Early on, decreased temperature and pain sensation occur in the dermatomes of the spinal segments occupied by the tumor and two to three segments caudal to the lesion. Other sensory modalities are not diminished while the tumor is confined to the central cord. This "dissociated" sensory loss is rarely seen with extramedullary tumors. Additionally, weakness and atrophy are early findings in the myotomes of the corresponding cord segments involved by tumor. As the tumor grows transversely, reflexes produced at the level of the tumor disappear, and spastic paralysis with hyperreflexia develops below the lesion. Eventually, all sensory modalities are affected. Cervical tumors can produce Horner syndrome by interrupting unilateral autonomic pathways.

Cauda Equina

Lesions can cause radicular pain in the thigh, weakness, and atrophy of muscles, including the glutei, hamstrings, gastrocnemius, and the anterior tibialis. Saddle anesthesia, absent ankle reflexes, impotence, urinary urgency or acute retention, and constipation are also commonly seen. Depending on the location of the lesion, other reflexes may be affected.

Conus Medullaris

Lesions can produce several symptoms including saddle anesthesia, acute urinary retention, incontinence of bowel and bladder, and impotence. If the lesion remains confined to the conus, it will not cause paralysis of the lower limbs, and the ankle reflexes are preserved. More commonly, tumors originating in the conus are diagnosed when they have enlarged enough to cause signs characteristic of intramedullary tumors. These findings can also be mixed with those caused by growth of the tumor in the direction of the cauda equine such as radicular pain.

By Sign or Symptom[6]

Flaccid weakness, atrophy, fasciculations, and reduced deep tendon reflexes are seen in corresponding myotomes with involvement of the anterior horn cells and the ventral roots (lower motor neuron lesions). A tumor involving the lateral corticospinal tracts can cause weakness, spasticity, hyperreflexia, and an extensor plantar response (Babinski sign). Motor weakness and spasticity are seen with tumors above the conus medullaris. Weakness and flaccidity are seen with tumors below the conus because they compress the peripheral nerve roots of the cauda equina. A tumor restricted to the conus should not cause weakness, although one also involving the cauda equina or the lumbar enlargement of the spinal cord will.

Sensory impairment often helps to localize the level of the tumor based on loss of dermatome function, although the upper level of impaired long tract function may be several segments below the actual tumor. A lesion involving the lateral spinothalamic tract will cause numbness, paresthesias, and decreased temperature sensation over the contralateral limb or trunk below the lesion. This produces the classic finding of a sensory level, which is best demonstrated with a pin or a metal or cold object to test temperature (cold) sensation and observation for absence of perspiration. A lesion in the posterior column causes an ataxic or tabetic gait. Standing posture is affected with the eyes closed (Romberg sign). Paresthesias can occur below the level of the lesion.

Because pain and temperature pathways cross over in the spinal cord and proprioceptive and motor pathways do not, a unilateral spinal cord lesion can result in ipsilateral paralysis and proprioceptive loss, as well as contralateral pain–temperature loss below the level of the lesion. Because light touch travels in two pathways, one that crosses in the spinal cord (spinothalamic tract) and one that does not (posterior columns), it is usually spared in unilateral lesions. This combination of findings is known as the Brown-Sequard syndrome.

Both bladder and bowel symptoms can result from a spinal cord tumor. Bladder symptoms include hesitancy, dribbling, incontinence, urgency with incontinence, or acute retention. Loss of bladder control is seen early in the presentation of tumors in or below the conus and later in tumors above the conus. If the bowel is affected, constipation occurs more frequently than incontinence. Cord lesions above L1 can lead to impotence or reflex priapism. Lesions involving S2–S4 may produce loss of erection and ejaculation ability. Decreased genital sensation can occur from lesions affecting the S2 nerve roots.

Pain from spinal canal tumors is caused by nerve root compression, bone destruction, or by pressure on the dura. The pain may be radicular, midline, or central. Radicular pain is secondary to involvement of the posterior roots and is typically described as shooting pain in a dermatomal distribution. The nerve can be compressed inside or outside the dura. Midline spinal pain causes discomfort localized to the area of the tumor, and is thought to arise from pain-sensitive structures in the dura and extradural tissues. Characteristically pain is more severe in extradural lesions. Sometimes with spinal cord compression, a dull or burning pain, more widespread than segmental spinal or radicular pain, occurs. This type of pain, relatively rare, has numerous designations including central pain, causalgia, and deafferentation pain. It involves a limb or trunk below the lesion. Pain is the most common presenting symptom in patients with sacrococcygeal tumors.

▶ NEURODIAGNOSTIC TESTS

Neuroimaging

In the evaluation of intramedullary and extramedullary spinal cord lesions, magnetic resonance imaging (MRI) is the diagnostic study of choice. A complete description of the fundamentals of MRI is beyond the scope of this chapter. Briefly, MRI provides excellent anatomic detail and spatial resolution in three dimensions, making it ideal for visualizing lesions in the spinal cord. Blood products, cystic regions, solid masses, and adjacent vessels can be differentiated with great accuracy. Contrast agents greatly enhance the sensitivity of these tests. Most spinal cord tumors enhance with contrast, the most common exception being World Health Organization (WHO) grade II gliomas. By differentially weighting images for different tissue-relaxation times, images sensitive for anatomic detail or water can be generated. On MRI, edema appears as an area of low signal intensity on T_1-weighted images and high signal intensity on T_2-weighted images. Fluid-attenuated inversion recovery (FLAIR) sequences can further improve contrast between abnormal lesions and cerebral spinal fluid (CSF). In cerebral astrocytic malignancies, tumor infiltration may be differentiated from edema by suppression of CSF signal using FLAIR sequences.[10] Magnetic resonance (MR) spectroscopy can help to differentiate tumor from cerebral necrosis by evaluating the regional distribution of chemicals associated with energy metabolism in the tumor.[11,12] However, the usefulness of FLAIR and spectroscopy has not yet been firmly established in spinal cord gliomas. Their utility in guiding radiation therapy treatment planning and response evaluation is currently under evaluation.[13–15]

Tumor and Cerebrospinal Fluid Markers

For patients with spinal tumors, examination of CSF may occasionally be useful for differential diagnosis and for monitoring of therapeutic response. Because of the risk of herniation as a result of increased intracranial pressure, neuroimaging studies, when indicated, should precede, rather than follow, lumbar puncture. When obstruction of CSF flow occurs as a consequence of tumor expansion, patients can develop hydrocephalus; thus, one should be especially wary of performing a lumbar puncture in a patient with a spinal cord tumor who presents with a headache.[16] With the exception of large tumors involving the foramen magnum, elevated intracranial pressure is unusual in those with primary spinal cord tumors. It can be produced by upward seeding of the tumor or by the development of carcinomatous meningitis from malignant tumors.

CSF examination is especially useful in the management of tumors that may seed the subarachnoid space and spread via the CSF, such as medulloblastoma and ependymoma. The CSF is examined for malignant cells (cytology), protein, and glucose. A high protein concentration with normal glucose levels and normal cytology is seen in spinal cord tumors, although if it has seeded the meninges, sugar may be low and cytology malignant. The appearance of xanthochromic CSF, caused by high protein content with an absence of erythrocytes, is characteristic of spinal cord tumors obstructing the subarachnoid space and producing stasis of the CSF in the caudal thecal sac.

Nonneoplastic Lesions Mimicking Spinal Cord Tumors

Various nonneoplastic conditions may mimic spinal cord tumors. These may include (in no particular order) infectious meningitis, acute transverse myelitis, *Angiostrongylus cantonensis* abscess, intradural disc herniation, sarcoidosis, and tuberculosis.[17–22] This should serve to emphasize the necessity of obtaining an accurate histologic diagnosis whenever possible.

▶ THERAPEUTIC MANAGEMENT: GENERAL PRINCIPLES

Surgery: General Principles

Surgery has traditionally been the mainstay of therapy for spinal cord tumors. The first successful resection of an intradural tumor was performed in 1887.[23] The first resection of an intramedullary tumor was performed in 1907,[24] and the first publication of the successful resection of an intramedullary tumor appeared in 1911.[25] Prior to contemporary neuroimaging and surgical technology, most patients underwent conservative management with biopsy and adjuvant radiation therapy.[26] As modern diagnostic and therapeutic technology such as MRI, the operating microscope, microsurgical tools, and intraoperative neurophysiology became available, more aggressive surgical intervention became a more prevalent treatment strategy.[27] This section discusses general principles of surgery for these lesions, depending on anatomic location within the spinal cord. The outcome of surgery and its role in multidisciplinary management are described in the sections for each individual type of tumor. Table 24-4 gives an overview of the outcomes of the most common spinal cord tumors by treatment modality.

Surgical Planning

Neuroimaging is the basis for preoperative planning of the surgical approach. MRI obtained both before and after the administration of intravenous gadolinium-based contrast agents is most often the imaging modality of choice as it is the most sensitive modality for detecting tumor and frequently best delineates tumor from reactive changes such as a syrinx. CT scans are most useful for delineating bony anatomy, acute blood, and intratumoral calcifications in the rarer instances (e.g., meningioma, hemorrhagic hemangioblastoma) when this is significant. When MRI is not available, CT, myelogram, and CT myelogram provide the best alternatives to MRI.

Spinal angiography is occasionally necessary to distinguish spinal cord tumors from vascular malformations such as dural arteriovenous malformation which may mimic them clinically and on MRI. Angiography is potentially useful for surgical planning when tumor resection may require sacrifice of radicular arteries. Identifying the primary radicular artery supplying the anterior spinal artery, that is, the artery of Adamkiewicz, is occasionally of concern, particularly in the lower thoracic spine. Resection of vascular tumors (such as hemangioblastoma) is occasionally made safer by preoperative endovascular embolization. Balanced against the potential benefits of spinal angiography are risks of embolic complications modestly greater than those for cerebral angiography.

The use of the operating microscope is essential for spinal cord tumor surgery. The availability of other surgical adjuncts, including image-guided navigation systems, intraoperative ultrasonography, CO_2 laser, and Cavitron Ultrasonic Surgical Aspirator (CUSA) are of value for selected tumors. Ultrasonography may be particularly useful for examining the spinal cord through an intact or open dura to assess the level of maximum tumor involvement and to differentiate solid tumors from tumor cysts.

Corticosteroids are routinely administered before, during, and after surgery to minimize edema of the spinal cord. Intravenous or oral dexamethasone or high-dose intravenous methylprednisolone are most often the agents of choice. One caveat is necessary: In the case of lymphoma, administration of preoperative steroids may result in disappearance of the tumor by the time of surgery (the "ghost-tumor" effect).[28–31] If lymphoma is suspected, corticosteroids should be withheld (if clinically appropriate) until the diagnosis is confirmed. In other cases, the length of time for which steroids are used and the speed of the corticosteroid taper is dictated by the clinical symptoms. Once maximum symptom resolution has occurred—usually approximately 7 days after beginning high-dose glucocorticoids—tapering steroids as rapidly as possible without resultant symptomatic worsening is the guiding principle as this minimizes the chance for and the extent of the numerous serious side effects of these agents.

Multiple modalities are available for intraoperative monitoring of physiologic function. The most commonly used are sensory-evoked response and electromyogram (EMG). Motor-evoked response is more difficult to monitor

▶ TABLE 24-4. OUTCOMES OF THE MOST COMMON SPINAL CORD TUMORS BY TREATMENT MODALITY

	Treatment	OS_3	OS_5	OS_{10}	CSS_5	CSS_{10}	CSS_{15}	DFS_5	DFS_{10}	DFS_{15}	LC_3	LC_5	LC_{10}	Overall LC
Low-grade glioma	GTR or STR + XRT		57%–88%	52%–83%				38%–44%	10%–26%					31%–100%
Ependymoma	Surgery		67%–100%	68%–100%	69%–96%	62%–93%								95%–100%
	Surgery + XRT		67%–100%	67%–100%	69%–97%	62%	46%	59%	59%					88%–100%
Meningioma	GTR or STR + XRT							93%	80%	68%				94%–99%
	STR alone							63%	45%	9%				
Chordoma	Surgery + XRT	88%–97%	75%–80%	54%							67%–71%	40%–75%	54%	
Chondro-sarcomas				90%				36%–72%	84%					97%

The numbers in subscript denote the number of years. References are found in the text.
CSS = cause-specific survival; DFS = disease-free survival; GTR = gross total resection; LC = local control; OS = overall survival; STR = subtotal resection; XRT = radiation therapy.

reliably as it is more sensitive to paralytic agents used in most anesthetic regimens and requires the use of sophisticated stimuli such as transcranial magnetic stimulation that may be difficult to calibrate in the operating room. Evoked responses monitor the long tracts. Outcome data are not available proving superiority of intraoperative-evoked response monitoring. However, for extramedullary tumors reversible vascular compromise can sometimes be identified before permanent damage results. For intramedullary tumors, compromise is less likely to be reversible by intraoperative maneuvers. EMG employs both recording of spontaneous or mechanically induced muscle activity and direct, intraoperative electrical stimulation of nerves. It is of particular use for cauda equina and foramen magnum tumors where monitoring of the extremity musculature, the anal, and sometimes the urinary, sphincter can reduce the risk of postoperative deficits.

Surgery of Intradural Extramedullary Tumors

Meningiomas and schwannomas (neurilemomas) occur in the intradural extramedullary spinal compartment.[32] Most of these tumors can be completely resected with curative intent because the normal spinal cord is not invaded by tumor.[33]

Meningiomas in most patients can be removed through a posterior (laminectomy) approach, because they are commonly lateral or anterolateral, and even the more anteriorly placed tumors cause enough lateral displacement of the spinal cord to allow access for resection without traction on the spinal cord. If the tumor is located anterior to the spinal cord, it may require an anterior approach including corpectomy—that is, removal of a vertebral body—with arthrodesis using cadaveric, locally harvested, anterolateral, or posterolateral approach. Anteriorly situated meningiomas are sometimes unresectable because of their encasement of the anterior spinal or at the foramen magnum of a vertebral artery.[33]

Schwannomas arise from spinal rootlets (most often the dorsal rootlets). Thus, resection requires removal of sections of the involved rootlets. Schwannomas may grow along the nerve root in a dumbbell fashion through a neural foramen. Some of these extraspinal tumor extensions can be removed by extending the initial laminectomy exposure laterally, while others must be resected at a separate or combined operation through a thoracotomy, a costotransversectomy, or a retroperitoneal approach.[33]

Surgery of Intramedullary Tumors

The most common intramedullary tumors are ependymomas and astrocytomas. Modern series advocate maximum safe resection of intramedullary spinal tumors. The ability to resect these tumors completely varies widely from less than 10% to as high as 86%.[34–43] This is dependent on histology: the gross total resection rates for ependymomas range from 19% to 100%, whereas 0 to 43% of astrocytomas are resectable. The majority of completely resectable lesions are WHO grade I because higher grades are defined by their infiltrative potential.[39,44–62] For infiltrative astrocytomas the role of surgery is most frequently limited to biopsy for diagnosis. Laminectomy also offers limited functional benefit by decompressing the spinal cord in the case of bulky, infiltrative tumors. Functional postoperative outcomes may be excellent in selected cases, with the majority of patients (72%–79%) experiencing either improvement or stabilization of their preoperative presenting symptoms after often transient postsurgical worsening.[34,35,42,43,58,63–65] The incidence of total, permanent, postoperative paralysis is reported to be 1%.[27] Paralysis is, unfortunately, often the result of unpredictable vascular events that occur sporadically and that cannot be eliminated by current technology.

Intramedullary tumors are almost always approached through a laminectomy exposure with the patient in the prone position.[27] For cervical tumors the head is generally secured using a three-point clamp affixed to the skull. After the dura is opened, a longitudinal myelotomy is made over the widened region of the spinal cord where imaging demonstrates the closest approximation of the tumor to the surface and the incision is deepened several millimeters until the tumor surface is reached. Preferred myelotomy routes include the midline and the dorsal root entry zones, as these minimize transaction of long tracts. Dissection planes around the tumor are sought microsurgically and, if found, are extended gradually around the tumor surface, because removal of the central tumor bulk (by CO_2 laser, the combination of bipolar cautery and suction, or CUSA) causes the tumor to collapse. Internal debulking may, however be necessary for larger tumors or those with a well-defined capsule. Usually, such tumors can be completely resected.

Infiltrative tumors with poorly defined dissection planes cannot be removed completely and, therefore, biopsy for diagnosis is often the safest course of action. When there is an exophytic component to the tumor, maximum safe debulking is typically performed, that is, resection of as much tumor as possible to alleviate any preoperative signs and symptoms, while preserving neurologic function.

Ependymomas offer particular challenges and opportunities for the surgeon because they arise near the center of the spinal cord and because complete removal has the potential to result in cure. The potential for cure may increase the severity of a hopefully transient deficit that surgeon and patient may be willing to incur. This illustrates the importance of preoperative communication between surgeon, other physicians, and patient to allow balancing short-term risks and longer-term potential benefits. Because ependymal cells are found lining the central canal, ependymomas are often found with an associated syrinx, most often inferior to the body of the tumor. Tumor removal may be aided by working within the syrinx cavity where the tumor appears as a nodule in the wall.

Hemangioblastomas are extremely vascular tumors occurring in the spinal intramedullary compartment. The dorsal location of most of these lesions and the commonly associated cyst help to simplify the removal somewhat as the cyst provides a safe route to approach the tumor. Removal of enhancing tumor is satisfactory to prevent reaccumulation of the cyst, and the remainder of the cyst wall may, therefore, be left intact. Tumor margins are addressed first and feeding arteries are coagulated. Then the tumor is dissected and removed en bloc.

Both intra- and, more rarely, extramedullary tumors can be associated with a CSF-filled syrinx dilating the central canal. The preferred treatment is tumor removal. If this is not possible, even modest shrinkage of the tumor as a result of radiation can stabilize or even reduce the size of a syrinx. Postoperatively a syrinx can form from scarring in the central canal. When an enlarging syrinx as demonstrated by serial neuroimaging studies correlates with progressive neurologic deficits, a syrinx drainage procedure may be warranted. Unfortunately, the resultant improvement in neurologic function is often less than hoped and the apparent benefit is stabilization or slowing of the decline in function. A choice of procedures is available to drain a syrinx. The first is simple marsupialization into the subarachnoid space. Stenting with a T- or K-shaped silastic tube can alternatively be performed through a smaller midline or dorsal root entry zone myelotomy. Finally, a syrinx to peritoneal shunt using a lumboperitoneal shunting system may be employed.

Complications of Surgery

In patients who are neurologically intact before surgery, the incidence of significant acute morbidity is generally below 5% for extramedullary tumors and is as low as 5% for carefully selected patients with intramedullary tumors.[27,66] Spinal deformities, including scoliosis and kyphosis, as well as infection and CSF leakage, can occur.[66–71] The development of postlaminectomy spinal deformities represents a serious postoperative complication, occurring in up to 40% of pediatric and adolescent patients and may be observed as soon as 8 months postoperatively.[72] Adult patients with paralysis from the combined effects of tumor and treatment are at particularly high risk of developing deformities warranting consideration of prophylactic arthrodesis with implanted titanium instrumentation.

If bladder function is compromised pre- or postoperatively, early neurourologic consultation is warranted. Improved management to prevent neurourologic complications of spinal cord tumors may, in fact, be responsible for much of the improvement in outcomes over the last 50 years. Intermittent self-catheterization is often the most desirable strategy until or unless bladder function returns as measured by urodynamic studies.

Radiation Therapy: General Principles

The intent of radiation therapy in the treatment of spinal cord tumors is to improve local control, possibly increase survival, and improve neurologic function.[73–75] This section discusses general principles of radiation therapy for lesions depending on anatomic location within the spinal cord. Outcomes of radiation therapy and its role in multidisciplinary management are described in the sections for each individual type of tumor. Because of the potential for growth and developmental side effects, the use of radiation therapy in children and infants with spinal cord tumors is controversial. Some authors do not recommend postoperative radiation therapy, suggesting that observation with close imaging followup, and re-resection at the time of second occurrence, is a better approach.[34,76] With this strategy, radiation therapy may be avoided or used only for children with multiply recurrent tumors.

Definitions of Treatment Volumes and Reporting of Dose

Treatment planning is based on three-dimensional volumes of interest, described by the International Commission on Radiation Units and Measurements (ICRU).[77,78] Gross tumor volume (GTV) represents the grossly visible disease burden.[78] Typically, this is the T_1-enhancing abnormality on MRI, or nonenhancing tumor seen on T_2 or FLAIR images. If there is no residual abnormality after a surgical resection, the tumor resection cavity is defined to be the GTV. Surrounding edema is not considered part of the GTV. Clinical target volume (CTV) is the T_2 or FLAIR abnormality (which does include edema) on MRI, as well as any areas potentially containing microscopic disease.[78] The planning target volume (PTV) adds a dosimetric margin, which takes into account variations in size, shape, and position of the CTV in relation to anatomic reference points, as well as uncertainties in daily treatment setup.[78] The target is usually considered to be appropriately treated if the PTV is enclosed within the 95% to 105% isodose lines. For plans emphasizing homogeneous dose delivery, the ICRU recommends that no more than 20% of the PTV should exceed 110% of the prescription dose.[77,78] However, because the spinal cord is exquisitely sensitive to both total dose and dose per fraction (Table 24-5), these factors must also be taken into consideration when deciding how much heterogeneity of dose is tolerable.

Organs at risk (OAR) are critical normal structures whose radiation sensitivity and proximity to the CTV may significantly influence the prescribed dose and the treatment-planning strategy. These typically include the thyroid and salivary glands, esophagus, lungs, heart, stomach, small bowel, liver, kidneys, bladder, ovaries, testicles, and the uninvolved portions of the spinal cord itself. The volume receiving more than the accepted tolerance dose should be evaluated from dose–volume histograms.

▶ TABLE 24-5. FRACTIONATION SCHEMES WITH A 5% RISK OF RADIATION-INDUCED SPINAL CORD MYELOPATHY

Dose Per Fraction (Gy)	Number of Fractions	Total Dose (Gy)
2.00	29	58.00
3.00	13	39.00
3.30	11	33.00
4.00	7	28.00
5.00	5	25.00
10.00	1	10.00

Source: From Marcus RB Jr, Million RR[86]; Cohen L, Creditor M[89]; Macbeth FR, et al[90]; Wara WM, et al[91]; Niewald M, et al[92]; Ang KK, et al[93]; Nieder C, et al[254]; McCunniff AJ, Liang MJ[255];Schultheiss TE[256]; Jeremic B, et al.[257]

Treatment Techniques

The most common treatment approaches include a single posterior (PA) field, opposed lateral fields, a PA field with opposed laterals, and oblique wedge-pair fields.[55,79] They are typically designed to treat the CTV and GTV. Table 24-6 gives suggested definitions of GTV and CTV by diagnosis.

For tumors in the cervicothoracic region, a split-beam approach is often used. The central axis is placed just above the shoulders. Opposed lateral fields are used to treat the upper spine, while a PA field is used for the area of the spine below. Tumors in the thoracic region are often treated with a three-field approach using a PA field and opposed lateral beams. In the lumbar region, care must be taken to minimize dose to the kidneys;

▶ TABLE 24-6. SUGGESTED DEFINITIONS OF ICRU VOLUMES BASED ON MRI

Diagnosis	Initial Treatment Field (CTV)	Final Field (to GTV)
WHO grade I glioma	(n/a)	Enhancing tumor (T_1 + C) 1-cm margin
WHO grade II glioma	Enhancing tumor (T_1 + C) Edema (T_2/FLAIR) 2-cm margin	Enhancing tumor (T_1 + C) 2-cm margin
WHO grades III–IV glioma	Enhancing tumor (T_1 + C) Edema (T_2/FLAIR) 2-cm margin	Enhancing tumor (T_1 + C) 2-cm margin
Ependymoma	Enhancing tumor (T_1 + C) Edema (T_2/FLAIR) 2-cm margin	Enhancing tumor (T_1 + C) 2-cm margin
Meningioma, benign/atypical	(n/a)	Enhancing tumor (T_1 + C) 1-cm margin
Meningioma, malignant	Enhancing tumor (T_1 + C) Edema (T_2/FLAIR) 2-cm margin	Enhancing tumor (T_1 + C) 2-cm margin
Chordoma	Enhancing tumor (T_1 + C) Tumor bed 2-cm margin	Enhancing tumor (T_1 + C) 2-cm margin
Chondrosarcoma	Enhancing tumor (T_1 + C) Tumor bed 2-cm margin	Enhancing tumor (T_1 + C) 2-cm margin
Sarcoma	Enhancing tumor (T_1 + C) Tumor bed Surgical track, including scar 2-cm margin	Enhancing tumor (T_1 + C) 2-cm margin
Vertebral hemangioma	Enhancing vascular lesion Entire involved vertebral body ≥1-cm margin	(n/a)
Metastasis	Enhancing tumor (T_1 + C) Tumor bed Surgical track, including scar One vertebral body above and below	(n/a)

+C = with contrast; CTV = clinical target volume; GTV = gross tumor volume; ICRU = International Commission on Radiation Units and Measurements.

a four-field approach using anterior/posterior (AP/PA) and opposed lateral beams with the AP/PA beams preferentially weighted may be useful. Comparison of differing treatment setups by means of dose–volume histograms (as described above) is strongly recommended.

Certain neoplasms, such as medulloblastomas and other primitive neuroectodermal tumors, as well as some ependymomas and germ cell tumors, require treatment to the entire craniospinal axis. Several modifications of this approach are used in clinical practice.[80] Patients may be treated either in the supine or prone position, often in an immobilization cast to ensure daily positional reproducibility. The intracranial contents, including the upper one or two segments of the cervical cord, are treated through opposed lateral fields. Customized blocks protect the normal head and neck tissues from the primary radiation beam. The spine is treated through one or two posterior fields, depending on the size of the patient. In one method, the collimator for the lateral cranial fields is angled to match the divergence of the upper border of the adjacent spinal field, and the treatment couch is angled so that the inferior border of the cranial field is perpendicular to the superior edge of the spinal field. Alternatively, one may dispense with collimator and couch angles by calculating appropriate gaps. The gap is calculated so that the 50% isodose lines meet at the level of the anterior spinal cord. All junction lines are moved 0.5 to 1.0 cm every 8 to 10 Gy to avoid overdosing or underdosing segments of the cord. This is accomplished by shortening the inferior margin of the lateral cranial fields, symmetrically lengthening the superior and inferior margins of the posterior spine field, and shortening the cranial margin of the caudal spinal field; a fixed block is placed at the inferior margin of the caudal spinal field to keep the lower margin of the irradiated volume at the same location (Fig. 24-2).

Intensity-modulated radiation therapy (IMRT) is a treatment delivery method that can be used to further optimize the dose distribution. There are two aspects of treatment that theoretically might benefit from the use of IMRT.

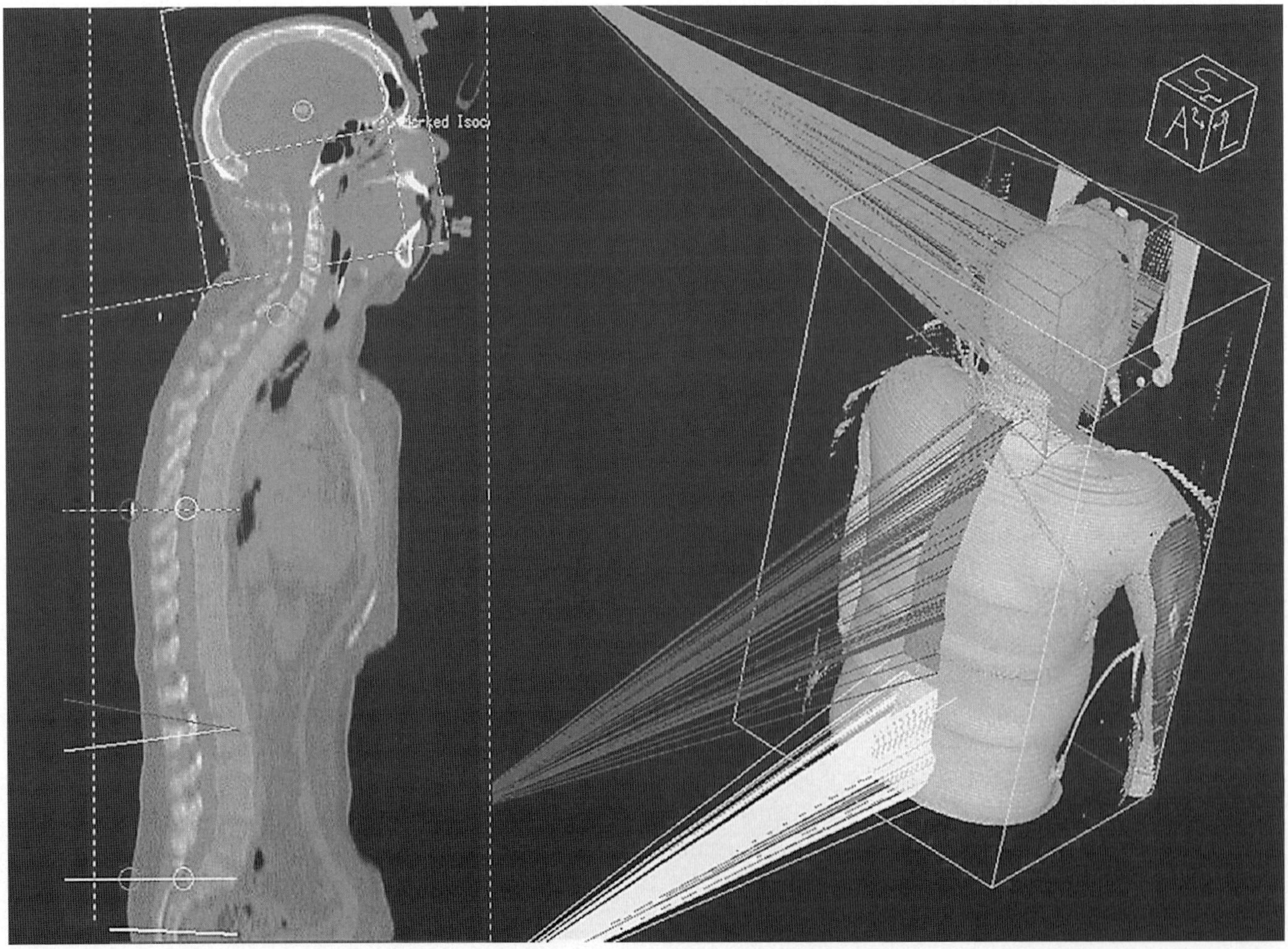

Figure 24-2. Two- and three-dimensional treatment planning images of craniospinal axis radiation therapy. Details of the treatment setup may be found in the accompanying text.

First, because multiple critical sensitive organs are located near the spinal cord, one may reason that improved dose distribution should allow the dose to these structures to be minimized. Second, because most spinal cord tumors typically recur locally, IMRT should allow the exploration of anatomic/biologic treatment planning and delivery in order to optimize different doses to different cell populations within heterogeneous volumes.[81] The use of IMRT is currently under investigation at multiple institutions.

Stereotactic radiosurgery (SRS) of spinal cord lesions remains experimental at this time.[82,83] The limiting factor is the dose per fraction that can be safely delivered to the normal spinal cord (see Table 24-5). Recent progress combining "live" tumor imaging[84] with stereotactic repositioning[85] makes single-fraction SRS or fractionated stereotactic radiosurgery a promising field of research.

Selecting Radiation Therapy Doses

Table 24-7 gives an overview of the typical doses delivered to the ICRU volumes by diagnosis. Details and references are given in the sections for each individual diagnosis.

Tolerance of the Spinal Cord and Lumbosacral Nerve Roots

A dose of 45 to 50.4 Gy in 25 to 28 fractions over 5 to 5.5 weeks usually is considered to be safe, with the risk of myelopathy less than 1%, well below the steep portion of the dose–response curve.[86–87] It is estimated that with conventionally fractionated irradiation (1.8 to 2.0 Gy per fraction, 5 fractions per week), at 5 years the incidence of myelopathy is 5% for doses in the range of 57 to 61 Gy (tolerance dose $[TD]_{5/5}$) and 50% for doses of 68 to 73 Gy ($TD_{50/5}$).[87] There is no convincing evidence that the cervical and thoracic cords differ in their radiosensitivity, and there appears to be little change in tolerance with variations in the length of cord irradiated.[87] Typically, half of the patients who develop radiation-induced myelopathy in the cervical or thoracic cord region will do so within 20 months of treatment, and 75% of the cases will occur within 30 months.[88] Table 24-5 shows a range of isomorbid fractionation schemes, all of which carry a 5% risk of radiation myelopathy.[86,89–93] There is no known consistently effective treatment for radiation myelitis.[94,95] The probability of dying from radiation myelopathy is approximately 70% in cervical lesions and 30% with thoracic spinal cord injury.[96]

The tolerance of the lumbosacral nerve roots appears to be somewhat higher than that of the spinal cord. Most series report a 0% complication rate if patients are treated to doses of 70 Gy (or equivalent) as long as fraction sizes are kept at or below 2 Gy.[97–99]

Complications of Treatment

Radiation myelopathy may present as a transient early delayed or as a late delayed reaction. Transient radiation myelopathy is clinically manifested by momentary, electrical shock–like paresthesias or numbness radiating from the neck to the extremities, precipitated by neck flexion (Lhermitte sign).[100] The syndrome typically develops 3 to 4 months after treatment, and spontaneously resolves over the following 3 to 6 months without therapy. It is attributed to transient demyelination caused by radiation-induced

▶ TABLE 24-7. SUGGESTED DOSE RANGES (IN GRAY) TO ICRU VOLUMES

Diagnosis	Clinical Target Volume	Gross Tumor Volume	Craniospinal Axis (if indicated)
WHO grade I glioma	(n/a)	45–50.4 Gy	(n/a)
WHO grade II glioma	45 Gy	50.4–54 Gy	(n/a)
WHO grades III–IV glioma	45–50.4 Gy	55.8–59.4 Gy	Leptomeningeal spread on MRI: 30–39.6 Gy Bulky disease: 55.8–59.4 Gy
Ependymoma	45 Gy	50.4–55.8 Gy	Negative CSF: 30 Gy Positive CSF: 36 Gy Leptomeningeal spread on MRI: 39.6 Gy Bulky disease: 54 Gy
Meningioma, benign/atypical	(n/a)	52.2–55.8 Gy	(n/a)
Meningioma, malignant	45–50.4 Gy	55.8–59.4 Gy	(n/a)
Chordoma	50 Gy	60–70 Gy	(n/a)
Chondrosarcoma	50 Gy	60–70 Gy	(n/a)
Sarcoma	50 Gy	60–70 Gy	(n/a)
Vertebral hemangioma	(n/a)	36–45 Gy	(n/a)
Metastasis	30–37.5 Gy	(n/a)	(n/a)

inhibition of myelin-producing oligodendroglial cells in the irradiated spinal cord segment.[100–102]

Irreversible radiation myelopathy typically is not seen earlier than 6 to 12 months after completion of treatment. It is thought to be multifactorial, involving demyelination and white matter necrosis, ultimately caused by oligodendroglial cell depletion and microvascular injury. The signs and symptoms are typically progressive over several months, but acute onset of plegia over several hours or a few days is possible. The diagnosis of radiation myelopathy is one of exclusion, which first requires a history of radiation therapy in doses sufficient to result in injury. The region of the irradiated cord must lie slightly above the dermatome level of expression of the lesion, the latent period from the completion of treatment to the onset of injury must be consistent with that observed in radiation myelopathy, and local tumor progression must be ruled out. There are no pathognomonic laboratory tests or imaging studies that conclusively diagnose radiation myelopathy. MRI findings include swelling of the spinal cord with hyperintensity on the T_2-weighted images with or without areas of contrast enhancement.[102,103]

Radiation side effects in children include growth abnormalities, such as decreased vertebral height, kyphosis, and scoliosis.[104] Secondary malignancies, including bone or soft-tissue sarcomas and glioblastomas multiforme, have been reported after irradiation of spinal cord tumors.[105–107] Radiation injury is discussed further in Chapter 32.

Treatment Toxicity Scoring

Several toxicity scoring systems are in use. The most commonly accepted are the National Cancer Institute's Common Terminology Criteria for Adverse Events (NCI CTCAE), version 3, and the Late Effects Toxicity Scoring of the EORTC, known as the LENT/SOMA (*l*ate *e*ffects on *n*ormal *t*issues, with four components: *s*ubjective, *o*bjective, *m*anagement, and *a*nalytical) scale.[108,109]

The purpose of the NCI CTCAE v3.0 is to standardize reporting of adverse events across groups and modalities by describing category, adverse event, grades, and attribution.[108] All adverse events are integrated into one document without distinguishing between acute, late, chronic, or permanent adverse events. This separates the definition of adverse events based on description and severity from the temporal component of the adverse event. Thus, serial evaluations of the presence and severity of an adverse event, instead of the grade of an adverse event, address the longevity of an adverse event. CTCAE v3.0, whenever possible, has also removed modality-based definitions for adverse events. The LENT-SOMA scale takes into account any interventions that attempt to treat a late effect.[109] It is designed to allow comparison between data sets of the clinical perception of injury, the patient's view of treatment efficacy, the medical measures that are available and implementable to correct the idiopathic injuries, and the underlying pathophysiology.

Chemotherapy: General Principles

The efficacy of chemotherapy agents may be limited by the intact blood–nervous system barrier. Regional drug delivery may be in the form of intra-CSF therapy, intraarterial infusion, and intratumoral therapy.[110] Extramedullary spinal tumors gain their blood supply from meningeal blood vessels that are significantly more permeable than those of the brain, and chemotherapy may be of more use for these tumors. Drugs with some efficacy in treating primary CNS malignancies,[111] and which are thought to cross the blood–brain barrier, have been used in the treatment of malignant glial tumors of the spinal cord; however, no clear benefit from the use of chemotherapy has been demonstrated thus far.[49,112–120]

▶ THERAPEUTIC MANAGEMENT: BY HISTOLOGY

Astrocytoma

General Background

Astrocytomas (Figs. 24-3 and 24-4) represent approximately 7% to 11% of all primary spinal tumors. They are the most common intramedullary spinal cord tumors and comprise 35% to 45% of all reported cases. The median age at presentation is approximately 35 years.[16,39,44,74] There does not appear to be a difference in the age of presentation between low- and high-grade tumors.[39] In children, 75% to 90% of intramedullary spinal cord tumors are astrocytomas and 85% to 95% of these are low-grade, fibrillary or juvenile pilocytic astrocytomas. Fewer than 10% of pediatric and 25% of adult spinal cord astrocytomas are malignant.[27,34–36,38,39,42,44,63,121–127]

Weakness is the most common presenting symptom in astrocytomas, occurring in up to 87% of patients. The median time from onset of symptoms to diagnosis ranges from 6 months to 2 years.[39,44,55,65,72,73,75] In general, high-grade astrocytomas tend to have a shorter prodrome (median duration: 1.6–7 months) than low-grade tumors (median duration: 2 years).[16,39,42] Tumor dissemination by spread along the subarachnoid space is reported in up to 58% of patients with high-grade astrocytomas.[16,128] Approximately 1% of WHO grades III to IV spinal cord astrocytomas have multifocal disease at presentation.[8]

Prognostic Factors

The most significant prognostic factors in patients with primary spinal cord astrocytomas are tumor histology, grade, and performance status.[34,36,40,51,53,74,126,129] High histopathologic grade is typically associated with a high risk of mortality and a short median survival time. The 10-year overall survival rate of patients with pilocytic astrocytomas is 81% in contrast to 15% for patients with diffuse fibrillary astrocytic tumors.[55] For patients with WHO grades I to II

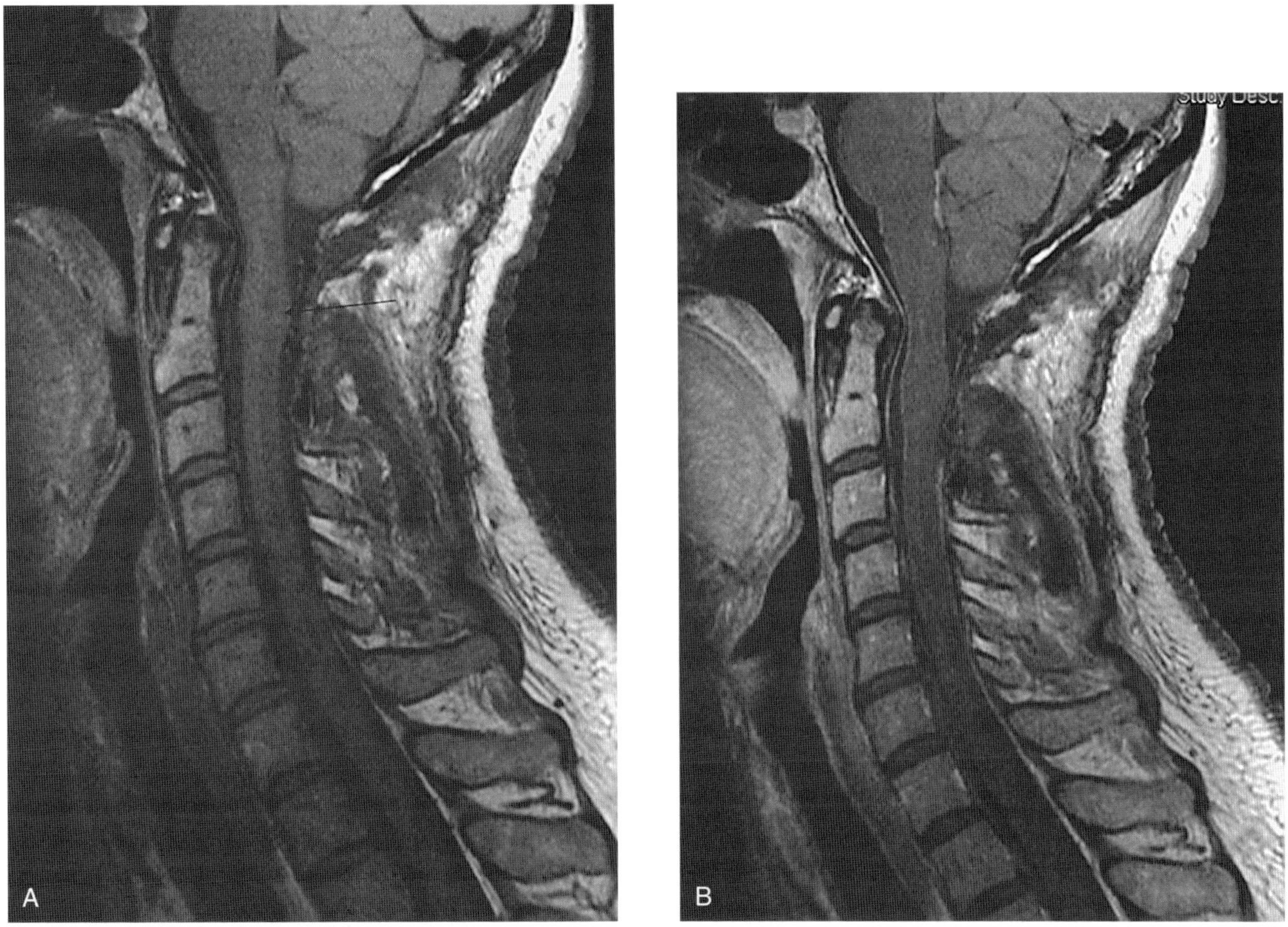

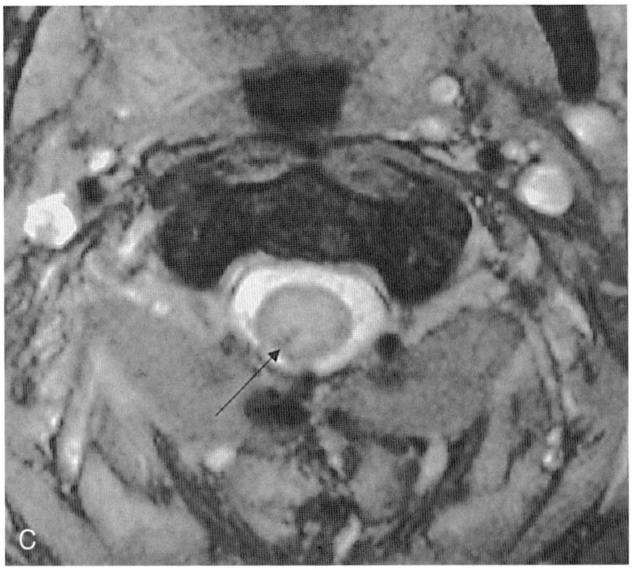

Figure 24-3. Diffuse fibrillary low-grade astrocytoma. A 50-year-old woman presented with a 2-year history of neck pain, left periscapular pain, and intermittent left arm weakness. Cervical MRI demonstrated a C2 intramedullary mass that was isointense on T_1-weighted imaging (A and B) and hyperintense on T_2-weighted imaging. There was focal expansion of the spinal cord (A, arrow) and minimal, if any, enhancement (B). A T_2-weighted axial image demonstrated a small biopsy defect just right of the midline (C, arrow).

spinal cord astrocytomas, the 5-year survival rates are 69% to 89%, but only 0% to 33% for WHO grades III to IV lesions;[73–75] the latter have a median survival time of approximately 6 months.[16] Other factors thought to be prognostic are young age (younger than age 18 years living the longest, whereas those older than age 40 years do poorly); the pattern of failure (local vs. disseminated, the latter developing in approximately 60% of all patients

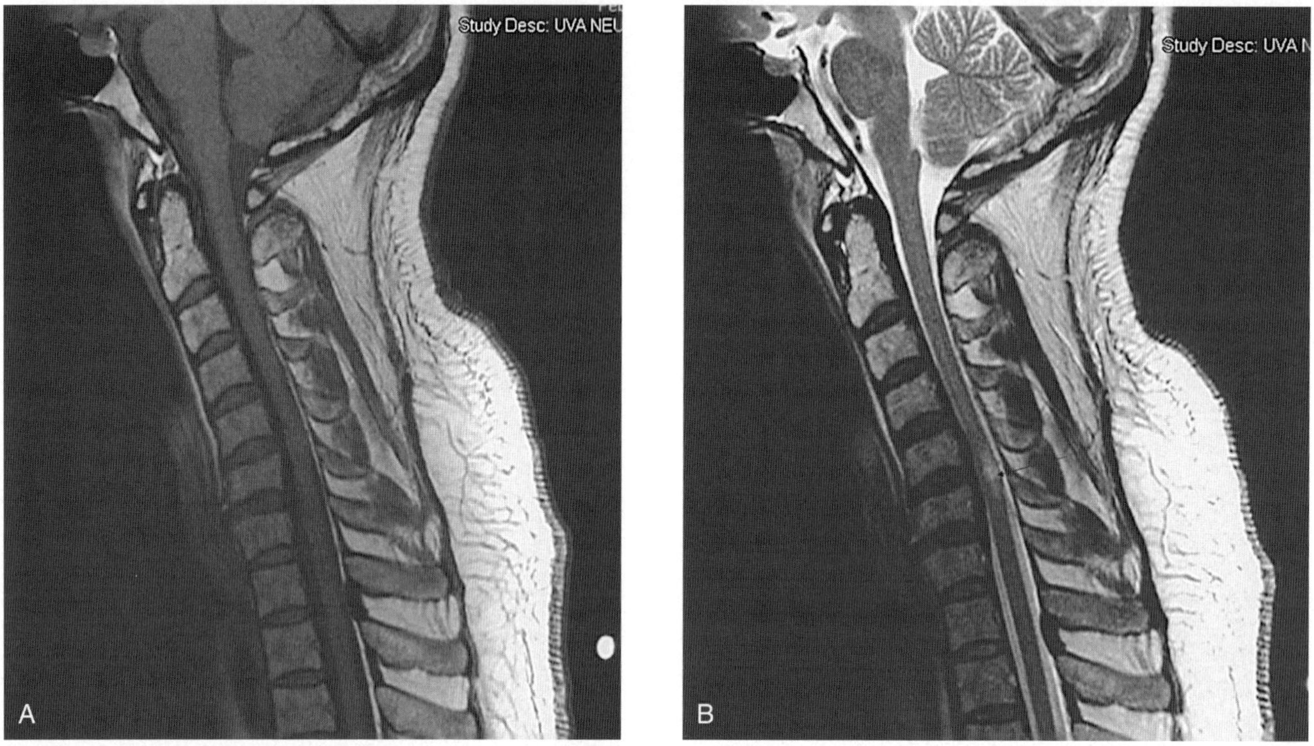

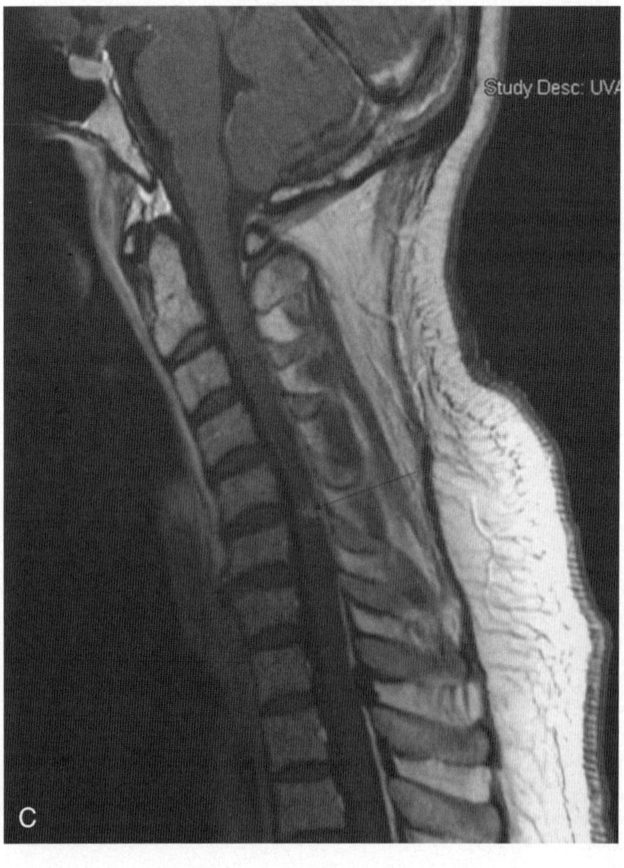

Figure 24-4. Cervical pilocytic astrocytoma. A 39-year-old male presented with sensory dysesthesias in all extremities. Cervical MRI demonstrates a paracentral intramedullary lesion at the C5–6 level (A and B). Some surrounding T_2-weighted hyperintensity suggesting mild edema was noted (B, arrow). There was intense, nodular contrast enhancement following intravenous gadolinium administration (C, arrow).

with high-grade tumors); and duration of symptoms prior to diagnosis (<6 months vs. >6 months, with short duration doing worse).[40,47–49,121,130] In most authors' series, neither extent of resection nor adjuvant radiation therapy appears to be prognostic,[27,47,48,51,52,55,74] although this is controversial and approaches statistical significance in some series.[54,55,74]

Treatment and Outcomes

Surgery

The treatment of choice for intramedullary astrocytomas is as complete an excision of the tumor as possible, providing this can be accomplished without a compromise in neurologic function. If this is not feasible, an incomplete excision is typically performed for grade I lesions and biopsy alone is the surgical strategy for the nonexophytic component of an infiltrative glioma. Gross total resection (GTR) is typically extremely difficult to achieve because of the infiltrative nature of all but the pilocytic lesions, with most authors reporting between 0% and 50% likelihood of GTR for spinal cord astrocytoma.[37,40,41,44,45,48–50,52,54,74,131]

In patients with favorable prognostic factors (low-grade histology, good performance status, and young age) observation with serial imaging studies, reserving radiation therapy for local recurrence, is an appropriate management option, particularly for young children.[27,125] In the remainder of patients, adjuvant radiation therapy is usually recommended.[34,39,40,45,126,129]

Radiation Therapy

Patients who undergo subtotal resection or biopsy of a low-grade glioma often receive subsequent radiation therapy, because progression of tumor in the spinal cord may lead to significant neurologic impairment. In the setting of intracerebral low-grade glioma, randomized trial data demonstrate that radiation therapy does not alter survival but increases the disease-free interval.[132] There does not appear to be a dose–response relationship between 45 and 64.8 Gy for cerebral low-grade glioma,[133,134] nor is there a suggestion of such in the treatment of spinal cord astrocytoma. Therefore, doses have traditionally been based on the experience with cerebral tumors.[133–136] The overall outcomes are similar for patients with low-grade gliomas of the spinal cord treated either by GTR or subtotal resection/biopsy followed by radiation therapy, with most series reporting overall survival rates at 5 and 10 years in the ranges of 57% to 88% and 52% to 83%, respectively, and disease-free survival rates of 38% to 44% and 26% at 5 and 10 years, respectively. Overall long-term local control rates range from 31% to 100%.[47,48,50,53–55,74,126,137] With high-grade tumors in adults and children, median survival time is quite poor (4–10 months) despite surgery and radiation therapy; approximately two-thirds of patients die of both local and disseminated disease.[16,46,49,52,55,74,130,138] One small series suggested a survival benefit for patients with high-grade tumors treated with craniospinal axis irradiation.[139] Table 24-4 compares survival and local control rates.

Chemotherapy

There is no established efficacy of chemotherapy in the setting of intracerebral low-grade glioma. Meta-analysis shows a small statistical benefit with high-grade cerebral tumors.[111] Data specific to adjuvant chemotherapy (after surgery and/or radiation therapy) for spinal cord astrocytomas are scant and composed mostly of small retrospective series.[49,112,114,115,130] In two small trials, children with high-grade spinal astrocytoma had a 5-year progression-free survival of 46% to 50% and a 5-year overall survival of 54% to 88% when chemotherapy was given either in the adjuvant setting or at time of relapse.[115,130] Overall, while there is no clear evidence of a difference in outcomes with or without chemotherapy for spinal cord tumors, chemotherapy is usually given for patients with malignant astrocytoma.

Ependymoma

General Background

These glial tumors (Fig. 24-5) are approximately equal in incidence to spinal astrocytomas.[66] The mean age at presentation for patients with ependymoma is 30 to 39 years. Ependymomas are more common in adults than in children,[39,60,126,140–142] and in males than in females.[57,60,75,140,142–145] The median duration of symptoms prior to presentation is 2 to 4 years.[39,44,58,131,143,145] Two-thirds occur in the lumbosacral regions, 40% from the filum terminale.[58,140,141,145] Because of the propensity of these tumors to seed the craniospinal axis, we favor CSF evaluation and craniospinal MRI for patients diagnosed with ependymoma. It is also important to note that 11% of patients with intracranial ependymomas have documented spinal metastases, so brain imaging may be indicated to rule out a primary brain tumor.[146]

The majority of tumors are low grade.[36,44,59,126,140] Most intradural–extramedullary ependymomas are myxopapillary and are often amenable to complete surgical resection if they are not multifocal.[143,147–150] Late failures may occur more than 4 years after curative surgery, particularly with the myxopapillary subtype, so long-term followup is warranted.[145,151–153] Myxopapillary ependymomas often progress slowly and cause more mild than expected neurological deficits as a function of size.

Pathology

Ependymomas arise from ependymomal cells and typically occur in the central canal of the spinal cord, the filum terminale, and white matter adjacent to a ventricular surface.[154] Histologically, ependymomas are either low-grade tumors or anaplastic tumors (which are more likely to disseminate via the CSF). Myxopapillary ependymomas are

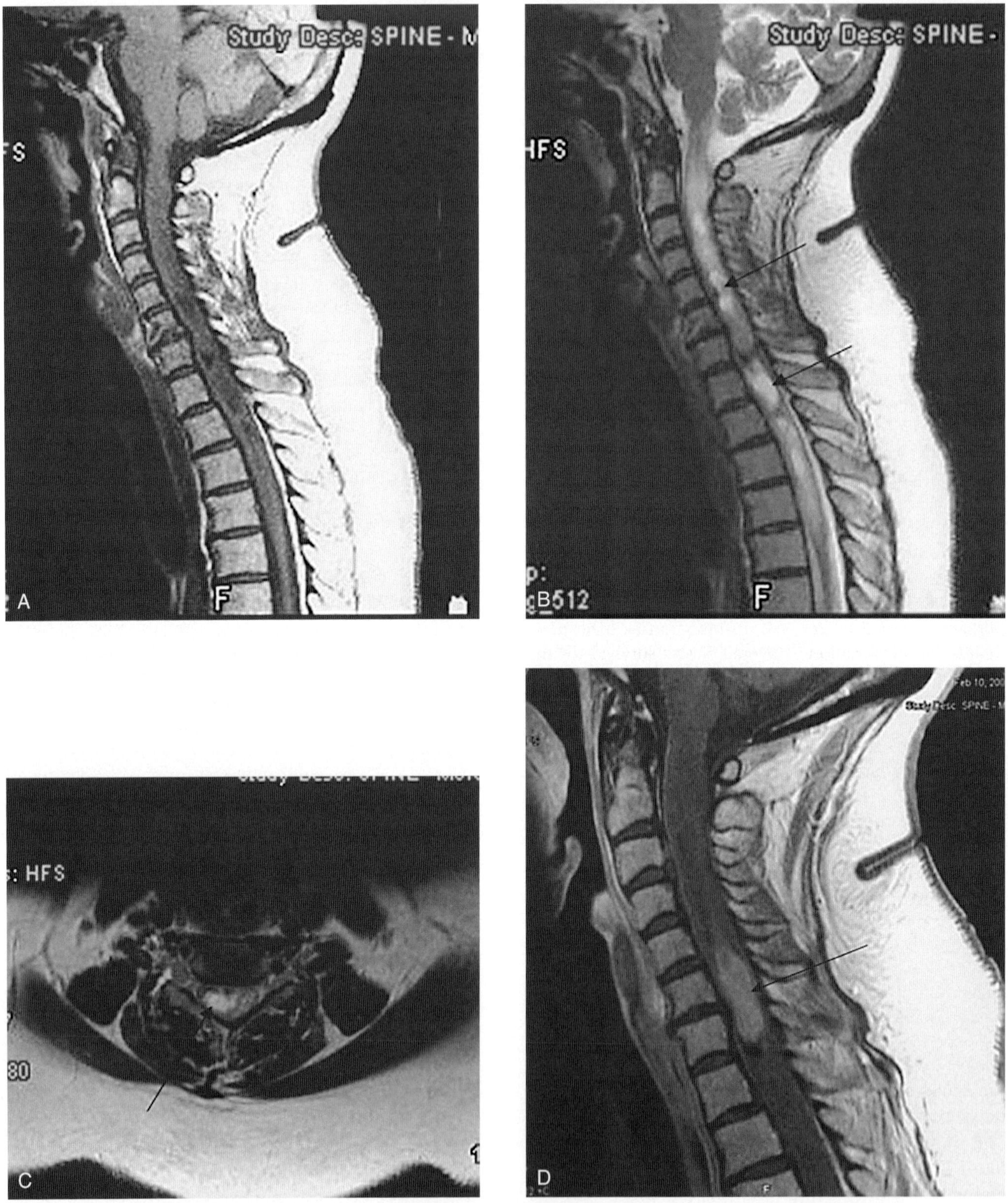

Figure 24-5. Cervical ependymoma. A 51-year-old woman presented with neck pain and right upper extremity pain. Cervical MRI demonstrated a 3.5-cm intramedullary lesion extending from the C5–6 to the C7–T1 levels (A) with perilesional cysts (B and C, arrows) associated cephalad and caudad to the lesion. A focal area of hypointensity on T_1- and T_2-weighted sequences may represent an area of hemorrhage (A, B, and C). The lesion enhanced homogeneously with intravenous gadolinium administration and appeared well-defined (D, arrow).

low-grade tumors that typically occur in the lumbosacral region (filum terminale), are well differentiated, and often encapsulated[145,150,155] but can seed the CSF,[156] typically going to the thecal sac.[150] Some series have included ependymoblastomas; however, these are primitive neuroectodermal tumors (PNETs), which have a high propensity to disseminate throughout the CNS, and therefore should be considered more in the medulloblastoma-PNET family of tumors.[157]

Prognostic Factors

Multiple potential prognostic factors for local recurrence and survival are reviewed in the literature. Factors prognostic for a favorable outcome include age (patients younger than 40 years of age), location (lumbosacral spine), histologic subtype (myxopapillary, although not all authors agree[143]), grade of the tumor (WHO grade I), extent of surgical resection (gross total or subtotal resection vs. biopsy only) and good preoperative function.[57,59,60,141,150,158–160] Whereas some authors believe that the volume of residual disease appears to correlate with a worse outcome after radiation therapy,[141,160,161] others have found no differences in outcomes when comparing complete excision to subtotal resection followed by radiation therapy.[59,159] Myxopapillary subtypes appear to be associated with a favorable prognosis perhaps because of the ease of resection as a result of their anatomic location.[57] Overall 5-year survival for the myxopapillary subtype and for WHO grade I tumors is 97% to 100%, and 5-year disease-specific survival is 97%.[158,159]

Therapy and Outcomes

Surgery

The goal of surgery is gross total resection. Every attempt should be made to remove myxopapillary tumors as a whole, as opposed to piecemeal, because of the risk of seeding, including upward seeding to the cranial nerves. Typically, complete resection is achievable in 79% to 100% of modern series.[43,45,56,58,60,62,63,131] Some authors report complete resection rates as low as 19%–50%, but these tend to be older series or those with a significant number of high-grade tumors.[37,39,44,57,141] Five and 10-year overall survival rates for all spinal cord ependymomas are 67%–100% and 68%–100%, respectively.[38,44,59–61,141,158,159] Disease-specific survival rates at 5 and 10 years are 69%–96% and 62%–93%, respectively.[39,57,126] Local control rates after gross total resection are 95% to 100%.[36,56,60] Radiation therapy is typically indicated in the case of incomplete resection, for all high-grade lesions, and for patients with craniospinal axis dissemination (positive CSF or MRI scan). In most series, the outcome for subtotal resection followed by radiation therapy appears to be similar to that of complete excision. As mentioned earlier, myxopapillary subtypes may be associated with a favorable prognosis because of their relative ease of resection.

Radiation Therapy

Postoperative radiation therapy appears to improve local control in patients with subtotally resected ependymomas.[44,57,107,141,143] In most series, the dose to the tumor bed has been 49 to 56 Gy, whereas the craniospinal axis (if indicated) has received 30 to 36 Gy.[56,59,61,158] Low-grade lesions with low risk of seeding are typically treated with limited fields to 50.4 to 55.8 Gy in 1.8 Gy daily fractions. In patients with tumors at high risk of seeding, and in those in whom pretreatment CSF cytology studies reveal malignant cells, or if the spinal MRI scan shows evidence of leptomeningeal disease, the craniospinal axis should be treated to 36 Gy in 1.5 to 1.8 Gy daily fractions. Subsequently, the primary tumor site is boosted to a total dose of 50.4 to 55.8 Gy. If gross leptomeningeal spread is evident, the craniospinal axis dose should be 39.6 Gy (1.8 Gy/fraction) or 40.5 Gy (1.5 Gy/fraction), with the same boost dose to primary as previously discussed.

In those patients undergoing incomplete resection followed by radiation therapy, overall survival rates at 5 and 10 years are 67% to 100% and 67% to 100%, respectively.[59–61,158,159] Cause-specific survival rates at 5, 10, and 15 years for all tumors are 69% to 93%, 62% to 93%, and 46%, respectively.[57,126] By tumor grade, cause-specific survival rates at 5 years are 87% to 97% for myxopapillary and low-grade lesions and 27% to 71% for high-grade tumors.[158,159] Disease-free survival rates at 5 and 10 years are 59% and 59%, respectively.[57] Local control rates are 88% to 100%.[56,59,61,159,162]

Chemotherapy

There is no strong body of evidence thus far demonstrating that the addition of chemotherapy to radiotherapy improves the outcome.[113,116–120] A single trial of etoposide for recurrent spinal ependymoma has shown a median response duration of 15 months with a median survival time of 16 months.[117] Patients who were responders had a median survival of 20 months, whereas those who did not respond lived only 4 months; the results approached statistical significance. Pediatric patients with anaplastic ependymoma or ependymoblastoma are routinely given chemotherapy, however.[163,164] Further clinical research in this area is necessary.

Meningioma

General Background

Spinal meningiomas (Fig. 24-6) make up only 8% of all meningiomas[165] but 25% to 46% of all spinal neoplasms.[68,69,165,166] They occur in females three to seven times more commonly than in males.[67,69,165–169] Most patients are older than age 40 years with the mean age at diagnosis being 49 to 63 years.[168,169] The incidence appears to be bimodal, the first peak being in the third decade of life, with a second larger peak seen after age

50 years, especially in the sixth and seventh decades of life.[168,169] In younger patients, 13% have neurofibromatosis type 2.[169] Younger patients (younger than 50 years of age) also have a recurrence rate of 23% versus a rate of 5% in older patients,[169] although not all authors agree that young age in and of itself carries a worse prognosis.[165]

The most common site is in the thoracic region, accounting for 55% to 80% of spinal meningiomas, whereas cervical lesions make up approximately 33% of all lesions.[68,69,165,167–171] The incidence by location varies with age: age 50 years and younger, 39%, 56%, and 5% occur in the cervical, thoracic, and lumbar spine, respectively; older than age 50 years, 16%, 80%, and 5% occur in the cervical, thoracic and lumbar spine, respectively.[169]

Treatment and Outcomes

Surgery

As in the brain, the mainstay of treatment of spinal meningiomas is surgical resection. Functional improvement of neurologic deficits is seen in 66% to 100% of patients.[67,68,167,168,171] Complete resection is achievable in 82% to 100% of cases, with a 1% to 6% late local failure rate.[68,69,171] With subtotal resection, late local recurrence rates range from 17% to 100%.[67–69] Local failures take place even decades after surgery: after complete resection, recurrence-free rates at 5, 10, and 15 years are 93%, 80%, and 68%, respectively; after subtotal resection, recurrence-free rates at 5, 10, and 15 years are 63%, 45%, and 9%,

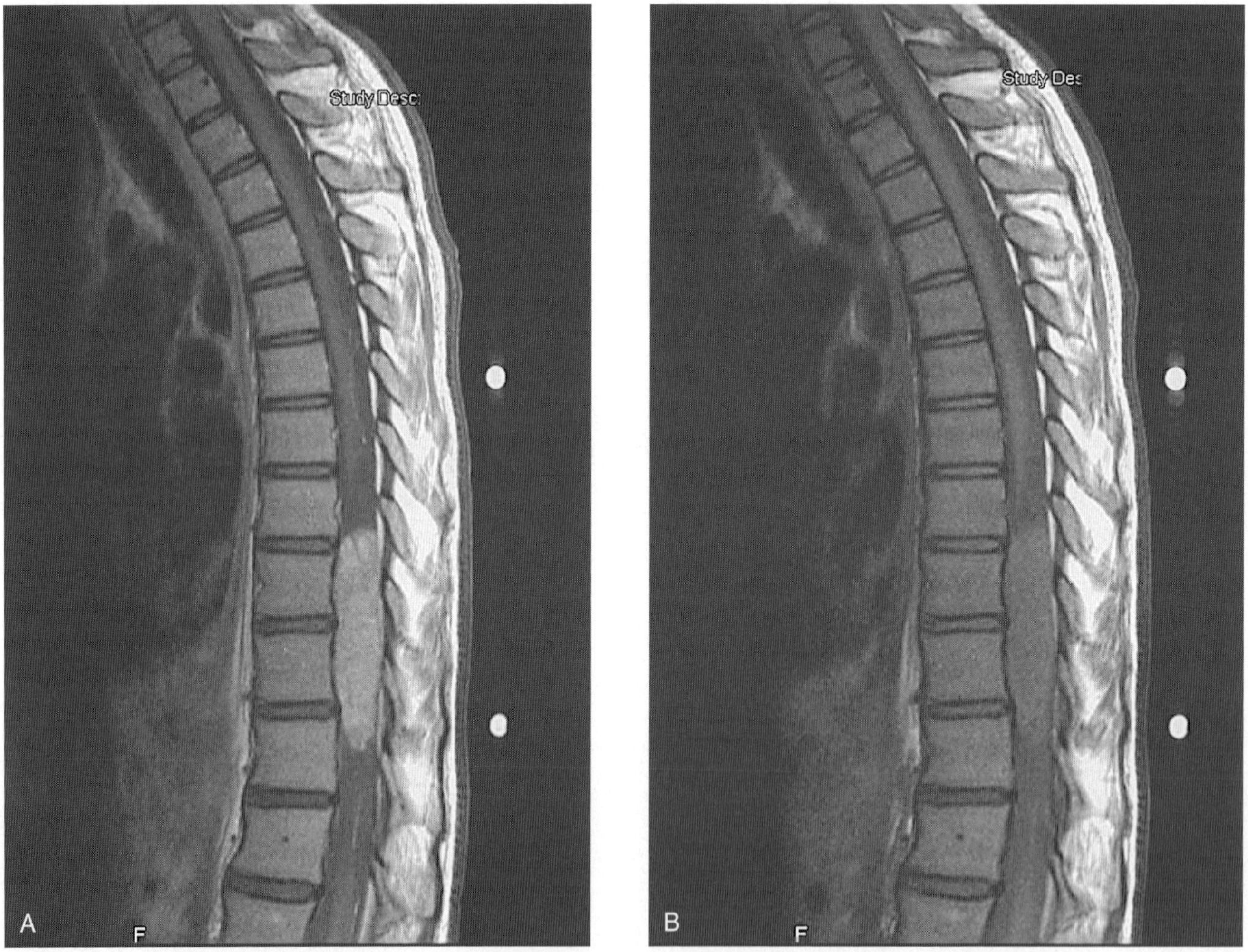

Figure 24-6. Clear-cell meningiomas. A 16-year-old female presented with back pain and mild bilateral lower-extremity weakness. Thoracic MRI demonstrated a large intradural, extramedullary mass extending from T8 to T11 (A). The mass was isointense on T_1-weighted images and inhomogeneously enhanced with intravenous gadolinium administration (A and B). Multiple additional lesions were seen on lumbar MRI, demonstrating the unique tendency for clear-cell meningiomas to disseminate via subarachnoid seeding, as opposed to their typical counterparts (C and D). (*Continued*)

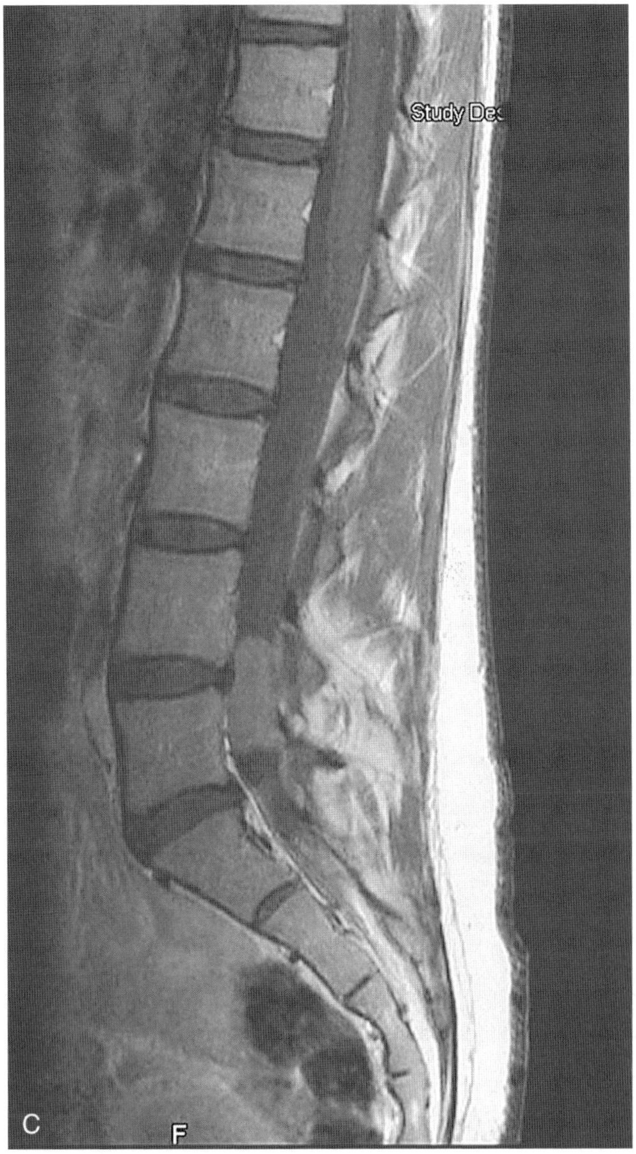

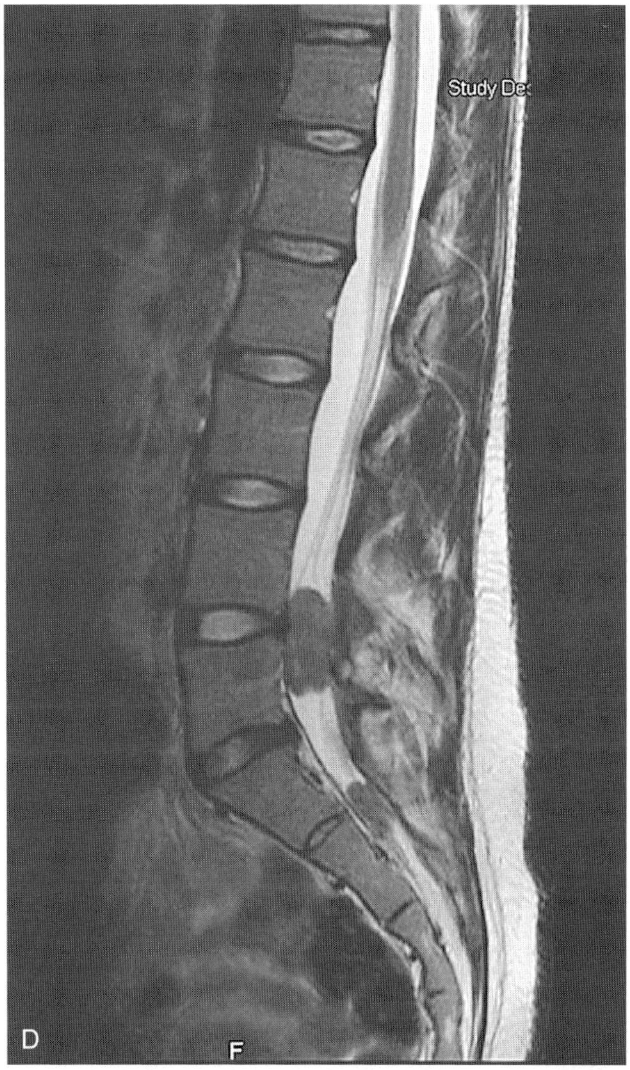

Figure 24-6. (*Continued*)

respectively.[165] Thus, the necessity for lifelong followup cannot be overemphasized. Because local failure rates in the spine are higher with subtotal resection, some authors recommend radiation therapy (see "Radiation Therapy and Chemotherapy," below).

Radiation Therapy and Chemotherapy

The role of radiation therapy is not well understood because of the small number of cases reported in the literature.[168,171,172] Most clinicians extrapolate from the data on irradiation of intracranial meningiomas. The expected outcome of radiation therapy is long-term stabilization of disease.[173] Patients who undergo complete resection should be observed. Even those with subtotally resected disease who either have improvement of their neurologic status or are asymptomatic postoperatively can be closely followed. When patients are irradiated, the dose delivered should be 52.2 Gy, based on the data from the treatment of intracranial meninigoma.[173] Single-fraction spinal stereotactic radiosurgery must be considered investigational at this time.[83] Hydroxyurea chemotherapy may also be of benefit in stabilizing postradiation disease progression.[174]

Schwannoma

Spinal schwannoma (Fig. 24-7) may present simultaneously in both the spinal canal and the thoracic cavity. These dumbbell-shaped tumors are typically benign and

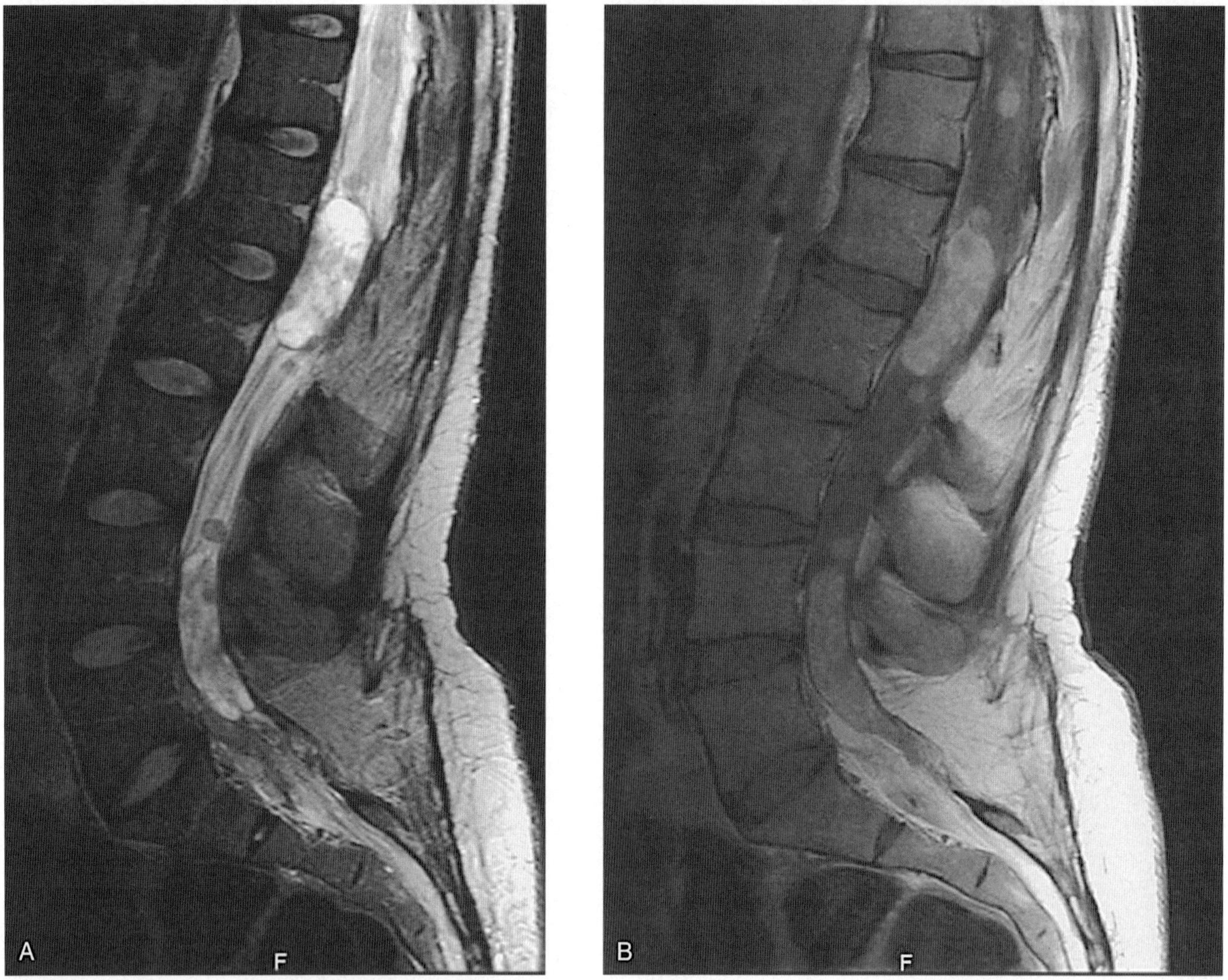

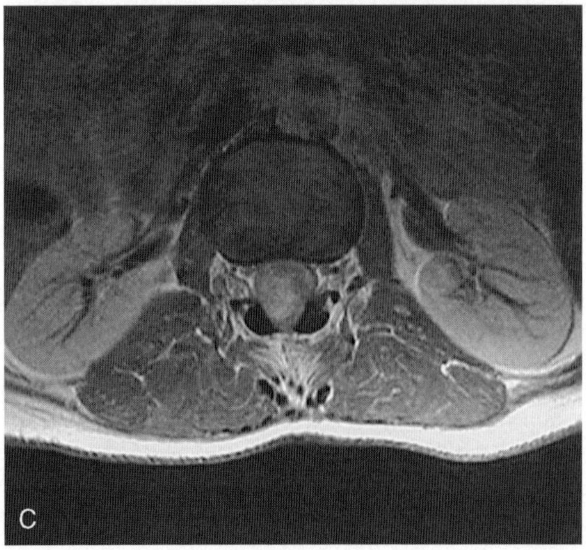

Figure 24-7. Multiple schwannomas. A 27-year-old woman with schwannomatosis presented with back pain and progressive lower-extremity motor weakness and sensory changes. Lumbar sagittal MRI revealed multiple intradural, extramedullary lesions that were hypointense on T_2-weighted imaging and heterogeneously enhanced following intravenous gadolinium administration (A and B). Lumbar axial imaging revealed that the tumor completely filled the thecal sac at the L-1 level, without recognizable CSF, nerve roots, or conus medullaris because of severe compression (C).

may involve the spinal cord and spinal nerves via the neural foramina. Surgical resection is the treatment of choice.[70,175,176] Only 3% are malignant,[177] in which case, adjuvant radiation therapy has been used. Outcomes are mixed.[176,177]

Chordoma

General Background

Chordomas are slow-growing neoplasms thought to be remnants of the embryonic notochord.[9] They make up approximately 4% of spinal tumors; 24% to 35% arise in the region of the base of skull (but in some series as many as 17% are thought to have originated in the cervical spine), 11% to 15% are known as chordomas of the mobile spine and arise in the true vertebral region (usually lumbar), and 50% to 58% in the sacrococcygeal region.[178–184] Most chordomas occur during the fourth decade of life with a 2:1 male-to-female ratio,[185] although sacrococcygeal chordomas tend to arise in the fifth and sixth decades.[98,186–189] Median survival is 6 years.[181]

Prognostic Factors

Several prognostic factors have been identified. Location is prognostic for survival,[190] with overall 5-year survival rates of 66% for sacrococcygeal tumors and 50% for vertebral lesions. Overall, 14% to 39% of patients develop metastases at a median of 5 years, most commonly to the lungs.[98,99,179–181,191–193] The incidence of metastases varies by location of the primary tumor: 26% to 44% of patients with sacrococcygeal lesions develop metastatic disease (usually to the thecal sac), whereas 61% of those with vertebral primaries metastasize, typically in a caudal direction. In some series, skull-base lesions are rarely reported to metastasize.[98,181,187] Gender may also be prognostic: 5- and 8-year local control rates are 81% and 75% for men and 65% and 17% for women, respectively.[194,195] The prognostic importance of age is controversial: in some series, children have higher incidence of metastases[196]; in other series, patients older than age 52 years have a worse local control rate.[178] Finally, residual microscopic disease after resection (either tumor spillage or positive margins) increases the risk of local relapse from 25% to 28% to 60% to 64% after a gross total resection.[188,197]

Treatment and Outcomes

Although en bloc gross total resection has traditionally been advocated for these lesions, it is rarely possible. As such, most patients undergo subtotal resection or biopsy, followed by radiation therapy. In most series, patients were treated with conventional photon radiation therapy, typically to doses of 55 to 70 Gy in 2-Gy fractions, with 5-year actuarial survival rates of 38% to 58%.[98,180,181,185,187,188,198,199] Although radiation therapy prolongs the disease-free interval,[185] the majority of tumors still recur unless they have also undergone complete resection,[181,185] and local progression is the most common cause of death. In one older series, the local control rate of sacrococcygeal tumors was 0% with either surgery or radiation therapy as monotherapy, but 40% when the two were combined.[180]

Some treatment series, using conventional photon radiation therapy, also suggest that local control rates improve with increasing radiation doses: with doses of <40, >48, <50, and >55 Gy, 5-year disease-free survival rates are approximately 0%, 13%, 31%, and 41%, respectively.[98,199] However, not all authors have found that increased dose improves outcome.[200] To improve the therapeutic ratio when treating residual or recurrent disease, most authors now advocate a combination of photon and charged-particle therapy (typically protons).[178,190,201–206] When patients are treated with charged-particle radiation therapy (with or without photons) delivering median doses of 65 to 76 Gy-equivalent, either immediately after maximum resection or at the time of recurrence, local control rates at 3, 5, and 10 years are 67% to 71%, 40% to 75%, and 54%, respectively, with overall survival rates at 3, 5, and 10 years of 88% to 97%, 75% to 80%, and 54%, respectively.[99,178,201,203,207] Radiosurgery has also been used in the treatment of residual and recurrent cervical spine chordoma. In one series, a mean dose of 19 Gy in a single fraction prescribed at the tumor margin resulted in a 4-year local control rate of 80% without neurologic sequelae.[208] The experience with interstitial irradiation is minimal and this modality is disfavored with the advent of charged-particle therapy and radiosurgery.[209–211] There is no known role for chemotherapy.

Chondrosarcoma

General Background

Primary chondrosarcoma of the spine is a rare, slow-growing tumor thought to originate from primitive mesenchymal cells or from the embryonal rests of the cranial cartilaginous matrix.[9] Of the axial skeleton chondrosarcomas, 33% occur in the mobile spine, most often in the thoracic region[212,213]; another 33% arise in the sacrum.[214] Spinal chondrosarcomas are slightly more common in men than in women.[215,216] The mean and median ages of presentation are 45 years and 51 years, respectively.[212,213,216]

Patients with spinal chondrosarcomas typically have a 25% to 54% overall long-term survival rate.[212,213,215,217,218] Adverse prognostic factors include positive surgical margins, high tumor grade, and older patient age.[214,218] Twelve percent to 19% of lesions may be high-grade tumors,[214,218] which carry a poor prognosis with an overall survival rate of only 14% at 3 years, a median survival time of 2.7 years, and a 75% to 86% incidence of metastases.[214,218]

Treatment and Outcomes

Surgery

Surgical resection is the mainstay of treatment of these lesions. Overall survival rates after any degree of resection are 55% to 72%, 67%, and 63% at 5, 10, and 15 years, respectively.[213,214] Median survival time is typically 6 years with local control rates ranging from 36% to 72%.[212–214,218] Patients with gross total resection have a better outcome than those with subtotal resection. After complete resection, the local control rate is 97%, with a 90% 10-year overall survival rate and an 84% disease-free survival rate.[214] Many chondrosarcomas have indolent courses, but others behave more aggressively.

Radiation Therapy and Chemotherapy

Radiation therapy after incomplete resection lengthened the disease-free interval from 16 to 44 months in one series.[212] Chemotherapy has not been shown to improve outcomes.[212,216]

Primary Sarcoma

General Background

Primary sarcomas of the spinal cord are exceedingly rare; sarcomas account for 0.7% of all central nervous system malignancies, and 5.6% of these are found in the spinal canal.[219] Malignant fibrous histiocytoma represents the most common histologic diagnosis,[219] arising from the nerve roots of the cauda equina, the spinal cord, or spinal blood vessels.[220]

Treatment and Outcomes

Surgical debulking and postoperative radiation therapy to approximately 60 Gy in 1.8- to 2.0-Gy fractions represent the typical treatment approach described in the literature.[219,220] The 5-year survival rate of patients with high-grade lesions is significantly worse at 28% than the 83% reported with low-grade lesions. The role of chemotherapy is not known.[221]

Hemangioblastoma

General Background

Intramedullary hemangioblastomas (Fig. 24-8) are slow-growing vascular tumors composed of endothelial and stromal components and account for 3% to 13% of all intramedullary spinal tumors.[9,222,223] The median age of presentation is 36 years for sporadic lesions, whereas patients with von Hippel-Lindau syndrome (VHLS) typically present a decade earlier and have multiple tumors.[224] The male-to-female ratio is 1.8:1.[224]

In the spinal cord, some authors report that 70% to 80% of hemangioblastomas occur as sporadic isolated lesions,[225,226] whereas other authors describe 80% of spinal cord hemangioblastomas as arising together with multiple cerebellar and retinal lesions as part of VHLS. In patients with VHLS, 51% of all neuraxis lesions are located in the spinal cord and only 29% are completely intramedullary, with the remainder having an extramedullary component[227]; 56% present in the cervical spine, and another 40% arise in the thoracic spine.[224,227] In the setting of VHLS, 83% of patients present with hypesthesia, 65% with weakness,

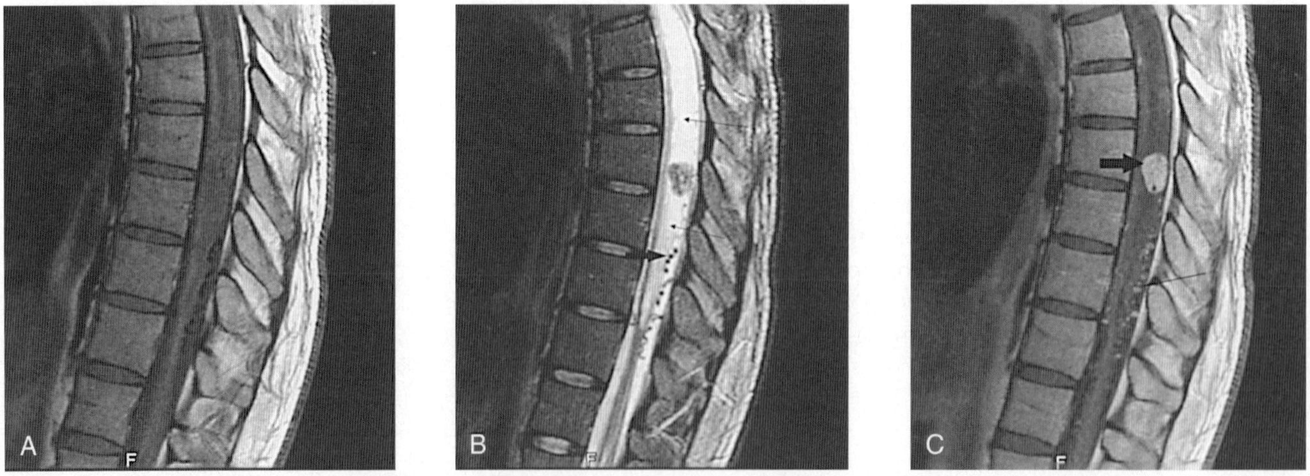

Figure 24-8. Thoracic hemangioblastoma. A 27-year-old male with a history of von Hippel-Lindau disease presented with a suspended sensory level at T-5. Thoracic MRI demonstrated an isointense intramedullary mass associated with a significant syrinx cavity (B, arrows). There was intense enhancement following administration of intravenous gadolinium (C, block arrow). Flow voids (B, block arrow) and blood vessel enhancement (C, line arrow) indicate the highly vascular nature of these lesions.

65% with gait ataxia, 52% with hyperreflexia, 17% with pain, and 14% with incontinence.[228]

Multiple central nervous system hemangioblastomas are diagnostic of VHLS. Multiply recurrent hemangioblastoma may also raise the suspicion of VHLS. Patients with isolated spinal hemangioblastoma should be screened for other manifestations of VHL by ophthalmologic evaluation, brain MRI, and abdominal CT scanning to rule out retinal and cranial hemangioblastoma and renal tumors, respectively.

Prognostic Factors

Factors prognostic for favorable outcome (defined as improvement or stabilization of neurologic function) are minimal or no preoperative neurologic deficits, lesions smaller then 0.5 cm^2, dorsally located lesions, and total surgical removal of the lesion.[227,229] Progressive syringomyelia is a negative prognostic factor with respect to preservation of neurologic function and is often recalcitrant to treatment attempts.

Treatment and Outcomes

Surgical resection is the mainstay of treatment for symptomatic lesions. After surgical resection, 41% to 68% of patients experience improvement of neurologic function and another 32% to 84% have stabilization of their preoperative function.[223,224,227] Although single-fraction stereotactic radiosurgery is an option for cerebellar hemangioblastoma,[230] it has not been properly evaluated for spinal hemangioblastoma because of concerns about the radiation tolerance of the spinal cord.

Vertebral Hemangioma

General Background

Vertebral hemangiomas are benign growths of endothelial origin, typically located in the thoracic and upper lumbar spine. They are the most common benign spinal column tumors with an incidence of approximately 11%.[231] Because vertebral body hemangiomas are most frequently stable over long periods of time, some authors consider them to be nonneoplastic. Growth causing progressive symptoms has been documented. Only 1% to 2% of patients develop clinically significant pain. New-onset back pain followed by subacute progression of a thoracic myelopathy, typically over a period of 4 to 5 months, is the most common presentation for patients with neurologic deficit.[232] These tumors also occasionally cause root and cord compression syndromes.

The diagnosis can be reliably made by preoperative radiographic imaging. Asymptomatic vertebral hemangiomas, when visible on plain films, are almost universally associated with prominent vertical trabeculation (PVT). Compressive vertebral hemangiomas have a much wider spectrum of radiologic appearances and many do not have any specific features. Plain-film radiography may reveal vertebral collapse, erosion of pedicles, osteopenia, or no abnormality. On CT imaging, asymptomatic vertebral hemangiomas classically consist of PVT surrounded by fat density. As with plain-film imaging, compressive vertebral hemangiomas have a less specific appearance than asymptomatic vertebral hemangiomas. Described CT features include stroma of soft-tissue density, an intraosseous polka-dot pattern, ballooning or lysis of the cortex, and extraosseous soft-tissue extension. MRI is less reliable in diagnosing these lesions. High signal intensity on T_1-weighted images is seen in 50% of compressive vertebral hemangiomas. Signal voids are the most useful additional MR sign. High signal intensity on T_2-weighted images and maintained vertebral height are frequently present, but are nonspecific, whereas other signs of vertebral hemangioma, such as intact cortex, a sharp margin with normal marrow and enlarged paraspinal vessels, are not commonly seen. Therefore, a preoperative diagnosis of compressive vertebral hemangioma can be made in 65% of plain-film and 80% of CT examinations, whereas asymptomatic vertebral hemangioma is much more easily recognized with this imaging combination.[233]

Treatment and Outcomes

Surgery

Treatment is initiated only when progressive symptoms, including focal pain or progressive neurologic deficit, develop. Historically, standard treatment consisted of surgical removal of the lesion. Endovascular embolization of these very vascular growths may also provide pain control. Vertebroplasty has high reported rates of success. The local control rate at 3 years is 70%. In those patients who experience regrowth of the lesion, 90% recur within the first 2 years.[234]

Radiation Therapy

Radiation therapy is an effective treatment alternative. A recent meta-analysis demonstrated that a total dose of 30 Gy given in 2-Gy fractions resulted in a 57% complete and 32% partial improvement of pain.[231] A second, smaller analysis showed an apparent dose–response relationship. Patients treated with the biologic equivalent of 36 to 44 Gy in 2-Gy fractions had significantly more complete pain relief than did those treated with 20 to 34 Gy (82% vs. 39%, respectively).[235]

Other Miscellaneous Tumors

Primary spinal lipomas are benign, congenital, intradural–extramedullary lesions located in the cervicothoracic region and account for approximately 1% of all spinal cord tumors.[236–241] The classic presentation is that of a slow-ascending spastic monoparesis or paraparesis with rapid late deterioration. Early surgical decompression is mandatory for preservation of existing neurologic function,[52,238,241] but complete surgical debulking is almost impossible because of their infiltrative nature.[52,236,237] There is no known role for radiation therapy or chemotherapy.

Epidermoid tumors are rare tumors of male preponderance, most commonly found in the lumbosacral region.[154] Complete surgical excision is usually curative. Incompletely excised tumors may recur, but because of their slow growth, this may take several years.

Primary intraspinal lymphomas, whether epidural or intramedullary, are uncommon lesions. Primary epidural lymphomas are almost always of B-cell origin.[242] At least half of such patients have favorable courses to either radiation therapy or chemotherapy. If recognized preoperatively they can be diagnosed by CT-guided needle biopsy. Treatment can commence without the "downtime" that follows decompressive laminectomy. Rapid responses may be seen with steroids, typical B-cell lymphoma chemotherapy, and radiation therapy to a median dose of 3800 cGy.[243] Lymphomas involving the spinal cord are seen in the context of primary central nervous system non-Hodgkin lymphoma (see Chapter 17).

Spinal canal chloroma (or granulocytic sarcoma) is defined as an extramedullary localized tumor mass of blasts of the granulocytic lineage.[244–247] This tumor can arise during the course of acute myeloid leukemia (AML) or myelodysplastic syndrome (MDS) synchronic with initial diagnosis or as relapse, as well as an isolated tumor without any signs of bone marrow involvement. Spinal chloromas can occasionally precede the development of systemic disease by weeks to years. Spinal complications of chloromas, such as cord compression secondary to epidural tumor or cauda equina syndrome, have been described but are uncommon. The median age at presentation is 22 years, with a 7.8:1 male-to-female ratio. The thoracic spine is most commonly involved (73%), followed by the lumbar (34%), sacral (23%), and cervical (5%) regions; 18% of patients exhibit multiple noncontiguous areas of involvement. Eighty percent of patients present with pain (generalized, localized, or radicular), with half of these reporting back pain. Sixty-six percent of patients present with motor deficits, ranging from lower-extremity weakness (34%) to paraplegia (30%). Numbness and bladder or bowel dysfunction are each seen in 27% of patients. The most effective treatment appears to be multimodality therapy in the setting of early diagnosis. Options include surgical decompression, intravenous and/or intrathecal chemotherapy, radiation therapy at doses of 2000 to 3000 cGy, or any combination of these treatments. Patient survival ranges from 18 days to 9.5 years after diagnosis. In a review of the literature, no clear relationship could be found between specific treatment modality and survival;[244] however, those receiving systemic therapy soon after diagnosis experienced the longest disease-free episodes.

True intramedullary teratoma is an extremely rare tumor, with only nine cases reported in the literature. Early surgical resection is recommended to preserve neurologic status. Because teratomas may adhere to the functional neural tissue of the spinal cord with no dissection plane, complete resection is often not possible. Low-grade histopathology predominates, so the symptomatic recurrence of incompletely resected mature teratomas is often slow and may eventually require a second surgical procedure.[248] Radiation therapy is generally reserved for multiply recurrent, subtotally resected disease.

Primary spinal melanoma must be distinguished from nonmalignant melanotic schwannoma. Primary nerve root melanomas have a prognosis more favorable than melanomas arising in other locations.[249]

Central neurocytoma has been reported to arise in the spine.[250–252] In the past, it may have often been mistaken for spinal oligodendroglioma. Staining for synaptophysin and neuron-specific enolase allows these tumors to be reliably distinguished. As in the brain, its behavior is variable. Because this tumor arises centrally in the spinal cord, observation or radiation may be primary management strategies with resection reserved for those with progressive neurologic deficits.

▶ CONCLUSION

Primary tumors of the spinal cord are uncommon lesions. Much of the literature groups these tumors together by location (intra- vs. extramedullary) when reporting outcomes. However, spinal cord tumors clearly behave differently depending upon histology, and this needs to be taken into account when making management decisions. Nonetheless, the primary treatment for most spinal cord tumors continues to be surgical resection, with radiation therapy recommended for those patients in whom a complete resection cannot be achieved and for those at high risk of recurrence. The role of chemotherapy in the management of spinal cord tumors remains unclear.

REFERENCES

1. National Cancer Institute, DCCPS Surveillance Research Program Cancer Statistics Branch. Surveillance, Epidemiology, and End Results (SEER) Program. SEER stat database: incidence—SEER 9 Regs Public-Use, Nov 2002 Sub (1973–2000) 2003;10–23–2003.
2. Central Brain Tumor Registry of the United States. 2002–2003 Primary brain tumors in the United States. Statistical report 1995–1999 years data collected. Chicago: CBTRUS, 2003.
3. Connoly ES. Spinal cord tumors in adults. In: Winn RH, ed. Youmans' Neurological Surgery. Philadelphia: WB Saunders, 1982:3196.

4. Sasanelli F, Beghi E, Kurland LT. Primary intraspinal neoplasms in Rochester, Minnesota 1935–1981. Neuroepidemiology 1983;2:156–163.
5. Preston-Martin S. Descriptive epidemiology of primary tumors of the spinal cord and spinal meninges in Los Angeles County 1972–1985. Neuroepidemiology 1990;9: 106–111.
6. Mumenthaler M. Diseases affecting mainly the spinal cord. In: Mumenthaler M, ed. Neurology, 3rd ed. New York: Thieme, 1990:181–232.
7. Hardison HH, Packer RJ, Rorke LB, et al. Outcome of children with primary intramedullary spinal cord tumors. Childs Nerv Syst 1987;3:89–92.
8. Choucair AK, Levin VA, Gutin PH, et al. Development of multiple lesions during radiation therapy and chemotherapy in patients with gliomas. J Neurosurg 1986;65:654–658.
9. International Agency for Research on Cancer. World Health Organization classification of tumours: pathology and genetics: tumours of the nervous system, 2nd ed. Lyon, France: Oxford University Press, 2000.
10. Essig M, Metzner R, Bonsanto M, et al. Postoperative fluid-attenuated inversion recovery MR imaging of cerebral gliomas: initial results. Eur Radiol 2001;11:2004–2010.
11. Li BS, Movsas B, Babb JS, et al. Quantifying injury to the brain from radiation therapy (RT) with whole brain N-acetylaspartate (WBNAA) proton magnetic resonance spectroscopy (1H-MRS). Int J Radiat Oncol Biol Phys 2000; 48:299–300.
12. Pirzkall A, Larson DA, McKnight TR, et al. MR-spectroscopy results in improved target delineation for high-grade gliomas. Int J Radiat Oncol Biol Phys 2000;48:115.
13. McKnight TR, dem Bussche MH, Vigneron DB, et al. Histopathological validation of a three-dimensional magnetic resonance spectroscopy index as a predictor of tumor presence. J Neurosurg 2002;97:794–802.
14. McKnight TR. Proton magnetic resonance spectroscopic evaluation of brain tumor metabolism. Sem Oncol 2004;31: 605–617.
15. Bourland JD, Shaw EG. The evolving role of biological imaging in stereotactic radiosurgery. Technol Cancer Res Treat 2003;2:135–139.
16. Cohen AR, Wisoff JH, Allen JC, et al. Malignant astrocytomas of the spinal cord. J Neurosurg 1989;70:50–54.
17. Aydin MV, Ozel S, Sen O, et al. Intradural disc mimicking: a spinal tumor lesion. Spinal Cord 2004;42:52–54.
18. Dhiwakar M, Buxton N. Acute transverse myelitis mimicking an intramedullary neoplasm. Br J Neurosurg 2004;18: 72–73.
19. Petjom S, Chaiwun B, Settakorn J, et al. Angiostrongylus cantonensis infection mimicking a spinal cord tumor. Ann Neurol 2002;52:99–101.
20. Yukawa Y, Kato F. Isolated spinal cord sarcoidosis mimicking an intramedullary tumor. J Spinal Disord 1999;12: 530–533.
21. Fouladi M, Heideman R, Langston JW, et al. Infectious meningitis mimicking recurrent medulloblastoma on magnetic resonance imaging. Case report. J Neurosurg 1999;91: 499–502.
22. Kilic G, Blankstein J, Kadanoff R. Vertebral tuberculosis presenting with elevated CA-125 and weight loss mimicking ovarian malignancy; case report. Eur J Gynaecol Oncol 2003;24:561–562.
23. Gowers WR, Horsley V. A case of tumour of the spinal cord. Removal and recovery. Med Chir Trans 1888;53:377–428.
24. Eiselsberg AV, Ranzi E. Über die chirugische Behandlung der Hirn- und Rückenmarkstumoren. Arch Klin Chir 1913; 102:309–468.
25. Elsberg CA, Beer E. The operability of intramedullary tumors of the spinal cord. A report of two operations with remarks upon the extrusion of intraspinal tumors. Am J Med Sci 1911;142:636–647.
26. Wood EH, Berne AS, Taveras JM. The value of radiation therapy in the management of intrinsic tumors of the spinal cord. Radiology 1954;63:11–24.
27. Jallo GI, Freed D, Epstein F. Intramedullary spinal cord tumors in children. Childs Nerv Syst 2003;19:641–649.
28. Heckmann JG, Druschky A, Kern PM, et al. "Ghost and mimicry-tumor"—primary CNS lymphoma. Nervenarzt 2000;71:305–310.
29. Vaquero J, Martinez R, Rossi E, et al. Primary cerebral lymphoma: the "ghost tumor." Case report. J Neurosurg 1984;60: 174–176.
30. Gray RS, Abrahams JJ, Hufnagel TJ, et al. Ghost-cell tumor of the optic chiasm. Primary CNS lymphoma. J Clin Neuro-ophthalmol 1989;9:98–104.
31. Coca A, Goday A, Font J, et al. Primary cerebral lymphoma: the "ghost tumor." J Neurosurg 1984;61:202–203.
32. el Mahdy W, Kane PJ, Powell MP, et al. Spinal intradural tumours: Part I—extramedullary. Br J Neurosurg 1999;13: 550–557.
33. McCormick PC, Stein BM. Spinal cord tumors in adults. In: Youmans JR, ed. Neurological surgery: a comprehensive reference guide to the diagnosis and management of neurosurgical problems, 4th ed. Philadelphia: Elsevier, 1996: 3111–3114.
34. Constantini S, Miller DC, Allen JC, et al. Radical excision of intramedullary spinal cord tumors: surgical morbidity and long-term follow-up evaluation in 164 children and young adults. J Neurosurg 2000;93:183–193.
35. Zileli M, Coskun E, Ozdamar N, et al. Surgery of intramedullary spinal cord tumors. Eur Spine J 1996;5:243–250.
36. Goh KY, Velasquez L, Epstein FJ. Pediatric intramedullary spinal cord tumors: is surgery alone enough? Pediatr Neurosurg 1997;27:34–39.
37. Lunardi P, Licastro G, Missori P, et al. Management of intramedullary tumours in children. Acta Neurochir (Wien) 1993;120:59–65.
38. Abdel-Wahab M, Corn B, Wolfson A, et al. Prognostic factors and survival in patients with spinal cord gliomas after radiation therapy. Am J Clin Oncol 1999;22:344–351.
39. Shirato H, Kamada T, Hida K, et al. The role of radiotherapy in the management of spinal cord glioma. Int J Radiat Oncol Biol Phys 1995;33:323–328.
40. Rodrigues GB, Waldron JN, Wong CS, et al. A retrospective analysis of 52 cases of spinal cord glioma managed with radiation therapy. Int J Radiat Oncol Biol Phys 2000; 48:837–842.
41. Weiner HL, Freed D, Woo HH, et al. Intra-axial tumors of the cervicomedullary junction: surgical results and long-term outcome. Pediatr Neurosurg 1997;27:12–18.

42. Cristante L, Herrmann HD. Surgical management of intramedullary spinal cord tumors: functional outcome and sources of morbidity. Neurosurgery 1994;35:69–74.
43. Xu QW, Bao WM, Mao RL, et al. Aggressive surgery for intramedullary tumor of cervical spinal cord. Surg Neurol 1996;46:322–328.
44. Hulshof MC, Menten J, Dito JJ, et al. Treatment results in primary intraspinal gliomas. Radiother Oncol 1993;29: 294–300.
45. Nishio S, Morioka T, Fujii K, et al. Spinal cord gliomas: management and outcome with reference to adjuvant therapy. J Clin Neurosci 2000;7:20–23.
46. Santi M, Mena H, Wong K, et al. Spinal cord malignant astrocytomas. Clinicopathologic features in 36 cases. Cancer 2003;98:554–561.
47. Sandler HM, Papadopoulos SM, Thornton AF Jr, et al. Spinal cord astrocytomas: results of therapy. Neurosurgery 1992;30:490–493.
48. Bouffet E, Pierre-Kahn A, Marchal JC, et al. Prognostic factors in pediatric spinal cord astrocytoma. Cancer 1998;83: 2391–2399.
49. Merchant TE, Nguyen D, Thompson SJ, et al. High-grade pediatric spinal cord tumors. Pediatr Neurosurg 1999; 30:1–5.
50. Rossitch E Jr, Zeidman SM, Burger PC, et al. Clinical and pathological analysis of spinal cord astrocytomas in children. Neurosurgery 1990;27:193–196.
51. Innocenzi G, Salvati M, Cervoni L, et al. Prognostic factors in intramedullary astrocytomas. Clin Neurol Neurosurg 1997;99:1–5.
52. Kim MS, Chung CK, Choe G, et al. Intramedullary spinal cord astrocytoma in adults: postoperative outcome. J Neurooncol 2001;52:85–94.
53. Lee HK, Chang EL, Fuller GN, et al. The prognostic value of neurologic function in astrocytic spinal cord glioma. Neuro-oncol 2003;5:208–213.
54. Przybylski GJ, Albright AL, Martinez AJ. Spinal cord astrocytomas: long-term results comparing treatments in children. Childs Nerv Syst 1997;13:375–382.
55. Minehan KJ, Shaw EG, Scheithauer BW, et al. Spinal cord astrocytoma: pathological and treatment considerations. J Neurosurg 1995;83:590–595.
56. Lee TT, Gromelski EB, Green BA. Surgical treatment of spinal ependymoma and post-operative radiotherapy. Acta Neurochir (Wien) 1998;140:309–313.
57. Whitaker SJ, Bessell EM, Ashley SE, et al. Postoperative radiotherapy in the management of spinal cord ependymoma. J Neurosurg 1991;74:720–728.
58. McCormick PC, Torres R, Post KD, et al. Intramedullary ependymoma of the spinal cord. J Neurosurg 1990;72: 523–532.
59. McLaughlin MP, Marcus RB Jr, Buatti JM, et al. Ependymoma: results, prognostic factors and treatment recommendations. Int J Radiat Oncol Biol Phys 1998;40: 845–850.
60. Hanbali F, Fourney DR, Marmor E, et al. Spinal cord ependymoma: radical surgical resection and outcome. Neurosurgery 2002;51:1162–1172.
61. Kochbati L, Nasr C, Frikha H, et al. Primary intramedullary ependymomas: retrospective study of 16 cases. Cancer Radiother 2003;7:17–21.
62. Ohata K, Takami T, Gotou T, et al. Surgical outcome of intramedullary spinal cord ependymoma. Acta Neurochir (Wien) 1999;141:341–346.
63. Hejazi N, Hassler W. Microsurgical treatment of intramedullary spinal cord tumors. Neurol Med Chir (Tokyo) 1998;38:266–271.
64. Fowler JF, Bentzen SM, Bond SJ, et al. Clinical radiation doses for spinal cord: the 1998 international questionnaire. Radiother Oncol 2000;55:295–300.
65. Cooper PR. Outcome after operative treatment of intramedullary spinal cord tumors in adults: intermediate and long-term results in 51 patients. Neurosurgery 1989;25: 855–859.
66. Constantini S, Allen JC, Epstein F. Pediatric and adult primary spinal cord tumors. In: Black PM, Loeffler JS, eds. Cancer of the nervous system. Cambridge: Blackwell, 1997:637–649.
67. Klekamp J, Samii M. Surgical results of spinal meningiomas. Acta Neurochir Suppl (Wien) 1996;65:77–81.
68. Levy WJ Jr, Bay J, Dohn D. Spinal cord meningioma. J Neurosurg 1982;57:804–812.
69. Solero CL, Fornari M, Giombini S, et al. Spinal meningiomas: review of 174 operated cases. Neurosurgery 1989;25: 153–160.
70. Seppala MT, Haltia MJ, Sankila RJ, et al. Long-term outcome after removal of spinal schwannoma: a clinicopathological study of 187 cases. J Neurosurg 1995;83:621–626.
71. Sim FH, Svien HJ, Bickel WH, et al. Swan-neck deformity following extensive cervical laminectomy. A review of twenty-one cases. J Bone Joint Surg Am 1974;56:564–580.
72. Reimer R, Onofrio BM. Astrocytomas of the spinal cord in children and adolescents. J Neurosurg 1985;63:669–675.
73. Jyothirmayi R, Madhavan J, Nair MK, et al. Conservative surgery and radiotherapy in the treatment of spinal cord astrocytoma. J Neurooncol 1997;33:205–211.
74. Huddart R, Traish D, Ashley S, et al. Management of spinal astrocytoma with conservative surgery and radiotherapy. Br J Neurosurg 1993;7:473–481.
75. Kopelson G, Linggood RM, Kleinman GM, et al. Management of intramedullary spinal cord tumors. Radiology 1980; 135:473–479.
76. Epstein F, Epstein N. Surgical treatment of spinal cord astrocytomas of childhood. A series of 19 patients. J Neurosurg 1982;57:685–689.
77. International Commission on Radiation Units and Measurements, Inc. ICRU Report 62: prescribing, recording and reporting photon beam therapy (supplement to ICRU report 50). Wambersie and Landberg Journal of the ICRU 62;1999. Bethesda, MD: Nuclear Technology Publishing, 1999.
78. International Commission on Radiation Units and Measurements, Inc. ICRU Report 50, prescribing, recording, and reporting photon beam therapy 50;1993. Bethesda, MD: Nuclear Technology Publishing, 1993.
79. Michalski JM. Spinal canal. In: Leibel SA, Phillips TL, eds. Textbook of radiation oncology, 1st ed. Philadelphia: WB Saunders, 1998:860–875.
80. Shiu AS, Chang EL, Ye JS, et al. Near simultaneous computed tomography image-guided stereotactic spinal radiotherapy: an emerging paradigm for achieving true stereotaxy. Int J Radiat Oncol Biol Phys 2003;57:605–613.

81. Stieber VW, Munley M. Central nervous system tumors. In: Mundt AJ, Roeske JC, eds. Intensity-modulated radiation therapy: a clinical perspective, 1st ed. Ontario, Canada: BC Decker, 2005;229–239.
82. Yin FF, Ryu S, Ajlouni M, et al. A technique of intensity-modulated radiosurgery (IMRS) for spinal tumors. Med Phys 2002;29:2815–2822.
83. Ryu SI, Chang SD, Kim DH, et al. Image-guided hypofractionated stereotactic radiosurgery to spinal lesions. Neurosurgery 2001;49:838–846.
84. Jaffray DA, Siewerdsen JH, Wong JW, et al. Flat-panel cone-beam computed tomography for image-guided radiation therapy. Int J Radiat Oncol Biol Phys 2002;53:1337–1349.
85. Blomgren H, Lax I, Naslund I, et al. Stereotactic high dose fraction radiation therapy of extracranial tumors using an accelerator. Clinical experience of the first thirty-one patients. Acta Oncol 1995;34:861–870.
86. Marcus RB Jr, Million RR. The incidence of myelitis after irradiation of the cervical spinal cord. Int J Radiat Oncol Biol Phys 1990;19:3–8.
87. Schultheiss TE, Kun LE, Ang KK, et al. Radiation response of the central nervous system. Int J Radiat Oncol Biol Phys 1995;31:1093–1112.
88. Schultheiss TE, Higgins EM, El Mahdi AM. The latent period in clinical radiation myelopathy. Int J Radiat Oncol Biol Phys 1984;10:1109–1115.
89. Cohen L, Creditor M. An iso-effect table for radiation tolerance of the human spinal cord. Int J Radiat Oncol Biol Phys 1981;7:961–966.
90. Macbeth FR, Wheldon TE, Girling DJ, et al. Radiation myelopathy: estimates of risk in 1048 patients in three randomized trials of palliative radiotherapy for non-small cell lung cancer. The Medical Research Council Lung Cancer Working Party. Clin Oncol (R Coll Radiol) 1996;8:176–181.
91. Wara WM, Phillips TL, Sheline GE, et al. Radiation tolerance of the spinal cord. Cancer 1975;35:1558–1562.
92. Niewald M, Feldmann U, Feiden W, et al. Multivariate logistic analysis of dose-effect relationship and latency of radio myelopathy after hyperfractionated and conventionally fractionated radiotherapy in animal experiments. Int J Radiat Oncol Biol Phys 1998;41:681–688.
93. Ang KK, Jiang GL, Feng Y, et al. Extent and kinetics of recovery of occult spinal cord injury. Int J Radiat Oncol Biol Phys 2001;50:1013–1020.
94. Feldmeier JJ, Lange JD, Cox SD, et al. Hyperbaric oxygen as prophylaxis or treatment for radiation myelitis. Undersea Hyperb Med 1993;20:249–255.
95. Liu CY, Yim BT, Wozniak AJ. Anticoagulation therapy for radiation-induced myelopathy. Ann Pharmacother 2001;35: 188–191.
96. Schultheiss TE, Stephens LC, Peters LJ. Survival in radiation myelopathy. Int J Radiat Oncol Biol Phys 1986;12: 1765–1769.
97. Pieters RS, O'Farrell D, Fullerton B. Cauda equina tolerance to radiation therapy [abstract]. Int J Radiat Oncol Biol Phys 1996;36(Suppl 1):359.
98. Fuller DB, Bloom JG. Radiotherapy for chordoma. Int J Radiat Oncol Biol Phys 1988;15:331–339.
99. Schoenthaler R, Castro JR, Petti PL, et al. Charged particle irradiation of sacral chordomas. Int J Radiat Oncol Biol Phys 1993;26:291–298.
100. Esik O, Csere T, Stefanits K, et al. A review on radiogenic Lhermitte's sign. Pathol Oncol Res 2003;9:115–120.
101. Okada S, Okeda R. Pathology of radiation myelopathy. Neuropathology 2001;21:247–265.
102. Nieder C, Ataman F, Price RE, et al. Radiation myelopathy: new perspective on an old problem. Radiat Oncol Invest 1999;7:193–203.
103. Wang PY, Shen WC, Jan JS. MR imaging in radiation myelopathy. AJNR Am J Neuroradiol 1992;13:1049–1055.
104. Mayfield JK. Postradiation spinal deformity. Orthop Clin North Am 1979;10:829–844.
105. Nadeem SQ, Feun LG, Bruce-Gregorios JH, et al. Post radiation sarcoma (malignant fibrous histiocytoma) of the cervical spine following ependymoma (a case report). J Neurooncol 1991;11:263–268.
106. Rappaport ZH, Loven D, Ben Aharon U. Radiation-induced cerebellar glioblastoma multiforme subsequent to treatment of an astrocytoma of the cervical spinal cord. Neurosurgery 1991;29:606–608.
107. Garcia DM. Primary spinal cord tumors treated with surgery and postoperative irradiation. Int J Radiat Oncol Biol Phys 1985;11:1933–1939.
108. CTEP and NCI. Common Terminology Criteria for Adverse Events v3.0 (CTCAE). Available at http://ctep.cancer.gov 2003. Accessed Sept 9, 2004.
109. Pavy J-J, Denekamp J, Letschert J, et al. Late effects toxicity scoring: The SOMA scale. Int J Radiat Oncol Biol Phys 1995;31:1043–1047.
110. Weingart J, Brem H, Grossman SA, et al. Gliadel followed by radiotherapy for newly diagnosed malignant glioma: Safety results, pathologic findings, and survival. Int J Radiat Oncol Biol Phys 2000;48:256.
111. Stewart LA. Chemotherapy in adult high-grade glioma: a systematic review and meta-analysis of individual patient data from 12 randomised trials. Lancet 2002;359:1011–1018.
112. Hassall TE, Mitchell AE, Ashley DM. Carboplatin chemotherapy for progressive intramedullary spinal cord low-grade gliomas in children: three case studies and a review of the literature. Neuro-oncol 2001;3:251–257.
113. Robertson PL, Zeltzer PM, Boyett JM, et al. Survival and prognostic factors following radiation therapy and chemotherapy for ependymomas in children: a report of the Children's Cancer Group. J Neurosurg 1998;88:695–703.
114. Fort DW, Packer RJ, Kirkpatrick GB, et al. Carboplatin and vincristine for pediatric primary spinal cord astrocytomas [abstract]. Childs Nerv Syst 1998:4;14.
115. Doireau V, Grill J, Zerah M, et al. Chemotherapy for unresectable and recurrent intramedullary glial tumours in children. Brain Tumours Subcommittee of the French Society of Paediatric Oncology (SFOP). Br J Cancer 1999;81: 835–840.
116. Evans AE, Anderson JR, Lefkowitz-Boudreaux IB, et al. Adjuvant chemotherapy of childhood posterior fossa ependymoma: cranio-spinal irradiation with or without adjuvant CCNU, vincristine, and prednisone: a Children's Cancer Group study. Med Pediatr Oncol 1996;27:8–14.
117. Chamberlain MC. Etoposide for recurrent spinal cord ependymoma. Neurology 2002;58:1310–1311.
118. Goldwein JW, Leahy JM, Packer RJ, et al. Intracranial ependymomas in children. Int J Radiat Oncol Biol Phys 1990;19:1497–1502.

119. Levin VA, Edwards MS, Gutin PH, et al. Phase II evaluation of dibromodulcitol in the treatment of recurrent medulloblastoma, ependymoma, and malignant astrocytoma. J Neurosurg 1984;61:1063–1068.
120. Goldwein JW, Glauser TA, Packer RJ, et al. Recurrent intracranial ependymomas in children. Survival, patterns of failure, and prognostic factors. Cancer 1990;66:557–563.
121. Epstein FJ, Farmer JP. Pediatric spinal cord tumor surgery. Neurosurg Clin North Am 1990;1:569–590.
122. McCormick PC, Stein BM. Intramedullary tumors in adults. Neurosurg Clin North Am 1990;1:609–630.
123. Guidetti B, Mercuri S, Vagnozzi R. Long-term results of the surgical treatment of 129 intramedullary spinal gliomas. J Neurosurg 1981;54:323–330.
124. Stein BM: Surgery of intramedullary spinal cord tumors. Clin Neurosurg 1979;26:529–542.
125. Mottl H, Koutecky J. Treatment of spinal cord tumors in children. Med Pediatr Oncol 1997;29:293–295.
126. Linstadt DE, Wara WM, Leibel SA, et al. Postoperative radiotherapy of primary spinal cord tumors. Int J Radiat Oncol Biol Phys 1989;16:1397–1403.
127. Miller DC. Surgical pathology of intramedullary spinal cord neoplasms. J Neurooncol 2000;47:189–194.
128. Chun HC, Schmidt-Ullrich RK, Wolfson A, et al. External beam radiotherapy for primary spinal cord tumors. J Neurooncol 1990;9:211–217.
129. McLaughlin MP, Buatti JM, Marcus RB Jr, et al. Outcome after radiotherapy of primary spinal cord glial tumors. Radiat Oncol Investig 1998;6:276–280.
130. Allen JC, Aviner S, Yates AJ, et al. Treatment of high-grade spinal cord astrocytoma of childhood with "8-in-1" chemotherapy and radiotherapy: a pilot study of CCG-945. Children's Cancer Group. J Neurosurg 1998;88:215–220.
131. Fornari M, Pluchino F, Solero CL, et al. Microsurgical treatment of intramedullary spinal cord tumours. Acta Neurochir Suppl (Wien) 1988;43:3–8.
132. Karim AB, Afra D, Cornu P, et al. Randomized trial on the efficacy of radiotherapy for cerebral low-grade glioma in the adult: European Organization for Research and Treatment of Cancer Study 22845 with the Medical Research Council study BR04: an interim analysis. Int J Radiat Oncol Biol Phys 2002;52:316–324.
133. Karim AB, Maat B, Hatlevoll R, et al. A randomized trial on dose-response in radiation therapy of low-grade cerebral glioma: European Organization for Research and Treatment of Cancer (EORTC) Study 22844. Int J Radiat Oncol Biol Phys 1996;36:549–556.
134. Shaw E, Arusell R, Scheithauer B, et al. Prospective randomized trial of low- versus high-dose radiation therapy in adults with supratentorial low-grade glioma: initial report of a North Central Cancer Treatment Group/Radiation Therapy Oncology Group/Eastern Cooperative Oncology Group Study. J Clin Oncol 2002;20:2267–2276.
135. Walker MD, Strike TA, Sheline GE. An analysis of dose-effect relationship in the radiotherapy of malignant gliomas. Int J Radiat Oncol Biol Phys 1979;5:1725–1731.
136. Chang CH, Horton J, Schoenfeld D, et al. Comparison of postoperative radiotherapy and combined postoperative radiotherapy and chemotherapy in the multidisciplinary management of malignant gliomas. A joint Radiation Therapy Oncology Group and Eastern Cooperative Oncology Group study. Cancer 1983;52:997–1007.
137. Cervoni L, Salvati M, Celli P, et al. Gliomas of the conus medullaris. Tumori 1996;82:249–251.
138. Epstein FJ, Farmer JP, Freed D. Adult intramedullary astrocytomas of the spinal cord. J Neurosurg 1992;77:355–359.
139. Ciappetta P, Salvati M, Capoccia G, et al. Spinal glioblastomas: report of seven cases and review of the literature. Neurosurgery 1991;28:302–306.
140. Chigasaki H, Pennybacker JB. A long follow-up study of 128 cases of intramedullary spinal cord tumours. Neurol Med Chir (Tokyo) 1968;10:25–66.
141. Sgouros S, Malluci CL, Jackowski A. Spinal ependymomas—the value of postoperative radiotherapy for residual disease control. Br J Neurosurg 1996;10:559–566.
142. Fine MJ, Kricheff II, Freed D, et al. Spinal cord ependymomas: MR imaging features. Radiology 1995;197:655–658.
143. Shaw EG, Evans RG, Scheithauer BW, et al. Radiotherapeutic management of adult intraspinal ependymomas. Int J Radiat Oncol Biol Phys 1986;12:323–327.
144. Di Marco A, Griso C, Pradella R, et al. Postoperative management of primary spinal cord ependymomas. Acta Oncol 1988;27:371–375.
145. Mork SJ, Loken AC. Ependymoma: a follow-up study of 101 cases. Cancer 1977;40:907–915.
146. Marks JE, Adler SJ. A comparative study of ependymomas by site of origin. Int J Radiat Oncol Biol Phys 1982;8:37–43.
147. Clover LL, Hazuka MB, Kinzie JJ. Spinal cord ependymomas treated with surgery and radiation therapy. A review of 11 cases. Am J Clin Oncol 1993;16:350–353.
148. Rivierez M, Oueslati S, Philippon J, et al. Ependymoma of the intradural filum terminale in adults: 20 cases. Neurochirurgie 1990;36:96–107.
149. Schiffer D, Chio A, Giordana MT, et al. Histologic prognostic factors in ependymoma. Childs Nerv Syst 1991;7:177–182.
150. Sonneland PR, Scheithauer BW, Onofrio BM. Myxopapillary ependymoma. A clinicopathologic and immunocytochemical study of 77 cases. Cancer 1985;56:883–893.
151. Chan HS, Becker LE, Hoffman HJ, et al. Myxopapillary ependymoma of the filum terminale and cauda equina in childhood: report of seven cases and review of the literature. Neurosurgery 1984;14:204–210.
152. Schweitzer JS, Batzdorf U. Ependymoma of the cauda equina region: diagnosis, treatment, and outcome in 15 patients. Neurosurgery 1992;30:202–207.
153. Stein BM. Intramedullary spinal cord tumors. Clin Neurosurg 1983;30:717–741.
154. Russell and Rubinstein's Pathology of Tumors of the Nervous System (7th ed). McLendon RE, et al. (eds). New York: Oxford University Press, 1998.
155. Kline MJ, Kays DW, Rojiani AM. Extradural myxopapillary ependymoma: report of two cases and review of the literature. Pediatr Pathol Lab Med 1996;16:813–822.
156. Rezai AR, Woo HH, Lee M, et al. Disseminated ependymomas of the central nervous system. J Neurosurg 1996;85:618–624.
157. Vanuytsel L, Brada M. The role of prophylactic spinal irradiation in localized intracranial ependymoma. Int J Radiat Oncol Biol Phys 1991;21:825–830.

158. Waldron JN, Laperriere NJ, Jaakkimainen L, et al. Spinal cord ependymomas: a retrospective analysis of 59 cases. Int J Radiat Oncol Biol Phys 1993;27:223–229.
159. Schild SE, Nisi K, Scheithauer BW, et al. The results of radiotherapy for ependymomas: the Mayo Clinic experience. Int J Radiat Oncol Biol Phys 1998;42:953–958.
160. Cervoni L, Celli P, Fortuna A, et al. Recurrence of spinal ependymoma. Risk factors and long-term survival. Spine 1994;19:2838–2841.
161. Healey EA, Barnes PD, Kupsky WJ, et al. The prognostic significance of postoperative residual tumor in ependymoma. Neurosurgery 1991;28:666–671.
162. Wen BC, Hussey DH, Hitchon PW, et al. The role of radiation therapy in the management of ependymomas of the spinal cord. Int J Radiat Oncol Biol Phys 1991;20:781–786.
163. Duffner PK, Horowitz ME, Krischer JP, et al. Postoperative chemotherapy and delayed radiation in children less than three years of age with malignant brain tumors. N Engl J Med 1993;328:1725–1731.
164. Grill J, Le Deley MC, Gambarelli D, et al. Postoperative chemotherapy without irradiation for ependymoma in children under 5 years of age: a multicenter trial of the French Society of Pediatric Oncology. J Clin Oncol 2001; 19:1288–1296.
165. Mirimanoff RO, Dosoretz DE, Linggood RM, et al. Meningioma: analysis of recurrence and progression following neurosurgical resection. J Neurosurg 1985;62:18–24.
166. Helseth A, Mork SJ. Primary intraspinal neoplasms in Norway 1955 to 1986. A population-based survey of 467 patients. J Neurosurg 1989;71:842–845.
167. Namer IJ, Pamir MN, Benli K, et al. Spinal meningiomas. Neurochirurgia (Stuttg) 1987;30:11–15.
168. Gezen F, Kahraman S, Canakci Z, et al. Review of 36 cases of spinal cord meningioma. Spine 2000;25:727–731.
169. Cohen-Gadol AA, Zikel OM, Koch CA, et al. Spinal meningiomas in patients younger than 50 years of age: a 21-year experience. J Neurosurg 2003;98:258–263.
170. Calogero JA, Moossy J. Extradural spinal meningiomas. Report of four cases. J Neurosurg 1972;37:442–447.
171. Roux FX, Nataf F, Pinaudeau M, et al. Intraspinal meningiomas: review of 54 cases with discussion of poor prognosis factors and modern therapeutic management. Surg Neurol 1996;46:458–463.
172. Schiebe ME, Hoffmann W, Kortmann RD, et al. Radiotherapy in recurrent malignant meningiomas with multiple spinal manifestations. Acta Oncol 1997;36:88–90.
173. Goldsmith BJ, Wara WM, Wilson CB, et al. Postoperative irradiation for subtotally resected meningiomas. A retrospective analysis of 140 patients treated from 1967 to 1990. J Neurosurg 1994;80:195–201.
174. Schrell UM, Rittig MG, Anders M, et al. Hydroxyurea for treatment of unresectable and recurrent meningiomas. II. Decrease in the size of meningiomas in patients treated with hydroxyurea. J Neurosurg 1997;86:840–844.
175. Konno S, Yabuki S, Kinoshita T, et al. Combined laminectomy and thoracoscopic resection of dumbbell-type thoracic cord tumor. Spine 2001;26:E130–E134.
176. Shadmehr MB, Gaissert HA, Wain JC, et al. The surgical approach to "dumbbell tumors" of the mediastinum. Ann Thorac Surg 2003;76:1650–1654.
177. Seppala MT, Haltia MJ. Spinal malignant nerve-sheath tumor or cellular schwannoma? A striking difference in prognosis. J Neurosurg 1993;79:528–532.
178. Noel G, Habrand JL, Jauffret E, et al. Radiation therapy for chordoma and chondrosarcoma of the skull base and the cervical spine. Prognostic factors and patterns of failure. Strahlenther Onkol 2003;179:241–248.
179. Chetiyawardana AD. Chordoma: results of treatment. Clin Radiol 1984;35:159–161.
180. Saxton JP. Chordoma. Int J Radiat Oncol Biol Phys 1981; 7:913–915.
181. Sundaresan N, Galicich JH, Chu FC, et al. Spinal chordomas. J Neurosurg 1979;50:312–319.
182. Mabrey RE. Chordoma: a study of 150 cases. Am J Cancer 1935;25:501–517.
183. Birrell JH. Chordomata: a review of nineteen cases of chordomata including five vertebral cases. Aust N Z J Surg 1953;22:258–267.
184. Dahlin DC, Maccarty CS. Chordoma. Cancer 1952;5:1170–1178.
185. Klekamp J, Samii M. Spinal chordomas—results of treatment over a 17-year period. Acta Neurochir (Wien) 1996; 138:514–519.
186. O'Neill P, Bell BA, Miller JD, et al. Fifty years of experience with chordomas in southeast Scotland. Neurosurgery 1985;16:166–170.
187. Rich TA, Schiller A, Suit HD, et al. Clinical and pathologic review of 48 cases of chordoma. Cancer 1985;56:182–187.
188. Kaiser TE, Pritchard DJ, Unni KK. Clinicopathologic study of sacrococcygeal chordoma. Cancer 1984;53:2574–2578.
189. Bethke KP, Neifeld JP, Lawrence W Jr. Diagnosis and management of sacrococcygeal chordoma. J Surg Oncol 1991; 48:232–238.
190. Benk V, Liebsch NJ, Munzenrider JE, et al. Base of skull and cervical spine chordomas in children treated by high-dose irradiation. Int J Radiat Oncol Biol Phys 1995;31: 577–581.
191. Chetty R, Levin CV, Kalan MR. Chordoma: a 20-year clinicopathologic review of the experience at Groote Schuur Hospital, Cape Town. J Surg Oncol 1991;46:261–264.
192. Markwalder TM, Markwalder RV, Robert JL, et al. Metastatic chordoma. Surg Neurol 1979;12:473–478.
193. Higinbotham NL, Phillips RF, Farr HW, et al. Chordoma. Thirty-five-year study at Memorial Hospital. Cancer 1967;20: 1841–1850.
194. Suit HD, Goitein M, Munzenrider J, et al. Definitive radiation therapy for chordoma and chondrosarcoma of base of skull and cervical spine. J Neurosurg 1982;56:377–385.
195. Terahara A, Niemierko A, Goitein M, et al. Analysis of the relationship between tumor dose inhomogeneity and local control in patients with skull base chordoma. Int J Radiat Oncol Biol Phys 1999;45:351–358.
196. Borba LA, Al Mefty O, Mrak RE, et al. Cranial chordomas in children and adolescents. J Neurosurg 1996;84:584–591.
197. Ozaki T, Hillmann A, Winkelmann W. Surgical treatment of sacrococcygeal chordoma. J Surg Oncol 1997;64:274–279.
198. Magrini SM, Papi MG, Marletta F, et al. Chordoma-natural history, treatment and prognosis. The Florence Radiotherapy Department experience (1956–1990) and a critical review of the literature. Acta Oncol 1992;31:847–851.

199. Romero J, Cardenes H, la Torre A, et al. Chordoma: results of radiation therapy in eighteen patients. Radiother Oncol 1993;29:27–32.
200. Cummings BJ, Hodson DI, Bush RS. Chordoma: the results of megavoltage radiation therapy. Int J Radiat Oncol Biol Phys 1983;9:633–642.
201. Hug EB, Loredo LN, Slater JD, et al. Proton radiation therapy for chordomas and chondrosarcomas of the skull base. J Neurosurg 1999;91:432–439.
202. Slater JM, Slater JD, Archambeau JO. Proton therapy for cranial base tumors. J Craniofac Surg 1995;6:24–26.
203. Munzenrider JE, Liebsch NJ. Proton therapy for tumors of the skull base. Strahlenther Onkol 1999;175(Suppl 2):57–63.
204. Austin-Seymour M, Munzenrider JE, Goitein M, et al. Progress in low-LET heavy particle therapy: intracranial and paracranial tumors and uveal melanomas. Radiat Res Suppl 1985;8:S219–S226.
205. Noel G, Habrand JL, Mammar H, et al. Combination of photon and proton radiation therapy for chordomas and chondrosarcomas of the skull base: the Centre de Protontherapie D'Orsay experience. Int J Radiat Oncol Biol Phys 2001;51:392–398.
206. Berson AM, Castro JR, Petti P, et al. Charged particle irradi ation of chordoma and chondrosarcoma of the base of skull and cervical spine: the Lawrence Berkeley Laboratory experience. Int J Radiat Oncol Biol Phys 1988;15:559–565.
207. Castro JR, Linstadt DE, Bahary JP, et al. Experience in charged particle irradiation of tumors of the skull base: 1977–1992. Int J Radiat Oncol Biol Phys 1994;29:647–655.
208. Chang SD, Martin DP, Lee E, et al. Stereotactic radiosurgery and hypofractionated stereotactic radiotherapy for residual or recurrent cranial base and cervical chordomas. Neurosurg Focus 2001;10(3):1–7.
209. Kumar PP, Good RR, Skultety FM, et al. Local control of recurrent clival and sacral chordoma after interstitial irradiation with iodine-125: new techniques for treatment of recurrent or unresectable chordomas. Neurosurgery 1988;22: 479–483.
210. Gutin PH, Leibel SA, Hosobuchi Y, et al. Brachytherapy of recurrent tumors of the skull base and spine with iodine-125 sources. Neurosurgery 1987;20:938–945.
211. Bernstein M, Gutin PH. Interstitial irradiation of skull base tumours. Can J Neurol Sci 1985;12:366–370.
212. York JE, Berk RH, Fuller GN, et al. Chondrosarcoma of the spine: 1954 to 1997. J Neurosurg 1999;90:73–78.
213. Shives TC, McLeod RA, Unni KK, et al. Chondrosarcoma of the spine. J Bone Joint Surg Am 1989;71:1158–1165.
214. Bergh P, Gunterberg B, Meis-Kindblom JM, et al. Prognostic factors and outcome of pelvic, sacral, and spinal chondrosarcomas: a center-based study of 69 cases. Cancer 2001; 91:1201–1212.
215. Camins MB, Duncan AW, Smith J, et al. Chondrosarcoma of the spine. Spine 1978;3:202–209.
216. Sim FH, Frassica FJ, Wold LE. Chondrosarcoma of the spine: Mayo Clinic experience. In: Sundaresan N, Schmidek HH, Schiller AL, et al., eds. Tumors of the spine: diagnosis and clinical management. Philadelphia: WB Saunders, 1990: 155–162.
217. Ozaki T, Hillmann A, Lindner N, et al. Chondrosarcoma of the pelvis. Clin Orthop 1997;337:226–239.
218. Sheth DS, Yasko AW, Johnson ME, et al. Chondrosarcoma of the pelvis. Prognostic factors for 67 patients treated with definitive surgery. Cancer 1996;78:745–750.
219. Oliveira AM, Scheithauer BW, Salomao DR, et al. Primary sarcomas of the brain and spinal cord: a study of 18 cases. Am J Surg Pathol 2002;26:1056–1063.
220. Merimsky O, Lepechoux C, Terrier P, et al. Primary sarcomas of the central nervous system. Oncology 2000;58: 210–214.
221. Sarcoma Meta-analysis Collaboration. Adjuvant chemotherapy for localised resectable soft-tissue sarcoma of adults: meta-analysis of individual data. Lancet 1997;350:1647–1654.
222. Ho VB, Smirniotopoulos JG, Murphy FM, et al. Radiologic-pathologic correlation: hemangioblastoma. AJNR 1992;13: 1343–1352.
223. Cristante L, Herrmann HD. Surgical management of intramedullary hemangioblastoma of the spinal cord. Acta Neurochir (Wien) 1999;141:333–339.
224. Roonprapunt C, Silvera VM, Setton A, et al. Surgical management of isolated hemangioblastomas of the spinal cord. Neurosurgery 2001;49:321–327.
225. Neumann HP, Eggert HR, Weigel K, et al. Hemangioblastomas of the central nervous system. A 10-year study with special reference to von Hippel-Lindau syndrome. J Neurosurg 1989;70:24–30.
226. Browne TR, Adams RD, Roberson GH. Hemangioblastoma of the spinal cord. Review and report of five cases. Arch Neurol 1976;33:435–441.
227. Lonser RR, Weil RJ, Wanebo JE, et al. Surgical management of spinal cord hemangioblastomas in patients with von Hippel-Lindau disease. J Neurosurg 2003;98:106–116.
228. Wanebo JE, Lonser RR, Glenn GM, et al. The natural history of hemangioblastomas of the central nervous system in patients with von Hippel-Lindau disease. J Neurosurg 2003;98:82–94.
229. Lee DK, Choe WJ, Chung CK, et al. Spinal cord hemangioblastoma: surgical strategy and clinical outcome. J Neurooncol 2003;61:27–34.
230. Jawahar A, Kondziolka D, Garces YI, et al. Stereotactic radiosurgery for hemangioblastomas of the brain. Acta Neurochir (Wien) 2000;142:641–644.
231. Heyd R, Strassmann G, Filipowicz I, et al. Radiotherapy in vertebral hemangioma. Rontgenpraxis 2001;53:208–220.
232. Fox MW, Onofrio BM. The natural history and management of symptomatic and asymptomatic vertebral hemangiomas. J Neurosurg 1993;78:36–45.
233. Cross JJ, Antoun NM, Laing RJ, et al. Imaging of compressive vertebral haemangiomas. Eur Radiol 2000;10:997–1002.
234. Djindjian M, Nguyen JP, Gaston A, et al. Multiple vertebral hemangiomas with neurological signs. Case report. J Neurosurg 1992;76:1025–1028.
235. Rades D, Bajrovic A, Alberti W, et al. Is there a dose–effect relationship for the treatment of symptomatic vertebral hemangioma? Int J Radiat Oncol Biol Phys 2003;55:178–181.
236. Dyck P. Intramedullary lipoma. Diagnosis and treatment. Spine 1992;17:979–981.
237. Kodama T, Numaguchi Y, Gellad FE, et al. Magnetic resonance imaging of a high cervical intradural lipoma. Comput Med Imaging Graph 1991;15:93–95.

238. Lee M, Rezai AR, Abbott R, et al. Intramedullary spinal cord lipomas. J Neurosurg 1995;82:394–400.
239. Kujas M, Sichez JP, Lalam TF, et al. Intradural spinal lipoma of the conus medullaris without spinal dysraphism. Clin Neuropathol 2000;19:30–33.
240. Timmer FA, van Rooij WJ, Beute GN, et al. Intramedullary lipoma. Neuroradiology 1996;38:159–160.
241. Razack N, Jimenez OF, Aldana P, et al. Intramedullary holocord lipoma in an athlete: case report. Neurosurgery 1998;42:394–396.
242. Chahal S, Lagera JE, Ryder J, et al. Hematological neoplasms with first presentation as spinal cord compression syndromes: a 10-year retrospective series and review of the literature. Clin Neuropathol 2003;22:282–290.
243. Lyons MK, O'Neill BP, Kurtin PJ, et al. Diagnosis and management of primary spinal epidural non-Hodgkin's lymphoma. Mayo Clin Proc 1996;71:453–457.
244. Mostafavi H, Lennarson PJ, Traynelis VC. Granulocytic sarcoma of the spine. Neurosurgery 2000;46:78–83.
245. Ugras S, Cirak B, Karakok M, et al. Spinal epidural granulocytic sarcoma (chloroma) in a non-leukemic child. Pediatr Int 2001;43:505–507.
246. Fiegl M, Rieger C, Braess J, et al. Isolated epidural chloroma with translocation t(15;17) successfully treated with chemotherapy and all-*trans*-retinoic acid. Br J Haematol 2003;122:688–689.
247. Landis DM, Aboulafia DM. Granulocytic sarcoma: an unusual complication of aleukemic myeloid leukemia causing spinal cord compression. A case report and literature review. Leuk Lymphoma 2003;44:1753–1760.
248. Hejazi N, Witzmann A. Spinal intramedullary teratoma with exophytic components: report of two cases and review of the literature. Neurosurg Rev 2003;26:113–116.
249. Schneider F, Putzier M. Primary leptomeningeal melanoma. Spine 2002;27:E545–E547.
250. Tatter SB, Borges LF, Louis DN. Central neurocytomas of the cervical spinal cord. Report of two cases. J Neurosurg 1994;81:288–293.
251. Tatter SB, Borges LF, Louis DN. Correction: central neurocytomas of the cervical spinal cord. J Neurosurg 1995;82:706.
252. Martin AJ, Sharr MM, Teddy PJ, et al. Neurocytoma of the thoracic spinal cord. Acta Neurochir (Wien) 2002;144: 823–828.
253. Sloof JL. Primary intramedullary tumors of the spinal cord and filum terminale. Philadelphia: WB Saunders, 1964.
254. Nieder C, Milas L, Ang KK. Tissue tolerance to reirradiation. Semin Radiat Oncol 2000;10:200–209.
255. McCunniff AJ, Liang MJ. Radiation tolerance of the cervical spinal cord. Int J Radiat Oncol Biol Phys 1989;16: 675–678.
256. Schultheiss TE. The radiation dose response of the human cervical spinal cord [abstract]. Int J Radiat Oncol Biol Phys 1999;45(Suppl):174.
257. Jeremic B, Djuric L, Mijatovic L. Incidence of radiation myelitis of the cervical spinal cord at doses of 5500 cGy or greater. Cancer 1991;68:2138–2141.

CHAPTER 25

Spinal Root and Peripheral Nerve Tumors

ASIS KUMAR BHATTACHARYYA / ABHIJIT GUHA

Spinal root and peripheral nerve tumors (PNTs) are derived from similar cellular and structural elements; hence, tumors that arise from them are quite similar in their histology and molecular pathogenesis. However, spinal root tumors differ from PNTs in several aspects of clinical presentation and management strategies because of their anatomic location. These include intra- and extradural extensions with spinal cord compromise, involvement or compression of paraspinal structures such as blood vessels, adjacent peripheral and sympathetic nerves, and visceral structures such as the esophagus and trachea. In addition, management strategies have to account for spinal column instability resulting from bony and ligamentous erosions caused by the tumor or surgery; lack of fascicular separation at such a proximal level, thereby increasing potential risks of a postoperative neurological deficit; and unique postoperative issues such as cerebrospinal fluid (CSF) leaks. In comparison, PNTs are often multiple and asymptomatic, especially in the context of predisposition syndromes such as neurofibromatosis type 1 (NF1) and neurofibromatosis type 2 (NF2), requiring judicious clinical appraisal regarding surgery versus conservative treatment.

This chapter highlights the clinical presentations, radiologic features, and management strategies of both spinal root and specific PNTs. In addition, it discusses the genetics and molecular biology of NF1 and NF2, the most common predisposition syndromes associated with these tumors, which, because of their multiplicity and more aggressive growth compared to their spontaneous counterparts, would benefit from biologically targeted therapies rather than multiple surgeries and potential associated morbidities. Although most of the spinal root and PNTs are benign with slow local growth, malignant transformation resulting in malignant peripheral nerve sheath tumor (MPNST) does occur. The goals of MPNST management are different from other spinal root or PNTs, but share the need for increased molecular understanding toward future biologically targeted therapies to prevent recurrence and systemic metastasis.

▶ CLASSIFICATION

The relative rarity of these tumors and a broad range of the primary transformed cell types, the nature of which is sometimes uncertain, have precluded the development of an all-encompassing classification. Tables 25-1 and 25-2 present a simplified classification, which, although excluding several rare pathologic subtypes, serves well toward the management of most spinal root and PNTs. Like with any organ system, these tumors can be divided

▶ TABLE 25-1. SPINAL ROOT TUMORS: CLASSIFICATION

Origin	Type
Nerve sheath	Neurofibroma, schwannoma, MPNST, lipoma, paragangliomas
Meninges	Meningioma
Blood vessel elements	Hemangioblastoma, hemangioma
Metastasis	Epidural, intradural
Developmental tumors	Epidermoid, dermoid, teratoma
Tumor-like lesions	Tarlov cyst, infectious granulomas

into benign and malignant forms, with a majority of tumors being the former and originating from the neural sheath. These include transformation of Schwann cells, which, depending on the primary genetic alterations, can result in schwannomas (mainly associated with loss of the *NF2* gene product merlin) or neurofibromas (mainly associated with the loss of the *NF1* gene product neurofibromin). In addition, other rarer transformed cellular elements of the neural sheath can lead to tumors located in either the spinal root or peripheral nerve, including pericytes (perineurioma), meninges (meningiomas), fibroblasts (desmoid tumors), endothelial cells (hemangiomas, hemangioblastomas, and angiomas), and lipocytes (lipomas). Aberrant differentiation and development can lead to another rare category of benign tumors, commonly associated with the axial spine: paragangliomas, epidermoids, and teratomas. Pseudotumors do not arise from cellular transformation, but rather from inflammation and include the "tumor-like lesions" listed in Tables 25-1 and 25-2. Metastasis to the spinal epidural space and along the neural foramina, or malignant tumors arising from adjacent soft-tissues or organs, such as Pancoast tumors from the lungs compressing the brachial plexus, are quite common. However, primary malignant tumors of spinal roots or peripheral nerves are relatively rare. These are collectively termed MPNSTs and arise from additional genetic alterations to the Schwann cells, especially those that are already transformed to neurofibromas.

▶ CLINICAL PRESENTATION

Spinal Root Tumor

Spinal root tumors present insidiously with progressive radiculopathy and/or myeloradiculopathy, although occasional acute exacerbations as a result of peritumoral

▶ TABLE 25-2. PERIPHERAL NERVE TUMORS: CLASSIFICATION

Benign	Malignant
Schwannoma (+/– NF2 or Schwannomatosis)	*Primary*
Typical	MPNST
Atypical	Primary CNS lymphoma
Ancient	Ganglioneuroblastoma
Psammomatous melanotic	
Cellular	*Secondary*
Benign epithelioid	Local spread
Neuroblastoma-like	Pancoast tumor
Plexiform	Soft tissue sarcoma
	Intraneural metastasis
Neurofibroma (+/– NF1)	**Tumor-like lesions**
Dermal	Ganglion cyst
Plexiform	Traumatic neuroma
	Inflammatory
	Pseudotumor
Perineuroma	Leprosy
Desmoid	Radiation neuritis
Palisaded encapsulated neuroma	Hypertrophic neuropathy
Neurothekoma (nerve sheath myxoma)	
Ganglioneuroma	
Lipoma	
Hemangioma	
Angiomatosis of peripheral nerve	
Meningioma	

edema, intratumoral hemorrhage, and/or necrosis may occur. The exact nature of the clinical presentation depends on the anatomic location and size of the tumor. Pain is the most common presentation, with a gradual and progressive onset and course, often characterized as increasing with recumbency, therefore triggering awakening at night. This differentiating feature on history is critical to delineate pain from a neoplastic origin versus the much more common radicular symptoms secondary to spinal degenerative disease. Radicular distribution of pain in the corresponding dermatome of the affected nerve root, with occasional hypesthesia, tingling, numbness, and burning sensation are frequent associations. Weakness, the second most common symptom of spinal root tumors, may either be a lower motor neuron type or occur in association with myelopathy, the latter being prevalent in cervical and thoracic locations. High cervical tumors may present with weakness, wasting, and fasciculation of the intrinsic muscles of the hand, perhaps reflecting the large contribution of the corticospinal fibers to supply the intrinsic muscle anterior horn pool. Sphincter dysfunction, of spastic variety, is the next common clinical presentation of spinal root tumors, except those arising from cauda equina, where hypotonic sphincter function is the rule. Impotence and the loss of sensation in the saddle distribution of the perineum provide additional diagnostic clues.

Less commonly, spinal root tumors may present with a wide variety of other features, including decreased sensation of face and impaired respiratory reserve in high cervical and foramen magnum lesions, band-like sensory alterations around the chest in thoracic lesions, Brown-Sequard syndrome with some lesions presenting with radiculomyelopathic symptoms, kyphoscoliosis as a consequence of induced skeletal abnormalities, especially in the developing child, and hydrocephalus from proteinaceous debris in the CSF.

Peripheral Nerve Tumors

A focused history and physical examination is the most vital component for arriving at the most probable diagnosis and best management strategy of a PNT. The history is directed toward (a) the onset, duration, and growth alterations of the mass; (b) any neurologic and nonneurologic symptoms, such as pain, numbness, and weakness; (c) any associated systemic complaints suggestive of an underlying cancer; (d) a family history suggestive of NF or other predisposition syndromes; and (e) a general medical inquiry of the patient. The physical exam is directed toward (a) the mass, which may be firm or soft, nonpulsatile, mobile perpendicular to, but not along, the long axis of a known peripheral nerve; (b) presence or absence of a Tinel sign, which may give a clue about the nerve of origin or one that is juxtaposed to the PNT; (c) fixed sensory or motor deficits, which are usually rare because of the slow growth rate of most PNTs; (d) examination of local structures that may be compressed by the PNT; and (e) a systemic examination with a focus on the absence or presence of clinical signs associated with NF1 as listed in Table 25-3.

▶ PREOPERATIVE INVESTIGATIONS

Spinal Root Tumors

Magnetic resonance imaging (MRI), including T_1 and T_2 gadolinium-enhanced images in both sagittal and axial planes, is the mainstay for the radiologic diagnosis and followup of spinal root tumors. Demonstration of a "dumbbell" tumor by MRI is very suggestive of a spinal root lesion (Fig. 25-1). Schwannomas and neurofibromas, the most common variety of spinal root neoplasms, are usually hypointense on T_1, hyperintense on T_2, and enhance homogeneously with gadolinium (Figs. 25-1 and 25-2). Meningiomas, very common spinal tumors, although not strictly lesions of spinal root, share similar characteristics except for a few subtle differences such as a more posterolateral location, more intense contrast enhancement, and a more frequent occurrence of adjacent dural enhancement, the so-called "dural-tail" sign.

Plain radiographs, although often ignored, are a useful imaging modality to demonstrate the bony outline, neural foraminal widening, posterior scalloping of the vertebral bodies, pathologic fractures, and, very rarely, calcification associated with meningiomas. Computerized tomography (CT), although better at identifying bony changes, has been largely superseded by MRI as the investigation instrument of choice. CT myelography is indicated in cases of significant canalicular encroachment by the spinal root tumor and when MRI is not available. Spinal angiography may be helpful for demonstrating vascular architecture of arteriovenous malformations (AVMs) or tumor blush of hemangioblastoma and paraganglioma, especially when they mimic spinal root tumors, and for providing an avenue for preoperative embolization when indicated. In addition, spinal angiography can demonstrate the origin, course, and distribution of the artery of Adamkiewicz, a potentially critical piece of information when dealing with a lower thoracic spinal root nerve tumor with a precarious blood supply to that region of the spinal cord.

Peripheral Nerve Tumors

Preoperative electrophysiologic examination is not routine in management of PNTs, because it does not add to the diagnosis or provide any information beyond that obtained from the history, physical examination, and radiologic workup of the PNT. Electrophysiology is most critical during intraoperative evaluation and to follow postoperative recovery if a deficit occurs. As with spinal

▶ TABLE 25-3. CLINICAL DIAGNOSTIC CRITERIA FOR NEUROFIBROMATOSIS TYPES 1 AND 2 AND SCHWANNOMATOSIS

Neurofibromatosis type 1

- Two or more of the following:
  - Six or more café-au-lait macules >5 mm in greatest diameter in prepubertal individuals or >15 mm in postpubertal individuals.
  - Two or more neurofibromas of any type or one plexiform neurofibroma.
  - Freckling in axillary or inguinal regions.
  - Optic nerve glioma.
  - Two or more Lisch nodules.
  - A distinct osseous lesion such as a sphenoid dysplasia or thinning of the long bone cortex with or without or without pseudoarthrosis.
  - A first-degree relative (parent, sibling, or offspring) with neurofibromatosis type 1 by the above criteria.

Neurofibromatosis type 2

- Definitive:
  - Bilateral vestibular schwannomas or
  - A family history of neurofibromatosis type 2 (first-degree relative) and either:
    - Unilateral vestibular schwannoma diagnosed at age younger than 30 years *or*
    - Any two of the following: meningioma, glioma, schwannoma, juvenile posterior subcapsular lenticular opacities/juvenile cortical cataract.
- Presumptive or probable neurofibromatosis type 2:
  - Unilateral vestibular schwanhoma at age younger than 30 years plus one of the following: meningioma, glioma, schwannoma, juvenile posterior subcapsular lenticular opacities/juvenile cortical cataract.
  - Multiple meningiomas (two or more) plus unilateral vestibular schwannoma at age younger than 30 years or one of the following: meningioma, glioma, schwannoma, juvenile posterior subcapsular lenticular opacities/juvenile cortical cataract.

Diagnostic criteria of schwannomatosis

- Definitive:
  - Two or more pathologically proven schwannomas; *plus*
  - Lack of radiographic evidences of vestibular nerve tumors, at age older than 18 years.
- Presumptive or probable schwannomatosis:
  - Two or more pathologically proven schwannomas, without symptoms of eighth nerve dysfunction, at age older than 30 years; *or*
  - Two or more pathologically proved schwannomas in an anatomically limited distribution (single limb or segment of the spine), without symptoms of eighth nerve dysfunction, at any age.

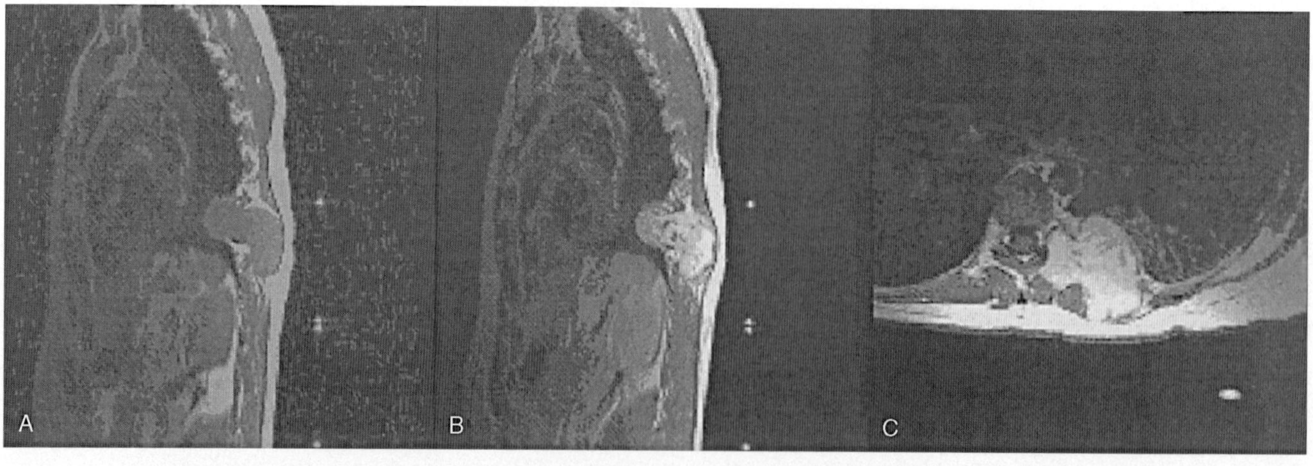

Figure 25-1. (A) Sagittal MRI demonstrating lower thoracic nerve sheath tumor with paraspinal extension. The tumor is isointense on T_1-weighted image. (B) Enhancement of the tumor with gadolinium. (C) Gadolinium-enhanced T_1-weighted axial image showing location of the tumor with dumbbell extension.

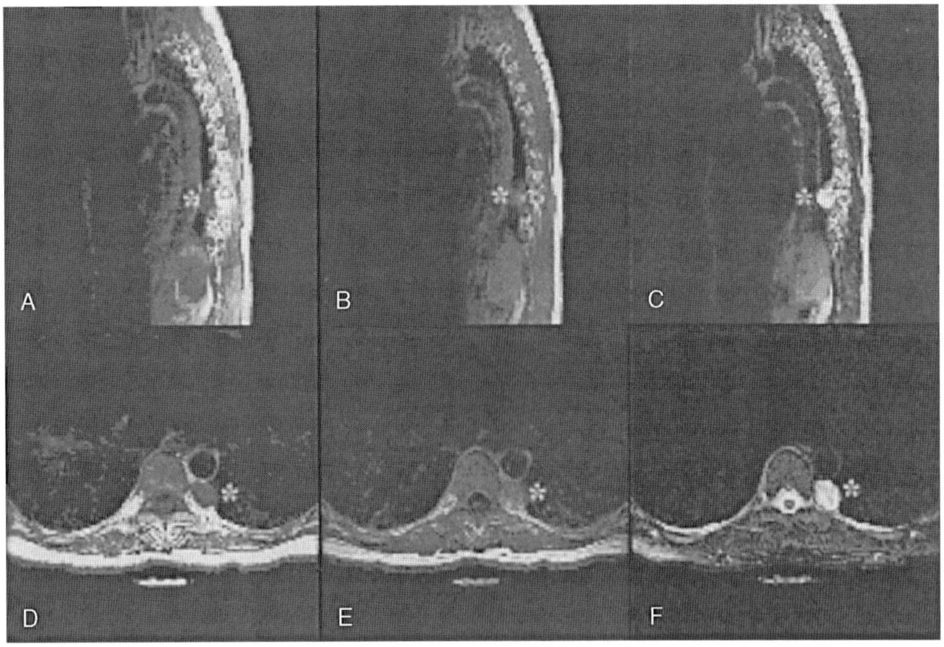

Figure 25-2. (A to F) Paraspinal location of the nerve sheath tumor (*) without intraforaminal extension. The tumor is isointense in sagittal and axial T_1 (A and D), enhances with gadolinium in sagittal and axial T_1 (B and E), and is hyperintense in sagittal and axial T_2 (C and F) imaging.

root lesions, MRI is the best investigation for PNTs; occasionally, however, CT scans are helpful, particularly in demonstrating remodeling of adjacent bony structures. There are no pathognomonic MRI features for PNTs and the various subtypes, although some features are highly suggestive. For example, a well-circumscribed elliptical or spherical tumor, with low T_1 and high T_2 signal and homogeneous or heterogeneous contrast enhancement, is highly suggestive of schwannoma (Fig. 25-3A). Demonstration of the nerves of origin or exit and displaced passer-by fascicles around the capsule, sometimes demonstrated by the preoperative MRI (see Fig. 25-3A), are highly suggestive of a schwannoma and its typical extrafascicular growth seen intraoperatively (Figs. 25-3B and 25-4B to F). This is in contrast to neurofibromas, which are usually fusiform or multinodular with intrafascicular growth (Figs. 25-3C and 25-5D and E). Another clue regarding the subtype of PNT is if the PNT occurs in the context of an NF1 patient, where the lesion will most certainly be a neurofibroma, in contrast with NF2 patients who harbor mainly schwannomas. Lipoma and ganglion cyst can usually be diagnosed on the basis of characteristic MR signals (Fig. 25-3D) and their relationship to the adjacent structures from which they originate, such as joint capsules in the case of ganglion cysts.

Preoperative imaging studies do not reliably demonstrate features of malignancy in a PNT. Nonhomogeneous contrast enhancement indicates intratumoral hemorrhage or necrosis, but correlation with malignancy is poor. There are no definitive radiologic features of MPNSTs, which are mainly suspected based on rapid clinical and radiologic growth, progressive neurologic deterioration, and pain, especially in the context of an NF1 patient with a symptomatic plexiform neurofibroma. [^{18}F]fluorodeoxyglucose positron emission tomography (FDG-PET) scanning has promise for distinguishing MPNST from benign plexiform neurofibromas, although further clinical verification is required.[1]

▶ OVERALL MANAGEMENT PEARLS

Spinal Root Tumors

The two main objectives for the surgical removal of a spinal root tumor are (a) to remove the tumor while sparing the nerve root and spinal cord if extending intradurally, and (b) to ensure that the patient is left with a stable spine. Special considerations are required for a high cervical tumor with canalicular extension, where a preoperative anesthesia evaluation for awake intubation may be required, with occasional need for postoperative ventilatory support. Muscle relaxants are often not used, to allow direct nerve root stimulation with audible intraoperative

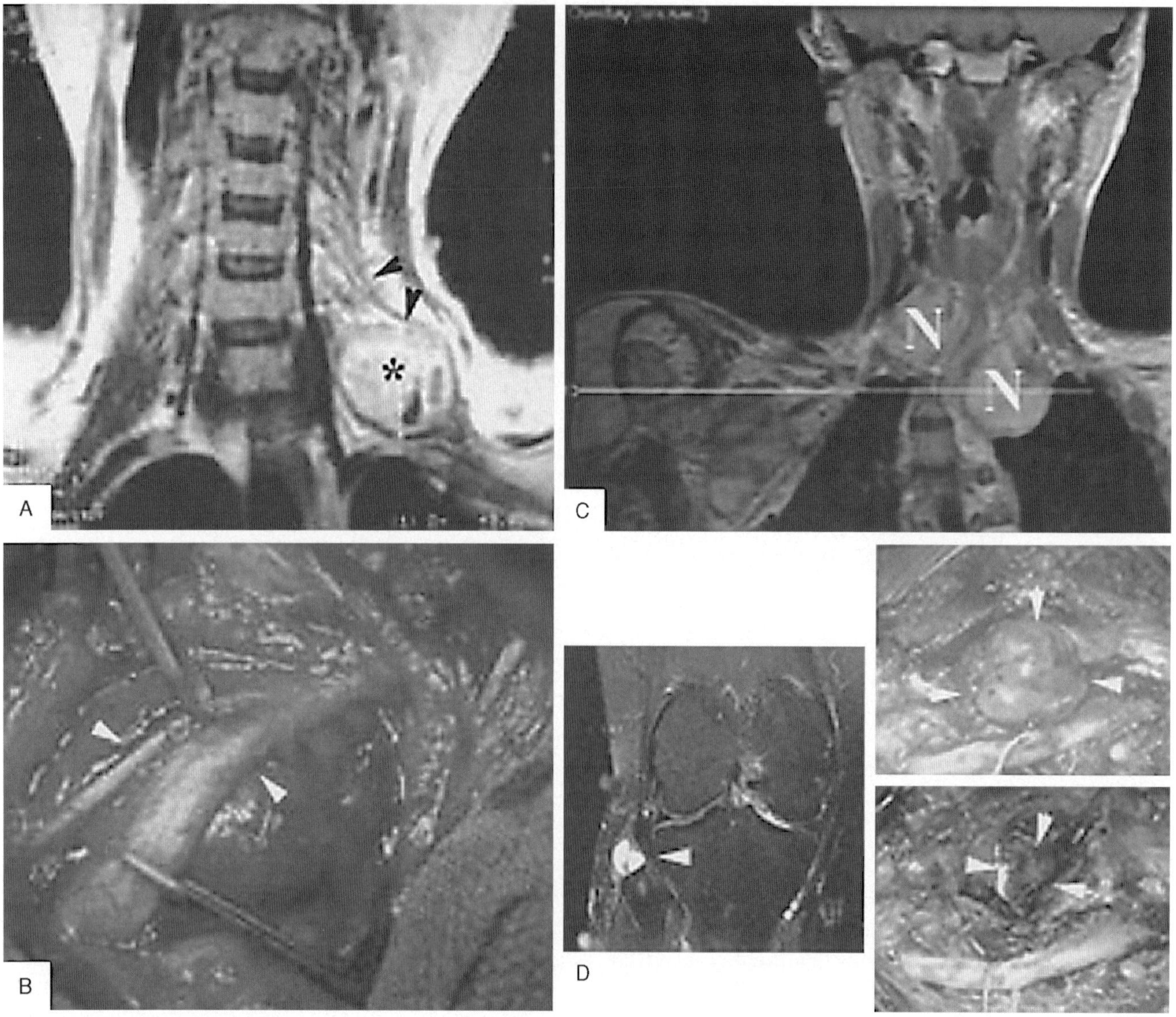

Figure 25-3. (A and B) Coronal MRI with gadolinium enhancement demonstrating typical features of a schwannoma arising from middle trunk of the brachial plexus (*). The lesion is discrete and spherical, with areas of heterogeneous enhancement with passerby fascicles displaced and draped around the tumor capsule, as demonstrated in the intraoperative picture (arrowhead), with vessel loop isolation of the upper trunk and suprascapular nerve from the underlying tumor capsule. (C) MRI with gadolinium coronal picture demonstrating the fusiform, heterogeneous multiple neurofibromas (N) in a NF1 patient. Note the local compression of the esophagus by the bilateral neurofibromas. (D) Coronal T_2 MRI image demonstrating a ganglion cyst arising from the tibia–fibula joint (arrowhead). Intraoperative images demonstrating isolation of the cyst from adjacent common peroneal nerve followed by removal of the entire cyst including the portion from within the joint (arrowhead), to minimize recurrence.

electromyography (EMG) monitoring, to minimize risk to nerve root injury. Somatosensory-evoked potentials (SSEPs) from the limbs are used for those tumors that also compress the spinal cord, with sphincter electrodes useful in tumors involving the cauda equina roots intradurally.

The majority of spinal root tumors are predominantly extradural and are safely removed by a midline posterior approach, often combined with medial facetectomy. If more than half of the facet is removed, consideration for fusion to prevent long-term spinal instability should be considered, though this issue is more critical in the cervical and lumbar regions than in the thoracic spine. Spinal root tumors with significant intradural extension require a concomitant laminectomy, dural opening, and initial removal of the intradural portion abutting the spinal cord. In these cases, dural reconstruction with fascia or dural substitute, supplemented by fibrin glue, and often a postoperative lumbar drain, are required to minimize risks of a CSF leak.

Dumbbell tumors with significant extraspinal extensions require complex surgical approaches, which at times are best staged after initial decompression of the portion of the tumor encroaching on the spinal canal. For example, in cervical dumbbell tumors with retropharyngeal extension, a separate anterior approach is often required after an adequate posterior decompression of the lesion. For tumors extending to the posterior mediastinum or retroperitoneum, a posterolateral transpedicular or costotransversectomy approach, or a staged transthoracic or retroperitoneal approach, may be needed.

Additional intraoperative pearls in the management of spinal root lesions include an adequate bony exposure to reach beyond the margins of the tumor and delineate normal nerve root at either tumor pole. In the lower thoracic region, care must be taken to preserve the radicular branches, because of the precarious blood supply of the spinal cord at this level, as previously mentioned. Whether one can spare the functioning fascicles depends on the nature of the tumor, as well as its anatomic importance. For example, in thoracic region nerve root tumors, the root can be sacrificed without significant deficits, as opposed to cervical and lumbosacral regions where a more conservative approach and preservation of the nerve root is mandatory. Like PNTs, fascicular-sparing surgery is achievable with both schwannomas and neurofibromas, but often to a limited extent and with difficulty in the latter. In root lesions with intradural extension, a midline durotomy with lateral extension over the nerve root sleeve is undertaken, with excision of the adjacent denticulate ligaments for tumors with a more anterior extension. The relationship of the tumor to corresponding nerve root and spinal cord is critical, with the primary objective in these cases to decompress the cord. A majority of intradural Schwann cell tumors will arise from the dorsal sensory rootlets, although a ventral origin is almost equally likely in those tumors associated with NF. Small tumors may be excised en bloc; for most larger tumors, however, intratumoral debulking with Cavitron Ultrasonic Surgical Aspirator (CUSA), followed by folding in of the tumor capsule, is required. Electrophysiologic monitoring of spinal cord function with SSEPs and nerve root function with direct electrical stimulation with audible EMG recordings from relevant muscles are crucial. Where available, motor-evoked potentials (MEPs) are also used, but are not part of the usual electrophysiologic monitoring paradigm at most centers.

The importance of steps to minimize CSF leaks was described above. The potential for acute or delayed spinal instability, resulting from primary bone remodeling by the tumor, or secondary to the requirement for adequate surgical exposure, must always be considered preoperatively. In children, laminoplasty may help to reduce spinal instability; in adults, however, spinal fusion procedure if needed usually includes some form of posterior fixation. As noted, this is rarely required in the thoracic region, because of the presence of the rib cage, but is often required in the cervical and lumbar regions. Details of the many forms of fixation are beyond the scope of this chapter and remain the province of spinal orthopedic or neurosurgeons.

Peripheral Nerve Tumors

Contrary to spinal root tumors where surgery is the treatment of choice, only a subset of patients suspected to have a PNT require operative intervention. For example, a suspected long-standing schwannoma in an elderly or medically compromised patient is best left alone if only minimal symptoms are present. Similarly, the multiple dermal or plexiform neurofibromas in an NF1 patient are best watched, unless local compressive symptoms or suspicion of malignant conversion supervene. If surgery is warranted, the preoperative goals (total excision vs. subtotal debulking vs. biopsy) and associated risks must be thoroughly discussed with the patient. Microneurosurgical techniques, intraoperative magnification, and electrophysiologic monitoring are essential prerequisites. Anesthesia should be without neuromuscular paralysis to allow intraoperative electrophysiologic evaluation. The affected limb should be positioned and draped to allow evaluation of the distal muscles supplied by the relevant nerve or audible EMG electrodes inserted into those muscles. The incision should be long enough to expose the proximal and distal normal nerve (see Fig. 25-4A). If the PNT is near a natural entrapment point such as the carpal tunnel or fibular head, prophylactic release of the nerve traversing through these regions should be undertaken to defray delayed entrapment syndromes.

Exposure commences with isolation of the proximal and distal segments of the nerve of origin, which are encircled in vessel loops and electrophysiologically confirmed (see Fig. 25-4B and C). Gross and microscopical examination of the PNT is then undertaken. Presence of passerby fascicles, which may be splayed across the tumor capsule, is highly suggestive of the extrafascicular growth of schwannomas (see Fig. 25-4D and E), with visual and electrical localization of these fascicles important to minimize deficits. An area devoid of any fascicles and one that is electrically silent, hence representing only tumor, is chosen to obtain a quick section to be interpreted by an

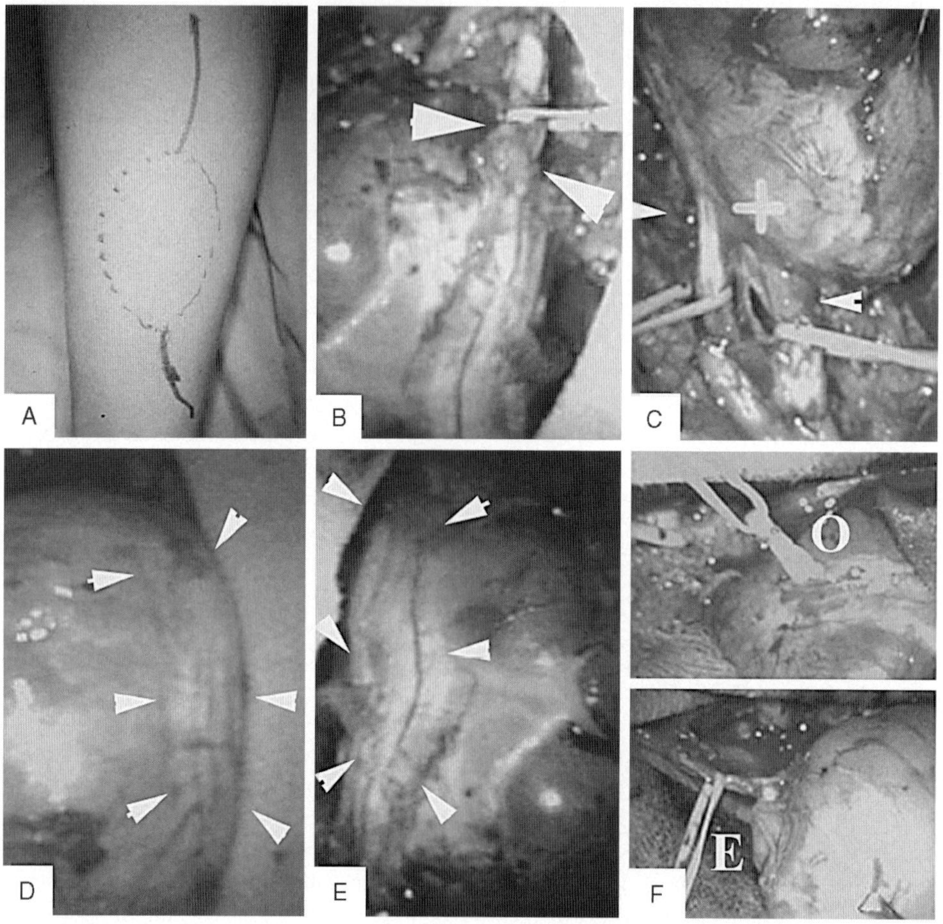

Figure 25-4. (A) Planning of the skin incision for safe removal should extend proximal and distal to the tumor mass itself, to isolate the nerve of origin. (B) Common sciatic nerve bundle in this mid-thigh schwannoma (arrowhead). (C) Distal nerve(s) isolated: posttibial and common peroneal nerve (arrowhead). (D and E) Passerby nerve fascicles attenuated and splayed by the tumor, recognized using microscopy and electrophysiological stimulation (arrowhead). (F) Microneurosurgical techniques with electrophysiologic stimulation are used to isolate the fascicle of origin (O) and exit (E), which, on stimulation, do not lead to any distal muscle activity.

experienced neuropathologist. If the macroscopic and pathologic examination is consistent with the diagnosis of a schwannoma, total removal is to be expected, whereas subtotal but radical debulking can be accomplished with neurofibromas. Often the exact differentiation of the PNT subtype cannot be made on the quick section, requiring use of good clinical judgment to maximize tumor removal with minimal deficits. The majority of small- to medium-size PNTs can be removed in total, although removal of larger tumors or those adjacent to vital structures such as the spinal canal first may require intratumoral decompression by CUSA, followed by resection of the capsule from adjacent functioning neural and nonneural structures. Microneurosurgical dissection, combined with electrophysiologic monitoring, is continued until the nerve fascicle of origin and exit is identified and electrically isolated and demonstrated to be nonfunctional (see Fig. 25-4F). Total capsular removal is often achievable, once the passerby-splayed fascicles are identified and able to be preserved by careful dissection using the microscope. The necessity of nerve grafts after resection of PNTs is extremely rare if good clinical judgment and microneurosurgical principles are used. The management of MPNST is considered separately, because the oncologic objectives are somewhat different from the more common benign schwannomas and neurofibromas. Similarly, intraoperative management goals and strategies also differ among some of the more rare PNT subtypes and are discussed in each section.

▶ SPECIAL CONSIDERATIONS

Schwannomas

Schwannomas (also called neurilemomas) are the most common PNTs in adults, affecting any nerve beyond the oligodendroglial–Schwann cell junction. Most of them are incidentally diagnosed; they are slow-growing solitary tumors on flexor surfaces of middle-aged patients without any gender predilection. Malignant transformation of a typical schwannoma does not occur, with only a small risk in some of the atypical varieties listed in Table 25-2. Spinal nerve sheath schwannomas may present with radiculomyelopathic symptoms as discussed. Microscopically, a typical schwannoma consists of alternating areas of cellular Antoni A and loosely arranged Antoni B regions, with palisading organization of nuclei termed *Verocay bodies* (see Fig. 25-5A to C). The cells are spindle-shaped with indistinct cytoplasm and elongated nuclei with blunt-point ends. Immunohistochemically, they demonstrate S100 and Leu-7 positivity and epithelial membrane antigen (EMA) negativity. Absence of intratumoral axons is a key point for differentiating them from neurofibromas. Electron microscopy may be helpful in difficult cases by demonstrating Schwann cell composition characterized by a completely surrounding basal lamina.

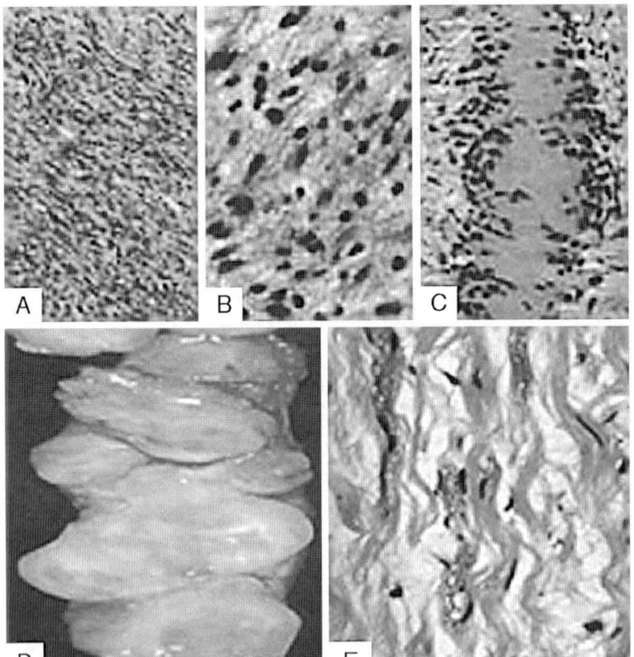

Figure 25-5 (PLATE 57). Histology of a typical schwannoma with (A) Antoni A hypercellular regions of transformed Schwann spindle-like cells. (B) Antoni B hypocellular loose myxoid regions. (C) Verocay bodies. (D) Gross picture of a neurofibroma with myxoid heterogeneous regions and intrafascicular growth. (E) Histopathology of a typical neurofibroma with loose myxoid architecture containing several cellular elements, including the transformed Schwann cells and axons, consistent with intrafascicular growth.

Atypical, relatively rare variants of schwannomas (see Table 25-2) include ancient, psammomatous melanotic, cellular, benign epithelioid, neuroblastoma-like, and plexiform schwannoma. The term *ancient* denotes aging and a degenerated appearance in histology, which is characterized by cyst formation, stromal edema, xanthomatous changes, and fibrosis. Although totally benign, rapid growth and heterogeneous contrast enhancement may falsely suggest malignancy. Psammomatous melanotic schwannomas are packed with melanin and lamellated calcospherules, and may occur sporadically or as a part of Carney syndrome.[2] Cellular schwannoma is another neuropathologic challenge, which may histologically mimic malignancy, although it has fewer mitotic figures than the usual MPNST.[3,4] Benign epithelioid schwannomas are characterized by epithelioid cells arranged in cords or nests with occasional features of degenerative changes.[5] Neuroblastoma-like schwannoma is a very rare, atypical variant, composed of giant rosettes, which histologically simulates a neuroblastoma.[6] Plexiform schwannomas are a rare morphologic variant, which may occur sporadically, with NF2, or with schwannomatosis, but unlike plexiform neurofibromas, do not have a propensity for malignant transformation.[7,8]

Neurofibromas

Neurofibromas may arise sporadically or as part of NF1 syndrome. There are at least three subtypes of neurofibromas: dermal, subcutaneous, and plexiform. Although varying in their biology and clinical behavior, the underlying transformed cell type in all is the Schwann cell. For example, dermal or subcutaneous neurofibromas do not become malignant, and hence removal should be rare and restricted to those lesions that are being abraded or causing gross cosmetic issues. Plexiform neurofibromas, in comparison, can cause problems by local but benign growth and pressure on adjacent vital structures, or, in approximately 10% to 15% of cases, by malignant transformation to MPNST.[9,10] Neurofibromas have intrafascicular growth, macroscopically involving the entire nerve (see Fig. 25-5D), with elongated wavy interlacing hyperchromatic spindle-shaped nucleated cells, in a disorderly loose mucoid background with collagenous fibrils (see Fig. 25-5E). The transformed cell has been shown to be the Schwann cell, but there are multiple cell types in a typical neurofibroma, including perineural cells, fibroblasts, lymphocytes, and mast cells. Intratumoral presence of axons is a cardinal and distinguishing feature of neurofibromas compared to schwannomas and is the main reason that attempts at radical resection may lead to deficits.[11]

Other Benign Peripheral Nerve Tumors

Perineuromas

These benign solitary circumscribed tumors of perineural cell origin clinically mimic schwannomas. Immunohistochemically, they are positive for EMA and negative for S100, Leu-7, and neurofilament staining.[12,13] Management and prognosis are similar to typical schwannomas.

Palisaded, Encapsulated Neuromas

These benign solitary dome-shaped tumors most commonly affect the face of middle-age persons. Immunohistochemistry reveals that they are composed of Schwann cells, perineural cells, and small axons.[14,15]

Neurothekeomas

These are benign tumors mainly affecting face, neck, shoulder, and arms of young women and are of two subtypes: myxomatous and cellular. Immunohistochemistry suggests that the myxomatous subtype is of Schwann cell origin, with the cellular subtype occasionally having atypical histologic features.[16]

Ganglion Cyst

Ganglion cysts, arising from joint or tendon sheaths, lead to extraneural compression and may recur even after resection (see Fig. 25-3D). They are most frequently located around the wrist, knee, elbow, and hip joints. Surgical treatment is aimed at removal of the cyst from both the nerve and the joint capsule to prevent recurrence. Rare intraneural ganglion cysts may arise like their extraneural counterparts and subsequently track along the sheath of small articular nerves into their final destinations.[17,18]

Lipoma

These lesions arise from adipocytes and fibrofatty tissues, and infiltrate adjacent nerves. They typically affect the median nerve and present with carpal tunnel syndrome and macrodactyly. MRI demonstrates the characteristic signals of fat, and intervention is not usually warranted unless progressive neurologic symptoms occur. Treatment, if indicated because of progressive symptoms or growth, depends on whether the lipoma is intrinsic or extrinsic to the nerve bundle. If intrinsic, attempts at removal of the lipoma from the nerve fascicles may lead to neurologic deficits, and hence surgery should be restricted to release of the entrapment and/or at most biopsy of the lesion.[19,20]

Desmoids

These locally aggressive tumors of adjacent fascial and musculoaponeurotic structures may invade nerves in the brachial or retroperitoneal plexus and cause significant progressive neurologic deficits. Although gross total removal is the goal, this is often challenging and associated with significant morbidity because of their invasive and infiltrative growth pattern. Many centers advocate postoperative radiotherapy to reduce recurrence, but radiation-induced neuritis prompts others to reserve radiation for recurrent disease after reoperation.[21,22] Biologic targeted therapies are being investigated in early clinical trials.

Pseudotumor of Peripheral Nerve

These lesions result from chronic inflammatory cell infiltration of peripheral nerve. A conservative microsurgical resection with neural sparing should be attempted.[23,24]

▶ MALIGNANT TUMORS OF PERIPHERAL NERVE

Malignant Peripheral Nerve Sheath Tumor

MPNSTs, also known as neurogenic sarcomas, account for 3% to 10% of all soft-tissue sarcomas. About half arise from NF1-associated plexiform neurofibromas. Patients with MPNSTs associated with NF1 tend to present at a younger age than those without NF1. Progressive enlargement, incapacitating pain, and increasing neurologic deficit are suggestive of malignant transformation of a preexisting plexiform neurofibroma, as discussed in section "Preoperative Investigations: Peripheral Nerve Tumors." MRI is the Investigation of choice, although it cannot distinguish MPNST from other PNTs or soft tissue sarcomas with certainty. Nonhomogeneous contrast enhancement, necrosis, and hemorrhage are suggestive, but not confirmatory, radiologic features. The cell of origin is the Schwann cell, although the mature Schwann cell S100 marker may be absent in approximately 50% of MPNSTs as a consequence of dedifferentiation. The classification of MPNSTs is based on the classification used for the much more common soft tissue sarcomas, from grades 1 to 3, depending on number of mitotic figures and the degree of nuclear and cellular atypia.[25]

The ideal management of MPNSTs remains problematic, with our institute recommending a multidisciplinary management strategy (Fig. 25-6A). Clinical suspicion is followed by biopsy; we recommend a four-quadrant open biopsy, rather than fine-needle or percutaneous biopsy, to maximize retrieval of representative tissue for a thorough pathologic examination with minimal morbidity and pain to the patient. We usually stage this and confirm our pathologic diagnosis. The implication of the pathology and the proposed management strategy is then discussed with the patient. We undertake a metastatic survey with CT/MRI of the chest and abdomen, and follow with definitive oncologic surgery. The goal of the surgery is to achieve an en bloc removal with tumor-free margins, even at the cost of major nerves and adjacent soft tissue structures (Fig. 25-6B). Nerve grafting is not

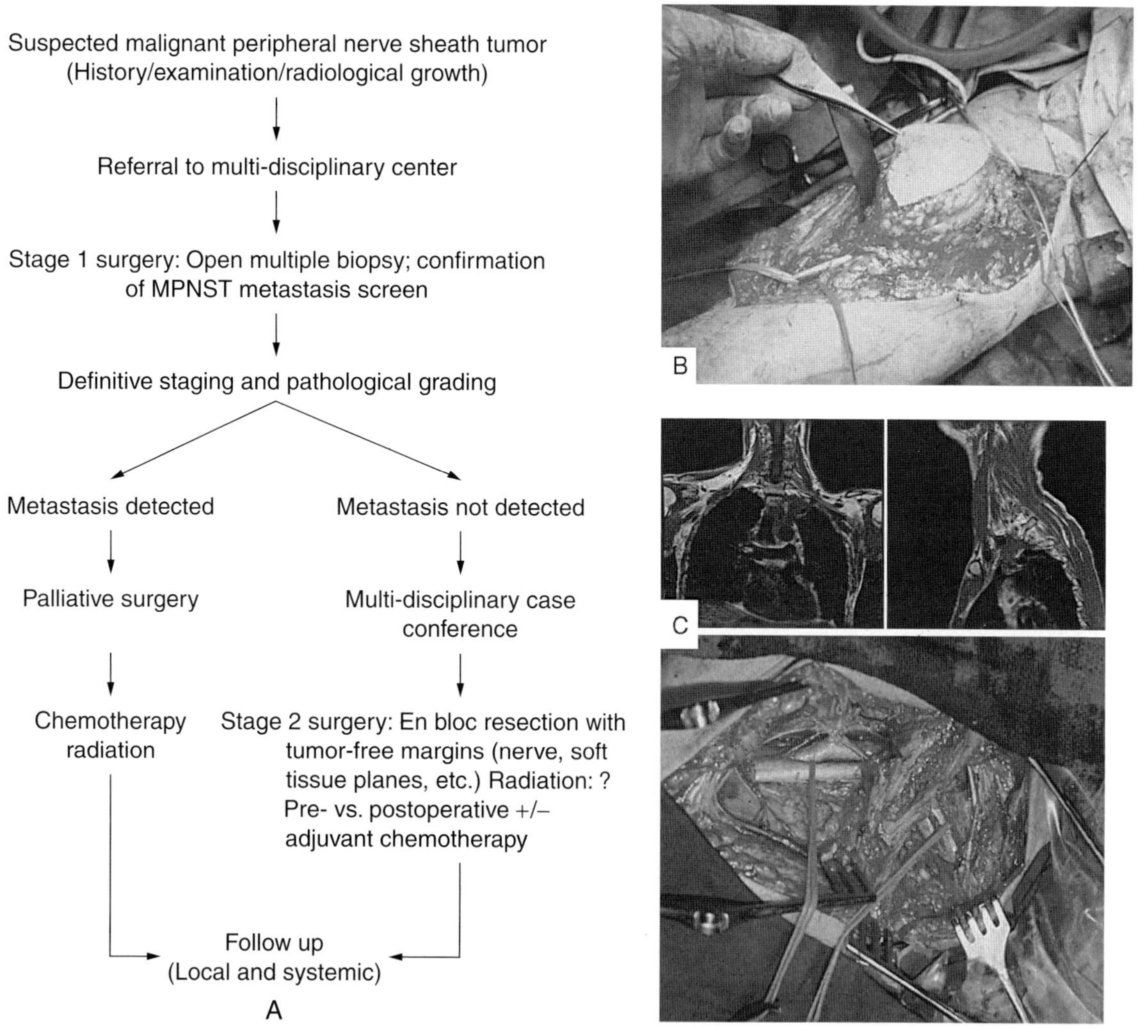

Figure 25-6. (A) Management strategy for MPNST (University of Toronto Multidisciplinary Sarcoma Group). (B) Stage 2 oncologic surgery of a MPNST arising from a plexiform neurofibroma of the musculocutaneous nerve in an NF1 patient. Pathologic diagnosis of MPNST was verified by open four-quadrant biopsy of the suspected MPNST at a prior stage 1 surgery. Note removal of both the MPNST, along with nerve of origin, and associated soft tissue structures (fascia, muscles, overlying subcutaneous tissue, and skin) in order to get tumor-free margins, which were verified by intraoperative quick sections. (C, top) Coronal and sagittal MRI images of left Pancoast lung cancer, confirmed on CT-guided needle biopsy. (C, bottom) After preoperative radiation, a supraclavicular and sternal thoracic opening facilitated en bloc resection of the tumor, with isolation of the lower trunk and vessels, which the tumor was abutting against, but not infiltrating.

considered because of the usual location of MPNSTs in the more proximal nerves; adjuvant radiation therapy and the natural history of MPNST often preclude effective reinnervation.

Adverse prognostic factors include large size (>5 cm), higher tumor grade, advanced histology, inability to achieve tumor-free surgical margins, and association with NF1. Preoperative versus postoperative radiation and adjuvant chemotherapy are controversial issues in MPNST, without any large-scale studies able to be conducted because of the few numbers of these patients, which are often managed outside of a multidisciplinary academic center. Metastasis, especially to the lungs, is the terminal event, and in spite of limited efficacy chemotherapy is indicated in that situation. Wedge resection of solitary pulmonary metastasis may sometimes be undertaken in a stable patient. The 5-year survival rate of MPNST is worse than other soft-tissue sarcomas and is generally approximately 34% to 51%, with our management strategy resulting in a 64% 5-year survival.[25]

Primary Lymphoma of Peripheral Nerve

Only 10 cases have been reported so far and the majority of them are of the B-cell type, affecting the sciatic nerve. This should be differentiated from neurolymphomatosis, which is a part of systemic manifestation of lymphoma. Treatment includes surgery and adjuvant therapies.[26,27]

Pancoast Tumor

Primary carcinomas of apex of lung involving or abutting against the lower elements of the brachial plexus, most prevalent in smokers, often warrants a combined neurosurgical and thoracic surgical procedure to obtain radical tumor removal. They present with progressive pain, weakness of the intrinsic muscles of the hand, and Horner syndrome, often accompanied by systemic signs from cancer burden. The subtype of lung cancer is often defined by needle biopsy or bronchoscopy, followed by a screen for systemic metastasis. In cases where metastasis to distant organs has not occurred and feasibility of local cure is still present, an aggressive approach is pursued. This involves preoperative radiation and several cycles of chemotherapy, to determine tumor responsiveness and to facilitate en bloc resection if regional nodes are positive or suspicious for tumor involvement. Although brachial plexopathy is often present, usually one cannot ascertain with certainty whether this is a result of compression from the apical lung cancer or a direct invasion of neural elements. The patient must be forewarned that the primary aim of surgery is to obtain tumor-free margins and whether this will involve sparing the brachial plexus elements or also require its removal can only be determined intraoperatively with gross and pathologic examination of the nerve roots. If both the upper and lower elements of the plexus are involved as determined by the preoperative clinical and MRI examinations, the chance that a total amputation of the limb may be required also should be discussed. This relatively aggressive approach to improve long-term survival is warranted in patients with localized disease and with a more favorable biology, such as a squamous carcinoma. Radiation followed by surgery results in 15% to 50% 5-year survival[28] in these patients. A supraclavicular exposure combined with sternotomy provides an open exposure to the great vessels, brachial plexus, and intrathoracic contents to facilitate resection (see Fig. 25-6C).

Intraneural Metastasis

Intraneural metastasis from breast carcinoma, malignant melanoma, and carcinoid have been described. The diagnostic dilemma resides in intraneural invasion versus radiation neuritis in the context of prior breast cancer or lung cancer patients treated with radiation, presenting with brachial plexopathy. In these cases, MRI may not reliably distinguish the two pathologies, which, on surgery, may both be present, leading to the progressive neurologic deterioration.[29]

Radiation-Induced Plexopathy

Immediate- or delayed-onset radiation-induced brachial plexopathy occurs in 1.5% to 35% of breast carcinoma patients, and differentiation from recurrence or metastasis is often difficult, as discussed above.[30] Focal compression by fibrosis and obliteration of the vasonervorum leading to chronic ischemia has been implicated in the etiology. Different surgical procedures, including neurolysis, omentoplasty, and muscle pedicle flap, have been attempted with variable results.[31] The surgical objective is to obtain pathology to rule in or out tumor recurrence (which may have significant implications in terms of additional chemotherapy/prognosis, etc.), and undertake limited neurolysis to help alleviate some of the neuropathic pain, which is often the most disabling symptom. Restoration of motor function, which is often lost in the intrinsics of the hand supplied by lower trunk elements, is not feasible.

▶ PREDISPOSITION SYNDROMES

Neurofibromatosis Type 1

NF1 and NF2 were initially known as von Recklinghausen disease, until modern genetics demonstrated that these represented two distinct syndromes caused by genetic alterations on two different genes. The term *von Recklinghausen syndrome* now is only equated with NF1, the most common cancer predisposition syndrome in humans. The incidence of NF1 is 1:2500 to 1:3600 of all live births, with about half caused by new mutations.[32,33] It is characterized by a myriad of abnormalities affecting almost all organs, thereby requiring lifelong followup.

NF1 patients tend to be of short stature with macrocephaly, but not necessarily hydrocephalus. The majority of NF1 patients have normal cognitive function; however, a significant number of NF1 children experience learning disabilities and attention deficits, which are possibly correlated to the number of unidentified bright objects on T_2-weighted MRI imaging, representing regions of heterotopia and CNS developmental abnormalities.[34] Cutaneous manifestations include café-au-lait spots, axillary freckling, dermal and plexiform neurofibromas, and xanthogranulomas. Café-au-lait spots may be present at birth or appear during the first 2 years of life and are detected in 95% of NF1 patients, making early diagnosis feasible on clinical criteria alone (see Table 25-3). Ophthalmologic signs include iris hamartomas or Lisch nodules and optic nerve gliomas, the latter presenting in approximately 15% of NF1 patients with decreased acuity, but only with rare clinical or radiologic growth requiring medical or surgical intervention. Osseous developmental anomalies include sphenoid-wing dysplasia, tibial pseudoarthrosis, scoliosis, and, rarely, hypophosphatemic osteomalacia. Cardiovascular manifestations include hypertension, a major complication of NF1, which may be secondary to associated pheochromocytomas or renal artery stenosis.[35,36]

NF1 is the most common cancer predisposition syndrome in humans; its associated malignancies are not restricted to peripheral nerves and the CNS. Other predisposed cancers include the pheochromocytomas, juvenile chronic myeloid leukemias, rhabdomyosarcomas, fibrosarcomas, squamous cell carcinomas, and carcinoid tumors.[37–39] Dermal and plexiform neurofibromas are the most common of all NF1-associated tumors. They can occur sporadically in non-NF1 patients, although they are usually restricted to one or two sites and hence are not pathognomic of the diagnosis of NF1 in the absence of other clinical signs, unlike bilateral vestibular schwannomas for NF2. They have a predominantly intrafascicular diffuse growth pattern along multiple branches of more proximal nerves, leading to a "string of onion" appearance (see Fig. 25-5D). The wrongly used term "elephantiasis," which is offensive to NF1 patients, is associated with a very large plexiform neurofibroma and accompanying massive soft tissue growth. Plexiform neurofibromas can occur anywhere in the body, with the trigeminal nerve being the most common cranial nerve to be affected.[40] Plexiform neurofibromas may be present at birth, with a majority manifesting within the first decade of life, followed by persistent slow growth throughout life, sometimes accentuated during early childhood, puberty, pregnancy, and, rarely, after traumatic intratumoral hemorrhage.[41,42] Surgical indications for removal of plexiform neurofibromas in NF1 patients have to be well defined because of their slow biologic growth, inherent risks of neurologic deficits as a consequence of intrafascicular growth, and multiplicity. These indications can include cosmesis, localized pain, progressive enlargement causing pressure effects on adjacent structures, increasing neurologic deficit, and suspected malignant transformation. The aim of surgery is debulking of the lesion with preservation of nerve function, which is often possible despite the intrafascicular growth, with microscopy and nerve stimulation intraoperatively. Spontaneous onset of unremitting pain, especially if documented by increased radiologic growth, is suggestive of malignant transformation of a plexiform neurofibroma. The cumulative lifetime risk in a NF1 patient may be as high as 10% to 15%.[1,9] As discussed above, current anatomic radiologic investigations fail to differentiate accurately between a benign plexiform neurofibroma and one that has undergone transformation to a MPNST, with biologic imaging strategies such as PET under investigation.

As a result of the multiplicity of plexiform neurofibromas, especially in NF1 patients, nonsurgical therapies have been sought. These include clinical trials of ketotifen fumarate (antihistamines because of the presence of mast cells in the tumors) and thalidomide (as an antiangiogenic agent), but with little success.[43,44] Chemotherapy for plexiform neurofibromas has not been beneficial because of the requirement for long-term therapy, which is associated with significant morbidity. Radiation therapy is used for tumors not surgically accessible, although with guarded efficacy and potential risk of malignant conversion. Biologic therapies aimed at rational molecular-based targets, such as activated p21-Ras resulting from loss of neurofibromin, are promising.

NF1 is a genetic disease with autosomal dominant inheritance pattern and full penetrance. Although the *NF1* gene has been identified, NF1 remains a clinical diagnosis based on National Institutes of Health (NIH) criteria (see Table 25-3) for some of the reasons discussed below. The *NF1* gene, located on the pericentromeric side of the long arm of chromosome 17 (17q11.2) is extremely large (350 kb) and has a high spontaneous mutation rate.[45,46] A wide variety of germ line mutations have been identified, including large deletions, microdeletions, single base-pair substitutions, duplications, insertions, splicing errors, and translocations.[47] Prenatal diagnosis or genetic screening of children, although conceptually very attractive, is prohibitively difficult because of lack of mutational hot spots, large size of the *NF1* gene, high rate of de novo mutation, and lack of genotype–phenotype correlation.[48,49] Hence, it has been reported mainly in familial cases, where specific mutations have already been characterized in the affected members of the family.

The gene product, called *neurofibromin*, is a large 220-kDa protein with 2818-amino-acid residues and multiple isoforms.[50,51] Neurofibromin is a cytosolic protein, with a central 360-amino-acid domain containing GTPase-activating protein (GAP) activity and hence called GAP-related domain (GRD). This GRD domain is critical in negatively regulating a key mitogenic signaling pathway mediated by p21-Ras, and as a result the loss of neurofibromin, leads to aberrant activation of p21-Ras (Fig. 25-7). The ensuing proliferative signals cause tumorigenesis, which has been demonstrated in NF1-associated PNTs and gliomas by our group as well as by others.[52] Farnesyltransferase inhibitors that block the posttranslational maturation, and thereby activation of p21-Ras, are of preclinical promise, and clinical trials are underway. Additional genetic alterations, such as involving loss of p53 and overexpression of epidermal growth factor receptor, are speculated to contribute toward malignant transformation to a MPNST.[53] It is hoped that increased molecular understanding of NF1

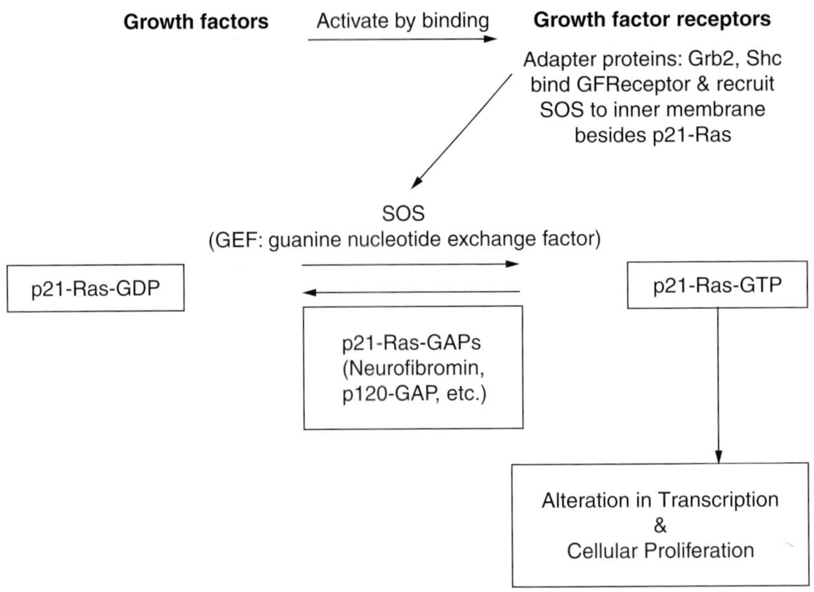

Figure 25-7. p21-Ras is a major mitogenic signaling pathway used by many growth factors in a variety of cells. On activation, the growth factor receptor recruits the mammalian son of sevenless (SOS), a p21-Ras GEF (gonadotropin-enhancing factor), to the inner cell membrane by adapter proteins such as Grb2 and Shc, through interactions of their protein modules, such as Sh2 and Sh3 (Src-homology) domains, with specific phosphorylated tyrosines on the receptor. SOS then can activate p21-Ras, which in its mature form is attached to the inner cell membrane, by exchanging GDP (guanine dinucleotide protein) for GTP (guanine trinucleotide protein). Activated p21-Ras-GTP interacts with downstream effectors to alter transcription and ultimately promote cell proliferation. p21-Ras-GAPs (GTPase-activating proteins), of which neurofibromin is a member, hydrolyze, thereby inactivating p21-Ras-GTP to p21-Ras-GDP. Consequently, loss of neurofibromin in NF1-associated tumors would result in aberrant p21-Ras-GTP activity and mitogenic tumor-promoting signals.

and spontaneous neurofibromas, which seem to share similar molecular pathogenetic mechanisms, will lead to targeted biologic therapies to enhance the current surgical management strategies.

Neurofibromatosis Type 2

NF2 is an autosomal-dominant disease affecting 1:40,000 to 1:87,000 live births, with about half resulting from new mutations.[54,55] The diagnosis is based on the NIH criteria[56] with subsequent modifications (see Table 25-3). Two distinct clinical subtypes are observed:[57] Wishart (early onset, more aggressive) and Gardner (late onset, more benign). Among clinical findings are bilateral vestibular schwannomas, meningiomas, astrocytomas, and ependymomas, affecting both the intracranial and spinal compartments.[58,59] The majority of NF2-associated PNTs are schwannomas, although dermal neurofibroma and plexiform schwannomas are also found.[7,60] Overlap with clinical signs associated with the more common NF1 syndrome, such as café-au-lait spots, is also found, although they are generally smaller in number compared to NF1. Segmental NF2 has a similar genetic basis compared to NF2, but varies from NF2 in its clinical manifestations with three subtypes: (a) a generalized form that is a milder manifestation of full-blown NF2; (b) a localized form that is a unilateral vestibular schwannoma with other ipsilateral tumors, or has features of NF2 localized to a particular segment of the body; and (c) a gonadal form, which is vertical transmission of full-blown disease from asymptomatic parents.[61,62]

The *NF2* gene is a typical tumor suppressor gene, located on long arm of chromosome 22 (22q12), encoding a protein called "merlin" or "schwannomin."[63,64] Merlin, which stands for "moesin-ezrin-radixin-like protein," derives its name from the corresponding members of the protein 4.1 family and is involved in linking cell membrane to the actin cytoskeleton. How the loss of merlin/schwannomin leads to cellular transformation is under study, but its normal function in regulating cellular cytoarchitecture is most likely disrupted. Like other cancer predisposition syndromes, the much more common sporadic tumors associated with NF2, such as schwannomas, meningiomas, and ependymomas, also harbor mutations and loss of the *NF2* gene with loss of merlin/schwannomin expression.[65,66]

Schwannomatosis

Schwannomatosis is characterized by multiple nonvestibular schwannomas without other features of NF2. It presents in an older age group (commonly middle-age) with infrequent familial occurrence.[8,67] Although diagnostic criteria have been proposed (see Table 25-3), it remains uncertain whether it is a separate form of neurofibromatosis or merely a subtype of NF2. Genetic analyses provide conflicting results, without a causative single gene yet to be found.

▶ CONCLUSION

Spinal root and peripheral nerve tumors have many overlapping features, including pathologic subtypes and their associated molecular basis. However, they do present differently and thereby require different management strategies. Not all of these tumors require surgery, as some may be best managed by observation alone, especially those associated with predisposition syndromes, where they are often multiple. A thorough history, physical examination, and radiologic examination, combined with sound clinical judgment, provide the best avenue for optimal management. Clinical and genetic studies are converging and opening hitherto unknown avenues for the understanding of these diseases. Scientists are striving hard to develop safe and effective biologically targeted therapies. Currently, however, the optimal management resides in a thorough knowledge of their biologic behavior, combined with expertise in microneurosurgical techniques when surgery is indicated.

REFERENCES

1. Ferner R, Gutmann D, Coffin C, et al. International consensus statement on malignant peripheral nerve sheath tumors in neurofibromatosis 1. Cancer Res 2002;62:1573–1577.
2. Carney JA. Psammomatous melanotic schwannoma. A distinctive, heritable tumor with special associations, including cardiac myxoma and the Cushing syndrome. Am J Surg Pathol 1990;14:206–222.
3. White W, Shiu MH, Rosenblum MK, et al. Cellular schwannoma. A clinicopathological study of 57 patients and 58 tumors. Cancer 1990;66:1266–1275.
4. Henke AC, Salomao DR, Hughes JH. Cellular schwannoma mimics a sarcoma: an example of a potential pitfall in aspiration cytodiagnosis. Diagn Cytopathol 1999;20:312–316.
5. Kindblom LG, Meis-Kindblom JM, Havel G, et al. Benign epithelioid schwannoma. Am J Surg Pathol 1998;22(6):762–770.
6. de Saint Aubain Somerhausen N, Valaeys V, Greets M, et al. Neuroblastoma-like schwannoma: a case report and review of the literature. Am J Dermatopathol 2003;25(1):32–34.
7. Ishida T, Kuroda M, Motoi T, et al. Phenotypic diversity of neurofibromatosis 2: association with plexiform schwannoma. Histopathology 1998;32(3):264–270.
8. Purcell SM, Dixon SL. Schwannomatosis. An unusual variant of neurofibromatosis or a distinct clinical entity? Arch Dermatol 1989;125(3):390–393.
9. Zoller ME, Rembeck B, Oden A, et al. Malignant and benign tumors in patients with neurofibromatosis type 1 in a defined Swedish population. Cancer 1997;79(11):2125–2131.
10. Sorensen SA, Mulvihill J, Nielsen A. A long-term follow-up of von Recklinghausen neurofibromatosis: survival and malignant neoplasm. N Engl J Med 1986;314(16):1010–1015.
11. Angelov L, Guha A. Peripheral nerve tumors. In: Bernstein M, Berger MS, eds. Neurooncology: the essentials. New York: Thieme, 2000:434–444.
12. Tsangn WY, Chan JK, Chow LT, et al. Perineurioma: an uncommon soft tissue neoplasm distinct from localized hypertrophic neuropathy and neurofibroma. Am J Surg Pathol 1992;16(8):756–763.
13. Ohno T, Park P, Akai M, et al. Ultrastructural study of a perineurioma [review]. Ultrastruct Pathol 1988;12(5):495–504.
14. Fletcher CD. Solitary circumscribed neuroma of the skin (so-called palisaded, encapsulated neuroma). A clinicopathologic and immunohistochemical study. Am J Surg Pathol 1989;13(7):574–580.
15. Megahed M. Palisaded encapsulated neuroma (solitary circumscribed neuroma). A clinicopathologic and immunohistochemical study. Am J Dermatopathol 1994;16(2):120–125.
16. Busam KJ, Mentzel T, Colpaert C, et al. Atypical or worrisome features in cellular neurothekeoma: a study of 10 cases. Am J Surg Pathol 1998;22(9):1067–1072.
17. Lowenstein J, Towers J, Tomaino MM. Intraneural ganglion of the peroneal nerve: importance of timely diagnosis. Am J Orthop 2001;30:816–819.
18. Spinner RJ, Atkinson JL, Harper CM Jr, et al. Recurrent intraneural ganglion cyst of the tibial nerve [case report]. J Neurosurg 2000;92(2):334–337.
19. Kameh DS, Perez-Berenguer JL, Pearl GS. Lipofibromatous hamartoma and related peripheral nerve lesions. South Med J 2000;93(8):800–802.
20. Babins DM, Lubahn JD. Palmar lipomas associated with compression of the median nerve. J Bone Joint Surg Am 1994;76(9):1360–1362.
21. Plukker JT, van Oort I, Vermey A, et al. Aggressive fibromatosis (non-familial desmoid tumour): therapeutic problems and the role of adjuvant radiotherapy. Br J Surg 1995;82(4):510–514.
22. Hoos A, Lewis JJ, Urist MJ, et al. Desmoid tumors of the head and neck—a clinical study of a rare entity. Head Neck 2000;22(8):814–821.
23. Perez-Lopez C, Gutierrez M, Isla A. Inflammatory pseudotumor of the median nerve. Case report and review of the literature. J Neurosurg 2001;95(1):124–128.
24. Beer T, Carr NJ, Weller RO. Inflammatory pseudotumor of peripheral nerve. Am J Surg Pathol 1998;22(8):1035–1036.
25. Angelov A, Davis A, O'Sullivan B, et al. Neurogenic sarcoma: experience at the University of Toronto. Neurosurgery 1998;43(1):56–64.

26. Misdraji J, Ino Y, Louis DN, et al. Primary lymphoma of peripheral nerve: report of four cases. Am J Surg Pathol 2000;24(9):1257–1265.
27. Roncaroli F, Poppi M, Riccioni L, et al. Primary non-Hodgkin's lymphoma of the sciatic nerve followed by localization in the central nervous system: case report and review of the literature [review]. Neurosurgery 1997;40(3):618–621; discussion 621–622.
28. Detterbeck FC. Pancoast (superior sulcus) tumors. Ann Thorac Surg 1997;63(6):1810–1818.
29. Cantone G, Rath SA, Richter HP. Intraneural metastasis in a peripheral nerve. Acta Neurochir (Wien) 2000;142(6): 719–720.
30. Olsen NK, Pfeiffer P, Mondrup K, et al. Radiation-induced brachial plexus neuropathy in breast cancer patients. Acta Oncol 1990;29(7):885–890.
31. LeQuang C. Postirradiation lesions of the brachial plexus. Results of surgical treatment. Hand Clin 1989;5(1):23–32.
32. Huson SM, Compston DA, Clark P, et al. A genetic study of von Recklinghausen neurofibromatosis in south east Wales. I. Prevalence, fitness, mutation rate, and effect of parental transmission on severity. J Med Genet 1989;26(11):704–711.
33. Riccardi V. Neurofibromatosis: phenotype, natural history and pathogenesis. Baltimore, MD: Johns Hopkins University Press, 1992.
34. North K. Neurofibromatosis type 1. Am J Med Genet 2000; 97(2):119–127.
35. Kalff V, Shapiro B, Lloyd R, et al. The spectrum of pheochromocytoma in hypertensive patients with neurofibromatosis. Arch Intern Med 1982;142(12):2092–2098.
36. Salyer WR, Salyer DC. The vascular lesions of neurofibromatosis. Angiology 1974;25(8):510–519.
37. Zvulunov A, Barak Y, Metzker A. Juvenile xanthogranuloma, neurofibromatosis, and juvenile chronic myelogenous leukemia. World statistical analysis. Arch Dermatol 1995; 131(8):904–908.
38. Griffiths DF, Williams GT, Williams ED. Duodenal carcinoid tumours, phaeochromocytoma and neurofibromatosis: islet cell tumour, phaeochromocytoma and the von Hippel-Lindau complex: two distinctive neuroendocrine syndromes. Q J Med 1987;64(245):769–782.
39. Crawford AH. Neurofibromatosis in children. Acta Orthop Scand Suppl 1986;218:1–60.
40. Gholkar A, Stack JP, Isherwood I. Plexiform trigeminal neurofibroma. Clin Radiol 1988;39(3):313–315.
41. Korf BR. Plexiform neurofibromas. Am J Med Genet 1999;89(1):31–37.
42. Krueger W, Weisberger E, Bllantyne AJ, et al. Plexiform neurofibroma of the head and neck. Am J Surg 1979; 138(4):517–520.
43. Riccardi VM. A controlled multiphase trial of ketotifen to minimize neurofibroma-associated pain and itching. Arch Dermatol 1993:129(5):577–581.
44. Gupta A, Cohen B, Ruggierri P, et al. A phase 1 study of thalidomide for the treatment of plexiform neurofibroma in neurofibromatosis 1. Neurology 2003:60(1):130–132.
45. Fountain JW, Wallace MR, Brereton AM, et al. Physical mapping of the von Recklinghausen neurofibromatosis region on chromosome 17. Am J Hum Genet 1989;44(1): 58–67.
46. Li Y, O'Connell P, Breidenbach HH, et al. Genomic organization of the neurofibromatosis 1 gene (NF1). Genomics 1995;25(1):9–18.
47. Lakkis MM, Tennekoon GI. Neurofibromatosis type 1. I. General overview. J Neurosci Res 2000;62(6):755–763.
48. Upadhyaya M, Shen M, Cherryson A, et al. Analysis of mutations at the neurofibromatosis 1 (NF1) locus. Hum Mol Genet 1992;1(9):735–740.
49. Hofman KJ, Boehm CED. Familial neurofibromatosis type 1: clinical experience with DNA testing. J Pediatr 1992; 120(3):394–398.
50. Nishi T, Lee PS, Oka K, et al. Differential expression of two types of the neurofibromatosis type 1 (NF1) gene transcripts related to neuronal differentiation. Oncogene 1991; 6(9):1555–1559.
51. Gutmann DH, Geist RT, Rose K, Wright DE. Expression of two new protein isoforms of the neurofibromatosis type 1 gene product, neurofibromin, in muscle tissues. Dev Dyn 1995;202(3):302–311.
52. Guha A, Lau N, Huvar I, et al. Ras-GTP levels are elevated in human NF1 peripheral nerve tumors. Oncogene 1996;12(3):507–513.
53. Menon AG, Anderson KM, Riccardi VM, et al. Chromosome 17p deletions and p53 gene mutations associated with the formation of malignant neurofibrosarcomas in von Recklinghausen neurofibromatosis. Proc Natl Acad Sci USA 1990; 87(14):5435–5439.
54. Evans DG, Huson SM, Donani D, et al. A genetic study of type 2 neurofibromatosis in the United Kingdom. I. Prevalence, mutation rate, fitness, and confirmation of maternal transmission effect on severity. J Med Genet 1992;29(12): 841–846.
55. Antiheimo J, Sankila R, Carpen O, et al. Population-based analysis of sporadic and type 2 neurofibromatosis-associated meningiomas and schwannomas. Neurology 2000;54(1): 71–76.
56. Gutmann DH, Aylsworth A, Carey JC, et al. The diagnostic evaluation and multidisciplinary management of neurofibromatosis 1 and neurofibromatosis 2. JAMA 1997;278(1): 51–57.
57. Evans DG, Huson SM, Donnai D, et al. A clinical study of type 2 neurofibromatosis. Q J Med 1992;84(304):603–618.
58. Martuza RL, Eldridge R. Neurofibromatosis 2 (bilateral acoustic neurofibromatosis). N Engl J Med 1988;318(11): 684–688.
59. Halliday AL, Sobel RA, Martuza RL. Benign spinal nerve sheath tumors: their occurrence sporadically and in neurofibromatosis types 1 and 2. J Neurosurg 1991;74(2): 248–253.
60. Kluwe L, Friedrich RE, Hagel C, et al. Mutations and allelic loss of the NF2 gene in neurofibromatosis 2-associated skin tumors. J Invest Dermatol 2000;114(5):1017–1021.
61. Bourn D, Carter SA, Evans DG, et al. A mutation in the neurofibromatosis type 2 tumor-suppressor gene, giving rise to widely different clinical phenotypes in two unrelated individuals. Am J Hum Genet 1994;55(1):69–73.
62. Parry DM, Eldridge R, Kaiser-Kupfer MI, et al. Neurofibromatosis 2 (NF2): clinical characteristics of 63 affected individuals and clinical evidence for heterogeneity. Am J Med Genet 1994;52(4):450–461.

63. Trofatter JA, MacCollin MM, Rutter JL, et al. A novel moesin-, ezrin-, radixin-like gene is a candidate for the neurofibromatosis 2 tumor suppressor. Cell 1993;19;75(4): 826.
64. Rouleau GA, Merel P, Lutchman M, et al. Alteration in a new gene encoding a putative membrane-organizing protein causes neuro-fibromatosis type 2. Nature 1993;363(6429): 515–521.
65. Gutmann DH, Giordano MJ, Fishback AS, et al. Loss of merlin expression in sporadic meningiomas, ependymomas and schwannomas. Neurology 1997;49(1):267–270.
66. Antiheimo J, Sallinen SL, Sallinen P, et al. Genetic aberrations in sporadic and neurofibromatosis 2 (NF2)-associated schwannomas studied by comparative genomic hybridization (CGH). Acta Neurochir (Wien) 2000;142(10):1099–1104; discussion 1104–1105.
67. Jacoby LB, Jones D, Davis K, et al. Molecular analysis of the NF2 tumor-suppressor gene in schwannomatosis. Am J Hum Genet 1997;61(6):1293–1302.

PART III

Metastatic Disease

CHAPTER 26

The Management of Brain Metastases

AMERICAN COLLEGE OF SURGICAL ONCOLOGY CNS WORKING GROUP

Central nervous system (CNS) metastatic disease from extracranial primary tumors is a common complication of systemic cancer and an important cause of morbidity and mortality in society. CNS metastases are the most common form of brain tumor in adults. Fifteen percent to 20% of all U.S. cancer patients will develop cerebral metastases. Because of the prevalence of CNS metastases, intense interest has been focused on the development of treatment strategies for these lesions. Although treatments for cerebral metastases have unquestionably extended survival in many patients, the majority of patients will ultimately succumb to their systemic disease. It is therefore unlikely that any *CNS-directed therapy or combination of therapies will likely impact overall survival in the vast majority of patients at this time. CNS therapies will, however, substantially impact the* quality *of survival of tens of thousands of patients. There is no consensus, however, about the optimal treatment strategy for most patients with CNS metastases and virtually no meaningful data exist regarding the factors that are most likely to be influenced by differing treatment strategies, namely quality of life (QOL) and neurocognition. This chapter reviews the existing data regarding the epidemiology, presentation, and treatment of cerebral metastases, and comments on current and proposed prospective analyses that could possibly address ongoing controversies in patient management. The chapter concludes with an outline for what we believe to be a rational treatment strategy for brain metastases, based on the existing literature.*

▶ EPIDEMIOLOGY OF BRAIN METASTASES

Approximately 1.3 million individuals are diagnosed with cancer each year in the United States.[1] It has been estimated that between 100,000 and 170,000 of those cancer patients will develop brain metastases.[2,3] Metastatic brain tumors represent the most common neurologic complication of systemic cancer,[4] and are taking on increasing significance in clinical neuro-oncology. Approximately 15% to 20% of cancer patients will actually be diagnosed with brain metastases during their lifetimes.[5] The annual incidence of brain metastases is approximately 4.1 to 11.1 per 100,000 population.[6] The incidence of brain metastases appears to be rising, and this increase has been variably attributed to improvements in systemic therapy leading to longer survival, an aging patient population, an increase in the incidence of lung cancer and melanoma, and the ability of magnetic resonance imaging (MRI) to detect small metastases.[5] Brain metastases are now considered to be the most common intracranial tumor, outnumbering primary brain tumors by a ratio as high as 10:1.[7]

The incidence of brain metastases is difficult to state precisely, as multiple sources of data have been used to define the scale of this particular clinical problem. Inadequate verification of tumor histology and underreporting of cases have limited epidemiologic studies from large patient populations, potentially the best source of data.[8] Surgical case series have suffered from significant selection biases. Large autopsy series, while also suffering from biases, probably provide us with the most accurate insight into the true incidence of this disease. Between 20% and 40% of all patients with all forms of metastatic cancer will have brain metastases at autopsy.[8] Although brain metastases may develop from any primary systemic cancer, specific sites have a particular predilection to metastasize to the brain. At autopsy, the frequency of brain metastases from a known primary site, when compared with the incidence of deaths expected from that specific primary tumor, allows one to estimate the incidence of brain metastases in patients dying of cancer for a particular primary cancer. In a recent review of multiple autopsy series, the probability of developing brain metastases from a specific primary tumor site in patients dying from lung, breast, melanoma, gastrointestinal, or renal cell primary tumor was calculated to be 32%, 21%, 48%, 6%, and 11%, respectively.[8] Malignant melanoma, which represents only 4% of all cancers, is the most likely histology to metastasize to brain, and various series have suggested that 40% to 50% of patients dying of this disease have intracranial involvement.[9] Other primary tumors, such as choriocarcinoma and renal cell carcinoma, also have a particularly high propensity to metastasize to the brain.[10,11] Histologies *within* individual organ sites can exhibit variable rates of brain metastasis. For example, 32% to 40% of patients with lung small cell carcinoma and adenocarcinoma will develop spread of their disease to the brain, a significantly greater rate in comparison to that of squamous cell carcinomas.[8,12,13] Diffuse infiltration of the leptomeninges, so-called neoplastic meningitis or meningeal carcinomatosis, is mostly associated with leukemias and lymphomas, followed by carcinomas of the lung and breast.[2,14]

Sixty percent to 80% of all brain metastases in adults are composed of tumors from lung, breast, melanoma, colon, and kidney primary sites. The most common primary site is the lungs, giving rise to approximately 40% to 60% of all brain metastases, followed by breast, melanoma, and, less frequently, colon, and kidney primary sites, with relative incidences of 10%, 3.5%, 2.8%, and 1.2%, respectively.[4,6,8,15] Lung metastases predominate in men, whereas breast metastases predominate in women. These approximations almost certainly underestimate the true relative incidence of brain metastases from breast cancer because of the overall incidence of this disease (greater than lung cancer)[16] and the longer anticipated survival of patients harboring this malignancy as compared with the other primary sites mentioned previously. Primaries of unknown origin may constitute 5% to 10% of the cases.[1,4,6,15] There is a lower overall incidence of brain metastases in children than in adults. Leukemia is the most common cause of brain metastases in children. Of solid tumors, sarcomas (in young children) and germ cell tumors (in children older than age 15 years) are the most common sources of brain metastases.[12,17]

The age at which a patient presents with a brain metastasis parallels the age at diagnosis of the primary systemic tumor. Brain metastases are most common in the fifth to seventh decades of life. Although brain metastases may be detected at the same time an extracranial malignancy is diagnosed (synchronous presentation), the majority (80%) of patients who develop brain metastases will already have been diagnosed with cancer (metachronous presentation).[18] Of these individuals, patients with a history of lung cancer will have the shortest latency period between the time of initial diagnosis and the diagnosis of brain metastases (median: 6–9 months). For renal cell carcinoma, the interval is approximately 1 year. Patients with breast, melanoma, and colon cancer typically experience spread of their disease to the brain at a median latency of about 2 years.[8]

The majority of brain metastases are multiple, although the reported percentage of patients with solitary or multiple lesions varies with the type of analysis made. In one large autopsy series of cancer patients who were found to harbor brain metastases, 40% had a solitary metastasis, 27% had two or three metastases, and 33% had four or more metastases. When computerized tomography (CT) was the primary diagnostic modality, 50% of lesions were thought to be solitary at the time of neurologic diagnosis.[19] With the widespread use of MRI, it has become apparent that the incidence of multiple metastases is greater than previously thought, perhaps occurring in up to 60% to 75% of patients.[20] Melanoma has the highest tendency to produce multiple lesions (75% of patients). Multiple lesions are also frequent in metastases from colon, breast and lung cancer. Renal cell metastases are more likely to be single.[21]

▶ THE BIOLOGY OF BRAIN METASTASES

Although most investigations of the biology of metastasis have focused on metastatic sites outside of the brain, many of the same principles and mechanisms appear to apply to metastatic brain tumors. For a tumor cell to form a clinically significant metastasis, it must complete a series of steps known as the metastatic cascade (Table 26-1). Any step missed or incomplete results in failure to form a metastasis.[22] Each step in the cascade represents a potential target for novel therapeutic approaches. The most promising targets for therapeutic intervention are steps that are most highly regulated, because of a prolonged amount of time available for targeting and treatment. The clinical window for identifying and delivering therapy in the less-regulated steps is too brief and unpredictable.[23]

Growth of tumor cells at secondary sites such as the brain is a highly regulated step in metastasis. In animal models, it has been found that the steps of local invasion, intravasation, survival and transport in the circulation, and extravasation occur rapidly and efficiently. In contrast, once cancer cells reach the target organ, fewer than 0.1% form metastatic deposits.[23] A delay of as long as several years may occur between the initial detection of disseminated cells and the clinical presentation of overt disease in the brain. In light of these observations, it has been hypothesized that there exists a mechanism of metastatic growth control at the secondary site.[24] Theoretically, if this mechanism is overcome, metastatic growth can occur much more rapidly. In support of this hypothesis is the report that when metastatic and nonmetastatic cancers were engrafted in mice, only the metastatic cancers were able to grow.[25]

Specific hypotheses for the mechanisms of metastatic growth control have been explored. The "seed and soil" hypothesis states that specific organs typically harbor metastases from one type of cancer but not from another type, by stimulating growth of these specific types of cancer. This interaction is further thought to be dynamic and reciprocal, as cancer cells have been observed to modify the environment that they encounter.[26–28] A second hypothesis, the "anatomic–chemical" hypothesis, argues that metastases develop in the capillary beds of any organ in which a disseminated cancer cell becomes mechanically lodged.[26] However, this theory fails to explain the occurrence of metastatic growth in only a single organ, which could be distant from the primary site, despite the existence of diffuse tumor cell dissemination.

▶ **TABLE 26-1.** STEPS IN THE METASTATIC CASCADE

- Cell division and growth within the primary tumor
- Cellular invasion of local tissue
- Cell entry into the bloodstream or lymphatic channels
- Survival of transit in the bloodstream or lymphatics
- Arrest in the microvasculature of the secondary site and invasion of the target tissue
- Proliferation of the cancer cell at the metastatic site

Recently, "metastasis suppressor genes" have been identified and characterized. These genes have the ability to suppress development of metastases in vivo; however, they have no effect on primary tumor growth. Seven metastasis suppressor genes have been identified to date.[29–35] The proteins coded for by the metastasis suppressor genes regulate a variety of functions, such as adhesion, migration, growth, and differentiation. Although most metastatic suppressor genes identified appear to impact growth at the secondary site, new approaches to metastasis treatment and prevention could potentially be based at several steps in metastatic cascade. For example, the suppressor genes that regulate the processes of adhesion and actin reorganization are possibly involved at multiple steps in the metastatic cascade; in contrast, genes involved in growth control probably only regulate the metastasis colonization step. It is hoped that further elucidation of the molecular mechanisms underlying the metastatic process will lead to additional targets for therapeutic intervention.

▶ PATHOLOGY AND DISTRIBUTION OF BRAIN METASTASES

CNS metastatic disease from extracranial primary tumors can involve skull, dura, leptomeninges, or brain parenchyma. Leptomeningeal carcinomatosis is found in up to 8% of patients autopsied with systemic cancer.[19] The most common primary tumors to involve the leptomeninges are breast, lung, and melanoma.[36] Parenchymal metastases are by far the most common CNS manifestation of systemic cancer. The most common route for metastasis to the brain parenchyma is by hematogeneous spread. Alternatively, the CNS may be involved secondarily by continuity with metastatic lesions to the adjacent bones. Most often, metastatic cancers enter the brain either via the internal carotid and vertebrobasilar arteries, or via Batson venous plexus.[37] Once within the brain, metastatic tumor cells tend to localize to the gray-white junction, as a consequence of the change in the size of the blood vessels in this zone, which trap the metastatic emboli.[38] A higher incidence of cerebral hemispheric metastases occur in the border zones of the arterial territories, with the middle and posterior cerebral arteries border zone being more involved than the anterior border zone between the anterior and middle cerebral arteries.

The relative distribution of brain metastases tends to occur in a pattern proportional to the blood flow to specific brain areas. In that regard, the great majority of brain metastases (approximately 80%) occur in the cerebral hemispheres, whereas the cerebellum and brainstem are less involved (10%–15% and 2%–3%, respectively).[39] Unlike the cerebrum, primary metastases into

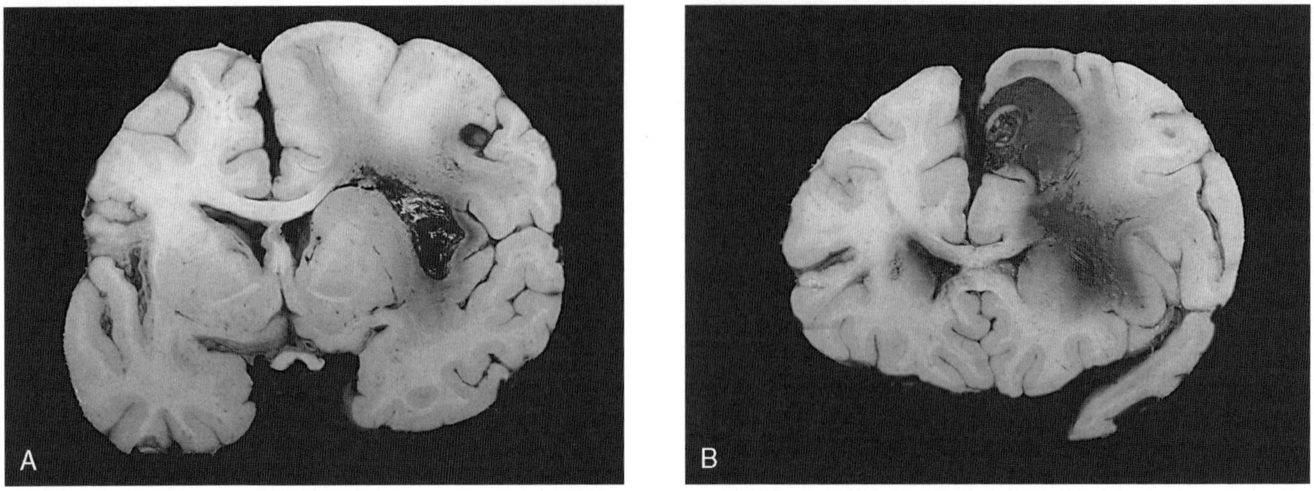

Figure 26-1. Gross pathologic specimen showing multiple brain metastases located in the right frontal lobe. Note the sharp demarcation between the hemorrhagic tumors and the surrounding brain parenchyma.

the spinal cord are rare. Most frequently, the spinal cord is involved secondarily as a result of metastases within the vertebral column.[40]

Metastatic lesions in the brain are usually discrete, spherical masses that displace rather than invade the surrounding brain parenchyma (Fig. 26-1). Metastases to the dura tend to form plaques, and infiltration of the cortical surface is not unusual. The lesions vary in size, ranging from microscopic to several centimeters in diameter. Some metastases may have a widespread distribution with multiple small lesions disseminated throughout the parenchyma. Cystic degeneration, necrosis, and areas of hemorrhage are not uncommon. Some specific tumors have a more characteristic gross appearance. For example, metastatic melanomas are likely to present as multiple pigmented lesions. Cysts filled with clear or mucoid fluid may be seen in metastases of mucus-secreting adenocarcinomas. Metastatic lesions of melanoma, choriocarcinoma and renal cell carcinoma have a high tendency to be hemorrhagic lesions.[41] Edema of the adjacent brain parenchyma is often prominent and sometimes disproportional to the small size of the lesions.[42]

Meningeal carcinomatosis presents as a diffuse opalescence of the leptomeninges. This is particularly prominent at the base of the brain and cranial and spinal nerve roots. Although in the great majority of cases the neoplastic infiltration is restricted to the leptomeninges, superficial infiltration of the brain parenchyma and small intraparenchymal nodules may also be present.

The histopathologic features of metastatic lesions are usually similar to those of the primary tumor from which they arise. Although the majority of metastatic lesions may appear clearly demarcated from the adjacent brain on both gross and microscopic examination, microinvasion of tumor cells is invariably present. This aspect is particularly evident in metastases of small cell lung carcinomas and melanomas.

Brain metastases elicit a number of reactions of the brain parenchyma (Fig. 26-2). Reactive astrocytosis is often present surrounding the metastatic nodules. Vascular proliferation with variable degree of endothelial/pericytic proliferation may be seen within and surrounding the tumor masses. Capillary endothelial cells in metastatic brain tumors often display morphologic and functional

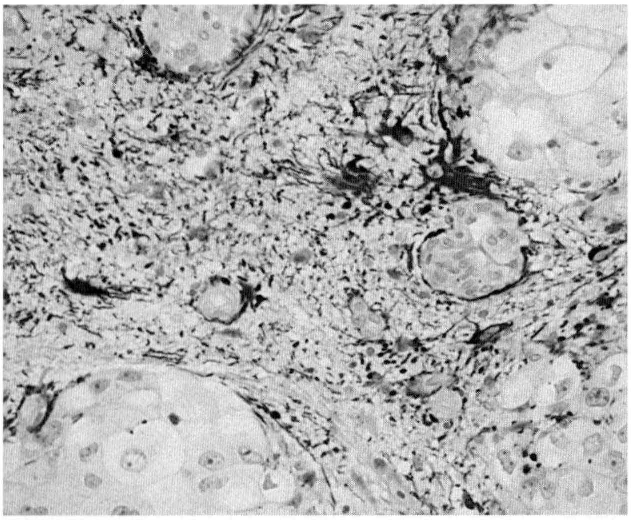

Figure 26-2 (PLATE 58). Histologic specimen with GFAP (glial fibrillary acidic protein) stain showing reactive astrocytosis adjacent to a metastasis (reactive astrocytes designated by arrow).

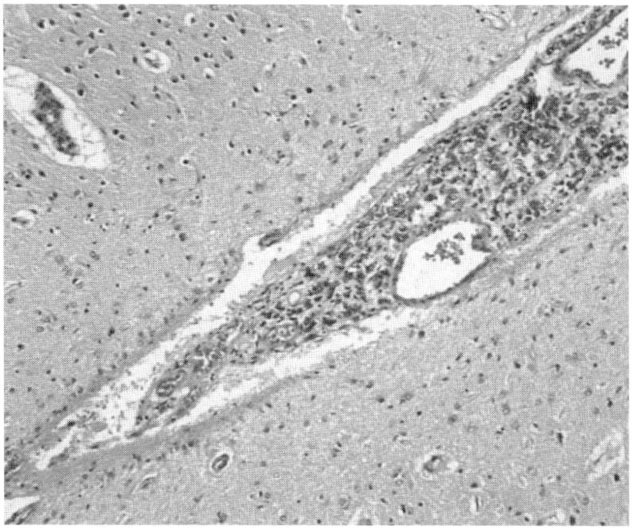

Figure 26-3 (PLATE 59). Microscopic view of leptomeningeal metastases. Note the invasion of the Virchow-Robin (perivascular) space (arrow) which is typical for this pathologic entity.

characteristics that are associated with the blood vessels of systemic neoplasms, having gap junctions and membrane fenestrations.[43] This rich neovasculature appears to play a significant role in the development and maintenance of the metastatic lesions. Additionally, tumor-induced angiogenesis gives rise to vessels with increased permeability, leading to blood–brain barrier disruption, and is thought to be a major contributory factor for the vasogenic edema that accompanies brain metastases.[8,40] Necrosis within tumors is frequent and macrophagic infiltration may be prominent around areas of necrosis.

Meningeal carcinomatosis is characterized by a diffuse infiltration of the subarachnoid space by the neoplastic cells, with significant accumulation of cells around the blood vessels (Fig. 26-3). Dissemination to the ventricles may be present, with small drop metastases of neoplastic cells within the ventricular walls.

▶ DIAGNOSIS

Brain metastases must be differentiated from other CNS pathologies such as primary brain tumors, abscesses, demyelination, and cerebrovascular accidents. The development of multiple cerebral lesions in a patient with a known history of cancer can generally be considered to be metastatic brain disease if typical radiographic findings are demonstrated. Solitary cerebral lesions can present a more challenging diagnostic dilemma. Although the majority of patients with a newly diagnosed brain mass and a known history of cancer can be assumed to have metastatic CNS involvement, one study showed that the false-positive rate, even when using contrast MRI for the diagnosis of a presumed single brain metastasis, is approximately 11%.[18] The diagnosis of a new brain mass in a patient with a remote history of cancer should always raise the possibility of a second primary. A classic example is the patient in her 50s with a history of breast cancer who presents with a single dural-based lesion. As the incidence of meningioma is increased in aging patients and in patients with a remote history of breast cancer, this histology should be considered in the differential.[44]

In most patients with a history of cancer, imaging studies can distinguish brain metastases from other CNS pathologies. MRI with gadolinium enhancement (generally T_1-weighted images) is by far the most sensitive imaging modality for both diagnosis and followup of patients with brain metastases.[45] T_2-weighted images are used to estimate the extent of peritumoral edema (Fig. 26-4). A metastasis itself may have various signal intensities, depending on the types of tissue present within the lesion (e.g., blood products, necrosis, melanin). The appearance of blood products on T_1-weighted images depends on the "age" of bleeding, and ranges from isointense in the first 24 hours to hyperintense after 24 to 72 hours. Melanin is paramagnetic and hyperintense on T_1-weighted images and hypointense on T_2-weighted images. Metastatic melanomas often have both components (blood and melanin), which appear bright on noncontrast T_1-weighted scans. In carcinomatous meningitis, the pial surface usually displays irregular, bright enhancement on T_1-weighted imaging with contrast. The arachnoidal surfaces, ventricular ependyma or dura may also enhance pathologically.

As stated previously, approximately 20% of patients presenting with brain metastases do not have a prior diagnosis of cancer.[46] When a patient without a history of systemic cancer presents with new neurologic findings and a brain mass is discovered on imaging studies, the lung should be the focus of the primary diagnostic evaluation. Because the majority of primary cancers that metastasize to the brain are from lung primaries, a plain chest radiograph and chest CT are always recommended. Patients presenting with a brain lesion as their first manifestation of systemic cancer are found to have lung primaries 53% to 68% of the time.[47] Breast primaries are relatively rare in these patients, most likely related to success of screening exams and the relative ease of early detection of the primary lesion.[47] During an initial evaluation, a chest CT allows reasonable screening of the breast tissue in females. CT of the abdomen and pelvis occasionally reveals an unknown primary cancer but also may allow the evaluation of the systemic disease burden by imaging the liver, adrenals, and lymph nodes, which are frequent sites of systemic metastases. When lesions are found on systemic imaging, percutaneous needle biopsy or, in the setting of suspected lung cancer, bronchoscopy, are often

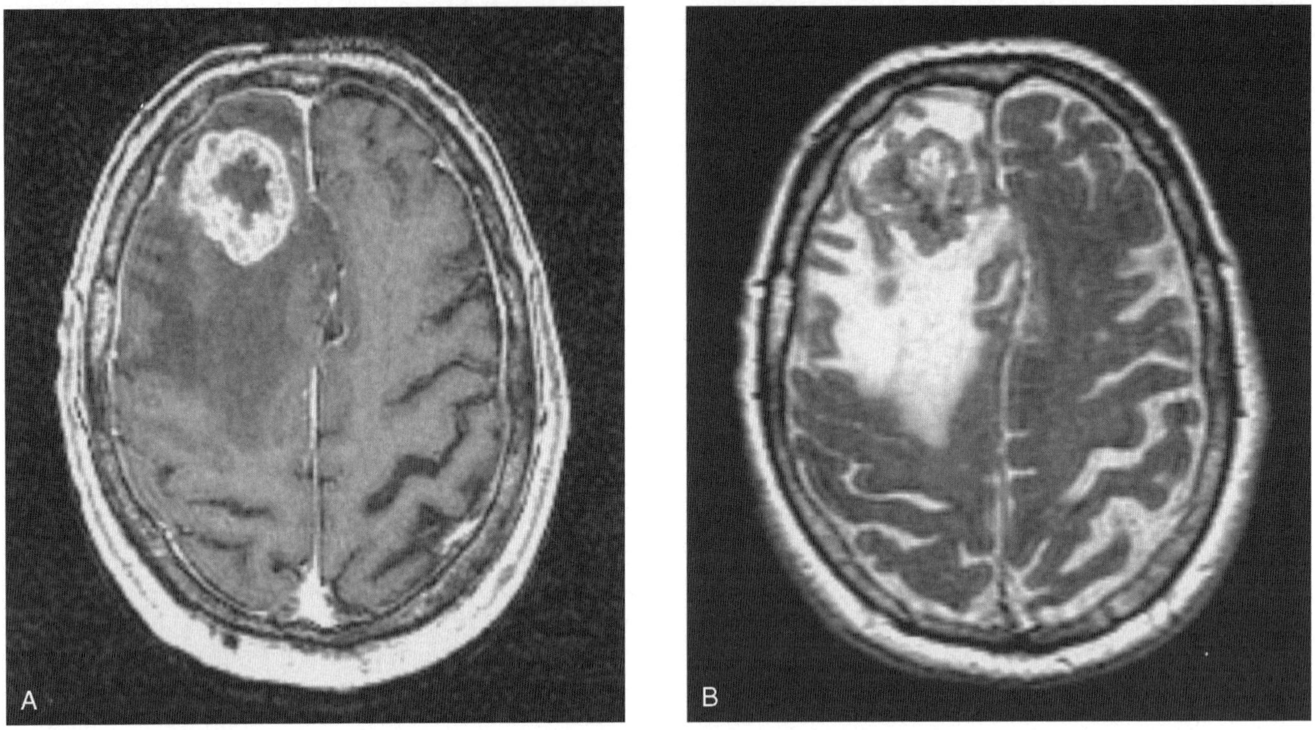

Figure 26-4. A typical brain metastasis is demonstrated in this 56-year-old man with a history of non–small cell lung cancer who presented with a seizure. (A) Axial, post-contrast, T_1-weighted image shows a discrete, contrast-enhancing mass in the right frontal lobe with a central area of low signal intensity, most likely representing necrosis. (B) Axial T_2-weighted image showing a mixed signal lesion with considerable associated edema (high signal intensity area in adjacent white matter).

used to obtain tissue for histopathologic analysis. The addition of [^{18}F]fluorodeoxyglucose positron emission tomography (FDG-PET) to the conventional radiologic testing for evaluation of brain metastases of unknown primary is of limited clinical relevance.[48] Further search for a primary cancer is rarely productive without positive features in the patient's history or localizing signs on physical examination that suggest primary tumor.[49]

Despite the most extensive workups, approximately 5% to 10% of patients with brain metastases may be expected to remain without a definite primary cancer site.[46] For these patients in particular, obtaining diagnostic tissue by biopsy or excision of a brain metastasis is essential in determining a treatment strategy. Once tissue is obtained, an important first step in evaluating such lesions is to determine if the metastasis fits into the small cell or the large polygonal cell group of tumors. In the first category, the differential diagnosis includes small cell lymphomas, leukemias, and small cell carcinoma of the lung in adults, and neuroblastoma, Ewing sarcoma, and embryonal rhabdomyosarcoma in children. In the category of large-cell metastatic neoplasm, carcinomas, large-cell non-Hodgkin lymphomas, and melanomas are the primary considerations in adults, whereas germ cell tumors should be considered in children. Once the determination regarding small- or large-cell tumor type is made, adjunctive morphologic techniques, such as immunohistochemistry, can be valuable methods for guiding the oncologists in their search of a primary site.[42] A large number of antibodies are now available for diagnostic identification of metastatic tumors of unknown origin. In many instances, immunohistochemistry, in conjunction with the clinical history, can define specific cell lineages.

In cases where light microscopy and immunohistochemistry are inconclusive, electron microscopy is a useful adjunctive tool in that subcellular structures may be diagnostic of cellular lineage, such as well-formed intercellular junctional complexes in carcinomas, premelanosomes in melanomas, and dense core granules in neuroendocrine tumors.

In summary, the majority of patients with a known history of cancer and characteristic brain imaging findings can be presumed to harbor CNS metastases. In any patient in whom the diagnosis of brain metastasis is in doubt, a biopsy or resection should be performed to confirm the diagnosis.

▶ CLINICAL PRESENTATION AND SYMPTOMATIC TREATMENT

The clinical presentation of brain metastases can be similar to that of any intracranial mass lesions, and two-thirds of patients with brain metastases will develop neurologic symptoms during the course of their illness.[50] Brain metastases should be suspected in any patient with a known primary cancer who has developed new neurologic signs or symptoms. Signs and symptoms of brain metastases can be roughly divided into a "generalized" category, typically related to cerebral edema and/or increased intracranial pressure (i.e., headaches, nausea/vomiting, cognitive problems), and a "focal" category that frequently results from localized compression or destruction of brain tissue (most often manifesting as weakness, numbness, speech disturbance, or seizures). Headaches are a presenting symptom in 30% to 50% of patients with brain metastases and are more frequent in patients with multiple metastases or posterior fossa lesions.[51–53] Headaches associated with brain metastases may be exacerbated by coughing, exertion, and/or change in posture. Up to 40% of patients will describe "morning headaches."[54] The character of these headaches, however, is insufficiently specific to reliably help distinguish brain metastases from a host of other potential etiologies. In the minority of cases when the headaches do localize to a particular region, the location of the tumor is found to correlate in approximately 70% of patients.[55] Headaches associated with brain metastases are a more common presenting complaint in patients with a prior history of benign headache.[56] Severe recurrent headaches in a patient without a previous history of such complaints should signal the physician to proceed with further investigation. Altered mental status, personality change, and impaired cognition may be seen in approximately one-third of patients and may be more prevalent with multiple metastases or raised intracranial pressure.[57] When there are bilateral lesions, the clinical picture may resemble a toxic or metabolic encephalopathy caused by bilateral hemispheric dysfunction.[52] Physical examination findings are more sensitive indicators of elevated intracranial pressure than any of the above-mentioned symptoms. Signs related to raised intracranial pressure secondary to cerebral metastases may include papilledema and cranial nerve dysfunction, particularly of cranial nerves III and VI. Papilledema is present in approximately 25% of patients on presentation.[52,54]

Patients with metastatic brain tumors can manifest progressive neurologic deficits in the form of sensory or motor loss, depending on the location of the lesion. Focal weakness is the presenting complaint in approximately 20% to 40% of patients.[52,54] Stroke-like symptoms are also observed in some patients and can be secondary to occlusion of blood vessels by tumor cells or hemorrhage into tumors. Five percent to 10% of patients experience sudden onset of focal neurologic symptoms associated with intratumoral hemorrhage, particularly from metastases originating from melanoma, choriocarcinoma, or renal cell carcinoma.[53] Even though a relatively small percentage of lung metastases present with hemorrhage, these lesions represent the most common source of hemorrhage as a consequence of their much greater overall occurrence.[58]

Seizures are common on initial presentation and are the first sign of brain metastasis in approximately 10% to 20% of patients.[52,54] Tumors that cause seizures are frequently located in the cerebral hemispheres and are often situated near or involve the cerebral cortex, as is often the case with brain metastases. Although direct compression or irritation of the neurons of the cerebral cortex is intuitively the most probable cause of seizure activity, cerebral edema, ischemia, and mechanical traction of the cerebral cortex may also play important roles in epileptogenesis.

Prolonged seizures in patients with brain tumors can elevate intracranial pressure and negatively impact oxygen delivery, blood pressure, and acid–base balance. Immediate control of seizure activity is of paramount importance, particularly in situations where further elevations in intracranial pressure might result in cataclysmic brain herniation syndromes. Benzodiazepines (e.g., lorazepam) are still the mainstay of treatment for patients who present in status epilepticus, (continuous seizure activity lasting longer than 30 minutes). For prophylaxis and maintenance therapy, phenytoin is the most frequently prescribed agent. Carbamazepine, phenobarbital, valproic acid, and levetiracetam are often added for breakthrough seizures or to replace phenytoin if allergic reactions occur. Although there is agreement that patients who present with seizures require antiepileptic drug therapy, the role of anticonvulsant therapy in patients with supratentorial brain metastases who have not had a seizure is controversial. A meta-analysis of 12 studies in patients with brain tumors of all etiologies (including brain metastases) resulted in the conclusion that there is no statistical evidence showing a significant benefit of prophylactic anticonvulsants in this patient population.[59]

Cerebral edema can contribute directly or indirectly to most of the signs and symptoms associated with cerebral metastases. Corticosteroids are the standard treatment for peritumoral edema associated with brain metastases. These agents produce their antiedema effect by reducing the permeability of tumor capillaries.[60] Most patients are treated initially with dexamethasone, a corticosteroid with relatively little mineralocorticoid activity (thus less risk of fluid retention). The effect of corticosteroids is often dramatic and may be evident within hours, but the benefit is generally short-lived in the absence of subsequent definitive therapy. A typical initial therapy would include the administration of a 10- to 20-mg intravenous bolus dose followed by 4 to 6 mg every 6 hours. Vigilance must be maintained for the unwanted side effects of corticosteroid treatment, such as hyperglycemia, gastritis, avascular necrosis, osteoporosis, immunosuppression, poor wound healing, and myopathy.

▶ DEFINITIVE THERAPY

Status of systemic disease dictates the survival of most patients with brain metastases. Overall survival associated with metastatic malignancy is generally poor. As such, clinical trials evaluating the efficacy of chemotherapy for various malignancies typically exclude patients with brain metastases as well as those with poor performance status. Even when one attempts to select more favorable patients with metastatic disease, long-term survival figures are poor.

Published studies evaluating the efficacy of platinum-based chemotherapy for extracranial metastatic non–small cell lung carcinoma report a median survival of approximately 8 months.[61,62] Melanoma is another malignancy that commonly spreads to the brain, but also is associated with short overall survivals in patients with extracranial metastatic disease. Most contemporary series that have evaluated patients with metastatic melanoma report a median survival of 8 to 12 months.[63,64] Metastatic breast carcinoma, unlike other cancers that make up the majority of brain metastases (such as non–small cell lung carcinoma), is associated with fairly effective systemic chemotherapy and hormonal therapy. A meta-analysis of 1430 breast cancer patients who developed extracranial metastases revealed a median survival of 19 months to 26 months, which varied depending on prior chemotherapy.[65] Two contemporary series report median survival in the range of 2 years following the development of extracranial metastases.[66,67] Some subsets of patients with metastatic breast carcinoma have even more favorable prognoses. Patients who present with metastases from breast carcinoma confined to the bones have a median survival of 33 months.[68]

The high overall mortality associated with metastatic malignancy (even in the absence of cerebral lesions) makes it difficult for therapies that are primarily focused on the control of brain metastases to have an appreciable impact on long-term survival in the majority of patients. Despite this fact, the prognosis of most patients with untreated cerebral metastases is exceedingly poor, with median survivals of 1 to 2 months reported.[69,70] Definitive therapies for many patients with brain metastases can extend survival by many months and sometimes much longer in selected patients. More importantly, definitive CNS therapies can impact the *quality* of survival in many patients. As most present therapies for brain metastases are inherently palliative, it is essential that the effect of these treatments on QOL, neurocognition, and functional survival be analyzed and considered by clinicians prescribing them. As the CNS is thought to act as a "sanctuary site" for metastatic lesions (partially related to difficulty of systemically administered agents crossing the blood–brain barrier) the relevance of definitive CNS therapies, with respect to both efficacy and impact on the quality of survival will inevitably increase as therapies for systemic malignancies continue to improve.

Definitive therapies for patients with brain tumors are directed at relieving neurologic symptoms and achieving long-term control. These therapies include whole-brain radiation therapy (WBRT), focused therapies (stereotactic radiosurgery, open resection, brachytherapy), chemotherapy, combination therapies, and experimental treatments. Our discussion of definitive therapies begins with WBRT, and then defines appropriate roles for focused therapies, alone and in combination with other treatments. Controversies in the use of various therapies are also addressed.

Whole-Brain Radiation Therapy

WBRT has been the mainstay of treatment for patients with cerebral metastases for almost 50 years. A great deal of effort has been expended examining the role of radiation therapy in brain metastases. Historically, the median survival of patients with brain metastases treated with steroids alone is 2 months, with whole-brain radiation therapy extending that survival to 3 to 6 months.[71] WBRT is effective in the palliation of neurologic symptoms and significantly decreases the likelihood of neurologic death (Fig. 26-5).[4]

Conventional techniques for the treatment of brain metastases with WBRT include the use of large, parallel-opposed, lateral beams with simple blocking or collimator rotation to avoid the eyes. All supratentorial and infratentorial contents are targeted, although simple techniques such as this may relatively underdose the frontal lobe at the cribriform plate and the inferior aspect of the temporal lobes.

Various dose and fractionation schedules have been studied for WBRT for brain metastases.[72–74] The largest studies have been conducted by the Radiation Therapy Oncology Group (RTOG). Borgelt reported the results of RTOG 69-01 and 73-61, which included more than 1812 patients treated in the early to mid 1970s. Seven different dose schedules delivering 30 to 40 Gy in 5 to 20 fractions were evaluated. All arms had equivalent survival, but the median time to neurologic progression was longer for more protracted schedules.[73] Kurtz subsequently studied dose fractionation in a more favorable subset of patients, but no survival benefit was seen with higher doses of

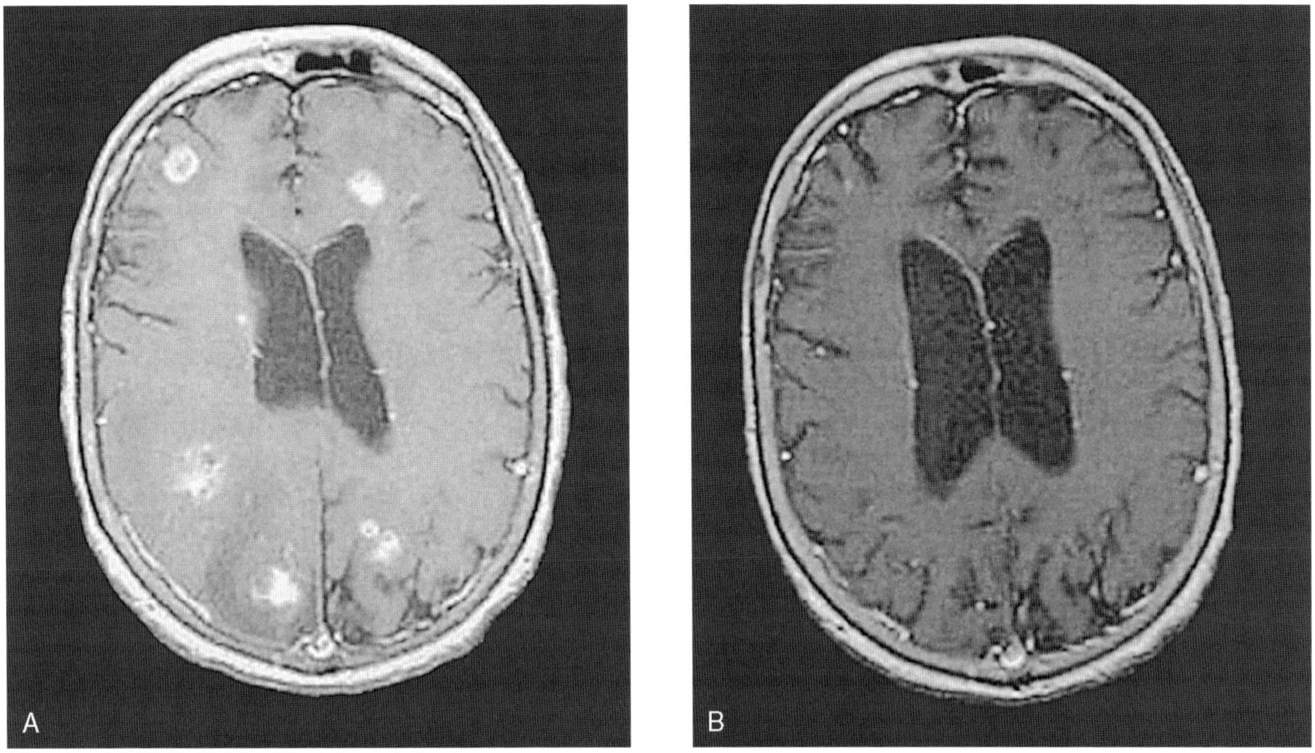

Figure 26-5. Contrast-enhanced T_1-weighted scans obtained pre- (A) and post- (B) WBRT are shown in a patient with metastatic non–small cell lung cancer who presented with progressive lethargy and confusion. Because of the multiplicity of his lesions, WBRT (3000 cGy in 12 fractions) was administered as primary therapy. WBRT resulted in complete radiographic resolution of all previously observed lesions. Additionally, the patient experienced good improvement in his neurologic symptoms. He ultimately succumbed to progressive systemic disease.

WBRT.[72] One specific finding in that analysis was that favorable patients with controlled primary tumors fared no better with an escalated WBRT dose (50 Gy in 20 fractions) than did patients receiving a dose of 30 Gy in 10 fractions. RTOG 79-16 randomized patients to 30 Gy in 10 fractions versus 30 Gy in 6 fractions.[75] There was a second randomization to misonidazole or no misonidazole. There was no survival difference between any of the four arms. One-third of patients experienced neurologic death, suggesting that further improvement in CNS control is required. Other studies examining accelerated fractionation and ultrarapid treatment schedules demonstrated no benefit over standard doses.[74,76,77]

On the basis of the above-mentioned analyses, 30 Gy in 10 fractions became the de facto regimen in the United States.

Common to other trials of brain metastases, it is difficult to impact overall survival with local therapies. Because no one WBRT dose schedule has been proven superior for overall survival, treating physicians must balance the length of treatment time with risk of neurologic sequelae that may be greater with shorter courses of WBRT. Although 30 Gy in 10 fractions remains a common regimen, many institutions have adopted the 2.5-Gy fraction size as the standard protocol for patients with a good prognosis since the publication of a long-term study from Memorial Sloan-Kettering Cancer Center that found an 11% risk of dementia in patients at 1 year following treatment with 3.0-Gy fraction sizes or greater.[78] The current RTOG standard dose for WBRT is 37.5 Gy in 15 fractions at 2.5 Gy per fraction.[79]

The dose necessary to control macroscopic disease is not entirely clear. It is apparent that when used as prophylactic treatment, lower doses are required. Prophylactic cranial irradiation (PCI) is standard therapy for many small cell lung carcinoma patients with an improvement in overall survival.[80] PCI is currently undergoing investigation in the setting of high-risk non–small cell carcinoma of the lung.

In an effort to improve local tumor control in patients receiving WBRT, several clinical trials have evaluated concurrent administration of radiation sensitizers. These have included randomized trials of halogenated pyrimidines, hypoxic cell sensitizers, and conventional chemotherapeutic agents.

RTOG 89-05 evaluated bromodeoxyuridine (BrdUrd) in patients with brain metastases. This randomized trial included various histologies and did not exclude patients with extracranial measurable tumor.[81] Seventy-two patients were randomized to 37.5 Gy in 15 fractions WBRT versus WBRT + BrdUrd administered 0.8 g/m^2 4 days per week during WBRT. Skin and hematologic toxicity was greater in patients who received BrdUrd, but there was no difference in overall survival between the arms.

Motexafin gadolinium (MGd) is an oxidative drug that sensitizes tumors cell to radiation in vitro, and by virtue of containing gadolinium, is visible on MRI. This agent showed promise in a phase I/II study and was subsequently tested in a phase III trial of newly diagnosed brain metastases.[82] Four hundred one patients were randomized to WBRT (30 Gy in 10 fractions) or WBRT + MGd concurrent with WBRT. MGd improved the time to neurologic progression and the neurocognitive function in the subset of lung cancer patients, but had no effect on overall survival. A confirmatory randomized trial of MGd in patients with brain metastases from non–small cell lung cancer is ongoing.

Temozolomide is an oral chemotherapy agent with CNS penetration and is structurally related to DTIC (dacarbazine). Studies of this agent in patients with refractory brain metastases demonstrate partial responses or disease stabilization.[83] Antonadou and associates performed a phase III randomized trial of this agent in patients receiving WBRT for previously untreated brain metastases. One hundred thirty-four patients were randomized to WBRT alone or to WBRT + temozolomide 75 mg/m^2 daily during WBRT followed by 200 mg/m^2 days 1 to 5 every 28 days for six cycles after completion of WBRT. Eighty-two percent of patients had lung cancer. The combination therapy improved the radiographic objective response rate (53.4% vs. 33.3%, $p = 0.039$). Although there was a trend toward a modest benefit in median survival with combination therapy, this did not reach statistical significance (8.3 months vs. 6.3 months, $p = 0.179$).[84] The RTOG is currently planning additional studies with this agent in combination with radiosurgery and WBRT.

Although WBRT can be associated with improved survival and palliation of neurologic symptoms, this therapy is associated with a number of short-term disadvantages, including alopecia, otitis, fatigue, and transient worsening of neurologic symptoms.[18] Local failure following WBRT is a persistent problem. Local control with WBRT has been described as 50% at 6 months, and 0% to 15% at 1 year.[85] Other studies have shown better control, with 70% of patients controlled at 1 year.[79] Long-term side effects of WBRT generally do not represent a significant issue because of the relatively short survival of most patients with brain metastases. Despite this, neurocognitive side effects have been described, particularly in long-term survivors. The available data on the neurocognitive effects of WBRT, however, are not compelling. The two most commonly quoted papers on the topic evaluated a total of 18 affected patients and were published in the late 1980s.[78,86] The patients evaluated in the larger series were treated in the late 1970s to the mid 1980s with radiation regimens that were generally not representative of present standards. In fact, 75% of the patients received daily fractions of 5 Gy or greater for some or all of their therapy.[78] Despite the widespread perception that WBRT inevitably results in worsened neurocognitive function, the contrary argument can be made that the *exclusion* of WBRT in patients with brain metastases can lead to inferior cognitive outcomes. Recently published data provide evidence that when patients treated with stereotactic radiosurgery (SRS) alone relapse, they are frequently symptomatic (71%) and the majority suffer a neurologic deficit (59%).[87] These authors also noted that the "successful" treatment of recurrent lesions often did not lead to an improvement in neurologic function. Similar data suggesting that patients with brain metastases who relapse have inferior neurocognitive function can also be found in the WBRT literature.[88] Taken together, these data suggest that the negative sequelae associated with recurrent brain metastases far outweigh the side effects of WBRT in the vast majority of patients with this disease. The significance of these observations is expanded on in the focused therapy sections below.

In summary, early clinical trials focused on various dose and timing schedules but no one schedule has proved superior in terms of overall survival. The recognition of *potential* late neurotoxicity with WBRT and the development of better imaging and focal therapies, such as microsurgical resection and radiosurgery, have shifted the research focus to study which patients are best treated with WBRT. Recent randomized trials suggest a potential benefit with new-generation radiation sensitizers.

Introduction to Focused Therapies: The Importance of Prognostic Factors

Although most patients with brain metastases succumb to systemic cancer progression, there are favorable subgroups of patients with good performance status and limited systemic disease who have a greater likelihood of surviving longer and therefore are at increased risk to experience neurologic deficits or die of neurologic progression if treated by WBRT alone. Aggressive focused therapies have the potential to improve local control in these patients and prolong survival. Patients most likely to benefit are those who are at significant risk of experiencing a decline in their QOL as a result of CNS progression or those (fewer) patients who are likely to die from CNS progression. How do we define these populations?

Patients who are likely to die from progression of their brain metastases make up the minority (approximately

20%) of those with metastatic brain cancer. Clearly, some of these patients, particularly those with large lesions that are imminently life-threatening and/or those with a longer anticipated survival, are candidates for aggressive local therapies. The majority of patients, however, will ultimately die of progressive systemic disease. As approximately 50% of patients will experience CNS progression with WBRT alone if they survive 6 or more months, patients whose predicted life expectancy exceeds 6 months appear to be most likely to benefit, either by means of prolonged survival or improved QOL, from the addition of focal therapies. Thus, the ability to predict which particular subset of patients is more favorable could help guide therapy as well as generate hypotheses for future studies.

Gaspar and associates performed the largest study examining prognostic variables in patients with cerebral metastases. These investigators performed a recursive partitioning analysis (RPA) of 1200 patients enrolled in RTOG WBRT trials conducted from 1979 to 1993.[89] If patients had a controlled primary tumor, age less than or equal to 65 years, Karnofsky performance status (KPS) of 70 or greater, and absence of non-CNS metastases (RPA Class I patients), median survival was 7.1 months. If KPS was less than 70 (RPA Class III patients), survival was only 2.4 months. Other patients (RPA Class II) had an intermediate median survival of 4.2 months. On the basis of this analysis, one might predict that RPA Class I patients are most likely to benefit from the addition of aggressive local therapies. Select patients in RPA Class II (particularly those with large and/or symptomatic lesions) might also be expected to benefit. Other prognostic factors that have been identified include number of metastases. A previous analysis by Swift of RTOG studies suggested the number of tumors (three or fewer vs. four or more) by CT was a predictor of survival.[90] Alexander and associates, however, suggested that patients with three or more cerebral metastases define a population with a lowered likelihood of prolonged survival.[91]

Surgery for Single Brain Metastases

The goals of surgery in patients with brain metastases are to provide rapid relief of symptoms that are secondary to mass effect of the tumor or adjacent edema, to improve local control and increase the likelihood of success of adjuvant therapies, to improve the chance for long-term survival, and, when necessary, to obtain tissue for histologic diagnosis. Most of the better data regarding the efficacy of surgery in the treatment of brain metastases comes from three randomized, prospective studies, all of which examined the value of surgery in the removal of a solitary brain metastasis. Patchell and colleagues were the first to examine this issue.[92] In their study, patients were randomized to biopsy plus WBRT versus WBRT plus open surgical resection for a single brain metastasis. These investigators reported a significant increase in survival in the surgical group (40 weeks vs. 15 weeks). Additionally, time to recurrence, freedom from death as a result of neurologic causes, and duration of functional independence were significantly longer in the surgery arm. No extra mortality from surgery was noted. A second study in Europe using similar treatment arms confirmed Patchell's conclusions regarding the benefit of surgery in extending survival in patients with single brain metastases (10 months vs. 6 months).[93] Combined modality treatment was also found to significantly increase functional survival in this study. Importantly, this study found that the greatest benefit of surgery plus WBRT was seen in patients with stable extracranial disease. Patients with active extracranial disease did not appear to benefit from the addition of surgery. This is consistent with the generally accepted principle that a patient's survival is primarily related to the status of systemic disease. A third analysis of WBRT versus WBRT plus surgical resection for treatment of single brain metastases failed to show a survival advantage related to the addition of surgery.[94] It should be noted that this study included a higher proportion of patients with lower performance scores and extensive systemic disease. Based on the evidence that that these two factors are known to predict poor survival in patients with brain metastases, one might expect that patient selection played a significant role in the failure of this study to detect a significant benefit from the addition of surgery.

Together, these studies provide support for the use of surgery in addition to WBRT in patients with a single brain metastasis and either no remaining systemic disease or stable extracranial disease. Even in the presence of uncontrolled primary or extracranial metastatic disease, resection of symptomatic single metastases that are the principal factor limiting quality of life is often indicated for palliation. Many surgeons would consider the use of surgery in select patients with progressive systemic disease, who are confronted with imminent loss of life or neurological function from an accessible, large, single metastasis. Patients whose symptoms cannot be successfully palliated with medical management (including high-dose steroids) and whose lesions can be excised without significant risk of producing or worsening a neurologic deficit are potential candidates for craniotomy. Although resection is not expected to prolong survival in these patients, it is probably indicated more often than it is performed.

In the case of single, asymptomatic brain metastases with an undiagnosed primary, the decision for surgery becomes more complex. For most patients, obtaining a tissue diagnosis is mandatory. If an extracranial lesion presents a target that is more safely biopsied, then biopsy of such a lesion is often recommended before the intracranial disease is addressed. For patients in whom a nonsurgical histology like small cell lung carcinoma (a highly radiation-sensitive histology) is diagnosed by such a biopsy, a potentially unnecessary craniotomy can be avoided. In other cases, knowledge of the putative histology of the single brain metastasis may lead to a recommendation for WBRT and/or SRS rather than craniotomy for tumor removal.

Stereotactic biopsy of single putative metastases in unresectable locations is indicated to obtain a tissue diagnosis in patients when no other lesion has been identified that can be more safely biopsied. Biopsy is also indicated when the chance of a coincidental nonmalignant intracranial lesion is greater than the probability of a significant biopsy-related complication. In most series the rate of such complications approximates 1%. Many specialists also strongly consider a stereotactic biopsy in patients whose primary and systemic malignant disease has been in remission for a length of time sufficient to raise the question of a new malignancy rather than a metastasis. For non–small cell lung cancers, for example, an interval of remission greater than 1 year and the absence of new systemic disease should raise the suspicion of a new primary when single or multiple brain lesions suggestive of metastasis are detected. Stereotactic or open biopsy of a single, putative brain metastasis may also be indicated after treatment to distinguish between recurrence and treatment effects such as radiation necrosis (see following sections). Single brain metastases from certain primary sites merit more in-depth discussion.

Surgery for Single Lung Metastases to Brain

The case for resection of single brain metastases was first and most convincingly made for non–small cell lung primaries.[95] The evidence for benefit from resection of single non–small cell lung cancer metastases is stronger than that for many other tumor types. Reported 5-year survival rates range from 0% to 45%.[96–98] This large variation is likely largely accounted for by two factors: (a) variation in the aggressiveness of treatment of the primary disease among the reported series and (b) variation in the incidence of systemic disease burden among those series.

Small cell lung cancer metastases to brain are rarely single. Responsiveness to chemotherapy and fractionated radiation coupled with a poor overall prognosis make small cell metastases among the least favorable candidates for resection. Occasional patients have small cell carcinoma that behaves more like non–small cell carcinoma in the brain with a single lesion and a more indolent course. Craniotomy may be indicated in such patients whose lesions have progressed after fractionated radiation and proven unresponsive to systemic chemotherapy.

Surgery for Single Breast Metastasis to Brain

Breast cancer metastases to brain are common with an even higher rate among patients treated with trastuzumab (Herceptin). This is likely to account for increasing incidence of brain metastases from breast in the future.[99] This may be either a result of predilection for the brain by HER-2-positive tumor cells and/or poor penetration of the CNS by trastuzumab or to improved visceral disease control leading to a longer life and onset of late tumor spread to the CNS. Single breast metastases to brain often follow a more indolent course than metastases from other primaries. Furthermore, increasingly successful treatment of systemic disease in these patients often warrants aggressive surgical treatment of single breast metastases to brain followed by adjuvant therapy expected to be effective against microscopic CNS disease (Fig. 26-6). Bony metastases are usually not a contraindication to resection of single breast metastases, whereas visceral metastases are a stronger relative contraindication because of poorer overall prognosis.

Surgery for Single Melanoma Metastasis to Brain

A single melanoma metastasis to the brain is not incompatible with long-term, high-quality survival in patients with systemic control of their primary disease.[100] Many

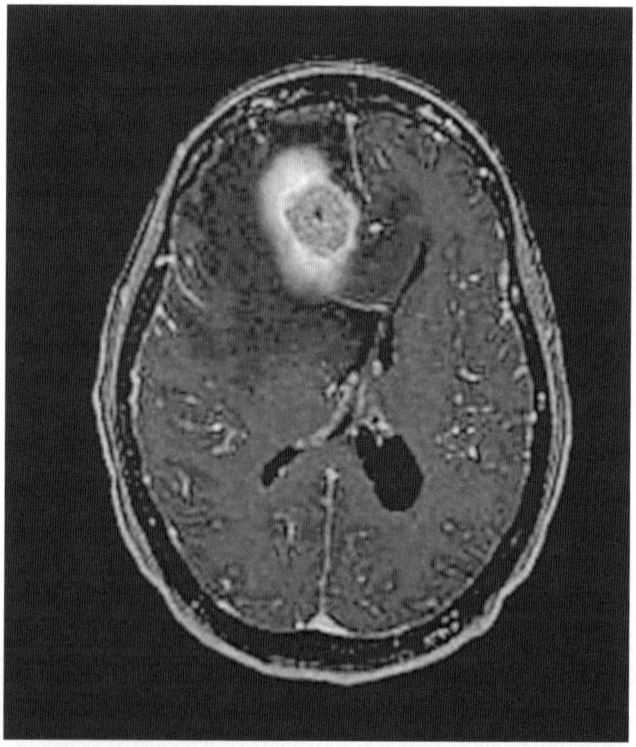

Figure 26-6. A single breast cancer metastasis to the right frontal lobe is seen in this contrast-enhanced, T_1-weighted, axial image. The patient had a history of breast cancer, diagnosed 5 years previously. She had evidence of progressive bone metastases, but no other systemic disease. She presented with progressive confusion. Because of the mass effect exerted by this mass and its associated edema, it was resected. The patient did well after surgery, with complete resolution of her neurologic symptoms.

patients whose primary melanoma is undetectable, or who present metachronously, may also hope for systemic disease control and therefore are often candidates for aggressive treatment of a single brain primary. Melanoma metastases, although radioresistant to fractionated radiation, have a high probability of being exquisitely sensitive to single-fraction stereotactic radiosurgery, leading some authors to prefer this modality. Resection of single metastases is indicated for symptomatic lesions. Randomized comparisons of radiosurgery versus craniotomy for single melanoma metastases to brain have not been performed. Both management strategies thus have proponents.

Surgery for Single Genitourinary Cancer Metastasis to Brain

Single renal cell carcinoma metastasis to brain is clinically nearly indistinguishable from melanoma metastasis with respect to neurosurgical management issues. In particular, this histology is very sensitive to single-fraction stereotactic radiosurgery and has a tendency to deteriorate by intratumoral hemorrhage. Again, resection of single metastases may be indicated for symptomatic lesions.

Prostate metastasis to brain parenchyma has a low incidence among patients with prostate cancer, but the prevalence of the primary tumor results in such metastases with sufficient frequency to warrant consideration. Most prostate metastases to the brain are single. Survival after metastasis of prostate cancer to the brain parenchyma is often short.[101] In contradistinction, McCutcheon and associates[102] report a median survival of 16 months in 9 patients treated with surgery and radiation versus 6 months in 29 patients with WBRT alone. Because bony metastases of prostate cancer often have an indolent course with systemic therapy, they are often not a contraindication to surgical treatment of a single prostate metastasis to brain parenchyma. In contrast to brain parenchymal metastases, calvarial metastases of prostate cancer are compatible with long survival. Thus, selected patients with single surgically accessible prostate carcinoma metastases who are symptomatic or have good performance status may be candidates for surgical resection.

Surgery for Single Gynecologic Metastasis to Brain

Single ovarian metastases have treatment considerations similar to many other primaries and often warrant surgical resection. As with many other primaries, the potential for resection of the brain lesion to contribute to long-term survival will be significantly influenced by the presence of extracranial metastases.[103] Single cervical cancer metastases to the brain warrant similar considerations.[104] Like single brain metastasis of most histologies, patients with surgically accessible, symptomatic lesions of putative ovarian or cervical origin generally benefit from resection of their brain lesion. Single choriocarcinoma metastases to brain are usually detected after delivery and are generally very sensitive to radiation and/or systemic chemotherapy. Single choriocarcinoma metastases, therefore, often do not require resection. Occurrence during pregnancy or lesions unresponsive to systemic therapy or radiotherapy may mandate resection of single choriocarcinoma metastases to brain.[105] Germ cell tumors, particularly those of testicular primary, are often very sensitive to focal or whole-brain radiation and systemic chemotherapy. Thus, even relatively large lesions may be successfully managed nonsurgically. Progressive symptoms in the face of medical management or presentation in extremis may, however, mandate surgical resection.

Surgery for a Single Gastrointestinal Metastasis to the Brain

Increased awareness of the possibility of brain metastases, early diagnosis, and aggressive therapy can provide increased survival time for patients with colorectal cancer with brain metastases.[106] Surgical removal of colorectal metastatic brain lesions results in substantially increased survival time with an average of 10 months.[107] Only the presence of cerebellar brain metastases is associated with decreased survival after surgical resection. It is very uncommon to have a survival more than 1 year after diagnosis of brain metastasis is made. However, most of the long-term survivors, which account for 16% of patients, have solitary lesions.[108] In patients with recurrent brain disease, repeated resection is a worthwhile consideration because it may prolong survival as compared with patients who do not undergo re-resection.[109]

Metastatic brain tumors from esophageal cancer are relatively rare. The median survival time of all patients from the treatment of brain metastases is around 2 months. These extremely poor treatment results reflect the fact that most patients at the time of diagnosis of brain metastasis had poor performance status and the presence of extracerebral metastases. Surgery for brain metastases from esophageal, gastric, pancreatic, and hepatocellular primary sites is rarely recommended because of poor overall survival when brain metastases are detected.[110,111]

In summary, exceptions to consideration of craniotomy for single brain lesions consistent with metastasis often include patients with small cell lung carcinoma, germ cell tumors, including particularly those of testicular primary, choriocarcinoma, and primary or secondary central nervous system lymphoma. These lesions generally respond dramatically to one or a combination of fractionated radiotherapy, focal radiation, or systemic chemotherapy, leading to very rapid resolution of symptoms.

Surgery for Multiple Metastases

Surgery to resect multiple brain metastases is a relatively new concept in neuro-oncology. Traditionally, the identification of multiple brain metastases was considered a contraindication to surgical intervention, and most patients with multiple brain metastases were treated exclusively with WBRT.[112,113] Resection of multiple metastases was undertaken only in the case of life-threatening lesions or in cases in which the diagnosis was in question.[39] Although WBRT is still a mainstay of treatment, recent data suggest that surgical resection of multiple brain metastases may provide a survival benefit in properly selected patients. This is important because the majority of patients with brain metastases have multiple lesions, especially those with common primaries such as lung cancer, breast cancer, and melanoma.[39,114] Indeed, MRI-based studies show that 60% to 85% of patients with intracranial metastases harbor multiple lesions. [115–117] As previously noted, melanoma has the highest frequency of metastasizing to multiple sites in the brain.[38,118–120]

To date, no prospective data exist to support the routine use of surgery for multiple brain metastases. Perhaps the most widely quoted retrospective analysis of this issue was presented by physicians from the University of Texas M. D. Anderson Cancer Center.[114] In this study, the results of 56 consecutive patients who underwent surgery for multiple brain metastases between 1984 and 1992 were examined. These 56 patients were divided into two groups. The first cohort (group A) consisted of 30 patients who underwent surgery for multiple metastases but in whom complete resection of all metastases was not possible. In contrast, the second cohort (group B) consisted of 26 patients who had all of their multiple brain metastases resected. No patient in either group had more than three lesions resected, and no patient had more than three craniotomies performed during the same operation. As a control cohort (group C), the authors identified 26 patients who had undergone resection of a single brain metastasis during the same time period and who were matched to group B patients in terms of their primary tumor type, the interval between the first diagnosis of cancer and the first diagnosis of a brain metastasis, and the presence or absence of systemic cancer at the time of surgery.

The most important result of this study was that the median survival for patients with multiple metastases who had all their lesions removed (group B, 14 months) was identical to the median survival of patients who had a single brain metastasis removed (group C, 14 months).[114] In contrast, patients with multiple metastases in whom all of the lesions could not be removed (group A) had a median survival of only 6 months. Multivariate analysis demonstrated that the only variables significantly affecting the survival durations were the group of the patient (A vs. B or C) and the extent of the systemic disease. A second finding reported in this study was that the morbidity associated with resecting multiple brain metastases was not significantly different from that of resecting a single brain metastasis. The authors concluded that, in properly selected patients, resection of multiple metastases appeared to be as effective as resection of a single metastasis, as long as all the lesions are removed.

A second retrospective analysis provides data to support surgical resection of multiple in selected patients. In a study of 138 patients, Iwadate and associates reported that the median survival after resecting multiple brain metastases (9.2 months) was comparable to that after resection of a single brain metastasis (8.7 months).[121] These authors found that the significant variables for shorter survival were age older than 60 years, KPS <70, incomplete surgical removal, and the presence of extensive systemic cancer. In contrast to the above-mentioned studies, Hazuka and associates found that surgery was of little benefit in patients with multiple metastases.[122] This study did support the use of surgery in patients with a single brain lesion. In conclusion, these retrospective analyses are intriguing but cannot be used as data to definitively support the routine use of surgery in patients with multiple brain metastases. Presently, most clinicians would consider surgery in patients with multiple brain metastases who present with a single life-threatening lesion. In this instance, resection of the dominant lesion would be performed with other therapies (SRS, WBRT) used on the remaining lesions. Based on the above analyses, a limited number of patients with controlled systemic disease, good functional status, a histology with an intermediate or low-radiation sensitivity and three or less surgically accessible lesions *might* be candidates for resection of all of their lesions.

Surgical Technique

A detailed discussion of surgical technique is found in Chapter 6. A few issues related to surgical considerations are, however, relevant to this discussion. Removal of single or multiple brain metastases can be accomplished safely with modern neurosurgical techniques and adjunctive technologies. These advances have reduced the operative morbidity and mortality rates to less than 10% (per craniotomy) and less than 5%, respectively.[114]

A surgeon must weigh the relative risks of operative intervention versus the risk of morbidity. Surgery should only be considered when an appropriate risk-to-benefit ratio is perceived. When considering the risk of surgery, tumor location is a critical variable to assess. Lesions located within eloquent cortex (primary motor area, language areas, brainstem) pose much greater risks to the patient with surgical resection than lesions in noneloquent brain (e.g., nondominant anterior frontal or temporal lobes). Although surgical excision of lesions is possible in these locations, the use of noninvasive therapies that may be associated with a more favorable toxicity profile, such as SRS, should be given consideration before open excision is attempted. When one does choose to remove lesions from these locations (e.g., large lesions or lesions producing severe symptoms from extensive associated edema, lesions with a broad cortical presentation, histologies poorly sensitive to other therapies, and recurrent or persistent lesions), adjuvant surgical techniques such as awake craniotomy and electrocorticography may reduce surgical morbidity. Note, however, that electrocorticography can lead to false reassurance in certain circumstances. For example, neurologic deficit can result from resection of lesions presenting below the brain surface even when the overlying cortex has been "cleared" by intraoperative motor mapping as descending fiber tracts do not always run perpendicular to the cortical surface. For lesions that do not arise to the cortical surface, brain dissection can often be minimized and morbidity decreased by approaching the tumor through an adjacent sulcus. Care must be taken to preserve all vessels that do not appear to terminate within the tumor. Image-guided surgery (IGS, frameless stereotaxis) can be used to localize lesions before a skin incision is made and during the ensuing surgery in a way that typically allows for a more minimally invasive dissection. Intraoperative ultrasonography is also commonly used to identify lesions below the cortical surface and confirm completeness of resection, particularly in lesions with poorly defined margins. Ultrasonography has the advantage of providing "real-time" imaging intraoperatively at a very small fraction of the cost of much more expensive techniques such as intraoperative MRI. Like MRI and unlike IGS, the reliability of ultrasonography is not affected by the brain shift that inevitably occurs after the liberation of CSF and tumor removal. In all cases, meticulous microsurgical technique employing the intraoperative microscope or other magnification tool, minimal tissue manipulation, and excellent hemostasis are critical to maximize tumor removal and minimize the potential for surgical complication.

In summary, surgery for brain metastases is a commonly employed treatment strategy. Most investigators agree that patients with controlled systemic disease and single, accessible lesions are optimally treated with surgical excision. Surgical resection is being employed at some centers in the treatment of patients with multiple (three or fewer) brain metastases although the value of surgery in these patients is still being debated. The use of other therapies in combination with surgery is discussed in subsequent sections.

Radiosurgery

SRS is a specialized technique that uses beams of high-energy photons to deliver a single, high-dose fraction of ionizing radiation to a small, precisely defined target volume while minimizing radiation delivered to the surrounding normal brain. Radiosurgery has become an important and prevalent form of therapy for cerebral metastases. Prospective analyses demonstrate the benefit of surgery in addition to WBRT in the treatment of single brain metastases. Many lesions, however, are not optimally treated with surgical therapy as a consequence of their location or other factors. SRS is a focused technique that offers many of the benefits of conventional open surgery without exposing patients to a number of the limitations associated with resection. For example, a number of published studies have reported local control rates for brain metastases that are equivalent or better than those reported for surgery plus WBRT. Additionally, SRS allows patients to avoid most of the risks of an open operation (surgical infection, intracerebral hemorrhage, exposure to anesthesia) and can be performed in the outpatient setting. Finally, SRS may be used to treat multiple lesions in widely disparate locations and can be employed in eloquent locations not amenable to open surgical approaches, such as the brainstem and deep nuclei (Fig. 26-7). Some data suggest that SRS is more cost-effective than open resection, although this will require further analysis.[123]

Most systems used for SRS presently depend upon the use of a stereotactic head-frame. The frame, a metal ring that is fixed to the patient's skull using a local anesthetic, serves two primary functions. First, the ring allows for the establishment of a fixed, three-dimensional stereotactic coordinate system to allow for accurate targeting.

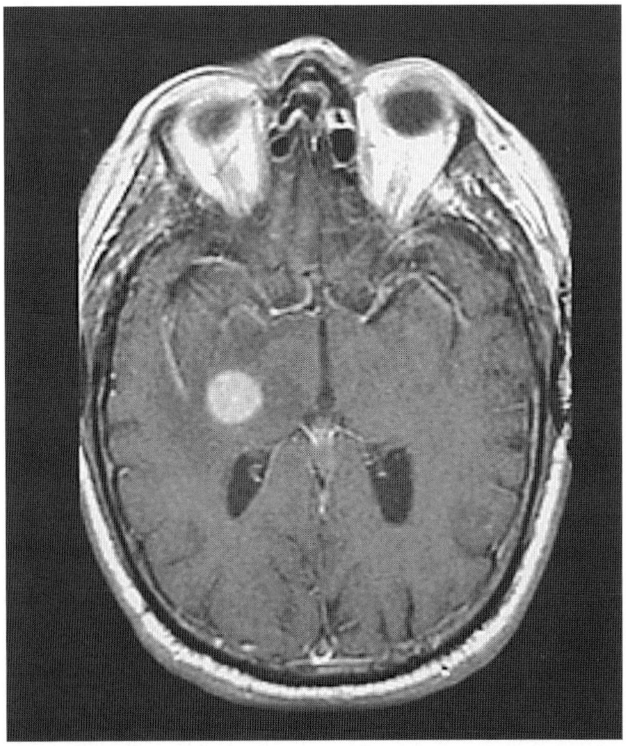

Figure 26-7. This postcontrast, T_1-weighted, axial image shows a solitary melanoma metastasis to the right basal ganglia region. Given the deep location of the lesion, it was elected to treat this patient with stereotactic radiosurgery.

Second, the frame also allows for immobilization of the patient during therapy to optimize treatment precision. Once the stereotactic head frame is applied, imaging studies are obtained to allow for treatment planning. Most institutions use MR scans for anatomic and spatial data. There is some evidence that CT studies fused with MRI may both enhance accuracy of planning and serve as an internal control for spatial accuracy by offsetting potential warping produced by an inhomogeneous MRI field. Imaging data are exported to a workstation where the contours of the lesion(s) are defined and the treatment planning is performed.

The first method developed to deliver SRS was the Leksell Gamma Knife (Elekta), which still operates using the original principle developed by Dr. Lars Leksell in the 1950s. This device consists of 201 concentrically aligned cobalt-60 sources, which emit gamma irradiation. Four different sizes of collimators are available and are placed into spherical "helmets" in alignment with the radiation sources. This multiple source configuration allows the vast majority of the radiation dose to be focused within a very precise volume while minimizing radiation to the surrounding normal brain. The epicenter of delivery of each dose (or "shot") of radiation is always in the center of the sphere defined by the helmet; the head position within the helmet is determined by the treatment planning system and is set using a stereotactic frame. SRS allows delivery of radiation to only a small volume of surrounding normal brain with a rapid falloff of the dose. Thus, brain tissue as close as 2 to 3 mm away from the lesion may receive less than 20% of the peak dose.

The second method for delivering SRS is by x-rays produced by a linear accelerator (LINAC), which is a machine that generates high-energy photons. The LINAC is the mainstay of a modern radiation oncology department and is typically used to deliver therapeutic radiation using a wide variety of techniques. Modified linear accelerators can be used for SRS by focusing the beams through a variety of fixed-shaped fields at the target, or by a variety of arcs with the same central point (isocenter) at the axis of rotation.

Unlike Gamma Knife therapy, in which the relationship between the patient's head and the treatment device remains fixed during the treatment of a specific area (isocenter), in most LINAC radiosurgery treatment algorithms the patient's head is maintained in a fixed position as the linear accelerator is moved along arcs of travel, or from point to point. The radiation beam remains fixed on a specific point during the arc of travel, maximizing the amount of radiation delivered to the target and minimizing exposure of adjacent tissue. LINAC radiosurgery can be used to treat lesions anywhere in the body as long as stereotactic localization can be performed accurately. In contrast, Gamma Knife SRS can be performed only on lesions above the foramen magnum. The most recent evidence shows that both the Gamma Knife and linear accelerators achieve similarly excellent clinical results.[124]

Although the theory behind radiosurgery was developed several decades ago, widespread clinical use began in earnest in the late 1980s and early 1990s spurred on by progression of computer technology and widespread availability of MRI. A multicenter phase I RTOG trial was initiated in 1990 to help determine which radiosurgery doses were safe in a group of patients previously treated with standard external beam radiation therapy.[125] The early publications showed good control rates and led to further investigation.[126–129] Large series have consistently revealed local control of the target lesions in the range of 80% to 85%, or even higher, with a very acceptable side-effect profile.[130,131] Interestingly, traditionally radioresistant histologies tend to be more sensitive to SRS than to conventional fractionated radiation treatment. The mechanism for this increased sensitivity is unclear; however, the effect may be related to the fact that SRS causes indirect vascular injury and subsequent sclerosis of the blood vessels and eventual compromise of blood supply and circulation within the tumor.[132]

Radiosurgery is not a replacement for traditional radiation therapy but it does offer a substitute for open surgery in certain circumstances. With the demonstration of the effectiveness of surgery for cerebral metastases (particularly single lesions) and the increasing application of radiosurgery, a number of clinicians have asked: "Is radiosurgery the therapeutic equivalent of open resection?" Before that question can be answered, one must define what is meant by "control" in both forms of therapy. Surgical control is easily defined. The optimal goal of resection is complete removal of the radiographic abnormality. Progression is defined as any evidence of tumor regrowth. In radiosurgery, treated lesions do not always disappear radiographically. Despite this, patients may still experience symptomatic improvement, and persistent lesions may remain stable on serial scans. Accordingly, radiosurgical control has been defined as the absence of tumor growth visualized on treatment imaging studies (tumor regression, tumor shrinkage, or stability) with no increase in clinical symptoms associated with the lesion. Edema refractory to medicines, symptomatic radiation necrosis, and tumor hemorrhage are also considered failures of local treatment.

To date, there are no completed randomized trials comparing radiosurgery to surgery. If one is willing to accept the above definitions of surgical and radiosurgical control, then the preponderance of retrospective data supports the equivalence of the modalities for small (<2.5–3 cm), single lesions with published local control rates generally ranging from 80% to 90%.[130,133] In particular, three retrospective analyses are worth studying in detail. Auchter and associates identified patients meeting Patchell's selection criteria and were treated with WBRT followed by an SRS boost.[131] Local control, survival, and functional independence were found to be comparable to the results of surgery and WBRT. Similarly, Muacevic and colleagues found in a retrospective matched comparison analysis of 108 patients that survival for patients with a single metastasis was similar whether they received SRS or surgery plus WBRT.[134] In contrast, Bindal and associates retrospectively compared consecutive patients treated with SRS or surgery. Local control and survival were considerably worse in the SRS patients. It should be mentioned, however, that in this analysis the low local control rates reported for the radiosurgery patients (61%) and differences in the extent of systemic disease between the two groups of patients examined may have accounted for the poor results of SRS.[114] Several authors have discussed the need to evaluate the equivalence of SRS and open surgical resection in a prospective fashion.[131] Unfortunately, as a result of the large number of patients required and very difficult randomization, this study is unlikely to be performed.

As mentioned previously, two randomized prospective studies demonstrated a benefit of surgery in addition to WBRT for the treatment of solitary brain metastases. In an attempt to address the question of the value of the addition of SRS to WBRT a multicenter retrospective analysis was carried out with 502 patients treated at 10 institutions in which all of the patients were treated with WBRT and SRS. The patients were stratified by RPA and compared to similar patients from the RTOG database who had been treated with WBRT alone.[124] The study revealed that patients with higher KPSs, controlled primary tumors, absence of extracranial metastases, and lower RPA classes had statistically superior survival. The addition of an SRS boost resulted in median survival of 16.1, 10.3, and 8.7 months, respectively, for RPA classes I, II, and III. This is in comparison to 7.1, 4.2, and 2.3 months for similar RPA class patients from the RTOG database. This improvement in overall survival stratified by RPA class with an SRS boost in addition to WBRT was statistically significant.[124] Although the retrospective data are compelling, these studies are limited, like all such studies, by confounding variables (including selection bias) that cannot be eliminated from the analysis. Accordingly, phase III prospective trials were necessary to more adequately assess whether the addition of SRS would be superior to WBRT alone.

Three randomized, prospective studies have now examined the role of SRS as an adjunct to WBRT for cerebral metastases. Kondziolka and associates reported a small (n = 25) series in which WBRT was compared to WBRT + SRS boost for patients with 2 to 4 metastases. Although no survival difference was observed, the authors reported a significant improvement in local control (100% vs. 8%) with SRS boost.[85] This paper has been criticized for using nonstandard end points. Similarly, a second prospective study, reported in abstract form, contained methodologic problems that prevent one from drawing firm conclusions from the data.[135] The largest series so far to examine the role of SRS in addition to WBRT has been performed by the RTOG (RTOG 95-08).[79] In RTOG 95-08, patients were randomized to WBRT alone or to WBRT + SRS. The patients with solitary metastases had a statistically significant improvement in overall survival from 4.9 months with WBRT alone to 6.5 months with WBRT + SRS ($p = 0.04$). In subset analysis, patients in RPA class I, age younger than 50 years, non–small cell lung carcinoma or any squamous histology, all had a statistically significant benefit in overall survival. Importantly, patients in the WBRT + SRS group were more likely to have a stable or improved performance status at 3 months (50% vs. 33%, $p = 0.02$) and 6 months (43% vs. 27%, $p = 0.03$).[79]

The presently available data appear to support the use of WBRT + SRS in patients with solitary metastases with good performance status. The evidence to date does not conclusively support the routine use of SRS as a boost therapy in patients with two to three metastases, but it appears that there are some subsets of patients that benefit, primarily patients who are RPA class I, young, or have non–small cell carcinoma of the lung. Patients with no extracranial disease or stable extracranial disease also seem more likely to benefit from improved control of the brain metastases afforded by the addition of SRS than will those patients with widespread, progressive, systemic disease. Radiosurgery plays an important role in salvage therapy after WBRT.

The use of radiosurgery in combination with open surgery is advocated in select patients with multiple metastases. This combined approach might be most logical for good functional status patients with limited systemic disease and histologies that are generally poorly sensitive to conventional radiation therapy (such as melanoma), particularly in the setting of a large symptomatic lesion. In this circumstance, an appropriate sequence of interventions might be resection of the dominant mass, followed by radiosurgery with or without WBRT for treatment to the resection cavity and any additional small or surgically inaccessible lesions. It should be noted, however, that no study to date has specifically examined the potential benefit of combined focused therapies in this subset of patients.

The overall side effects of SRS are limited, but can occasionally be serious. There are very few acute side effects of SRS related to the radiation, but the head frame can result in discomfort as well as a small risk of bleeding and infection. SRS does not result in hair loss or nausea and in general results only in mild fatigue. There is a risk of late side effects, the most common and serious of which is radionecrosis. Radionecrosis is damage to the substance of the brain in the high-dose area that can result in edema and subsequent side effects that can occasionally require surgical intervention, or on rare occasions even death. Fortunately, the risk of symptomatic radionecrosis is usually less than 5% and most frequently can be managed with steroids.[79,85,131] The risk of side effects increases with the treated volume; thus, SRS is generally only utilized for lesions 3.0 cm in diameter or less.

In summary, SRS is an established technology with substantial published literature supporting its use in the treatment of brain metastases. SRS offers a very high control rate with a low risk of serious side effects.

Focused Therapies and Adjuvant Whole-Brain Radiation Therapy

In light of data suggesting that both surgery and radiosurgery are efficacious in the treatment of brain metastases (particularly single lesions), some investigators have begun to question whether WBRT is necessary after these focused therapies have been employed. A number of individuals advocate sole use of focused therapies with the intent of limiting the potential negative neurocognitive effects of WBRT.

A single prospective study has evaluated the role of adjuvant radiation with focused therapy. Patchell and associates examined 95 patients with a single brain metastasis who underwent complete surgical excision of their tumors. After surgery, the patients were randomized to WBRT (50.4 Gy) for observation. These investigators reported that the addition of WBRT to surgery for a single lesion markedly reduced the incidence of local recurrence (46% vs. 10%), distant brain recurrence (37% vs. 14%), and the likelihood of death from neurologic cause (44% vs. 14%). There was no difference in overall survival or duration of functional independence (possibly related to salvage therapies in the surgery arm). The authors concluded that WBRT was necessary as an adjunct to surgical therapy to help improve local control and decrease risk of distant brain recurrence.[136]

No prospective data exist regarding the use of adjuvant SRS, with or without WBRT. In a randomized trial evaluating the role of WBRT following surgical resection, patients treated with conventional open surgical resection without WBRT had a 46% risk of failure at the site of the resection.[136] In contrast, some authors retrospectively examined the efficacy of SRS alone in the treatment of brain metastases (without WBRT) and found excellent local control, all greater than 70% at 1 year, but most on the order of 80%.[137–139] Of note, other published series of patients treated with SRS alone have reported significant risk of distant brain failure at 1 year ranging from 43% to 57%.[137–140]

Despite a relatively high risk of distant failure for many patients with brain metastases treated with SRS alone, retrospective studies have not confirmed a survival benefit to adjuvant WBRT.[137,141,142] In one of the studies, freedom from local recurrence in the brain at 1 year was significantly superior in the patients receiving WBRT in addition to SRS (28% vs. 69%), although the overall survival was not significantly different.[137] A retrospective, multiinstitutional study in which 268 patients were treated with SRS alone and 301 received SRS + WBRT has also been published, and after adjustment for known prognostic factors there was not a significant difference in overall surviva1.[141] Despite the high rate of new lesions developing in patients treated with SRS alone, however, overall survival appears to be equivalent to SRS + WBRT as salvage therapies are fairly effective and patients' extracranial disease is frequently the cause of death.[137,141] Pirzkall and associates did report a trend toward improved survival with adjuvant WBRT in a subset of patients with no extracranial tumor (15.4 months vs. 8.3 months; $p = 0.08$), but no benefit for a overall group of 236 patients.[142] Chidel and associates reported the experience from the Cleveland Clinic with 78 patients managed initially with SRS alone and 57 patients treated with SRS and adjuvant WBRT. WBRT did not improve overall survival but was useful in preventing the progression of the treated tumor and in protecting against the development of new brain metastases (74% vs. 48%, $p = 0.06$).[143] These retrospective studies do suggest that WBRT will improve local and distant control in the brain, but do not clearly demonstrate a survival advantage.

The net conclusion that some have drawn from the surgical and radiosurgical studies discussed is that as WBRT does not appear to confer a survival benefit to patients, it can be dispensed with. The perception that WBRT leads to unacceptable neurocognitive complications in a significant number of patients has further fueled this conclusion. As discussed earlier in the "Whole Brain Therapy" subsection however, the frequency of serious long-term complications related to WBRT using contemporary radiation doses is unknown and is almost certainly overestimated. Furthermore, the negative consequences of recurrent brain metastases are almost certainly *underestimated*. Because of the uncertainties created by the various retrospective analyses regarding the need for adjuvant WBRT with SRS discussed above, many investigators have suggested the need for a prospective analysis of SRS vs. SRS + WBRT for the treatment of cerebral metastases.

There are two ongoing randomized trials by the European Organization for Research and Treatment of Cancer (EORTC) and the American College of Surgeons of Oncology Group (ACOSOG) to determine the role of adjuvant WBRT following radiosurgical treatment of brain metastases. Table 26-2 shows the design of the ACOSOG study. Patients with one to three metastases receive radiosurgery and are randomized to adjuvant WBRT (30 Gy in 12 fractions) versus initial observation with salvage therapy at the time of progression. The primary end point of the study is overall survival, but secondary end points include neurocognitive function and quality of life. This trial is currently open and accruing patients. The primary end point of the study is overall survival because the previous retrospective analyses referenced all suffered from unavoidable selection bias. Perhaps equally important, however, are secondary end points that include prospective evaluation of quality of life and neurocognitive function. The ACOSOG trial is the first prospective multiinstitutional trial to evaluate the neurocognitive effects of WBRT in which one arm does not receive WBRT. This feature should allow accurate conclusions to be drawn regarding the role of WBRT in the optimal management of patients with one to three brain metastases for not only survival, but also quality of life and neurocognitive effects (Table 26-2). Again, because most patients will succumb to their systemic disease, it is believed that the prospective accumulation of data regarding QOL is essential in developing rational treatment strategies in the future.

In summary, the available data indicate that SRS and open surgical resection are both excellent treatment options for patients with solitary brain metastases, and possibly for select patients with multiple lesions. The need for, and optimal timing of, WBRT in patients treated with these focused therapies is undergoing evaluation in a randomized, prospective fashion.

Chemotherapy for Brain Metastases

Intuitively, the notion of chemotherapy for brain metastases offers appeal. Most patients who develop brain metastases have active systemic cancer, which focal brain-directed strategies do not address. Systemic failure is the cause of death in the majority of patients with brain metastases. Therefore, the development of agents that might have activity against systemic and brain metastases is highly desirable. Additionally, the great majority of patients with brain metastases have multiple lesions. Like WBRT, chemotherapy has the potential to treat all brain metastases, including microscopic disease.

The first issue that arises in considering the role of chemotherapy for brain metastases is the blood–brain barrier. Tight intercellular junctions inhibit the passage of drugs into brain parenchyma and CSF. Drugs that cross the intact blood–brain barrier tend to be lipophilic and small (<400–500 daltons). Specific carrier mechanisms also play a role, particularly for hydrophobic molecules like the anthracyclines, taxanes, vinca alkaloids, and podophyllotoxins. These are substrates of P-glycoprotein, the product of the MDR (multi-drug resistance) gene, which is prominent in brain capillary endothelium and presumably helps exclude these drugs from the CNS. As noted in previous sections, however, the blood–brain barrier in brain metastases is generally disrupted. This is obvious histologically and is evidenced clinically by the invariable enhancement

▶ **TABLE 26-2.** SCHEMA FOR ACOSOG TRIAL Z0300

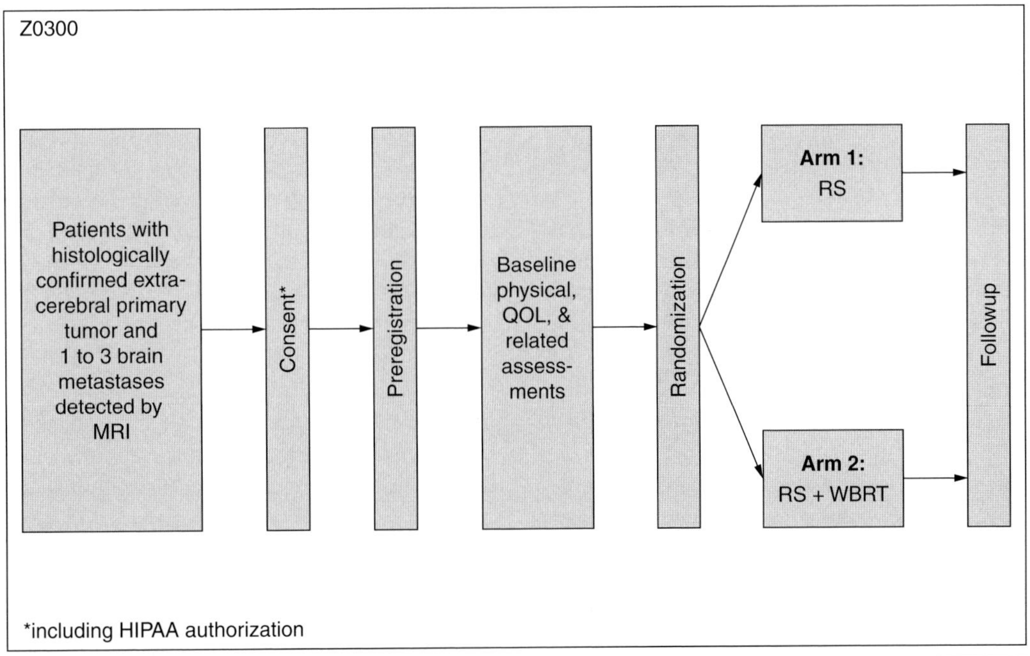

HIPAA = Health Insurance Portability and Accountability Act; MRI = magnetic resonance imaging; QOL = quality of life; RS = radiosurgery; WBRT = whole-brain radiation therapy.

of macroscopic lesions with intravenous contrast agents on CT and MR scans. In addition, chemical analysis of primary and metastatic brain tumors resected shortly after administration of chemotherapy commonly show high intratumoral concentrations of chemotherapy that would not have been predicted to cross the blood–brain barrier. Furthermore, radiographic responses of brain metastases to blood–brain barrier–impenetrable chemotherapy are very well documented.

In contrast to these observations, the development of brain metastases while patients are undergoing systemic chemotherapy producing systemic remission highlights the fact that the blood–brain barrier makes the brain a sanctuary from certain chemotherapeutic agents that do not cross the blood–brain barrier effectively. In breast cancer, this is commonly seen while patients are receiving paclitaxel or trastuzumab, a monoclonal antibody treatment. Similarly, in small cell lung cancer (SCLC), the high incidence of CNS failure following systemic chemotherapy has resulted in the use of prophylactic cranial irradiation in patients who have achieved systemic remission.

The most plausible interpretation of the above data is that the blood–brain barrier is a relative but not an absolute factor in excluding large and water-soluble chemotherapies from brain metastases. The intact blood–brain barrier likely plays a role in allowing development of micrometastases, but the blood–brain barrier in bulky brain metastases does not preclude entry of many chemotherapeutic agents.

Despite these uncertainties about the significance of the blood brain barrier in inhibiting responses of brain metastases to certain systemically administered agents, there are certain drugs that are believed to cross the intact blood–brain barrier fairly well. Among DNA-alkylating agents, the nitrosoureas (e.g., BCNU and CCNU), thiotepa, and temozolomide achieve high CSF levels. Topotecan, irinotecan, and hydroxyifosfamide also get in well. High-dose methotrexate and cytarabine, etoposide, and idarubicin do not cross well but may still achieve cytotoxic CSF concentrations.

Innumerable studies have examined the use of chemotherapy in brain metastases. Unfortunately, many factors hamper the interpretation and comparison of results of these studies. Patient populations are often incompletely specified, or heterogeneous in terms of underlying tumor, whether patients have had prior WBRT, and how intensive prior chemotherapy has been. All of these factors likely impact on response rates. Definition of response rates has not been standardized. Some studies have used the standard Macdonald criteria for radiographic response, although most have not required radiographic response to persist on a second study 1 month later. Others have included "stable disease" as a positive response to treatment—a practice fraught with problems given variable growth rates of tumors. The impact of corticosteroids in reducing contrast enhancement is well known, and rarely have studies controlled for the possibility that dexamethasone could be accounting for favorable radiographic responses.

Even with the above-mentioned caveats in mind, the majority of studies presented to date have not suggested an impressive response of most brain metastases to systemic chemotherapy.[144,145] This is particularly true with the most common source of brain metastasis, non–small cell lung cancer. Despite these observations, brain metastases of certain histologies have shown good responses to systemic therapy. These have generally been the more chemosensitive tumors, such as breast, small cell lung cancer (SCLC), and germ cell tumors. The results of some of these analyses are discussed below.

Some of the strongest data supporting a role for chemotherapy come from the experience managing brain metastases from SCLC. Multiple studies have demonstrated that the podophyllotoxins teniposide (VM-26, used primarily in Europe), high-dose etoposide (VP16), and standard-dose VP16 are active in patients with previously untreated brain metastases, with complete response (CR) and partial response (PR) rates of approximately 40%.[146] Response of CNS metastases tends to parallel the response of systemic metastases.[147] Response rates are lower in patients who previously received WBRT than in radiation-naive patients.[148] Platinum, topotecan, and cyclophosphamide-based regimens—all active against systemic SCLC—also show activity against SCLC brain metastases.

Although chemotherapy has not been compared to WBRT for SCLC brain metastases in a randomized trial, comparison of data from the two modalities suggests that they are roughly equally effective.[147,149,150] Chemotherapy has the added advantage of potentially treating the active systemic metastases that most of these patients harbor. The question then becomes whether the addition of WBRT adds significantly to results with chemotherapy alone. To address this, a European cooperative group randomized patients with brain metastases from SCLC to teniposide alone versus teniposide + WBRT. The combined modality group had a significantly higher brain response rate (57% vs. 22%). However, the systemic response rates and overall survival were similar between the two groups, reflecting the fact that the prognosis from systemic disease often dominates the outcome.[147]

Chemotherapy can be useful in management of brain metastases from breast cancer. Two phase II studies using regimens including cyclophosphamide and fluorouracil have demonstrated radiographic response rates of approximately 50% and median survival of approximately 6 months in patients who have not previously received whole-brain radiotherapy.[151] Response of systemic disease has typically mirrored response of brain metastases. The combination of cisplatin + etoposide is also active, with a 35% CR/PR rate in previously nonirradiated patients.[152] Certain hormonal agents, such as tamoxifen, cross the blood–brain barrier very well,[153] and complete responses of brain metastases from breast cancer have been reported with both tamoxifen and megestrol acetate.[154,155]

Chemotherapy appears to play a role in the management of brain metastases from germ cell tumors, which is not surprising considering the chemosensitivity of these tumors when situated extracranially. Patients with brain metastases treated with both chemotherapy and radiation have a median survival of 12 months, compared to 2 to 3 months with single-modality management. One series used chemotherapy as the sole treatment modality for brain metastases.[151] In this report, 10 patients with brain metastases from nonseminomatous germ cell tumors were treated with combination chemotherapy. Eight were alive without evidence of active disease 3 to 54 months (mean: 32 months) after therapy. Five patients were without evidence of relapse after 18 months, suggesting these patients were cured. Nine of these patients had very high serum human chorionic gonadotropin (hCG) supporting the diagnosis of choriocarcinoma. The authors suggested that WBRT might be unnecessary for long-term control of brain metastases; no confirmatory series have been published.[151]

Despite temozolomide's lack of substantial single-agent activity against brain metastases from various primary sites, one study suggests that it may add significantly to the results obtained with WBRT. A recent phase II trial randomized 52 patients with brain metastases (31 non–small cell lung cancer, 9 SCLC, 5 breast, and 7 with other primary sites) to whole-brain radiotherapy ± temozolomide. Temozolomide was given in small daily doses during radiotherapy and then on a standard schedule. Patients were assessed at 2 months following completion of radiation with scans reviewed by blinded central radiologists. The CR/PR rate was significantly higher in the combined modality group (96% vs. 67%), and fewer patients still required steroids. Median survival results insignificantly favored the combined modality group (8.6 months vs. 7 months).[84] This study, which requires replication, raises the questions of why median survival on both arms was so good, and why an agent with little or no single-agent activity would add substantially to WBRT.

In summary, chemotherapy has not yet emerged as a standard therapy for the treatment of most brain metastases. Certain patients, however, may benefit from chemotherapy. Specifically, select patients with small, asymptomatic tumors from chemosensitive primaries may be adequately treated with systemic therapy, based on the available data. Newer agents appear to have some promise in the treatment of patients with brain metastases.

Other Adjuvant Therapies

The importance of focused therapies in the treatment of brain metastases is discussed elsewhere in this chapter. Surgery and SRS are frequently used treatment modalities and can significantly prolong survival in many patients with metastatic brain cancer. Although patients who undergo surgical resection are thought to benefit from subsequent treatment with radiation, concerns about potential neurotoxicities associated with WBRT have led clinicians to consider other forms of adjuvant therapies. Although SRS has been used in combination with open resection, the treatment planning around a resection cavity can be complex, and this modality is not universally available.[156] SRS has sometimes been used as a sole-treatment modality for brain metastases, but the technique has limitations, including the inability to treat lesions larger than 3 cm in diameter effectively.

Local radiation therapy modalities, like brachytherapy with permanent ^{125}I seeds and inflatable balloon catheter and liquid ^{125}I radiation source (GliaSite radiation therapy system), are currently being evaluated for efficacy in the setting of brain metastases. GliaSite is a novel local radiotherapy for management of recurrent or newly diagnosed resectable brain metastasis. GliaSite consists of an inflatable balloon catheter that is inserted into resection cavities at the time of surgery. Excellent conformance has been observed between the balloon surface and the surrounding brain parenchyma. Internal radiation is delivered with an aqueous solution of organically bound ^{125}I (Iotrex [sodium 3-(125I)-iodo-4-hydroxybenzenesulfonate]), which is temporarily introduced into the balloon portion of the device via a subcutaneous port approximately 5 to 14 days following surgery. The ^{125}I is uniformly distributed within the treatment balloon, allowing for a uniform and very predictable dose of radiation to the surrounding brain parenchyma. The Iotrex is typically allowed to dwell in the device for 3 to 6 days, after which time the device is explanted. GliaSite has several advantages that relate to the uniform distribution of ^{125}I including simplified treatment planning and a theoretically diminished risk of radiation necrosis compared with other focal forms of radiation. By delivering a high dose of radiation to the resection margin, the potential side effects associated with WBRT can be deferred until new peripheral lesions appear and additional radiotherapy for those lesions is required. Complications associated with GliaSite have included pseudomeningocele, wound infection, and meningitis in humans. Another possible complication reported in animal studies is device failure with resultant leak of radiotherapy solution.[157] Additionally, we have noticed a radiation necrosis rate associated with the device that significantly exceeds that seen with radiosurgery. The GliaSite system remains an option for the treatment of newly diagnosed or potentially recurrent metastases when other forms of treatment have failed.[158] GliaSite can be particularly useful when tumors present with volumes too large to permit radiosurgery (the maximal treatment balloon diameter is 4 cm).

As discussed previously in the "Chemotherapy for Brain Metastases" subsection, most of the systemically administered chemotherapeutics have poor central nervous system penetration. BCNU biodegradable polymer wafers (Gliadel) were developed as a method of optimizing drug delivery into the central nervous system with satisfactory safety and efficacy without producing undesirable systemic side effects. The chemotherapy wafers are implanted in the tumor resection cavity at the time of surgery. The neurologic morbidity of implanting polymers in the brain is minimal, as has been observed in treatment of primary brain tumors.[159] Gliadel is effective in animal models for melanoma, renal cell, colon, and lung carcinomas in combination with radiotherapy. Interestingly, Gliadel was effective in breast cancer without subsequent administration of radiotherapy.[160,161] A phase I-II study of surgery, Gliadel, and WBRT showed no local recurrences with a prolonged median surviva1.[161] Local BCNU administration in another study for patients with brain metastases showed an improvement of the mean survival rate to 14.9 months in 29 patients who harbor different types of tumors and had a life expectancy of less than 12 weeks.[162]

One of two ongoing Phase III trials is studying the efficacy of Gliadel in preventing local recurrence of brain metastases when added to surgery and radiation therapy. The other is a NABTT (New Approaches to Brain Tumor Therapy) consortium study of patients with one or two metastases; patients receive surgery plus Gliadel, with radiation held in reserve. In summary, local therapies delivered at the time of surgical resection of brain metastases hold promise but have yet to be rigorously proven to provide benefit for patients with metastatic brain disease.

▶ A TREATMENT ALGORITHM FOR PATIENTS WITH CEREBRAL METASTASES

Based on the information outlined above, a treatment algorithm that is practiced in our institutions and one that the authors believe is rational based on the available data is offered in the following paragraphs.

Patients with single or multiple brain lesions and disseminated systemic disease with poor treatment options, poor functional status or highly radiation-sensitive histologies, such as small cell lung cancer, lymphoma, and germ cell neoplasms, are generally offered WBRT if palliative care is indicated. Patients with solitary, accessible brain lesions and a known history of cancer are offered surgical resection followed by either WBRT or focal irradiation such as a radiosurgical boost or brachytherapy. Inaccessible solitary lesions, if less than 3 cm, are generally treated with SRS with or without WBRT. On occasion, we find that WBRT allows for at least partial regression of larger lesions that are not deemed to be good surgical targets. In this situation, the remaining lesions are sometimes treated with a subsequent radiosurgical boost, particularly in good functional status patients.

We believe that the guidelines for treatment of patients with multiple lesions and a known history of cancer are less clear. In our institutions, patients with one to three lesions are presently offered radiosurgery, with or without WBRT, generally on protocol (Z0300). Patients with more than three lesions are generally offered WBRT. Based on the results of RTOG 95-08, patients with persistent lesions status after WBRT (particularly RPA Class I patients with non–small cell carcinoma of the lung) are offered a radiosurgical boost to the remaining lesions. Occasionally, we encounter a patient with a single, large, symptomatic lesion and a few additional smaller lesions located elsewhere in the brain. In these circumstances, we have sometimes offered resection of the dominant mass followed by radiosurgical boost to the remaining lesions and resection cavity or adjuvant WBRT. Alternatively, some patients have been offered participation in a phase II protocol, which calls for resection of the dominant lesion with insertion of a brachytherapy balloon in the resection cavity. Following brachytherapy, the remaining lesions are treated with SRS. End points of this study include survival, progression-free survival, and QOL measures. Again, these more aggressive local therapies are generally reserved for patients with a good functional status and/or limited systemic disease/reasonable systemic treatment options. We do not routinely advocate the resection of multiple lesions as we believe that other less invasive and equally efficacious treatment options exist.

Patients with single or multiple CNS lesions and no history of cancer require a systemic workup. At a minimum, a complete blood cell count and chest radiography are performed. Generally, a chest and abdominal CT scan are obtained. Nuclear medicine studies are employed in some cases when traditional tests are negative, but they rarely allow for the identification of a metastatic focus suitable for biopsy when other tests are negative. Positron emission tomography in particular is more useful in helping clinicians decide which treatment options to pursue after CNS metastases have been addressed. If a readily accessible mass is identified on imaging, then percutaneous biopsy (or, in the case of certain lung cancers, bronchoscopy) is attempted. If diagnostic tissue is obtained, the patients are treated according to the algorithm outlined above. If no other readily accessible tumor is available for biopsy, or if nondiagnostic tissue is obtained, then stereotactic/open biopsy or resection of the suspect brain lesion is performed. Again, if evidence of metastatic cancer is identified, patients are treated according to the above guidelines. Although followup imaging is tailored for individual patients, repeat MRI scans approximately every 3 months are obtained.

Treatment options for patients with recurrent CNS disease are based on the patient's histology, extent of systemic disease, and functional status. Patients with systemic disease progression or poor systemic options who have not had WBRT receive that therapy. Patients who have already had prior WBRT may be candidates for salvage SRS or, on occasion, surgical resection. A rare patient who has already received WBRT may be a candidate for re-irradiation if a positive response was observed previously. Some patients with chemosensitive tumors (breast, small cell lung, germ cell) may be candidates for chemotherapy.

Most of our treatment plans are devised in a multidisciplinary forum. Our treatment pathways are continually reassessed and altered according to the best available data.

▶ CONCLUSION

Brain metastases are the most common form of cerebral malignancy, outnumbering primary brain tumors by a ratio of almost 10:1. Although many effective therapeutic options are available for cerebral metastases, significant controversy exists regarding the optimal treatment of these lesions. As most patients will ultimately succumb to their systemic disease, it is imperative that any treatment strategy for brain metastases takes into account potential effects on parameters other than survival, including neurocognition, QOL, and functional independence. Presently, many treatment paradigms are based on outdated and/or retrospective data. Randomized, prospective clinical trials comparing different treatment strategies that include QOL end points are required to help develop rational treatment strategies for this clinically important and increasingly prevalent disorder.

▶ ACKNOWLEDGMENT

The authors would like to acknowledge the expert technical assistance of Mr. Joseph Taylor, who helped prepare this manuscript. We also are indebted to M. Beatriz S. Lopes, M.D., Associate Professor of Pathology at the University of Virginia, who kindly provided the pathology photomicrographs shown in this chapter.

REFERENCES

1. Cancer Society 2002, http://www.cancer.org/downloads/STT/CancerFacts&Figures2002TM.pdf. Accessed August 2004.
2. Landis SH, Murray T, Bolden S, et al. Cancer statistics 1998. CA Cancer J Clin 1998;48:6–29.
3. Chang SD, Lee E, Sakamoto GT, et al. Stereotactic radiosurgery in patients with multiple brain metastases. Neuro Focus 2000;9:2.
4. Posner JB. Management of brain metastases. Rev Neurol 1992;148:477–487.
5. Wen PY, Loeffler JS. Management of brain metastases. Oncology (Huntington) 1999;13:941–957.
6. Nelson JS, von Deimling A, Petersen I, et al. Metastatic tumours of the CNS. In: Kleihues P, Cavenee WK, eds. Pathology and genetics of tumours of the nervous system. World Health Organization classification of tumours. Lyon, France: IARC Press, 2000:250–253.
7. Sawaya R, Ligon BL, Bindal RK. Management of metastatic brain tumors. Ann Surg Oncol 1994;1:169–178.
8. Sawaya R, Bindal RK, Lang FF, et al. Metastatic brain tumors. In: Kaye AH, Laws ER Jr, eds. Brain tumors: an encyclopedic approach, 2nd ed. New York: Churchill Livingstone, 2001:999–1026.
9. Lavine SD, Petrovich Z, Cohen-Gadol AA, et al. Gamma knife radiosurgery for metastatic melanoma: an analysis of survival, outcome, and complications. Neurosurgery 1999; 44:59–66.
10. Culine S, Bekradda M, Kramar A, et al. Prognostic factors for survival in patients with brain metastases from renal cell carcinoma. Cancer 1998;83:2548–2553.
11. Vogelzang NJ, Stadler WM. Kidney cancer. Lancet 1998;352:1691–1696.
12. Takakura K, Sano K, Hojo S, et al. Metastatic tumors of the central nervous system. New York: Igaku-Shoin, 1982.
13. Sen M, Demiral AS, Cetingoz R, et al. Prognostic factors in lung cancer with brain metastasis. Radiother Oncol 1998;46: 33–38.
14. Nakagawa H, Murasawa A, Nakajima S, et al. Study of meningeal carcinomatosis: diagnosis and treatment. Neurol Surg 1992;20:31–37.
15. Lagerwaard FJ, Levendag PC, Nowak PJCM, et al. Identification of prognostic factors in patients with brain metastases: a review of 1292 patients. Int J Radiat Oncol Biol Phys 1999;43:795–803.
16. American Cancer Society. Cancer facts and figures, 2003. www.cancer.org. Accessed August 2004.
17. Graus F, Walker RW, Allen JC. Brain metastases in children. J Pediatr 1983;103:558–561.
18. Patchell RA. The management of brain metastases. Cancer Treat Rev 2003;29:533–540.
19. Patchell RA, Posner JB. Neurologic complications of systemic cancer. Neurol Clin 1985;3:729–750.
20. Sze G, Johnson C, Kawamura Y, et al. Comparison of single- and triple-dose contrast material in the MR screening of brain metastases. AJNR 1998;19:821–828.
21. Decker DA, Decker VL, Herskovic A, et al. Brain metastases in patients with renal cell carcinoma: prognosis and treatment. J Clin Oncol 1984;2:169–173.
22. Kauffman EC, Robinson VL, Stadler WM, et al. Metastasis suppression: the evolving role of metastasis suppressor genes for regulating cancer cell growth at the secondary site. J Urol 2003;169:1122–1133.
23. Chambers AF, MacDonald IC, Schmidt EE, et al. Clinical targets for anti-metastasis therapy. Adv Cancer Res 2000;79:91–121.
24. Yoshida BA, Sokoloff MM, Welch DR, et al. Metastasis-suppressor genes: a review and perspective on an emerging field. J Natl Cancer Inst 2000;92:1717–1730.

25. Kuo TH, Kubota T, Watanabe M, et al. Liver colonization competence governs colon cancer metastasis. Proc Natl Acad Sci USA 1995;92:12,085–12,089.
26. Nicolson GL. Cancer metastasis: tumor cell and host organ properties important in metastasis to specific secondary sites. Biochim Biophys Acta 1988;948(2):175–224.
27. Chackal-Roy M, Niemeyer C, Moore M, et al. Stimulation of human prostatic carcinoma cell growth by factors present in human bone marrow. J Clin Invest 1989;84:43–50.
28. Aslakson CJ, Rak JW, Miller BE, et al. Differential influence of organ site on three subpopulations of a single mouse mammary tumor at two distinct steps in metastasis. Int J Cancer 1991;47(3):466–472.
29. Leone A, Flatow U, King CR, et al. Reduced tumor incidence, metastatic potential, and cytokine responsiveness of nm23-transfected melanoma cells. Cell 1991;65:25–35.
30. Dong JT, Lamb PW, Rinker-Schaeffer CW, et al. KAI1, a metastasis suppressor gene for prostate cancer on human chromosome 11p11.2. Science 1995;268:884–886.
31. Lee JH, Miele ME, Hicks DJ, et al. KiSS-1, a novel human malignant melanoma metastasis-suppressor gene [erratum in J Natl Cancer Inst 1997;89:1549]. J Natl Cancer Inst 1996;88(23):1731–1737.
32. Gao AC, Lou W, Dong JT, et al. CD44 is a metastasis suppressor gene for prostatic cancer located on human chromosome 11p13. Cancer Res 1997;57:846–849.
33. Yoshida BA, Dubauskas Z, Chekmareva MA, et al. Mitogen-activated protein kinase kinase 4/stress-activated protein/Erk kinase 1 (MKK4/SEK1), a prostate cancer metastasis suppressor gene encoded by human chromosome 17. Cancer Res 1999;59:5483–5487.
34. Bhujwalla ZM, Aboagye EO, Gillies RJ, et al. Nm23-transfected MDA-MB-435 human breast carcinoma cells form tumors with altered phospholipid metabolism and pH: a ^{31}P nuclear magnetic resonance study in vivo and in vitro. Magn Reson Med 1999;41:897–903.
35. Seraj MJ, Samant RS, Verderame MF, et al. Functional evidence for a novel human breast carcinoma metastasis suppressor, BRMS1, encoded at chromosome 11q13. Cancer Res 2000;60:2764–2769.
36. Wilkins RH, Rengachary SS, eds. Neurosurgery. New York: McGraw-Hill, 1985.
37. Weiss L, Grundmann E, Torhorst J, et al. Haematogenous metastatic patterns in colonic carcinoma: an analysis of 1541 necropsies. J Pathol 1986;150:195–203.
38. Delattre JY, Krol G, Thaler HT, et al. Distribution of brain metastases. Arch Neurol 1988;45:741–744.
39. Patchell RA. Brain metastases. Neurol Clin 1991;9:817–824.
40. Russell DS, Rubinstein LJ. Pathology of tumours of the nervous system, 5th ed. London: Edward Arnold, 1989: 825–854.
41. Nutt SH, Patchell RA. Intracranial hemorrhage associated with primary and secondary tumors. Neurosurg Clin North Am 1992;3:591–599.
42. DeYoung BR, Wick MR. Immunohistologic evaluation of metastatic carcinomas of unknown origin: an algorithmic approach. Semin Diagn Pathol 2000;17:184–193.
43. Long D. Capillary ultrastructure in human metastatic brain tumors. J Neurosurg 1983;51:53–58.
44. Wen P, Loeffler J. Management of brain metastases. Oncology 1999;13:941–965.
45. Healy ME, Hesselink JR. Increased detection of intracranial metastases with intravenous Gd-DTPA. Radiology 1987;165:619–624.
46. Merchut MP. Brain metastases from undiagnosed systemic neoplasms. Arch Intern Med 1989;149:1076–1080.
47. Sawaya R, Bindal RK. Metastatic brain tumors. In: Kaye AH, Laws ER Jr, eds. Brain tumors: an encyclopedic approach. Edinburgh, UK: Churchill Livingstone, 1995:923–946.
48. Kole AC, Niewig OE, Pruim J, et al. Detection of unknown primary tumors using positron emission tomography. Cancer 1998;82:1160–1166.
49. Van de Pol M, van Aalst VC, Wilmink JT, et al. Brain metastases from an unknown primary tumor: which diagnostic procedures are indicated? J Neurol Neurosurg Psychiatry 1996;61:321–323.
50. Cairncross JG, Posner JB. The management of brain metastases. In: Walker MD, ed. Oncology of the central nervous system: cancer treatment and research, vol 12. Boston: Martinus Nijhoff, 1983:341–377.
51. Hendrickson FR. The optimum schedule for palliative radiotherapy for metastatic brain cancer. Int J Radiat Oncol Biol Phys 1977;2:165–168.
52. Lassman AB, DeAngelis, LM. Brain metastases. Neurol Clin North Am 2003;21:1–23.
53. Soffietti R, Ruda R, Mutani R. Management of brain metastases. J Neurol 2002;249:1357–1369.
54. Tikhtman AJ, Patchell RA. Brain metastases. In: Morantz RA, Walsh JW, eds. Brain tumors: a comprehensive text. New York: Marcel Dekker, 1994:533–566.
55. Simionescu MD. Metastatic tumors of the brain. A follow-up study of 195 patients with neurosurgical considerations. J Neurosurg 1960;17:361–373.
56. Forsyth PA, Posner JB. Headaches in patients with brain tumors: a study of 111 patients. Neurology 1993;43:1678–1683.
57. Posner JB. Clinical manifestations of brain metastasis. In: Weiss L, Gilbert H, Posner J, eds. Brain metastasis. Boston: GK Hall, 1980:189–207.
58. Salcman M. Intracranial hemorrhage caused by brain tumors. In: Kaufman H, ed. Intracerebral hematomas. New York: Raven Press, 1992:95–106.
59. Glantz MJ, Cole BF, Forsyth PA, et al. Practice parameter: anticonvulsant prophylaxis in patients with newly diagnosed brain tumors. Report of the Quality Standards Subcommittee of the American Academy of Neurology. Neurology 2000;54:1886–1893.
60. Batchelor T, DeAngelis LM. Medical management of cerebral metastases. Neurosurg Clin North Am 1996;7:435–446.
61. Wozniak AJ, Crowley JJ, Balcerzak SP, et al. Randomized trial comparing cisplatin with cisplatin plus vinorelbine in the treatment of advanced non-small-cell lung cancer: a Southwest Oncology Group study. J Clin Oncol 1998; 16:2459–2465.
62. Sandler AB, Nemunaitis J, Denham C, et al. Phase III trial of gemcitabine plus cisplatin versus cisplatin alone in patients with locally advanced or metastatic non–small-cell lung cancer. J Clin Oncol 2000;18:122–130.

63. Eton O, Legha SS, Bedikian AY, et al. Sequential biochemotherapy versus chemotherapy for metastatic melanoma: results from a phase III randomized trial. J Clin Oncol 2002;20(8):2045–2052.
64. Danson S, Lorigamp P, Arance A, et al. Randomized phase II study of temozolomide given every eight hours or daily with either interferon alpha-2B or thalidomide in metastatic malignant melanoma. J Clin Oncol 2003;21(13):2551–2557.
65. Pierga J, Asselain B, Jouve M, et al. Effect of adjuvant chemotherapy on outcome in patients with metastatic breast carcinoma treated with first line doxorubicin-containing chemotherapy. Cancer 2001;91:1079–1089.
66. Perez EA, Geeraerts L, Suman V, et al. A randomized phase II study of sequential docetaxel and doxorubicin/cyclophosphamide in patients with metastatic breast cancer. Ann Oncol 2002;13:1225–1235.
67. Paulicki M, Rolski J, Zaluski J, et al. A phase II study of intravenous Navelbine and doxorubicin combination in previously untreated advanced breast carcinoma. Oncologist 2002;7:205–209.
68. Sherry M, Greco F, Johnson D, et al. Breast cancer with skeletal metastases at initial diagnosis. Distinctive clinical characteristics and favorable prognosis. Cancer 1986;58:178–182.
69. Markesbery W, Brooks W, Gupta G, et al. Treatment for patients with cerebral metastases. Arch Neurol 1978;35:754–756.
70. Ruderman N, Hall T. Use of glucocorticoids in the palliative treatment of metastatic brain tumors. Cancer 1965;18:298–306.
71. Cairncross JG, Chernick NL, Kim J-H, et al. Sterilization of cerebral metastases by radiation therapy. Neurology 1979;29:1195–1202.
72. Kurtz JM, Gelber R, Brady LW, et al. The palliation of brain metastases in a favorable patient population: a randomized clinical trial by the Radiation Therapy Oncology Group. Int J Radiat Oncol Biol Phys 1981;7:891–895.
73. Borgelt B, Gelber R, Kramer S, et al. The palliation of brain metastases: final results of the first two studies by the Radiation Therapy Oncology Group. Int J Radiat Oncol Biol Phys 1980;6:1–9.
74. Murray KJ, Scott C, Greenberg HM, et al. A randomized phase III study of accelerated hyperfractionation versus standard in patients with unresected brain metastases: a report of the Radiation Therapy Oncology Group (RTOG) 9104. Int J Radiat Oncol Biol Phys 1997;39:571–574.
75. Komarnicky LT, Phillips TL, Martz K, et al. A randomized phase III protocol for the evaluation of misonidazole combined with radiation in the treatment of patients with brain metastases (RTOG-7916). Int J Radiat Oncol Biol Phys 1991;20:53–58.
76. Fu KK, Pajak TF, Trotti A, et al. A Radiation Therapy Oncology Group (RTOG) phase III randomized study to compare hyperfractionation and two variants of accelerated fractionation to standard fractionation radiotherapy for head and neck squamous cell carcinomas: first report of RTOG 9003. Int J Radiat Oncol Biol Phys 2000;48:7–16.
77. Epstein BE, Scott CB, Sause WT, et al. Improved survival duration in patients with unresected solitary brain metastasis using accelerated hyperfractionated radiation therapy at total doses of 54.4 gray and greater. Results of Radiation Therapy Oncology Group 85-28. Cancer 1993;71:1362–1367.
78. DeAngelis LM, Delattre JY, Posner JB. Radiation-induced dementia in patients cured of brain metastases. Neurology 1989;39:789–796.
79. Andrews DW, Scott CB, Sperduto PW, et al. Whole brain radiation therapy with or without stereotactic radiosurgery boost for patients with one to three brain metastases: phase III results of the RTOG 9508 randomized trial. Lancet 2004;363:1665–1672.
80. Auperin A, Arriagada R, Pignon JP, et al. Prophylactic cranial irradiation for patients with small-cell lung cancer in complete remission. Prophylactic Cranial Irradiation Overview Collaborative Group. N Engl J Med 1999;341:476–484.
81. Phillips TL, Scott CB, Leibel SA, et al. Results of a randomized comparison of radiotherapy and bromodeoxyuridine with radiotherapy alone for brain metastases: report of RTOG trial 89-05. Int J Radiat Oncol Biol Phys 1995;33:339–348.
82. Mehta MP, Rodrigus P, Terhaard CH, et al. Survival and neurologic outcomes in a randomized trial of motexafin gadolinium and whole-brain radiation therapy in brain metastases. J Clin Oncol 2003;21:2529–2536.
83. Abrey LE, Christodoulou C. Temozolomide for treating brain metastases. Semin Oncol 2001;28:34–42.
84. Antonadou D, Paraskevaidis M, Sarris G, et al. Phase II randomized trial of temozolomide and concurrent radiotherapy in patients with brain metastases. J Clin Oncol 2002;20:3644–3650.
85. Kondziolka D, Patel A, Lunsford LD, et al. Stereotactic radiosurgery plus whole brain radiotherapy versus radiotherapy alone for patients with multiple brain metastases. Int J Radiat Oncol Biol Phys 1999;45:427–434.
86. Asai A, Matsutani M, Kohno T, et al. Subacute brain atrophy after radiation therapy for malignant brain tumor. Cancer 1989;63:1962–1974.
87. Regine WF, Huhn JL, Patchell RA, et al. Risk of symptomatic brain tumor recurrence and neurologic deficit after radiosurgery alone in patients with newly diagnosed brain metastases: results and implication. Int J Radiat Oncol Biol Phys 2002;52:333–338.
88. Regine WF, Scott C, Murray K, et al. Neurocognitive outcome in brain metastases patients treated with accelerated-fractionation vs. accelerated-hyperfractionated radiotherapy: an analysis from radiation therapy oncology group study 91-04. Int J Radiat Oncol Biol Phys 2001;51:711–717.
89. Gaspar L, Scott C, Rotman M, et al. Recursive partitioning analysis (RPA) of prognostic factors in three Radiation Therapy Oncology Group (RTOG) brain metastases trials. Int J Radiat Oncol Biol Phys 1997;37:745–751.
90. Swift PS, Phillips T, Martz K, et al. CT characteristics of patients with brain metastases treated in RTOG study 79-16. Int J Radiat Oncol Biol Phys 1993;25:209–214.
91. Alexander E, Moriaty TM, Davis RB et al. Stereotactic radiosurgery for the definitive non-invasive treatment of brain metastases. J Natl Cancer Inst 1995;87:34–40.

92. Patchell RA, Tibbs PA, Walsh JW, et al. A randomized trial of surgery in the treatment of single metastases to the brain. N Engl J Med 1990;322:494–500.
93. Vecht CJ, Haaxma-Reich H, Noordjik E, et al. Treatment of single brain metastasis: radiotherapy alone or combined with neurosurgery. Ann Neurol 1993;33:583–590.
94. Mintz AH, Kestle J, Rathbone MP, et al. A randomized trial to assess the efficacy of surgery in addition to radiotherapy in patients with a single cerebral metastasis. Cancer 1996;78:1470–1476.
95. Magilligan DJ Jr, Duvernoy C, Malik G, et al. Surgical approach to lung cancer with solitary cerebral metastasis: twenty-five years' experience. Ann Thorac Surg 1986;42: 360–364.
96. Hankins JR, Miller JE, Salcman M, et al. Surgical management of lung cancer with solitary cerebral metastasis. Ann Thorac Surg 1988;46:24–28.
97. Smalley SR, Laws ER Jr, O'Fallon JR, et al. Resection for solitary brain metastasis. Role of adjuvant radiation and prognostic variables in 229 patients. J Neurosurg 1992;77: 531–540.
98. Wronski M, Arbit E, Burt M, et al. Survival after surgical treatment of brain metastases from lung cancer: a follow-up study of 231 patients treated between 1976 and 1991. J Neurosurg 1995;83:605–616.
99. Bendell JC, Domchek SM, Burstein HJ, et al. Central nervous system metastases in women who receive trastuzumab-based therapy for metastatic breast carcinoma. Cancer 2003;97:2972–2977.
100. Buchsbaum JC, Suh JH, Lee SY, et al. Survival by radiation therapy oncology group recursive partitioning analysis class and treatment modality in patients with brain metastases from malignant melanoma: a retrospective study. Cancer 2002;94:2265–2272.
101. Tremont-Lukats IW, Bobustuc G, Lagos GK, et al. Brain metastasis from prostate carcinoma: the M. D. Anderson Cancer Center experience. Cancer 2003;98:363–368.
102. McCutcheon IE, Eng DY, Logothetis CJ. Brain metastasis from prostate carcinoma: antemortem recognition and outcome after treatment. Cancer 1999;86:2301–2311.
103. Cormio G, Maneo A, Colamaria A, et al. Surgical resection of solitary brain metastasis from ovarian carcinoma: an analysis of 22 cases. Gynecol Oncol 2003;89:116–119.
104. Tajran D, Berek JS. Surgical resection of solitary brain metastasis from cervical cancer. Int J Gynecol Cancer 2003;13:368–370.
105. Mamelak AN, Withers GJ, Wang X. Choriocarcinoma brain metastasis in a patient with viable intrauterine pregnancy. Case report. J Neurosurg 2002;97:477–481.
106. Ko FC, Liu JM, Chen WS, et al. Risk and patterns of brain metastases in colorectal cancer: 27-year experience. Dis Colon Rectum 1999;42:1467–1471.
107. Hammoud MA, McCutcheon IE, Elsouki R, et al. Colorectal carcinoma and brain metastasis: distribution, treatment, and survival. Ann Surg Oncol 1996;3:453–463.
108. Farnell GF, Buckner JC, Cascino TL, et al. Brain metastases from colorectal carcinoma. The long-term survivors. Cancer 1996;78:711–716.
109. Wronski M, Arbit E. Resection of brain metastases from colorectal carcinoma in 73 patients Cancer 1999;85:1677–1685.
110. Sueyama H, Yamanoi T, Uematu T, et al. Brain metastases from esophageal cancers: clinical features and treatment results [Japanese]. Nippon Igaku Hoshasen Gakkai Zasshi 2001;61:534–539.
111. York JE, Stringer J, Ajani JA, et al. Gastric cancer and metastasis to the brain. Ann Surg Oncol 1999;6:771–776.
112. Ransohoff J. Surgical management of metastatic tumors. Semin Oncol 1975;2:21–27.
113. Patchell RA. Metastatic brain tumors. Neurol Clin 1995;13: 915–925.
114. Bindal RK, Sawaya R, Leavens ME, et al. Surgical treatment of multiple brain metastases. J Neurosurg 1993;79:210–216.
115. Davis P, Hudgins P, Peterman S, et al. Diagnosis of cerebral metastases: double-dose delayed CT vs. contrast-enhanced MR imaging. AJNR 1991;12:293–300.
116. Sze G, Milano E, Johnson C, et al. Detection of brain metastases: comparison of contrast-enhanced MR with unenhanced MR and enhanced CT. AJNR 1990;11:785–791.
117. Nussbaum ES, Djalilian HR, Cho KH, et al. Brain metastases. Histology, multiplicity, surgery, and survival. Cancer 1996;78:1781–1788.
118. Madajewicz S, Karakousis S, West C, et al. Malignant melanoma brain metastases. Review of Roswell Park Memorial Institute experience. Cancer 1984;53:2550–2552.
119. Byrne T, Cascino T, Posner J. Brain metastases from melanoma. J Neurooncol 1983;1:313–317.
120. Konstadoulakis MM, Messaris E, Zografos G, et al. Prognostic factors in malignant melanoma patients with solitary or multiple brain metastases. Is there a role for surgery? J Neurosurg Sci 2000;44:211–219.
121. Iwadate Y, Namba H, Yamaura A. Significance of surgical resection for the treatment of multiple brain metastases. Anticancer Res 2000;20:573–577.
122. Hazuka MB, Burleson WD, Stroud DN, et al. Multiple brain metastases are associated with poor survival in patients treated with surgery and radiotherapy. J Clin Oncol 1993;11:369–373.
123. Mehta M, Noyes W, Craig B, et al. A cost-effectiveness and cost-utility analysis of radiosurgery vs. resection for single brain metastases. Int J Radiat Oncol Biol Phys 1997;39: 445–454.
124. Sanghavi SN, Miranpuri SS, Chappell R, et al. Radiosurgery for patients with brain metastases: a multi-institutional analysis, stratified by the RTOG recursive partitioning analysis method. Int J Radiat Oncol Biol Phys 2001;51:426–434.
125. Shaw E, Scott C, Souhami L, et al. Single dose radiosurgical treatment of recurrent previously irradiated primary brain tumors and brain metastases: final report of RTOG protocol 90-05. Int J Radiat Oncol Biol Phys 2000;47:291–298.
126. Sturm V, Kober B, Hover KH, et al. Stereotactic percutaneous single dose irradiation of brain metastases with a linear accelerator. Int J Radiat Oncol Biol Phys 1987;13: 279–282.
127. Loeffler JS, Kooy HM, Wen PY, et al. The treatment of recurrent brain metastases with stereotactic radiosurgery. J Clin Oncol 1990;8:571–573.
128. Coffey RJ, Flickinger JC, Bissonette DJ, et al. Radiosurgery for solitary brain metastases using the cobalt-60 gamma unit: methods and results in 24 patients. Int J Radiat Oncol Biol Phys 1991;20:1287–1295.

129. Mehta MP, Rozental JM, Levin AB, et al. Defining the role of radiosurgery in the management of brain metastases. Int J Radiat Oncol Biol Phys 1992;24:619–625.
130. Flickinger JC, Kondziolka D, Lunsford LD, et al. A multi-institutional experience with stereotactic radiosurgery for solitary brain metastasis. Int J Radiat Oncol Biol Phys 1994;28:797–802.
131. Auchter RM, Lamond JP, Alexander E, et al. A multiinstitutional outcome and prognostic factor analysis of radiosurgery for resectable single brain metastasis. Int J Radiat Oncol Biol Phys 1996;35:27–35.
132. Szeifert GT, Massager N, DeVriendt D, et al. Observations of intracranial neoplasms treated with gamma knife radiosurgery. J Neurosurg 2002;97:623–626.
133. Tsao M, Sneed P, McDermott M, et al. Radiosurgery and radiotherapy for non–small-cell lung cancer metastatic to brain. Clin Lung Cancer 2001;2(3):197–203.
134. Muacevic A, Kreth FW, Horstmann GA, et al. Surgery and radiotherapy compared with gamma knife radiosurgery in the treatment of solitary cerebral metastases of small diameter. J Neurosurg 1999;91:35–43.
135. Chougule PB, Burton-Williams M, Zheng Z. Randomized treatment of brain metastases with gamma knife radiosurgery, whole brain radiotherapy or both. Int J Radiat Oncol Biol Phys 2000;48(S):114.
136. Patchell RA, Tibbs PA, Regine WF, et al. Postoperative radiotherapy in the treatment of single metastases to the brain: a randomized trial. JAMA 1998;4;280(17):1485–1489.
137. Sneed PK, Lamborn KR, Forstner JM, et al. Radiosurgery for brain metastases: Is whole brain radiotherapy necessary? Int J Radiat Oncol Biol Phys 1999;43:549–558.
138. Lutterbach J, Cyron D, Henne K, et al. Radiosurgery followed by planned observation in patients with one to three brain metastases. Neurosurgery 2003;52:1066–1073.
139. Chitapanarux I, Goss B, Vongama R, et al. Prospective study of stereotactic radiosurgery without whole brain radiotherapy in patients with four or less brain metastases: incidence of intracranial progression and salvage radiotherapy. J Neurooncol 2003;61:143–149.
140. Hasegawa T, Kondziolka D, Flickinger JC, et al. Brain metastases treated with radiosurgery alone: an alternative to whole brain radiotherapy? Neurosurgery 2003;52:1318–1326.
141. Sneed PK, Suh JH, Goetsch SJ, et al. A multi-institutional review of radiosurgery alone vs. radiosurgery with whole brain radiotherapy as the initial management of brain metastases. Int J Radiat Oncol Biol Phys 2002;53:519–526.
142. Pirzkall A, Debus J, Lohr F, et al. Radiosurgery alone or in combination with whole-brain radiotherapy for brain metastases. J Clin Oncol 1998;16:3563–3569.
143. Chidel MA, Suh JH, Reddy CA, et al. Application of recursive partitioning analysis and evaluation of the use of whole brain radiation among patients treated with stereotactic radiosurgery for newly diagnosed brain metastases. Int J Radiat Oncol Biol Phys 2000;47:993–999.
144. Korfel A, Thiel E. Chemotherapy of brain metastases. Front Radiat Ther Oncol 1999;33:343–348.
145. Lesser GJ. Chemotherapy of cerebral metastases from solid tumors. Neurosurg Clin North Am 1996;7:527–536.
146. Grossi F, Scolaro T, Tixi L, et al. The role of systemic chemotherapy in the treatment of brain metastases from small-cell lung cancer. Crit Rev Oncol Hematol 2001;37: 61–67.
147. Postmus PE, Smit EF. Chemotherapy for brain metastases of lung cancer: a review. Ann Oncol 1999;10:753–759.
148. Twelves CJ, Souhami RL. Should cerebral metastases be treated by chemotherapy alone? Ann Oncol 1991;2:15–17.
149. Pronzato P, Bruna F, Neri E, et al. Radiotherapy plus carboplatin and teniposide in patients with brain metastases from non small cell lung cancer. Anticancer Res 1995;15:517–519.
150. Landonio G, Sartore-Bianchi A, Giannetta L, et al. Controversies in the management of brain metastases: the role of chemotherapy. Forum 2001;11:59–74.
151. Schiff D, Wen PY, eds. Cancer neurology in clinical practice. Totowa, NJ: Humana Press, 2002.
152. Franciosi V, Cocconi G, Michiara M, et al. Front-line chemotherapy with cisplatin and etoposide for patients with brain metastases from breast carcinoma, nonsmall cell lung carcinoma, or malignant melanoma: a prospective study. Cancer 1999;85:1599–1605.
153. Lien EA, Wester K, Lonning PE, et al. Distribution of tamoxifen and metabolites into brain tissue and brain metastases in breast cancer patients. Br J Cancer 1991;63:641–645.
154. Pors H, von Eyben FE, Sorensen OS, et al. Long-term remission of multiple brain metastases with tamoxifen. J Neurooncol 1991;10:173–177.
155. Stewart DJ, Dahrouge S. Response of brain metastases from breast cancer to megestrol acetate: a case report. J Neurooncol 1995;24:299–301.
156. Gerosa M, Nicolato A, Foroni R, et al. Gamma knife radiosurgery for brain metastases: a primary therapeutic option J Neurosurg 2002;97(Suppl 5):515–524.
157. Stubbs JB, Strickland AD, Frank RK, et al. Biodistribution and dosimetry of an aqueous solution containing sodium 3-(125I)iodo-4-hydroxybenzenesulfonate (Iotrex) for brachytherapy of resected malignant brain tumors. Cancer Biother Radiopharm 2000;15:645–656.
158. McDermott MW, Cosgrove GR, Larson DA, et al. Interstitial brachytherapy for intracranial metastases. Neurosurg Clin North Am 1996;7:485–495.
159. Brem H, Piantadosi S, Burger PC, et al: Placebo-controlled trial of safety and efficacy of intraoperative controlled delivery by biodegradable polymers of chemotherapy for recurrent gliomas. The Polymer-Brain Tumor Treatment Group. Lancet 1995;345:1008–1012.
160. Ewend MG, Sampath P, Williams JA, et al. Local delivery of chemotherapy prolongs survival in experimental brain metastases from breast carcinoma. Neurosurgery 1998;43: 1185–1193.
161. Ewend MG, Williams JA, Tabassi K, et al. Local delivery of chemotherapy and concurrent external beam radiotherapy prolongs survival in metastatic brain tumor models. Cancer Res 1996;56:5217–5223.
162. Brem S, Snodgrass S, Staller A, et al. Implantation of BCNU chemotherapeutic wafers to prevent recurrence of brain metastases. Poster in AANS 2003 Annual Meeting. San Diego, CA; 4/26/03–5/1/03.

CHAPTER 27

Spinal Metastases

TALI SIEGAL / TZONY SIEGAL

Metastases to the spine most frequently involve the vertebral elements and the epidural space.[1–4] In a small proportion of patients neurologic symptoms and signs may arise from spinal metastases that spread to the intradural spinal compartment. They may be located either extramedullary or intramedullary (Table 27-1).[5–7] The approach to treatment depends on correct diagnosis of the affected site and ideally requires a shared decision of a multidisciplinary team. The specific treatment should be integrated into patient's overall treatment program and may include various combinations of steroids, irradiation, surgery, chemotherapy, hormone therapy, and bisphosphonates, as appropriate for the type of malignancy inducing spinal involvement.

▶ VERTEBRAL METASTASES

The skeletal system is the third most common site of cancer metastases, following the lung and liver. Bone metastases are a significant cause of morbidity as a result of pain, pathologic fractures, hypercalcemia, and spinal cord compression.[3,4,8] The vertebral column is the most common site for skeletal metastases,[9] and in autopsy series, 60% of patients dying of neoplasia were found to have spinal and epidural metastases.[10]

Destructive vertebral lesions are a common source of morbidity in patients with metastatic disease and multiple myeloma, with pain the presenting complaint in the majority of cases.

All patients with vertebral metastases are at potential risk of developing spinal instability and neurologic impairment. Therefore, it is useful to classify vertebral metastases according to biomechanical stability and the presence or absence of dural sac displacement or neural element compression (see Table 27-1). This classification allows for early recognition of potential complications. Treatment can then be adjusted to meet the potential risks and preserve or restore normal function.

Assessment of the extent of vertebral metastases is based on imaging findings that can be obtained by spine radiography, bone scintigraphy, positron emission tomography (PET) using [^{18}F]fluorodeoxyglucose (FDG), computerized tomography (CT), and magnetic resonance imaging (MRI). It is important to note that MRI is sensitive to both focal vertebral lesions and bone marrow involvement in hematologic malignancies, as well as in solid tumors.[11]

Even in patients with diffuse marrow involvement, the spine may not be defined as mechanically unstable. The criteria for spinal stability in neoplastic disease are complex and differ from those established for trauma. Unfortunately, no validated system exists for making this determination.

Clinical and Imaging Criteria for Spinal Stability in Neoplastic Disease

Determining spinal stability is of paramount importance in choosing the appropriate form of management for

▶ **TABLE 27-1.** SPINAL METASTASES

Vertebral metastases
- Biomechanically stable
- Potentially unstable
  - Without compression fracture
  - With compression fracture
- Biomechanically unstable
  - Without compression fracture
  - With compression fracture

Vertebral metastases with epidural extension
- Without root/neural element displacement ± instability
- With nerve root displacement/encasement ± instability
- With spinal cord displacement/compression ± instability
- With cauda equina displacement ± instability

Epidural metastases without vertebral lesion
- Paravertebral mass with an epidural extension
- Epidural mass without a paravertebral tumor

Intradural metastases
- Intradural extramedullary mass
- Intramedullary spinal mass

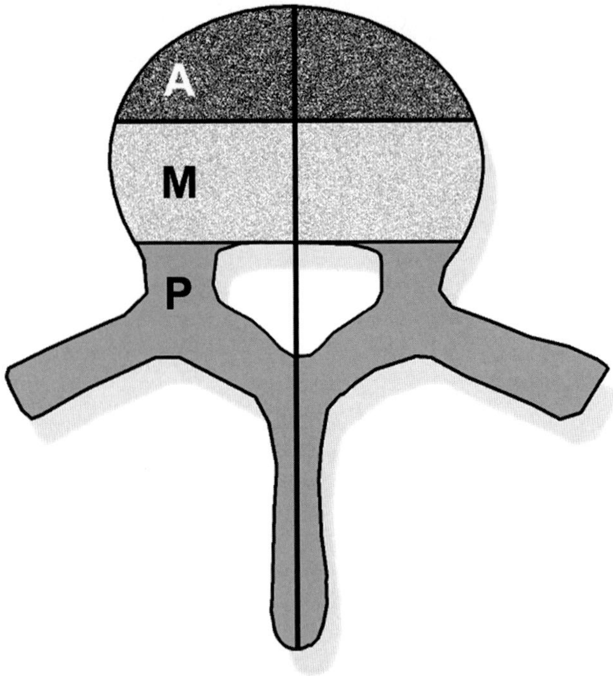

Figure 27-1. Classification system for the evaluation of spinal stability. The three-column system of Denis[12] was devised for assessment of spinal column stability in trauma. The system divides the spine into the anterior (A), middle (M), and posterior (P) columns. The spine is considered unstable if two of the three columns are disrupted. The six-column system of Kostuik and Errico[13] was devised for evaluating stability in spine tumors. Here the three columns, as defined by Denis, are subdivided into left and right halves. The spine is unstable if three to four of the columns are destroyed.

patients with metastatic disease to the spine, because a major goal of treatment is restoration or maintenance of spine stability. In trauma, the accepted biomechanical model for determination of thoracolumbar stability in fractures is the three-column concept of the spine (Fig. 27-1)[12] in which:

- The anterior column consists of the anterior half of the vertebral body, the anterior longitudinal ligament, and the anterior annulus fibrosus;
- The middle column includes the posterior longitudinal ligament, the posterior half of the vertebral body, and the posterior annulus; and
- The posterior column consists of the neural arch (laminae and pedicles), facets, the ligamentum flavum, and the supraspinous and interspinous ligaments.

The spine is considered unstable if two of the three columns are disrupted. Spinal fractures are classified according to the mechanism of injury and involvement of the columns.

In neoplastic destruction of the spine these concepts may not always be applicable, because trauma and tumors are quite different conditions in terms of the disruption of bone, disc, and ligament; the quality of surrounding bone stock; and the ability of the spine to heal.

A set of criteria, which requires validation, has been developed for spinal tumors.[13] The spine is divided into six columns: the three columns defined above[12] subdivided into left and right halves (see Fig. 27-1). The spine is considered to be stable if fewer than three of the six columns are destroyed, unstable if three to four of the columns are destroyed, and markedly unstable if five to six of the columns are involved. Angulation of 20 degrees or more adds to the consideration of instability.

Instability does not usually develop when involvement is limited to the vertebral spongy bone core or to the anterior column. When the posterior half (middle column) of the vertebral body is also involved (cortical bone included), pathologic compression fracture can occur, producing kyphosis and extrusion of bone, tumor, or disc into the spinal canal, with resulting neural compromise. Tumor involvement of the middle and posterior column may produce forward shearing deformity. In addition, segmental instability is probably present when the clinical syndrome is characterized by pain that is aggravated by movement (in the absence of significant neural encroachment), and it is associated with progressive collapse of vertebral bodies or localized kyphosis on imaging studies. Figure 27-2 schematically describes the various patterns of vertebral collapse. The MRI appearance of acute vertebral fractures was studied in a series of 100 patients evaluated for suspected spinal cord compression.[14] Pathologic fracture

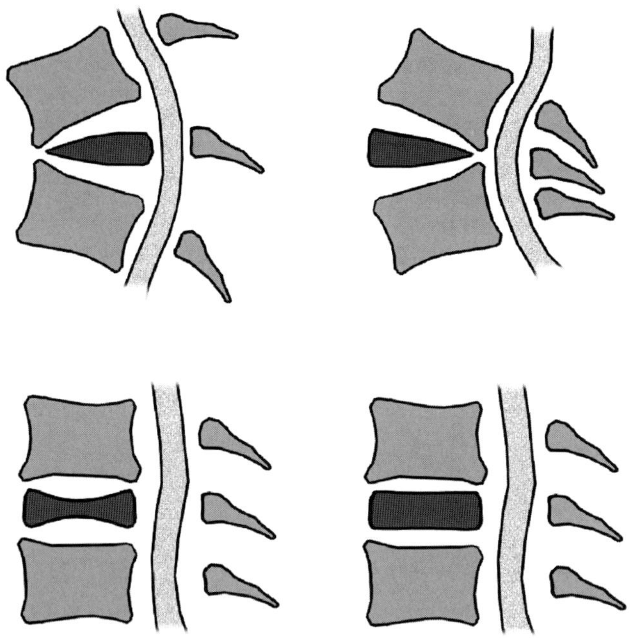

Figure 27-2. Patterns of vertebral collapse identified in neoplastic vertebral fractures. Central collapse is the most common type. Uniform and anterior collapses are detected with similar frequency. Posterior collapse is uncommon.

of the vertebral body was present in 51% of compressive levels. Of these, 68% had loss of height greater than 50%. The most common pattern of collapse was central compression fracture; anterior and uniform compressions were equally distributed, and posterior compression was relatively rare. Vertebral bodies in the lower thoracic region were more likely to have pathologic fractures and, in the authors' experience, prostatic lesions were least likely to give rise to collapse of the vertebral body.

A systematic approach to determine the clinical instability of the spine should include anatomic, biomechanical, symptomatic, and therapeutic considerations.[15,16] Apart from neuroimaging studies that define anatomic details used in the three-column spinal model (see Fig. 27-1),[14] the concept of clinical instability should be accounted for. Clinical instability is defined as "loss of the ability of the spine under physiologic loads to maintain relationships between vertebrae in such a way that there is either damage or subsequent irritation to the spinal cord or nerve roots, and in addition there is development of incapacitating deformity or pain due to structural changes."[16]

Treatment of Vertebral Metastases

Biomechanically Stable Vertebral Metastases

Although some vertebral metastases are painless, many cause significant and debilitating pain. Besides pain, vertebral metastases can also give rise to pathologic fracture and spinal cord compression—two important complications that result in significant morbidity. Treatment of vertebral metastases often requires a multimodality approach, with the main aims of alleviating pain and preventing future complications. It is important to base the treatment plan on the overall clinical situation, because vertebral metastases represent only one aspect of the disease process. Treatment of biomechanically stable vertebral metastases usually includes analgesic medication and focal radiotherapy as the immediate modalities to alleviate pain. In certain tumor types, hormone therapy, cytotoxic drugs, and bisphosphonates are added in view of the likelihood of further skeletal involvement.

Radiation Therapy

Radiotherapy is a frequently used treatment modality for bone metastases. It is effective in reducing metastatic bone pain and, in some instances, causing tumor shrinkage or growth inhibition.[17–19] There is, as yet, no consensus regarding the most appropriate way of delivering radiotherapy for metastatic bone pain. The practice differs significantly between countries and even between treatment centers within the same country. One controversy is whether single-fraction radiotherapy is as effective as multifraction radiotherapy. Single-fraction radiotherapy is more convenient for the patient, as well as less costly when compared with multifraction radiotherapy. However, there are some important concerns relating to single-fraction radiotherapy. The equivalent biologic dose of single-fraction treatment is usually smaller than the total multifraction treatment dose. As a result, the pain response to a single dose may be inferior to the multifraction radiotherapy response. Even if the initial pain response is similar, it may not be durable enough to ensure that the patient remains asymptomatic. In addition, with a potentially reduced tumoricidal effect, single-fraction radiotherapy may not be as effective in preventing complications such as pathologic fractures and spinal cord compression. A systematic review of randomized studies examining the effectiveness of single-fraction radiotherapy versus multifraction radiotherapy pooled the results and used meta-analysis to estimate the effect of treatment on pain response, retreatment rate, and complications.[17] There was no difference between the two radiotherapy schedules for either overall or complete pain-response rates; however, patients treated by single-fraction radiotherapy had a higher retreatment rate and a higher rate of pathologic fractures than did patients treated by multifraction schedule. The spinal cord compression rates were similar for both arms of the treatment schedules. But it should be noted that there was a trend of increasing spinal cord compression rates for patients treated by single-fraction radiotherapy, although the number of events was too small to allow sufficient statistical power to test the differences.

Based on the above analysis of the two treatment schedules, multifraction radiotherapy is recommended for most vertebral metastases. Still, for those patients whose life expectancy is considered to be extremely short, a single-fraction schedule may be appropriate when radiotherapy is used primarily for the immediate pain control. The treatment schedule should be tailored for each patient based on the type of palliative therapy required and the complications that might develop.

Bisphosphonates

These agents work by several different mechanisms to reduce both bone resorption and bone formation.[20,21] In vitro, bisphosphonates may have a direct effect on tumor cells by inducing apoptosis, inhibiting matrix metalloproteinase-1, and inhibiting adhesion of tumor cells within the bone. Bisphosphonates can be divided into two groups. Those resembling pyrophosphate (for example, clodronate, etidronate) act as analogues of adenosine triphosphate (ATP) and inhibit ATP-dependent intracellular enzymes. The second group, aminobisphosphonates (e.g., pamidronate, zoledronic acid), inhibits enzymes of the mevalonate pathway, disrupting the signaling function of key regulatory proteins. The net effect in both groups is inhibition of osteoclast function, which leads to a decrease in bone resorption. Systematic review of the impact of bisphosphonates in metastatic cancer patients showed that bisphosphonates significantly decrease skeletal morbidity and significantly reduce the probability of vertebral fracture[3,4,8]; however, the incidence of spinal cord compression is not reduced. This may be related to the fact that studies examining skeletal events were insufficiently powered to show a difference between bisphosphonates and controls for spinal cord compression, which is a relatively rare skeletal event. Based on the systematic review, the recommendation is that treatment with bisphosphonate medications should start when bone metastases are diagnosed and continue until they are no longer clinically relevant.[3]

Vertebral Metastases with Biomechanical Potential or Overt Instability

Vertebral metastases that lead to biomechanical spine instability, or potential instability, produce a range of symptoms and signs that should direct therapeutic consideration. Patients with localized kyphosis, collapsed vertebra, fracture dislocation, retropulsion of a bone fragment, or segmental instability may require various surgical procedures tailored to meet decompression, stabilization, or pain-relief requirements, depending on symptomatology (Fig. 27-3). However, not every case defined by the criteria for unstable spine requires surgical intervention. If the tumor is relatively radiosensitive, radiotherapy may result in satisfactory axial settling and pain relief over a period of weeks or months (Fig. 27-3). These patients should be

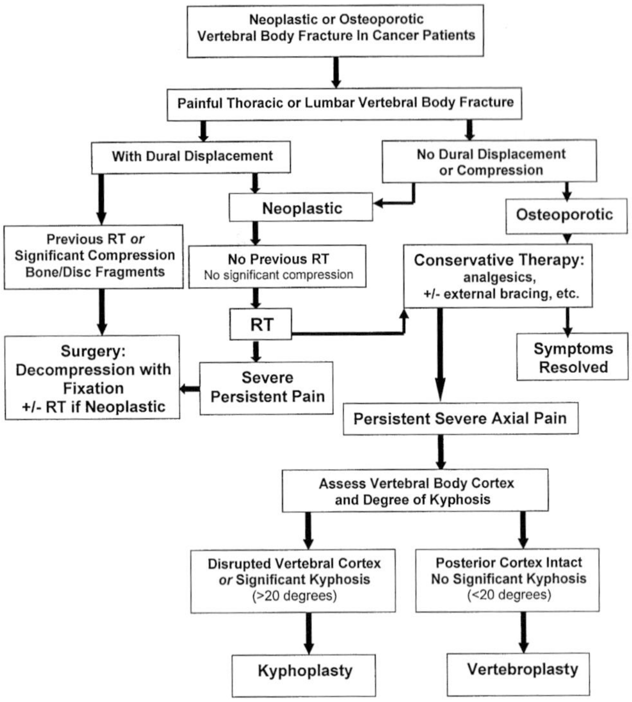

Figure 27-3. Treatment algorithm for painful thoracic or lumbar vertebral body fractures. The fracture can be either osteoporotic or secondary to disruption of the vertebral cortical shell by metastatic tumor.

carefully followed because they are potentially unstable. Surgical procedures are reserved for symptomatic cases, because preventive surgery is probably unjustified in the management of metastatic disease of the spine.

When the anterior and middle columns are destroyed by tumor, treatment considerations should include decompression as well as restoration of stability by instrumentation and vertebral replacement constructs. If the posterior column structures are involved, then the treatment plan is to replace or substitute for the support role of these structures by posterior decompression combined with posterior instrumentation to maintain stability. Recommendations for patient selection and optimal methods of decompression and stabilization are constantly evolving. Table 27-2 summarizes the criteria for spinal instability that should lead to consideration of spinal stabilization.

Vertebral Compression Fracture in Cancer Patients

Acute vertebral compression fractures are common and may occur because of osteoporosis, neoplastic infiltration of the vertebral body, or trauma (Fig. 27-4). Patients seen in neuro-oncology practice may present with osteoporotic fracture secondary to various precipitating factors such as age, steroid therapy, immobility, and prolonged use of low-molecular-weight heparin. At the same time neoplastic

▶ **TABLE 27-2.** CATEGORIES OF SPINAL INSTABILITY IN METASTATIC DISEASE THAT REQUIRE CONSIDERATION OF SPINAL FIXATION*

- Anterior + middle column involvement or collapse with loss of more than 50% of vertebral body height
- Middle + posterior column involvement or shearing deformity
- Three-column involvement
- Involvement of two or more adjacent vertebrae in the same column
- Iatrogenic
  - Laminectomy in face of anterior and/or middle column disease
  - Prospective resection of more than 50% of cut surface of the vertebral body

*Definition of potential instability relies on imaging studies and is valid only if the vertebral cortical shell is involved.

vertebral compression is a common occurrence in both hematologic malignancies and systemic solid tumors.[11,22–24] The differential diagnosis may be difficult. Imaging findings are suggestive, but often nonconclusive. It has been reported, for example, that osteoporotic fractures may accumulate FDG to varying degrees, and false-positive findings may occur when FDG-PET imaging is performed to assess whether metastases are present.[25] A differential pattern of FDG uptake, clinical correlation, and MRI findings, when used together, usually allow accurate differentiation of osteoporotic fracture from neoplastic process.

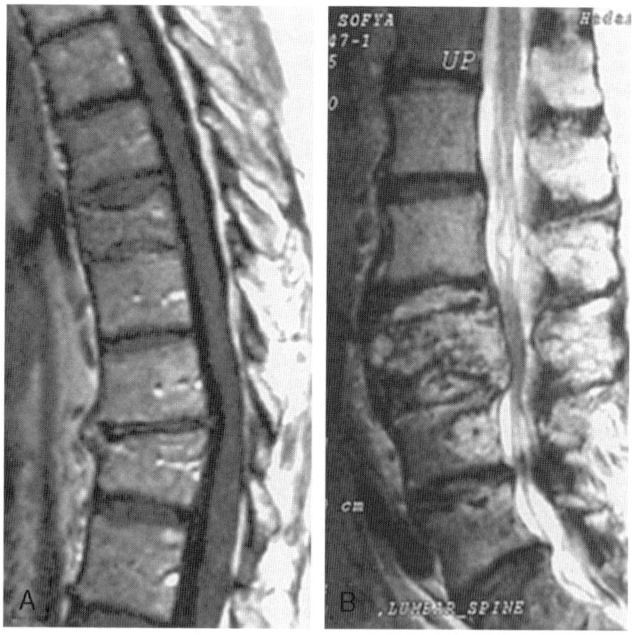

Figure 27-4. MRI of vertebral fractures in cancer patients. (A) Osteoporotic collapse of thoracic vertebra in a female patient with primary central nervous system (CNS) lymphoma. The patient had been treated with dexamethasone for several months to control increased intracranial pressure induced by the brain tumor, and subsequently received additional steroids as part of the treatment schedule. She presented with a new incapacitating back pain. MRI revealed central collapse of the sixth thoracic vertebra. (B) Neoplastic collapse of the third lumbar vertebra associated with compression of the thecal sac. Note that the tumor (prostatic carcinoma) also involves the fourth and fifth lumbar vertebrae.

MRI findings may be useful for differentiation between metastatic and acute osteoporotic compression fracture of the spine (see Fig. 27-4). A convex posterior border of the vertebral body, abnormal signal intensity of the pedicle or posterior elements, epidural mass, focal paraspinal mass, and other spinal metastases are suggestive for metastatic compression fractures. Conversely, imaging findings suggestive of acute osteoporotic compression fractures are a low-signal-intensity band on T_1- and T_2-weighted images, spared normal bone marrow signal intensity of the vertebral body, retropulsion of a posterior bone fragment, multiple compression fractures, and fluid collection (the fluid sign) that results from bone marrow edema.[22,23]

Treatment Options for Vertebral Compression Fracture

Vertebral compression fracture (see Fig. 27-3) is associated with severe pain and is frequently the cause of immobility. A multidisciplinary approach to patient selection and management is essential (see Fig. 27-4). Once vertebral body fracture is diagnosed, it is important to evaluate whether dural displacement or significant neural compression is present. In cases with significant compression of neural elements secondary to impingement of bone, disc fragments, or tumor mass, early consideration of surgical decompression combined with stabilization should take place. In neoplastic vertebral fractures where dural displacement is present, but the compression is not significant, radiotherapy followed by conservative therapy can form the initial treatment approach. Conservative treatment of thoracic or lumbar vertebral fracture includes analgesic medications with or without external bracing and encouragement to maintain weight-bearing activities. Radiotherapy is also added to metastatic vertebral fractures that are not associated with dural displacement. None of these latter modalities is uniformly effective in relieving pain or improving ambulatory status.

For patients who fail to improve with conservative management and who have no evidence of cord or thecal sac compression, a minimally invasive procedure that involves the percutaneous injection of polymethylmethacrylate (PMMA), a surgical bone cement, under imaging guidance can be offered.[26,27] Precise indications for these techniques are still evolving.

The goal of vertebroplasty is to provide pain relief and bone strengthening in painful vertebral body compression fracture. Selected patients with focal, intense, and intractable midline spinal pain at the level of the fracture, or within two vertebral levels below it, and who failed conservative management, are candidates for this minimally invasive procedure. Vertebroplasty does not reexpand a collapsed vertebra, but it provides a certain degree of reinforcement and stabilization of the fracture, which alleviates pain. However, the procedure is only suitable for patients with no evidence of dural displacement or compression, and no significant radicular pain. Contraindications for the procedure include bleeding disorder, unstable fracture as a consequence of posterior element involvement, and lack of a definable level of collapse. Procedural complications are relatively rare; most are related to PMMA leakage through cortical defects.[27–29] Cement leakage rates range from 9% to 88%, and, in most cases, leakage is asymptomatic. Neural element compression resulting from cement extravasation remains a rare event.

Percutaneous balloon kyphoplasty, a recent modification of vertebroplasty, involves inflation of a balloon within a collapsed vertebral body to restore height and reduce kyphotic deformity prior to stabilization with PMMA. The risk of cement extravasation is theoretically reduced because inflation of the balloon creates a void within the vertebral body into which the cement can be injected under relatively low pressure. Therefore, this procedure is indicated once there is evidence for disrupted posterior cortex of the collapsed vertebra and in cases where significant kyphotic deformity contributes to the pathophysiology of spinal pain.

Current experience with percutaneous vertebroplasty and kyphoplasty for painful vertebral fractures in cancer patients remains limited, but favorable results can be obtained with careful selection of appropriate patients.[26,27,30,31] Marked or complete pain relief is reported in 70% to 84% of procedures performed in neoplastic vertebral fractures, and the rate exceeds 90% in osteoporotic fractures. No change in the level of pain is reported in approximately 9% of neoplastic fractures. Pain relief and increased mobility are expected within 24 hours after the procedure, but occasionally these responses occur after a few days. Reduction in pain score is significant and remains so for up to 1 year. As a result, analgesic consumption is also significantly reduced in the majority of treated patients.[27]

In conclusion, these procedures can be applied with good safety profile in well-selected patients with osteoporotic fractures and in patients with multiple myeloma or metastatic cancer who have refractory spinal pain.

▶ VERTEBRAL METASTASES WITH EPIDURAL EXTENSION

Breast, lung, and prostate cancer account for approximately 60% of cases of metastatic vertebral lesions associated with epidural extension in adults.[1,32–35] Other common primary cancers that can result in epidural extension include lymphoma, renal cell carcinoma, sarcoma, and multiple myeloma. The origin of metastases cannot be identified in 7% to 12% of cases.[11,34,36,37]

All patients with vertebral metastases are at potential risk of developing compression of the neural roots, cauda equina, and/or the spinal cord. Epidural metastases are the most common cause of spinal cord and cauda equina dysfunction in cancer patients. The term *spinal cord compression* (SCC) is used in this chapter to include cauda equina compression, unless otherwise noted.

Frequency

SCC incidence is unknown. Retrospective clinical studies suggest that 2% to 20% of patients with vertebral metastases develop myelopathy secondary to SCC.[9,34,38] A recent population-based study of malignant SCC in Ontario, Canada, found that the cumulative probability of experiencing at least one episode of SCC in the last 5 years preceding death from cancer was 2.5% overall, and ranged from 0.2% in cancer of the pancreas to 7.9% in myeloma.[34] An autopsy study estimated that 5% of cancer patients develop spinal epidural tumor deposits,[39] but a proportion may remain clinically silent. Although spinal metastases generally occur in patients with known malignancy, they are the initial manifestation of malignancy in approximately 8% to 20% of patients with SCC.[40,41] Carcinoma of the lung, cancer of unknown primary site, multiple myeloma, and non-Hodgkin lymphoma are disproportionately represented in series of epidural metastases occurring as initial manifestation of malignancy, accounting for 78% of all episodes of SCC. These primary tumors account for only 26% of SCC in patients with previously established diagnosis of malignancy.

The incidence of SCC secondary to lymphoma, breast, and prostate cancer has decreased over the years.[42] Declining incidence probably reflects a shift in oncologic treatment policies toward the early use of radiotherapy or more effective and earlier treatment of the primary tumor reducing the rate of metastatic complications. The routine use of advanced imaging techniques (CT and MRI) also contributes to early detection and treatment of clinically silent spinal metastases[1,2,14,36,37] because imaging of the whole spine is feasible with these techniques. When performed, for example, in patients with clinical symptomatology suggestive of SCC, whole-spine images often reveal that two or more levels of compression are present, affecting more than one region of the spine. Multiple levels of neural element compression are detected in 25% to 43% of suspected SCC.[2,14,36,37,43]

The incidence of clinical SCC in children is approximately 5%. Tumor types leading to SCC in these young patients are different from those encountered in adults and include sarcomas, neuroblastomas, and lymphomas.[44–47] Sarcoma and neuroblastoma comprise more than 80% of all cases of pediatric SCC, and Ewing sarcoma has the highest propensity for epidural extension. Most pediatric tumors invade the spinal canal via the neural foramen rather than via vertebral metastases (Fig. 27-5).

Tumor Location

Level of Spinal Cord Compression

The thoracic spine is the most common site of SCC.[14,37] The involvement of a specific region of the spine by metastatic deposits is thought to relate to the number of vertebrae contained therein. In a review of 2977 cases of SCC, cervical involvement occurred at a lower-than-expected rate (11%–13% vs. the 27% expected rate), whereas involvement in the lumbar and thoracic areas was close to the predicted figures.[48] The lower incidence of SCC in the cervical spine may be related to two factors. The bone volume of the cervical spine is smaller than that of other regions, and therefore hematogenous vertebral colonization by a metastatic tumor is less likely to occur. The spinal canal is more capacious in the upper cervical area relative to the thoracic canal, allowing more space for an expanding epidural tumor, and thus a lesser likelihood of epidural deposits becoming clinically evident.

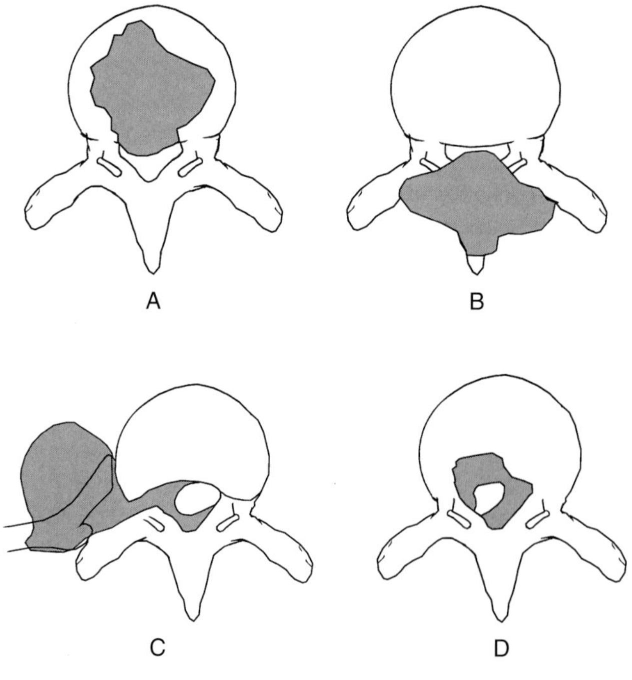

Figure 27-5. Modes of invasion into the spinal canal by metastatic tumors. Epidural metastases usually arise from extension of metastases located in the adjacent vertebral column into the spinal canal (A and B), or from paravertebral masses penetrating through the intervertebral foramina (C). The extension of the tumor into the spinal canal produces variable involvement of the anterior (ventral) compartment (A), the posterior compartment (B), the lateral gutter (C), or any combination of these conditions (D).

Location of Epidural Tumor in Relation to the Spinal Cord and the Yield of Diagnostic Imaging

Epidural SCC usually results from metastases to one of three sites: the vertebrae, the paravertebral tissue, or the epidural space itself. Extension of the tumor into the spinal canal may produce variable involvement of the anterior (ventral) compartment, the lateral gutters, the posterior compartment, or any combination of these sites (see Fig. 27-5).

Because the vertebral column is the most common site for metastases resulting in epidural SCC, it is not surprising that spinal radiography is predictive of epidural disease[49] and that an epidural mass is identified at 86% of symptomatic spinal segments. However, radiographic results require 30% to 70% bony destruction before they become positive. An MRI study demonstrated that although an absent pedicle is often the first radiographic sign of metastatic disease, the pedicle is involved by direct extension from either the vertebral body or the posterior elements, and is therefore a late occurrence in the disease process.[50] The region of the vertebral column that is most often involved is the vertebral body, probably because of its extensive vascular supply; thus, most epidural tumors arise in a vertebral body and invade the epidural space anteriorly.[14,48] MRI evaluation of acute SCC caused by metastases showed that metastatic disease was present in the bodies of all 160 vertebral levels that were studied.[14] Structural vertebral involvement evaluated by the vertebral quadrants (one anterior, two lateral, and one posterior column) showed that 97% of the vertebrae had more than 50% involvement. Four-column involvement was seen in 52% of affected vertebrae that were evaluated, and three columns were affected in 30%. Single-column involvement was seen only in the anterior column, and accounted for 3% of affected vertebrae. Coexisting anterior and posterior column disease was observed in 75%. These findings of extensive structural vertebral involvement associated with acute neoplastic SCC are evidence that any attempt to perform decompressive surgery should always be combined with measures to stabilize the spine.

Normal spinal roentgenograms, seen in 6% of SCC, do not exclude epidural metastases. For example, normal radiographs may be found in 89% of lymphoma patients with epidural compression,[42] in whom a paravertebral tumor mass usually invades the epidural space through the intervertebral foramina, rather than via vertebral extension (see Fig. 27-5). This mode of epidural invasion is seen in patients with lymphomas, renal cell cancer, superior sulcus tumors (Pancoast syndrome), and neuroblastoma and accounts for approximately 10% of all SCC.[42] Up to 36% of patients with paraspinal tumor have epidural metastases on myelography.[51] With the advent of CT scanning and MRI, which adequately demonstrate paravertebral soft tissues, these lesions are being more frequently recognized. A paraspinal mass is detected by MRI at the site of extradural SCC in 28% of patients. Only one-third of these masses were detected on plain radiography.[37] Pure, exclusively epidural lesions are rare, and their incidence is unknown. In a consecutive series of 100 patients with acute SCC evaluated by MRI, no isolated epidural lesion was noted.[14]

The location of the extradural metastases within the vertebral canal has important surgical implications. Accurate definition of the epidural mass as posterior, lateral, cuff, or anterior requires CT-myelography or a noninvasive MRI study (Fig. 27-6). MRI is the procedure of choice to evaluate the vertebral column, spinal cord, and soft-tissue parts, and usually eliminates the need for other imaging studies. MRI is equivalent to myelography in detecting epidural disease, and superior in detecting vertebral metastases and paravertebral masses.[36,44,52,53] MRI is the imaging method of choice both as a screening tool and as the ultimate diagnostic test to evaluate SCC.[2,14,36,37,54,55] Thus, whenever MRI is readily available, it has become the preferred imaging method. Still, spinal CT is an excellent screening method to diagnose patients at risk and to verify presence of an epidural mass in an emergency setting.[1] In a study of 342 episodes of suspected SCC in cancer patients evaluated with spinal CT, additional MRI assessment was required because of diagnostic uncertainty in only 5% of patients.[1]

MRI, however, has broader impact on management. It detects unexpected vertebral and epidural lesions that lead to a change in treatment in up to 50% of patients.[2,14,36,54,55] Thus, when SCC is suspected, a complete spine evaluation is indicated. MRI provides significant economic benefits compared with other imaging modalities for spine evaluation.[56] Myelography combined with CT should be performed when diagnosis and treatment are delayed by the inability to perform MRI, when patients are unable to undergo MRI (because of pacemakers or claustrophobia), or when a technically adequate MRI cannot be obtained (e.g., presence of spinal instrumentation at the investigated level or extreme obesity).

Symptoms and Signs

Onset of SCC symptoms may be acute or insidious, and symptom duration varies widely. Pain is the initial symptom in 96% of cases, preceding other symptoms by approximately 2 to 3 months.[32,57] Pain can be localized close to the site of the lesion or can be radicular. Pain generally results from nerve root compression or infiltration, compression fractures, segmental instability, displacement of the dura, or dural invasion. The site of pain may not correspond to the site of epidural compression on imaging.[32] In cancer patients with symptoms and signs of spinal metastases, it is difficult to distinguish those with vertebral metastases alone purely on the basis of the clinical presentation. Therefore, all patients with symptomatic spinal metastases must be considered at risk for SCC.

Although pain should alert the clinician to the potential diagnosis, it may be nonspecific or referred to other sites, frequently leading to a delay in diagnosis.[32,57] This is especially true in patients without a previous history of cancer. At the time of diagnosis, neurologic signs are common[32,42,44,57] and include various degrees of muscle weakness in 76%, bladder and bowel dysfunction in more than 50%, and sensory deficit in approximately 50% of patients with SCC. However, weakness and sensory abnormalities are often reported late and identified even later, despite patients having reported pain for a considerable time. Nearly half of severely affected patients develop a complete deficit (no residual spinal cord function) after diagnosis and before undergoing any treatment. Of the paraparetic patients, 28% become paraplegic in less than 24 hours and before initiation of treatment.[58] Consequently, SCC should be treated as soon as possible, and early diagnosis is crucial as functional outcome largely depends on the neurologic function before treatment.[42,58–60]

Apart from the typical manifestations of SCC symptoms, several unusual clinical presentations may be seen. Patients may present with an atypical facial pain and numbness, with Brown-Sequard syndrome, with ataxia secondary to posterior column dysfunction, or with herpetic rash along the affected dermatomes.[42,44,61]

Pathophysiology

The mechanisms that determine the degree of irreversible tissue damage are poorly understood, but appear to be associated with endogenous neurochemical changes resulting from the initial event of compressive injury. Therefore, it is imperative to try to link therapeutic strategies that alleviate compressive mechanical injury with tactics designed to limit the secondary autodestructive processes operating in the compressed spinal cord that lead to neuronal cell death

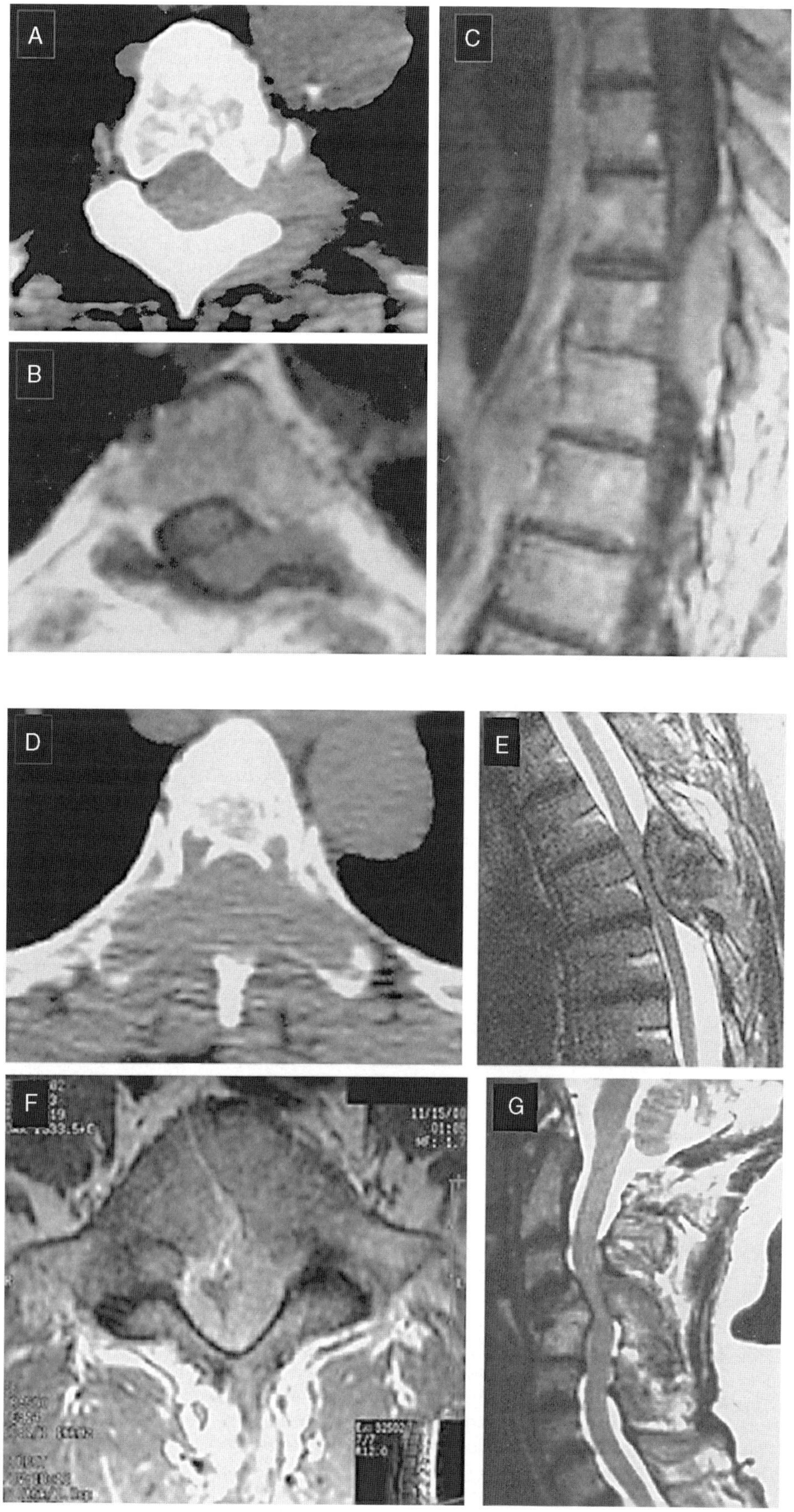

Figure 27-6. Imaging tumors with epidural extension. (A) CT of a thoracic paravertebral mass penetrating through the intervertebral foramen into the spinal canal. The tumor extends within the canal and forms a posterior lateral mass that compresses the spinal cord. Biopsy revealed an aggressive non-Hodgkin lymphoma. (B) Axial MRI view from the same patient as in A. The tumor mass fills the intervertebral foramen and penetrates into the spinal canal. Note that MRI reveals that the vertebral body is involved by the tumor, although no epidural extension of the tumor affects the anterior aspect of the canal. (C) Sagittal MRI view (enhanced T_1-weighted image) in the same patient as in B. The tumor is forming an enhancing posterior mass that extends within the spinal canal across three vertebral levels and compresses the spinal cord. Note adjacent vertebral bodies are affected by tumor. (D) CT study of a lytic lesion that involves the posterior elements of the vertebra in a patient with multiple myeloma. A soft-tissue mass is obliterating the spinal canal and compressing the spinal cord. (E) Sagittal MRI view (T_2-weighted image) of the same patient as in D. A posterior tumor mass is compressing the spinal cord. The vertebral bodies are intact. (F) MRI (enhanced T_1-weighted image) of non-Hodgkin lymphoma that penetrates into the spinal canal via the intervertebral foramen at the L5 vertebra level. The tumor encases the thecal sac, inducing severe circumferential compression of the cauda equina. (G) MRI of the cervical spine (T_2-weighted image) demonstrating pathologic fractures of the C4 and C5 vertebrae associated with retropulsion of tumor and bone into the spinal canal. The tumor is a metastatic breast carcinoma that also involves the posterior elements at the same vertebral levels. The spinal cord is compressed by both the anterior and the posterior epidural tumors.

and permanent loss of function. Comprehension of the neurochemical cascade activated by the neoplastic compression has increased with the use of well-characterized animal models that enable better understanding of tissue injury at a cellular level.[62–76] These laboratory studies demonstrate that pharmacologic treatments modify neurochemical changes, attenuate secondary events such as spinal cord edema, ameliorate structural neuronal destruction such as neurofilament disintegration, and significantly delay neurologic deterioration, even if the compressing tumor is not removed. Figure 27-7 summarizes the paradigm of secondary events operating in neoplastic SCC, and the pharmacologic strategies used to ameliorate them in experimental animal models.

The mechanism of injury induced by the expanding extradural tumors is complex and multifactorial. The enlarging extradural tumor causes early obstruction of the spinal epidural venous plexus, and also induces arteriolar dilatation via local spinal autoregulatory mechanisms such as activation of endothelial nitric oxide (NO) synthase.[64,65,77] These changes in vascular tone and drainage enhance production of a vasogenic type of edema. The edema initially involves the white matter, and, in the late stages, also the gray matter. At the end stage there is a rapid decrease in spinal cord blood flow at the site of compression.

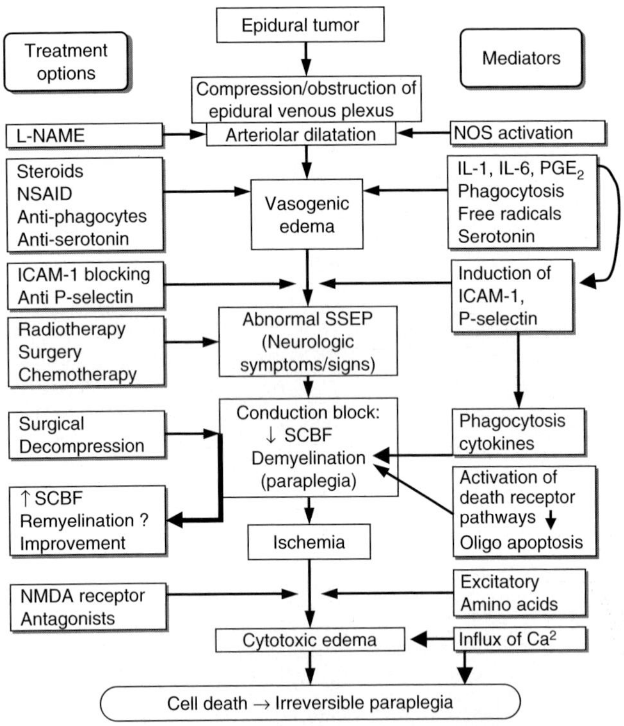

Figure 27-7. An algorithm of the recognized mechanisms involved in the pathophysiology of spinal cord compression. Pharmacologic treatment options may reduce neural tissue damage. Data related to pharmacologic manipulations are derived from investigation of animal models of neoplastic SCC. The relationship of the currently used therapeutic modalities in humans (corticosteroids, radiotherapy, surgery, and chemotherapy) to the specific stage of spinal cord injury is also shown.
L-NAME = L-nitro-arginine methyl ester; NOS = nitric oxide synthase; Oligo = oligodendrocyte; SCBF = spinal cord blood flow; SSEP = somatosensory evoked potentials.

Ischemia may play the final deleterious role, leading to cell death if compression is not promptly alleviated. In an animal model, abnormalities in spinal somatosensory-evoked responses preceded neurologic signs of myelopathy.[76] The conduction block may be related to myelin destruction, as has been demonstrated by an electron microscopic study.[76] The disruption of myelin is probably caused by both mechanical compression and ischemia, and by activation of death receptor pathways associated with oligodendroglial apoptosis.[78] Although demyelination can occur at sites of spinal compression,[79,80] remyelination may take place after transient compression,[81] thereby providing a possible morphologic correlate for recovery of function after prompt decompression.

Local production of cytokines such as prostaglandins, as well as interleukin (IL)-1 and IL-6, may promote an inflammatory response with associated physiologic changes of vasodilation, plasma exudation, and edema formation.[75,82] In fact, elevation in prostaglandin E_2 (PGE_2) synthesis is demonstrated in the compressed segments concomitantly with the development of spinal cord edema. In keeping with that concept, a rapid antiedema effect is achieved only when partial or marked reduction of PGE_2 synthesis is accomplished, either by steroidal or by nonsteroidal antiinflammatory drugs (e.g., indomethacin),[67,69,70] or by inhibitors of phagocytic activity.[75,82] Recently, the possible role of the inflammatory tissue response that upregulates endothelial adhesion molecules such as P-selectin and intercellular adhesion molecule (ICAM)-1 was investigated in animal models. It was demonstrated that cytokines such as IL-1 induce upregulation of these adhesion molecules and that blockage of this process resulted in white matter preservation and improved neurologic outcome.[83,84]

Other studies looked at the microglia and their phagocytic activity. Immunohistochemical studies showed that in tumor-bearing paraplegic rats, the normal population of resting microglia was replaced by activated amoeboid cells, probably engaged in phagocytosis.[75] At onset of paraplegia, marked disruption of normal neurofilament cytoarchitecture was evident. In vivo pharmacologic inhibition of phagocytosis (using chloroquine and colchicine) blocked lysosomal activity and cell migration. The ratio of amoeboid microglia was reduced, marked preservation of neurofilament structure was achieved, the enhanced synthesis of cytokines (PGE_2, IL-1, IL-6) observed in untreated rats was markedly diminished, and significant attenuation in spinal cord edema was evident. Initiating this treatment at the first sign of neurologic dysfunction significantly delayed onset of paraplegia, and protracted the course of neurologic deterioration toward paraplegia. These results suggest that inhibition of phagocytosis may delay structural damage, enhancing the chance of recovery following decompression by antitumor therapy. It provides the scientific background for the clinical use of steroids, and it also explains the favorable neurologic outcome in patients with neoplastic SCC treated by radiotherapy who receive high-dose dexamethasone.[85] Although dexamethasone is incapable of blocking phagocytosis, it does inhibit the associated inflammatory responses and production of some cytokines that play a role in the phagocytic cascade.

In addition to phagocytosis, a marked increase in serotonin use is present in the compressed cord segments. Inhibition of serotonin receptors results in attenuated vascular permeability and a protracted clinical course toward paraplegia, similar to the favorable effect produced by steroids or nonsteroidal antiinflammatory agents.[73–75,82] Receptor-activated serotonergic mechanisms distinct from the mechanism associated with the inflammatory response probably participate in the disruption of the blood–spinal cord barrier in the subacutely developing compression injury. These mechanisms can be separately manipulated pharmacologically to yield measurable effects in the experimental model. However, it is unclear whether a combined pharmacologic regimen will result in an additive effect.

In end-stage SCC, when conduction block and ischemia are present, cytotoxic edema may also develop. The glutamate receptor antagonists ketamine and MK-801 produce an antiedema effect in SCC that is not associated with either inhibition of the inflammatory cytokines (PGE_2) or reduction of vascular permeability. Cytotoxic edema may therefore be present, and excitotoxins (such as glutamate) probably mediate its evolution.[71,72]

The experimental findings indicate that early pharmacologic intervention may offer the potential to delay neurologic deterioration and may attenuate neuronal damage. However, given the complexity of the pathophysiologic mechanisms, pharmacologic manipulations should be carefully assessed in animal models before their extrapolation to human clinical studies.

Survival and Spinal Cord Compression

The magnitude of the clinical problem of spinal epidural metastases is usually underestimated. The best evidence suggests that approximately 5% of patients dying of cancer have suffered from epidural metastases.[34,39] This calculated incidence exceeds the annual rate of traumatic spinal cord injury. However, because of the high mortality among these patients (50%–70% at 1 year), the socioeconomic impact of neoplastic SCC is less than traumatic injury. The overall median survival following the first episode of SCC is short, ranging from 3 to 4 months.[33,34,86] As a result, neoplastic SCC accounts for only 10% to 14% of all spinal cord injury admissions to rehabilitation units.[87] It was demonstrated that pretreatment ambulatory function is the main determinant for posttreatment gait function, and the survival of nonambulatory patients can only be improved by restoration of gait function by immediate treatment.[33,35,88] In spite of the poor prognosis of the disease, most patients should receive active treatment[33,44,89] to preserve or restore mobility and continence and to alleviate intractable pain. SCC in itself is usually not the direct cause of death, except when it occurs in the upper portion of the cervical spine. The survival in SCC is related to the natural history of the systemic malignancy. Only approximately 30% of patients are expected to survive beyond 1 year and rarely as long as 4 to 9 years.[40,90–92]

Factors Influencing Recovery of Function

Tumor Biology and Cell Type

The biologic activity of the primary neoplasm determines the aggressiveness of both local and systemic disease, the success of therapy, and the posttreatment survival rate.[34,58,93] Patients with myeloma, lymphoma, Ewing sarcoma, neuroblastoma, or carcinoma of the breast have a favorable prognosis for recovery of function, and they survive longer after the first episode of SCC.[34] The outlook for patients with metastatic bronchogenic carcinoma, or metastatic disease of an unknown primary site, is generally poor. Overall, high tumor radiosensitivity and chemosensitivity are associated with a more favorable prognosis and functional outcome, whereas radioresistant tumors tend to have worse results.[34,58,94]

Pretreatment Neurologic Status

SCC outcome depends in good part on the patient's neurologic status at the time of treatment. A positive correlation exists between the pretreatment mobility and the functional outcome.[44,58,93,95–99] From 80% to 90% of the patients who can walk at the time of diagnosis remain ambulant after treatment, 35% to 45% of those who are initially paraparetic become ambulatory, and only 5% to 7% of paraplegic patients regain the ability to walk. The success of therapy in paraplegic patients depends on whether the patient has complete functional cord transection, or whether there is preservation of some neurologic function, with motor function the most significant. Only 2% of patients with complete transection recover ambulation, compared to 20% of patients with residual neurologic function. Regardless of the mode of therapy, complete paraplegia carries a bad functional prognosis and paraplegic patients rarely recover ambulation. The value of early diagnosis is clear, and with the advent of modern imaging techniques the percentage of patients diagnosed while still able to walk is steadily increasing. Series in which modern imaging techniques were used to diagnose SCC contain 42% to 56% ambulatory patients,[85,98–100] unlike previous reports in which only 25% of patients were ambulatory at diagnosis.[59,94,101,102] Nevertheless, an unacceptable delay in diagnosis, investigation, and referral occurs in most patients with malignant SCC, with a median delay of 14 days from the onset of symptoms. This delay results in preventable loss of function before treatment.[32,103,104]

Progression Rate of Symptoms

It has been suggested that a rapid onset and progression of neurologic symptoms is associated with a worse prognosis compared to gradual onset and slow progression of neurologic deficit.[58,88,105–107] The importance of the rate of symptom progression was emphasized in a study of 15 paraplegic patients treated with radiation therapy.[108] Five of the 15 patients regained ambulation after a delay of 3 months or more. The median time from the initial motor symptoms to total paralysis was longer (45 days) in patients who recovered than in those who remained paralyzed (9 days). The relevance of progression rate of motor deficit prior to diagnosis and treatment of SCC was further evaluated by using multiple logistic regression analysis of variables, which showed that this is an independent prognostic factor for posttreatment functional outcome.[88,106,107] A slower development of motor dysfunction predicted a better outcome and was found to be a stronger predictor than other prognostic factors, such as the type of tumor (favorable vs. unfavorable histology) or the pretreatment ambulatory status.

However, if the degree of spinal cord damage is taken into account, the neurologic grade still has a great influence on prognosis in patients with rapidly developing symptoms (less than 24 hours).[58] In patients with rapidly evolving deficit, 20% of paraparetic patients recover, compared with none of the paraplegic patients. Therefore, residual cord function should also be taken into account as an important prognostic variable in the rapidly evolving deficit. Once paraplegia has set in, the duration of paralysis does have prognostic significance, although anecdotal recovery has been reported even after periods of 4 to 8 weeks.[108]

Administration of High-Dose Dexamethasone

The use of steroids in the treatment of SCC is widely accepted.[58,60,85,94,102,109] The scientific basis for steroid use stems from animal models of SCC, in which reduction of spinal cord edema and delayed onset of paraplegia were observed after treatment with dexamethasone.[62,64,66,67,69,75] The clinical basis for steroid use of high-dose steroids is the rapid symptom relief noted in some patients receiving initial doses of 100 mg of dexamethasone, although the outcome was not superior compared to historical controls who received lower doses of steroids.[94] In a prospective study, patients with SCC were randomly assigned to receive initial treatment with either high-dose dexamethasone (100 mg) or a conventional intravenous bolus dose (10 mg) of dexamethasone followed by 16 mg/d orally.[109] No dose effect was observed on neurologic outcome, but a substantial effect on pain was noted within 24 hours after high-dose treatment. There is only one well-designed randomized controlled trial that compared high-dose dexamethasone to no steroids in 57 patients with metastatic SCC treated with radiotherapy alone.[85] There was a statistically and clinically significant difference between the steroid-treated and control arms. Of patients receiving steroids, 81% were ambulatory after treatment, compared to only 63% of patients in the control arm. However, steroid treatment was associated with significant side effects in 11%.

Several investigators observed a dramatic resolution of symptoms after treatment with steroids alone.[42,110,111] Such steroid-related improvement is probably related to the type of tumor and most likely represents a direct oncolytic effect, such as the response in lymphomas and leukemias. This response differs from the above-described pharmacologic effect, produced by high doses of steroids, that protracts the cascade of deleterious events leading to irreversible spinal cord damage, which are demonstrated in Fig. 27-7.

Principles of Management

Although spinal canal compression caused by metastatic malignancy is relatively common, SCC management remains controversial.[58–60,93,98,99,112,113] Controversy stems from the lack of prospective, well-designed, controlled clinical studies directly comparing various treatment modalities and from an absence of standard criteria for evaluation of response. Patients with metastatic SCC have, by definition, tumors that have spread from a primary site and thus are no longer curable by local measures. The therapeutic modalities of surgery and radiotherapy are palliative, and preservation or restoration of ambulation and bladder control are the criteria for successful therapy. Pain relief is also an important, but secondary, goal. Because the treatment is not curative, its effect on the quality of further survival is particularly important. Table 27-3 lists the therapeutic modalities currently available for the treatment of patients with epidural SCC. Figure 27-8 is an algorithm for treatment selection in the various categories of SCC.

Pharmacotherapy

Specific Chemotherapy

Epidural metastases arising from chemoresponsive primary tumors are likely to respond to chemotherapy, particularly early in the course of the disease. The response of lymphomas affecting the spine to corticosteroid treatment[42] may serve as an example. Because corticosteroids are used in almost all patients as nonspecific chemotherapy, their occasional specific effect may be indistinguishable from the effect of radiotherapy.

▶ TABLE 27-3. THERAPEUTIC MODALITIES IN SPINAL EPIDURAL METASTASES

Pharmacotherapy
- Specific (antineoplastic; combination chemotherapy)
- Nonspecific (antiedema, analgesia)

Radiation Therapy
- External beam radiotherapy—conventional fields
- Image-guided intensity-modulated radiosurgery
- Fractionated stereotactic conformal radiotherapy

Surgery
- Laminectomy (posterior decompression) + spinal fixation
- Vertebral body resection (anterior decompression) + spinal fixation
- Combined anterior and posterior decompression + spinal fixation (may be staged as sequential procedures)

The usual policy is not to use specific chemotherapy alone as the primary treatment of patients with SCC caused by malignancy with limited chemoresponsiveness, because of the uncertainty of response and the irreversibility of severe spinal cord dysfunction. Instead, specific chemotherapy is usually combined with other therapeutic modalities. However, several reports suggest that good recovery of neurologic function can be obtained by chemotherapy alone in chemosensitive neoplasms such as lymphoma, myeloma, Ewing sarcoma, germ cell tumors, and neuroblastoma.[113–118] The published experience of chemotherapy alone is limited and large-scale studies are not available.

Chemotherapy should be considered for treating spinal metastases with epidural components in the following settings:

- In some patients with lymphoma, neuroblastoma, germ cell tumors, or Ewing sarcoma with SCC as the presenting manifestation of malignancy, or when SCC is recognized during evaluation of the extent of disease. The best approach to treatment in these settings is still unclear. We believe that in SCC diagnosed early in the course of the disease, with mild neurologic dysfunction and no sign of rapid deterioration, chemotherapy can be used first.
- Patients with SCC whose level of neural compression was previously irradiated, and who are not candidates for further radiation or surgical therapy should be considered for chemotherapy.
- Chemotherapy can be used in chemosensitive tumors in conjunction with either surgery or radiotherapy in the acute treatment of symptomatic SCC.

Nonspecific Pharmacotherapy

Corticosteroids Glucocorticoids rarely achieve the dramatic relief from neurologic disability that is seen in patients with brain metastases. When high doses of corticosteroids are used to treat SCC, most patients experience

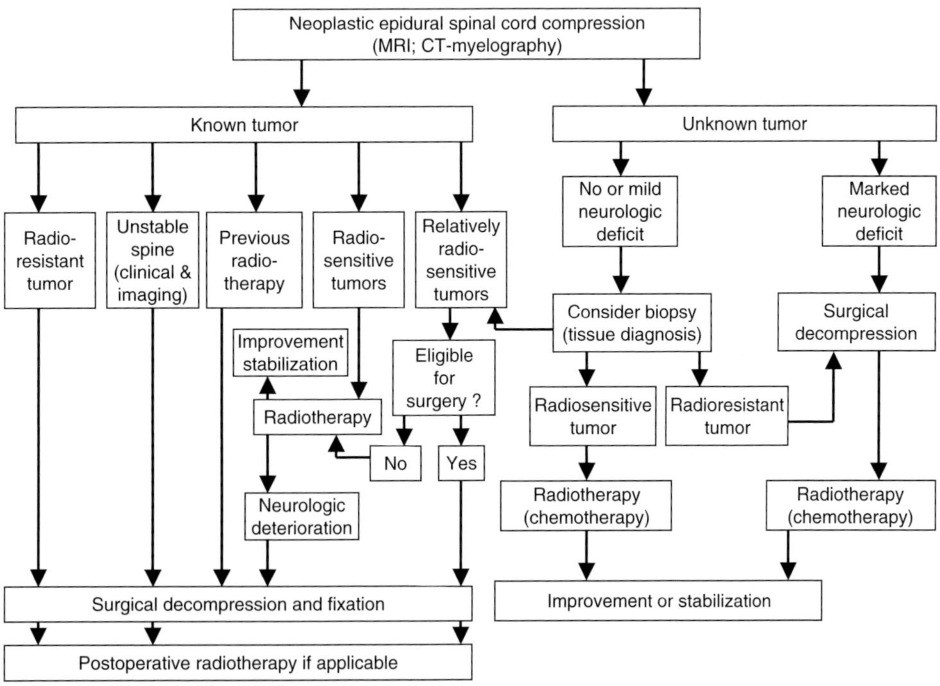

Figure 27-8. An algorithm for evaluating and selecting the preferred therapeutic approach in patients with neoplastic SCC.

dramatic relief of pain.[94,109] Some experience an arrest of progressively deteriorating neurologic function, and a few may improve from corticosteroids alone. Although high doses of steroids are frequently used in SCC, apart from pain relief, no clear advantage over conventional doses has been demonstrated.[60,94,109] However, the associated side effects that can arise with the use of corticosteroids should be an important consideration. The incidence of serious steroid-related complications in neuro-oncology patients has been the subject of several studies.[119–121] At least one steroid-related side effect was observed in 51% of treated patients, and 19% required hospital admission. Both the duration and the total dose of steroid therapy predicted toxicity. A significant increase in severe complications, including fatal sepsis, was noted when dexamethasone was used for more than 40 days to treat SCC.[122] In addition, intestinal perforation and gastrointestinal bleeding occurred with equal frequency, and significantly more rectosigmoid perforation occurred in neurologic (nononcologic) patients manifesting steroid toxicity.[119,121] Patients with SCC present fewer signs and symptoms of peritonitis than patients not treated with steroids who develop intestinal perforation. Because major complications occur in patients who receive steroids for more than 1 month, they must be used judiciously and should be discontinued as rapidly as possible, or tapered down to the lowest possible level that is compatible with clinical benefit. The following recommendations apply for the use of steroids:

- For patients with imaging evidence of SCC, but without signs of myelopathy, dexamethasone does not need to be given during treatment by radiotherapy.[60,123]
- Patients with SCC and moderate pain, but without myelopathy, may be treated with standard dose (16 mg/d) of dexamethasone for pain relief. Nonsteroidal antiinflammatory agents may serve as substitutes.
- Patients with SCC and signs of myelopathy should be treated initially with high doses of dexamethasone to increase their chance for posttreatment ambulation.[85]

This comes with moderate risk of serious toxicity, which has to be accepted in view of the expected benefit. The drug should be tapered off as soon as treatment with definitive modalities has been initiated.

Analgesia Because pain is the presenting symptom in more than 95% of patients with epidural SCC,[32,42,89,94] the principles of good analgesic management must be applied. In most patients, treatment with either radiotherapy alone or resection of tumor and restoration of stability frequently results in pain relief.[42,44,48] Neurosurgical procedures directed at pain control (e.g., cordotomy, rhizotomy) can be considered in patients with intractable pain from plexus or nerve root invasion, especially in those patients with limited life expectancy.[124]

Radiation Therapy

Table 27-4 summarizes the results of radiation therapy in patients with a variety of metastatic tumors. Between 28% and 50% of irradiated patients either regain or maintain ambulation at the end of therapy, and of those who survive 1 year, 50% maintain that improvement.[42,94] The proportion of patients who are ambulatory at diagnosis is increasing, and they comprise 42% to 64% of patients diagnosed with SCC.[33,42,85,98,100] Between 80% and 96% of patients who are ambulatory at diagnosis are likely to maintain mobility. However, 4% to 20% of patients who can walk at the start of treatment will deteriorate to nonambulatory status during or soon after completion of radiotherapy. Radiation therapy also results in pain relief in 50% to 80% of patients treated for SCC.[33,42,44,48,93,97,98]

The efficacy of radiation therapy depends on the radiosensitivity of the tumor, the patient's neurologic status at the time radiation therapy is undertaken, and maintenance of spinal stability. Patients with highly radiosensitive tumors (such as lymphoma, Ewing sarcoma, neuroblastoma, seminoma, and myeloma) are more likely to regain or maintain ambulation than are those with less radiosensitive tumors (overall 60%–80% vs. 40%).[48,58,102,111,113] Improvement after the initiation of radiation therapy may be delayed for a few days before it becomes evident, even in patients with radiosensitive tumors. This is of some concern, because 28% of severely paraparetic patients are expected to become paraplegic within 24 hours.[58] Radiotherapy should also be considered as primary therapy for moderately radiosensitive neoplasms, such as breast carcinoma. However, the need for surgical intervention should be critically reviewed for each patient. Radiotherapy is considered as the treatment of first choice for patients who are ambulatory at presentation, and whose spinal stability is maintained. However, in nonambulatory patients, surgical decompression should be considered as the primary avenue of therapy because radiotherapy requires a time interval that may cause an irreversible delay in the reduction of spinal cord damage. A randomized study assigned patients with SCC to primary treatment with either radiotherapy alone or to surgical decompression with stabilization followed by postoperative radiotherapy.[125] Patients treated by immediate direct surgical decompressive surgery plus radiotherapy retained the ability to walk longer and regained the ability to walk more often than patients treated by radiotherapy alone. Radiotherapy alone should be employed if surgery is contraindicated because of the patient's poor general medical status, multiple compression levels, or long-standing paraplegia.

The indication for primary radiotherapy is less clear for tumors generally regarded as poorly radioresponsive.

▶ **TABLE 27-4.** RESULTS OF TREATMENT FOR SPINAL CORD COMPRESSION: RADIOTHERAPY ALONE

First Authors	Year	Patients (n)	Improved (%)*	Worse (%)
Greenberg[94]	1980	83	57	7
Stark[168]	1982	31	35	—
Constans[95]	1983	108	39	26
Obbens[139]	1984	83	28	23
Harrison[140]	1985	33	27	36
Bach[40]	1990	149	35	18
Sorensen[85]	1994	27 (dexa)	50	0
		30 (no dexa)	18	12
Posner[42]	1995	54 (nonamb)	28	—
		96 (amb)	—	10
Helweg-Larsen[98]	1996	74 (nonamb)	28	—
		79 (amb)		
Huddart[100]	1997	69	52	—
Maranzano[141]	1997	41	38	8
Kovner[169]	1999	79	33	13
Brown[170]	1999	35 (colorectal cancer)	—	8.5
Zaidat[33]	2002	139	47	3
Mean		—	35	14
Total		1210	—	—

*Improvement was judged by motor-function criteria.
amb = ambulatory; dexa = dexamethasone; nonamb = nonambulatory.

Nevertheless, radiotherapy should be tried as a primary modality if the patient's neurologic deficit is not severe, and if the rate of progression of the deficit is such that there would be time to resort to surgical decompression should radiotherapy fail. Still, if the odds are that surgery will be required, the increased rate of postoperative complications observed in previously irradiated patients should be carefully weighed against the benefit of early surgical intervention. Where surgery is the primary therapy, postoperative radiation is traditionally employed to prevent regrowth of residual tumor and to contribute to pain relief.

No controlled studies have compared the various dose and fractionation schedules of radiation therapy given to patients with SCC.[60] Single-arm studies (see Table 27-4) and retrospective reviews of nonrandomized studies[107,126–128] suggest that neither the dose nor the fractionation schedule have major impact on outcome. The chosen treatment schedule should be a short palliative regimen at doses below spinal cord tolerance. The frequently used schedules are 20 Gy in 5 fractions, 28 Gy in 7 fractions, and 30 Gy in 10 fractions, prescribed to a depth of 5 to 8 cm using 4- to 8-megavolt (MV) photons. The treatment is given by single posterior field that should encompass the site of compression and the tumor causing it, with a 2- to 4-cm margin.

Surgery

Surgical treatment of SCC has been a subject of debate for a long time. A randomized trial compared direct decompressive surgical resection plus radiotherapy to treatment with radiotherapy alone.[125] This trial proved that primary treatment with surgical decompression and stabilization yields better outcome than treatment with radiotherapy alone. Prior to this study, surgical series suggested that a high proportion of nonambulatory patients regain ambulation.[99,102,129–138] However, the risk associated with operative morbidity and mortality should be carefully weighed against the expected gain from surgery (Table 27-5). Surgery is usually indicated for patients with SCC who have an expected survival that exceeds 3 to 6 months. This expected survival is longer than the overall median survival of patients with SCC, which ranges between 3 and 4 months.[33,34,86]

The traditional approach to the treatment of neoplastic SCC has been decompressive laminectomy, with or without postoperative radiation therapy.[38,40,42,85,94,95,98,100,101,111,135,139–141] Ambulation is maintained or regained in 35% to 50% of treated patients, a result similar to that achieved by radiation therapy alone (see Table 27-4). Pain is improved in 50% to 70% of patients after laminectomy, a rate that is also similar to radiation therapy. Patients treated by radiotherapy can deteriorate (see Table 27-4), which is also true following surgery. Approximately 15% of the patients are reported to have worse neurologic outcome after laminectomy. These results of laminectomy used as a decompressive surgery are similar to those reported for radiation therapy

TABLE 27-5. RESULTS OF TREATMENT FOR SPINAL CORD COMPRESSION: SURGERY—CASE-DEPENDENT APPROACH—VERTEBRAL BODY RESECTION, POSTERIOR DECOMPRESSION, AND COMBINED APPROACH WITH FIXATION AND RADIOTHERAPY BEFORE OR AFTER SURGERY*

Authors	Year	Patients (n)	Improved (%)†	Improved Pain (%)	Morbidity (%)	Operative Mortality (%)
Harrington[129]	1984	52	55	77	8	4
Siegal[130]	1985	61	80 ambulatory	91	11	6
Sundaresan[96]	1985	101	80 ambulatory	80	10	6
Ominus[171]	1986	36	72	97	—	6
Cooper[131]	1993	33	88 ambulatory	97	42	0
Posner[42]	1995	71	50 83 ambulatory	—	39	8
Sundaresan[99]	1995	110	82	90	48	5
Onimus[132]	1996	100	79	62	—	—
Walsh[172]	1997	61	75	90	30	8
Sapkas[173]	1997	20	80	—	25	—
Gokaslan[174]	1998	72	76	92	33	3
Wise[138]	1999	80	24	—	25	0
Hirabayashi[136]	2003	81	70 ambulatory	77	20	4
Mean		—	74	85	14	4.5
Total		878	—	—		

*Before or after radiotherapy.
†Improvement was judged by motor-function criteria.

alone; consequently, oncology literature favors initial radiotherapy in the majority of the patients, reserving surgery for salvage or diagnosis.

Laminectomy via the midline posterior approach is technically easy and safe, and allows for tissue diagnosis, but provides adequate decompression only when the tumor mass lies dorsolateral to the dura. Laminectomy also destabilizes the spine if the vertebral body and the pedicles are destroyed by tumor, and only allows a limited access to tumor lying ventral to the cord.

The reasons for surgical failures in the past were (a) nonselective use of one surgical approach, (b) inadequate tumor resection, (c) ineffective stabilization, and (d) poor patient selection. To obtain an effective decompression the surgical approach should be selected according to the location of the main compressing mass within the spinal canal. Spinal fixation should follow as an integral part of the decompressive procedure in order to establish spinal stability and restore ambulation.

Indications for Surgical Intervention

Figure 27-8 specifies the circumstances in which surgery should be considered, and although some of them are clear-cut, others need further evaluation.

Diagnosis in Doubt

In 8% to 20% of patients with neoplastic SCC, spinal involvement is the initial presentation of cancer.[41,101] When the etiology of the spinal lesion is in doubt, surgical decompression should be considered to obtain a tissue diagnosis and to achieve rapid decompression. Current image-assisted percutaneous needle biopsy of vertebral lesions is diagnostic in 95% of patients with no previous history of malignancy,[41,142] and has a reported complication rate of less then 1%. Therefore, surgery is rarely needed simply to establish the diagnosis of malignancy. If the biopsy shows a chemosensitive tumor (e.g., lymphoma), the patient can immediately proceed to treatment without the delay imposed by surgery. If the biopsy results are not diagnostic, or if the patient's ability to walk is already impaired and the neurologic status is unstable with rapidly evolving signs, surgical decompression is advisable to achieve an accurate prompt diagnosis and to initiate treatment without delay.

Spinal Instability or Bone Compression

A major goal of treatment is the restoration or maintenance of spinal stability. The determination of spinal instability is of paramount importance in choosing the appropriate form of management for patients with metastatic disease of the spine. The criteria for spinal stability in neoplastic disease of the spine are specified in "Clinical and Imaging Criteria for Spinal Stability in Neoplastic Disease" above. Apart from the neuroimaging studies that define anatomic details used in the three-column spinal model (see Fig. 27-1), the concept of clinical instability should be taken into account.[16] Clinical instability should be suspected whenever an incapacitating pain under physiologic loads develops and is associated with structural changes identified on imaging. Symptoms and signs should direct therapeutic consideration. Patients with fracture dislocation, localized kyphosis, collapsed vertebra with retropulsion of a bone fragment, or segmental instability, may require surgical decompression and stabilization if either pain or neurologic symptomatology is present. Not every case defined by the criteria for unstable spine requires surgical intervention. If the tumor is relatively radiosensitive, and no neurologic deficit is present, a course of radiotherapy may result in satisfactory axial settling and pain relief over a period of weeks or months. Bracing is optional in these patients, but in our experience it is rarely helpful. These patients should be carefully followed because they are potentially unstable.

When the anterior and middle columns are destroyed by tumor, treatment considerations should include decompression by the anterior approach to the spine as well as restoration of stability by vertebral body replacement constructs. If the posterior column structures are involved, then the treatment plan is to replace (or substitute) for the support role of these structures by posterior decompression combined with posterior instrumentation for maintenance of stability. Table 27-2 summarizes the criteria of spinal instability that should bring about consideration for spinal stabilization. Table 27-5 summarizes the results of surgical treatment in which decompression is combined with spinal stabilization. The criteria for patient selection, the surgical approach for decompression, and the methods of stabilization vary. Recommendations for patient selection and optimal methods of decompression and stabilization are undergoing constant development.

Previous Radiation Exposure

When radiotherapy cannot be used because of previous irradiation, surgical decompression is indicated as the primary therapeutic modality, even in highly radiosensitive tumors, because of the risk of exceeding spinal cord tolerance by further irradiation. Surgery is warranted for relapse occurring months or even years after a successful previous treatment, in the hope of preserving neurologic function. In many patients, however, life expectancy at the time of relapse of SCC is short. Re-treatment with radiotherapy often preserves ambulation with a low risk of radiation myelopathy during the remaining life span.[126,143–145]

Radioresistant Tumors

In radioresistant tumors, for example, renal cell carcinoma, decompressive surgery might be considered as the primary mode of therapy. Postoperative radiotherapy is administered with the hope of retarding tumor regrowth. However, this indication is not generally accepted, and sometimes, especially in neurologically stable patients, radiotherapy may be tried first.

Neurologic Deterioration During Radiotherapy

Neurologic deterioration occurring during radiotherapy of a relatively radiosensitive tumor should prompt an early consideration for surgical decompression. The decline in neurologic function may reflect radioresistance, progressive spinal instability, or bone compression secondary to vertebral collapse, all of which may be most effectively treated by spinal decompression and stabilization.

There has been concern that radiation therapy may result in neurologic deterioration, presumably by inducing radiation edema in the tumor, spinal cord, or both. So far, experimental studies do not support this concept[112]; therefore, deterioration represents treatment failure, prompting consideration of surgery as the alternative treatment.

Selection of Surgical Approach

The goal of surgery is the optimal removal of the compressing epidural mass and restoration and maintenance of spinal stability. Therefore, the selection of the surgical approach should be determined by variables such as the location of the tumor inside and outside the spinal canal, the main cause of the instability, and feasible options for stabilization. Table 27-6 details the preoperative assessment required for determining the surgical approach.

TABLE 27-6. PRETREATMENT ASSESSMENT OF TUMOR LOCATION AND EXTENT OF PATHOLOGY IN SPINE TUMORS

Bone involvement (CT, MRI)
- Vertebral body and pedicles, posterior elements, or a combination of both
- Number of vertebrae involved
- Percentage of bone mass loss of the vertebral cut surface

Epidural mass (CT myelography, MRI)
- Epidural mass related or unrelated to the bone lesion
- Number of spinal levels involved
- Position of the epidural mass: anterior, lateral, posterior, and/or encircling

Spinal stability (spinal radiography, CT, and MRI)
- Involvement of two or more adjacent vertebrae
- Involvement of two or more spinal columns as well as the vertebral cortical shell
- Loss of more than 50% of the vertebral width
- Shearing deformity
- Any combination of the above

Retroperitoneal and/or paravertebral mass (CT, MRI)
- Location
- Extent
- Involvement of adjacent structures or organs (kidneys, uterus, large vessels)
- Involvement of posterior chest or abdominal wall

The location of epidural compression should dictate the approach for decompression. Primary spinal tumors are classified based on tumor location and according to the zones of involvement (McLain and Weinstein classification),[146] and this information is used to determine the optimal surgical approach (Fig. 27-9). These guidelines are also applicable to metastatic spine lesions.

- Zone 1 includes the spinous process to the pars interarticularis and inferior facets and is best approached posteriorly.
- Zone 2 encompasses the superior articular facets, transverse process, and pedicle; tumors in this zone may be resected via a posterior or posterolateral approach.
- Zone 3 includes the anterior three-fourths of the vertebral body; tumors here are best approached anteriorly.
- Zone 4 is defined as the posterior fourth of the vertebral body, and is the most inaccessible region of the spine; a combined anterior and posterior approach is recommended for these lesions.

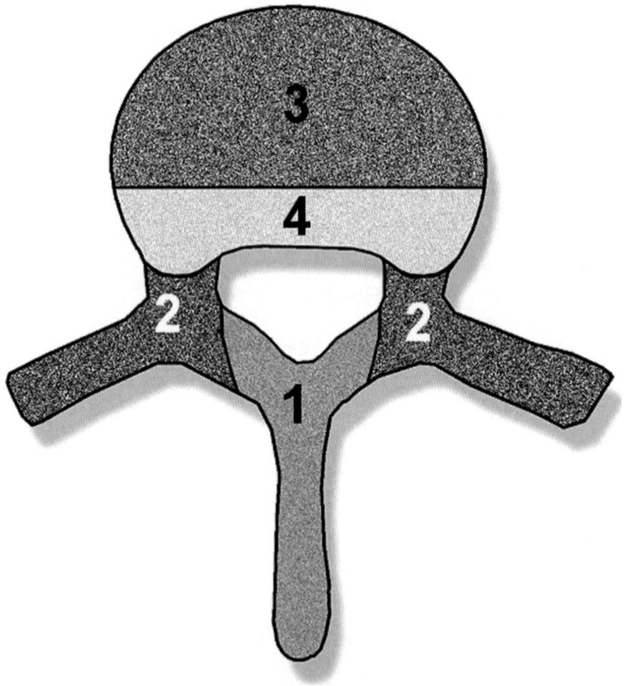

Figure 27-9. Classification system of McLain and Weinstein[146] suggested for determining the optimal surgical approach for resection of spinal tumors. The spine is divided into four zones of possible tumor involvement. Zone 1 is best approached posteriorly. Zone 2 tumors may be resected via a posterior or posterolateral approach. Zone 3 tumors are best approached anteriorly. Zone 4 is the most inaccessible region, hence a combined anterior and posterior approach may be recommended.

However, in patients with metastatic spine disease and limited life expectancy, radical excision of the vertebral tumor is not always the main goal; therefore selection of surgical approach also requires other considerations. In patients with progressive kyphosis without anterior cord compression, or in patients with thoracic or lumbar pathologic fracture or dislocation without significant soft-tissue or bony neural compromise, posterior realignment and stabilization may relieve pain and most cord impingement. In patients for whom the anterior approach is not feasible for technical reasons, poor medical status, or widespread disease, partial decompression and stabilization via a posterior approach may be a useful palliative procedure.[147]

Complications

Radiotherapy

Palliative radiotherapy to the spine is not a known cause of mortality. Most papers dealing with radiotherapy alone do not comment on complications of therapy or mortality. Death in the first month after radiotherapy is most likely the result of active primary or metastatic disease. The main determinants of survival are performance status and tumor burden; 70% of patients considered severely ill at the time of SCC diagnosis are reported to die within 30 days after diagnosis.[102] The risk of radiation myelopathy is related to dose/fractionation parameters, which, in palliative treatment, are below the level of spinal cord tolerance. The proportion of patients surviving for more than 2 years after diagnosis of neoplastic SCC is less than 3%, and these patients are at risk of developing radiation-induced myelopathy.[126] Of patients who survive for more than 18 months, 5% may develop symptomatic myelopathy.[126]

Surgical Complications

Mortality

The incidence of death within the first month after decompressive laminectomy ranges from 3% to 19%, with an average mortality rate of 8%.[42,148–151] The surgical mortality rate after vertebral body resection, 4% to 8%, falls within the same range (see Table 27-5).

Morbidity

The risk of neurologic deterioration as a result of surgery is a major concern in patients who present while they are still able to walk. It occurred in 5% to 30% of patients undergoing laminectomy (mean of 14%).[42,92,152,153] Neurologic deterioration is rare after vertebral body resection, and occurs in only 2% to 6% of patients.[96,102,129,154]

In patients undergoing laminectomy combined with radiotherapy, nonneurologic complications include wound infection, wound dehiscence, spinal epidural hematoma, cerebrospinal fluid leak, and spinal instability. The frequency

▶ TABLE 27-7. NONNEUROLOGIC SURGERY-RELATED MORBIDITY IN NEOPLASTIC SPINAL CORD DECOMPRESSION

	Morbidity (%)	
Surgical Procedure	**Range**	**Average**
Laminectomy	8–54	15
Laminectomy and fixation	1–21	11
Vertebral body resection and fixation	8–41	23
Patient-specific approach (anterior, posterior, or both) and fixation	25–48	37

of these complications ranges from 8% to 54%, with a mean of 12%.[42,59] Only a few authors mentioned the problem of instability,[42,101] which amounts to approximately 9% of cases.

As the use of instrumentation increases, nonneurologic complications, especially instrumentation-related complications such as dislodgment and infections, are increasing (Table 27-7). Preoperative protein depletion and perioperative administration of corticosteroids are risk factors for wound infection in patients undergoing surgery for spine metastases.[138,155] The likelihood of postoperative complications is significantly increased in patients with poor neurologic outcome, and in patients who develop severe motor deficit prior to surgery.[138] Spinal radiation before surgical decompression is associated with a significantly higher rate of major wound complications.[156,157] Patients with preoperative irradiation had a 32% major wound complication rate that was threefold higher than the 12% rate observed in patients who underwent de novo surgery.[157] It should be noted that a tailored, patient-specific approach, including vertebral body resection and spinal instrumentation techniques, requires considerable expertise. These procedures should be undertaken only by a surgeon familiar with the specific techniques for posterior and anterior spinal instrumentation, with different options to suit specific levels along the spine.

Recurrent Epidural Spinal Cord Compression

Approximately 10% of patients will eventually develop local recurrence of spinal epidural metastasis. Most of these patients have received radiotherapy and some have had previous surgery. Little attention has been paid to this subgroup of patients. For the majority, no reliably effective chemotherapy option remains at this stage of their disease. Spinal surgery should be considered in these patients, although many have advanced visceral disease limiting their life expectancy to a few months, or widespread spinal metastases, which limit surgical feasibility. Surgical decompression after previous radiotherapy is associated with an increased rate of morbidity.[156,157] A retrospective study of 51 patients undergoing a second course of spinal radiation found that re-irradiation was highly successful in preserving neurologic function and rarely resulted in radiation myelopathy.[143]

Conclusions for Epidural Metastases

This chapter is a plea for early diagnosis and treatment of neoplastic SCC secondary to epidural extension of metastases. A high index of suspicion is essential, especially in patients known to harbor a neoplastic process. Wider acceptance and judicious use of modern and novel surgical techniques for spinal decompression and stabilization may improve the quality of life of subgroups of patients too often denied such treatment. Early consideration of surgery in patients with life expectancy greater than 6 months may bring about improved mobility, better quality of life, fewer surgical complications, and longer survival. Prospective randomized clinical trials are highly needed to identify patients most likely to benefit from advanced surgical techniques.

▶ INTRADURAL METASTASES

Metastatic disease within the confines of the dura constitutes less than 5% of all metastatic spinal tumors. Intradural metastases that affect the spinal cord can be categorized into those that involve the subarachnoid space, causing intradural spinal cord compression (Fig. 27-10), and into intramedullary metastasis that invade the cord substance (Fig. 27-11).

Intradural Extramedullary Metastases

Metastatic tumors involving the subarachnoid space are by definition leptomeningeal metastases. Unlike the multifocal manifestations produced by diffuse seeding of the subarachnoid space, this form of spinal metastatic spread may present as a single intradural extramedullary mass lesion compressing the spinal cord.[158–160] The clinical features of these metastases are essentially identical to those of patients with epidural spinal cord compression. Primary tumors in a series of 10 patients included breast,

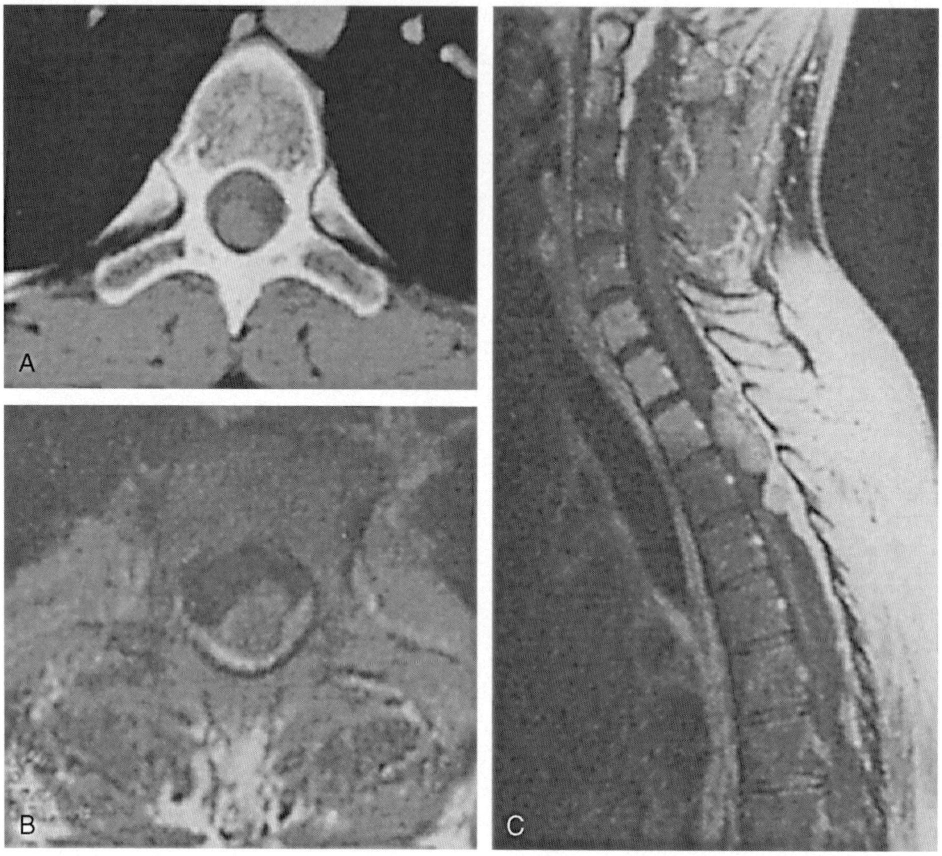

Figure 27-10. Intradural extramedullary metastases of a malignant melanoma. (A) A nonenhanced CT study reveals a posterior hyperdense mass lesion within the spinal canal at T3. The patient presented with severe localized upper back pain with no signs of myelopathy. (B) Axial MRI view (enhanced T_1-weighted image) confirms the intradural extramedullary position of the tumor mass. (C) The MRI study (enhanced T_1-weighted image with fat suppression, sagittal view) reveals a multilobulated enhancing posterior intradural extramedullary mass. Note the enhancing irregular dural tails extending both rostral and caudal.

lung, melanoma, and uterine neoplasm, in a descending order of frequency.[159] Of the 10 tumors, 9 appeared to have spread from a brain metastasis via the cerebrospinal fluid pathway. In another series of 10 patients, brain metastases preceded the spinal spread in 80% of cases.[158] The intradural location of the tumor can be identified by MRI evaluation (see Fig. 27-10). The treatment of choice is probably radiotherapy. However, if neurologic deterioration is relentless and there is no evidence for diffuse spread of metastatic disease in the subarachnoid space, then surgical intervention may be justified.

Intramedullary Metastases

Intramedullary spinal metastases arise either from direct hematogenous spread to the parenchyma of the spinal cord, or by growth of subarachnoid tumor along nerve roots directly into the spinal cord.[161] Intramedullary metastases comprise 8.5% of all central nervous system (CNS) metastases, and 2% of cancer cases who had autopsy. Lung cancer is a common primary tumor, and accounts for approximately 50% of these metastasis, equally dividing between small cell and non–small cell tumors.[5,7,42,161,162] Breast cancer accounts for approximately 15% of these metastases, with lymphoma and melanoma each contributing another 10% of cases.[5,42,161,162] Intramedullary spinal cord metastases were the initial manifestation of malignancy for approximately 30% of cases in two series, although this was considered a rare presentation of cancer.[5,163]

Disease at other levels of the neuraxis is common in patients with intramedullary metastases[5,6,162]; approximately 50% of patients have brain metastases and 30% have multiple spinal cord metastases. Brain metastases are almost invariably diagnosed prior to the intramedullary lesion, although in some patients the diagnosis is simultaneous. Leptomeningeal seeding coexists in 15% to 44% of

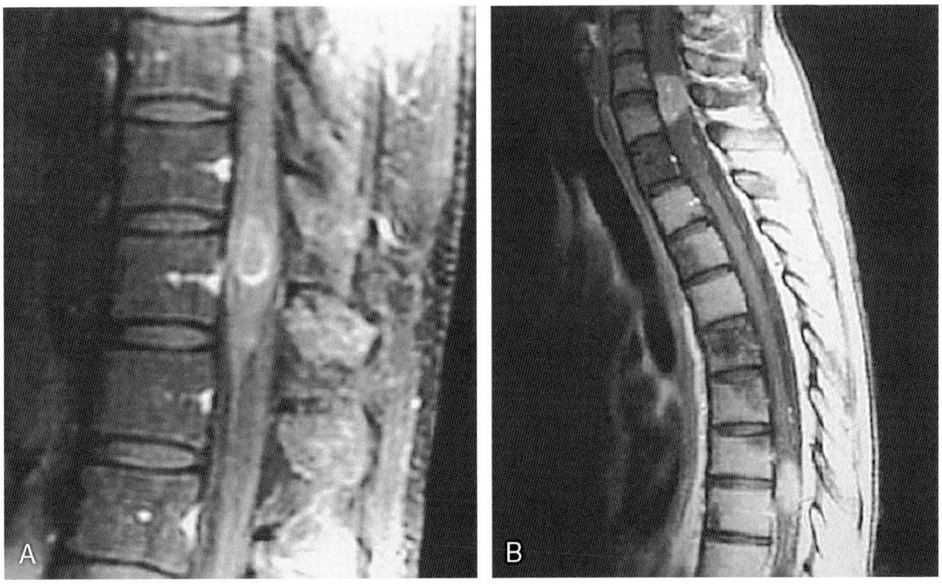

Figure 27-11. Intramedullary metastases. (A) MRI (enhanced T_1-weighted image) shows an enhancing intramedullary metastasis at the T11 vertebral level. The patient had a known metastatic breast carcinoma. Note the associated spinal cord swelling. (B) A patient with a metastatic non–small cell lung carcinoma with a previous history of brain metastases presented with back pain and myelopathy. MRI (enhanced T_1-weighted image) reveals two enhancing intradural lesions. The lesion at the level of C7-T1 is located intradurally, but it is an extramedullary metastasis. The second lesion at the T8-T9 vertebral level is an intramedullary metastasis with an oval-shaped enhancement. Note the vertebral body metastases at multiple levels.

patients, and one autopsy study showed that seeding was associated with focal or multifocal direct extension of the leptomeningeal tumor across the pia into the parenchyma of the spinal cord.[161]

The clinical features of intramedullary metastases at diagnosis include pain in approximately 50% of patients, sensory deficit in more than 80%, weakness in 90%, and urinary incontinence in more than 60%.[5,42,162] None of these features reliably differentiates intramedullary metastases from malignant epidural SCC. However, markedly asymmetric dysfunction of the spinal cord (Brown-Sequard or pseudo–Brown-Sequard syndrome), reported in approximately 30% of cases, is suggestive of intramedullary rather than extramedullary lesion.

Contrast-enhanced MRI is the ultimate diagnostic examination, but when contraindicated, CT-myelography should be performed.[5,6] Myelography is less sensitive than MRI and yields a positive diagnosis in only 50% to 80% of symptomatic cases.[5,42] MRI findings show that intramedullary metastases are most commonly isolated, small oval-shaped lesions, without or with slight deformation of the spinal profile (see Fig. 27-11). The lesions are isointense on spin-echo T_1-weighted images, with significant homogenous nodular contrast enhancement, and pencil-shaped hyperintensity, frequently extending cranially to the lesion, on spin-echo proton density and T_2-weighted sequences.[6] Lumbosacral myelomeres are the most frequently affected segments, but involvement of the thoracic and cervical myelomeres is often encountered. Because multiple spinal lesions are found in approximately 33% of patients, the MRI study should be extended to encompass the entire spine or the whole neuraxis.

Differential diagnoses include primary intramedullary tumors such as glioma or ependymoma, radiation myelopathy in previously irradiated patients, spinal cord infarction from embolus or vascular occlusion, and paraneoplastic necrotic myelopathy. In patients with no previous history of malignancy, the differential diagnosis also includes myelitis or acute demyelinating plaque. Imaging evaluation of the whole neuraxis combined with careful history and neurologic examination may aid in the differential diagnosis.

Intramedullary metastases commonly develop late in the course of a widespread cancer. The median survival from diagnosis of the intramedullary lesion is approximately 4 months.[5] Patients with radiosensitive or relatively radiosensitive neoplasms may respond to radiotherapy. Most patients who are ambulatory when diagnosed will experience durable stabilization of function when given treatment with dexamethasone and radiotherapy.

In a small subset of patients, surgical resection of an intramedullary lesion should be considered. This is frequently the case if the diagnosis is doubtful, or when the intramedullary lesion is the first manifestation of malignancy. As with brain metastases, the intramedullary deposits are frequently circumscribed with little invasion of the surrounding spinal medulla, thus amenable for gross total resection. In patients with a known diagnosis of cancer, radiation may be considered when the metastasis is isolated, and when the mode of spread is likely to be hematogenic rather than via the subarachnoid space. A few patients who underwent surgical removal of intramedullary metastases are reported to have long-term survival with good neurologic function after treatment.[164–167]

REFERENCES

1. Talcott JA, Stomper PC, Drislane FW, et al. Assessing suspected spinal cord compression: a multidisciplinary outcomes analysis of 342 episodes. Support Care Cancer 1999;7(1):31–38.
2. Cook AM, Lau TN, Tomlinson MJ, et al. Magnetic resonance imaging of the whole spine in suspected malignant spinal cord compression: impact on management. Clin Oncol 1998;10(1):39–43.
3. Ross JR, Saunders Y, Edmonds PM, et al. Systematic review of role of bisphosphonates on skeletal morbidity in metastatic cancer. BMJ 2003;327(7413):469.
4. Pavlakis N, Stockler M. Bisphosphonates for breast cancer. Cochrane Database Syst Rev 2002(1):CD003474.
5. Schiff D, O'Neill BP. Intramedullary spinal cord metastases: clinical features and treatment outcome. Neurology 1996;47(4):906–912.
6. Crasto S, Duca S, Davini O, et al. MRI diagnosis of intramedullary metastases from extra-CNS tumors. Eur Radiol 1997;7(5):732–736.
7. Potti A, Abdel-Raheem M, Levitt R, et al. Intramedullary spinal cord metastases (ISCM) and non-small cell lung carcinoma (NSCLC): clinical patterns, diagnosis and therapeutic considerations. Lung Cancer 2001;31(2–3):319–323.
8. Rosen LS, Gordon D, Tchekmedyian S, et al. Zoledronic acid versus placebo in the treatment of skeletal metastases in patients with lung cancer and other solid tumors: a phase III, double-blind, randomized trial—the Zoledronic Acid Lung Cancer and Other Solid Tumors Study Group. J Clin Oncol 2003;21(16):3150–3157.
9. Schaberg J, Gainor BJ. A profile of metastatic carcinoma of the spine. Spine 1985;10(1):19–20.
10. Abrams HL, Spiro R, Goldstein N. Metastases in carcinoma. Analysis of 1000 autopsied cases. Cancer 1950;3:74–85.
11. Vande Berg BC, Lecouvet FE, Michaux L, et al. Magnetic resonance imaging of the bone marrow in hematological malignancies. Eur Radiol 1998;8(8):1335–1344.
12. Denis F. Spinal instability as defined by the three-column spine concept in acute spinal trauma. Clin Orthop 1984(189): 65–76.
13. Kostuik JP, Errico JN. Differential diagnosis and surgical treatment of metastatic spine tumors. In: Frymoyer JW, ed. The adult spine. New York: Raven Press, 1991:861–888.
14. Khaw FM, Worthy SA, Gibson MJ, et al. The appearance on MRI of vertebrae in acute compression of the spinal cord due to metastases. J Bone Joint Surg Br 1999;81(5):830–834.
15. Bradford DS. Spinal instability: orthopedic perspective and prevention. Clin Neurosurg 1980;27:591–610.
16. White AAI, Panjabi MM. Clinical biomechanics of the spine. Philadelphia: JB Lippincott, 1987:191–276.
17. Sze WM, Shelley MD, Held I, et al. Palliation of metastatic bone pain: single fraction versus multifraction radiotherapy—a systematic review of randomised trials. Clin Oncol (R Coll Radiol) 2003;15(6):345–352.
18. Saarto T, Janes R, Tenhunen M, et al. Palliative radiotherapy in the treatment of skeletal metastases. Eur J Pain 2002;6(5):323–330.
19. Jeremic B. Single fraction external beam radiation therapy in the treatment of localized metastatic bone pain [a review]. J Pain Symptom Manage 2001;22(6):1048–1058.
20. Fleisch H. Development of bisphosphonates. Breast Cancer Res 2002;4(1):30–34.
21. Fleisch H. Bisphosphonates in osteoporosis. Eur Spine J 2003:(Suppl 2):142–146.
22. Baur A, Stabler A, Arbogast S, et al. Acute osteoporotic and neoplastic vertebral compression fractures: fluid sign at MR imaging. Radiology 2002;225(3):730–735.
23. Jung HS, Jee WH, McCauley TR, et al. Discrimination of metastatic from acute osteoporotic compression spinal fractures with MR imaging. Radiographics 2003;23(1):179–187.
24. Kim JK, Learch TJ, Colletti PM, et al. Diagnosis of vertebral metastasis, epidural metastasis, and malignant spinal cord compression: are T(1)-weighted sagittal images sufficient? Magn Reson Imaging 2000;18(7):819–824.
25. Shon IH, Fogelman I. F-18 FDG positron emission tomography and benign fractures. Clin Nucl Med 2003;28(3): 171–175.
26. Peh WC, Gilula LA. Percutaneous vertebroplasty: indications, contraindications, and technique. Br J Radiol 2003; 76(901):69–75.
27. Fourney DR, Schomer DF, Nader R, et al. Percutaneous vertebroplasty and kyphoplasty for painful vertebral body fractures in cancer patients. J Neurosurg 2003;98(Suppl 1): 21–30.
28. Yeom JS, Kim WJ, Choy WS, et al. Leakage of cement in percutaneous transpedicular vertebroplasty for painful osteoporotic compression fractures. J Bone Joint Surg Br 2003;85(1):83–89.
29. Mousavi P, Roth S, Finkelstein J, et al. Volumetric quantification of cement leakage following percutaneous vertebroplasty in metastatic and osteoporotic vertebrae. J Neurosurg 2003;99(Suppl 1):56–59.
30. Alvarez L, Perez-Higueras A, Quinones D, et al. Vertebroplasty in the treatment of vertebral tumors: postprocedural outcome and quality of life. Eur Spine J 2003;12(4): 356–360.
31. Coumans JV, Reinhardt MK, Lieberman IH. Kyphoplasty for vertebral compression fractures: 1-year clinical outcomes from a prospective study. J Neurosurg 2003;99(Suppl 1): 44–50.
32. Levack P, Graham J, Collie D, et al. Don't wait for a sensory level—listen to the symptoms: a prospective audit of

the delays in diagnosis of malignant cord compression. Clin Oncol (R Coll Radiol) 2002;14(6):472–480.
33. Zaidat OO, Ruff RL. Treatment of spinal epidural metastasis improves patient survival and functional state. Neurology 2002;58(9):1360–1366.
34. Loblaw DA, Laperriere NJ, Mackillop WJ. A population-based study of malignant spinal cord compression in Ontario. Clin Oncol (R Coll Radiol) 2003;15(4):211–217.
35. Helweg-Larsen S, Sorensen PS, Kreiner S. Prognostic factors in metastatic spinal cord compression: a prospective study using multivariate analysis of variables influencing survival and gait function in 153 patients. Int J Radiat Oncol Biol Phys 2000;46(5):1163–1169.
36. Schiff D, O'Neill BP, Wang CH, et al. Neuroimaging and treatment implications of patients with multiple epidural spinal metastases. Cancer 1998;83(8):1593–1601.
37. Husband DJ, Grant KA, Romaniuk CS. MRI in the diagnosis and treatment of suspected malignant spinal cord compression. Br J Radiol 2001;74(877):15–23.
38. Cobb CA 3rd, Leavens ME, Eckles N. Indications for nonoperative treatment of spinal cord compression due to breast cancer. J Neurosurg 1977;47(5):653–658.
39. Barron KD, Hirano A, Araki S, et al. Experiences with metastatic neoplasms involving the spinal cord. Neurology 1959;9(2):91–106.
40. Bach F, Larsen BH, Rohde K, et al. Metastatic spinal cord compression. Occurrence, symptoms, clinical presentations and prognosis in 398 patients with spinal cord compression. Acta Neurochir 1990;107(1–2):37–43.
41. Schiff D, O'Neill BP, Suman VJ. Spinal epidural metastasis as the initial manifestation of malignancy: clinical features and diagnostic approach. Neurology 1997;49(2):452–456.
42. Posner JB. Spinal metastases. In: Posner JB, ed. Neurologic complications of cancer. Philadelphia: FA Davis, 1995: 111–142.
43. Chamberlain MC, Kormanik PA. Epidural spinal cord compression: a single institution's retrospective experience. Neuro-oncol 1999;1(2):120–123.
44. Byrne TN. Spinal cord compression from epidural metastases. N Engl J Med 1992;327(9):614–619.
45. Raffel C, Neave VC, Lavine S, et al. Treatment of spinal cord compression by epidural malignancy in childhood. Neurosurgery 1991;28(3):349–352.
46. Klein SL, Sanford RA, Muhlbauer MS. Pediatric spinal epidural metastases. J Neurosurg 1991;74(1):70–75.
47. Bouffet E, Marec-Berard P, Thiesse P, et al. Spinal cord compression by secondary epi- and intradural metastases in childhood. Childs Nerv Syst 1997;13(7):383–387.
48. Siegal T, Siegal T. Spinal epidural metastases from solid tumors. In: Twijnstra A, Keyser A, Ongerboer de Visser BW, eds. Clinical diagnosis and management. Amsterdam, The Netherlands: Elsevier Science, 1993:283–305.
49. Portenoy RK, Galer BS, Salamon O, et al. Identification of epidural neoplasm. Radiography and bone scintigraphy in the symptomatic and asymptomatic spine. Cancer 1989; 64(11):2207–2213.
50. Asdourian PL, Weidenbaum M, DeWald RL, et al. The pattern of vertebral involvement in metastatic vertebral breast cancer. Clin Orthop 1990;(250):164–170.
51. Graus F, Krol G, Foley KM. Early diagnosis of spinal epidural metastases: correlation with clinical and radiological findings. Proc Am Soc Clin Oncol 1985;4:269.
52. Carmody RF, Yang PJ, Seeley GW, et al. Spinal cord compression due to metastatic disease: diagnosis with MR imaging versus myelography. Radiology 1989;173(1):225–229.
53. Colletti PM, Dang HT, Deseran MW, et al. Spinal MR imaging in suspected metastases: correlation with skeletal scintigraphy. Magn Reson Imaging 1991;9(3):349–355.
54. Heldmann U, Myschetzky PS, Thomsen HS. Frequency of unexpected multifocal metastasis in patients with acute spinal cord compression. Evaluation by low-field MR imaging in cancer patients. Acta Radiol 1997;38(3):372–375.
55. Colletti PM, Siegel HJ, Woo MY, et al. The impact on treatment planning of MRI of the spine in patients suspected of vertebral metastasis: an efficacy study. Comput Med Imaging Graph 1996;20(3):159–162.
56. Jordan JE, Donaldson SS, Enzmann DR. Cost effectiveness and outcome assessment of magnetic resonance imaging in diagnosing cord compression. Cancer 1995;75(10): 2579–2586.
57. Solberg A, Bremnes RM. Metastatic spinal cord compression: diagnostic delay, treatment, and outcome. Anticancer Res 1999;19(1B):677–684.
58. Barcena A, Lobato RD, Rivas JJ, et al. Spinal metastatic disease: analysis of factors determining functional prognosis and the choice of treatment. Neurosurgery 1984;15(6): 820–827.
59. Findlay GF. Adverse effects of the management of malignant spinal cord compression. J Neurol Neurosurg Psychiatry 1984;47(8):761–768.
60. Loblaw DA, Laperriere NJ. Emergency treatment of malignant extradural spinal cord compression: an evidence-based guideline. J Clin Oncol 1998;16(4):1613–1624.
61. Hainline B, Tuszynski MH, Posner JB. Ataxia in epidural spinal cord compression. Neurology 1992;42(11):2193–2195.
62. Ushio Y, Posner R, Kim JH, et al. Treatment of experimental spinal cord compression caused by extradural neoplasms. J Neurosurg 1977;47(3):380–390.
63. Ushio Y, Posner R, Posner JB, et al. Experimental spinal cord compression by epidural neoplasm. Neurology 1977; 27(5):422–429.
64. Ikeda H, Ushio Y, Hayakawa T, et al. Edema and circulatory disturbance in the spinal cord compressed by epidural neoplasms in rabbits. J Neurosurg 1980;52(2):203–209.
65. Kato A, Ushio Y, Hayakawa T, et al. Circulatory disturbance of the spinal cord with epidural neoplasm in rats. J Neurosurg 1985;63(2):260–265.
66. Delattre JY, Arbit E, Thaler HT, et al. A dose–response study of dexamethasone in a model of spinal cord compression caused by epidural tumor. J Neurosurg 1989;70(6):920–925.
67. Siegal T, Shapira Y, Sandbank U, et al. Indomethacin and dexamethasone treatment in experimental neoplastic spinal cord compression: Part 1. Effect on water content and specific gravity. Neurosurgery 1988;22(2):328–333.
68. Siegal T, Shohami E, Shapira Y. Indomethacin and dexamethasone treatment in experimental neoplastic spinal cord compression: Part 2. Effect on edema and prostaglandin synthesis. Neurosurgery 1988;22(2):334–339.

69. Siegal T, Shohami E, Shapira Y. Comparison of soluble dexamethasone sodium phosphate with free dexamethasone and indomethacin in treatment of experimental neoplastic spinal cord compression. Spine 1988;13(10):1171–1176.
70. Siegal T, Siegal T, Shapira Y, et al. The early effect of steroidal and non-steroidal anti-inflammatory agents on neoplastic epidural cord compression. Ann NY Acad Sci 1989;559:488–490.
71. Siegal T, Lossos F. Experimental neoplastic spinal cord compression: effect of anti-inflammatory agents and glutamate receptor antagonists on vascular permeability. Neurosurgery 1990;26(6):967–970.
72. Siegal T, Shohami E, Lossos F. Experimental neoplastic spinal cord compression: effect of ketamine and MK-801 on edema and prostaglandins. Neurosurgery 1990;26(6): 963–966.
73. Siegal T. Participation of serotonergic mechanisms in the pathophysiology of experimental neoplastic spinal cord compression. Neurology 1991;41(4):574–580.
74. Siegal T. Serotonergic manipulations in experimental neoplastic spinal cord compression. J Neurosurg 1993;78(6): 929–937.
75. Siegal T. Spinal cord compression: from laboratory to clinic. Eur J Cancer 1995;31A(11):1748–1753.
76. Siegal T, Siegal TZ, Sandbank U, et al. Experimental neoplastic spinal cord compression: evoked potentials, edema, prostaglandins, and light and electron microscopy. Spine 1987;12(5):440–448.
77. Ishikawa M, Sekizuka E, Krischek B, et al. Role of nitric oxide in the regulation of spinal arteriolar tone. Neurosurgery 2002;50(2):371–377; discussion 377–378.
78. Casha S, Yu WR, Fehlings MG. Oligodendroglial apoptosis occurs along degenerating axons and is associated with FAS and p75 expression following spinal cord injury in the rat. Neuroscience 2001;103(1):203–218.
79. Blight AR, Decrescito V. Morphometric analysis of experimental spinal cord injury in the cat: the relation of injury intensity to survival of myelinated axons. Neuroscience 1986;19(1):321–341.
80. Waxman SG. Demyelination in spinal cord injury. J Neurol Sci 1989;91(1–2):1–14.
81. Gledhill RF, McDonald WI. Morphological characteristics of central demyelination and remyelination: a single-fiber study. Ann Neurol 1977;1(6):552–560.
82. Siegal T, Shezen E, Siegal T. The effect of in vivo inhibition of phagocytic activity in experimental neoplastic spinal cord compression: Immunohistochemistry, vascular permeability and neurologic function [abstract P269]. J Neurooncol 1994;21:68.
83. Farooque M, Isaksson J, Olsson Y. Improved recovery after spinal cord injury in neuronal nitric oxide synthase-deficient mice but not in TNF-alpha-deficient mice. J Neurotrauma 2001;18(1):105–114.
84. Farooque M, Isaksson J, Olsson Y. White matter preservation after spinal cord injury in ICAM-1/P-selectin-deficient mice. Acta Neuropathol (Berl) 2001;102(2):132–140.
85. Sorensen S, Helweg-Larsen S, Mouridsen H, et al. Effect of high-dose dexamethasone in carcinomatous metastatic spinal cord compression treated with radiotherapy: a randomised trial. Eur J Cancer 1994;30A(1):22–27.
86. Guo Y, Young B, Palmer JL, et al. Prognostic factors for survival in metastatic spinal cord compression: a retrospective study in a rehabilitation setting. Am J Phys Med Rehabil 2003;82(9):665–668.
87. McKinley WO, Huang ME, Tewksbury MA. Neoplastic vs. traumatic spinal cord injury: an inpatient rehabilitation comparison. Am J Phys Med Rehabil 2000;79(2):138–144.
88. Rades D, Heidenreich F, Bremer M, et al. Time of developing motor deficits before radiotherapy as a new and relevant prognostic factor in metastatic spinal cord compression: final results of a retrospective analysis. Eur Neurol 2001; 45(4):266–269.
89. Schiff D. Spinal cord compression. Neurol Clin 2003;21(1): 67–86, viii.
90. Podd TJ, Carpenter DS, Baughan CA, et al. Spinal cord compression: prognosis and implications for treatment fractionation. Clin Oncol (R Coll Radiol) 1992;4(6):341–344.
91. Tatsui H, Onomura T, Morishita S, et al. Survival rates of patients with metastatic spinal cancer after scintigraphic detection of abnormal radioactive accumulation. Spine 1996;21(18):2143–2148.
92. Bauer HC, Wedin R. Survival after surgery for spinal and extremity metastases. Prognostication in 241 patients. Acta Orthop Scand 1995;66(2):143–146.
93. Maranzano E, Latini P. Effectiveness of radiation therapy without surgery in metastatic spinal cord compression: final results from a prospective trial. Int J Radiat Oncol Biol Phys 1995;32(4):959–967.
94. Greenberg HS, Kim JH, Posner JB. Epidural spinal cord compression from metastatic tumor: results with a new treatment protocol. Ann Neurol 1980;8(4):361–366.
95. Constans JP, de Divitiis E, Donzelli R, et al. Spinal metastases with neurological manifestations. Review of 600 cases. J Neurosurg 1983;59(1):111–118.
96. Sundaresan N, Galicich JH, Lane JM, et al. Treatment of neoplastic epidural cord compression by vertebral body resection and stabilization. J Neurosurg 1985;63(5):676–684.
97. Turner S, Marosszeky B, Timms I, et al. Malignant spinal cord compression: a prospective evaluation. Int J Radiat Oncol Biol Phys 1993;26(1):141–146.
98. Helweg-Larsen S. Clinical outcome in metastatic spinal cord compression. A prospective study of 153 patients. Acta Neurol Scand 1996;94(4):269–275.
99. Sundaresan N, Sachdev VP, Holland JF, et al. Surgical treatment of spinal cord compression from epidural metastasis. J Clin Oncol 1995;13(9):2330–2335.
100. Huddart RA, Rajan B, Law M, et al. Spinal cord compression in prostate cancer: treatment outcome and prognostic factors. Radiother Oncol 1997;44(3):229–236.
101. Gilbert RW, Kim JH, Posner JB. Epidural spinal cord compression from metastatic tumor: diagnosis and treatment. Ann Neurol 1978;3(1):40–51.
102. Siegal T. Surgical decompression of anterior and posterior malignant epidural tumors compressing the spinal cord: a prospective study. Neurosurgery 1985;17(3):424–432.
103. Husband DJ. Malignant spinal cord compression: prospective study of delays in referral and treatment. BMJ 1998; 317(7150):18–21.
104. Helweg-Larsen S, Sorensen PS. Symptoms and signs in metastatic spinal cord compression: a study of progression

from first symptom until diagnosis in 153 patients. Eur J Cancer 1994;30A(3):396–398.
105. Rades D, Blach M, Bremer M, et al. Prognostic significance of the time of developing motor deficits before radiation therapy in metastatic spinal cord compression: one-year results of a prospective trial. Int J Radiat Oncol Biol Phys 2000;48(5):1403–1408.
106. Rades D, Heidenreich F, Karstens JH. Final results of a prospective study of the prognostic value of the time to develop motor deficits before irradiation in metastatic spinal cord compression. Int J Radiat Oncol Biol Phys 2002;53(4):975–979.
107. Rades D, Karstens JH, Alberti W. Role of radiotherapy in the treatment of motor dysfunction due to metastatic spinal cord compression: comparison of three different fractionation schedules. Int J Radiat Oncol Biol Phys 2002; 54(4):1160–1164.
108. Helweg-Larsen S, Rasmusson B, Sorensen PS. Recovery of gait after radiotherapy in paralytic patients with metastatic epidural spinal cord compression. Neurology 1990;40(8): 1234–1236.
109. Vecht CJ, Haaxma-Reiche H, van Putten WL, et al. Initial bolus of conventional versus high-dose dexamethasone in metastatic spinal cord compression. Neurology 1989;39(9): 1255–1257.
110. Clarke PR, Saunders M. Steroid-induced remission in spinal canal reticulum cell sarcoma. Report of two cases. J Neurosurg 1975;42(3):346–348.
111. Marshall LF, Langfitt TW. Combined therapy for metastatic extradural tumors of the spine. Cancer 1977;40(5):2067–2070.
112. Siegal T. Current considerations in the management of neoplastic spinal cord compression. Spine 1989;14(2):223–228.
113. Siegal T, Siegal T. Spinal epidural involvement in haematological tumors: clinical features and therapeutic options. Leuk Lymphoma 1991;5:101–110.
114. Wong ET, Portlock CS, O'Brien JP, et al. Chemosensitive epidural spinal cord disease in non-Hodgkin's lymphoma. Neurology 1996;46(6):1543–1547.
115. Cooper K, Bajorin D, Shapiro W, et al. Decompression of epidural metastases from germ cell tumors with chemotherapy. J Neurooncol 1990;8(3):275–280.
116. Gale GB, O'Connor DM, Chu JY, et al. Successful chemotherapeutic decompression of epidural malignant germ cell tumor. Med Pediatr Oncol 1986;14(2):97–99.
117. Gale J, Mead GM, Simmonds PD. Management of spinal cord and cauda equina compression secondary to epidural metastatic disease in adults with malignant germ cell tumours. Clin Oncol (R Coll Radiol) 2002;14(6):481–490.
118. Hayes FA, Thompson EI, Hvizdala E, et al. Chemotherapy as an alternative to laminectomy and radiation in the management of epidural tumor. J Pediatr 1984;104(2): 221–224.
119. Fadul CE, Lemann W, Thaler HT, et al. Perforation of the gastrointestinal tract in patients receiving steroids for neurologic disease. Neurology 1988;38(3):348–352.
120. Weissman DE. Glucocorticoid treatment for brain metastases and epidural spinal cord compression: a review. J Clin Oncol 1988;6(3):543–551.
121. Weiner HL, Rezai AR, Cooper PR. Sigmoid diverticular perforation in neurosurgical patients receiving high-dose corticosteroids. Neurosurgery 1993;33(1):40–43.
122. Martenson JA Jr, Evans RG, Lie MR, et al. Treatment outcome and complications in patients treated for malignant epidural spinal cord compression (SCC). J Neurooncol 1985;3(1): 77–84.
123. Maranzano E, Latini P, Beneventi S, et al. Radiotherapy without steroids in selected metastatic spinal cord compression patients. A phase II trial. Am J Clin Oncol 1996; 19(2):179–183.
124. Sundaresan N, DiGiacinto GV. Antitumor and antinociceptive approaches to control cancer pain. Med Clin North Am 1987;71(2):329–348.
125. Regine WF, Tibbs PA, Young A, et al. Metastatic spinal cord compression: a randomized trial of direct decompressive surgical resection plus radiotherapy vs. radiotherapy alone. Int J Radiat Oncol Biol Phys 2003;57(Suppl 2): S125.
126. Maranzano E, Bellavita R, Floridi P, et al. Radiation-induced myelopathy in long-term surviving metastatic spinal cord compression patients after hypofractionated radiotherapy: a clinical and magnetic resonance imaging analysis. Radiother Oncol 2001;60(3):281–288.
127. Hoskin PJ, Grover A, Bhana R. Metastatic spinal cord compression: radiotherapy outcome and dose fractionation. Radiother Oncol 2003;68(2):175–180.
128. Rades D, Karstens JH. A comparison of two different radiation schedules for metastatic spinal cord compression considering a new prognostic factor. Strahlenther Onkol 2002;178(10):556–561.
129. Harrington KD. Anterior cord decompression and spinal stabilization for patients with metastatic lesions of the spine. J Neurosurg 1984;61(1):107–117.
130. Siegal T, Tiqva P. Vertebral body resection for epidural compression by malignant tumors. Results of forty-seven consecutive operative procedures. J Bone Joint Surg Am 1985;67(3):375–382.
131. Cooper PR, Errico TJ, Martin R, et al. A systematic approach to spinal reconstruction after anterior decompression for neoplastic disease of the thoracic and lumbar spine. Neurosurgery 1993;32(1):1–8.
132. Onimus M, Papin P, Gangloff S. Results of surgical treatment of spinal thoracic and lumbar metastases. Eur Spine J 1996;5(6):407–411.
133. Tomita K, Kawahara N, Kobayashi T, et al. Surgical strategy for spinal metastases. Spine 2001;26(3):298–306.
134. Durr HR, Wegener B, Krodel A, et al. Multiple myeloma: surgery of the spine: retrospective analysis of 27 patients. Spine 2002;27(3):320–324; discussion 325–356.
135. Schoeggl A, Reddy M, Matula C. Neurological outcome following laminectomy in spinal metastases. Spinal Cord 2002;40(7):363–366.
136. Hirabayashi H, Ebara S, Kinoshita T, et al. Clinical outcome and survival after palliative surgery for spinal metastases: palliative surgery in spinal metastases. Cancer 2003;97(2):476–484.
137. Hatrick NC, Lucas JD, Timothy AR, et al. The surgical treatment of metastatic disease of the spine. Radiother Oncol 2000;56(3):335–339.

138. Wise JJ, Fischgrund JS, Herkowitz HN, et al. Complication, survival rates, and risk factors of surgery for metastatic disease of the spine. Spine 1999;24(18):1943–1951.
139. Obbens EA, Kim JH, Thaler H, et al. Metronidazole as a radiation enhancer in the treatment of metastatic epidural spinal cord compression. J Neurooncol 1984;2(2):99–104.
140. Harrison KM, Muss HB, Ball MR, et al. Spinal cord compression in breast cancer. Cancer 1985;55(12):2839–2844.
141. Maranzano E, Latini P, Perrucci E, et al. Short-course radiotherapy (8 Gy × 2) in metastatic spinal cord compression: an effective and feasible treatment. Int J Radiat Oncol Biol Phys 1997;38(5):1037–1044.
142. Fyfe IS, Henry AP, Mulholland RC. Closed vertebral biopsy. J Bone Joint Surg Br 1983;65(2):140–143.
143. Schiff D, Shaw EG, Cascino TL. Outcome after spinal reirradiation for malignant epidural spinal cord compression. Ann Neurol 1995;37(5):583–589.
144. Grosu AL, Andratschke N, Nieder C, et al. Retreatment of the spinal cord with palliative radiotherapy. Int J Radiat Oncol Biol Phys 2002;52(5):1288–1292.
145. Milker-Zabel S, Zabel A, Thilmann C, et al. Clinical results of retreatment of vertebral bone metastases by stereotactic conformal radiotherapy and intensity-modulated radiotherapy. Int J Radiat Oncol Biol Phys 2003;55(1):162–167.
146. McLain RF, Weinstein JN. Tumors of the spine. Semin Spine Surg 1990;2:157–180.
147. Shimizu K, Shikata J, Iida H, et al. Posterior decompression and stabilization for multiple metastatic tumors of the spine. Spine 1992;17(11):1400–1404.
148. Levy WJ, Latchaw JP Jr, Hardy RW, et al. Encouraging surgical results in walking patients with epidural metastases. Neurosurgery 1982;11(2):229–233.
149. Dunn RC Jr, Kelly WA, Wohns RN, et al. Spinal epidural neoplasia. A 15-year review of the results of surgical therapy. J Neurosurg 1980;52(1):47–51.
150. DeWald RL, Bridwell KH, Prodromas C, et al. Reconstructive spinal surgery as palliation for metastatic malignancies of the spine. Spine 1985;10(1):21–26.
151. Perrin RG, McBroom RJ. Anterior versus posterior decompression for symptomatic spinal metastasis. Can J Neurol Sci 1987;14(1):75–80.
152. Heller M, McBroom RJ, MacNab T, et al. Treatment of metastatic disease of the spine with posterolateral decompression and Luque instrumentation. Neuroorthopedics 1986;2:70–74.
153. Sherman RM, Waddell JP. Laminectomy for metastatic epidural spinal cord tumors. Posterior stabilization, radiotherapy, and preoperative assessment. Clin Orthop 1986(207):55–63.
154. Slatkin NE, Posner JB. Management of spinal epidural metastases. Clin Neurosurg 1983;30:698–716.
155. McPhee IB, Williams RP, Swanson CE. Factors influencing wound healing after surgery for metastatic disease of the spine. Spine 1998;23(6):726–732; discussion 732–733.
156. Sundaresan N, Rothman A, Manhart K, et al. Surgery for solitary metastases of the spine: rationale and results of treatment. Spine 2002;27(16):1802–1806.
157. Ghogawala Z, Mansfield FL, Borges LF. Spinal radiation before surgical decompression adversely affects outcomes of surgery for symptomatic metastatic spinal cord compression. Spine 2001;26(7):818–824.
158. Chow TS, McCutcheon IE. The surgical treatment of metastatic spinal tumors within the intradural extramedullary compartment. J Neurosurg 1996;85(2):225–230.
159. Perrin RG, Livingston KE, Aarabi B. Intradural extramedullary spinal metastasis. A report of 10 cases. J Neurosurg 1982;56(6):835–837.
160. Mirimanoff RO, Choi NC. Intradural spinal metastases in patients with posterior fossa brain metastases from various primary cancers. Oncology 1987;44(4):232–236.
161. Costigan DA, Winkelman MD. Intramedullary spinal cord metastasis. A clinicopathological study of 13 cases. J Neurosurg 1985;62(2):227–233.
162. Grem JL, Burgess J, Trump DL. Clinical features and natural history of intramedullary spinal cord metastasis. Cancer 1985;56(9):2305–2314.
163. Dunne JW, Harper CG, Pamphlett R. Intramedullary spinal cord metastases: a clinical and pathological study of nine cases. Q J Med 1986;61(235):1003–1020.
164. Schijns OE, Kurt E, Wessels P, et al. Intramedullary spinal cord metastasis as a first manifestation of a renal cell carcinoma: report of a case and review of the literature. Clin Neurol Neurosurg 2000;102(4):249–254.
165. Gasser TG, Pospiech J, Stolke D, et al. Spinal intramedullary metastases. Report of two cases and review of the literature. Neurosurg Rev 2001;24(2–3):88–92.
166. Ogino M, Ueda R, Nakatsukasa M, et al. Successful removal of solitary intramedullary spinal cord metastasis from colon cancer. Clin Neurol Neurosurg 2002;104(2):152–156.
167. Findlay JM, Bernstein M, Vanderlinden RG, et al. Microsurgical resection of solitary intramedullary spinal cord metastases. Neurosurgery 1987;21(6):911–915.
168. Stark RJ, Henson RA, Evans SJ. Spinal metastases. A retrospective survey from a general hospital. Brain 1982;105(Pt 1): 189–213.
169. Kovner F, Spigel S, Rider I, et al. Radiation therapy of metastatic spinal cord compression. Multidisciplinary team diagnosis and treatment. J Neurooncol 1999;42(1):85–92.
170. Brown PD, Stafford SL, Schild SE, et al. Metastatic spinal cord compression in patients with colorectal cancer. J Neurooncol 1999;44(2):175–180.
171. Onimus M, Schraub S, Bertin D, et al. Surgical treatment of vertebral metastasis. Spine 1986;11(9):883–891.
172. Walsh GL, Gokaslan ZL, McCutcheon IE, et al. Anterior approaches to the thoracic spine in patients with cancer: indications and results. Ann Thorac Surg 1997;64(6): 1611–1618.
173. Sapkas G, Kyratzoulis J, Papaioannou N, et al. Spinal cord decompression and stabilization in malignant lesions of the spine. Acta Orthop Scand Suppl 1997;275:97–100.
174. Gokaslan ZL, York JE, Walsh GL, et al. Transthoracic vertebrectomy for metastatic spinal tumors. J Neurosurg 1998;89(4):599–609.

CHAPTER 28

Leptomeningeal Metastases and Dural/Skull Metastases

SUSAN M. BLANEY / DAVID G. POPLACK

Tumors of the meninges include leptomeningeal metastases and dural or skull-based metastases. The leptomeninges, which are comprised of the arachnoid membrane and the pia mater, are a site of metastatic spread for many malignancies, including leukemias, lymphomas and a wide variety of intracranial and extracranial tumors. The dura mater, a dense membrane composed of an outer fibrous layer (the connective tissue membrane of the skull bone) and an inner meningeal layer, is also a site of metastatic spread for a wide variety of intracranial and extracranial tumors. The incidences of leptomeningeal leukemia and lymphoma have dramatically decreased over the past four decades as a consequence of the routine incorporation of central nervous system (CNS) preventive therapy into frontline treatment regimens. However, leptomeningeal tumor dissemination is an increasingly recognized complication of both intracranial and extracranial solid tumors; a consequence of more effective primary therapy that has led to an increase in overall disease-free survival.[1,2] Treatment of leptomeningeal metastases, particularly those resulting from solid tumors, and dural or skull-based metastases poses a unique treatment challenge for the clinician. These challenges result from the limitations of systemically administered chemotherapy imposed by the blood–brain barrier, as well as the potential for severe neurocognitive and neuroendocrine sequelae resulting from the tumor or as a consequence of therapy. This chapter provides an overview of the clinical presentation, diagnosis, and treatment for patients with leptomeningeal or dural-based metastases.

▶ LEPTOMENINGEAL METASTASES

Leptomeningeal metastases, a general term used to describe the dissemination of a multitude of different tumor types to the leptomeninges, are also referred to in the literature by a variety of other names, including neoplastic meningitis, carcinomatous meningitis, lymphomatous meningitis, and leukemic meningitis. Although leptomeningeal metastasis may start in a focal area within the CNS, it is a diffuse disease of the neuraxis because the cerebrospinal fluid (CSF) within the leptomeninges circulates throughout the entire ventricular system and subarachnoid space.[3]

Incidence and Prognosis

It is estimated that the leptomeninges are a clinically recognized site of tumor spread in approximately 5% to 10% of patients with solid tumors; most commonly those with advanced systemic or primary CNS disease.[1,2] Several factors, including institutional referral patterns and the exclusion of patients with primary intracranial neoplasms or CNS leukemia/lymphoma, bias the reported frequency of leptomeningeal metastases by cancer type. Thus, the exact incidence of leptomeningeal metastases is unknown; however, they probably occur more frequently than is clinically recognized as evidenced by the fact that the reported incidence of leptomeningeal disease in autopsy series is as high as 25%.[4]

Leptomeningeal Metastases from Solid Tumors

In adults, the extracranial tumors most commonly associated with leptomeningeal metastases include cancers of the breast and lung,[4–6] as well as melanomas and carcinomas with an unknown primary.[7,8] Leptomeningeal dissemination occurs less frequently in patients with ovarian carcinomas,[9] cancers of the gastrointestinal tract,[10] or as a result of primary intracranial tumors, such as high-grade gliomas.[11,12] Table 28-1 lists the prevalence of leptomeningeal metastases by tumor type. The prognosis for adults with leptomeningeal metastases from a solid tumor is dismal, with an overall median survival of approximately 4 to 6 weeks in those who are not treated.[13] Factors associated with a particularly poor prognosis include poor baseline cognitive performance status; low Karnofsky performance status (KPS); multiple, serious, fixed neurologic deficits; and extensive systemic disease.[14,15]

Solid extracranial tumors of childhood associated with leptomeningeal metastases include rhabdomyosarcoma,[16,17] Ewing sarcoma,[18,19] neuroblastoma,[20,21] and retinoblastoma.[22] Primary intracranial tumors with a predilection for leptomeningeal dissemination include medulloblastomas, atypical teratoid/rhabdoid tumors, germinomas, ependymomas, high-grade and low-grade gliomas,[23] and carcinomas of the choroid plexus.

The overall survival for children with medulloblastoma and neuraxis dissemination following multimodality therapy (surgery, radiation therapy, and chemotherapy) is as high as 60% to 80%. However, their prognosis with regard to long-term permanent sequelae is poor with the majority of children having neuroendocrine and neuropsychological deficits. Children with recurrent leptomeningeal medulloblastoma may have a clinically protracted course, with tumor stabilization or regression for many months to several years, or a rapidly progressive course over a period of 4 to 8 weeks. However, there are no known clinical or biologic characteristics to prospectively determine which disseminated medulloblastomas will behave indolently versus aggressively. In contrast, leptomeningeal tumor dissemination from low-grade gliomas does not appear to negatively impact children's long-term clinical outcome.[23] Unfortunately, with the exceptions noted above, the overall prognosis for the majority of children with leptomeningeal metastases from extracranial or intracranial solid tumors is dismal, with rapid progression over weeks to several months.

▶ TABLE 28-1. PREVALENCE OF LEPTOMENINGEAL DISSEMINATION BY TUMOR TYPE

Tumor Type	Range of Prevalence
Breast cancer	22%–64%
Lung cancer	10%–26%
Malignant melanoma	7%–15%
Gastrointestinal tract tumors	4%–14%
Carcinomas of unknown primary	1%–7%
Primary CNS tumors	10%–32%
Lymphomas (AIDS-related)	20%–25%

Leptomeningeal Metastases from Leukemias and Lymphomas

In contrast to solid tumors, leukemias and lymphomas have a marked propensity for leptomeningeal dissemination. Leptomeningeal tumor involvement, as evidenced by positive CSF cytology or cranial nerve palsy(ies), is present at diagnosis in approximately 5% to 10% of patients with acute lymphocytic leukemia (ALL). Prior to the routine incorporation of CNS-directed therapy into frontline leukemia treatment regimens, the leptomeninges were the most frequent site of leukemic relapse, with a cumulative incidence of leptomeningeal leukemia of approximately 35% in adults[24] and exceeding 50% in children.[25,26] However, since the routine use of CNS-preventive therapy in the treatment of ALL, the cumulative incidence of CNS relapse is now less than 5% for children and approximately 7% for adults.[27] In some series, patients with T-cell phenotype ALL have a higher risk of CNS relapse than do patients with B-cell progenitor ALL.[28]

The prognosis for adults with ALL and an initial CNS recurrence is dismal, with a median survival from CNS recurrence of 6 months, a 28% survival at 1 year, and a 6% survival at 4 years.[27] In contrast, the prognosis for children with ALL and an initial CNS recurrence is better with an overall 4-year event-free survival (EFS) of 71.1% ± 5.3% for children with an initial complete response (CR) of less than 18 months and 83.3% ± 5.3% for those children with an initial CR of 18 months or longer.[29] These survival rates were achieved using a treatment strategy that delayed definitive craniospinal irradiation (CSI) for at least 6 months following the relapse to facilitate administration of more intensive systemic and intrathecal therapy. This is a marked improvement from earlier series where the median survival from the time of CNS relapse was 25 months with a 5-year overall survival of 25%.[30] The important prognostic factor concerning survival in children with ALL and a CNS relapse appears to be duration of the first CR.

Unfortunately, the prognosis for children with second or greater relapse is dismal, with a 17% survival at 22 months for children in second relapse and a 9% survival in those in third or greater relapse.[31]

In children with acute non-lymphocytic leukemias (ANLL), the incidence of CNS involvement at diagnosis is less than 5%, with a higher probability in patients with myelomonocytic (M4) or monocytic (M5) phenotypes or an initial leukocyte count of >25,000/mm.[32–34] In some series, children younger than 2 years of age also had a higher incidence of CNS disease either at diagnosis or relapse.[35,36] Interestingly, M4 and M5 phenotypes confer a favorable prognosis in infants with ANLL, despite the higher rate of CNS involvement.[35] In adults with ANLL, the incidence of CNS metastases at diagnosis is as high as 35% for patients with the acute myelomonocytic subtypes.[37,38] Similar to ALL, the incidence of recurrent CNS disease is extremely low for children and adults with ANLL because of the routine use of CNS-directed therapy.[39]

The incidence of leptomeningeal dissemination for patients with non-Hodgkin lymphoma is highly dependent on histology. Although the overall incidence of leptomeningeal involvement in children with non-Hodgkin lymphoma is approximately 8%, it is as high as 13% in small non–cleaved cell lymphomas and as low as 1% in large cell lymphomas.[40] In adults with systemic non-Hodgkin lymphoma the incidence of meningeal involvement has been reported to range from 10% to 25% in patients with unfavorable histologies.[41–43] The incidence of leptomeningeal involvement with non-Hodgkin lymphoma and AIDS appears to be similar.[43] Since the routine incorporation of CNS preventive therapeutic strategies into the frontline treatment of high-grade non-Hodgkin lymphoma, the incidence of recurrent CNS lymphoma in most modern pediatric and adult series is generally less than 5%.[44–48]

Pathogenesis

Tumor cells may reach the leptomeninges in a variety of ways including hematogeneous dissemination, CSF dissemination, or direct invasion or extension into the subarachnoid space.[49–51] Other postulated mechanisms include tracking along peripheral nerves and direct invasion through the choroids plexus.[13]

Hematogeneous dissemination is believed to be the most common mechanism for leptomeningeal metastases, particularly for extracranial solid tumors and leukemias.[50,51] Less commonly, direct extension of solid tumors to the subarachnoid space may occur when there is an underlying parameningeal, paraspinal, or vertebral tumor.[49] Similarly, in patients with leukemia, particularly those with leukostasis, there may be direct extension to the leptomeninges from the involved bone marrow within the calvarium.[51] Leptomeningeal metastases may also result from malignant cells that are shed directly into the CSF and then circulate freely throughout the CSF. This happens most commonly with intracranial malignancies, particularly in tumors that arise within the cerebellum or that are adjacent to the ventricles. Inadvertent spillage of tumor cells into the CSF during surgical resection of isolated cerebellar metastases may increase the risk of leptomeningeal metastases.[52,53] This same phenomenon may also occur in patients with leukemia who have a traumatic lumbar puncture. Clinical evidence suggests that there is an increased cumulative incidence of leptomeningeal metastases following a traumatic diagnostic lumbar puncture (≥10 erythrocytes/μL of CSF with identifiable blasts on cytospin), as a result of the presence of blood containing leukemic blasts in the CSF.[54]

As previously noted, the incidence of leukemic leptomeningeal involvement varies with histologic or immune phenotype, suggesting that inherent genetic or molecular characteristics may impact tumor cell motility or invasiveness. Further studies to confirm these hypotheses will be facilitated by the recent advances in molecular cytogenetics and biology.

Clinical Presentation

Because leptomeningeal metastases affect the entire neuraxis, clinical signs and symptoms of leptomeningeal dissemination are quite variable (Table 28-2).[2,7,8,55–59] In many instances, the clinical recognition of leptomeningeal metastases are delayed because of unfamiliarity with the diversity of the presenting signs and symptoms.[60]

The initial signs and symptoms of leptomeningeal metastases are commonly grouped according to the sites of CNS involvement, that is, cerebral hemispheres, cranial nerve, or spinal cord.[59,61,62] Most patients with leptomeningeal metastases from a solid tumor have multifocal signs and symptoms at diagnosis. In contrast, patients with CNS leukemia or lymphoma are frequently asymptomatic because the diagnosis is made at the time of a surveillance lumbar puncture.

Headache or cranial nerve dysfunction, particularly cranial nerve (CN) VI, are the most common signs and symptoms of leptomeningeal involvement in the patients with hematologic malignancies. In contrast, cerebral or spinal/radicular symptoms are the most common presenting signs and symptoms in solid-tumor patients with leptomeningeal metastases.

Signs and Symptoms of Cerebral Hemisphere Involvement

Headaches, the most common symptom of leptomeningeal tumor spread to the cerebral hemispheres, may be focal but are generally nonspecific in location. Nausea and vomiting, other common symptoms, typically result from increased intracranial pressure because of either an obstructive or communicating hydrocephalus.[49]

TABLE 28-2. SYMPTOMS AND SIGNS OF LEPTOMENINGEAL DISEASE BY SITE AND DECREASING ORDER OF FREQUENCY

	Symptom	Signs
Cerebral hemisphere	Headache Mental status change Nausea/vomiting Hemibody weakness Seizures	Mental status change Seizures Papilledema Focal weakness Hemiparesis
Cranial nerves	Diplopia Hearing loss Facial numbness Decreased vision	Ophthalmoplegia (III, IV, VI) Facial weakness (VII) Decreased hearing (VIII) Facial neuropathy (V) Hypoglossal weakness (XII)
Spinal cord and roots	Limb weakness Pain Gait instability Bladder dysfunction Bowel dysfunction	Extremity weakness Dermatomal/segmental sensory loss Deep tendon reflex abnormality Nuchal rigidity (meningismus) Gait ataxia Pain on straight-leg raising

Less common signs and symptoms include hemiparesis, papilledema, seizures, and mental status changes.[59] The latter may initially be quite subtle, ranging from slowing of thought processes to loss of recent memory. However, with progressive leptomeningeal spread, mental status changes may become quite striking, ranging from overt confusion, to a depressed level of consciousness, or frank encephalopathy.[63] Weakness and seizures, less common manifestations of leptomeningeal spread, are most likely to occur in patients with concomitant intraparenchymal tumor or bulky subarachnoid tumor.

Signs and Symptoms of Cranial Nerve Involvement

Leptomeningeal dissemination should be considered in the differential diagnosis of any cancer patient who presents with any new cranial nerve palsy. Diplopia, the most common symptom of leptomeningeal metastases to the cranial nerves, generally results from involvement of CN VI; however, CN III and/or CN IV may also be affected. Less commonly, leptomeningeal tumor spread may result in unilateral or bilateral hearing loss[64] as a result of involvement of CN VIII, facial weakness resulting from involvement of CN VII, decreased facial sensation in the distribution of the trigeminal nerve, or hypoglossal weakness as a consequence of involvement of CN XII.

Signs and Symptoms of Spinal Cord Involvement

Signs and symptoms of leptomeningeal dissemination to the spinal cord or exiting nerve roots reflect the level of tumor involvement and most commonly include weakness, numbness, pain, and/or gait instability. Weakness may be manifest as either a polyradiculoneuropathy or a myelopathy.[65] The former, which results from involvement of multiple exiting nerve roots or the cauda equina, is characterized by decreased limb tone, diminished or absent deep tendon reflexes, and dermatomal or root-referable sensory loss (lower motor neuron findings). The latter, which results from spinal cord or conus medullaris involvement, is characterized by increased limb tone, exaggerated deep tendon reflexes, extensor plantar response, and segmental or fixed-level sensory loss (upper motor neuron findings).[2,60]

Bowel or bladder dysfunction may also occur when there is leptomeningeal dissemination to the canal. Symptoms of bowel or bladder dysfunction typically occur early with spinal cord or conus medullaris dysfunction, and late with cauda equina dysfunction in conjunction with other neurologic signs and symptoms.[60]

Diagnosis

Clinicians must have a high index of suspicion for leptomeningeal involvement in patients with neurologic signs or symptoms and tumors with the potential for leptomeningeal spread because of the wide heterogeneity in the presenting signs and symptoms of leptomeningeal metastases. Prior to advances in neuroimaging, the presence of malignant cells in the CSF was a prerequisite for the diagnosis of leptomeningeal disease. However, in patients with solid tumors there was frequently discordance between clinical findings and CSF cytology results. This discrepancy further widened with the widespread availability of advanced magnetic resonance imaging

(MRI); many solid tumor patients with clinical and imaging findings suggestive of leptomeningeal metastases had negative CSF cytology results. It is now feasible, and standard practice, to establish a diagnosis of leptomeningeal metastases based on imaging findings in patients with an underlying solid tumor in whom serial CSF cytology findings are negative. In such situations, the patient must have clinical signs and symptoms for which there is no other explanation and MRI findings consistent with leptomeningeal metastases.[14] Specific considerations in evaluating CSF cytology and MRI results in patients with known or suspected leptomeningeal metastases are discussed below.

Cerebrospinal Fluid Examination

Laboratory evaluation of the CSF remains an important diagnostic tool in patients with suspected leptomeningeal metastases. Essential elements of the laboratory CSF evaluation include a cell count, protein level, glucose concentration, and cytologic examination. Because leptomeningeal metastases may cause hydrocephalus or be accompanied by bulky intraparenchymal metastases, a CNS MRI or computerized tomography (CT) scan is recommended in all patients with solid tumors and as clinically indicated in patients with leukemia/lymphoma, prior to obtaining CSF for diagnostic purposes. In addition to evaluating the MRI for evidence of leptomeningeal metastases or parenchymal disease, the preprocedure MRI should specifically be evaluated for evidence of hydrocephalus or other lesions that may be a contraindication to CSF collection.

In patients with Ommaya reservoirs, CSF for diagnostic purposes should be collected from both lumbar and ventricular sites because there may be discordant cytologic results depending on the sample site. In adults the presence of spinal signs or symptoms of leptomeningeal metastases, the lumbar CSF cytology is more likely to be positive than ventricular; in contrast, in the presence of cranial signs or symptoms, ventricular CSF cytology is more likely to be positive than lumbar.[66] Discordance between paired CSF samples obtained from ventriculoperitoneal (VP) shunt taps and lumbar puncture in children with primary CNS tumors has also been reported. Gajjaar and associates evaluated 90 paired CSF samples and found discordant results in 14; with malignant cells detected at a significantly higher rate than in lumbar versus ventricular shunt CSF.[67] Therefore, in children with intracranial tumors, CSF obtained for staging purposes should ideally be collected from the lumbar CSF.[67] The higher yield of malignant cells in CSF obtained from lumbar CSF is postulated to be a direct result both of the caudad flow of CSF and of the effect of gravity; that is, the malignant cells circulating throughout the CSF tend to have a tendency to preferentially flow to the lumbar space.[67]

Other important considerations when obtaining CSF for diagnostic purposes include the volume for cytologic evaluation, the promptness of CSF processing, and the number of CSF evaluations.[68] Greater CSF volumes and prompt sample processing minimize the chance of a false-negative result. In addition, several investigators have shown that serial CSF samples may be required to detect malignant cells, particularly in solid tumor patients. For example, Wasserstrom and associates demonstrated that only 55% of initial lumbar punctures were positive in a series of adult patients with suspected leptomeningeal metastases. The incidence of positive results increased to 80% following a second lumbar puncture and by an additional 2% with each subsequent CSF evaluation.[55] In a similar series, Kaplan and associates found that 71% of patients had positive cytology after an initial lumbar puncture, whereas 92% had positive results after the second lumbar puncture.[2] Thus, if there is a high index of suspicion for leptomeningeal metastases, CSF should be collected on a minimum of two occasions if the initial CSF cytology result is negative.

In addition to elevations in white blood cell (WBC) count, there are other nonspecific CSF abnormalities in patients with leptomeningeal metastases including elevations in protein concentration and decreases in glucose concentration (Table 28-3).[55] High CSF protein levels may also be observed in patients with VP shunts caused by

▶ **TABLE 28-3.** LABORATORY EVALUATION OF CSF IN PATIENTS WITH LEPTOMENINGEAL METASTASIS SECONDARY TO SOLID TUMORS

Variable	Initial (n = 90)	Subsequent (n = 90)
CSF pressure >160 mm Hg	45 (50%)	64 (71%)
Cells >5/μL	51 (57%)	65 (72%)
Protein >50 mg/dL	73 (81%)	80 (89%)
Glucose <40 mg/dL	28 (31%)	37 (41%)
Positive cytology	49 (54%)	82 (91%)
Normal	3 (3%)	1 (1%)

Source: From DeAngelis L.[56]

alterations in CSF flow dynamics. Therefore, an isolated elevation in CSF protein may not be useful in diagnosing or assessing response of leptomeningeal metastases to therapy. Likewise, low CSF glucose concentrations or high CSF WBC counts are nonspecific findings that support, but do not confirm, a diagnosis of leptomeningeal metastases.

CSF Findings in Solid Tumors

In patients with underlying primary extracranial or intracranial solid tumors, the finding of malignant cells in the CSF provides unequivocal evidence of leptomeningeal metastases. The one exception is cytology-positive CSF obtained in children with posterior fossa tumors during the immediate postoperative period. In this situation, false-positive cytology results may occur in the early postoperative period as a consequence of tumor cell dissemination throughout the CSF following surgical manipulation of the primary tumor. In such situations, cytology for diagnostic staging purposes should not be obtained until at least 10 to 14 days after surgery.[69]

Specific immunohistochemical studies or biochemical markers, including carcinoembryonic antigen, α-fetoprotein, and β-human chorionic gonadotropin, may be abnormal in selected cases of leptomeningeal metastases. Biochemical markers should be evaluated simultaneously in serum and CSF to ascertain whether an abnormal CSF result is a result of underlying leptomeningeal disease or a result of passive diffusion from the systemic circulation.[56] Although these and other markers are not of prognostic significance, they may be useful in establishing a diagnosis or in monitoring response to therapy.

Other potentially useful CSF analyses include cytogenetic analyses for tumor-specific clonal abnormalities, and polymerase chain reaction,[70] or fluorescence *in situ* hybridization studies for tumor-specific abnormalities. In the future, mitochondrial DNA mutations in the CSF may also provide a potential means of monitoring disease progression and predicting the potential for leptomeningeal metastases. In a preliminary report of eight medulloblastoma cases, mitochondrial DNA (mtDNA) mutations were found in both the CSF and primary tumor of seven. One patient without evidence of leptomeningeal disease, but with persistent CSF mtDNA mutations from the time of initial diagnosis, experienced a leptomeningeal relapse 5 months after the completion of therapy. Patients without detectable mtDNA mutations at the end of therapy, or in whom mutations were different from the primary tumor, remained disease free at the time of the report.[71] Although such tumor-specific analyses are yet known to be of prognostic significance, they may be useful in monitoring an individual patient's response to therapy. There are also ongoing studies evaluating other nonspecific markers that may play a role in leptomeningeal metastases including vascular endothelial growth factor (VEGF)[72] and matrix metalloproteinases. To date, none of these markers has been shown to be of prognostic significance.

▶ TABLE 28-4. CNS STAGING IN CHILDHOOD LEUKEMIA

Category	CSF WBC Cell Count	CSF Cytology
CNS 1	<5/μL	Negative
CNS 2	<5/μL	Positive
CNS 3	≥5/μL	Positive

CSF Findings in CNS Leukemia

The traditional definition of CNS leukemia required a minimum CSF WBC count of 5/μL plus the presence of leukemic blasts on a cytospin preparation of CSF. However, in separate studies performed by St. Jude Children's Research Hospital and the Pediatric Oncology Group (POG), the subgroup of patients with leukemic blasts in their CSF but a WBC count of <5/μL were found to be at higher risk for a subsequent leptomeningeal relapse.[73,74] As a result, a new CNS classification system, which incorporated an intermediate category (CNS2) to distinguish this patient subgroup, was developed (Table 28-4). Using this new classification schema, CNS2 patients in subsequent studies receive more doses of intrathecal chemotherapy than patients who are CNS negative (CNS1), but fewer than those with overt CNS involvement (CNS3). In contrast, in analyses performed by the Children's Cancer Group (CCG) and the Berlin-Franklin-Munster (BFM) Consortium, patients who were retrospectively characterized as CNS2 did not appear to have an adverse prognosis.[75,76] These apparently discordant findings are best explained by differences in intensity of early CNS-directed therapy between the St. Jude and POG studies versus the CCG and BFM studies.[54] Similar subset analyses have not been reported for adults with ALL.

Specific flow cytometric and cytogenetic studies of CSF may provide additional information in select cases of CNS leukemia or lymphoma. However, CSF flow cytometric studies are generally of limited value because of an inadequate number of cells for analyses.[77] In patients with suspected lymphomatous meningitis, polymerase chain reaction assays to identify immunoglobulin gene rearrangements, such as clonal V-J arrangements, may also be considered.[78] However, it is not standard practice to employ these specialized studies for routine surveillance CSF evaluations in patients with leukemia.

Radiographic Evaluation

Neuroimaging studies in patients with suspected leptomeningeal disease are helpful in establishing a diagnosis, defining the extent of disease, providing information to guide the clinician in making treatment recommendations for an individual patient, and facilitating evaluation of treatment response. The extent and type of neuraxis imaging employed will vary with individual patient circumstance(s). In patients with advanced systemic disease, the primary purpose of imaging studies is to facilitate lesion identification or localization prior to palliative radiotherapy; as a result imaging studies in this circumstance may be quite focal. In contrast, neuroimaging studies in less advanced patients should include an assessment of the entire brain and spine. In addition, because leptomeningeal metastases may become quite large and impair or obstruct normal CSF flow, studies to evaluate the integrity of normal CSF flow may be required if intrathecal drug administration is a potential treatment option.

Magnetic Resonance Imaging Scans

MRI scans with and without gadolinium (Gd) enhancement are the imaging studies of choice for suspected leptomeningeal metastases. Although contrast-enhanced CT scans of the head may show abnormalities consistent with leptomeningeal metastases, they are relatively insensitive compared to Gd-enhanced MRIs.[79,80] Similarly, MRI imaging of the spine (with and without Gd) is preferred over CT myelography because it is noninvasive and is at least comparable in the detection of leptomeningeal metastases.[81,82] In fact, in some studies, Gd-enhanced MRI was superior to CT myelography in demonstrating extramedullary nodules, focal spinal cord enlargement, clumping of nerve roots, and pial enhancement ("sugar-coating").[81] As with CSF cytology studies, a negative Gd-enhanced MRI does not preclude the diagnosis of leptomeningeal metastases. One report suggests that high-dose Gd-enhanced MRI may be useful in situations where a strong clinical suspicion of leptomeningeal metastases remains despite negative imaging and cytology studies.[83] Further investigations are required to establish the clinical utility of this approach.

MRI findings in patients with solid tumor leptomeningeal metastases include enhancement of the leptomeninges, dura, subependyma, and/or cranial nerves. These findings are not specific to leptomeningeal metastases[84] and must be placed in the appropriate clinical context prior to initiation of treatment for leptomeningeal metastases. Because leptomeningeal metastases typically occur in patients with advanced systemic disease, cranial MRIs may also reveal concomitant bulky intraparenchymal or leptomeningeal-based lesions (Figs. 28-1 to 28-4), or findings consistent with communicating hydrocephalus.[85] In contrast to solid tumors, the initial evidence of leukemic leptomeningeal involvement is usually the result of routine surveillance CSF studies obtained in asymptomatic patients. As a result, in most instances there is no radiographic evidence of leptomeningeal spread at initial diagnosis in patients with CNS leukemia. In symptomatic leukemia patients, there may be isolated enhancement of a cranial nerve(s). Patients with acute nonlymphocytic leukemia may also present with chloromas, which are collections of myeloid leukemic cells. Although chloromas most commonly involve the orbit or periorbital area, they may also involve the spinal cord or cause other lesions within the CNS.[32] In advanced or refractory cases of CNS

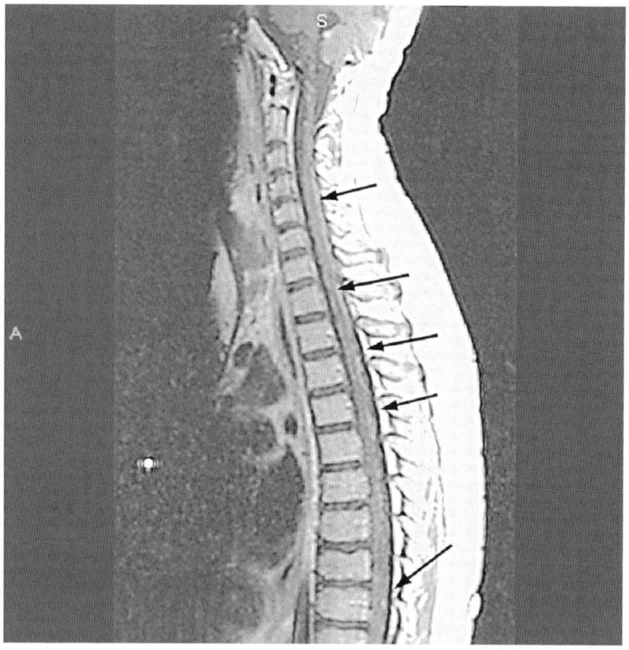

Figure 28-1. Multiple leptomeningeal metastases of the spinal cord in a patient with recurrent medulloblastoma.

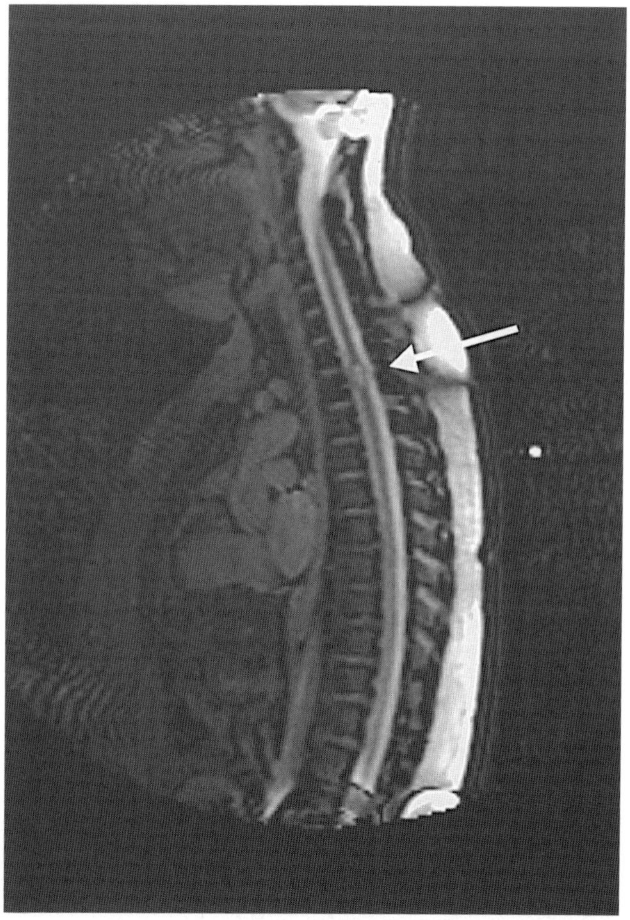

Figure 28-2. Leptomeningeal involvement of the spinal cord from an underlying medulloblastoma.

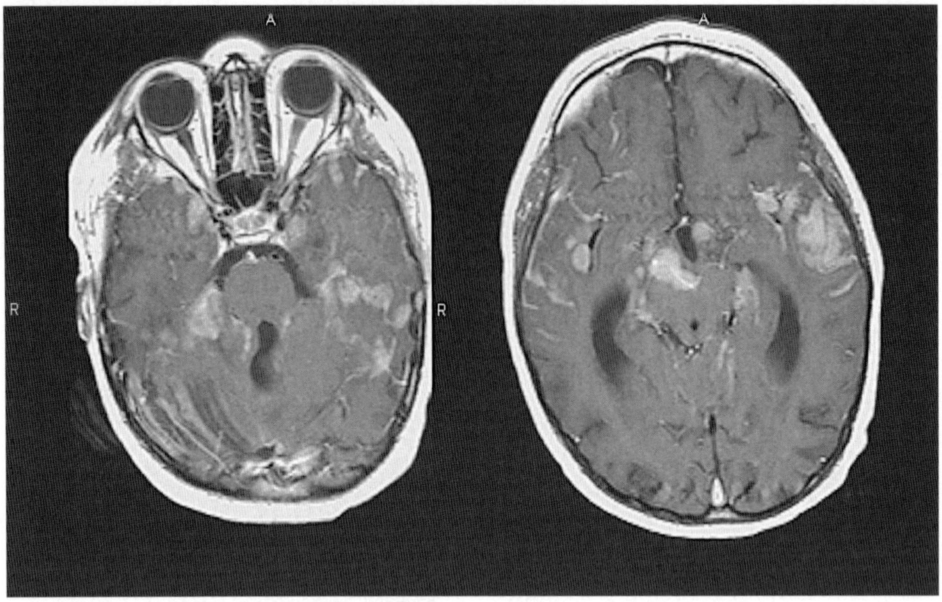

Figure 28-3. Diffuse leptomeningeal disease with bulky intraparenchymal metastases in a patient with a supratentorial primitive neuroectodermal tumor.

acute lymphocytic or nonlymphocytic leukemia, there may be diffuse leptomeningeal enhancement (Fig. 28-5).

Ideally, MRI imaging of the spine in patients with CNS tumors (primary or metastatic) should be obtained prior to any neurosurgical procedure in order to avoid confusion that may result from postoperative artifact or blood. If preoperative spinal imaging is not possible, a minimum of 14 days should elapse after surgery to minimize any imaging changes that are related to the surgery. Spinal imaging should also be performed prior to acquisition of CSF for

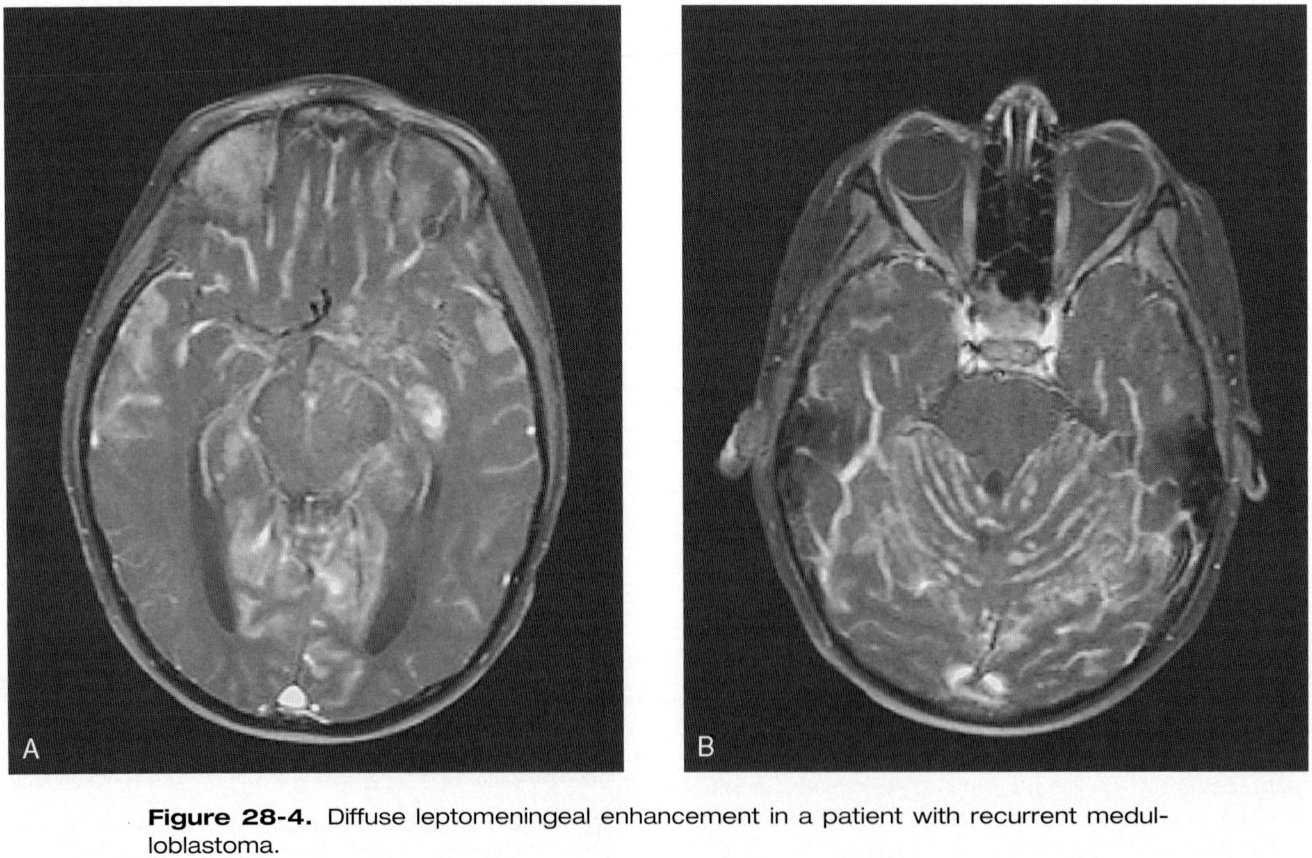

Figure 28-4. Diffuse leptomeningeal enhancement in a patient with recurrent medulloblastoma.

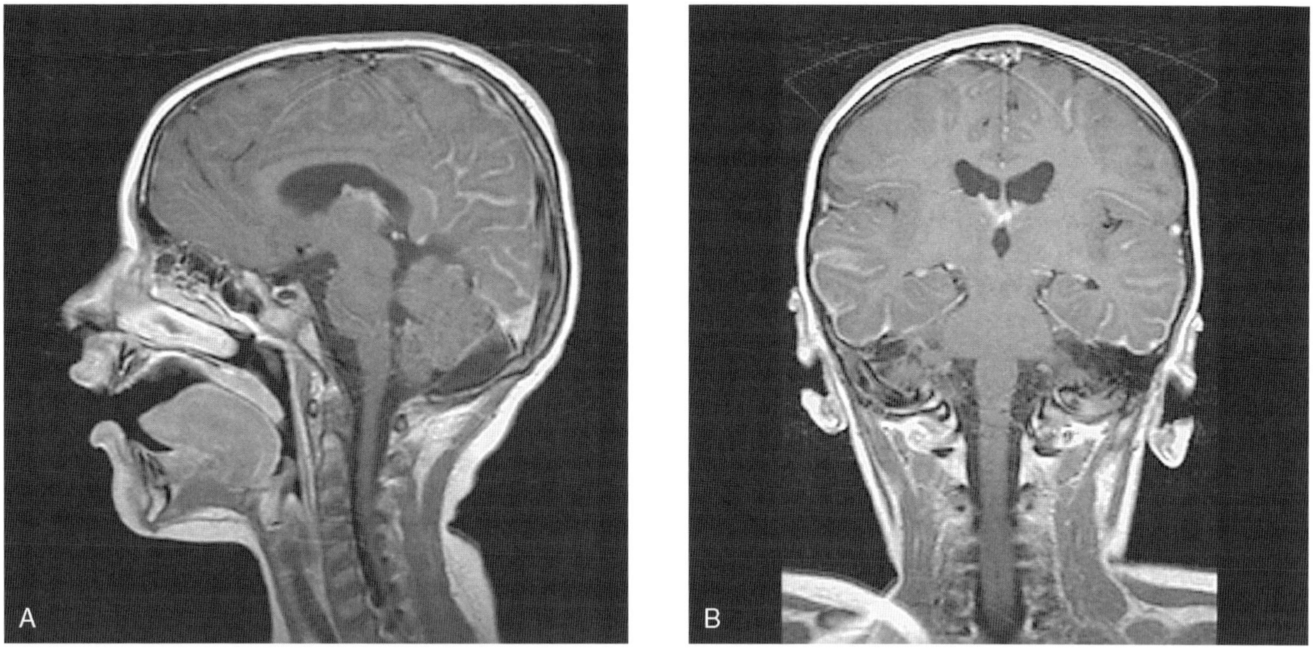

Figure 28-5. Diffuse leptomeningeal enhancement in a patient with refractory CNS leukemia. The patient's CSF cytology and radiographic evidence of disease resolved after placement of an Ommaya reservoir for "C × T" therapy.

cytologic studies in order to avoid local imaging changes that may result from the lumbar puncture.

A variety of MRI sequences, including fat-saturation and fast fluid-attenuated inversion recovery (FLAIR) imaging sequences, have been evaluated by several groups in an attempt to define the optimal MRI sequence for the detection and evaluation of leptomeningeal metastases. Some investigators hypothesized that contrast-enhanced FLAIR imaging sequences were better than standard contrast-enhanced T_1-weighted MRI sequences in screening for leptomeningeal disease because FLAIR suppresses the signal intensity from normal vascular structures on the surface of the brain.[86–89] Although a small evaluation of 10 children at high risk of leptomeningeal metastases supported this hypothesis,[88] a larger study of 68 adults with suspected leptomeningeal metastases demonstrated that standard contrast-enhanced, T_1-weighted MRI sequences were more sensitive than FLAIR imaging sequences in detecting intracranial leptomeningeal metastases.[86]

CSF Flow Studies

Nuclear medicine CSF flow studies (radionuclide cisternograms), usually performed with indium-111 (^{111}In) diethylenetriamine pentaacetic acid (DTPA), or less commonly with technetium-99 (^{99}Tc) DTPA, are more sensitive than CT or MRI scans in providing a physiologic assessment of the clinical anatomy of the CSF spaces.[57,90,91] Clinical series in adults with leptomeningeal metastases reveal evidence of functional CSF flow blocks in up to 70% of patients with leptomeningeal metastases, most commonly in patients with skull base lesions[57,92,93] Therefore, CSF flow studies are routinely recommended prior to initiation of intrathecal therapy in patients with leptomeningeal metastases from an underlying extra- or intracranial solid tumor.[80,92] Because CNS leukemias are less likely to cause alterations in CSF flow dynamics, decision(s) regarding the need for a CSF flow study prior to intrathecal therapy should be made on a patient-by-patient basis. However, if there is any imaging evidence of hydrocephalus or obstruction to CSF flow, a CSF flow study should be performed prior to intrathecal therapy regardless of the diagnosis.

Prospective identification of patients with abnormal CSF flow is crucial to minimizing the risk for acute or delayed toxicity(ies) of intrathecal therapy (see below). CSF flow obstructions essentially compartmentalize the CSF space, resulting in uneven drug distribution and high local drug concentrations. Thus, an agent administered proximal to an obstruction increases the risk of leukoencephalopathy, and an agent administered distal to an obstruction increases the risk of an acute or subacute myelopathy. Another adverse consequence of abnormal or obstructed CSF flow is that it compromises potential efficacy because of uneven or suboptimal drug exposure throughout the neuraxis. Normal CSF flow can be restored in approximately one-third of patients following involved field radiation therapy.[57] Patients in whom CSF flow is not successfully restored following radiotherapy are not candidates for intrathecal drug administration and have an extremely poor prognosis.[14,92]

Principles of Treatment of Leptomeningeal Metastases

The ideal treatment for leptomeningeal metastases is preventive therapy. This strategy has been successfully used in the treatment of leukemias and lymphomas through the routine incorporation of CNS-directed therapy into frontline treatment regimens. Likewise, therapy directed at the entire neuraxis, through the use of craniospinal, rather than focal, radiotherapy and adjuvant chemotherapy, has been successful in preventing disseminated CNS disease in the majority of children with medulloblastomas.

Unfortunately, there are no known effective preventive therapies for extra- or intracranial solid tumors that have a predilection for leptomeningeal spread. Furthermore, only a relatively small percentage of solid tumor patients develop leptomeningeal dissemination and, in most instances, one cannot prospectively predict which solid tumor patients are at increased risk for leptomeningeal dissemination.

Once the diagnosis of leptomeningeal disease has been confirmed, patients with leptomeningeal disease from solid tumors must be carefully evaluated to enable appropriate selection of therapy. Important considerations include: the patient's underlying diagnosis and disease status, the patient's performance status, and the extent of neurologic and/or cognitive deficits. Patients who have advanced systemic disease, a poor performance status, or symptoms in multiple CNS sites have a relatively poor prognosis and a limited life expectancy (Table 28-5).[14] These poor-prognosis patients are generally not candidates for therapeutic clinical trials, and palliative therapy is recommended. Potential treatment options for patients with less advanced disease, or in the preventive setting, include radiation therapy and/or chemotherapy, both of which are discussed in more detail below. In addition, the reader can refer to the National Comprehensive Cancer Network guidelines for adult patients with "carcinomatous/lymphomatous meningitis."[15]

Radiotherapy

Role in Adults with Leptomeningeal Metastases

In adults with leptomeningeal tumor spread, the primary indication for radiotherapy is palliation. This typically involves administration of 25 to 30 cGy in 10 to 20 fractions to the focal lesions(s).[56,94–96] In some instances radiotherapy results in improvement in or resolution of recent onset neurologic deficits, but more typically provides local disease control of limited duration. Deficits that have been present for days or weeks are unlikely to improve or resolve with radiotherapy.

Whole brain radiotherapy may be administered to patients with CNS leukemia or extensive intracranial leptomeningeal disease, particularly those with hydrocephalus, increased intracranial pressure, significant cortical deficits, or cranial neuropathies.[13] Lumbosacral radiation may be considered in patients with lower extremity weakness or dysfunction of their bowels or bladder.[13]

Radiotherapy may also be administered in an attempt to alleviate a CSF obstruction. If radiotherapy successfully restores normal CSF flow, which occurs in approximately 33% of cases, consideration can be given to initiating intrathecal therapy.[57] If CSF flow is not restored, the patient is considered to be "poor risk" and supportive/palliative care is recommended.

Role in Children

Radiotherapy has successfully been used in children for the prevention and treatment of leptomeningeal disease, as well as for palliation of symptoms related to leptomeningeal metastases. Historically, cranial or craniospinal irradiation were used for the prevention of CNS leukemias and lymphomas.[97] However, in addition to the potential for severe neuroendocrine and neuropsychological sequelae, preventive radiation therapy has been associated with an increased risk of developing second malignant neoplasms.[98] As a result, intrathecal therapy has generally been replaced in frontline treatment regimens for childhood leukemias and lymphomas except for a small subgroup of patients who are at extremely high risk of developing a CNS relapse.

CSI therapy is routinely employed in the postsurgical treatment of children older than 3 years of age with newly diagnosed medulloblastoma. Standard therapy for "standard-risk" patients is reduced-dose CSI therapy (25 Gy to the neuraxis and 54 Gy to the posterior fossa) followed by adjuvant chemotherapy. Children with overt leptomeningeal metastases at diagnosis or with other high-risk prognostic features typically receive standard-dose

▶ TABLE 28-5. RISK STATUS IN CARCINOMATOUS/LYMPHOMATOUS MENINGITIS IN ADULTS[14]

Risk Factor	Good Risk	Poor Risk
Karnofsky performance status	>60	≤60
Extent of neurologic deficit	None or minimal	Multiple, serious, fixed deficits
Status of systemic disease	Minimal	Extensive
Treatment options for systemic disease	Available	None or few

Source: Adapted from Grossman S, with permission.[14]

CSI therapy (36 Gy to the neuraxis and 54 Gy to the posterior fossa) followed by adjuvant chemotherapy. Clinical trials to evaluate the feasibility of further decreasing radiation therapy doses are in progress.

Radiation therapy also plays an important role in the treatment of children with ALL and an initial CNS relapse. As previously noted, the prognosis of children with an isolated CNS relapse is markedly improved when definitive CSI therapy (24 Gy cranial/15 Gy spinal) is delayed by at least 6 months to facilitate the delivery of more intensive systemic and intrathecal therapy.[29] These results were confirmed in a followup study designed to assess the impact of further intensification of systemic chemotherapy, delay of radiation therapy to 12 months, and reduction of the radiotherapy volume (cranial only) and dose (18 Gy) to low-risk patients (complete initial remission duration of >18 months).[99]

Adverse Effects of Radiotherapy

Adverse effects of radiotherapy may be acute or long-term. The major acute adverse effects include myelosuppression, mucositis, and esophagitis.[13] Long-term sequelae include neuroendocrine and neuropsychological deficits, leukoencephalopathy, and second malignancies.[98,100–107] Variables that may impact the incidence and severity of these adverse events include the treatment field and dose, the timing relative to systemically or intrathecally administered chemotherapy, particularly methotrexate, and the age at the time of therapy.

Chemotherapy

General Considerations

The primary limitation of systemic chemotherapy in the treatment of leptomeningeal metastases is that the blood–brain and blood–CSF barriers limit the CNS drug exposure of most commonly used antineoplastic agents (Table 28-6). As a result, malignant cells within the CNS are protected from the cytotoxic effects of the systemically administered therapy. This limitation can be circumvented through (a) the use of high-dose systemic chemotherapy with or without autologous stem cell rescue, (b) systemic administration of agents with good CSF penetration, (c) direct intra-CSF drug administration (via a lumbar puncture, ventricular access device, or lumbar reservoir), or (d) the use of pharmacokinetically guided dosing of systemic therapy to achieve a minimum target CSF drug exposure.[108]

An important consideration in determining the optimal route of drug administration, that is, systemic versus intrathecal, is the extent of leptomeningeal disease. Patients with "bulky" or nodular leptomeningeal metastases are less likely to derive benefit from intrathecal therapy than patients with either an isolated positive CSF cytology or minimal radiographic evidence of leptomeningeal enhancement. This is a result of the limited tissue (intratumoral and intraparenchymal) penetration of cytotoxic agents following intrathecal administration.[109] As a result, the optimal chemotherapeutic approach for patients with extensive leptomeningeal disease may include systemic chemotherapy, preferably with high-dose chemotherapy or an agent that effectively penetrates the blood–CSF barrier or systemic chemotherapy with or without an intrathecal agent.

▶ TABLE 28-6. CNS PENETRATION OF COMMONLY USED ANTICANCER AGENTS

Agent	CSF: Plasma Ratio (%)
Alkylating agents	
Cyclophosphamide	
Total drug	50
Active metabolite	15
Ifosfamide	
Total drug	30
Active metabolite	15
Thiotepa	>95
Carmustine	>90
Cisplatin	
Free platinum	40
Total platinum	<5
Carboplatin	
Free platinum	30
Total platinum	<5
Antimetabolites	
Methotrexate	3
6-Mercaptopurine	25
Cytarabine	15
5-Fluorouracil	
Bolus	50
Infusion	15
Antitumor antibiotics	
Anthracyclines	ND
Dactinomycin	ND
Plant alkaloids	
Vinca alkaloids	5
Epipodophyllotoxins	<5
Topoisomerase I inhibitors	
Topotecan	32
Irinotecan	
CPT-11 lactone	14
SN-38 lactone	<8
Miscellaneous	
Prednisolone	<10
Dexamethasone	15
L-Asparaginase	ND*

*Although drug is ND in CSF, CSF L-asparagine is depleted by systemic administration of L-asparaginase.
CSF = cerebrospinal fluid; ND = not detectable.
Source: Modified with permission from Balis F, Poplack D. Cancer chemotherapy. In: Nathan DG, Oski FA, eds. Hematology of infancy and childhood, 4th ed. Philadelphia: WB Saunders, 1993:1207–1238.

Another consideration for patients with leptomeningeal metastases is to determine whether or not they require additional concomitant therapy for the treatment of their underlying neoplasm or sites of bulky leptomeningeal disease. Patients with CNS leukemia or lymphoma routinely require systemic therapy to treat or prevent a subsequent bone marrow relapse. In contrast, patients with solid tumors frequently have advanced systemic disease and a limited life expectancy when their leptomeningeal metastases are diagnosed. Nevertheless, these patients may derive benefit from local radiotherapy to sites of bulky disease in terms of either palliation or restoration of CSF flow. Therefore, decisions about the need for or goals of concomitant systemic or radiotherapy therapy in solid tumor patients with leptomeningeal metastases must be individualized.

High-Dose Systemic Chemotherapy

In theory, cytotoxic concentrations of anticancer agents with limited CNS penetration can be achieved in the CSF through administration of very high systemic doses. Unfortunately, the systemic toxicity of most anticancer agents precludes the routine use of this approach. Nevertheless, it is feasible to administer very high-dose chemotherapy for agents where an effective systemic rescue strategy exists, for example, leucovorin rescue for methotrexate or autologous stem cell rescue for agents where myelosuppression is dose limiting. In practice, this strategy is most commonly used for patients with leukemia and a CNS relapse because high-dose chemotherapy may provide therapeutic benefit for the leptomeningeal disease and may be useful in preventing a subsequent bone marrow relapse.

This approach has been successfully used in a pilot study of adults with lymphomatous or solid-tumor neoplastic meningitis. Administration of high-dose intravenous methotrexate, 8 g/m^2 over 4 hours, and leucovorin rescue resulted in prolonged exposure in serum and CSF to methotrexate concentrations known to be cytotoxic and comparable to those achieved with intrathecal methotrexate. Cytologic clearing of CSF and survival appeared to be better than a historical control of patients who received intrathecal methotrexate. Prospective trials are required to confirm these preliminary results.[110]

Other authors have suggested that there should be a greater role for systemic therapy in the treatment of leptomeningeal metastases. In a comprehensive, retrospective review of the literature, Siegal and associates found that the response rate and survival of patients with leptomeningeal metastases were similar in patients treated with radiotherapy combined with systemic therapy versus patients who also received intrathecal therapy.[111] Again, prospective trials to confirm these observations are required. In addition, further studies will be required as new intrathecal agents, particularly combinations of agents for intrathecal administration, are developed.

Intrathecal Chemotherapy

The primary advantage of intrathecal chemotherapy is that it provides a direct means of circumventing the limited penetration of most antineoplastic agents across the blood–brain and blood–CSF barriers (see Table 28-6). In addition, intrathecal administration takes advantage of the tremendous difference in the volumes of distribution between the systemic circulation (3500 mL for plasma) and the CSF space (approximately 140 mL).[112–114] As a result, much higher concentrations of drug can be achieved in the CSF, that is, the target tumor site, with a fraction of the dose that would be required if administered via the systemic route. Systemic drug exposure after intrathecal administration is minimal, if any, thereby decreasing the potential for drug-related systemic toxicity.

In adults, intrathecal agents are frequently administered using a surgically implanted ventricular access device (Fig. 28-6) such as an Ommaya reservoir. The primary advantage of a ventricular access device is that it overcomes some of the limitations of intralumbar drug delivery, including the potential technical difficulties associated with lumbar punctures in patients with degenerative changes of their spine or abnormal coagulation profiles, the pain and inconvenience associated with lumbar punctures, and the potential for epidural drug administration or leakage in up

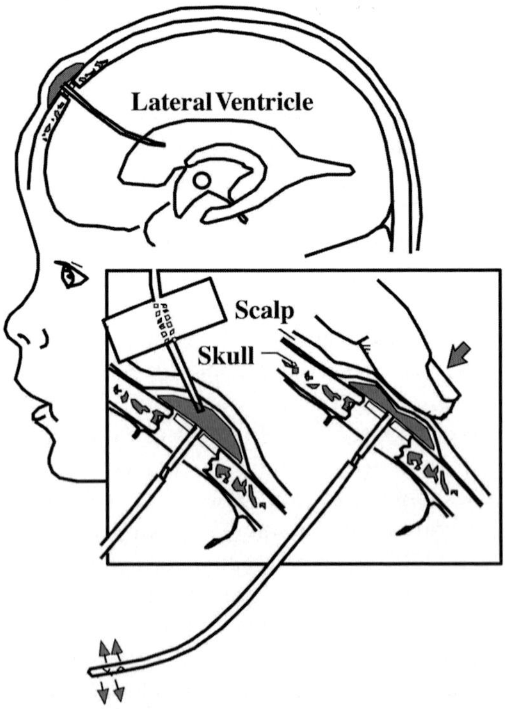

Figure 28-6. Diagram of an intraventricular drug delivery system. A subcutaneously implanted Ommaya reservoir is attached to a catheter, the tip of which sits in the lateral ventricle. (*Reproduced with permission from Balis F, Poplack D. Central nervous system pharmacology of antileukemia drugs. Am J Pediatr Hematol Oncol 1989; 11:74–86.*)

to 10% of cases.[115] Another advantage of an Ommaya reservoir is the more homogeneous drug distribution throughout the neuraxis after intraventricular administration because the CSF flow is with and not against gravity. Preclinical studies in nonhuman primates showed that drug exposure in ventricular CSF after an intralumbar injection was much greater when the animals remained prone for 1 hour after drug administration versus immediate placement in an upright position.[116] Intraventricular access devices also facilitate drug delivery on a frequent-dosing schedule. This is particularly important in optimizing the antitumor effect of cell-cycle–specific anticancer agents.

The primary disadvantage of an intraventricular access device is that it requires a neurosurgical procedure. In addition, as with the placement of any foreign catheter, there is a potential risk of infection, bleeding, or obstruction. The risk of infection can be minimized by meticulous adherence to strict antiseptic procedures for accessing the reservoir. A very uncommon complication is migration or misplacement of the catheter tip. Therefore, postoperative coronal sections of a postoperative scan should be closely scrutinized for catheter placement prior to initial use of the reservoir. Despite these potential complications, the advantages of an intraventricular access device generally outweigh the risks, particularly in adults with leptomeningeal metastases. Intraventricular access devices are also very useful in children with leptomeningeal metastases because of an underlying solid tumor or who have CNS leukemia in second or greater relapse.

Principles of Dosing There is a disproportionate increase in CSF volume versus the body surface area during infancy, which results in a relatively fixed CSF volume after 3 years of age.[117] Therefore, in contrast to body surface area or weight-based dosing practices for systemically administered chemotherapy, dosing for intrathecal agents is based on patient age (Table 28-7 and Fig. 28-7). Because dosing strategies based on body surface area effectively overdosed adults and undertreated young children and infants, routine implementation of age-based dosing strategies for intrathecal methotrexate resulted in less neurotoxicity in adults and a lower CNS relapse rate for young children and infants with ALL.[118,119] Dosing older patients or adults on the basis of body surface area is likely to lead to increased toxicity and is contraindicated.

Intrathecal Methotrexate Methotrexate, the most commonly administered intrathecal anticancer agent, is usually administered as a single agent to adults, whereas in children with ALL, it may be administered alone or in combination with cytarabine and hydrocortisone. Table 28-7 lists typical age-based dosing recommendations for intralumbar methotrexate.

Intraventricular methotrexate regimens in adults are somewhat variable. Many neuro-oncologists routinely administer 12 mg weekly for 4 weeks and less frequently thereafter. However, intraventricular methotrexate administration using a "concentration versus time" ("C × T") approach increases the duration of CSF exposure to cytotoxic methotrexate concentrations, which is particularly

▶ TABLE 28-7. AGE-BASED DOSING FOR INTRALUMBAR METHOTREXATE, CYTARABINE, AND HYDROCORTISONE BASED ON PATIENT AGE

Age (Years)	Methotrexate (mg)	Hydrocortisone (mg)	Cytarabine (mg)
<1	6	6	12
≥1 and <2	8	8	16
>2 and <3	10	10	20
≥3 and ≤10	12	12	24
≥10	15*	15	30–50

*Some investigators do not exceed doses of 12 mg for patients ≥3 years of age.

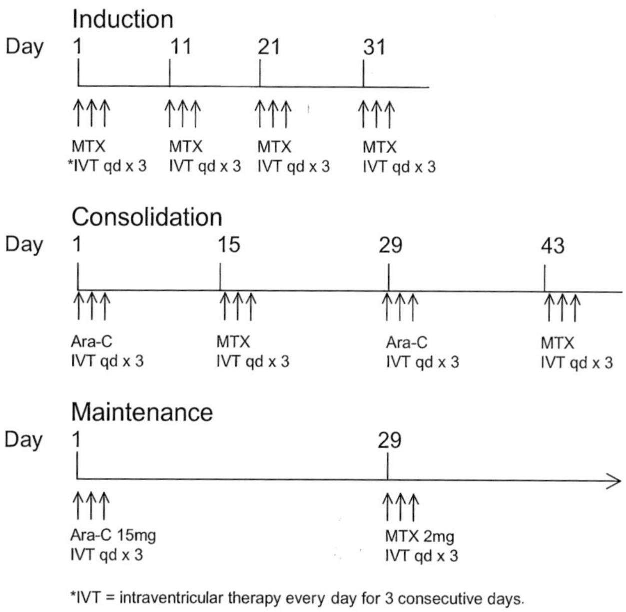

Age-based dosing for intraventricular methotrexate or cytarabine using the "C x T" dosing schedule

Age (years)	Daily Dose: Methotrexate (mg)	Daily Dose: Cytarabine (mg)
≥1 and <2	1.3	10
≥2 and <3	1.6	12.5
≥3	2	15

Figure 28-7. Diagram of the concentration times time ("C × T") regimen used for the treatment of patients with recurrent meningeal leukemia or lymphoma. The recommended age-based doses for methotrexate and cytarabine are shown in Table 28-7. (*Adapted from Moser A, Adamson PC, Gillespie A, et al. Intraventricular concentration times time [C × T] methotrexate and cytarabine for patients with recurrent meningeal leukemia and lymphoma. Cancer 1999;85:511–516.*)

important because it is a cell-cycle–specific cytotoxic agent. Figure 28-7 shows age-based dosing recommendations for intraventricular methotrexate using a "C × T" dosing schedule. The "C × T" approach induces remission in patients who were refractory to standard-dosing practices and decreases acute methotrexate-related neurotoxicity.[120,121] In theory, "C × T" dosing also decreases the potential for long-term methotrexate-related toxicity because an overall lower total drug dose is administered.[122]

Pharmacokinetic studies after intralumbar methotrexate show that elimination is biphasic with a terminal half-life of approximately 14 hours.[123] CSF methotrexate clearance occurs via bulk CSF resorption, as well as via a nonspecific transport system.[124] Low concentrations of methotrexate can be measured in plasma after standard intrathecal drug dosing. As a result, some physicians routinely administer oral leucovorin (10 mg BID × 6 doses) to minimize the risk of myelosuppression or mucositis.[13] Leucovorin does not interfere with the CNS cytotoxicity of methotrexate because it does not effectively penetrate the blood–brain barrier.

The most common acute adverse event associated with intrathecal methotrexate administration is a self-limiting chemical arachnoiditis that typically occurs within 24 hours of dosing.[125] Signs and symptoms include headache, nausea, vomiting, neck or back pain, and CSF pleocytosis. Subacute methotrexate-related toxicities occur within days to weeks of administration. These rare toxicities, which are reported to occur in less than 0.5% of patients, include paraplegia, an ascending myelopathy, and encephalopathy.[126–129] Characteristic signs and symptoms of subacute toxicities include limb weakness, which is initially distal and then ascends, ataxia, cranial nerve palsies, visual impairment, seizures, and coma. Leukoencephalopathy, which may occur months to years following therapy, is the primary late neurologic adverse event associated with intrathecal methotrexate.[130] In addition, patients who received cranial irradiation and intrathecal methotrexate are at increased risk for additional long-term neuropsychological sequelae, including impairments in nonverbal intelligence, perceptual abilities, and susceptibility to distraction.[125]

Intrathecal Cytarabine Cytarabine, the second most commonly used anticancer agent for intrathecal administration, is cleared more slowly from CSF than from plasma because CSF levels of cytidine deaminase, the enzyme that converts cytarabine to uracil arabinoside (ara-U), are much lower than in plasma.[131] CSF elimination of cytarabine is biphasic, with a terminal half-life of 3.4 hours. CSF cytarabine concentrations following a 30-mg intraventricular dose exceed 1 μM for longer than 24 hours.[132]

Cytarabine, like methotrexate, is a cell-cycle–specific anticancer agent. Therefore, the duration of tumor cell exposure to concentrations that exceed those required for cytotoxicity is an important determinant of efficacy.[113] As a result, the potential advantages of the "C × T" dosing regimen for cytarabine are similar to those for methotrexate. Extended CSF exposure to cytarabine can also be achieved using a liposomal formulation of cytarabine (see "Intrathecal cytarabine liposome injection [DepoCyt]," below). Table 28-7 and Fig. 28-7, respectively, show the recommended age-based dosing for cytarabine after intralumbar and intraventricular dosing.

The most common acute adverse event associated with intrathecal cytarabine is arachnoiditis.[125] Other much less commonly observed adverse events include seizures,[133] transient paraplegia,[134] peripheral neuropathy,[135] myelopathy, and encephalopathy.[125]

Intrathecal Cytarabine Liposome Injection (DepoCyt) DepoCyt, a sustained-release formulation of cytarabine, is approved by the U.S. Food and Drug Administration (FDA) for the treatment of adults with lymphomatous meningitis. The recommended DepoCyt dosage for adults is 50 mg,[136] whereas the maximum tolerated dose in children is 35 mg.[137] Patients treated with DepoCyt must receive concomitant dexamethasone (4 mg BID in adults or 0.15 mg/kg BID in children) to minimize the risk of arachnoiditis. Dexamethasone, which minimizes the risk of arachnoiditis, should be initiated with the first dose of DepoCyt and continues for 5 consecutive days thereafter. Tables 28-8 and 28-9 show the dosing schedules that evaluated for DepoCyt in adults and children, respectively.

CSF pharmacokinetic of intrathecal DepoCyt in adults showed that the terminal half-life of free cytarabine was more than 40 times longer than that of the standard (unencapsulated) cytarabine formulation (3.4 hours vs. 141 hours). As a result, cytotoxic concentrations of free cytarabine were maintained for an average of 9 days following intrathecal DepoCyt[138] versus 24 hours for cytarabine.[139] Limited CSF pharmacokinetic studies of intrathecal

▶ TABLE 28-8. RECOMMENDED DEPOCYT DOSING SCHEDULE IN ADULTS WITH LYMPHOMATOUS MENINGITIS

	Dosing Frequency	Week of Therapy
Induction	Every 14 days × 2 doses	Weeks 1, 3
Consolidation	Every 14 days × 3 doses, then every 28 days × 1 dose	Weeks 5, 7, 9, 13
Maintenance	Every 28 days for 4 doses	Weeks 17, 21, 25, 29

Source: From Glantz M, et al.[136]

▶ **TABLE 28-9.** SCHEDULE OF DEPOCYT EVALUATED IN CHILDREN WITH LEPTOMENINGEAL METASTASES

	Dosing Frequency	Week of Therapy
Induction	Every 14 days × 2 doses	Weeks 1, 3
Consolidation	Every 28 days × 2 doses	Weeks 7, 11, 15, 19
Maintenance	Every 56 days for 8 doses	Weeks 23, 31, 39, 47, 55, 63, 71, 79

Source: From Bomgaars L, et al.[140]

DepoCyt in children revealed that the terminal half-life of free cytarabine ranged from 50 to 57 hours. Similar to adults, cytotoxic CSF concentrations of free cytarabine in children were maintained for a prolonged period of time with a reported average of 8 days.[137]

The toxicity profile of DepoCyt plus concomitant dexamethasone appears to be similar to that of unencapsulated cytarabine. Adverse events related to intrathecal DepoCyt include headache, back pain, neck pain, fever, nausea, and encephalopathy.[136,138,140]

Intrathecal Thiotepa Thiotepa, a lipid-soluble alkylating agent that readily crosses the blood–brain barrier after intravenous dosing, is occasionally administered by the intrathecal route. Despite the fact that CSF exposure is enhanced following systemic administration of lipid-soluble agents, this physicochemical characteristic is not advantageous after intrathecal dosing because it leads to rapid drug egress from the CSF. As a result, the CSF clearance of thiotepa is approximately 9 times faster than the CSF bulk flow rate.[141] TEPA, an active lipid-soluble metabolite of thiotepa that is formed after systemic thiotepa administration, readily penetrates into the CSF. The clearance of TEPA from plasma and CSF is slower than that of thiotepa. As a result, after systemic thiotepa administration, the CSF exposure to TEPA exceeds that of thiotepa.[141] Unfortunately, thiotepa is not converted to TEPA after intrathecal dosing. Because TEPA is the active metabolite of the drug, there is no apparent rationale to administering thiotepa by the intrathecal route.

Results of clinical studies of intrathecal thiotepa confirm the limited utility of this route of drug administration. In a randomized prospective study evaluating intrathecal thiotepa versus intrathecal methotrexate for adults with leptomeningeal metastases, the median survival was 14.1 weeks in the thiotepa arm versus 15.1 weeks in the methotrexate arm.[142] Likewise, the median survival for children with leptomeningeal metastases who received intrathecal thiotepa therapy was also only 15 weeks.[143]

▶ TREATMENT RECOMMENDATIONS

Treatment of CNS Leukemic or Lymphomatous Meningitis

Methotrexate and/or cytarabine are the most commonly used intrathecal agents for patients with an initial CNS relapse. Although they are routinely administered via a lumbar puncture in the preventive setting, a "C × T" schedule (see Fig. 28-7), which requires the use of an intraventricular access device, may increase efficacy and decrease toxicity of the intrathecal therapy.[120,121] DepoCyt, a sustained-release formulation of cytarabine (see "Intrathecal Cytarabine Liposome Injection [DepoCyt]," above), is another potential treatment option for adults with lymphomatous meningitis. A randomized multicenter controlled trial of intrathecal DepoCyt versus intrathecal cytarabine in adults with lymphomatous meningitis demonstrated a significantly higher response rate in the DepoCyt arm (41% vs. 6%, $p = 0.04$).[144] There was also a trend of improvement in time to neurologic progression (median: 78.5 vs. 42 days) and median survival (median: 99.5 vs. 63 days) in the DepoCyt arm. Thus, the better response rate and comparable toxicity profile of DepoCyt (plus concomitant dexamethasone) versus cytarabine supports the use of DepoCyt in adults with lymphomatous meningitis. The sustained-release nature of DepoCyt appears to provide the same benefits of "C × T" dosing, but with much less frequent dosing. Patients with subsequent isolated CNS relapses and a good performance status are excellent candidates for trials of investigational agents for intrathecal administration.

Patients with CNS leukemia routinely receive systemic chemotherapy to prevent a subsequent bone marrow relapse whether or not they have evidence of a simultaneous systemic relapse. In some situations, this includes administration of high-dose systemic chemotherapy. Thus, the timing of the CNS-directed intrathecal therapy, relative to the systemic therapy, must be carefully orchestrated to minimize the potential for CNS toxicity.

The primary difference in the treatment of leptomeningeal metastases caused by CNS leukemia in children versus in adults is the approach for children with an initial CNS relapse. As previously discussed, substantial improvement in the event-free and overall survival rates of children with an initial CNS relapse have been realized through strategies to delay delivery of CSI for a minimum of 6 to 12 months in order to facilitate administration of early intensive chemotherapy.[29,99]

Treatment considerations for children with a second or greater leptomeningeal relapse should include the "C × T" approach or intrathecal DepoCyt. Patients with subsequent isolated CNS relapses and a good performance status are excellent candidates for trials of investigational agents for intrathecal administration.

The role of bone marrow transplantation in children and adults with a CNS leukemic relapse has not been established. There are an inadequate number of patients to prospectively evaluate this approach. However, there are anecdotal reports of patients with a history of CNS disease and prolonged disease-free survival after bone marrow transplantation.[145–148] There is a substantial risk for treatment-related adverse events, particularly CNS toxicity, in patients with a history of CNS disease who undergo a bone marrow transplantation.[148]

Patients with CNS leukemia or lymphoma and the onset of symptoms of cranial nerve involvement should receive systemic steroid therapy and have an urgent referral to a radiation oncologist. In addition, focal radiotherapy may also benefit patients with symptomatic CNS chloromas with the potential to cause significant morbidity, such as vision loss or spinal cord compression.[32,149]

Treatment of Leptomeningeal Metastases from Solid Tumors

Intrathecal chemotherapy should be considered for patients with a good performance status. It is reasonable to consider an investigational agent in patients with leptomeningeal metastases from underlying solid tumors who have ready access to clinical trials because there are no known effective therapies for the majority of these patients. The exceptions to this consideration include leptomeningeal dissemination from germinomas or medulloblastomas at initial diagnosis. Concomitant administration of radiotherapy and/or systemic chemotherapy must be addressed on a case-by-case basis, in part depending on the extent and severity of the underlying primary malignancy. For patients without access to a clinical trial, methotrexate is a reasonable option, although the potential for benefit is relatively limited. Clinical trials of intrathecal DepoCyt, gemcitabine, and topotecan are in progress.

Palliative Therapy

An important consideration in the management of patients with leptomeningeal metastases is palliative therapy. Pain is one of the most difficult challenges and may require treatment with narcotic analgesics or focal radiotherapy. Neuropathic pain may respond to a tricyclic antidepressant or an anticonvulsant.[63] Symptoms of increased intracranial pressure may be ameliorated with dexamethasone. However, because many patients find the long-term side effects of dexamethasone intolerable, the risks and benefits should be carefully discussed prior to initiation. Patients with obstructive hydrocephalus secondary to tumor may also benefit from focal or whole-brain radiotherapy. Seizures generally respond to anticonvulsant therapy; use of a nonsedating anticonvulsant is best.[63] Cortical symptoms resulting from the tumor or as a sequelae of therapy, for example, decreased attention or somnolence, may be improved through the use of psychostimulants.[63] Optimal palliation of pleomorphic symptoms associated with leptomeningeal metastases and the potential for extremely rapid disease progression require substantial communication between the patient and health care team.

Investigational Agents for the Treatment of Leptomeningeal Metastases

The paucity of new agents for intrathecal administration has prevented clinicians from developing effective combination strategies for intrathecal administration. Multidrug combinations, the mainstay of treatment for systemic malignancies, must also be developed for the treatment of leptomeningeal metastases. The use of a nonhuman primate model with a chronically indwelling lateral and fourth ventricular Pudenz catheters attached to subcutaneously implanted Ommaya reservoirs has resulted in the preclinical development of several new cytotoxic agents for intrathecal administration.[150] It is hoped that the ongoing development of active new cytotoxic agents will result in the development and identification of effective combinations for intrathecal administration.

Topotecan

Topotecan, a water-soluble topoisomerase I poison, has substantial antitumor activity after systemic administration in a wide variety of adult and pediatric tumors, including carcinomas of the lung and ovary, leukemia, neuroblastoma, rhabdomyosarcoma, and medulloblastoma. A recently completed phase I trial of intrathecal topotecan demonstrated the safety and feasibility of this route of administration in patients with leptomeningeal metastases.[151] Phase II trials of topotecan in adults and children with leptomeningeal metastases are in progress.

Gemcitabine

Gemcitabine, a fluorinated deoxycytidine analogue, has a broad spectrum of antitumor activity in solid tumors and leukemias. Gemcitabine is triphosphorylated in tumor cells by deoxycytidine kinase. Gemcitabine triphosphate subsequently inhibits DNA polymerase, whereas gemcitabine diphosphate inhibits ribonucleotide reductase. The feasibility of intrathecal gemcitabine was demonstrated in preclinical studies.[152] A phase I trial of intrathecal gemcitabine in children and adults with leptomeningeal metastases is in progress.

Mafosfamide

Mafosfamide is a preactivated analogue of cyclophosphamide that does not require hepatic metabolism to have a cytotoxic effect. Phase I trials and clinical series have demonstrated the feasibility of intrathecal mafosfamide administration in children and adults with leptomeningeal metastases.[153] A Pediatric Brain Tumor Consortium (PBTC) trial is currently evaluating the feasibility of intrathecal drug administration using mafosfamide in children younger than 3 years of age with newly diagnosed CNS embryonal tumors.[154] It is hypothesized that if feasible, this strategy may eliminate the need for CSI in infants and young children with embryonal CNS tumors who are at high risk of leptomeningeal tumor spread.

Other Strategies

A variety of other strategies for the treatment of leptomeningeal metastases have been evaluated in the phase I or II clinical settings, including a variety of monoclonal antibodies,[155–158] immunotoxins,[159–162] interferons,[163] and gene therapy.[164–166]

▶ DURAL AND SKULL-BASED METASTASES

The dura mater, a dense membrane composed of an outer fibrous layer, which is actually the connective tissue membrane of the skull bone, and an inner meningeal layer, is a site of metastatic spread for a wide variety of intracranial and extracranial tumors, including carcinomas of the prostate, lung, and breast in adults.[167] In children, a variety of sarcomas, including rhabdomyosarcoma, hemangiopericytoma, fibrosarcoma, malignant fibrous histiocytoma, extraskeletal myxoid chondrosarcoma, mesenchymal chondrosarcoma, and Ewing sarcoma, and a variety of acute leukemias and lymphomas may disseminate to the dura or skull.[168] Other malignant tumors that have been reported to metastasize to the skull or dura include squamous cell carcinomas,[169] parotid gland oncocytomas,[170] solitary fibrous tumors,[171] and colon carcinoma.[172]

Solitary dural metastases are very uncommon and frequently resemble meningiomas. Other differential diagnoses include Rosai-Dorfman disease,[173] benign pituitary adenomas,[174] melanocytomas, inflammatory pseudotumor, and a variety of histiocytic disorders, such as juvenile xanthogranuloma and Langerhans cell histiocytosis.[168]

The treatment approach for dural or skull-based metastases is similar to that for patients with leptomeningeal metastases in that the approach to each patient must be individualized based on the underlying histopathologic diagnosis and the status of the underlying systemic or primary CNS malignancy. In those patients with advanced systemic disease and a poor performance status, the recommended treatment may be palliative. In contrast, in patients with stable systemic disease, treatment may include surgery, radiation therapy, or systemic chemotherapy depending on the location and extent of the metastatic dural or skull-based metastases.

▶ CONCLUSION AND FUTURE DIRECTIONS

Tremendous progress has been made in the treatment and prevention of leptomeningeal metastases in patients with leukemias and lymphomas. As a result of this success we have learned a tremendous amount about appropriate dosing strategies for intrathecal agents and the adverse sequelae associate with CNS-targeted therapies. Similar strides have not yet been realized in the treatment of leptomeningeal metastases resulting from underlying solid (extra- or intracranial) tumors. Ongoing clinical efforts for solid tumor leptomeningeal metastases must focus on the development of combination chemotherapy strategies for intrathecal administration and optimal delivery of systemic therapy. These efforts must be closely lined with basic biology and correlative laboratory studies evaluating tumor genes and markers that may predict which patients are at highest risk for leptomeningeal dissemination because the optimal treatment for leptomeningeal metastases is preventive. Well-designed clinical trials, which focus on efficacy, disease-free progression, and quality of life, are prerequisites for critically evaluating the success of new treatment strategies for leptomeningeal metastases.

REFERENCES

1. Grossman S, Moynihan T. Neurologic complications of systemic cancer; neoplastic meningitis. Neurol Clin 1991;9:843–856.
2. Kaplan JG, DeSouza TG, Farkash A, et al. Leptomeningeal metastases: comparison of clinical features and laboratory data of solid tumors, lymphomas and leukemias. J Neurooncol 1990;9:225–229.
3. Pansky B, Allen DJ. Review of neuroscience. New York: Macmillan, 1980.
4. Rosen S, Aisner J, Makuch R, et al. Carcinomatous leptomeningitis in small cell lung cancer: a clinicopathologic review of the National Cancer Institute experience. Medicine (Baltimore) 1982;61:45–53.
5. Nugent J, Bunn PJ, Matthews M, et al. CNS metastases in small cell bronchogenic carcinoma: increasing frequency and changing pattern with lengthening survival. Cancer 1979;44:1885–1893.
6. Kosmas C, Malamos NA, Tsavaris NB, et al. Leptomeningeal carcinomatosis after major remission to taxane-based front-line therapy in patients with advanced breast cancer. J Neurooncol 2002;56:265–273.
7. Little J, Dale A, Okazaki H. Meningeal carcinomatosis: clinical manifestations. Arch Neurol 1974;30:138–143.
8. Theodore W, Gendelman S. Meningeal carcinomatosis. Arch Neurol 1981;38:696–699.
9. Mayer R, Berkowitz R, Griffiths C. Central nervous system involvement by ovarian carcinoma: a complication of prolonged survival with metastatic disease. Proc Ann Meet Assoc Cancer Res Am Soc Clin Oncol 1978;19:318.

10. Lisenko Y, Kumar AJ, Yao J, et al. Leptomeningeal carcinomatosis originating from gastric cancer: report of eight cases and review of the literature. Am J Clin Oncol 2003;26: 165–170.
11. Saito R, Kumabe T, Jokura H, et al. Symptomatic spinal dissemination of malignant astrocytoma. J Neurooncol 2003; 61:227–235.
12. Endo H, Kumabe T, Jokura H, et al. Leptomeningeal dissemination of cerebellar malignant astrocytomas. J Neurooncol 2003;63:191–199.
13. Glantz M. Carcinomatous and lymphomatous meningitis. In: Rose B, ed. UpToDate. Welleseley, MA: 2003.
14. Grossman S. Clinical practice guidelines in oncology: central nervous system cancers, vol. 1. On-line reference, Version 1, 2002, 6/25/02. National Comprehensive Cancer Network, 2002.
15. Shlomit R, Ayala AG, Michal D, et al. Gains and losses of DNA sequences in childhood brain tumors analyzed by comparative genomic hybridization. Cancer Genet Cytogenet 2000;121:67–72.
16. Littman P, Raney B, Zimmerman R, et al. Soft-tissue sarcomas of the head and neck in children. Int J Radiat Oncol Biol Phys 1983;9:1367–1371.
17. Wharam MJ. Rhabdomyosarcoma of parameningeal sites. Semin Radiat Oncol 1997;7:212–216.
18. Trigg M, Glaubiger D, Nesbit M. The frequency of isolated CNS involvement in Ewing's sarcoma. Cancer 1982;49: 2404–2409.
19. Yu L, Craver R, Baliga M, et al. Isolated CNS involvement in Ewing's sarcoma. Med Pediatr Oncol 1990;18:354–358.
20. Kramer K, Kushner B, Heller G, et al. Neuroblastoma metastatic to the central nervous system. Cancer 2001;91: 1510–1519.
21. Shaw P, Eden T. Neuroblastoma with intracranial involvement: an ENSG study. Med Pediatr Oncol 1992;20:149–155.
22. Meli F, Boccaleri C, Manzitti J, et al. Meningeal dissemination of retinoblastoma: CT findings in with patients. Am J Neuroradiol 1990;11:983–986.
23. Perilongo G, Garre ML, Giangaspero F. Low-grade gliomas and leptomeningeal dissemination: a poorly understood phenomenon. Childs Nerv Syst 2003;19:197–203.
24. Scheinberg D, Maslak P, Weiss M. Acute leukemias. In: DeVita V, Hellman S, Rosenberg S, eds. Cancer: principles and practice of oncology, 6th ed. Philadelphia: Lippincott Williams & Wilkins, 2001:2404–2433.
25. Evans A, Gilbert E, Zandstra R. The increasing incidence of central nervous system leukemia in children. Cancer 1970;26:404–407.
26. Price R, Johnson W. The central nervous system in childhood leukemia. I. The arachnoid. Cancer 1973;31:520–533.
27. Surapeneni U, Cortes J, Thomas DG, et al. Central nervous system relapse in adults with acute lymphoblastic leukemia. Cancer 2002;94:773–779.
28. Goldberg JM, Silverman LB, Levy DE, et al. Childhood T-cell acute lymphoblastic leukemia: the Dana-Farber Cancer Institute acute lymphoblastic leukemia consortium experience. J Clin Oncol 2003;21:3616–3622.
29. Ritchey A, Pollock B, Lauer S, et al. Improved survival of children with isolated CNS relapse of acute lymphoblastic leukemia. J Clin Oncol 1999;17:3745–3752.
30. Behrendt H, Leeuwen E, Schuwirth C, et al. The significance of an isolated central nervous system relapse, occurring as first relapse in children with acute lymphoblastic leukemia. Cancer 1989;63:2066–2072.
31. Morris EC, Harrison G, Bailey CC, et al. Prognostic factors and outcome for children after second central nervous system relapse of acute lymphoblastic leukaemia. Br J Haematol 2003;120:787–789.
32. Golub T, Arceci R. Acute myelogenous leukemia. In: Pizzo PA, Poplack DG, eds. Principles and practice of pediatric oncology, 4th ed. Philadelphia: Lippincott Williams & Wilkins, 2002:545–590.
33. Pui CH, Dahl GV, Kalwinsky DK, et al. Central nervous system leukemia in children with acute nonlymphoblastic leukemia. Blood 1985;66:1062–1067.
34. Dusenbery KE, Howells WB, Arthur DC, et al. Extramedullary leukemia in children with newly diagnosed acute myeloid leukemia: a report from the Children's Cancer Group. J Pediatr Hematol Oncol 2003;25: 760–768.
35. Pui CH, Raimondi SC, Srivastava DK, et al. Prognostic factors in infants with acute myeloid leukemia. Leukemia 2000;14:684–687.
36. Pui CH, Kalwinsky DK, Schell MJ, et al. Acute nonlymphoblastic leukemia in infants: clinical presentation and outcome. J Clin Oncol 1988;6:1008–1013.
37. Glass JP, Van Tassel P, Keating MJ, et al. Central nervous system complications of a newly recognized subtype of leukemia: AMML with a pericentric inversion of chromosome 16. Neurology 1987;37:639–644.
38. Holmes R, Keating MJ, Cork A, et al. A unique pattern of central nervous system leukemia in acute myelomonocytic leukemia associated with inv(16)(p13q22). Blood 1985;65: 1071–1078.
39. Ghaddar HM, Plunkett W, Kantarjian HM, et al. Long-term results following treatment of newly-diagnosed acute myelogenous leukemia with continuous-infusion high-dose cytosine arabinoside. Leukemia 1994;8:1269–1274.
40. Sandlund J, Murphy S, Santana V, et al. CNS involvement in children with newly diagnosed non-Hodgkin's lymphoma. J Clin Oncol 2000;18:3018–3024.
41. Levitt L, Dawson D, Rosenthal D, et al. CNS involvement in the non-Hodgkin's lymphomas. Cancer 1980;45:545–552.
42. Weizsaecker M, Koelmel HW. Meningeal involvement in leukemias and malignant lymphomas of adults: incidence, course of disease, and treatment for prevention. Acta Neurol Scand 1979;60:363–370.
43. Sarker D, Thirwell C, Nelson M, et al. Leptomeningeal disease in AIDS-related non-Hodgkin's lymphoma. AIDS 2003;11:861–865.
44. Spreafico F, Massimino M, Luksch R, et al. Intensive, very short-term chemotherapy for advanced Burkitt's lymphoma in children. J Clin Oncol 2002;20:2783–2788.
45. Millot F, Suciu S, Philippe N, et al. Value of high-dose cytarabine during interval therapy of a Berlin-Frankfurt-Munster-based protocol in increased-risk children with acute lymphoblastic leukemia and lymphoblastic lymphoma: results of the European Organization for Research and Treatment of Cancer 58881 randomized phase III trial. J Clin Oncol 2001;19:1935–1942.

46. Hollender A, Kvaloy S, Nome O, et al. Central nervous system involvement following diagnosis of non-Hodgkin's lymphoma: a risk model. Ann Oncol 2002;13:1099–1107.
47. Haioun C, Besson C, Lepage E, et al. Incidence and risk factors of central nervous system relapse in histologically aggressive non-Hodgkin's lymphoma uniformly treated and receiving intrathecal central nervous system prophylaxis: a GELA study on 974 patients. Groupe d'Etudes des Lymphomes de l'Adulte. Ann Oncol 2000;11: 685–690.
48. Linassier C, Desablens B, Lefrancq T, et al. Stage I-IIE primary non-Hodgkin's lymphoma of the testis: results of a prospective trial by the GOELAMS Study Group. Clin Lymphoma 2002;3:167–172.
49. Kokkoris CP. Leptomeningeal carcinomatosis. How does cancer reach the pia-arachnoid? Cancer 1983;51:154–160.
50. Groves MD. The pathogenesis of neoplastic meningitis. Curr Oncol Rep 2003;5:15–23.
51. Bleyer W. Biology and pathogenesis of CNS leukemia. Am J Pediatr Hematol Oncol 1989;11:57–63.
52. Norris LK, Grossman SA, Olivi A. Neoplastic meningitis following surgical resection of isolated cerebellar metastasis: a potentially preventable complication. J Neurooncol 1997;32:215–223.
53. DeAngelis LM, Mandell LR, Thaler HT, et al. The role of postoperative radiotherapy after resection of single brain metastases. Neurosurgery 1989;24:798–805.
54. Pui CH. Toward optimal central nervous system-directed treatment in childhood acute lymphoblastic leukemia. J Clin Oncol 2003;21:179–181.
55. Wasserstrom W, Glass J, Posner J. Diagnosis and treatment of leptomeningeal metastases from solid tumors: experience with 90 patients. Cancer 1982;49:759–772.
56. DeAngelis L. Current diagnosis and treatment of leptomeningeal metastasis. J Neurooncol 1998;38:245–252.
57. Chamberlain M, Corey-Bloom J. Leptomeningeal metastases: 111 indium-DTPA CSF flow studies. Neurology 1991;41:1765–1769.
58. Olson M, Chernik N, Posner J. Infiltration of leptomeninges by systemic cancer: a clinical and pathologic study. Arch Neurol 1974;30:122–137.
59. Demopoulos A, DeAngelis LM. Neurologic complications of leukemia. Curr Opin Neurol 2002;15:691–699.
60. Bomgaars L, Chamberlain MC, Poplack DG, et al. Leptomeningeal metastases. In: Levin VA, ed. Cancer in the nervous system. New York: Oxford University Press, 2002: 375–393.
61. Chamberlain MC. New approaches to and current treatment of leptomeningeal metastases. Curr Opin Neurol 1994;7:492–500.
62. van Oostenbrugge RJ, Twijnstra A. Presenting features and value of diagnostic procedures in leptomeningeal metastases. Neurology 1999;53:382–385.
63. Berg SL, Chamberlain MC. Systemic chemotherapy, intrathecal chemotherapy, and symptom management in the treatment of leptomeningeal metastasis. Curr Oncol Rep 2003;5:29–40.
64. Shen T, Young Y. Meningeal carcinomatosis manifested as bilateral progressive sensorineural hearing loss. Am J Otol 2000;21:510–512.
65. Dunne JW, Harper CG, Pamphlett R. Intramedullary spinal cord metastases: a clinical and pathological study of nine cases. Q J Med 1986;61:1003–1020.
66. Chamberlain MC, Kormanik PA, Glantz MJ. A comparison between ventricular and lumbar cerebrospinal fluid cytology in adult patients with leptomeningeal metastases. Neuro-oncol 2001;3:42–5.
67. Gajjar A, Fouladi M, Walter AW, et al. Comparison of lumbar and shunt cerebrospinal fluid specimens for cytologic detection of leptomeningeal disease in pediatric patients with brain tumors. J Clin Oncol 1999;17:1825–1828.
68. Bigner S, Johnston W. The cytopathology of cerebrospinal fluid. Acta Cytol 1981;25:461–477.
69. Meyers SP, Wildenhain SL, Chang JK, et al. Postoperative evaluation for disseminated medulloblastoma involving the spine: contrast-enhanced MR findings, CSF cytologic analysis, timing of disease occurrence, and patient outcomes. AJNR 2000;21:1757–1765.
70. Gleissner B, Siehl J, Korfel A, et al. CSF evaluation in primary CNS lymphoma patients by PCR of the CDR III IgH genes. Neurology 2002;58:390–396.
71. Wong L, Lueth M, Li X, et al. Detection of mitochondrial DNA mutations in the tumor and cerebrospinal fluid of medulloblastoma patients. Cancer Res 2003;63: 3866–3371.
72. Stockhammer G, Poewe W, Burgstaller S, et al. Vascular endothelial growth factor in CSF: a biological marker for carcinomatous meningitis. Neurology 2000;54:1670–1676.
73. Mahmoud H, Rivera G, Hancock M, et al. Low leukocyte counts with blast cells in cerebrospinal fluid of children with newly diagnosed acute lymphoblastic leukemia. N Engl J Med 1993;329:314–319.
74. Lauer S, Shuster J, Kirchner P, et al. Prognostic significance of cerebrospinal fluid (CSF) lymphoblasts (LB) at diagnosis (dx) in children with acute lymphoblastic leukemia (ALL). Proc Am Soc Clin Oncol 1994;13:317.
75. Gilchrist G, Tubergen D, Sather H, et al. Low numbers of CSF blasts at diagnosis do not predict for the development of CNS leukemia in children with intermediate-risk acute lymphoblastic leukemia: a Children's Cancer Group Report. J Clin Oncol 1994;12:2594–2600.
76. Burger B, Zimmermann M, Mann G, et al. Diagnostic cerebrospinal fluid examination in children with acute lymphoblastic leukemia: significance of low leukocyte counts with blasts or traumatic lumbar puncture. J Clin Oncol 2003;21:184–188.
77. Moriarty AT, Wiersema L, Snyder W, et al. Immunophenotyping of cytologic specimens by flow cytometry. Diagn Cytopathol 1993;9:252–258.
78. Rhodes C, Glantz M, Callanan H, et al. A comparison of polymerase chain reaction examination of cerebrospinal fluid and conventional cytology in the diagnosis of lymphomatous meningitis. Cancer 1996;77:543–548.
79. Jaeckle K, Krol G, Posner J. Evolution of computed tomographic abnormalities in leptomeningeal metastases. Ann Neurol 1985;17:85–89.
80. Chamberlain M, Sandy A, Press G. Leptomeningeal metastasis: a comparison of gadolinium-enhanced MR and contrast-enhanced CT of the brain. Neurology 1990;40: 435–438.

81. Chamberlain M. Comparative spine imaging in leptomeningeal metastases. J Neurooncol 1995;23:233–238.
82. Chamberlain M. A review of leptomeningeal metastases in pediatrics. J Child Neurol 1995;10:191–199.
83. Kallmes D, Gray L, Glass J. High-dose gadolinium-enhanced MRI for diagnosis of meningeal metastases. Neuroradiology 1998;40:23–26.
84. Schumacher M, Orszagh M. Imaging techniques in neoplastic meningosis. J Neurooncol 1998;38:111–120.
85. Freilich RJ, Krol G, DeAngelis LM. Neuroimaging and cerebrospinal fluid cytology in the diagnosis of leptomeningeal metastasis. Ann Neurol 1995;38:51–57.
86. Sze S, Leeds NE, Ginsberg LE. MR imaging of leptomeningeal metastases: comparison of three sequences. Am J Neuroradiol 2002;23:745–746.
87. Singh SK, Leeds NE, Ginsberg LE. MR imaging of leptomeningeal metastases: comparison of three sequences. AJNR 2002;23:817–821.
88. Griffiths P, Coley S, Romanowski C, et al. Contrast-enhanced fluid-attenuated inversion recovery imaging for leptomeningeal disease in children. Am J Neuroradiol 2003;24:719–723.
89. Mathews V, Caldemeyer K, Lowe M, et al. Brain: gadolinium-enhanced fast fluid-attenuated inversion-recovery MR imaging. Radiology 2000;215:922–924.
90. Grossman S, Trump D, Chen D, et al. Cerebrospinal fluid flow abnormalities in patients with neoplastic meningitis: an evaluation using ^{111}Indium-DTPA ventriculography. Am J Med 1982;73:641–647.
91. Korkmaz M, Kim EE, Wong FC, et al. In-111 DTPA Ommaya grams in leptomeningeal carcinomatosis. Clin Nucl Med 1995;20:610–612.
92. Glantz M, Hall W, Cole B, et al. Diagnosis, management, and survival of patients with leptomeningeal cancer based on cerebrospinal fluid-flow status. Cancer 1995;75:2919–2931.
93. Chamberlain M, Kormanik P. Prognostic significance of ^{111}indium-DTPA CSF flow studies in leptomeningeal metastases. Neurology 1996;46:1674–1677.
94. Chang CH, Housepian EM, Herbert C Jr. An operative staging system and a megavoltage radiotherapeutic technic for cerebellar medulloblastomas. Radiology 1969;93:1351–1359.
95. Zachariah B, Zachariah SB, Varghese R, et al. Carcinomatous meningitis: clinical manifestations and management. Int J Clin Pharmacol Ther 1995;33:7–12.
96. Cokgor I, Friedman AH, Friedman HS. Current options for the treatment of neoplastic meningitis. J Neurooncol 2002;60:79–88.
97. Margolin J, Poplack D. Acute lymphoblastic leukemia. In: Pizzo PA, Poplack DG, eds. Principles and practice of pediatric oncology, 4th ed. Philadelphia: Lippincott Williams & Wilkins, 2002:489–544.
98. Pui CH, Cheng C, Leung W, et al. Extended follow-up of long-term survivors of childhood acute lymphoblastic leukemia. N Engl J Med 2003;349:640–649.
99. Barredo J, Lauer S, Billet AL, et al. Isolated CNS relapse of acute lymphoblastic leukemia (ALL) treated with intensive systemic chemotherapy and delayed CNS radiation: a Pediatric Oncology Group study. Proc Am Soc Clin Oncol 2003;22:796.
100. Voorhess M, Brecher M, Glickman A, et al. Hypothalamic pituitary function of children with acute lymphocytic leukemia after three forms of central nervous system prophylaxis. Cancer 1986;57:1287–1291.
101. Pasqualini T, McCalla J, Berg S, et al. Subtle primary hypothyroidism in patients treated for acute lymphoblastic leukemia. Acta Endocrinol (Copenh) 1991;124:375–380.
102. Blatt J, Bercu B, Gillen C, et al. Reduced pulsatile growth hormone secretion in children after therapy for acute lymphoblastic leukemia. J Pediatr 1984;104:182–186.
103. Moss H, Nannins E, Poplack D. The effects of prophylactic treatment of the central nervous system on the intellectual function of children with acute lymphocytic leukemia. Am J Med 1981;71:47–52.
104. Paolucci G, Rosito P. Adverse sequelae of central nervous system prophylaxis in acute lymphoblastic leukemia. In: Mastrangelo R, Poplack D, Riccardi R, eds. Central nervous system leukemia. Boston: Martinus Nijhoff, 1983:105–111.
105. Poplack D. Evaluation of adverse sequelae of central nervous system prophylaxis in acute lymphoblastic leukemia. In: Mastrangelo R, Poplack D, Riccardi R, eds. Central nervous system leukemia. Boston: Martinus Nijhoff, 1983:95–103.
106. Radcliff J, Packer R, Atkins T, et al. Prospective study of cognitive function in children with medulloblastoma receiving whole brain radiotherapy and chemotherapy. Ann Neurol 1992;32:551–555.
107. Johnson D, McGabe M, Nicholson H, et al. Quality of long-term survival in young children with medulloblastoma. J Neurosurg 1994;80:1004–1010.
108. Bomgaars L, Poplack D, Blaney S. Intrathecal chemotherapy. In: Yaksh, TL, ed. Spinal drug delivery. Amsterdam: Elsevier Science BV, 1999:503–512.
109. Blasberg R, Patlak C, Fernstermacher J. Intrathecal chemotherapy. Brain tissue profiles after ventriculo-cisternal perfusion. J Pharm Exp Therap 1975;195:73–83.
110. Glantz MJ, Cole BF, Recht L, et al. High-dose intravenous methotrexate for patients with nonleukemic leptomeningeal cancer: is intrathecal chemotherapy necessary? J Clin Oncol 1998;16:1561–1567.
111. Siegal T. Leptomeningeal metastases: rationale for systemic chemotherapy or what is the role of intra-CSF chemotherapy? J Neurooncol 1998;38:151–157.
112. Collins J. Regional therapy: an overview. In: Poplack DG, Massimo L, Cornaglia-Ferraris P, eds. The role of pharmacology in pediatric oncology. Boston: Martinus Nijhoff, 1987:125–135.
113. Chabner B. The role of drugs in cancer treatment. In: Chabner B, Collins J, eds. Pharmacologic principles of cancer treatment. Philadelphia: WB Saunders, 1982:3–14.
114. Poplack D, Riccardi R. Pharmacologic approaches to the treatment of central nervous system malignancy. In: Poplack DG, Massimo L, Cornaglia-Ferraris P, eds. The role of pharmacology in pediatric oncology. Boston: Martinus Nijhoff, 1987:125–135.
115. Larson S, Schall G, DiChiro G. The influence of previous lumbar puncture and pneumoencephalography on the

incidence of unsuccessful radioisotope cisternography. J Nucl Med 1971;12:555–557.

116. Blaney S, Poplack D, Godwin K, et al. The effect of body position on ventricular cerebrospinal fluid methotrexate concentration following intralumbar administration. J Clin Oncol 1995;13:177–179.
117. Bleyer W. Clinical pharmacology of intrathecal methotrexate. II. An improved dosage regimen derived from age-related pharmacokinetics. Cancer Treat Rep 1977;61:1419–1425.
118. Bleyer W, Coccia P, Sather H, et al. Reduction in central nervous system leukemia with a pharmacokinetically derived intrathecal methotrexate dosage regimen. J Clin Oncol 1983;1:317–325.
119. Bleyer W, Savitch J, Holcenberg J. An improved regimen for intrathecal chemotherapy. Clin Pharm Ther 1976;19:103.
120. Bleyer W, Poplack D, Simon R. "Concentration-time" methotrexate via a subcutaneous reservoir: a less toxic regimen for intraventricular chemotherapy of central nervous system neoplasms. Blood 1978;51:835–842.
121. Moser A, Adamson PC, Gillespie A, et al. Intraventricular concentration times time (C × T) methotrexate and cytarabine for patients with recurrent meningeal leukemia and lymphoma. Cancer 1999;85:511–516.
122. Sagar S. Carcinomatous meningitis: it does not have to be a death sentence. Oncology 2002;16:237–242.
123. Bleyer W, Poplack D. Clinical studies on the central-nervous-system pharmacology of methotrexate. Amsterdam: Elsevier/North-Holland Biomedica, 1978.
124. Bode U, McGrath I, Bleyer W, et al. Active transport of methotrexate from cerebrospinal fluid in humans. Cancer Res 1980;40:2184–2187.
125. Kaplan R, Wiernik P. Neurotoxicity of antineoplastic drugs. Semin Oncol 1982;9:103–130.
126. Saiki J, Thompson S, Smith F, et al. Paraplegia following intrathecal chemotherapy. Cancer 1972;29:370–374.
127. Gagliano R, Costanzi J. Paraplegia following intrathecal methotrexate. Cancer 1976;37:1663–1668.
128. Koh S, Nelson MD Jr, Kovanlikaya A, et al. Anterior lumbosacral radiculopathy after intrathecal methotrexate treatment. Pediatr Neurol 1999;21:576–578.
129. Hirschfeld S, Flowers C, Smith M. Toxicity from intrathecal therapy in pediatric hematologic neoplasms: is the incidence increasing? Proc Am Soc Clin Oncol 1998;17:539a.
130. Butler R, Hill J, Steinherz P, et al. Neuropsychologic effects of cranial irradiation, intrathecal methotrexate, and systemic methotrexate in childhood cancer. J Clin Oncol 1994;12:2621–2629.
131. Camiener G, Smith C: Studies of the enzymatic deamination of cytosine arabinoside. I. Enzyme distribution and species specificity. Biochem Pharmacol 1965;14:1405–1416.
132. Zimm S, Collins J, Miser J, et al. Cytosine arabinoside cerebrospinal fluid kinetics. Clin Pharmacol Therap 1984;35: 826–830.
133. Kay H, Knapton P, O'Sullivan J, et al. Encephalopathy associated with methotrexate therapy. Arch Dis Child 1972;47: 344–354.
134. Wolff L, Zighelboim J, Gale R. Paraplegia following intrathecal cytosine arabinoside. Cancer 1979;43: 83–88.
135. Russell J, Powles R. Neuropathy due to cytosine arabinoside. Br Med J 1974;4:652–653.
136. Glantz M, LaFollette S, Jaeckle K, et al. Randomized trial of a slow-release versus a standard formulation of cytarabine for intrathecal treatment of lymphomatous meningitis. J Clin Oncol 1999;17:3110–3116.
137. Bomgaars L, Geyer J, Franklin J, et al. A phase I trial of intrathecal liposomal cytarabine in children with neoplastic meningitis. J Clin Oncol 2004;22:3916–3921.
138. Kim S, Chatelut E, Kim J, et al. Extended CSF cytarabine exposure following intrathecal administration of DTC 101. J Clin Oncol 1993;11:2186–2193.
139. Kim S, Khatibi S, Howel S, et al. Prolongation of drug exposure in cerebrospinal fluid by encapsulation into DepoFoam. Cancer Res 1993;53:1596–1598.
140. Bomgaars L, Geyer J, Franklin J, et al. A phase I dose escalation study of intrathecal DepoFoam™ encapsulated cytarabine (DTC101) in pediatric patients with advanced malignancies. Pediatr Hematol Oncol 1998;20:683.
141. Strong J, Collins J, Lester C, et al. Pharmacokinetics of intraventricular and intravenous *N,N,'N''*-triethylenethiophosphoramide (thiotepa) in rhesus monkeys and humans. Cancer Res 1986;46:6101–6104.
142. Grossman S, Finkelstein D, Ruckdeschel J, et al. Randomized prospective comparison of intraventricular methotrexate and thiotepa in patients with previously untreated neoplastic meningitis. Eastern Cooperative Oncology Group. J Clin Oncol 1993;11:561–569.
143. Fisher P, Kadan-Lottick N, Korones D. Intrathecal thiotepa: reappraisal of an established therapy. Pediatr Hematol Oncol 2002;24:274–278.
144. Glantz M, Jaeckle K, Chamberlain M, et al. A randomized controlled trial comparing intrathecal sustained-release cytarabine (DepoCyt) to intrathecal methotrexate in patients with neoplastic meningitis from solid tumors. Clin Cancer Res 1999;5:3394–3402.
145. Messina C, Valsecchi MG, Arico M, et al. Autologous bone marrow transplantation for treatment of isolated central nervous system relapse of childhood acute lymphoblastic leukemia. AIEOP/FONOP-TMO group. Associzione Italiana Emato-Oncologia Pediatrica. Bone Marrow Transplant 1998;21:9–14.
146. van Besien K, Forman A, Champlin R. Central nervous system relapse of lymphoid malignancies in adults: the role of high-dose chemotherapy. Ann Oncol 1997;8:515–524.
147. Classen CF, Debatin KM, Friedrich W, et al. Long-term remission of APL with a second allogeneic BMT after CNS relapse following HLA-identical allogeneic BMT. Bone Marrow Transplant 2003;32:843–846.
148. van Besien K, Przepiorka D, Mehra R, et al. Impact of preexisting CNS involvement on the outcome of bone marrow transplantation in adult hematologic malignancies. J Clin Oncol 1996;14:3036–3042.
149. Mostafavi H, Lennarson PJ, Traynelis VC. Granulocytic sarcoma of the spine. Neurosurgery 2000;46:78–83; discussion 83–84.
150. McCully C, Balis F, Bacher J, et al. A rhesus monkey model for continuous infusion of drugs into cerebrospinal fluid. Lab Anim Sci 1990;40:520–525.

151. Blaney SM, Heideman R, Berg S, et al. Phase I clinical trial of intrathecal topotecan in patients with neoplastic meningitis. J Clin Oncol 2003;21:143–147.
152. Egorin MJ, Zuhowski EG, McCully CM, et al. Pharmacokinetics of intrathecal gemcitabine in nonhuman primates. Clin Cancer Res 2002;8:2437–2442.
153. Blaney S, Balis F, Murphy R, et al. A phase I study of intrathecal mafosfamide in patients with refractory meningeal malignancies. J Clin Oncol 2005;23:1555–1563.
154. Blaney S, Boyett J, Friedman H, et al. Phase 1 trial of intrathecal mafosfamide in infants with embryonal CNS tumors: a Pediatric Brain Tumor Consortium Study. J Clin Oncol 2005;23:525–531.
155. Brown MT, Coleman RE, Friedman AH, et al. Intrathecal ^{131}I-labeled antitenascin monoclonal antibody 81C6 treatment of patients with leptomeningeal neoplasms or primary brain tumor resection cavities with subarachnoid communication: phase I trial results. Clin Cancer Res 1996;2:963–972.
156. Coakham HB, Garson JA, Brownell B, et al. Use of monoclonal antibody panel to identify malignant cells in cerebrospinal fluid. Lancet 1984;1:1095–1098.
157. Kemshead JT, Hopkins K, Pizer B, et al. Dose escalation with repeated intrathecal injections of ^{131}I-labelled MAbs for the treatment of central nervous system malignancies. Br J Cancer 1998;77:2324–2330.
158. Pizer BL, Kemshead JT. The potential of targeted radiotherapy in the treatment of central nervous system leukaemia. Leuk Lymphoma 1994;15:281–289.
159. Zovickian J, Youle RJ. Efficacy of intrathecal immunotoxin therapy in an animal model of leptomeningeal neoplasia. J Neurosurg 1988;68:767–774.
160. Gunther R, Chelstrom LM, Tuel-Ahlgren L, et al. Biotherapy for xenografted human central nervous system leukemia in mice with severe combined immunodeficiency using B43 (anti-CD19)-pokeweed antiviral protein immunotoxin. Blood 1995;85:2537–2545.
161. Herrlinger U, Schmidberger H, Buchholz R, et al. Intrathecal therapy of leptomeningeal CEM T-cell lymphoma in nude rats with anti-CD7 ricin toxin A chain immunotoxin. J Neurooncol 1998;40:1–9.
162. Laske DW, Muraszko KM, Oldfield EH, et al. Intraventricular immunotoxin therapy for leptomeningeal neoplasia. Neurosurgery 1997;41:1039–1049d,e.
163. Chamberlain MC. A phase II trial of intra-cerebrospinal fluid alpha interferon in the treatment of neoplastic meningitis. Cancer 2002;94:2675–2680.
164. Oldfield EH, Ram Z, Chiang Y, et al. Intrathecal gene therapy for the treatment of leptomeningeal carcinomatosis. GTI 0108. A phase I/II study. Hum Gene Ther 1995;6:55–85.
165. Ram Z, Walbridge S, Oshiro EM, et al. Intrathecal gene therapy for malignant leptomeningeal neoplasia. Cancer Res 1994;54:2141–2145.
166. Driesse MJ, Vincent AJ, Sillevis Smitt PA, et al. Intracerebral injection of adenovirus harboring the HSVtk gene combined with ganciclovir administration: toxicity study in nonhuman primates. Gene Ther 1998;5:1122–1129.
167. Possner J, Chernik N. Intracranial metastases from systemic cancer. Adv Neurol 1978;19:579–592.
168. Perry A, Dehner LP. Meningeal tumors of childhood and infancy. An update and literature review. Brain Pathol 2003;13:386–408.
169. Moffat DA, Grey P, Ballagh RH, et al. Extended temporal bone resection for squamous cell carcinoma. Otolaryngol Head Neck Surg 1997;116:617–623.
170. Maiuri F, Esposito F, Del Basso De Caro M, et al. Dural cerebellopontine angle metastasis from malignant parotid oncocytoma. J Neurooncol 2003;61:69–72.
171. Martin AJ, Fisher C, Igbaseimokumo U, et al. Solitary fibrous tumours of the meninges: case series and literature review. J Neurooncol 2001;54:57–69.
172. Higuchi M, Fujimoto Y, Miyahara E, et al. Isolated dural metastasis from colon cancer. Clin Neurol Neurosurg 1997;99:135–137.
173. Natarajan S, Post KD, Strauchen J, et al. Primary intracerebral Rosai-Dorfman disease: a case report. J Neurooncol 2000;47:73–77.
174. Kumar K, Kelly M. Benign pituitary adenoma with multiple dural metastases: a case report. Surg Neurol 2000;54:380–383; discussion 384.
175. Balis F, Poplack D. Cancer chemotherapy. In: Nathan DG, Oski FA, eds. Hematology of infancy and childhood, 4th ed. Philadelphia: WB Saunders, 1993:1207–1238.
176. Balis F, Poplack D. Central nervous system pharmacology of antileukemia drugs. Am J Pediatr Hematol Oncol 1989;11:74–86.

CHAPTER 29

Cancer Metastasis to the Peripheral Nervous System

NAGANAND SRIPATHI / LISA R. ROGERS

Metastasis of cancer to the peripheral nervous system is less common than to the central nervous system, and the clinical syndromes and treatment results in metastatic neuropathy have not been explored to the same extent. Similarly, researchers have paid comparatively little attention to the mechanisms by which tumor metastasizes to nerve and the resultant peripheral nerve injury. The best characterized nerve dysfunction is brachial or lumbar plexopathy that occurs from compression (and, less frequently, invasion) of the plexus by adjacent primary or metastatic systemic cancer. Metastatic plexopathy presents a diagnostic challenge to the clinician, especially when patients have received therapeutic radiation to the plexus region, because of the difficulty in differentiating metastasis from radiation-induced plexopathy or the rare radiation-induced tumor. Using a clinical algorithm that includes the type of cancer and cancer treatment, neurologic symptoms and signs, imaging abnormalities of neural tissue and adjacent structures, and electrophysiologic testing, the diagnosis can usually be established so that appropriate antineoplastic therapy can be administered. In many instances, however, treatment results for metastatic plexopathy are not satisfactory, and persistent pain and limb weakness require aggressive supportive therapy. When cancer metastasis results in a distal mononeuropathy or peripheral polyneuropathy, the differential diagnosis includes other common neuropathic syndromes associated with cancer, including radiculopathy, treatment-related polyneuropathy and paraneoplastic syndromes. An aggressive approach to diagnosis is warranted in this setting, because early diagnosis and treatment can be rewarding.

▶ PATHOPHYSIOLOGY OF METASTATIC NEUROPATHY

The method by which cancer cells directly affect the plexus or peripheral nerves is deduced from both clinical material and experimental studies. Figure 29-1 depicts the mechanisms by which tumor interfaces with peripheral nerves.[1] Nerve tissue is most commonly displaced or compressed by local tumor growth. The epineurium and perineurium form an effective barrier against tumor cell invasion of nerve, and the clinical signs of nerve dysfunction result from indirect nerve damage. Nerve compression can occur at the primary site of cancer, such as in compression of the brachial plexus by a primary superior sulcus lung tumor, or at the site of metastatic cancer, such as brachial or lumbosacral plexus compression

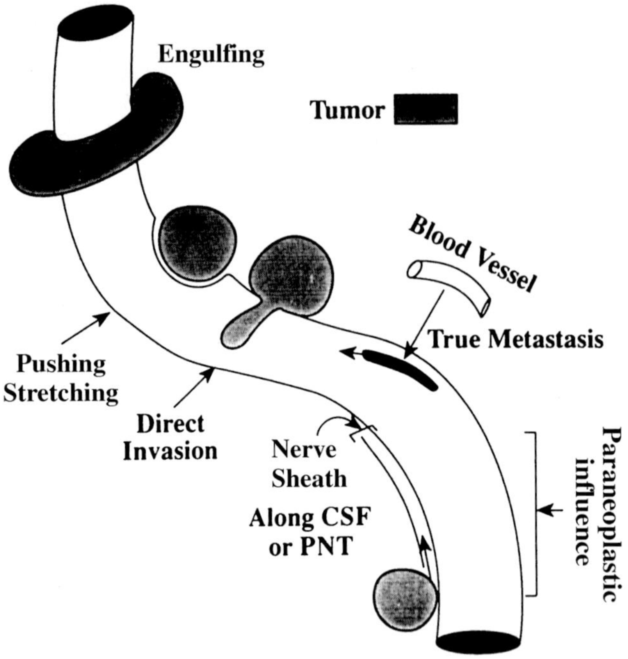

Figure 29-1. Mechanisms of peripheral nerve involvement by cancer. (*Reproduced from Cancer 1995;76: 1829–1832, with permission of Wiley-Liss, Inc., a subsidiary of John Wiley & Sons, Inc. Copyright © 1995 American Cancer Society.*)

by lymph node or other metastasis arising from a regional or distant cancer. Individual peripheral nerves are typically compressed by soft tissue or bone metastasis. Less commonly, nerves are damaged by cancer which spreads contiguously along the nerve. One setting for this is cancer in the leptomeninges that extends from the spinal root into peripheral nerves, as Ushio's experimental model suggests.[2] In other instances, the primary tumor arises in the limb. In a pathologic study of 98 amputated limbs containing a sarcoma, Barber and associates[3] identified 4 cases in which the perineurium was diffusely infiltrated by sarcoma, which extended long distances from the original site of tumor, including 1 case of tumor in the wrist that spread along the median nerve to the brachial plexus.

Experimental animal models of nerve compression by cancer confirm the rarity of tumor invasion of nerve. Vega and associates[4] developed an experimental model of carcinomatous brachial plexopathy by implanting thyroid carcinoma into the immediate vicinity of the brachial plexus in Fisher rats. Morphologic studies revealed that the tumor surrounded the branches of the brachial plexus, as well as the overlying muscles and subcutaneous spaces, in each of 30 animals. On histologic examination, tumor cells were found in the epineurium of all nerve specimens; however, invasion of the intrafascicular area was uncommon. Forty-one of the brachial plexus specimens showed pathologic changes, most commonly segmental demyelination with endoneurial edema and variable amounts of axonal degeneration at the site of compression. Distal axonal degeneration also developed with prolonged survival of the animal. Similarly, in an experimental rat model of limb nerve metastasis, Kashef and associates[5] injected Walker 256 carcinoma cells into muscles near the sciatic nerve of rats. In the early phase, tumor cells were seen in the perineurium. In the intermediate phase, they were identified in the endoneurium, and at the latest stage macrophages and hypertrophied fibroblasts were seen in the nerve, but there was no nerve invasion by tumor. Segmental demyelination, with occasional distal wallerian degeneration, was identified in the nerves.

A third and rare mechanism of neoplastic nerve involvement is presumably direct hematogeneous spread of tumor to the nerves. Single or multiple nerves can be affected, including cases of symmetric polyneuropathy. Meller and associates[1] define an isolated metastatic deposit by an open biopsy revealing metastatic infiltration beneath the nerve sheath and between the fascicles, the absence of tumor material in soft tissue and nodes around the nerve and its close vicinity, and no previous surgical manipulation of the area. This method of tumor spread can also be suspected clinically when there is plexopathy or peripheral neuropathy and neuroimaging fails to identify the tumor in or near the nerve, and when nonneoplastic conditions have been excluded. Although isolated nerve metastasis is reported in few types of carcinoma,[1] the preponderance of cases are in lymphoma. When it develops in lymphoma in the setting of a complete response to chemotherapy, it suggests that there is a selection of chemoresistant clones with a specific neurotropism or that the peripheral nerves are a sanctuary site for chemotherapy because of the blood–nerve barrier.[6]

▶ METASTATIC BRACHIAL PLEXOPATHY

Clinical Setting

The brachial plexus is more commonly involved by cancer than is the lumbosacral plexus. Plexus damage typically results from tumor growth adjacent to the plexus that arises from direct extension, as in superior sulcus lung cancer, or from drainage into the adjacent lymph nodes, as in breast cancer. In distant cancers, metastasis to the soft tissues or lymph nodes adjacent to the plexus compresses the plexus. Rarely, metastasis is by hematogeneous spread to the plexus, without adjacent tumor or adenopathy. Many clinical reports of metastatic brachial plexopathy fail to differentiate the clinical setting, symptoms and signs, and treatment results that are unique to that arising from adjacent lung cancer or from cancer metastatic to adjacent nodes or soft tissue, which confounds the interpretation of clinical findings and treatment results. When possible, we separate these neoplastic plexopathies according to the primary site of origin.

Pancoast Tumors

Pulmonary superior sulcus tumors comprise 3% to 5% of all lung cancers.[7] They are more common in men and in smokers. The average age at presentation is the sixth decade of life. The most common tumor is a non–small cell lung cancer. They are usually unilateral, but rarely bilateral. Uncommonly, the tumors are of nonpulmonary histologies, such as other carcinomas or lymphoma.

Hare published the first report of a superior sulcus tumor causing neurologic signs in 1838.[8] Pancoast subsequently reported seven patients with a superior sulcus tumor and clinical and neuroimaging findings that comprise the "Pancoast syndrome," including arm pain and Horner syndrome in association with destruction of the upper ribs or adjacent vertebrae.[9] A formal definition has not been proposed, but usually Pancoast syndrome refers to this constellation of clinical findings and radiologic evidence of involvement of the brachial plexus, subclavian vessels, sympathetic chain, uppermost ribs, and/or vertebral bodies. Pancoast tumor typically refers to a tumor in the superior sulcus, although some authors use this to refer to the entire symptom and imaging complex. Because of the nonpulmonary nature of the symptoms, there is often a considerable delay in the diagnosis, often up to 1 year or more.

Metastatic Brachial Plexopathy

It is difficult to estimate the incidence of metastatic brachial plexopathy caused by cancers other than lung. The most common tumor underlying metastatic brachial plexopathy is breast cancer. Fulton[10] identified 32 patients with definite or probable metastatic brachial plexopathy from breast cancer in a 5-year interval at an institution averaging 391 new cases of breast cancer per year. The mode of spread to the plexus region in breast cancer is speculated to be drainage into the axillary lymph nodes, the lateral group of nodes which drain the majority of the breast tissue and are in close proximity to the plexus. Figure 29-2 shows the lymphatic drainage of breast tissue and the proximity of the axillary nodes to the plexus. However, many women undergo mastectomy and lymph node removal at the diagnosis of

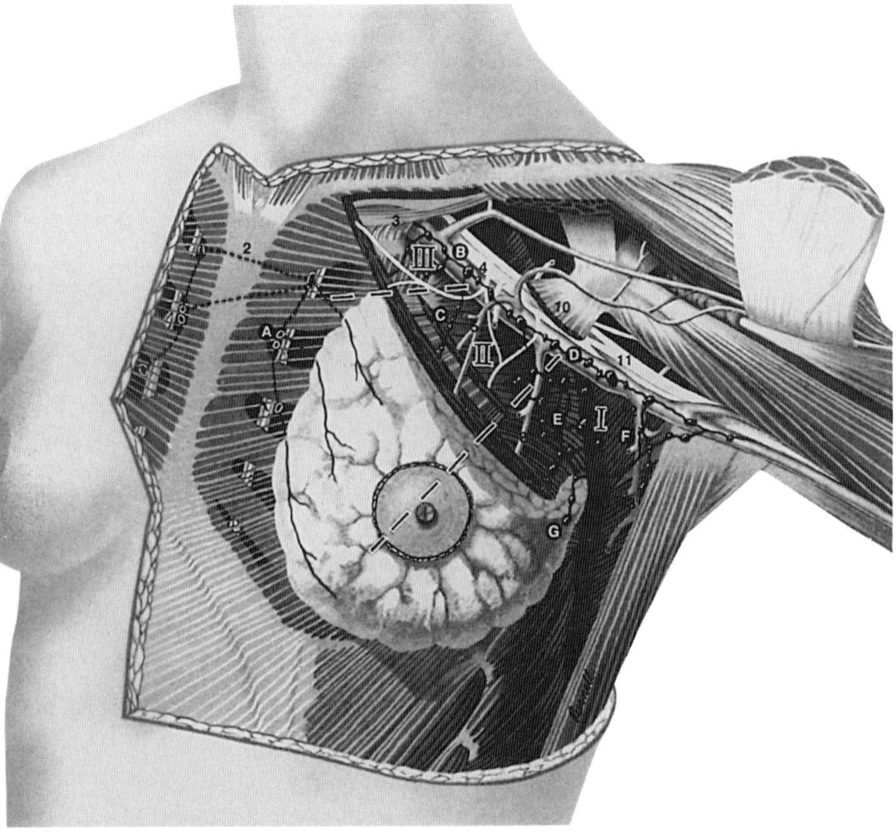

Figure 29-2. Lymphatic drainage of the breast and the relationship of the nodes to the brachial plexus. (*Reproduced with permission from Harris JR, et al. Diseases of the breast. Philadelphia: Lippincott-Raven, 1996.*)

breast cancer and the precise mechanism of late brachial plexus metastasis spread is disputed. A wide variety of other cancers are reported to metastasize to the nodes or soft tissue of the plexus region, including melanoma, sarcoma, non-Hodgkin lymphoma, myeloma, and genitourinary, gastrointestinal, cutaneous, and head and neck carcinomas.[11–23] One surgical series of five cases of isolated hematogeneous metastasis to the brachial plexus included breast and laryngeal cancer and non-Hodgkin lymphoma.[1] Others have also reported non-Hodgkin lymphoma directly infiltrating the plexus without adjacent lymphadenopathy.[14,24,25] Brachial plexopathy from lymphoma may occur in conjunction with a diffuse peripheral neuropathy (neurolymphomatosis) and be the first manifestation of this process.[12] The interval between the detection of malignancy and the initial symptoms of metastatic brachial plexopathy varies, with a median onset around 1.5 years.[11,26]

Clinical Signs

PANCOAST TUMORS

Figure 29-3 shows the relationship of Pancoast tumor to the adjacent neural structures. The most common symptom of Pancoast syndrome is pain in the shoulder, resulting from involvement of the brachial plexus, endothoracic fascia, parietal pleura, uppermost ribs, and adjacent vertebral bodies, singly or in combination. When pain radiates down the arm, it is typically felt along the distribution of the lower trunk (see Fig. 29-3). Pain and abnormal sensation in the axilla and medial aspect of the upper arm in the distribution of the intercostobrachial nerve (T2) may also herald Pancoast syndrome. The pain may also extend to the scapula, axilla, anterolateral chest, neck and face. Cough, dyspnea, and hemoptysis are rare because the lung involvement is peripheral. Weakness and atrophy of the intrinsic muscles of the hand occur as a result of progressive involvement of the lower trunk. Horner syndrome occurs in 20% of people because of involvement of the sympathetic chain.[27] Ipsilateral facial flushing and hyperhidrosis may herald the classical features of Horner syndrome (ipsilateral miosis, ptosis, and anhidrosis).[28] Epidural spinal cord compression resulting from tumor extension through the intervertebral foramen is present in about 5% of patients on initial presentation and up to 25% of patients experience this complication during the course of the disease. Reflex sympathetic dystrophy is a rare occurrence.[29]

Metastatic Brachial Plexopathy

The cardinal symptom of tumor compression of the brachial plexus is pain. The distribution of pain is dependent upon what portion of the plexus is affected by tumor. Kori and associates[11] reported signs of a lower plexopathy in the majority of patients with neoplastic involvement. Twenty-nine of the 78 patients in this series had lung cancer and it is possible that many of these cases involved a Pancoast tumor that would be expected to produce signs of a lower plexopathy. They identified signs of panplexopathy in 19 other patients. Fulton[10] reported panplexopathy or upper plexopathy in the majority of patients with metastatic plexopathy from breast cancer.

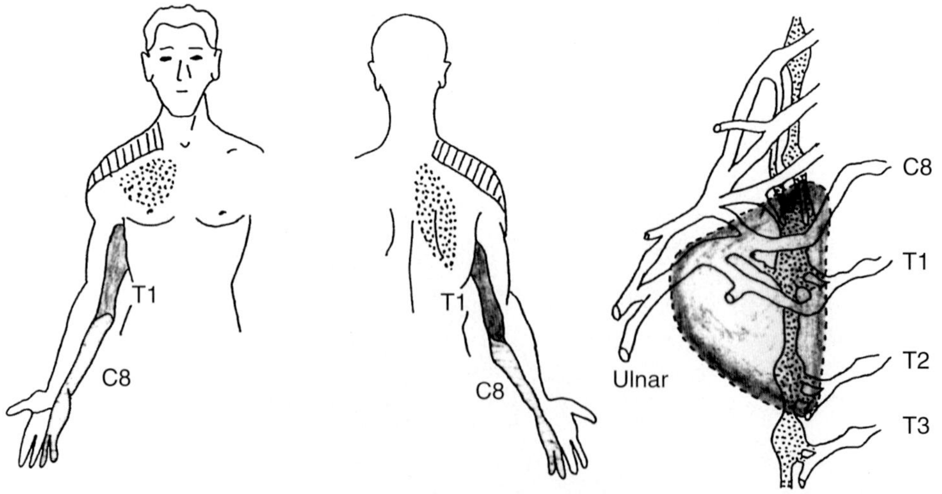

Figure 29-3. Nerve involvement in a typical Pancoast tumor (C8, T1, T, lower trunk of the brachial plexus, sympathetic chain). The dermatomes of C8 and T1 are illustrated, as well as areas of referred pain in the scapular and pectoral regions (mediated through afferent fibers of the sympathetic chain). (*Reproduced from Detterbeck FC. Pancoast (superior sulcus) tumors. Ann Thorac Surg 1997;63:1810–1818, with permission of the Society of Thoracic Surgeons.*)

The clinical series by Thomas and Colby[30] demonstrated that any portion of the plexus could be affected by metastatic tumor and that the clinical pattern of pain and weakness was indistinguishable from radiation-induced plexopathy. Occasionally, a complex regional pain syndrome of the upper extremity precedes the neurologic deficit or the detection of the tumor spread to the axilla, by 4 to 6 months.[31] Some patients may complain of a freezing and burning sensation. The limb may be tender to touch, and any manipulation may produce the radiating pain and paresthesias.

When the patient presents with pain and paresthesias, the neurologic examination may be normal except for the presence of a mass in the supra- or infraclavicular fossa. A Tinel sign may be elicited by palpation in the supraclavicular fossa or axilla. Bilateral loss of the finger flexor reflex with otherwise brisk reflexes indicates T1 vertebral body, root, and spinal cord involvement. Horner syndrome suggests paraspinal and epidural extension of the tumor. Lymphedema and swelling of the arm may be seen. A mass will not be palpable in patients with hematogeneous spread of cancer to the plexus.[1] A prominent venous pattern may be seen over the anterior chest wall from collateral circulation that develops from axillary or subclavian vein compression. There is focal weakness and muscle atrophy that depends upon the portion of the plexus affected.

▶ DIAGNOSIS

Electrophysiology

Electrodiagnostic studies may aid in establishing the diagnosis of metastatic plexopathy and also in differentiating it from radiation plexopathy in difficult cases. The findings depend on the type of injury: axonal loss, demyelination, or conduction block.

Electrodiagnostic studies in Pancoast tumor demonstrate a lower brachial plexopathy. However, this may present as C8 or T1 radiculopathy.[32] Kori and associates[11] reported clinical signs of predominantly lower trunk involvement in metastatic brachial plexopathy, but electrodiagnostic studies have found that the involvement may more often be generalized with lower trunk predominance.[33]

When the lesion is mild, the only electrical abnormality may be fibrillation potentials on needle electrode examination in the appropriate muscles.[34] With more severe involvement, the amplitude of sensory nerve action potentials (ulnar and medial antebrachial sensory potentials in a lower trunk lesion) may decrease, followed by a decrease in the compound muscle action potentials of median and ulnar motor nerves. Reduced median and ulnar motor amplitudes indicating axonal loss in the lower trunk and medial cord of the brachial plexus is more common in neoplastic than in radiation-induced brachial plexopathy.

Some reports indicate that the upper trunk of the plexus is more affected in radiation-induced rather than tumor-induced plexopathy. Even in generalized plexopathy, the most frequent abnormality seen in radiation plexopathy is reduced median sensory amplitude (especially to the first digit) followed by the lateral cutaneous nerve of forearm.[34] Denervation potentials and reduced recruitment with high amplitude, long duration, polyphasic motor unit potentials are seen in most patients, and fasciculations and myokymia best characterize radiation plexopathy.[34] The paraspinal muscles are more commonly involved in radiation (23% of patients) than in metastatic plexopathy.[26] Serial investigations may be needed to demonstrate all the changes. The three distinct electrographic features of radiation plexopathy include low sensory nerve action potentials before the appearance of fibrillation potentials; spontaneous activity other than fibrillations, such as myokymia, repetitive fasciculations, grouped repetitive discharges, and complex repetitive potentials; and conduction block as a consequence of demyelination.[35] A problem that can be encountered when searching for a conduction block with supraclavicular stimulation is a "pseudoconduction block" caused by inexcitable plexus fibers because of overlying scar tissue.[33]

Imaging

Pancoast Tumor

When a superior sulcus tumor is suspected, routine chest radiographs may reveal the upper lung tissue density abnormality and bone destruction. Abnormal or normal chest radiographs should be followed by chest computerized tomography (CT) to better delineate the tumor and to stage the cancer. Magnetic resonance imaging (MRI) is excellent for visualizing the relationship of a superior sulcus tumor to adjacent vascular structures, the plexus, and upper thoracic neural foramina (Fig. 29-4). Both CT and MRI can also demonstrate destruction of upper thoracic ribs and vertebral bodies.

Metastatic Brachial Plexopathy

MRI is superior to CT in detecting tumor associated with neoplastic brachial plexopathy.[36] MRI has direct multiplanar imaging capability and superior soft tissue resolution, allowing differentiation of nerve tissue from adjacent fat, muscle, blood vessel, and tumor (Fig. 29-5). Unlike CT, intravenous contrast is not required. A minimum of two planes should be imaged with T_1 and T_2 images. Coronal and axial planes display the brachial plexus bilaterally from its origin to the axilla and allow assessment of asymmetry. In the series of metastatic plexopathy by Bilbey,[37] MRI correctly identified tumor in 10 of 12 cases. The only two false-negative cases had microscopic recurrence

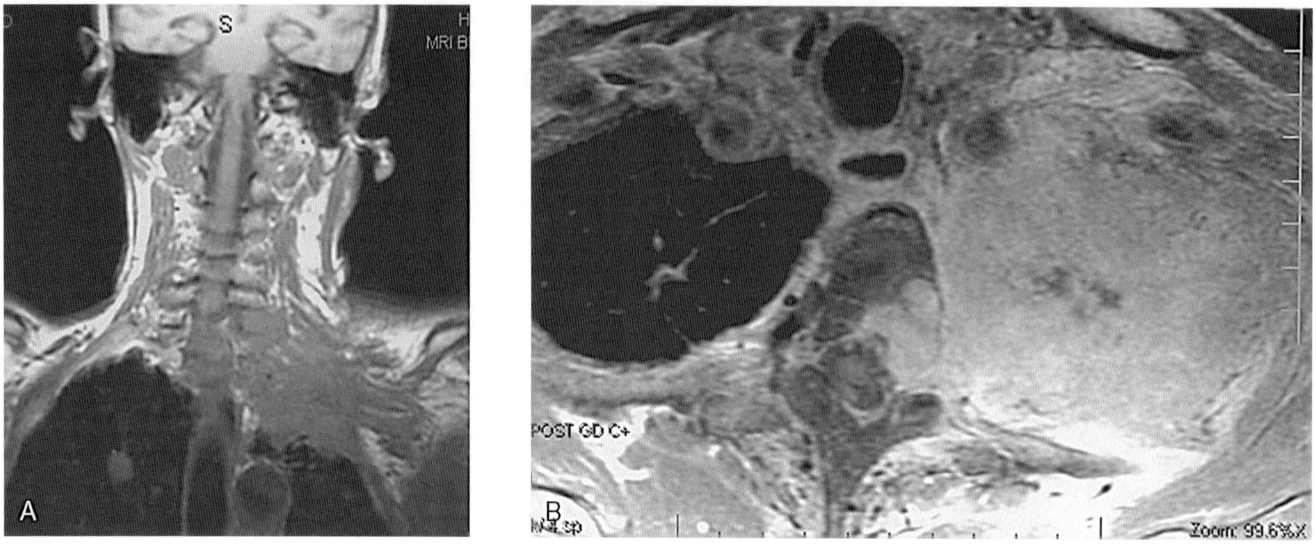

Figure 29-4. A large left superior sulcus lung tumor (Pancoast tumor) is visualized on coronal MRI. (A) The tumor invades the brachial plexus and extends posteriorly into the upper thoracic spine. (B) The axial contrast-enhanced image demonstrates the tumor extending into the adjacent intervertebral foramina and vertebral bodies, resulting in spinal cord compression.

obscured by fibrosis. MRI is expected to be negative when the tumor is microscopic within the plexus, especially when tumor has spread hematogeneously and there is no adjacent adenopathy or soft tissue mass. In one large series the discordance between the MRI findings and clinicopathologic diagnosis was 18% when MRI failed to detect a mass in or near brachial plexus.[38] Castagno and Suhman[39] correctly identified tumor in 15 patients and excluded it in 25 others. Soft tissue changes with low signal intensity, similar to muscle on both T_1- and T_2-weighted images,

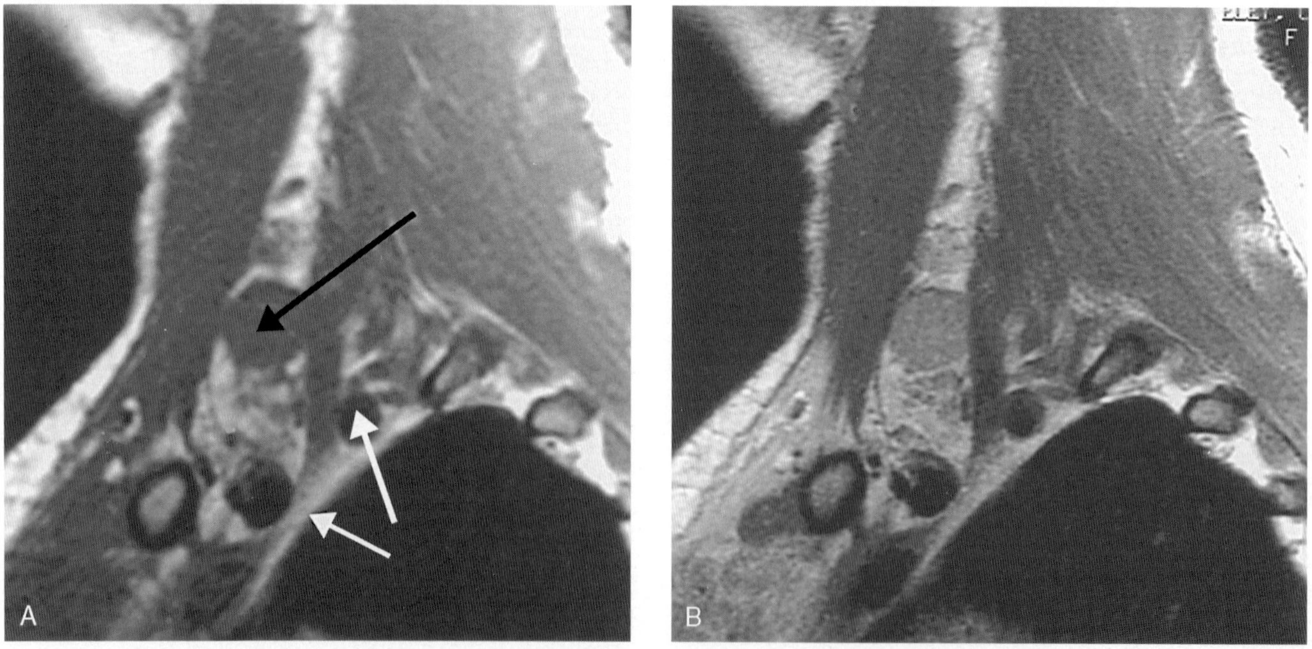

Figure 29-5. Sagittal T_1-weighted MRI in a patient with metastatic breast cancer and signs of brachial plexopathy shows isointense lymphadenopathy (dark arrow) compressing the brachial plexus. (A) The subclavian vessels are indicated with light arrows. (B) The tumor enhances diffusely following contrast injection.

are more consistent with radiation fibrosis. Tumor infiltration shows a low signal intensity on T_1-weighted images and increased intensity on T_2-weighted images. Metastatic tumors are hypointense with respect to fat and isointense with respect to muscle.[40,41] Detection of adjacent lymphadenopathy, bone metastasis, and intrathoracic and chest wall masses favor tumor infiltration of the brachial plexus.[38] Gallium-67 scintigraphy can be an adjunct to MRI detection of tumor infiltrating the plexus from lymphoma.[14,24,25] [^{18}F]fluorodeoxyglucose positron emission tomography (FDG-PET) can assist in identifying the axillary nodes and brachial plexus in breast cancer patients, and is complementary to CT or MRI. In one study, 14 of 19 cancer patients had abnormal uptake of FDG in the region of the symptomatic brachial plexus. Six of these patients had either normal or minimal thickening of the brachial plexus on CT, but had positive FDG-PET scans indicating metastatic plexopathy.[42] FDG-PET may also be useful for distinguishing between radiation-induced and metastatic plexopathy.

Surgery

Bronchoscopy and sputum cytology are ineffective in diagnosing Pancoast tumor because of the peripheral location of the tumor. A CT-guided percutaneous needle biopsy of the mass is the procedure of choice. A CT-guided biopsy to obtain tumor tissue may also be necessary in patients with other cancers who are suspected to have metastatic plexopathy when the imaging and electrophysiology findings are not diagnostic. It may be particularly useful in those patients with radiation fibrosis who are suspected of also having microscopic tumor recurrence.[43] The subclavian vessels are valuable landmarks for locating the plexus from the C5 vertebral level through the inferior axillary level and a high-resolution contrast-enhanced axial CT maximizes vascular enhancement. Cole and associates[44] reported obtaining diagnostic tissue with no morbidity using this procedure in three patients. If tumor infiltration is strongly suspected and neuroimaging changes are equivocal, surgical exploration may be required and is often diagnostic.[1] There is a risk of increased neurologic morbidity with brachial plexus biopsy and it should be performed by a surgeon skilled in this technique. Kori and associates[11] found that the initial biopsy may be negative in some cases and a repeat biopsy months later can be diagnostic.

Differential Diagnosis

In patients who have received therapeutic radiation to the plexus region, the major differential is radiation-induced plexopathy. There is a wide range of incidence of radiation-induced brachial plexopathy in different series. The risk of damage may be influenced by different factors, including patient age, nerve length exposed, cumulative radiation dose, fraction size and number, field technique, and adjuvant chemotherapy.[45,46] Reducing the radiation dose from 63 Gy to 57.75 Gy reduced the rate of brachial plexus involvement from 73% to 15% in one series.[47] The interval from treatment and signs of plexopathy is typically longer with radiation damage than with tumor compression, but it may depend upon the dose of radiation. In Kori and associates' series,[11] if the dose was less than 60 Gy, 82% of symptomatic plexopathy cases within the first year were a consequence of tumor recurrence. If the dose was more than 60 Gy, 70% of tumor recurrences were symptomatic after 1 year. They suggest that if a patient receives more than 60 Gy and is symptomatic within the first year, it is more likely to be radiation-induced. If the dose is less than 60 Gy and the patient is symptomatic within the first year, it is more likely to be tumor. Patients developing plexopathy more than 1 year after receiving >60 Gy may have either.

It is not always possible, however, to distinguish radiation-induced plexopathy from neoplastic brachial plexopathy by clinical signs. Kori and associates[11] suggest that neoplastic plexopathy predominantly involves the lower trunk with neurologic dysfunction in the distribution of C8 and T1 roots and radiation plexopathy typically affects the upper trunk, involving fibers derived from the C5, C6, and C7 roots.[11] This clinical series included patients with lung cancer, thus there may be an overrepresentation of lower plexopathies. Lederman and Wilbourn[34] found that lower trunk involvement was not uncommon in radiation plexopathy. Horner syndrome is very common with neoplastic brachial plexopathy, and also more common in patients with epidural cord compression than in those with radiation-induced plexopathy. Shoulder or arm pain suggests neoplastic brachial plexopathy. Weakness is rarely a presenting symptom in either group, but numbness and paresthesias are common presenting symptoms in radiation plexopathy. Fasciculations and myokymia on electromyography (EMG) are virtually pathognomonic of radiation plexopathy.[34,35] A well-defined mass lesion near the plexus on imaging studies is suggestive of neoplastic plexopathy. MRI in radiation fibrosis typically shows thickening of the plexus with or without enhancement and low signal intensity on T_1- and T_2-weighted images. T_2-weighted images help differentiate changes of radiation fibrosis from early tumor infiltration, because tumor usually shows a higher signal intensity. Occasionally, however, metastasis may demonstrate low signal on T_2.[41] Table 29-1 provides clinical, electrophysiological, and imaging findings to aid in the differentiation of tumor from radiation plexopathy. It may be necessary to resort to surgical exploration for definitive diagnosis in difficult cases.

Acute ischemic plexopathy associated with involvement of the subclavian artery more than 20 years after radiation has been described.[48] A sudden painless paresis of the arm with distal numbness may follow radiation-induced

▶ **TABLE 29-1.** FEATURES USEFUL TO DIFFERENTIATE NEOPLASTIC AND RADIATION BRACHIAL PLEXOPATHY

	Favoring Neoplastic BP	Favoring Radiation BP
Pain		
Incidence of pain	Common (80%)	Uncommon (20%)
Location of pain	Shoulder, upper arm, elbow, 4th and 5th fingers	Shoulder, wrist, hand
Onset	Rapid	Gradual
Horner syndrome	Frequent	Rare
Electrodiagnostics: (abnormal nerve conductions)		
Median SNAP	Rare	Frequent
Lateral antebrachial SNAP	Rare	Frequent
Median CMAP	Rare	Frequent
Ulnar CMAP	Rare	Frequent
Myokymia	Absent	Present
MRI abnormality		
Mass	Frequent	Rare
T_2 signal	Increased	Decreased
Enhancement	Frequent	Uncommon
Loss of fat planes	Uncommon	Common

BP = brachial plexopathy; CMAP = compound muscle action potential; SNAP = sensory nerve action potential.
Source: Adapted from Lederman, et al. Neurology 1984;34:1331 and Thyagarajan, et al. Neurology 1995;45:421.

occlusion of the subclavian artery. An acute reversible radiation plexopathy occurs in some patients treated for breast cancer. The symptoms typically occur within the first few months of radiation.

Conditions that are unrelated to cancer and should be included in the differential diagnosis are thoracic outlet syndrome, neuralgic amyotrophy, and cervical radiculopathy. These can be distinguished by the clinical presentation, time course, EMG, and imaging studies.

Radiation-induced malignant plexus tumors are reported most often after therapeutic radiation for Hodgkin disease and breast cancer.[49–53] The histologies are typically malignant schwannoma or sarcoma, and the interval from radiation usually exceeds 10 years. The symptoms and signs are typical of tumor, not radiation fibrosis. The tumors are usually large enough to be seen on CT or MRI.

▶ TREATMENT/PROGNOSIS

The goals of therapy for metastatic brachial plexopathy differ depending on the tumor type and stage of disease. Therapy for superior sulcus tumors is primarily designed to achieve local tumor control. Many of these patients ultimately die from distant brain or systemic metastasis. When other cancers, such as breast cancer, metastasize to the plexus, therapy is usually palliative. For the purpose of this chapter, we limit the results of therapy to the neurologic symptoms and signs for each of these conditions.

Pancoast Tumors

Surgical resection of superior sulcus tumors is usually performed by a high posterolateral thoracotomy (Paulson technique). When there is a significant anterior component and when the subclavian vessels are involved, an anterior transcervical–thoracic approach (Dartevelle) is preferred. If there is extension to the vertebrae, a variety of additional procedures can be performed to alleviate or prevent spinal nerve or cord dysfunction, including partial or complete vertebrectomy or resection of the neural foramina or transverse processes.[54,55] These techniques are technically feasible and the results are encouraging, but the true benefit has not been established. Radiation combined with surgery is more effective than surgery alone in obtaining local tumor control and induction radiotherapy followed by surgical resection is currently the standard treatment. The addition of chemotherapy to preoperative radiation may be even more effective.[56–58] Details of improvement in neurologic function after therapy for Pancoast syndrome are not provided in many published series, but aggressive tumor treatment appears to reduce pain in the majority of patients. With combined radiation and surgical treatment in series comprised of 10 to 60 patients, durable and significant (defined as complete or moderate) pain relief is reported in 80% to 88% of patients.[59–62] Shahian also described that posttreatment arm function was excellent in 30%, good in 60%, and fair in 10%.[59]

Metastatic Brachial Plexopathy

For patients with breast or other cancer that metastasizes to the plexus, therapy is palliative and surgery is rarely performed, unless a biopsy is required to establish the diagnosis. There are conflicting reports regarding the effectiveness of radiation therapy alone in relieving neurologic symptoms and signs from metastatic brachial plexopathy, and the results are confounded because some authors have included lung cancer (which most likely included Pancoast tumor) with other tumor types. In addition, varying doses of radiation were employed, which may lead to different outcomes. In general, pain relief is a more likely benefit than improvement in arm function. Ampil[63] reported that 77% of 22 patients with lung or breast cancer or sarcoma had significant pain relief for 1 to 17 months (median: 3 months). Kori and associates[11] reported that only 46% of patients with lung, breast, or other cancers experienced pain relief. Son[64] reported excellent recovery of pain and motor signs in only 4 of 22 cases of plexopathy, including 3 of 15 with lung cancer and 1 of 7 with breast cancer. Isolated case reports attest to exceptional effectiveness and prolonged durability of aggressive therapy in some cases.[22] Meller and associates[1] reported that radiotherapy for hematogeneous spread of cancer to the plexus in five patients with a variety of cancers resulted in complete resolution of pain in each, and stable, but not improved, neurologic signs.

Clinical series that include only breast cancer also give conflicting results with radiation therapy. Nisce and Chu[65] reported the largest series of metastatic plexopathy from breast cancer (47 patients) and found that 25% of patients had complete relief of pain for a mean of 15 months (range: 3 months to 6 years) and 49% had a partial relief for a mean of 6 months (range: 1 month to 6 years); 25% had no relief. Complete motor and sensory recovery also occurred in 15% of patients, ranging from 4 months to 4 years and partial recovery occurred in 32% for 3 months to 3 years. They found that relief of pain and sensorimotor deficit was greater if no radiation had been administered previously, a factor that is not described in other reports. Fulton[10] reported that 9 of 17 breast cancer patients had pain relief but it was usually not durable. Two patients had improved arm function and others showed improved neurologic examination but not arm function.

Most studies found that clinical improvement is correlated with higher doses of radiation administered. Ampil[63] reported that 92% of patients improved when the dose was >40 Gy, compared to 55% when it was less than 40 Gy. Son[64] found that doses between 30 and 60 Gy responded better than doses between 20 and 30 Gy, and Nisce and Chu[65] reported that doses between 40 and 50 Gy produced better results than doses between 30 and 40 Gy.

Radiation therapy is not a viable option for many patients who have already received radiation to the plexus region. Chemotherapy and hormonal therapy are options in this setting, but have not been studied to the same extent as radiation. Fulton[10] reported that 2 of 7 patients with breast cancer showed definite or probable improvement with chemotherapy alone, and 1 of 6 others showed definite or probable improvement with hormonal therapy alone.

Persistent and disabling arm pain posttreatment is the most common symptom requiring symptomatic management in patients with metastatic brachial plexopathy. Steroids can provide temporary analgesia. Analgesics in accordance with the World Health Organization Analgesia Ladder should be instituted. Tricyclic antidepressants, anticonvulsants, and other nonopiate medications can be used to reduce neuropathic pain. A variety of anesthetic and neurosurgical techniques are also reported to provide prolonged pain relief, especially brachial plexus blocks and cordotomy.[11,66–70] Intrapleural analgesia and dorsal root entry zone surgery are reported to be effective in small numbers of patients treated.[71–73] Paravertebral blocks, dorsal rhizotomy, and hypophysectomy are less effective.[11] Supportive measures such as transdermal electrical nerve stimulation[11] and physical and occupational therapy help to improve the quality of life. When there is severe intractable pain with loss of limb function, no response to radiation or chemotherapy, and local tumor-related complications (such as tumor fungation, hemorrhage, sepsis, severe lymphedema, and venous gangrene), palliative forequarter amputation is effective in reducing pain and eliminating the above-mentioned complications.[74] This is performed rarely and should be considered only in this highly select group of patients because of the risk of complications, including phantom pain.

Lumbosacral Plexus

The mechanism of tumor-related lumbosacral plexopathy is inferred from imaging studies. The largest series of neoplastic lumbosacral plexopathy includes 85 patients reported by Jaeckle and associates.[75] They identified direct extension of a primary intraabdominal tumor, most commonly colorectal carcinoma or sarcoma, to be the most common mechanism of plexus involvement, as visualized on CT. Typically this was in association with adjacent invasion of soft tissues (61%), bone (6%), or both (33%). Adjacent bone metastasis in the sacrum is particularly common when the sacral plexus is affected, and here plexopathy may be bilateral. Roughly another 25% of the reported patients had metastatic plexopathy from a tumor that was originally extraabdominal, including breast, lung, thyroid, and gastric cancer and melanoma. In another series of 31 patients studied by MRI, direct involvement of the plexus was visualized in 23, and 6 others had widespread metastatic disease in the region of the plexus.[76] In the other two cases no mass was seen, although they were clinically suspected of having tumor in the plexus, and the mechanism of tumor-related plexopathy in these cases is not certain.

The mechanism of plexus involvement may differ with tumor type. In a review of 50 cases of metastatic lumbosacral plexopathy in cervical cancer, the most common cause was retroperitoneal lymph node metastasis.[77] In another review of bladder cancer patients with lumbosacral plexopathy, direct extension of the cancer was the cause in 5 of 7 cases, and retroperitoneal adenopathy was the cause in only 2 cases.[78]

Clinical Setting

In the series by Jaeckle and associates[75] of patients with metastatic lumbosacral plexopathy, there were an equal number of men and women where the median age was 52 years in men and 53 years in women. Taylor's series from the Mayo Clinic included 31 cases, 20 of whom were men. The mean age was 62 years. It usually occurs in the setting of widespread disease, and the interval to the development of plexopathy is relatively short. It can develop in the setting of prior radiation to the pelvis.[76,79] In the series by Jaeckle and associates,[75] the majority of diagnoses of plexopathy were made within 1 year of cancer diagnosis and in 66% within 3 years of diagnosis. In 15% of patients, the symptoms of plexopathy were the presenting sign of cancer. In Taylor's series,[76] plexopathy developed at an average of 56 months (range: 11–216 months) from cancer diagnosis. In 50 cases of cervical cancer, the interval ranged from 0 to 86 months (median: 20 months).[77] In seven cases of bladder cancer, all had locally advanced or disseminated disease and the tumor was diagnosed after 5 to 204 months (median: 23 months).[78] Colorectal cancer is the most common underlying tumor.[75,76,80,81] Retroperitoneal sarcomas were also common in the series by Jaeckle and associates[75] from a tertiary care cancer center, but are not reported by others. Saphner and associates[77] reported an incidence of 50 cases among 2261 patients with cervical cancer. Lymphoma, myeloma, and leukemia are rare causes.

Clinical Signs

Pain is the first symptom of metastatic plexopathy in the majority of patients and it can be the only sign of plexopathy. The pain is described as aching, pressure-like, stabbing or burning. Jaeckle and associates[75] divided the clinical syndromes based on the level of involvement in 34 patients who were prospectively examined: lower plexus (L5-S3) was present in 51%, upper plexus (L1-L4) in 31%, and panplexopathy (L1-S3) in 18% of patients. Table 29-2 shows the symptoms and signs in these patients of which local and radicular pain are the most common. Pain is felt at the costovertebral angle if the upper lumbar plexus is involved. Radicular pain may overshadow the local pain, and the resulting pain is felt in the groin or anterolateral aspect of the thigh. Pain may be referred to the flank or iliac crest. If the lower lumbar and sacral plexus are involved, the pain is lower and mostly situated in the buttock and perineum. Radicular pain extends onto the posterolateral thigh and leg. Pain may be

▶ TABLE 29-2. LUMBOSACRAL PLEXOPATHY: SYMPTOMS AND SIGNS BY THE LEVEL OF PLEXUS INVOLVEMENT BY TUMORS

Clinical Level	Upper	Lower	Pan
Most common tumor	Colorectal	Sarcoma	Genitourinary
Clinical level	Upper	Lower	Pan
# of patients	12	16	6
Pain distribution			
Local	Lower abdomen	Buttock, perineum	Lumbosacral
Radicular	Anterolateral thigh	Posterolateral thigh, leg	Variable
Referred	Flank, iliac crest	Hip and ankle	Variable
Numbness/paresthesias	Anterior thigh	Perineum, thigh, sole	Anterior thigh, leg, foot
Motor and reflex changes	L2-L4	L5-S1	L2-S2
Sensory loss	Anterolateral thigh	Posterior thigh, sole	Especially anterior thigh, leg
Tenderness	Lumbar	Sciatic notch and sacrum	Lumbosacral
Positive SLRT*			
Direct	6/12	8/16	5/6
Reverse	2/12	8/16	5/6
Leg edema	5/12	6/16	5/6
Rectal mass	3/12	7/16	1/6
Sphincter weakness	0/12	8/16	0/6

*Straight-leg raising test.

Source: Adapted from Jaeckle KA, Young DF, Foley KM. The natural history of lumbosacral plexopathy in cancer. Neurology 1985;35:8–15.

referred to the hip and ankle. In panplexopathy, there is pain in the lumbosacral area, and the location of radicular and referred pain is variable. In Jaeckle and associates' series,[75] the plexopathy was left-sided in 46%, right-sided in 27%, and bilateral in 27% of patients. Lower plexopathy is more common with metastatic spread of tumor, often because of metastasis to the sacrum. A primary intraabdominal tumor more often results in upper plexopathy or panplexopathy.

Pain is usually continuous and is commonly exacerbated by sudden movement. In a smaller number of patients, pain is worse with lying supine and is relieved by standing or walking. Pain can sometimes be relieved by either lying on one side with the knees flexed or flexing the affected leg at the hip. A hot and dry foot associated with local and referred pain with minimal abnormalities on neurologic examination was the only sign in 3 of 15 patients in one series.[82] The vegetative foot symptoms are presumed to be caused by involvement of the lumbar sympathetic nerves near the anterolateral aspect of the vertebrae. Limb pain in many patients may be elicited by hyperextending the leg while the patient is in the lateral decubitus position (reverse straight-leg raising test). The straight-leg raising test is positive in a smaller number, and more often when there is bilateral plexus disease.[75] Even if the straight-leg raising test is negative, there may be pain when the leg descends, because of stretching of the iliopsoas muscle. Within weeks to months after the onset of pain, leg weakness, numbness, or paresthesias may ensue. There may be some impairment of bowel, bladder, and sexual function if the sacral roots are involved, especially when this is bilateral. When the upper plexus is involved, abnormalities on examination include weakness of the iliopsoas and quadriceps muscles with loss of the patellar reflex. Sensory changes are not as pronounced, but there may be decreased sensation on the anterolateral thigh. Metastasis to the lower lumbar and sacral plexus causes weakness of the hamstrings and the ankle dorsiflexors and plantar flexors. There is loss of the Achilles reflex, and numbness may be present in the posterior thigh and sole.

Leg edema is present in many patients as a consequence of obstruction of the venous or lymphatic systems, and is more common in bilateral plexopathies. Rectal examination may reveal a mass.[75,79]

Electrophysiologic Diagnosis

There are very few published reports reviewing electrodiagnostic studies in metastatic lumbosacral plexopathy. Nerve conduction studies show unilateral reduction in the compound muscle action potential and sensory nerve action potential amplitudes in the clinically involved segments compared to the uninvolved limb. Only limited sensory nerve conduction studies can be performed in the lower extremities, adding to the difficulties in distinguishing lumbosacral polyradiculopathy from lumbosacral plexus lesions. Twenty-five of 26 patients in Jaeckle and associates' series had active and chronic denervation on electromyography. Denervation was bilateral in 8 of the 17 patients who underwent bilateral EMG. Paraspinal involvement, suggesting radiculopathy, is seen in some patients and can add to the diagnostic difficulty.[75,81]

Imaging

MRI and CT findings may include a soft tissue mass involving the plexus, with or without lymphadenopathy, thickening of the plexus, and tumor within the adjacent bony structures without direct involvement of the plexus (Fig. 29-6).[75,76,81] A detailed study of CT findings correlated with clinical findings is provided by Vock and associates.[83] MRI offers better contrast resolution and is more sensitive than CT in detecting neoplastic plexopathy. In one study, MRI detected metastatic plexopathy when the CT results were either normal or equivocal.[76] Vertebral or sacral erosion is often present, and spinal epidural extension of tumor was present in 23 of 51 patients who underwent a myelogram in the series by Jaeckle and associates.[75] Thus it is prudent to include MRI or CT of the lower thoracic and upper lumbar spine routinely in patients evaluated for metastatic lumbosacral plexopathy.

Surgery

Surgical exploration is rarely performed but is indicated if imaging studies are normal and neoplastic plexopathy is suspected.

Differential Diagnosis

Radiation-induced plexopathy usually develops a year or more after treatment. Indolent distal leg weakness, sometimes with leg numbness, occurs initially, and in the majority of patients there is no pain. Pain may develop over time.[81] The weakness is typically bilateral, accompanied by lymphedema. This is in contrast to tumor invasion of lumbosacral plexus, which is usually unilateral with severe pain and less often has lymphedema.[81] Abnormal EMG finding in some patients following radiation therapy may be a result of involvement of the anterior horn cells, the lower spinal cord, or the caudal nerve roots. As in brachial plexus radiation-induced plexopathy, myokymia is characteristic. Pelvic CT is usually normal with radiation-induced lumbosacral plexopathy.[81]

Radiation therapy may also result in an acute lumbosacral plexopathy. Acute bilateral lower extremity weakness with pelvic pain is a rare complication of pelvic radiotherapy for cervical cancer, especially when intracavitary radiation is used.[84–86] Epidural cord compression and

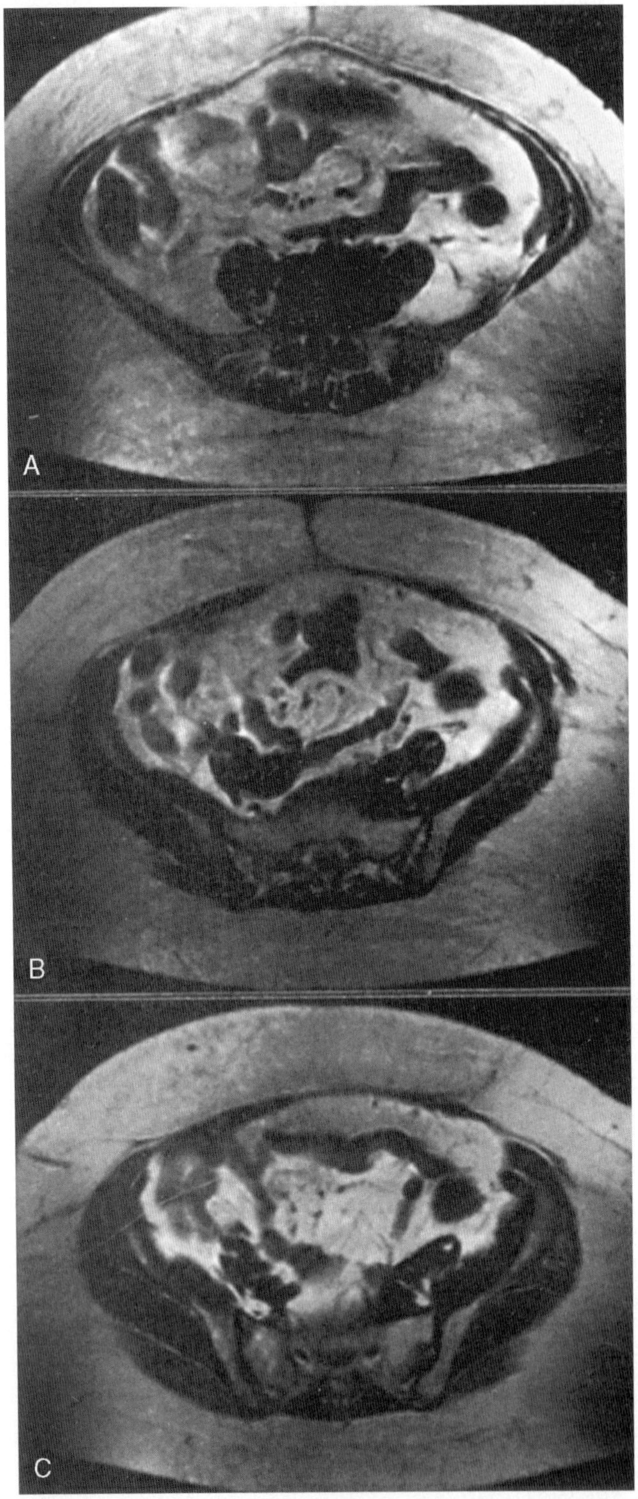

Figure 29-6. (A, B, and C) T_1-weighted axial MRI of lower abdomen and pelvis shows a soft-tissue mass obliterating the prevertebral fat to the left of L4, the sacrum, and also around the left lumbosacral plexus. *(Reproduced from Taylor BV, et al. Magnetic resonance imaging in cancer-related lumbosacral plexopathy. Mayo Clin Proc 1997;72:823–829, with permission of Elsevier Science.)*

radiculopathies from epidural or leptomeningeal metastasis can be confused with plexopathy. Leptomeningeal metastasis is often bilateral and is characterized by less pain. Spine imaging and cerebrospinal fluid examination can be diagnostic. Osteitis pubis can mimic plexus involvement. Metastasis, avascular necrosis, or osteoporotic fracture of the hip can produce leg pain that suggests upper plexopathy. Radiation-induced lumbosacral plexus sarcomas and malignant triton tumors are rare complications of pelvic radiation that can be confused with metastatic plexopathy.[87,88]

▶ TREATMENT/PROGNOSIS

Therapy is palliative. The results of treatment are generally poor and patient survival is short. The subjective and objective response to treatment varies among different series. In Jaeckle and associates' series,[75] 25 patients underwent debulking of the tumor and 52 received radiation, typically external beam radiation. A wide range of radiation doses were employed; the median dose was 35.5 Gy. Fifty-three patients received chemotherapy, sometimes in combination with radiation. Sixty-five patients were evaluable for pain relief; only 10 patients (15%) showed pain improvement, 20% were stable, and 65% had worse pain. Fifty-nine patients were reexamined and 10 (17%) showed improved strength that persisted for 1 to 17 months (median: 10 months), 24% remained stable, and 59% worsened. Posttreatment CT scans were obtained in 46 patients and 28% showed a decrease in tumor size. The most responsive tumor was lymphoma. The median survival was 5.5 months (range: 1–34 months). In the series by Taylor and associates,[76] the prognosis was almost identical, with a median survival of 5 months (range: 1–45 months). Ampil[80] reported the results of radiotherapy for metastatic lesions of the lumbosacral plexus, although it is not apparent if some of the 30 patients had additional involvement of adjacent spinal nerve roots. A complete subjective response to radiation occurred in 23 patients (85%) and correlated with administration of at least 30 Gy radiation. Complete objective response occurred in 30% and also correlated with at least a 30-Gy dose. Pain relief lasted an average of 4 months. Pettigrew and associates[79] reported that treatment with radiation or chemotherapy resulted in reduction of pain in each of five patients and mild to moderate improvement in strength in three. In 19 evaluable patients with cervical cancer,[77] treatment of metastatic lumbosacral plexopathy resulted in pain relief only in 9 patients and there was no relief or worsening of pain in the others. None had improvement in neurologic signs and the survival was poor, with a range of 0 to 17 months (median: 5 months). The reason for the wide discrepancy in subjective treatment response in different series is unknown and cannot be explained by tumor type or radiation dose.

Systemic chemotherapy can be effective for plexus invasion or compression by lymphoma and also diffuse peripheral nerve infiltration by lymphoma.[89] Pettigrew also reported that high-dose intravenous steroids gave temporary, but clinically significant, relief. As in patients with neoplastic brachial neuropathy, pain should be managed initially with systemic or transcutaneous opioids, but they are often ineffective. When pain persists, spinal opioids or other methods of pain relief, such as cordotomy, should be considered.

▶ PERIPHERAL NEUROPATHY

Clinical Setting

Peripheral nerve infiltration by metastatic tumor is rare. In most reported cases occurring from solid tumors, compression of the nerve by metastasis to adjacent soft tissue or bone is the mechanism. The most common individual nerves affected are those that supply the lower extremity. The site of compression is more often the pelvis than the limb. As is the case with plexus involvement, the mononeuropathy usually occurs in the setting of widespread metastatic tumor, but there are some reports of individuals who have limited stage disease, and the mononeuropathy can even be the presenting sign of malignancy. In one series of six patients with symptomatic obturator neuropathy, the obturator neuropathy was the sole presenting sign of new pelvic cancer in three cases.[90] In a series of 2261 cervical cancer patients undergoing surgery, Saphner[77] reported obturator nerve and genitofemoral nerve impingement from cervical cancer in one patient each. Five patients with isolated pelvic recurrence of colorectal cancer that resulted in inferior gluteal and posterior femoral cutaneous neuropathy are reported by LaBan and associates.[91] The sites of entrapment were presumed to be within the pelvis, the piriform foramen, and the sciatic notch. Sciatic mononeuropathy resulting from gluteal metastasis with nerve compression and infiltration is also reported. Tumor types include colorectal carcinoma (one of which was contralateral to the original site of cancer) and malignant melanoma.[92–94]

Hematogeneous spread of cancer to a nerve is rare in solid tumors.[93,95] This mode of peripheral nerve metastasis occurs most commonly in lymphoma, and in this setting, single or multiple nerves can be affected. Neurolymphomatosis is a term used to describe metastasis of lymphoma to peripheral nerves, often in association with other sites of lymphoma in the nervous system. Baehring and associates[6] define four clinical presentations, including painful involvement of peripheral nerves or spinal nerve roots, painless or painful cranial neuropathies, painless involvement of peripheral nerves, and painless or painful involvement of a single peripheral nerve. Mononeuropathies from lymphoma are reported in all major nerves of the upper and lower limbs.[6,96–104]

Diffuse involvement of peripheral nerves by lymphoma, producing a symmetric or asymmetric sensorimotor polyneuropathy, is rare. This pattern of nerve involvement is also reported rarely in leukemia and myeloma.[105–110] Metastatic polyneuropathy from hematologic tumors is likely to be more common than is reported, because it is difficult to diagnose antemortem. It typically occurs in non-Hodgkin lymphoma, usually of B-cell origin. T-cell lymphoma is a rare cause.[101,111]

In neurolymphomatosis, there is often systemic or brain lymphoma.[6,112–115] The syndrome may begin in the peripheral nerves or plexus and predate the onset of signs of systemic or CNS lymphoma, develop concurrently, or occur when other sites of tumor are in remission.[96,99,100,106,113,116–121] In the latter situation, it is speculated that the blood–nerve barrier forms a sanctuary from systemic chemotherapy.[6]

Clinical Signs

The clinical presentation of a metastatic mononeuropathy may be localized pain or pain and sensory loss in the cutaneous distribution of the nerve. Weakness may result if the nerve compression or infiltration is severe. A Tinel sign and a mass in close proximity of the site of limb tumor involvement may be observed. Ipsilateral leg edema can be seen with obturator neuropathy from pelvic tumors, presumably as a consequence of lymphatic obstruction.[90]

Polyneuropathy is often painful, but in some patients there are paresthesias, numbness, and loss of stretch reflexes without significant pain. The polyneuropathy is usually symmetric, but can be asymmetric. The onset of symptoms is usually slowly progressive but may be rapid, mimicking mononeuritis multiplex or Guillain-Barré syndrome.[122,123]

Diagnosis

Mononeuropathies can be confused with radiculopathy or with pain solely caused by bone or soft tissue metastasis. It is also difficult to distinguish polyneuropathy caused by tumor infiltration from paraneoplastic, idiopathic, or treatment-related polyneuropathies in the cancer patient on clinical grounds alone.

The widespread distribution of neuropathy can also suggest leptomeningeal metastasis.

Electrophysiology

EMG can localize a mononeuropathy caused by tumor.[90,91,99] An axonal polyneuropathy, rarely a demyelinating one, is characteristic of diffuse lymphoma nerve involvement.[121]

Imaging

Pelvic CT or MRI is usually sensitive in detecting pelvic tumor in the cases reported, but due to the rarity of metastatic mononeuropathy, the true sensitivity is not known. Rogers and associates[90] reported that pelvic CT was sensitive in demonstrating tumor affecting the obturator nerve in each case identified clinically. The site of tumor was the posterolateral wall of the upper or midpelvis, the anterior wall of the lower pelvis, or muscles extrinsic to the bony pelvis (Fig. 29-7). MRI of the buttock or limb in the suspected region of nerve involvement can detect sites of peripheral nerve compression or invasion.[93] Individual fascicles of large nerves can be seen with fat-suppressed T_2-weighted, thin-section MRI. Signal-intensity changes, enlargement, and enhancement of the nerve can be seen with metastatic involvement (Fig. 29-8).[6,96,99,100,114,120] Other useful modalities for detecting nerve metastasis are gallium scan and PET-CT fusion imaging, but their specificity and sensitivity are unknown.[14,120,124]

Biopsy

MRI can identify involved nerve segments and possible sites for biopsy (see Fig. 29-8). A biopsy of a symptomatic nerve has the greatest yield in diffuse neuropathy. The standard sural nerve biopsy may be negative because of the patchy nature of the nerve involvement.[104,112,125]

Treatment/Prognosis

Optimal therapy is not defined for mononeuropathy caused by cancer because of the small number of reported cases. Resection of a solitary tumor mass can improve symptoms in some patients. It appears that other antineoplastic therapy can relieve symptoms in the majority of patients. Treatment with radiation, chemotherapy, or both provided symptomatic relief that lasted 11 months to 10 years in 4 of 6 patients with obturator neuropathy caused by cancer. The clinical response correlated with tumor response on CT.[90] In each of the reported cases of sciatic neuropathy from metastatic cancer or melanoma, pain was improved with subtotal resection, which in one case was followed by radiation. Local nerve blocks should also be considered for symptomatic therapy.

Steroids are palliative in lymphoma and provide short-term benefit only. Chemotherapy alone is usually effective for neurolymphomatosis and it can be used again at relapse.[89,96,101,111,121,126] The first clinical response is usually resolution of pain, followed by improved motor and sensory function. The optimal chemotherapy regimen is not known; a variety of combination chemotherapies or single-agent high-dose methotrexate are used effectively.[6]

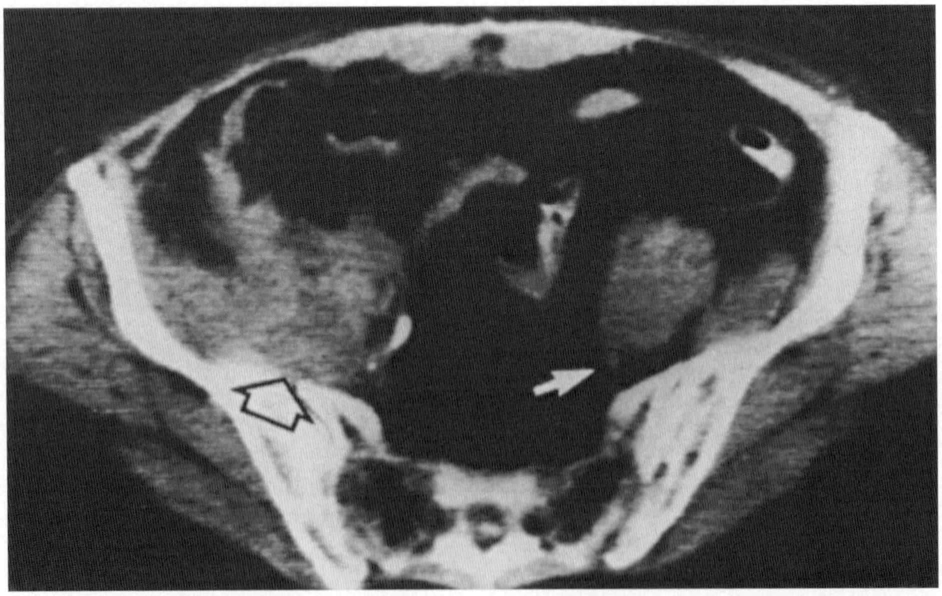

Figure 29-7. CT in the midpelvis shows a tumor in the right iliac fossa region (left in figure, open arrow). The normal fat plane separating the psoas and iliacus muscles is obliterated. The solid arrow shows the obturator nerve on the contralateral side. (*Reproduced from Rogers LR, Borkowski GP, Albers JW, et al. Obturator mononeuropathy caused by pelvic cancer: six cases. Neurology 1993;43:1489–1492, with permission of Lippincott Williams & Wilkins.*)

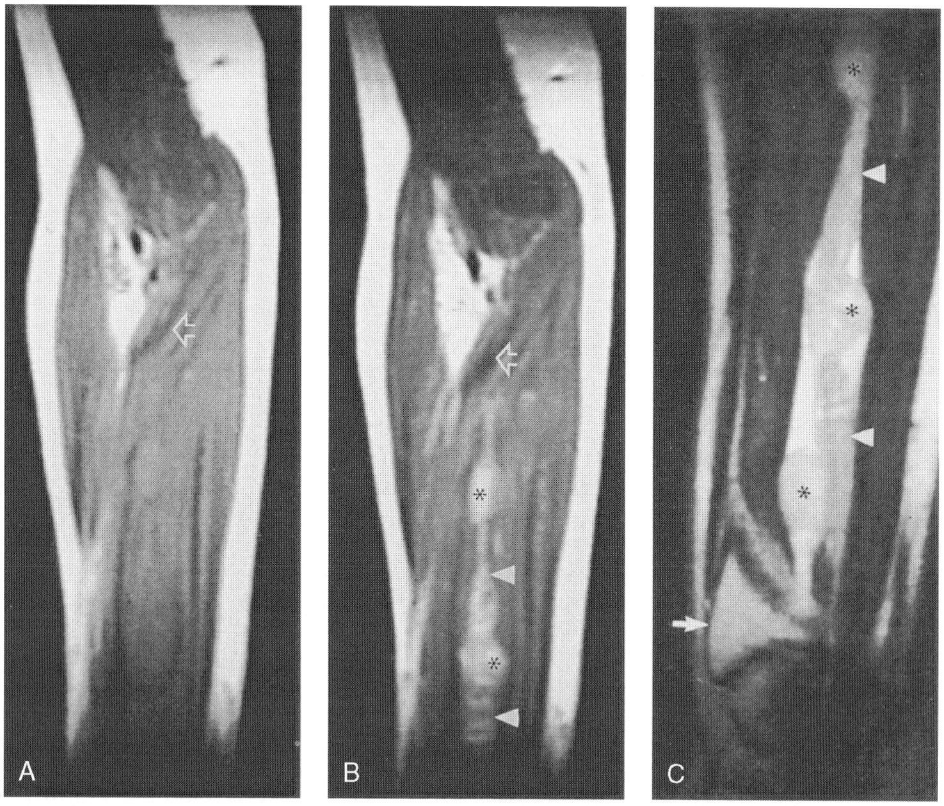

Figure 29-8. T_1-weighted coronal slice of the proximal right forearm before (A) and after (B) intravenous gadolinium administration; after repositioning (C): T_2-weighted coronal slice through the distal right forearm, showing a swollen median nerve (arrowheads) with enhancement following gadolinium administration and swollen lymph nodes(*). Open arrow = pronator teres muscle; closed arrow = distal part of the radial bone. *(Reproduced from van den Bent MJ, deBruin HG, Beun GDM, et al. Neurolymphomatosis of the median nerve. Neurology 1995;45:1403–1405, with permission of Lippincott Williams & Wilkins.)*

Peripheral nerve, CNS, or systemic relapse can occur after chemotherapy is discontinued, so patients should be observed clinically after treatment.[99,100,127–129]

REFERENCES

1. Meller I, Alkalay D, Mozes M, et al. Isolated metastases to peripheral nerves. Cancer 1995;76:1829–1832.
2. Ushio Y, Chernik NL, Posner JB, et al. Meningeal carcinomatosis: development of an experimental model. J Neuropathol Exp Neurol 1977;36:228–244.
3. Barber JR, Coventry MB, McDonald JR. The spread of soft-tissue sarcomata of the extremities along peripheral nerve trunks. J Bone Joint Surg Am 1957;39:534–540.
4. Vega F, Davila L, Delattre JY, et al. Experimental carcinomatous plexopathy. Neurology 1993;240:54–58.
5. Kashef R, Das Gupta TK. Segmental demyelination of peripheral nerves in the presence of malignant tumors. Br J Cancer 1967;21:411–417.
6. Baehring JM, Damek D, Martin EC, et al. Neurolymphomatosis. Neuro-oncology 2003;5:104–115.
7. Vallieres E, Karmay-Jones R, Mulligan MS, et al. Pancoast tumors. Curr Probl Surg 2001;38:306–307.
8. Hare ES. Tumor involving certain nerves [letter]. London Med Gaz 1838;1:16–18.
9. Pancoast HK. Superior pulmonary sulcus tumor: tumor characterized by pain, Horner's syndrome, destruction of bone and atrophy of hand muscles. JAMA 1932;32:99:1391–1396.
10. Fulton DS. Brachial plexopathy in patients with breast cancer. In: Paterson AHF, Lees AW, eds. Fundamental problems in breast cancer. Proceedings of the Second International Symposium on Fundamental Problems in Breast Cancer held at Banff, Alberta, Canada, April 26–29, 1986. Boston: Martinus Nijoff, 1987:249–257.
11. Kori SH, Foley KM, Posner JB. Brachial plexus lesions in patients with cancer: 100 cases. Neurology 1981;31:45–50.
12. Pietrangeli A, Milella M, DeMarco S, et al. Brachial plexus neuropathy as unusual onset of diffuse neurolymphomatosis. Neurol Sci 2000;21:241–245.

13. Mills PR, Han LY, Dick R, et al. Pancoast syndrome caused by a high grade B cell lymphoma. Thorax 1994;49:92–93.
14. Liang R, Kay R, Maisey MN. Brachial plexus infiltration by non-Hodgkin's lymphoma. Br J Radiol 1985;58:1125–1127.
15. Rao R, Robins HI. Non-Hodgkin's tumor and Pancoast's syndrome. Oncol Rep 2001;8:165–166.
16. Savas MC, Celik I, Benekli M, et al. Renal cell carcinoma presenting as solitary cervical node metastasis compressing the brachial plexus. Nephron 1998;79:107–108.
17. Kodama T, Satoh H, Homma S, et al. Pancoast's syndrome due to metastatic carcinoma from the stomach. Can Respir J 2003;10:330.
18. Chang C, Su W, Chou T, et al. Hepatocellular carcinoma with Pancoast's syndrome as an initial symptom: a case report. Jpn J Clin Oncol 2001;31:119–121.
19. Usuki K, Yuo A, Muto Y, et al. Primary malignant lymphoma of the left brachial plexus. Jpn J Clin Hematol 1988;29:1125–1128.
20. Omenn GS. Pancoast syndrome due to metastatic carcinoma from the uterine cervix. Chest 1971;60:268–270.
21. Amin R. Bilateral Pancoast's syndrome in a patient with carcinoma of the cervix. Gynecol Oncol 1986;24:126–128.
22. Hans S, Lindner DW, Webster JD. Brachial plexus neuropathy from metastatic testicular seminoma. Urology 1985;25:398–400.
23. Ampil FL. Brachial plexus neuropathy from prostatic carcinoma metastasis. J La State Med Soc 1986a;138:38–40.
24. Suzuki M, Watanabe T, Mogi G. Primary non-Hodgkin's lymphoma of brachial plexus. Auris Nasus Larynx 1999;26:337–342.
25. Ohta H. A case of non-Hodgkin's lymphoma infiltrating the brachial plexus detected by Ga-67 scintigraphy. Ann Nucl Med 2002;16:297–298.
26. Harper CM, Thomas JE, Cascino TL, et al. Distinction between neoplastic and radiation-induced brachial plexopathy. Neurology 1989;39:502–506.
27. Detterbeck FC. Pancoast (superior sulcus) tumors. Ann Thorac Surg 1997;63:1810–1818.
28. Kanner R, Martini N, Foley K. Incidence of pain and other clinical manifestations of the superior pulmonary sulcus (Pancoast) tumors, vol. 4. New York: Raven Press, 1982.
29. Derbekyan V, Novales-Diaz J, Lisbona R. Pancoast tumor as a cause of reflex sympathetic dystrophy. J Nucl Med 1993;34:1992–1994.
30. Thomas JE, Colby MY. Radiation-induced or metastatic brachial plexopathy? JAMA 1972;222:1392–1395.
31. Ku A, Lachman E, Tunkel R, et al. Upper limb reflex sympathetic dystrophy associated with occult malignancy. Arch Phys Med Rehabil 1996;77:726–772.
32. Vargo MM, Flood KM. Pancoast tumor presenting as cervical radiculopathy. Arch Phys Med Rehabil 1990;71:606–609.
33. Wilbourn AJ. Electrodiagnosis of plexopathies. Neurol Clin 1985;3:511–529.
34. Lederman RJ, Wilbourn AJ. Brachial plexopathy: recurrent cancer or radiation? Neurology 1984;34:1331–1335.
35. Albers JW, Allen AA, Bastron JA, et al. Limb myokymia. Muscle Nerve 1981;4:494–550.
36. Rapoport S, Blair DN, McCarthy SM, et al. Brachial plexus: correlation of MR imaging with CT and pathologic findings. Radiology 1988;167:161–165.
37. Bilbey JH, Lamond RG, Mattrey RF. MR imaging of disorders of the brachial plexus. J Magn Reson Imag 1994;4:13–18.
38. Thyagarajan D, Cascino T, Harms G. Magnetic resonance imaging in brachial plexopathy of cancer. Neurology 1995;45:421–427.
39. Castagno AA, Shuman WP. MR imaging in clinically suspected brachial plexus tumor. AJR 1987;149:1219–1222.
40. Wittenberg KH, Adkins MC. MR imaging of the nontraumatic brachial plexopathies: frequency and spectrum of findings. Radiographics 2000;20:1023–1032.
41. Swarnkar A, Fukui MB, Fink DJ, et al. MR imaging of brachial plexopathy in neurolymphomatosis. AJR 1997;169:1189–1190.
42. Ahmad A, Barrington S, Maisey M, et al. Use of positron emission tomography in evaluation of brachial plexopathy in breast cancer patients. Br J Cancer 1999;79:478–482.
43. Hoang P, Ford DJ, Burke FD. Post mastectomy pain after brachial plexus palsy: metastases or radiation neuritis? J Hand Surg 1986;11:441–443.
44. Cole JW, Quint DJ, McGillicuddy JE, et al. CT-guided brachial plexus biopsy. Am J Neuroradiol 1997;18:1420–1422.
45. Olsen NK, Pfiffer P, Johannsen L, et al. Radiation-induced brachial plexopathy: neurological follow-up in 161 recurrence-free breast cancer patients. Int J Radiat Oncol 1993;26:43–49.
46. Bagley FH, Walsh JW, Cady B, et al. Carcinomatous versus radiation-induced brachial plexus neuropathy in breast cancer. Cancer 1978;41:2154–2157.
47. Stoll BA, Andrews JT. Radiation induced peripheral neuropathy. Br Med J 1966;1:834–837.
48. Gerard JM, Franck N, Moussa Z, et al. Acute ischemic brachial plexus neuropathy following radiation therapy. Neurology 1989;39:450–451.
49. Fisher PM, Dodwell DJ, Bridges LR, et al. Malignant schwannoma following treatment for Hodgkin's disease. Clin Oncol 1994;6:204–205.
50. Newbould MJ, Wilkinson N, Mene A. Post-radiation malignant peripheral nerve sheath tumor: a report of two cases. Histopathology 1990;17:263–265.
51. Grudera-Popova J, Goranov S, Kumchev I. Third malignancy after treatment of Hodgkin's disease. Folia Medica (Plovdiv) 1999;41:13–15.
52. Borman H, Safak T, Erty D. Fibrosarcoma following radiotherapy for breast carcinoma: a case report and review of the literature. Ann Plast Surg 1998;41:201–204.
53. Hussussian CJ, Mackinnon SE. Postradiation neural sheath sarcoma of the brachial plexus: a case report. Ann Plast Surg 1999;43:313–317.
54. Gandhi S, Walsh G L, Komaki R, et al. A multidisciplinary surgical approach to superior sulcus tumors with vertebral invasion. Ann Thorac Surg 1999;68:1778–1785.
55. Bilsky MH, Vitaz TW, Boland PJ, et al. Surgical treatment of superior sulcus tumors with spinal and brachial plexus involvement. J Neurosurg Spine 2002;97:301–309.
56. Rusch VW, Giroux DJ, Kraut MJ, et al. Induction chemoradiation and surgical resection for non-small cell lung carcinomas of the superior sulcus: initial results of Southwest Oncology Group Trial 9416 (Intergroup Trial 0160). J Thorac Cardiovasc Surg 2001;121:472–483.

57. Wright CD, Menard MT, Wain JC, et al. Induction chemoradiation compared with radiation for lung cancer involving the superior sulcus. Ann Thorac Surg 2002;73:1541–1544.
58. Evans TL, Donahue DM, Mathisen DJ, et al. Building a better therapy for stage IIIA non-small cell lung cancer. Clin Chest Med 2002;23:191–207.
59. Shahian DM, Neptune WB, Ellis FH. Pancoast tumors: improved survival with preoperative and postoperative radiotherapy. Ann Thorac Surg 1987;43:32–38.
60. Maggi G, Casadio C, Pischedda F, et al. Combined radiosurgical treatment of Pancoast tumor. Ann Thorac Surg 1994;57:198–202.
61. Komaki R, Roth JA, Walsh GL, et al. Outcome predictors for 143 patients with superior sulcus tumors treated by multidisciplinary approach at the University of Texas M. D. Anderson Cancer Center. Int J Rad Oncol Biol Phys 2000;48:347–354.
62. Ahmad K, Fayos JV, Kirsh MM. Apical lung carcinoma. Cancer 1984;54:913–917.
63. Ampil FL. Radiotherapy for carcinomatous brachial plexopathy. Cancer 1985;56:2185–2188.
64. Son YH. Effectiveness of irradiation therapy in peripheral neuropathy caused by malignant disease. Cancer 1967;9: 1447–1451.
65. Nisce LZ, Chu FCH. Radiation therapy of brachial plexus syndrome from breast cancer. Radiology 1968;91:1022–1025.
66. Mullin V. Brachial plexus block with phenol for painful arm associated with Pancoast's syndrome. Anesthesiology 1980;53:431–433.
67. Wang MY, Teitelbaum GP, Loskota WJ, et al. Brachial plexus catheter reservoir for the treatment of upper-extremity cancer pain: technical case report. Neurosurgery 2000;46:1009–1012.
68. Fischer HBJ, Peters TM, Fleming IM, et al. Peripheral nerve catheterization in the management of terminal cancer pain. Reg Anesth 1996;21:482–485.
69. Vranken JH, Zuurmond WWA, de Lange JJ. Continuous brachial plexus block as treatment for the Pancoast syndrome. Clin J Pain 2000;16:327–333.
70. Kanpolat Y, Savas A, Ucar T, et al. CT-guided percutaneous selective cordotomy for treatment of intractable pain in patients with malignant pleural mesothelioma. Acta Neurochir (Wien) 2002;144:595–599.
71. Dionne C. Tumor invasion of the brachial plexus: management of pain with intrapleural analgesia. Can J Anaesth 1992;39:520–521.
72. Myers DP, Lema MJ, de Leon-Casasola OA, et al. Interpleural analgesia for the treatment of severe cancer pain in terminally ill patients. J Pain Symptom Manage 1993;8:505–510.
73. Sindon M. Microsurgical DREZotomy (MDT) for pain, spasticity and hyperactive bladder: a 20-year experience. Acta Neurochir (Wien) 1995;137:1–5.
74. Wittig JC, Bickels J, Kollender Y, et al. Palliative forequarter amputation for metastatic carcinoma to the shoulder girdle region: indications, preoperative evaluation, surgical technique, and results. J Surg Oncol 2001;77:105–113.
75. Jaeckle KA, Young DF, Foley KM. The natural history of lumbosacral plexopathy in cancer. Neurology 1985;35:8–15.
76. Taylor BV, Kimmel DW, Krecke KN, et al. Magnetic resonance imaging in cancer-related lumbosacral plexopathy. Mayo Clin Proc 1997;72:823–829.
77. Saphner T, Gallion HH, Van Nagell JR, et al. Neurologic complications of cervical cancer. Cancer 1989;64:1147–1151.
78. Anderson TS, Regine WF, Kryscio R, et al. Neurological complications of bladder cancer: a review of 359 cases. Cancer 2003;97:2267–2272.
79. Pettigrew LC, Glass JP, Maor M, et al. Diagnosis and treatment of lumbosacral plexopathies in patients with cancer. Arch Neurol 1984;41:1282–1285.
80. Ampil FL. Palliative irradiation of carcinomatous lumbosacral plexus neuropathy. Int Radiat Oncol Biol Phys 1986b;12:1681–1686.
81. Thomas JE, Cascino TL, Earle JD. Differential diagnosis between radiation and tumor plexopathy of the pelvis. Neurology 1985;35:1–7.
82. Dalmau J, Graus F, Marco M. "Hot and dry foot" as initial manifestation of neoplastic lumbosacral plexopathy. Neurology 1989;39:871–872.
83. Vock P, Mattle H, Studer M, et al. Lumbosacral plexus lesions: correlations of clinical signs and computed tomography. J Neurol Neurosurg Psychiatr 1988;51:72–79.
84. Frykholm GJ, Sintorn K, Montelius A, et al. Acute lumbosacral plexopathy during and after preoperative radiotherapy of rectal adenocarcinoma. Radiother Oncol 1996; 38:121–130.
85. Abu-Rustum NR, Rajbhandari D, Glusman S, et al. Acute lower extremity paralysis following radiation therapy for cervical cancer. Gynecol Oncol 1999;75:152–154.
86. Georgiou A, Grigsby PW, Perez CA. Radiation-induced lumbosacral plexopathy in gynecologic tumors: clinical findings and dosimetric analysis. Int Radiat Oncol Biol Phys 1993;26:479–482.
87. Woodruff JM, Perino G. Non-germ cell or teratomatous malignant tumors showing additional rhabdomyoblastic differentiation, with emphasis on the malignant Triton tumor. Semin Diagn Pathol 1994;11:69–81.
88. Yakulis R, Manack L, Murphy AI. Postradiation malignant triton tumor. A case report and review of the literature. Arch Pathol Lab Med 1996;120:541–548.
89. Krendel DA, Stahl RL, Chan WC. Lymphomatous polyneuropathy. Arch Neurol 1991;48:330–332.
90. Rogers LR, Borkowski GP, Albers JW, et al. Obturator mononeuropathy caused by pelvic cancer: Six cases. Neurology 1993;43:1489–1492.
91. LaBan MM, Meerschaert JR, Taylor RS. Electromyographic evidence of isolated inferior gluteal nerve compromise: an early representation of recurrent colon carcinoma. Arch Phys Med Rehabil 1982;63:33–35.
92. Stulc JP, Petrelli NJ, Herrera L, et al. Isolated metachronous metastases to soft tissues of the buttock from a colonic adenocarcinoma. Dis Colon Rectum 1985;28:117–121.
93. Cantone G, Rath SA, Richter HP. Intraneural metastasis in a peripheral nerve. Acta Neurochir (Wien) 2000;142:719–720.
94. Rao BK, Lange TA, Hafez GR, et al. Extension of recurrent rectal carcinoma through sciatic foramen: diagnosis by computed tomography. Comput Radiol 1982;6:193–197.
95. Grisold W, Jellinger K, Lutz D. Human neurolymphomatosis in a patient with chronic lymphatic leukemia. Clin Neuropathol 1990;9:224–230.
96. Van den Bent MJ, deBruin HG, Beun GDM, et al. Neurolymphomatosis of the median nerve. Neurology 1995;45: 1403–1405.

97. Teisser J. A case of primary malignant lymphoma confined to the trunk of the ulnar nerve in the elbow. Ann Chir Main Memb Super 1992;11:170–172.
98. Eusebi V, Bondi A, Cancellieri A, et al. Primary malignant lymphoma of sciatic nerve. Report of a case. Am J Surg Pathol 1990;14:881–885.
99. Purohit DP, Dick DJ, Perry RH, et al. Solitary extranodal lymphoma of sciatic nerve. J Neurol Sci 1986;74:23–34.
100. Pillay PK, Hardy RW Jr, Wilbourn AJ, et al. Solitary primary lymphoma of the sciatic nerve: case report. Neurosurgery 1988;23:370–371.
101. Gherardi R, Gaulard P, Prost C, et al. T-cell lymphoma revealed by a peripheral neuropathy. Cancer 1986;58: 2710–2716.
102. Brohi SR. Neurolymphomatosis of peroneal nerve. J Coll Phys Surg Pakistan 1999;9:199–200.
103. Van Bolden V, Kline DG, Garcia CA, et al. Isolated radial nerve palsy due to metastasis from a primary malignant lymphoma of the brain. Neurosurgery 1987;21:905–909.
104. Walk D, Handelsman A, Beckmann E, et al. Mononeuropathy multiplex due to infiltration of lymphoma in hematologic remission. Muscle Nerve 1998;21:823–826.
105. Kuroda Y, Nakata H, Kakigy R, et al. Human neurolymphomatosis by adult T-cell leukemia. Neurology 1989;39: 144–146.
106. Krendel DA, Albright RE, Graham DG. Infiltrative polyneuropathy due to monoblastic leukemia in hematologic remission. Neurology 1987;37:474–477.
107. Dufour C, Garaventa A, Brisigotti M, et al. Massively diffuse multifocal granulocytic sarcoma in a child with acute myeloid leukemia. Tumori 1995;81:222–224.
108. Lekos A, Katirji MB, Cohen ML, et al. Mononeuritis multiplex: a harbinger of acute leukemia in relapse. Arch Neurol 1994;51:618–622.
109. Grisold W, Piza-Katzer H, Jahn R, et al. Intraneural nerve metastasis with multiple mononeuropathies. J Periph Nerv Sys 2000;5:163–167.
110. Dayan AD, Urich H, Gardner-Thorpe C. Peripheral neuropathy and myeloma. J Neurol Sci 1971;14:21–35.
111. Atiq OT, Deangelis LM, Rosenblum M, et al. Cutaneous T-cell lymphoma presenting with diffuse lymphomatous infiltration of the peripheral nerves response to combination chemotherapy. Am J Clin Oncol 1992;15:212–215.
112. Guberman A, Rosenbaum H, Braciale T, et al. Human neurolymphomatosis. J Neurol Sci 1978;36:1–12.
113. Diaz-Arrastia R, Younger DS, Hair L, et al. Neurolymphomatosis: a clinicopathologic syndrome re-emerges. Neurology 1992;42:1136–1141.
114. Quinones-Hinojosa A, Friedlander RM, Boyer PJ, et al. Solitary sciatic nerve lymphoma as an initial manifestation of diffuse neurolymphomatosis. Case report and review of the literature. J Neurosurg 2000;92:165–169.
115. Rosner LJ, Lucia M, Verity MA. Progressive bilateral lower limb weakness and cranial mononeuritis multiplex. Bull LA Neurol Soc 1974;39:30–38.
116. Shoenfeld Y, Aderka D, Sandbank U, et al. Fatal peripheral neurolymphomatosis after remission of histiocytic lymphoma. Neurology 1983;33:243–245.
117. Gemignani F, Marchesi G, DiGiovanni G, et al. Low-grade non-Hodgkin B-cell lymphoma presenting as sensory neuropathy. Eur Neurol 1996;36:138–141.
118. Grisold W, Drlicek M, Jellinger K. Neurolymphomatosis. Neurology 1993;43:1628.
119. Gordon PH, Younger DS. Neurolymphomatosis. Neurology 1996;46:1191–1192.
120. Kanamori M, Matsui H, Yudoh K. Solitary T-cell lymphoma of the sciatic nerve: case report. Neurosurgery 1995;36: 1203–1205.
121. Ince PG, Shaw PJ, Fawcett PRW, et al. Demyelinating neuropathy due to primary IgM kappa B cell lymphoma of peripheral nerve. Neurology 1987;37:1231–1235.
122. Vallat JM, De Mascarel HA, Bordessoule D, et al. Non-Hodgkin's malignant lymphomas and peripheral neuropathies—13 cases. Brain 1995;118:1223–1245.
123. Vital C, Vital A, Brustet A, et al. Neurolymphomatosis. Neurology 1993;43:1627–1628.
124. Trojan A, Jermann M, Taverna C, et al. Fusion PET-CT imaging of neurolymphomatosis. Ann Oncol 2002;13:802–805.
125. Van den Bent MJ, deBruin HG, Bos GM, et al. Negative sural nerve biopsy in neurolymphomatosis. J Neurol 1999;246: 1159–1163.
126. Dubas F, Penisson-Besnier I, Fazi S, et al. Infiltration of the peripheral nerve by a T-cell lymphoma mycosis fungoides: report of a case with improvement after chemotherapy. J Neurol 1990;237:S25.
127. Misdraji J, Ino Y, Louis DN, et al. Primary lymphoma of peripheral nerve: report of four cases. Am J Surg Pathol 2000;24:1257–1265.
128. Roncaroli F, Poppi M, Riccioni L, et al. Primary non-Hodgkin's lymphoma of the sciatic nerve followed by localization in the central nervous system: case report and review of the literature. Neurosurgery 1997;40: 618–622.
129. Wulff EA, Simpson DM. Peripheral neuropathy associated with acquired immunodeficiency syndrome (AIDS)-related Burkitt's lymphoma. Muscle Nerve 2000;23:1764–1766.

PART IV

Indirect Complications of Cancer

CHAPTER 30
Paraneoplasia

Setareh Shams'ili / Peter Sillevis Smitt

By definition, paraneoplastic neurologic syndromes (PNS) are remote effects of cancer that are not caused by invasion of the tumor or its metastases nor by infection, cerebrovascular complications, surgery, or other forms of tumor treatment.[1] *Some clinical syndromes, such as subacute cerebellar degeneration,*[2] *subacute sensory neuronopathy,*[3] *opsoclonus/myoclonus,*[4] *and limbic encephalitis,*[5] *are relatively often paraneoplastic and are preferentially associated with certain tumors (Tables 30-1 and 30-2). In these cases a careful and directed search for an underlying neoplasm should be conducted. When more common neurologic syndromes such as mixed somatic polyneuropathy*[6] *and chronic inflammatory demyelinating polyneuropathy (CIDP)*[7] *occur in close temporal relation with a relatively frequent event as cancer, a chance association should be considered. A paraneoplastic etiology depends in these instances on the relative frequencies of tumor and nontumor cases. In an individual patient, a paraneoplastic etiology is strongly suggested when improvement of the neurologic syndrome coincides with treatment of the tumor. The discovery of paraneoplastic antineuronal autoantibodies has facilitated the diagnosis of a neurologic syndrome as paraneoplastic. The paraneoplastic or onconeural antibodies are associated with specific clinical syndromes and tumor types. The high specificity of these antibodies helps diagnose a syndrome as paraneoplastic and directs the search toward an underlying neoplasm. The discovery of paraneoplastic autoantibodies has also led to the autoimmune hypothesis of paraneoplastic disorders. This hypothesis postulates that an immune response directed against neuronal antigens expressed by the tumor cross-reacts with the same or similar antigens in the nervous system.*[8] *Intrathecal synthesis of the paraneoplastic antibodies and the finding that the antibodies are directed against antigens expressed in affected parts of the nervous system support the autoimmune hypothesis of paraneoplasia.*[9] *Despite the presumed autoimmune etiology of the paraneoplastic neurologic syndromes, the results of various forms of immunotherapy with some exceptions have been generally disappointing. Detection and subsequent treatment of the underlying tumor appears to offer the best chance of preventing neurologic deterioration.*

▶ TABLE 30-1. PARANEOPLASTIC NEUROLOGIC SYNDROMES*

Central nervous system
- *Subacute cerebellar ataxia*
- *Limbic encephalitis*
- *Encephalomyelitis*
- *Opsoclonus–myoclonus*
- Stiff-person syndrome
- Chorea
- Cancer and melanoma-associated retinopathy
- Optic neuritis
- Subacute motor neuronopathy/motor neuron disease

Peripheral nervous system
- *Subacute sensory neuronopathy*
- Sensorimotor neuropathy
- Sensorimotor neuropathy associated with M protein
- Subacute autonomic neuropathy
- Vasculitis of nerve and muscle
- Neuromyotonia

Neuromuscular Junction and Muscle
- *Lambert-Eaton myasthenic syndrome*
- Myasthenia gravis
- Dermatomyositis/polymyositis
- Acute necrotizing myopathy
- Paraneoplastic carcinoid myopathy
- Cachectic myopathy

*In *italic* are clinical syndromes that are relatively often paraneoplastic. Because these syndromes are preferentially associated with certain tumors, a careful and directed search for an underlying neoplasm should be conducted.

▶ SPECIFIC CLINICAL PRESENTATIONS

PNS are characterized by the association of specific neurologic syndromes with typical paraneoplastic antibodies and tumor types. The most common associations are summarized in Tables 30-2 and 30-3. Characteristic clinical presentations are discussed below.

Central Nervous System

Subacute Cerebellar Ataxia

Paraneoplastic cerebellar degeneration (PCD) is one of the most common and characteristic paraneoplastic syndromes.[10,11] In a study of 137 consecutive patients with PNS associated with a paraneoplastic antibody, 50 (37%) presented with subacute cerebellar ataxia.[11] Brouwer first described PCD in 1919,[12] but the association with cancer was not recognized until 1938.[13] PCD usually starts with slight incoordination of walking, but evolves rapidly over weeks to a few months with progressive appendicular, truncal, and gait ataxia, dysarthria, and often nystagmus with oscillopsia. The disease reaches its peak within months and then stabilizes. By this time, most patients are severely debilitated. They are generally unable to walk without support and may be unable to sit unsupported. Handwriting is often illegible and feeding oneself difficult. The neurologic signs are always bilateral but may be asymmetric. Diplopia is common at presentation, although the investigator usually cannot detect abnormalities of ocular movement. Symptoms and signs are limited to the cerebellum and cerebellar pathways, but other mild neurologic abnormalities may be found on careful examination. These include hearing loss, dysphagia, pyramidal and extrapyramidal tract signs, mental status change, peripheral neuropathy, and Lambert-Eaton myasthenic syndrome (LEMS).[14–17] Magnetic resonance imaging (MRI) and computerized tomography (CT) scan are initially normal but often reveal cerebellar atrophy later in the course of the disease. Cerebral spinal fluid (CSF) examination, carried out to exclude leptomeningeal metastases, shows mild lymphocytic pleocytosis with elevation of protein and immunoglobulin (Ig) G levels in the first weeks to months. Oligoclonal bands may be present.

Underlying Tumor

PCD can be associated with any cancer but the most common tumors are lung cancer (usually small cell lung cancer (SCLC)), ovarian cancer, and lymphomas (particularly Hodgkin disease). In 60% to 70% of the patients, the neurologic symptoms precede the diagnosis of the cancer by a few months to 2 to 3 years and lead to its detection.[11,17,18]

Diagnostic Evaluation

PCD is a rare disorder in cancer patients. Conversely, 50% of patients presenting with acute or subacute nonfamilial ataxia are estimated to have an underlying malignancy.[10] The diagnosis of PCD is established by demonstration of specific antineuronal antibodies. The type of antibody directs the search for an underlying neoplasm (see Table 30-2).

Antineuronal Antibodies

PCD can be associated with various antineuronal autoantibodies. Anti-Yo, anti-Tr, anti-voltage-gated calcium channel (VGCC), anti-Ri, and anti-mGluR1 are associated with relatively "pure" cerebellar syndromes (Fig. 30-1).[11,19,20] Approximately 50% of patients presenting with PCD and an underlying SCLC have high titer anti-Hu antibodies.[14] In these patients, PCD is part of the paraneoplastic encephalomyelitis (PEM)/sensory neuronopathy (SN) syndrome, and more widespread neurologic symptoms and signs are usually found. In patients with SCLC and PCD without additional neurologic manifestations, anti-VGCC antibodies are more common (41%) than anti-Hu antibodies (16%).[20] Approximately half of the patients with PCD and anti-VGCC antibodies have additional clinical or electrophysiologic signs of LEMS.[14,20] Anti-Ri (ANNA-2) antibodies combine PCD and paraneoplastic opsoclonus

▶ TABLE 30-2. NEUROLOGIC SYNDROMES AND THE ROLE OF SPECIFIC AUTOANTIBODIES IN ESTABLISHING A PARANEOPLASTIC ETIOLOGY AND DIRECTING THE SEARCH FOR AN UNDERLYING NEOPLASM

Syndrome	Antibody	Paraneoplastic Antibody	Cancer (Most Common)
Central nervous system			
Subacute cerebellar degeneration		Anti-Yo	Ovary, breast
		Anti-Hu	SCLC
		Anti-Tr	Hodgkin disease
		Anti-Ri	Breast, gynecologic
		Anti-VGCC	SCLC
		Anti-mGluR1	Hodgkin disease
		PCA-2	SCLC
		ANNA-3	SCLC
		Anti-Ma	Miscellaneous
		Anti-Zic4	SCLC
Limbic encephalitis		Anti-Hu	SCLC
		Anti-Ta/Ma2	Testicular seminoma
		Anti-Ma	Lung cancer and other cancers
		ANNA-3	Lung cancer
		Anti-CRMP5/CV2	SCLC, thymoma
Encephalomyelitis		Anti-Hu	SCLC
		Anti-amphiphysin	SCLC, breast
		Anti-CRMP5/CV2	SCLC
		ANNA-3	Lung cancer
		PCA-2	SCLC
Opsoclonus–myoclonus (infant)		Anti-Hu	Neuroblastoma
Opsoclonus–myoclonus (adult)		Anti-Hu	SCLC
		Anti-Ri	Breast, gynecologic, bladder, SCLC
Stiff-person syndrome	Anti-GAD	Anti-amphiphysin	Breast, SCLC
Extrapyramidal syndrome		Anti-CRMP5/CV2	SCLC, lymphoma, renal cancer
		Anti-Hu	SCLC
Cancer-associated retinopathy		Anti-recoverin	SCLC
Cancer-associated melanoma		Antibodies against retinal bipolar cells	Melanoma
Optic neuritis		Anti-CRMP5/CV2	SCLC, thymoma
		Anti-Hu	SCLC
Motor neuronopathy (MND)		Anti-Hu	SCLC
Peripheral nervous system			
Subacute sensory neuronopathy		Anti-Hu	SCLC
		Anti-amphiphysin	SCLC
		Anti-CRMP5/CV2	SCLC, thymoma
		ANNA-3	Lung cancer
		PCA-2	SCLC
Sensorimotor neuropathy		Anti-Hu	SCLC
		Anti-CRMP5/CV2	SCLC, thymoma
Sensorimotor neuropathy-associated M protein		IgG or IgM M proteins	Multiple myeloma, osteosclerotic myeloma, B-cell NHL, B-cell CLL
		Anti-MAG IgM	Waldenström macroglobulinemia
Autonomic neuropathy	Anti-nAchR	Anti-Hu	SCLC
Neuromyotonia	Anti-VGKC	NA	Thymoma, lung cancer
Neuromuscular junction and Muscle			
Lambert-Eaton myasthenic syndrome	Anti-VGCC	NA	SCLC
Myasthenia gravis	Anti-AchR Anti-MuSK	Anti-titin	Thymoma
Dermatomyositis, polymyositis	Anti-Jo-1 Anti-Mi-2 Anti-PM-Sc1	NA	Various

ANNA = antineuronal nuclear antibody; CLL = chronic lymphocytic leukemia; GAD = glutamic acid decarboxylase; MAG = myelin-associated glycoprotein; mGluR1 = metabotropic glutamate receptor type 1; MuSK = muscle specific kinase; NA = not applicable; nAChR = nicotinic acetylcholine receptor; NHL = non-Hodgkin lymphoma; PCA = Purkinje cytoplasmic antibody; SCLC = small cell lung cancer; VGCC = voltage-gated calcium channels; VGKC = voltage-gated potassium channel.

▶ **TABLE 30-3.** PARANEOPLASTIC ANTIBODIES

Antibody	Clinical Syndromes	Associated Cancer	Neuronal Immunoreactivity	Protein Antigens	Genes	Protein Function	Reference
Anti-Hu (ANNA-1)	Paraneoplastic encephalomyelitis, paraneoplastic limbic encephalitis, paraneoplastic sensory neuronopathy, paraneoplastic cerebellar degeneration, autonomic neuropathy	SCLC, neuroblastoma, prostate cancer	Nucleus more than cytoplasm of all neurons, nucleolar sparing	35–40 kDa	*HuD, HuC, Hel-N1*	RNA binding	36, 173
Anti-Yo (PCA-1)	Paraneoplastic cerebellar degeneration	Ovarian, breast, and lung cancer	Cytoplasm of Purkinje cells and large brainstem neurons	34 and 62 kDa	*cdr34, cdr62*	DNA binding	174, 175
Anti-Ri (ANNA-2)	Cerebellar ataxia with or without opsoclonus and myoclonus	Breast, gynecologic, and bladder cancer and SCLC	Nucleus more than cytoplasm of all central neurons, nucleolar sparing	55 and 80 kDa	*Nova*	RNA binding	176, 177
Anti-Tr (PCA-Tr)	Paraneoplastic cerebellar degeneration	Hodgkin lymphoma	Cytoplasm and dendrites of Purkinje cells	?	Unknown	Unknown	18, 178, 179
Anti-CRMP5 (anti-CV2)	Paraneoplastic encephalomyelitis, paraneoplastic limbic encephalitis, paraneoplastic sensory neuronopathy, sensorimotor neuropathy, chorea, optic neuritis, paraneoplastic cerebellar degeneration, autonomic neuropathy	SCLC, thymoma	Cytoplasm of oligodendrocytes and neurons	60 kDa	*CRMP5* (*POP66*)	Neuronal development	21, 22
Anti-VGCC	Lambert-Eaton myasthenic syndrome, paraneoplastic cerebellar degeneration	SCLC	Presynaptic neuromuscular junction	64 kDa (P/Q type VGCC)	*CACNA1A, MysB*	Transmission at the nerve–muscle synapse	14, 20
Anti-amphiphysin	Stiff-person syndrome, paraneoplastic encephalomyelitis, paraneoplastic sensory neuronopathy, paraneoplastic cerebellar degeneration	Breast cancer, SCLC	Presynaptic nerve terminals	128 kDa	Amphiphysin	Synaptic vesicle endocytosis	39, 57, 60

PCA-2	Paraneoplastic encephalomyelitis, paraneoplastic cerebellar degeneration, motor neuropathy, autonomic neuropathy	SCLC	Cytoplasm of Purkinje cells and other neurons	280 kDa	—	—	23
Anti-retinal	Cancer-associated retinopathy Melanoma-associated retinopathy	SCLC Melanoma	Photoreceptors, ganglion cells Retinal bipolar cells	23, 65, 145, and 205 kDa	Recoverin	Light-dark adaptation by regulating Ca-dependent rhodopsin phosphorylation	77 74
Anti-Ma	Limbic brainstem encephalitis, paraneoplastic cerebellar degeneration	Lung cancer and other cancers	Nuclei and cytoplasm of neurons	40 kDa	*Ma1-3*	Unknown	29
Anti-Ta/Ma2	Limbic brainstem encephalitis	Testicular cancer	Nuclei and cytoplasm of neurons	40 kDa	*Ma2*	Unknown	26, 29
ANNA-3	Paraneoplastic encephalomyelitis, paraneoplastic sensory neuronopathy	Lung cancer	Nuclei of Purkinje cells and other neurons	170 kDa	—	—	40
Anti-mGluR1	Paraneoplastic cerebellar degeneration	Hodgkin lymphoma	Cytoplasm of Purkinje cells and brush cells, climbing fibers	160 kDa	*mGluR1*	Signal transmission by coupling G proteins in the cytoplasm, motor learning	19
Anti-Zic4	Paraneoplastic cerebellar degeneration	SCLC	Nuclei of cerebellar granule cells and other neurons	55, 50, 48, and 35–38 kDa	*Zic4*	Zinc-finger protein, cerebellar development	180
Anti-nAChR	Subacute autonomic neuropathy	SCLC	Postsynaptic, autonomic ganglia	Neuronal ganglionic nicotinic acetylcholine receptor	Neuronal ganglionic nicotinic acetylcholine receptor	Fast synaptic transmission through autonomic ganglia	120, 181

(*Continued*)

▶ **TABLE 30-3.** PARANEOPLASTIC ANTIBODIES (*CONTINUED*)

Antibody	Clinical Syndromes	Associated Cancer	Neuronal Immunoreactivity	Protein Antigens	Genes	Protein Function	Reference
Anti-VGKC	Limbic encephalitis, peripheral nerve hyperexcitability (neuromyotonia)	Thymoma, SCLC	Peripheral nerve	VGKC	Potassium channels	Controlling neuronal excitability	128, 182
Anti-MAG	Peripheral neuropathy	Waldenström macroglobulinemia	Peripheral nerve	107 kDa	MAG	Glia–axon interactions	183, 184

ANNA = antineuronal nuclear antibody; MAG = myelin-associated glycoprotein; mGluR1 = metabotropic glutamate receptor type 1; nAChR = nicotinic acetylcholine receptor; PCA = Purkinje cytoplasmic antibody; SCLC = small cell lung carcinoma; VGCC = voltage-gated calcium channels; VGKC = voltage-gated potassium channel.

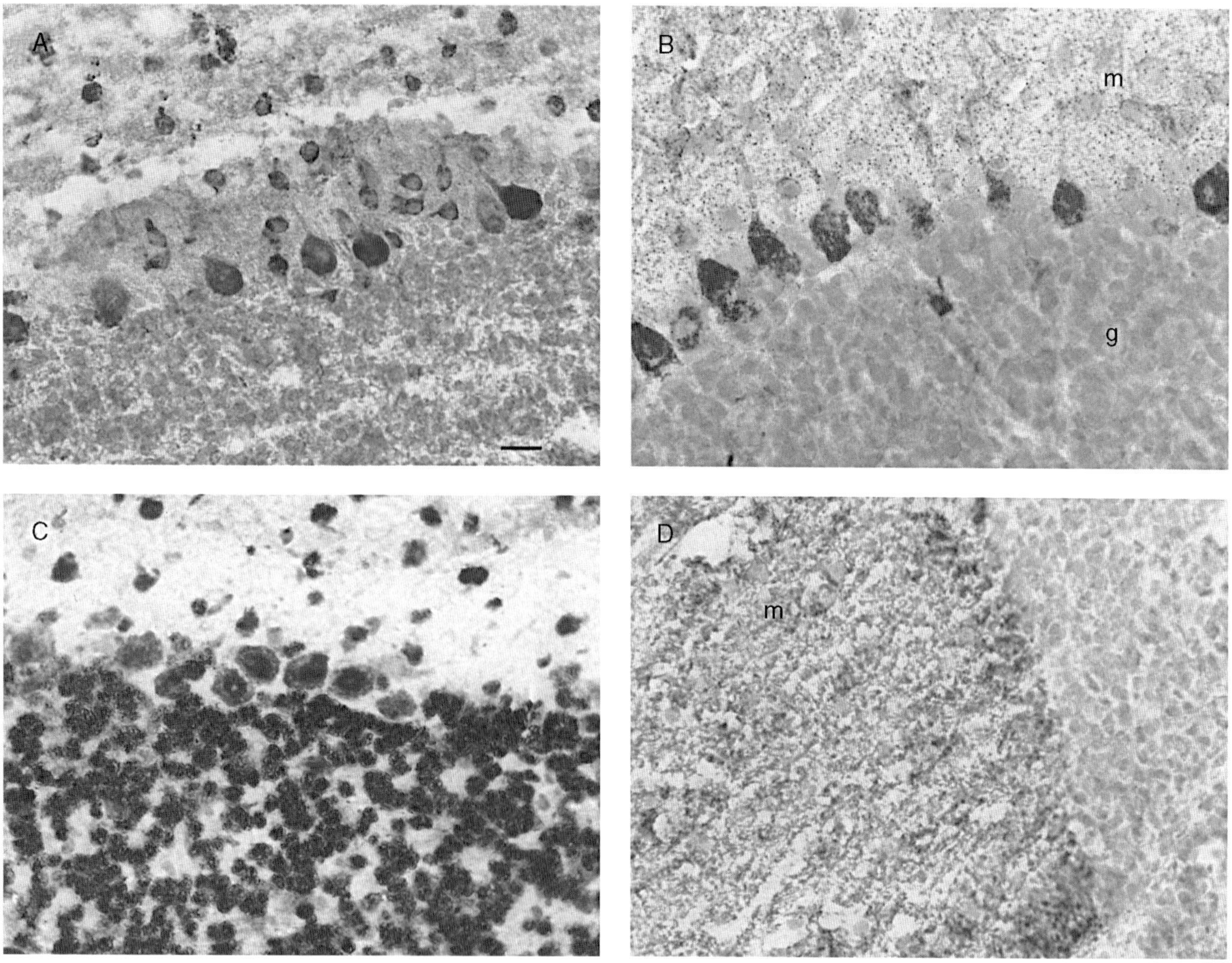

Figure 30-1 (PLATE 60). Paraneoplastic antibodies associated with "pure" PCD. (A) Anti-Yo antibodies label cytoplasm of Purkinje cells. (B) Incubation with anti-Tr antibodies results in strong immunoreactivity of Purkinje cell cytoplasm and dot-like labeling of the molecular layer. (C) Anti-Ri antibodies stain nuclei more than cytoplasm of all central neurons with sparing of the nucleolus. (D) Anti-mGluR1 strongly stains molecular layer and, to a lesser extent, the Purkinje cells. Frozen sections of rat cerebellum were incubated with the patients' sera after acetone fixation. The scale bar represents 20 μm; m = granular layer; g = molecular layer.

and myoclonus (see below). Patients with antibodies directed against amphiphysin and CRMP-5 (anti-CV2) usually do not present with symptoms of PCD, although cerebellar ataxia may become part of the paraneoplastic syndrome later in the course of the disease in 25% of patients.[21,22] The more recently discovered Purkinje cell antibody (PCA-2) is associated with lung cancer and a variety of neurologic syndromes, including PCD.[23]

Differential Diagnosis

The differential diagnosis of PCD includes alcohol intake, vitamin E deficiency, multiple sclerosis, cerebral vasculitis, chronic central nervous system (CNS) infection, systemic autoimmune diseases, celiac disease, metabolic and endocrine encephalopathies, hereditary spinocerebellar degenerations, and primary neurodegenerative disorders. In patients with cancer, intracerebral and leptomeningeal metastases and infections should be excluded.

Treatment and Prognosis

The outcome of PCD is generally poor and no recommended treatment exists. Incidental improvement has been reported either spontaneously, in response to tumor excision, or in association with plasma-exchange, steroids, intravenous immunoglobulin (IVIg), or cyclophosphamide. In a recent report of 34 women with anti-Yo–associated

PCD, the only independent predictor for survival was the type of associated tumor.[17] The median survival was 100 months for patients with breast cancer and 22 months for those with gynecologic cancer. Although PCD leads to the diagnosis of cancer in 60% to 70% of patients, cancer progression is the cause of death in approximately 50% of patients.[11,15–17] The neurologic outcome in anti-Yo–associated PCD is grim: 80% to 94% of patients become bed- or chair-bound, and neurologic improvement rarely occurs.[11,17] The picture is somewhat less gloomy in anti-Ri–, anti-mGluR1–, and anti-Tr–associated PCD. With successful treatment of the tumor and/or immunotherapy, symptoms may disappear.[11,18,19]

Limbic Encephalitis

Paraneoplastic limbic encephalitis (PLE) is a rare disorder characterized by the subacute onset (in days to a few months) of short-term memory loss, seizures, confusion, and psychiatric symptoms, suggesting involvement of the limbic system.[10,24] Selective impairment of recent memory is a hallmark of the disease but may not be evident in patients presenting with severe confusion or multiple seizures.[5] More than half of patients presenting with limbic encephalitis may have PLE.[5] Clinically three groups of patients with PLE can be identified.[5] The first group consists of patients with anti-Hu antibodies and lung cancer (usually SCLC). The PLE is part of PEM, and these patients have involvement of other areas outside the limbic system and brainstem. They are older (median age: 62 years), usually smoke, and are more often female.[5,25] The second group consists of young males with testicular cancer and anti-Ta antibodies.[26] The median age of the second group of patients is 34 years. Symptoms are usually confined to the limbic system, hypothalamus, and brainstem. The third group has no antineuronal antibodies (approximately 40% of patients with PLE).[5,27] In these patients, the symptoms are more often confined to the limbic system, the median age is around 57 years, and the associated tumor is often located in the lung.[5,25] MR and CT scan are abnormal in 65% to 80% of patients.[5,27] Abnormalities consist of increased signal on T_2-weighted and fluid-attenuated inversion recovery (FLAIR) images of one or both medial temporal lobes, hypothalamus, and brainstem (Fig. 30-2). Early in the course of the disease, the MRI may be normal and repeat imaging may be indicated. Coregistration of [^{18}F]fluorodeoxyglucose positron emission tomography (FDG-PET) may further improve the imaging sensitivity.[28] CSF examination is abnormal in 80% of PLE patients, showing transient mild lymphocytic pleocytosis with increased protein, IgG, or oligoclonal bands.[5,27]

Underlying Tumor

SCLC is present in 40% to 55% of patients; testicular cancer is present in approximately 20% of patients.[5,25,27] Other tumors include non-SCLC, breast cancer, Hodgkin disease, and immature teratomas, as well as many other cancers.[5,27]

Diagnostic Evaluation

The diagnosis is often difficult because there are no specific clinical markers and symptoms that usually precede the diagnosis of cancer.[5] MRI and CSF examination help to exclude other diagnoses. Detection of paraneoplastic antibodies will direct a tumor search that should include the lung, breasts, and testicles in the absence of paraneoplastic antibodies.

Antineuronal Antibodies

In 60% of patients with PLE, antineuronal antibodies are found.[5,27] These include anti-Hu (36%), anti-Ta (20%), and anti-Ma (4%) antibodies.[5] Patients with anti-Ta antibodies show reactivity to Ma2 only, whereas patients with anti-Ma antibodies harbor additional reactivity with Ma1 and Ma3. Patients with anti-Ma antibodies develop additional cerebellar and more intense brainstem symptoms and have tumors other than testicular cancer.[29] Approximately 10% of patients with anti-Hu–associated PNS present with limbic encephalitis.[30–32] More recently, voltage-gated potassium channel (VGKC) antibodies were demonstrated in 4 of 15 patients with both idiopathic and paraneoplastic limbic encephalitis.[33]

Differential Diagnosis

In patients without known cancer, the differential diagnosis includes primary degenerative dementia, viral encephalitis, Creutzfeldt-Jakob disease, primary tumors (including CNS lymphoma), and psychiatric disorders. In patients with known cancer, cerebral and leptomeningeal metastases, metabolic or toxic encephalopathies, and disseminated intravascular coagulation (DIC) are the main considerations.[5]

Treatment and Prognosis

Spontaneous complete recovery has been described, albeit very rarely.[25,34] Immunotherapy is largely ineffective,[5] but multiple cases benefiting from antitumor treatment have been reported.[5,25,29] Therefore, all efforts should be directed at identifying and treating the underlying tumor. If no tumor is found, the search should be repeated every 3 months for 2 to 3 years. Irrespective of treatment, partial neurologic recovery was seen in 38% of anti-Hu, 30% of anti-Ta (Ma2), and 64% of patients without antibodies.[5]

Encephalomyelitis

Henson and colleagues introduced the term *encephalomyelitis with cancer* to define patients with clinical or pathologic evidence of severe and multiple involvement of two or more areas of the nervous system, excluding the neuromuscular junction or muscle.[35] In PEM, at least one area of the central nervous system must be involved, including

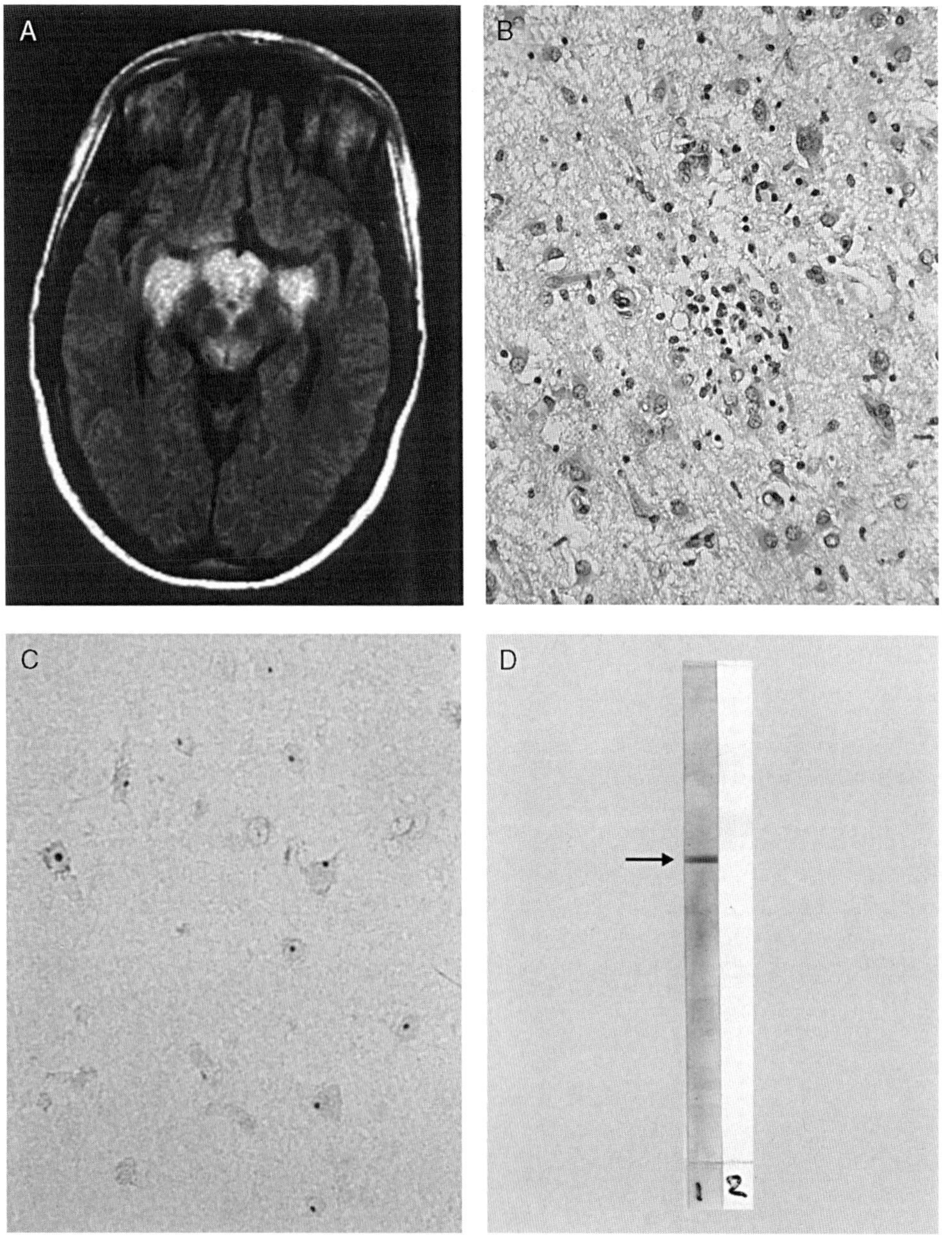

Figure 30-2 (PLATE 61). Paraneoplastic limbic encephalitis and anti-Ma2 antibodies. (A) MRI shows increased signal intensities in the medial temporal lobes, diencephalon and brainstem (FLAIR). (B) At autopsy, the medial temporal lobe showed parenchymal inflammatory infiltrates, consisting mostly of mononuclear cells. (C) The patient's serum, when reacted with human cortex, showed strong immunoreactivity against neuronal nucleoli. (D) The patient's serum (lane 1) contains immunoreactivity against purified Ma2 fusion protein (arrow). Control serum (lane 2) is negative.

the temporal lobes and cortex (limbic encephalitis), brainstem (brainstem encephalitis), cerebellum (subacute cerebellar ataxia), or spinal cord (motor neuronopathy).[10,36] Peripheral involvement affects the dorsal root ganglia (subacute sensory neuronopathy), peripheral nerves (sensorimotor polyneuropathy), or myenteric plexus (autonomic neuropathy). Patients with predominant involvement of one area but clinical evidence of only mild involvement of other areas are usually classified according to the predominant clinical syndrome. Symptoms of paraneoplastic *limbic encephalomyelitis* and *subacute cerebellar ataxia* are described above. Symptoms of *brainstem encephalitis* can include diplopia, dysarthria, dysphagia, gaze abnormalities (nuclear, internuclear, or supranuclear), facial numbness, and subacute hearing loss. The symptoms of *myelitis* usually result from inflammatory degeneration of anterior horn lower motor neurons. Symptoms of *subacute sensory neuronopathy* and *autonomic neuropathy* are described below.

UNDERLYING TUMOR

A lung tumor is identified in 85% of PEM patients, which is SCLC in 60%.[10,30] However, a wide range of other tumors is associated less frequently with PEM.[10,30] When anti-Hu antibodies are detected, or when the patient is at risk for lung cancer (smoking, age older than 50 years), a careful and repeated search for an underlying SCLC is warranted. When CT scan and bronchoscopy are negative, a total body FGD-PET scan might detect the neoplasm.[37,38] Tumors other than SCLC detected in a patient with anti-Hu antibodies may unexpectedly express the Hu-antigen,[30] or may be unrelated secondary neoplasms.[31] When the tumor tissue is available for analysis and expresses the Hu antigen, a further workup for a second tumor (SCLC) can probably be safely deferred.[30]

DIAGNOSTIC EVALUATION

MR or CT brain scan is normal or demonstrates nonspecific changes in most PEM patients with two exceptions.[36] In 65% to 80% of patients with predominant limbic encephalitis, MR and CT scan reveal temporal lobe abnormalities.[5,27] Patients with a predominant cerebellar syndrome develop cerebellar atrophy in the chronic stage. CSF is abnormal in most patients, showing elevated protein, mild mononuclear pleocytosis, elevated IgG index, or oligoclonal bands.[36]

ANTINEURONAL ANTIBODIES

Patients with PEM and SCLC often have anti-Hu antibodies in their serum and CSF.[30–32,36] Other antibodies associated with PEM include anti-CRMP5/CV2,[21] anti-amphiphysin,[39] and the less-well-characterized ANNA-3[40] and PCA-2.[23]

DIFFERENTIAL DIAGNOSIS

The differential diagnosis of PEM will vary with the most involved areas of the nervous system and is discussed more extensively with the individual syndromes. In cancer patients, leptomeningeal and parenchymal metastases can, like PEM, result in widespread and patchy involvement of the nervous system. CSF cytology and craniospinal MRI will generally rule out leptomeningeal metastases and structural lesions of the central nervous system. Vasculitis (systemic or confined to the nervous system), sarcoid and other granulomatous disorders, and infections and inflammatory disorders, including multiple sclerosis and related conditions, can all mimic PEM.

TREATMENT AND PROGNOSIS

Tumor treatment offers the best chance of stabilizing the patient's neurologic status, whereas immunotherapy does not appear to modify the outcome of PEM.[30,32,41] Because of incidental reports of spectacular neurologic improvement following various forms of immunosuppressive treatment, a trial of one or two immunosuppressive modalities may be warranted in a single patient. The overall functional outcome is bad, and more than 50% of patients are confined to bed or chair in the chronic phase of the disease.[30,32,41] In one study, the only independent predictor of improvement or stabilization of PEM was antineoplastic treatment.[30] Another study also identified younger age and better functional status at diagnosis as predictors of improved functional outcome.[32] The median survival of patients is approximately 1 year from diagnosis.[30,32] Mortality is predicted by worse functional status at diagnosis, age greater than 60 years, involvement of more areas of the nervous system, and absence of treatment.[30] The median time from onset of symptoms to diagnosis is approximately 4 months, and is shorter in patients with a poor functional status. Early diagnosis is facilitated by demonstration of paraneoplastic antibodies and is important to arrest the disease process before more damage is done.

Opsoclonus–Myoclonus

Opsoclonus consists of involuntary, arrhythmic, multidirectional, high-amplitude conjugate saccades and is often associated with diffuse or focal myoclonus and truncal titubation with or without cerebellar signs.[2,42] An excessive startle response reminiscent of hyperekplexia may also occur in opsoclonus–myoclonus (OM).[43] OM occurs primarily in children as a self-limited illness and is probably the result of a viral infection of the brainstem. OM may be paraneoplastic (POM) in children with neuroblastoma.

UNDERLYING TUMOR

In adult cancer patient, POM is a rare symptom. Conversely, approximately 20% of patients with OM may have a previously undiscovered malignancy.[42] The most commonly associated neoplasms are SCLC and breast and gynecologic cancers.[4,43] Many other tumors, including thyroid cancer and bladder cancer, have been reported in association with POM.[44] Approximately 2% to 3% of children with neuroblastoma have POM.[45,46]

DIAGNOSTIC EVALUATION

CT and MRI are normal, while examination of the CSF may show mild pleocytosis and protein elevation. In some patients, POM resembles PCD. The prominent opsoclonus and truncal, rather than appendicular, ataxia distinguish this syndrome from anti-Yo– and anti-Hu–associated PCD.[2] Patients with POM are older (median age: 66 years) than patients with idiopathic OM (median age: 40 years).

ANTINEURONAL ANTIBODIES

Specific antibodies are found in only a minority of patients with POM.[4] In adults, anti-Ri antibodies are mostly associated with breast cancer and gynecologic tumors. Anti-Ri occasionally has been found in bladder cancer and SCLC, and may occur in male patients.[2,44] POM can also be associated with anti-Hu antibodies, usually as part of a more widespread PEM. Bataller and associates[47] screened a brainstem complementary DNA (cDNA) library with sera from 21 patients with OM or POM. Twenty-five proteins were identified, recognized by one or two sera each, demonstrating that immunity to neuronal autoantigens in OM is both frequent and heterogenous.

In children presenting with OM, the detection of anti-Hu antibodies is diagnostic of an underlying neuroblastoma.[48] Combining several studies, the frequency of anti-Hu antibodies in neuroblastoma with POM is approximately 10%.[48–50] This finding differs little from the 4% to 15% of anti-Hu positive sera in children with neuroblastoma who do not have POM.[48,49]

Differential Diagnosis

The differential diagnosis of OM includes structural lesions in the posterior fossa, infections and other inflammatory conditions, including multiple sclerosis, and toxic and metabolic disorders. POM is more likely than idiopathic OM in patients older than 50 years of age who have additional encephalopathy.[4]

Treatment and Prognosis

In contrast to most of the other paraneoplastic syndromes, POM may remit either spontaneously, following treatment of the tumor, or in association with clonazepam or thiamine treatment. Most patients with idiopathic OM make a good recovery that seems to be accelerated by steroids or IVIg. Usually POM has a more severe clinical course, and treatment with steroids or IVIg appears ineffective. In a series of 14 patients with POM, 8 patients whose tumors were treated showed complete or partial neurologic recovery. In contrast, 5 of 6 patients whose tumors were not treated died of POM despite steroids, IVIg, or plasma exchange.[4]

In children, immunotherapy of POM includes corticotropin (ACTH), prednisone, azathioprine, and IVIg.[51] Treatment of the tumor with chemotherapy is the most important predictor of good neurologic recovery.[51]

Children with neuroblastoma and POM have a better survival rate than do patients without POM. Despite the excellent survival, more than two-thirds of POM patients display some sort of developmental or neurologic abnormality.[46,51]

Stiff-Person Syndrome

Stiff-person syndrome (SPS) is a clinically, electrophysiologically, and serologically heterogeneous disorder that is paraneoplastic in a subset of patients. Typically, SPS begins insidiously with gradual onset of painful rigidity and spasms in the axial muscles, spreading slowly to proximal extremity muscles.[52] Persistent contraction of the axial muscles leads to truncal rigidity, characteristic lumbar hyperlordosis, and restriction of movement of the hips and spine. Superimposed on this background rigidity are extremely painful muscle spasms that are often precipitated by psychological factors or by auditory or tactile stimuli. The spasms disappear during sleep and with localized, spinal, or general anesthesia. Electromyogram (EMG) studies show continuous motor unit activity in agonist and antagonist muscles that disappears following diazepam injection. Clinically, three categories of patients with a less typical course have been identified. One is progressive encephalomyelitis with rigidity that is often paraneoplastic.[53] It shares features with SPS but the course is relentlessly progressive, resulting in death within a few months. Additional signs of brainstem and spinal cord dysfunction are often present. The second variant is "jerking stiff-man syndrome" with prominent additional myoclonic jerking.[54] The third clinical group is the stiff-limb syndrome.[55] Clinically, these patients have painful spasms, rigidity, and posturing of the distal limb, usually the leg. The response to treatment is less favorable, and half go on to develop brainstem or sphincter involvement.

Underlying Tumor

The most common tumors associated with SPS are lung and breast cancer, but a variety of other tumors have been reported, including thymoma, Hodgkin disease, and colon cancer.[56–58] The neurologic symptoms generally precede the diagnosis of the tumor.[57]

Diagnostic Evaluation

MRI studies are normal in the majority of patients with only some reports of spinal MRI abnormalities in patients with a stiff-limb syndrome. Half of the patients with the classic form have CSF oligoclonal bands. Progressive lymphocytosis may be seen in patients with encephalomyelitis. The diagnosis is confirmed by the characteristic EMG findings and requires a high level of clinical suspicion.

Antineuronal Antibodies

Approximately 60% of patients with classic, nonparaneoplastic, SPS have antibodies against glutamic acid decarboxylase (GAD65).[59] The majority of these have coexisting diabetes mellitus or another autoimmune disorder (hyperthyroidism, vitiligo, myasthenia gravis). Anti-amphiphysin antibodies are present in the serum and CSF from female patients with paraneoplastic SPS and breast cancer.[57] Anti-amphiphysin antibodies are not specific for SPS because they are also associated with PEM and paraneoplastic sensory neuronopathy (PSN) in breast cancer and SCLC. Anti-amphiphysin antibodies have also been reported in SCLC without an associated paraneoplastic neurologic syndrome.[39,60,61] Recently anti-gephyrin antibodies were detected in a patient with SPS and an associated mediastinal tumor.[62]

Differential Diagnosis

The differential of SPS includes tetanus, neuromyotonia (see "Neuromyotonia"), strychnine intoxication, rigid spine syndrome, dystonia musculorum deformans, generalized fibrosing myositis, and psychiatric disorders.

Treatment and Prognosis

Rigidity and spasms often respond to treatment with baclofen, diazepam, valproate, vigabatrin, and carbamazepine.[63] Responses to treatment with steroids, plasma exchange, and IVIg have been reported.[64] When all these fail, methylprednisolone and cyclophosphamide pulse therapy can be tried.[65] Patients with atypical presentations, including encephalomyelitis and stiff-limb syndrome, respond less favorably to treatment.

In patients with paraneoplastic SPS, treatment of the tumor generally improves the neurologic symptoms.[66,67]

Chorea

Vernino and associates[68] describe 16 patients with paraneoplastic chorea associated with anti-CRMP5 (anti-CV2) antibodies. In 11 patients, the chorea was the initial or most prominent symptom. The chorea may be asymmetric and affects the face in most patients. Dystonic posturing is noted in a minority. Fourteen patients (88%) had other neurologic manifestations, including loss of vision as a consequence of optic neuritis (n = 5), progressive peripheral neuropathy (n = 5), limbic encephalitis (n = 5), cerebellar ataxia (n = 3), LEMS (n = 1), or myelitis (n = 1). The widespread involvement of multiple areas of the central nervous system suggests that anti-CRMP5-associated chorea is part of PEM.

Underlying Tumor

Paraneoplastic chorea is closely associated with SCLC but has also been reported with lymphoma and renal cell carcinoma.[68–70]

Diagnostic Evaluation

Most patients (83%) have mild CSF abnormalities, including lymphocytosis and elevated protein levels. Cranial MRI shows increased T_2 and FLAIR signals in the caudate and putamen which may resolve. MRI is essential to rule out other causes of chorea.

Antineuronal Antibodies

In 12% of patients with anti-CRMP5/CV2 antibodies the basal ganglia are involved, manifesting as chorea (10%), athetosis, or parkinsonism (1%).[21,68] Chorea has also been described in pathologically proven anti-Hu–associated PEM in a patient with SCLC.[71]

Differential Diagnosis

Autoimmune forms of chorea occur following streptococcal infections (Sydenham chorea) and as rare manifestations of systemic lupus erythematosus and antiphospholipid syndrome.[72] Hereditary neurologic disorders (Huntington disease, benign familial chorea, familial paroxysmal choreoathetosis, dentatorubral-pallidoluysian atrophy [DRPLA], Wilson disease, neuroacanthosis), vascular causes (basal ganglia infarction or hemorrhage, polycythemia vera, essential thrombocythemia, vasculitis), metabolic and hormonal causes (e.g., oral contraceptives, pregnancy, thyrotoxicosis, hypocalcemia, kernicterus), toxic causes (many drugs and carbon monoxide can cause chorea), and, rarely, tumors of the basal ganglia must be excluded.

Treatment and Prognosis

Chorea improves in half of patients with symptomatic treatment and in two-thirds of the patients following either chemotherapy for SCLC or intravenous methylprednisolone.[68]

Cancer- and Melanoma-Associated Retinopathy

Autoantibodies have defined two paraneoplastic visual disorders related to small cell lung cancer: retinopathy (antirecoverin antibodies) and optic neuritis (anti-CRMP5/CV2 antibodies).[73] The disorders are discussed separately in the following sections.

Cancer-associated retinopathy (CAR) results from dysfunction of the retinal photoreceptors. The incidence is equal among women and men. CAR is a subacute, progressive, autoimmune retinopathy in which the patient develops bilateral, but often asymmetric, loss of visual acuity and impaired color vision. Many patients develop night blindness and may have positive symptoms such as glaring, distortions, sparkles, and shimmering or bizarre images.

Melanoma-associated retinopathy (MAR) is a related entity in which bipolar cell function is affected.[74] Patients with MAR typically present with sudden onset of night blindness and flickering or pulsating photopsias followed by progressive loss of vision.[75] Unlike CAR, MAR is more common in men than in women.

Underlying Tumor

SCLC is the tumor most frequently associated with CAR, followed at a distance by breast cancer, non-SCLC, a variety of gynecologic tumors, and colon cancer.[76] CAR usually heralds the onset of a malignancy with an interval varying from months to 2 years or more. Conversely, MAR commonly presents after the melanoma is diagnosed with a mean latency of 3.6 years.[75]

Diagnostic Evaluation

The responses in the electroretinogram (ERG) are typically reduced as a consequence of loss of the rod and cone cells. Perimetry may show paracentral and midperipheral scotomas. Cerebrospinal fluid reveals a nonspecific mild lymphocytic pleocytosis and an increased concentration of protein.

Antineuronal Antibodies

Many CAR patients have antibodies against the 23-kDa calcium-binding protein recoverin.[77] Approximately 90% of patients with antirecoverin antibodies harbor a SCLC. Many other autoantibodies have been described in patients with CAR, including antibodies against the 70 kDa heat-shock cognate protein, enolase-α, polypyrimidine tract-binding (PTB)-like protein, and photoreceptor cell-specific nuclear receptor. Sera from patients with MAR contain antibodies reactive with bipolar cells and other retinal elements.[74,75]

Differential Diagnosis

The differential diagnosis includes metastatic tumor and side effects of antitumor treatment. Breast, lung, and gastrointestinal carcinomas metastasize most commonly to the eye, usually to the choroid. In patients suspected of MAR, melanoma metastasis should be excluded. Approximately one-third of patients have no history of a primary tumor at the time of ocular diagnosis.

Treatment and Prognosis

Spontaneous recovery of CAR has not been reported and the symptoms generally deteriorate over weeks to months, leaving the patient with severely impaired vision. Stabilization and minimal visual improvement has been reported following immunotherapy with steroids, plasma exchange or IVIg.[78] However, once cell death has occurred, therapy is no longer of any benefit. Treatment of the tumor does not alter the course of the neurologic dysfunction in most cases. In a Lewis rat model of CAR, the retinopathy could be improved by administration of a calcium antagonist.[79] In MAR, treatment with IVIg or cytoreductive surgery (metastasectomy), improves vision in some cases.[75]

Optic Neuritis

All patients present with painless subacute loss of vision that becomes bilateral in weeks to months.[73] Bilateral optic disc swelling and nerve fiber layer hemorrhages are common.[73,80] Some patients develop concomitant symptoms of myelopathy, superficially resembling Devic disease. In the majority of patients, abundant cells are present in the posterior vitreous. Fluorescein angiography shows vascular leakage at and remote from the disc. In addition, most tested patients have abnormal retinograms. Vitrectomy shows reactive lymphocytosis, predominantly CD4+. Most patients presenting with optic neuritis develop a variety of other neurologic symptoms suggestive of PEM.

Underlying Tumor

In a series of 16 anti-CRMP5–positive patients with paraneoplastic optic neuritis, 69% had SCLC whereas in 2 patients no active cancer was detected.[73] Renal cell and thyroid carcinoma appear associated with the Devic-like disease.[73]

Antineuronal Antibodies

Anti-CRMP5/CV2 antibodies are associated with paraneoplastic optic neuritis and SCLC.[21,22,73] Demonstration of anti-CRMP5/CV2 antibodies obviates the need of vitrectomy to exclude ocular lymphoma and directs the search of an underlying malignancy to the lung.

Treatment and Prognosis

Treatment of the tumor may result in stabilization or even improvement of the optic neuritis.[81,82] Steroids alone may also improve vision in paraneoplastic optic neuritis.[83]

Subacute Motor Neuronopathies/Motor Neuron Disease

Weakness without sensory symptoms can be caused by paraneoplastic disorders that involve the lower motor neuron anywhere along its course from the anterior horn cells to the neuromuscular junction. Although some axonal and demyelinating paraneoplastic neuropathies are clinically predominantly motor, they are considered below under "Sensorimotor Neuropathy." Although most associations between motor neuron disease (MND) and cancer are based on chance, some syndromes may be paraneoplastic. A paraneoplastic etiology is suggested (but not proven) by common association of a characteristic motor neuron syndrome with a typical tumor, by improvement of MND following treatment of the tumor, and by the association with an onconeural antibody.[84]

Characteristic Associations of Motor Neuron Syndromes with a Typical Tumor

A disorder called subacute motor neuronopathy is associated with Hodgkin and non-Hodgkin lymphoma and may be a variant of MND.[85,86] Characteristically, a patient already known to harbor a lymphoma develops subacute painless and often patchy lower motor neuron weakness. The proximal legs are more affected than the arms, while the bulbar muscles usually remain spared. Atrophy is present, but fasciculations are not prominent. Upper motor neuron and sensory signs are usually absent. Although the disease can result in death, the course is usually benign and independent of the activity of the underlying neoplasm. Unlike MND, the neurologic defect often stabilizes or improves spontaneously after months or years without incapacitating the patient. Electroneurophysiology demonstrates signs of denervation with intact conduction velocities. Pathology shows loss of anterior horn motor neurons while the lateral columns of the spinal cord, unlike in MND, are typically spared. Indirect evidence suggests a viral etiology but a specific virus has never been isolated.

A different lower motor neuron syndrome can occur as a complication of radiotherapy to the spinal cord. In this disorder, the legs are affected with more distal than proximal weakness. Spontaneous improvement does not occur.[87,88] A slowly evolving lower motor neuron syndrome may also complicate mantle irradiation for Hodgkin lymphoma. These patients develop weakness and atrophy of predominantly proximal muscles including the neck, paraspinal, and shoulder musculature.

One prospective series of 37 MND patients shows a higher-than-expected incidence of lymphoma.[89] The main clinical implication is that patients with MND should probably be screened by immunofixation for the presence of a paraprotein. Bone marrow biopsy should be considered in patients with paraproteinemia, CSF oligoclonal bands, or an increased CSF protein (>0.75 g/L).

The third association is an upper motor neuron syndrome resembling primary lateral sclerosis in patients with breast cancer.[90] The symptoms usually develop in close temporal relationship (months) with the tumor diagnosis. The syndrome is slowly progressive and some patients remain free from lower motor neuron involvement.

Improvement of MND Following Treatment of the Tumor

MND, including amyotrophic lateral sclerosis (ALS), has been reported in association with cancer.[91,92] Systematic reviews suggest that the association is coincidental in most patients.[91] However, reports of stabilization, or even remission, of motor neuron symptoms in some patients,[1,93] and unusual pathologic findings, including inflammatory changes in others,[94] suggest that some cases of MND may have a paraneoplastic origin.

MND Associated with Paraneoplastic Antibodies

Predominant motor neuron dysfunction can occur as part of PEM.[35] When the underlying tumor is a SCLC, the anti-Hu antibody is often present.[30–32,36,84] In these patients, the symptoms have an acute or subacute onset with rapid progression and eventual involvement of other areas of the nervous system, differentiating this syndrome from ALS. Incidentally, other antibodies have been described in combination with pure motor syndromes. One patient developed ophthalmoplegia and subacute motor axonal neuropathy in association with anti-GQ1b antibodies and recurrent malignant melanoma. Response to immunotherapy (steroids) and expression of the GQ1b antigen in her tumor strongly suggested a paraneoplastic etiology.[95] Berghs and associates[96] reported the case of a woman with breast cancer and a paraneoplastic lower motor neuron syndrome whose serum contained autoantibodies directed against axon initial segments and nodes of Ranvier of myelinated axons, including the axons of motor neurons. The major targets of these autoantibodies were beta-IV spectrin isoforms.

Peripheral Nervous System

Subacute Sensory Neuronopathy

The clinicopathologic description of PSN was established by Denny-Brown in 1948.[97] He first described two patients with "spreading numbness and sensory loss of the extremities (in one the face was also involved) and severe and progressive ataxia associated with carcinoma." The pathologic hallmark is reflected in the name and consists of inflammatory infiltrates with neuronal cell loss in the dorsal root and corresponding cranial nerve (Gasserian) ganglia.[97,98] Although all ganglia are affected, the distribution may be patchy. Subacute sensory neuronopathy is an uncommon disorder of middle age, equally affecting males and females. Subacute sensory neuronopathy is probably paraneoplastic in approximately 20% of patients.[3,99] The symptoms begin with painful paresthesias and dysesthesias. Clumsiness and unsteady gait then develop and usually become predominant. Initially symptoms are usually distal and may be very asymmetric, although sometimes the distribution is more proximal in the limbs, trunk, and, occasionally, the face. In most patients, the disease progresses rapidly over weeks to months, leaving the patient severely disabled. In a few patients, the neuronopathy remains stable for months, with mild neurologic deficits.[100] On examination, all sensory modalities are affected, but the most striking abnormality is sensory ataxia with pseudoathetosis of the hands. Tendon reflexes are depressed or absent.

Underlying Tumor

Two-thirds of patients with PSN have lung cancer, in particular SCLC.[3,31,36] Other associated tumors include breast cancer and Hodgkin disease.[3,99] Usually the neuronopathy precedes the tumor diagnosis by an average of about 1 year.

Diagnostic Evaluation

Electrophysiologic studies demonstrate small or absent sensory action potentials in the presence of normal motor nerve conduction velocity and F waves. Early in the course of the disease there is a mild pleocytosis, with an elevated IgG and oligoclonal bands.[3,32,99] Assessment of paraneoplastic antineuronal antibodies in the serum of patients with subacute sensory neuronopathy is a useful test.

Antineuronal Antibodies

Associated paraneoplastic antibodies include anti-Hu, anti-amphiphysin, and anti-CRMP5/CV2.[6,21,30–32,36,39] The most frequent antineuronal antibody in PSN is anti-Hu.[30–32,36] In a series of 126 patients presenting with subacute sensory neuronopathy, anti-Hu antibodies were detected in 40 patients (32%) with PSN. One patient with anti-Hu antibodies had idiopathic sensory neuronopathy. The specificity of anti-Hu detection was 99% and the sensitivity was 82%.[101]

Differential Diagnosis

The pain and marked asymmetry in the beginning may lead to a diagnosis of (poly)radiculopathy or mononeuritis multiplex.[3] PSN is not always a purely sensory syndrome, and patients may demonstrate various involvement of motor nerves, autonomic nervous system, spinal cord, or brain (paraneoplastic encephalomyelitis). In a patient without cancer, the differential diagnosis of subacute sensory neuropathy includes collagen-vascular disease (e.g., Sjögren syndrome), idiopathic sensory neuronopathy, toxins, and primary biliary cirrhosis.[102] For patients undergoing active cancer treatment, the main differential diagnosis is chemotherapy-induced neuropathy, particularly by cisplatin and taxanes.[103]

Treatment and Prognosis

The course of the disorder is mostly independent of the tumor; neurologic symptoms usually progress rapidly and then stabilize. Immunotherapy consisting of plasma exchange, steroids, IVIg, and cyclophosphamide is ineffective in most cases.[41] Nevertheless, individual case reports suggest that some patients may benefit from immunotherapy. Treatment of the underlying neoplasm, usually SCLC, often results in complete remission of the tumor. On average, patients receiving antitumor treatment have a better neurologic outcome.[104] Interestingly, patients with SCLC and anti-Hu antibodies respond better to antitumor treatment than do SCLC patients without a paraneoplastic syndrome.[105] In patients with an identifiable tumor, antitumor treatment is recommended. In the absence of a tumor, antitumor treatment may be considered in patients with anti-Hu antibodies, age older than 50 years, and a history of smoking. In patients not receiving antitumor therapy, a short course of immunotherapy can be considered. Based on the literature, it is impossible to recommend one form of immunotherapy over another.

Sensorimotor Neuropathy

Paraneoplastic sensorimotor neuropathies are clinically and electrophysiologically heterogenous and are associated with many different tumor types.[106]

Because of this heterogeneity the association of the tumor and the neuropathy will be coincidental in many cases. A relatively mild sensorimotor neuropathy develops in approximately 15% of cancer patients in the terminal stage of the disease and may be related to cachexia.[106] Another group of paraneoplastic neuropathies is much more severe and develops rapidly, often before the cancer diagnosis is made. Antoine and associates[6] studied 26 patients with a severe neuropathy preceding the tumor diagnosis in most patients. Seven patients had paraneoplastic antibodies (6 anti-Hu; 1 anti-CRMP5/CV2), whereas 19 did not. All six patients with anti-Hu antibodies had signs of sensory neuronopathy, which was combined with motor neuropathy in two. Electrophysiologic studies were consistent with a mild axonal motor neuropathy in three of the six patients. In fact, these patients can better be classified as sensory neuronopathy with motor involvement. The patient with anti-CRMP5/CV2 antibodies had a mild axonal motor neuropathy. The 19 antibody-negative patients could be divided into four groups: (a) four patients with sensory neuronopathy or sensory neuronopathy with motor involvement as part of rapidly progressive PEM; (b) two patients with mononeuritis multiplex who had systemic or nerve-restricted nonnecrotizing vasculitis; (c) seven patients with an axonal sensorimotor polyneuropathy without inflammatory changes in their nerve biopsies and who showed stabilization after several months or years of followup; and (d) six patients with a demyelinating neuropathy, which was acute in one patient, who presented as a typical Guillain-Barré syndrome. The other patients had a CIDP-like neuropathy.[7]

Associated Tumors

The associated tumors are very heterogenous.

Paraneoplastic Antibodies

Anti-Hu antibodies and anti-CRMP5/CV2 are most commonly associated with sensorimotor neuropathies.[6,30–32,36,107] Of 20 patients with anti-Hu antibodies and predominant peripheral neuropathy, 14 (70%) had sensory neuronopathy, 5 (25%) had sensorimotor neuropathy, and 1 (5%) had motor neuronopathy.[108] The electrophysiologic patterns in the five patients with sensorimotor neuropathy were sensory axonal/neuronal and motor mixed axonal/demyelinating.

Differential Diagnosis

In patients with cancer, the development of a peripheral neuropathy usually represents a side effect of therapy (taxanes, vinca alkaloids, cisplatin), infiltration of nerves or spinal roots by the tumor, or metabolic and nutritional deficits. The diagnosis of a rapidly progressive debilitating neuropathy is a challenge for the neurologist and requires extensive examinations. Demonstration of paraneoplastic antibodies defines the neuropathy as paraneoplastic and directs the search to an underlying neoplasm.

Sensorimotor Neuropathy Associated with M Proteins

The malignancies that are associated with malignant monoclonal (or M) proteins include disorders that produce

IgG or IgA proteins (osteosclerotic myeloma and multiple myeloma) and disorders that produce IgM proteins (Waldenström macroglobulinemia, B-cell lymphoma, and chronic B-cell lymphocytic leukemia).

Osteosclerotic Myeloma

Osteosclerotic myeloma is a rare (1%–2%) and relatively benign variant of multiple myeloma. The disorder is characterized by single or multiple sclerotic bone lesions that are commonly located in the long bones of the arms and legs, the spine, or the pelvis. The lesions are not found in the skull where osteolytic lesions commonly occur in typical myeloma. More than 50% of patients with osteosclerotic myeloma develop a characteristic polyneuropathy.[109,110] Deficits are predominantly motor and often slowly progressive over months to years. The neuropathy is sometimes mistaken for a slowly progressive form of CIDP. All or some features of the POEMS (polyneuropathy, organomegaly, endocrinopathy, monoclonal protein, and skin changes) syndrome can be present. Correct diagnosis is important because these patients may improve with treatment of the myeloma. Patients with single lesions do best. Radiation or excision of the osteosclerotic lesion results in the elimination of the M protein and in gradual recovery in the ensuing months. Patients with multiple lesions are more difficult to treat and generally require chemotherapy (usually consisting of alkylating agents combined with high doses of steroids).[111] Immunotherapy is generally ineffective in these patients.

Multiple Myeloma

Although approximately 30% of patients with multiple myeloma have electrophysiologic signs of peripheral neuropathy, only a few percent develop clinical symptoms.[112–114] The neuropathy usually precedes the diagnosis of the myeloma. Weakness and sensory symptoms in the distal limbs appear over a period of weeks. In typical cases, neurophysiologic studies demonstrate axonal damage whereas biopsies often show destruction of both axons and myelin. Approximately 30% to 40% of patients with multiple myeloma and neuropathy develop amyloid deposits. In these patients, atypical features including carpal tunnel syndrome, mononeuritis multiplex, and autonomic features occur, superimposed on the symptoms of mild axonal sensorimotor neuropathy. Sensory neuropathy and a CIDP-like neuropathy are also associated with multiple myeloma. No specific treatment exists for these neuropathies, and treatment of the myeloma does not influence the neurologic symptoms.

Waldenström Macroglobulinemia

Waldenström macroglobulinemia may arise from IgM–MGUS (monoclonal gammopathy of unknown significance), and similar polyneuropathy syndromes affect these two groups of patients. Approximately 10% of patients with Waldenström macroglobulinemia develop a symptomatic polyneuropathy.[115] The neuropathies can be separated into demyelinating polyneuropathy associated with IgM anti-MAG (myelin-associated glycoprotein) antibodies, demyelinating polyneuropathies with IgM antibodies reactive to gangliosides (but not with MAG), polyneuropathies with monoclonal IgM proteins nonreactive with a known antigen, cryoglobulinemic neuropathy, and amyloid polyneuropathy. Approximately 50% of patients with Waldenström macroglobulinemia and a demyelinating polyneuropathy have IgM anti-MAG antibodies and present with a progressive distal symmetric sensorimotor polyneuropathy. Predominant involvement of large sensory fibers results in postural tremor and pseudoathetosis. The CSF often shows increased protein concentration, and electrophysiologic studies demonstrate slow conduction velocities and prolonged distal motor and sensory latencies. Biopsies show widening between lamellae of myelin sheaths caused by intercalation of anti-MAG antibodies. The treatment should be directed at the tumor and symptomatic sensorimotor neuropathy may be reason to start treatment of Waldenström macroglobulinemia.[116,117] Occasionally, patients with IgM anti-MAG respond to treatment with plasma exchange or IVIg. A promising new agent for polyneuropathies associated with IgM M proteins is the anti-CD20 monoclonal antibody rituximab.[118,119]

Subacute Autonomic Neuropathy

In a series of 157 patients presenting with symptoms of autonomic failure, 18 (12%) had paraneoplastic subacute autonomic neuropathy.[120] In subacute autonomic neuropathy, sympathetic failure is manifested as severe orthostatic hypotension and anhydrosis, and parasympathetic failure as dry mouth, sexual dysfunction, impaired pupillary response to light and accommodation, and a fixed heart rate. Many patients have gastrointestinal dysmotility varying from anorexia and early satiety to diarrhea or chronic pseudo-obstruction. In LEMS, autonomic signs or symptoms are ultimately present in 80%.[121]

Underlying Tumor

In 12 of 18 patients with paraneoplastic subacute autonomic neuropathy, the underlying tumor was SCLC. Ten of these patients had anti-Hu antibodies.[120] Other tumors included thymoma in four and rectal and bladder cancer in one. In a series of 12 patients with paraneoplastic gastric motility disorders, 9 had an underlying SCLC, and 8 of these harbored anti-Hu antibodies.[122]

Antineuronal Antibodies

Vernino and associates found anti-Hu antibodies in 56% of patients with paraneoplastic subacute autonomic neuropathy. Previously, autonomic involvement has been reported in up to 25% of patients with PEM/SN and anti-Hu antibodies.[30–32,36] Autoantibodies that bind or block specifically with the nicotinic acetylcholine receptors in the autonomic ganglia are present in 40% of patients with idiopathic or paraneoplastic subacute autonomic neuropathy.[120]

Differential Diagnosis
The differential diagnosis includes idiopathic subacute autonomic neuropathy, postural tachycardia syndrome, idiopathic gastrointestinal dysmotility, diabetic and amyloid autonomic neuropathy, nondiabetic sensorimotor and autonomic neuropathy, pure autonomic failure, and multiple system atrophy.[123] In familial cases, a form of hereditary sensory and autonomic neuropathy (HSAN) I to V should be excluded.[123]

Treatment and Prognosis
The disease is usually monophasic with slow and incomplete or no recovery. Stabilization may be achieved by treatment of the tumor.[124] Palliation of the debilitating symptoms of pseudo-obstruction may be achieved by repeated administration of neostigmine.[125]

Vasculitis of Nerve and Muscle
Patients often present with a painful asymmetric or symmetric polyneuropathy or, less commonly, with a mononeuritis multiplex. The neuropathy may antedate the diagnosis of the neoplasm. The neuropathy is subacute and progressive and usually affects older men.[126] Some patients with paraneoplastic vasculitic neuropathy also suffer from LEMS or PEM.

Underlying Tumor
A localized vasculitis of the nerve and muscle is found most commonly with lung cancer and lymphomas.[126] It is also reported in association with malignancies of prostate, breast, endometrium, kidney, and bile duct. In 50% of patients, the vasculitic symptoms precede the cancer diagnosis.

Diagnostic Evaluation
Two helpful laboratory abnormalities are a high erythrocyte sedimentation rate and high CSF protein content. Electrophysiologic studies show axonal degeneration involving both sensory and motor nerves. The diagnosis is confirmed by a nerve or muscle biopsy showing intramural and perivascular inflammatory infiltrates that are mainly composed of CD8+ T-lymphocytes.[127]

Antineuronal Antibodies
When the vasculitic neuropathy is associated with SCLC, anti-Hu antibodies have been described.[36]

Treatment and Prognosis
Recognition of this syndrome is important, because the disorder may respond to both antineoplastic and immunosuppressive treatment. Combination of steroids and cyclophosphamide may offer better results than steroids alone.[126]

Neuromyotonia
Acquired neuromyotonia (Isaac syndrome, cramp-fasciculation syndrome, undulating myokymia) is characterized by spontaneous and continuous muscle fiber activity. Symptoms include muscle cramps in proximal and distal muscles, made worse by exercise and stiffness. Examination reveals myokymia, pseudomyotonia (slow relaxation) and excessive sweating. The rippling and twitching of muscles sometimes lead to sustained abnormal posture. Paraneoplastic neuromyotonia can be part of PEM. In patients with neuromyotonia, other autoimmune disorders such as myasthenia gravis occur more frequently than expected.[128]

Underlying Tumor
In a series of 60 patients with neuromyotonia, an underlying neoplasm was identified in 15 (25%).[128] Paraneoplastic neuromyotonia is most often associated with thymoma or lung cancer.[128] Other reported tumors include Hodgkin lymphoma and plasmocytoma.

Diagnostic Evaluation
EMG shows fibrillation, fasciculation, myokymic discharges, doublets, triplets, and high-frequency neuromyotonic discharges.[129] This abnormal muscle activity continues during sleep and general anesthesia, is abolished by curare, and may be unaffected or reduced by peripheral nerve block.[130]

Antineuronal Antibodies
Both paraneoplastic and idiopathic neuromyotonia are associated with autoantibodies to VGKC.[128] This antibody increases the release of quanta of acetylcholine and prolongs the action potential, which may explain the peripheral nerve hyperexcitability in the patients.[131,132]

Treatment and Prognosis
Symptoms of neuromyotonia may improve with carbamazepine, phenytoin, or other antiepileptic drugs.[129] When the disease is immune-mediated, steroids, plasma exchange, and IVIg may be effective.[129] Because of the small number of reported cases, the impact of tumor treatment on neuromyotonia is not known.

Differential Diagnosis
Muscle cramps are common complications of cancer and are most often related to electrolyte imbalances. Disorders

of the central nervous system such as stiff-person syndrome, tetanus, and neuroleptic malignant syndrome can be confused with neuromyotonia. Stiff-person syndrome is characterized by prominent rigidity and continuous contraction of paraspinal muscles with intermittent paroxysmal painful muscle spasms. The distinguishing feature is the disappearance of abnormal muscle activity during sleep or anesthesia with stiff-person syndrome (but not with neuromyotonia).

Neuromuscular Junction and Muscle

Lambert-Eaton Myasthenic Syndrome

Most patients present with proximal weakness of the lower extremities and fatigability, but unlike myasthenia gravis, the symptoms do not significantly affect the bulbar musculature. Respiratory weakness can occur. Deep tendon reflexes, especially those in the legs, are diminished or absent but may reappear after exercise. Autonomic features, particularly dry mouth, impotence, and mild/moderate ptosis, ultimately develop in 80%.[121,133] In some patients, LEMS may develop in association with other paraneoplastic syndromes, including PCD and PEM/SN.[14]

Underlying Tumor

Sixty percent of patients have a SCLC.[121] Other tumors include small cell carcinomas of the prostate and cervix, lymphomas, and adenocarcinomas. The prevalence of LEMS in SCLC is estimated to be approximately 3%.[133,134] Clinically and serologically, the 40% without identifiable tumor are indistinguishable from the paraneoplastic LEMS patients.

Diagnostic Evaluation

The typical pattern of electromyographic abnormalities is the hallmark of LEMS (Fig. 30-3). This includes a low, compound muscle action potential at rest with a decreased response at low rates of repetitive stimulation (3 Hz) and an incremental response at high rates of repetitive stimulation (50 Hz) or 15 to 30 seconds of maximal voluntary contraction.[135]

Antineuronal Antibodies

Most patients with LEMS have antibodies against VGCC that are located presynaptically in the neuromuscular junction.[135] Approximately 20% have anti-MysB antibodies reactive with the β-subunit of neuronal calcium channels.[136]

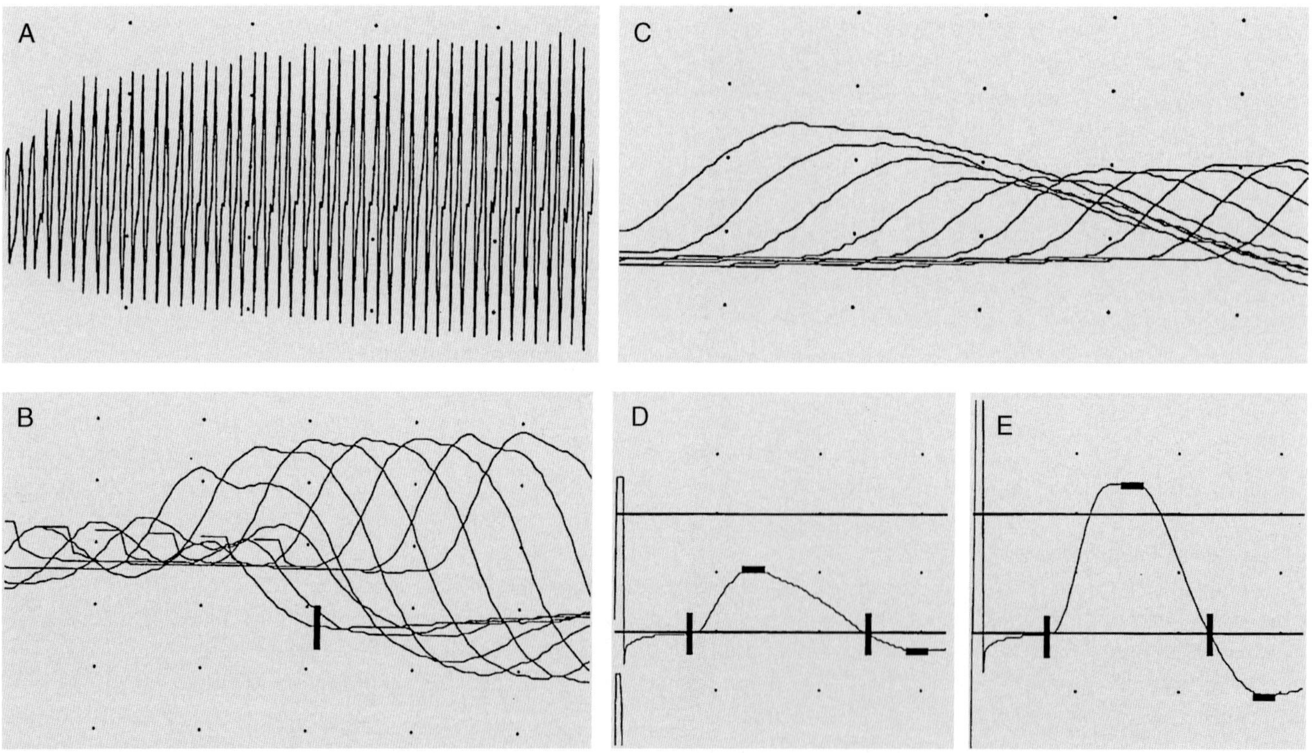

Figure 30-3. Electrophysiological testing in a patient with LEMS. (A,B) Repetitive nerve stimulation (50 Hz) of the ulnar nerve registering over the musculus abductor digiti minimi results in an increment of the amplitude of 100% between the first and the 10th stimulus. (C) Repetitive nerve stimulation at a frequency of 3 Hz results in a >50% decrement of the amplitude. (D) After a single stimulus, the CMAP of the musculus abductor digiti minimi is decreased (2.8 mV). (E) Following maximal voluntary contraction, the CMAP significantly increases (7.2 mV). (*Courtesy Marjan Scheltens, MD.*)

Differential Diagnosis

Proximal weakness in cancer patients can have many neoplastic and treatment-related causes. The characteristic clinical picture (including autonomic dysfunction) in combination with EMG findings and anti-VGCC antibodies is diagnostic of LEMS.

Treatment and Prognosis

Treatment of LEMS must be tailored to the individual based on severity of the symptoms, underlying disease, life expectancy, and previous response to treatment. In patients with paraneoplastic LEMS, treatment of the tumor frequently leads to neurologic improvement.[137] Symptomatic treatment is with drugs such as 3,4-diaminopyridine (DAP) that facilitate the release of acetylcholine from motor nerve terminals.[138] In a placebo-controlled randomized trial, DAP (5–20 mg TID-QID) was effective for long-term treatment, alone or in combination with other treatments.[139] The maximum recommended daily dose of DAP is 80 mg; at higher doses seizures occur.[139] Cholinesterase inhibitors (pyridostigmine, 30–60 mg q6h) may improve dryness of mouth but rarely relieve weakness. If these treatments are not effective enough, immunosuppressive therapy with steroids, azathioprine or cyclosporine may be considered. Removal of antibodies by plasma exchange[140] and IVIg can provide quick, but transient, relief.[121,141] LEMS responds less favorably to immunotherapy than myasthenia gravis.

Myasthenia Gravis

Myasthenia gravis (MG) is a postsynaptic disorder of neurotransmission caused by antibodies reacting with the nicotinergic acetylcholine receptors at the neuromuscular junction. In ocular MG, diplopia and ptosis as a result of weakness of extraocular and levator palpebrae muscles predominate. In generalized MG, the patient has additional facial, oropharyngeal, and limb muscle weakness. The weakness fluctuates over time and increases with repeated efforts of the affected muscles. There are no sensory symptoms or signs of denervation.

Underlying Tumor

MG occurs in approximately 30% of patients with a thymoma and, conversely, approximately 10% of patients with MG harbor a thymoma. Symptoms do not differ between patients with or without thymoma.

Diagnostic Evaluation

The diagnostic evaluation may include EMG, autoantibody assay, and pharmacologic testing. The EMG shows characteristic decrement of the compound muscle action potential (CMAP; >10%) during repetitive nerve stimulation.[142] EMG is diagnostic in 50% to 80% of patients with ocular MG and in 90% to 100% of patients with generalized MG. Autoantibodies against the nicotinic acetylcholine receptor (anti-AChR) are present in 70% to 80% of patients with ocular MG and in 90% to 100% of patients with generalized MG. Single-fiber EMG is more sensitive than repetitive nerve stimulation.[142] Temporal reversion of weakness by acetylcholinesterase inhibitors (neostigmine) is a useful diagnostic test.

Antineuronal Antibodies

Anti-AChR antibodies are present in approximately 85% of all MG patients. All MG patients with a thymoma have anti-AChR antibodies.[143] Antibodies to striated muscle proteins, including the titin protein, are present in 85% of patients with MG and thymoma, and in 30% of patients with either MG or thymoma.[144] In young patients, the anti-striated muscle antibodies help diagnose an underlying thymoma. Recently, an IgG antibody against the muscle-specific kinase (MuSK) was identified.[145] The antibody is present in approximately 40% of seronegative MG patients.[143] The presence of antibodies against MuSK defines a subgroup of patients with seronegative MG who have predominantly localized, in many cases bulbar, muscle weakness and reduced response to conventional immunosuppressive treatments. Moreover, muscle wasting may be present, which prevents complete response to these therapies.[143]

Treatment and Prognosis

Symptomatic treatment of MG relies on cholinesterase inhibitors. Immunotherapy comprises thymectomy, immunosuppressive drugs, plasma exchange, and IVIg.[143]

Differential Diagnosis

The differential diagnosis of MG includes other disorders of the neuromuscular junction (e.g., LEMS, congenital myasthenic disorders, botulism, and snakebite poisoning), MND, inflammatory neuropathies, myopathies, and oculopharyngeal muscular dystrophy.

Dermatomyositis/Polymyositis/Inclusion Body Myositis

Clinical, electromyographic, and pathologic findings of the inflammatory myopathies are similar in patients with and without cancer. The course is usually subacute and slowly progressive. In dermatomyositis, the characteristic heliotrope rash (purplish discoloration of the eyelids) often precedes the appearance of proximal muscle weakness. Other manifestations include arthralgia, myocarditis and congestive heart failure, and interstitial lung disease. Polymyositis presents with subacute or insidious weakness of neck flexors and proximal limb muscles. Involvement of distal muscles varies. Inclusion-body myositis (IBM) is characterized by a gradual but relentlessly progressing weakness of both proximal and distal muscles. A distinctive clinical feature is atrophy of the volar forearm muscles.[146]

Underlying Tumor

The most recent evidence from population-based cohort studies confirms the association between malignancy and dermatomyositis, polymyositis, and IBM.[147–149] An underlying malignancy is more common in patients older than age 50 years, but can occur in children.[150] In contrast to other more typical paraneoplastic neurologic syndromes, the underlying tumors are very heterogenous. Buchbinder and associates[147] found that the highest risk for a malignant disease is associated with dermatomyositis (standardized incidence ratio, 6.2 [95% confidence interval (CI), 3.9–10.0]). The risk is also increased in polymyositis (standardized incidence ratio, 2.0 [5% CI, 1.4–2.7]), whereas the excess risk for malignancy in IBM is 2.4 (95% CI, 2.7–7.1). The excess risk for cancer diminishes with the time from diagnosis. Dermatomyositis is associated with a higher risk for cancer of the ovary, lung, pancreas, non-Hodgkin lymphoma, stomach, colorectal, and breast.[148] In polymyositis, non-Hodgkin lymphoma and tumors of the lung and bladder are overrepresented.[148]

Diagnostic Evaluation

Most patients with dermatomyositis/polymyositis have elevated serum creatine kinase (CK) levels and electromyographic evidence of myopathy. In IBM, CK levels are lower than in polymyositis and may be normal. Usually CK levels in IBM are two- to fivefold elevated. Muscle imaging (CT or MRI) may help in confirming the diagnosis, determining the type of inflammatory myopathy, and selecting an appropriate biopsy site. Muscle biopsy is the definitive diagnostic procedure and shows inflammatory infiltrates.[150]

Associated Antibodies

Anti-Jo-1 (an antibody against histidyl-transfer RNA synthetase) is present in approximately 30% of patients with polymyositis and is associated with interstitial lung disease.[151]

Antibodies to the Mi-2 protein complex are highly specific for dermatomyositis and are present in high titers in approximately 35% of cases, including cases of juvenile dermatomyositis.[151] Antibodies to the polymyositis (PM)-Scl nucleolar antigen (anti-PM-1) are present in 50% of patients with the scleroderma-myositis overlap syndrome.[150]

Treatment and Prognosis

Treatment of paraneoplastic dermatomyositis/polymyositis is generally the same as for patients without tumor. Nearly all patients with dermatomyositis/polymyositis respond to corticosteroids.[146] Refractory patients and patients requiring steroid-sparing agents may be treated with azathioprine. Methotrexate and cyclophosphamide can also be considered.[146]

Acute Necrotizing Myopathy

Acute necrotizing myopathy manifests as muscle pain and proximal weakness. The course of the disease is rapidly progressive, involves the pharyngeal and respiratory muscles, and can lead to death within a few weeks to months.[152] Many solid tumors can accompany this syndrome, including SCLC, gastrointestinal tract cancers, and malignancies of breast, kidney, and prostate.[153] The serum creatine kinase is markedly increased, and muscle biopsy shows prominent necrosis with little or absent inflammation. No specific autoantibody is reported. Some patients improved after successful antineoplastic therapy.[153] The differential diagnosis includes polymyositis and rhabdomyolysis related to chemotherapy and combination treatment including interleukin (IL)-2 and interferon-α.[154]

Paraneoplastic Carcinoid Myopathy

Paraneoplastic carcinoid myopathy is found in only 0.5% of patients with carcinoid tumors and may present years before tumor detection. The muscle enzymes are mildly elevated, and muscle biopsy shows nonspecific changes, including type II atrophy, necrosis of fibers, central nuclei, and mitochondrial changes. Symptoms may improve with serotonin antagonists such as cyproheptadine or the somatostatin analogue octreotide.[155]

Cachectic Myopathy

Cachexia is defined as a significant involuntary weight loss that complicates debilitating diseases, including cancer. The cancer cachexia syndrome may be present in up to 80% of patients with cancer.[156] Despite diffuse muscle wasting, the strength of cancer patients with cachectic myopathy is often preserved until late in the course of the disease. Biopsy shows muscle atrophy involving both types of fibers without evidence of inflammation or nerve degeneration. Malnutrition resulting from cancer cachexia is a significant cause of morbidity and mortality.[156] Recent studies suggest that growth factors and host cytokines produced in response to the tumor play a role in the pathogenesis of paraneoplastic cachexia.[156] The host cytokines include tumor necrosis factor-α, IL-1, IL-6, interferon-γ, and D-factor.[156] The efficacy of nutritional support in cancer related cachexia has not been adequately studied.[156]

▸ PARANEOPLASTIC AUTOANTIBODIES

Many patients with paraneoplastic neurologic syndromes have in their serum (and CSF) antibodies that react with both the tumor and with neuronal elements in

▶ **TABLE 30-4.** TUMOR SPECIFICITY OF PARANEOPLASTIC ANTIBODIES

Well-Characterized (Typical) Paraneoplastic Antibodies	Partially Characterized Paraneoplastic Antibodies	Antibodies that Also Occur Without Cancer
Anti-Hu (ANNA-1)	Anti-mGluR1	Anti-Tr (PCA-Tr)
Anti-Yo (PCA-1)	ANNA-3	Anti-VGCC
Anti-Ri (ANNA-2)	PCA-2	Anti-VGKC
Antiamphiphysin	Anti-Zic4	Anti-nAChR
Anti-CRMP5 (anti-CV2)		Anti-MAG
Antirecoverin		
Anti-Ma/Ta		

ANNA = antineuronal nuclear antibody; MAG = myelin-associated glycoprotein; mGluR1 = metabotropic glutamate receptor type 1; PCA = Purkinje cytoplasmic antibody; VGCC = voltage-gated calcium channels; VGKC = voltage-gated potassium channel.

affected parts of the nervous system. These onconeural or paraneoplastic antibodies are most important diagnostically because of their high specificity and association with certain tumor types (see Table 30-3). In the past 15 years, many paraneoplastic antibodies have been described. The typical paraneoplastic antibodies have been studied in large series and are now well characterized (Table 30-4). The association of anti-Yo, anti-Hu, anti-Ri, anti-amphiphysin, anti-CRMP5/CV2, anti-recoverin, and anti-Ma/Ta antibodies with both cancer and severe neurologic syndromes is firmly established. In patients with these antibodies, the likelihood of developing a tumor is almost 100%. With other, more recently discovered antibodies, the association is less robust because the antibody specificity has not yet been confirmed in another laboratory or too few patients have been studied (Table 30-4). A third group consists of autoantibodies that are associated with both the idiopathic and paraneoplastic variant of the neurologic syndrome. Examples include LEMS with anti-VGCC that is associated with lung cancer in 60% of cases.[121] Anti-Tr antibodies that are associated with Hodgkin lymphoma or other tumors in 90% of cases provide another example. Ten percent of the cases are idiopathic and, in contrast to the typical paraneoplastic antibodies, the target antigen could not be demonstrated in most tumors.[18]

Although there is considerable overlap, each of the antibodies is associated with a restricted spectrum of clinical syndromes and tumors. In most cases, the target antigen has been cloned and identified (see Table 30-3). Expression of the onconeural antigen by both the tumor and in affected parts of the nervous system supports an autoimmune etiology. Some of the paraneoplastic antigens are expressed by all tumors of a certain histology regardless of the presence of an autoimmune response. For example, Hu antigens are expressed by most SCLC, whereas only 16% of patients will develop low-titer anti-Hu antibodies and <1% will develop high-titer antibodies and a paraneoplastic syndrome.[105,157] Other tumors rarely express onconeural antigens unless the cancer causes a paraneoplastic neurologic disorder.[158]

Unfortunately, approximately 50% to 60% of patients with a paraneoplastic syndrome have no detectable onconeural antibodies in their serum. Therefore, the absence of paraneoplastic antibodies does not exclude PNS.

The detection of paraneoplastic antibodies is carried out in specialized academic laboratories and in more limited settings using commercially available kits. The quality of commercial kits varies widely and consist of a dot-blot assay reactive with four of the most common onconeural antigens (HuD, CDR62, Nova, Amphiphysin). However, the wide variety of clinical findings in patients with paraneoplastic antibodies necessitates a wide screening approach using immunohistochemistry rather than looking for a few specific antibodies; positive results can then be confirmed with more specific tests, such as Western blotting. The paraneoplastic antibodies can be detected both in CSF and serum. However, a positive CSF test in the absence of detectable antibodies in the serum is only rarely reported.[18] Therefore, for diagnostic screening purposes, serum detection suffices.

▶ DIAGNOSTIC EVALUATION

Clinical syndromes are never pathognomonic for a paraneoplastic etiology, and a high index of clinical suspicion is important. Symptoms can be atypical, psychiatric, or even fluctuating. PNS should often be in the differential diagnosis of otherwise unexplained neurologic syndromes. Detection of a typical antineuronal autoantibody (see Table 30-4) is very helpful because it proves the paraneoplastic etiology. Once a paraneoplastic diagnosis has

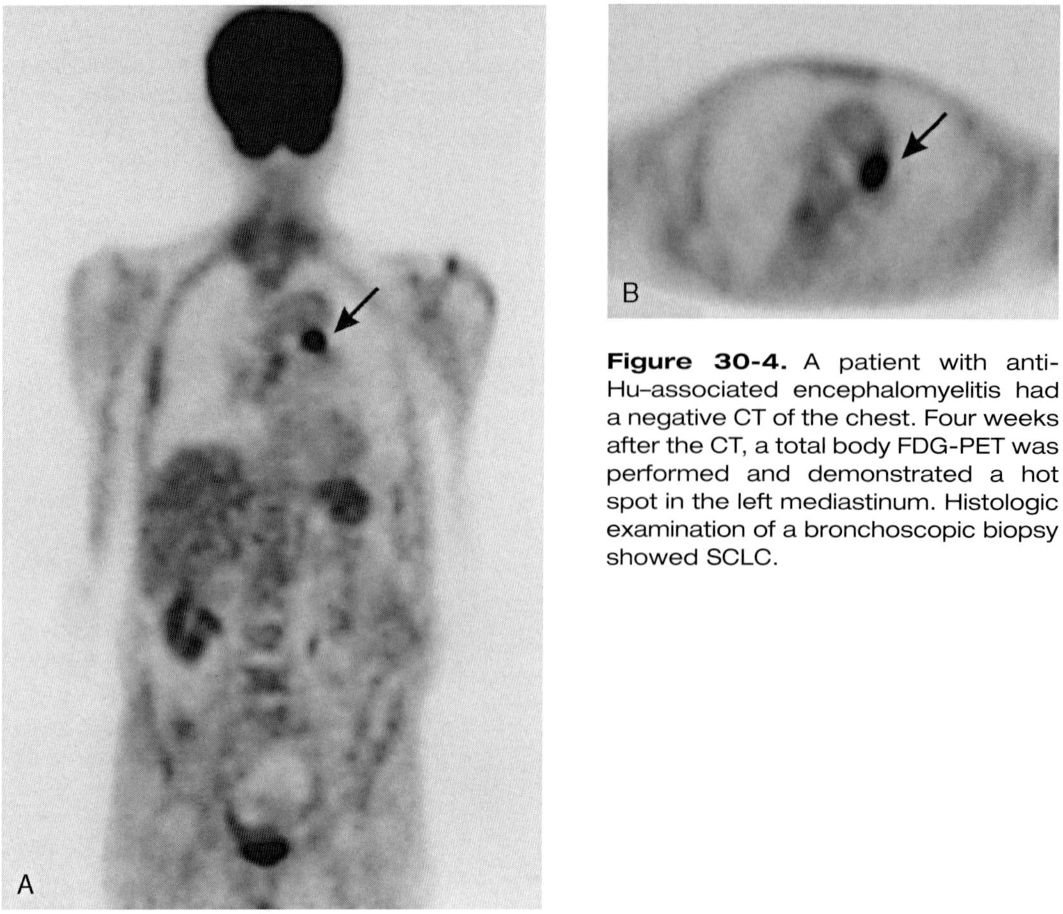

Figure 30-4. A patient with anti-Hu–associated encephalomyelitis had a negative CT of the chest. Four weeks after the CT, a total body FDG-PET was performed and demonstrated a hot spot in the left mediastinum. Histologic examination of a bronchoscopic biopsy showed SCLC.

been established or is suspected (in the absence of antibodies), rapid identification of the tumor becomes essential, but may be difficult. The type of antineuronal antibody will, in combination with the clinical syndrome, help direct the search for the underlying neoplasm (see Tables 30-2 and 30-3).

The workup for an underlying tumor starts with a detailed history including smoking habits, weight loss, night sweats, and fever. A thorough physical examination should include palpation for pathologic lymph nodes, rectal and pelvic examination, and palpation of breasts and testes. Routine laboratory tests including erythrocyte sedimentation rate should be carried out, and tumor markers can be added depending on the site under suspicion. The search for an underlying SCLC should further include chest CT. If the CT remains negative, FDG-PET is recommended (Fig. 30-4).[37] The workup for underlying breast cancer includes mammography (may be replaced by MRI) and cancer antigen (CA)-15-3 tumor marker. Gynecologic tumors are detected by a skilled pelvic examination, appropriate imaging studies, CA-125 tumor marker, and sometimes laparoscopy or laparotomy.[2] Testicular cancer is diagnosed on the basis of serum markers, physical and ultrasonography examination of the testes, and abdominal CT scan. Suspicion of prostate cancer leads to a determination of serum prostate-specific antigen levels and subsequent rectal examination. When the initial tumor workup is negative, a repeat workup is recommended at 3- to 6-month intervals for 2 to 3 years.

▶ NEUROPATHOLOGY AND PATHOGENESIS

Neuropathology

Denny-Brown, who described the first two patients with PSN, provided the earliest report of the pathologic changes in PNS.[97] The pathology demonstrated loss of dorsal root ganglion cells with heavy inflammatory infiltration in the dorsal root ganglia. In the Hu syndrome, the infiltrating cells have been further characterized as CD4+ T-helper cells and B-cells in the perivascular spaces and cytotoxic CD8+ T-cells in the interstitial spaces.[159] Further immunohistochemical analysis showed that a great number of T cells express the cytotoxic protein TIA-1. By contrast, Fas, FasL, C9neo, and activated caspase-3 immunoreactivities were negative in pathologic areas. These data indicate that neuronal death in anti-Hu–associated PEM is cytotoxic and nonapoptotic.[160] To further elucidate the pathogenic role of the anti-Hu antibody, elution of Hu-specific IgG from the affected regions of the brain has been attempted.[159,161] Although Hu-specific IgG could be eluted from involved brain areas, an artifact could not be excluded. In addition, complement activation was lacking.[159,161]

In contrast, in anti-Yo– and anti-Tr–associated PCD there is complete loss of Purkinje cells, with minimal or no identifiable inflammatory changes.[18,162] Lack of inflammatory cells in these patients most likely reflects a final, burned-out stage of the immune disorder.[162] More remarkably, in some patients with paraneoplastic opsoclonus–myoclonus, autopsy revealed an entirely normal brain. Even the omnipause neurons that are responsible for opsoclonus were normal.[163]

PATHOGENESIS

The discovery of paraneoplastic antineuronal autoantibodies resulted in the general belief that these are immune-mediated disorders triggered by aberrant expression of "onconeural" antigens in the tumor. Support for this hypothesis comes from the fact that the target paraneoplastic antigens are expressed both in the tumor and in the affected parts of the nervous system. Furthermore, the tumors are usually small, heavily infiltrated with inflammatory cells, and have a better prognosis; spontaneous remission at the time of neurologic presentation has even been described.[164,165] In addition, the paraneoplastic antibodies are synthesized intrathecally and antigen-specific T cells have been demonstrated in the blood.[166–168] A pathogenic role could, however, only be proven for paraneoplastic autoantibodies directed against easily accessible antigens located at the cell surface. Examples of such antigens are the acetylcholine receptor (anti-AChR muscle type in myasthenia gravis and neuronal ganglionic type in autonomic neuropathy), anti-VGCC in LEMS, anti-VGKC in neuromyotonia, and anti-mGluR1 in PCD. Most paraneoplastic antigens are located in the cytoplasm (e.g., Yo) or nucleus (e.g., Hu and Ri) of the cell, and a pathogenic role for the respective antibodies could not be demonstrated.[169] In these disorders, indirect lines of evidence support the view that the cellular immune response against these antigens is responsible for the neurologic damage.[166,170] The paraneoplastic antibodies may, in these cases, be surrogate markers for T-lymphocyte activation.[21] Another unanswered question is why only a small proportion of patients with SCLC develop an "anti-Hu syndrome," whereas all SCLC express the Hu antigens. Development of the "anti-Hu syndrome" is not associated with human leukocyte antigen (HLA) alleles, rendering a genetic "autoimmune" disposition unlikely.[171] Careful examination of SCLC samples from anti-Hu–positive patients showed markedly increased major histocompatibility complex expression compared to tumor samples from seronegative patients.[48] Recent findings in LEMS also indicate that SCLC can trigger a strong autoimmune reaction in the absence of the proper HLA genotype.[172]

A totally different mechanism seems at work in PCD in Hodgkin disease because the target antigens of the associated anti-Tr and anti-mGluR1 autoantibodies are not expressed in the Hodgkin tumor tissue.[18] Dysregulation of the immune system in Hodgkin lymphoma and an etiologic role for (viral?) infections have been postulated in this disorder.

▶ TREATMENT AND PROGNOSIS

Treatment of PNS is directed at suppression of the autoimmune reaction and eradication of the underlying tumor (see Table 30-5). Despite the immunologic etiology of most PNS, the results of immunosuppressive treatment are disappointing.[41] Exceptions are the neurologic syndromes caused by functional interference of the paraneoplastic antibodies with the target receptor or channel. These include not only disorders of the peripheral nervous system (LEMS, myasthenia gravis, neuromyotonia, autonomic neuropathy), but also anti-mGluR1–associated PCD.[19] In paraneoplastic syndromes where the target antigen is cytoplasmic or nuclear, the nervous dysfunction is probably not caused by functional interference of antibodies with the antigen. Immunotherapy modalities that are recommended for disorders associated with antibodies against cell surface receptor or membrane antigens include plasma exchange, immunoadsorption (extraction of patient IgG over a protein A column), steroids, and IVIg. In disorders associated with intracellular target antigens and a strong cellular immune reaction, plasma exchange and immunoabsorption are not expected to give much benefit. In these cases, a trial of a treatment that modulates the activation and function of effector T cells makes more sense. Based on the literature, it is not possible to recommend either steroids with or without cyclophosphamide, IVIg, or any other treatment.

The first goal of antitumor treatment is control of the tumor. In addition, successful treatment of the tumor stops the paraneoplastic neurologic deterioration and leaves the patients, on average, in a better condition.[104] In severely debilitated patients, for example, the elderly and bedridden, treatment of an underlying tumor is often withheld because of the very small chance of clinically relevant neurologic improvement.

TABLE 30-5. TREATMENT SUMMARY OF PARANEOPLASTIC NEUROLOGIC SYNDROMES

Syndrome	Antibody	Immunotherapy	Antitumor Treatment	Comments
PCD	Anti-Yo	No established effect	No effect on neurologic outcome	
	Anti-Tr	May improve	May improve	PCD associated with Hodgkin lymphoma may also improve spontaneously
	Anti-mGluR1	May improve	No data	
PEM	Anti-Hu	No established effect	Stabilizes the patient in better condition	In limbic encephalitis, partial improvement may occur spontaneously or during treatment
POM	Anti-Ri (adults)	No established effect	Partial neurologic recovery	Thiamine, baclofen, and clonazepam may be effective
	No antibody (children)	ACTH, steroids	Partial neurologic recovery	
SPS	Antiamphiphysin	IVIg, steroids, PE, pulse cyclophosphamide/steroids effective	No data	Responds to baclofen, diazepam, valproate, vigabatrine, and carbamazepine; Painful spasms may require opioids
CAR	Antirecoverin	No established effect	No established effect	
LEMS	Anti-VGCC	IVIg, steroids, PE effective	Improves neurologic condition	3,4-Diaminopyridine effective symptomatic treatment; immunotherapy less effective than in MG

CAR = cancer-associated retinopathy; IVIg = intravenous immunoglobulins; LEMS = Lambert-Eaton myasthenic syndrome; PCD = paraneoplastic cerebellar degeneration; PE = plasma exchange; PEM = paraneoplastic encephalomyelitis; POM = paraneoplastic opsoclonus–myoclonus; SPS = stiff-person syndrome; VGCC = voltage-gated calcium channels.

REFERENCES

1. Brain WR, Norris F. The remote effects of cancer on the nervous system. New York: Grune & Stratton, 1965.
2. Posner JB. Paraneoplastic syndromes. Neurologic complications of cancer. Philadelphia: FA Davis, 1995:353–385.
3. Chalk CH, Windebank AJ, Kimmel DW, et al. The distinctive clinical features of paraneoplastic sensory neuronopathy. Can J Neurol Sci 1992;19:346–351.
4. Bataller L, Graus F, Saiz A, et al. Clinical outcome in adult onset idiopathic or paraneoplastic opsoclonus-myoclonus. Brain 2001;124:437–443.
5. Gultekin SH, Rosenfeld MR, Voltz R, et al. Paraneoplastic limbic encephalitis: neurological symptoms, immunological findings and tumour association in 50 patients. Brain 2000;123:1481–1494.
6. Antoine JC, Mosnier JF, Absi L, et al. Carcinoma associated paraneoplastic peripheral neuropathies in patients with and without anti-onconeural antibodies. J Neurol Neurosurg Psychiatry 1999;67:7–14.
7. Antoine JC, Mosnier JF, Lapras J, et al. Chronic inflammatory demyelinating polyneuropathy associated with carcinoma. J Neurol Neurosurg Psychiatry 1996;60: 188–190.
8. Darnell RB, Posner JB. Paraneoplastic syndromes involving the nervous system. N Engl J Med 2003;349:1543–1554.
9. Furneaux HF, Reich L, Posner JB. Autoantibody synthesis in the central nervous system of patients with paraneoplastic syndromes. Neurology 1990;40:1085–1091.
10. Henson RA, Urich H. Cancer and the nervous system: the neurologic complications of systemic malignant disease. Oxford: Blackwell Scientific, 1982.
11. Shams'ili S, Grefkens J, de Leeuw B, et al. Paraneoplastic cerebellar degeneration associated with antineuronal antibodies: analysis of 50 patients. Brain 2003;126:1409–1418.
12. Brouwer B. Beitrag zur Kenntnis der chronischen diffusen Kleinhirnerkrankungen. Mendels neurologisches Zentralblatt 1919;38:674–682.
13. Brouwer B, Biemond A. Les affections parenchymateuse du cervelet et leur signification du point de vue de l'anatomie et la physiologie de cet organe. J Belge Neurol Psychiatrie 1938;38:691–757.
14. Mason WP, Graus F, Lang B, et al. Small-cell lung cancer, paraneoplastic cerebellar degeneration and the Lambert-Eaton myasthenic syndrome. Brain 1997;120:1279–1300.
15. Hammack J, Kotanides H, Rosenblum MK, et al. Paraneoplastic cerebellar degeneration. II. Clinical and immunologic findings in 21 patients with Hodgkin disease. Neurology 1992;42:1938–1943.
16. Posner JB. Paraneoplastic cerebellar degeneration. Can J Neurol Sci 1993;20:S117–S122.

17. Rojas I, Graus F, Keime-Guibert F, et al. Long-term clinical outcome of paraneoplastic cerebellar degeneration and anti-Yo antibodies. Neurology 2000;55:713–715.
18. Bernal F, Shams'ili S, Rojas I, et al. Anti-Tr antibodies as markers of paraneoplastic cerebellar degeneration and Hodgkin's disease. Neurology 2003;60:230–234.
19. Sillevis Smitt P, Kinoshita A, DeLeeuw B, et al. Paraneoplastic cerebellar ataxia due to autoantibodies against a glutamate receptor. N Engl J Med 2000;342:21–27.
20. Graus F, Lang B, Pozo-Rosich P, et al. P/Q type calcium-channel antibodies in paraneoplastic cerebellar degeneration with lung cancer. Neurology 2002;59:764–766.
21. Yu Z, Kryzer TJ, Griesmann GE, et al. CRMP-5 neuronal autoantibody: marker of lung cancer and thymoma-related autoimmunity. Ann Neurol 2001;49:146–154.
22. Honnorat J, Antoine JC, Derrington E, et al. Antibodies to a subpopulation of glial cells and a 66 kDa developmental protein in patients with paraneoplastic neurological syndromes. J Neurol Neurosurg Psychiatry 1996;61:270–278.
23. Vernino S, Lennon VA. New Purkinje cell antibody (PCA-2): marker of lung cancer-related neurological autoimmunity. Ann Neurol 2000;47:297–305.
24. Corsellis JAN, Goldberg GJ, Norton AR. "Limbic encephalitis" and its association with cancer. Brain 1968;91:481–496.
25. Alamowitch S, Graus F, Uchuya M, et al. Limbic encephalitis and small cell lung cancer. Clinical and immunological features. Brain 1997;120:923–928.
26. Voltz R, Gultekin SH, Rosenfeld MR, et al. A serologic marker of paraneoplastic limbic and brain-stem encephalitis in patients with testicular cancer. N Engl J Med 1999;340: 1788–1795.
27. Lawn ND, Westmoreland BF, Kiely MJ, et al. Clinical, magnetic resonance imaging, and electroencephalographic findings in paraneoplastic limbic encephalitis. Mayo Clin Proc 2003;78:1363–1368.
28. Kassubek J, Juengling FD, Nitzsche EU, et al. Limbic encephalitis investigated by 18FDG-PET and 3D MRI. J Neuroimaging 2001;11:55–59.
29. Rosenfeld MR, Eichen JG, Wade DF, et al. Molecular and clinical diversity in paraneoplastic immunity to Ma proteins. Ann Neurol 2001;50:339–348.
30. Graus F, Keime-Guibert F, Rene R, et al. Anti-Hu-associated paraneoplastic encephalomyelitis: analysis of 200 patients. Brain 2001;124:1138–1148.
31. Lucchinetti CF, Kimmel DW, Lennon VA. Paraneoplastic and oncologic profiles of patients seropositive for type 1 antineuronal nuclear autoantibodies. Neurology 1998;50: 652–657.
32. Sillevis Smitt P, Grefkens J, De Leeuw B, et al. Survival and outcome in 73 anti-Hu positive patients with paraneoplastic encephalomyelitis/sensory neuronopathy. J Neurol 2002; 249:745–753.
33. Pozo-Rosich P, Clover L, Saiz A, et al. Voltage-gated potassium channel antibodies in limbic encephalitis. Ann Neurol 2003;54:530–533.
34. Taylor RB, Mason W, Kong K, et al. Reversible paraneoplastic encephalomyelitis associated with a benign ovarian teratoma. Can J Neurol Sci 1999;26:317–320.
35. Henson RA, Hoffman HL, Urich H. Encephalomyelitis with carcinoma. Brain 1965;88:449–464.
36. Dalmau J, Graus F, Rosenblum MK, et al. Anti-Hu-associated paraneoplastic encephalomyelitis/sensory neuronopathy. A clinical study of 71 patients. Medicine (Baltimore) 1992;71: 59–72.
37. Antoine JC, Cinotti L, Tilikete C, et al. [18F]fluorodeoxyglucose positron emission tomography in the diagnosis of cancer in patients with paraneoplastic neurological syndrome and anti-Hu antibodies. Ann Neurol 2000;48:105–108.
38. Rees JH, Hain SF, Johnson MR, et al. The role of [18F]fluoro-2-deoxyglucose-PET scanning in the diagnosis of paraneoplastic neurological disorders. Brain 2001;124:2223–2231.
39. Dropcho EJ. Antiamphiphysin antibodies with small-cell lung carcinoma and paraneoplastic encephalomyelitis. Ann Neurol 1996;39:659–667.
40. Chan KH, Vernino S, Lennon VA. ANNA-3 anti-neuronal nuclear antibody: marker of lung cancer-related autoimmunity. Ann Neurol 2001;50:301–311.
41. Keime-Guibert F, Graus F, Fleury A, et al. Treatment of paraneoplastic neurological syndromes with antineuronal antibodies (Anti-Hu, anti-Yo) with a combination of immunoglobulins, cyclophosphamide, and methylprednisolone. J Neurol Neurosurg Psychiatry 2000;68:479–482.
42. Digre KB. Opsoclonus in adults. Report of three cases and review of the literature. Arch Neurol 1986;43:1165–1175.
43. Wirtz PW, Sillevis Smitt PA, Hoff JI, et al. Anti-Ri antibody positive opsoclonus-myoclonus in a male patient with breast carcinoma. J Neurol 2002;249:1710–1712.
44. Prestigiacomo CJ, Balmaceda C, Dalmau J. Anti-Ri-associated paraneoplastic opsoclonus-ataxia syndrome in a man with transitional cell carcinoma. Cancer 2001;91:1423–1428.
45. Altman AJ, Baehner RL. Favorable prognosis for survival in children with coincident opso-myoclonus and neuroblastoma. Cancer 1976;37:846–852.
46. Rudnick E, Khakoo Y, Antunes NL, et al. Opsoclonus-myoclonus-ataxia syndrome in neuroblastoma: clinical outcome and antineuronal antibodies-a report from the Children's Cancer Group Study. Med Pediatr Oncol 2001; 36:612–622.
47. Bataller L, Rosenfeld MR, Graus F, et al. Autoantigen diversity in the opsoclonus-myoclonus syndrome. Ann Neurol 2003;53:347–353.
48. Dalmau J, Graus F, Cheung NK, et al. Major histocompatibility proteins, anti-Hu antibodies and paraneoplastic encephalomyelitis in neuroblastoma and small cell lung cancer. Cancer 1995;75:99–109.
49. Antunes NL, Khakoo Y, Matthay KK, et al. Antineuronal antibodies in patients with neuroblastoma and paraneoplastic opsoclonus-myoclonus. J Pediatr Hematol Oncol 2000;22: 315–320.
50. Pranzatelli MR, Tate ED, Wheeler A, et al. Screening for autoantibodies in children with opsoclonus-myoclonus-ataxia. Pediatr Neurol 2002;27:384–387.
51. Russo C, Cohn SL, Petruzzi MJ, et al. Long-term neurologic outcome in children with opsoclonus-myoclonus associated with neuroblastoma: a report from the Pediatric Oncology Group. Med Pediatr Oncol 1997;28:284–288.
52. Lorish TR, Thorsteinsson G, Howard FM. Stiff-man syndrome updated. Mayo Clin Proc 1989;64:629–636.
53. Whiteley AM, Swash M, Urich H. Progressive encephalomyelitis with rigidity. Brain 1976;99:27–42.

54. Leigh PN, Rothwell JC, Traub M, et al. A patient with reflex myoclonus and muscle rigidity: "jerking stiff-man syndrome." J Neurol Neurosurg Psychiatry 1980;43:1125–1131.
55. Barker RA, Revesz T, Thom M, et al. Review of 23 patients affected by the stiff man syndrome: clinical subdivision into stiff trunk (man) syndrome, stiff limb syndrome, and progressive encephalomyelitis with rigidity. J Neurol Neurosurg Psychiatry 1998;65:633–640.
56. Bateman DE, Weller RO, Kennedy P. Stiff-man syndrome: a rare paraneoplastic syndrome? J Neurol Neurosurg Psychiatry 1990;53:695–696.
57. Folli F, Solimena M, Cofiell R, et al. Autoantibodies to a 128-kd synaptic protein in three women with the stiff-man syndrome and breast cancer. N Engl J Med 1993;328: 546–551.
58. Grimaldi LM, Martino G, Braghi S, et al. Heterogeneity of autoantibodies in stiff-man syndrome. Ann Neurol 1993;34:57–64.
59. Solimena M, Folli F, Aparisi R, et al. Autoantibodies to GABA-ergic neurons and pancreatic beta cells in stiff-man syndrome. N Engl J Med 1990;322:1555–1560.
60. Saiz A, Dalmau J, Butler MH, et al. Anti-amphiphysin I antibodies in patients with paraneoplastic neurological disorders associated with small cell lung carcinoma. J Neurol Neurosurg Psychiatry 1999;66:214–217.
61. Antoine JC, Absi L, Honnorat J, et al. Antiamphiphysin antibodies are associated with various paraneoplastic neurological syndromes and tumors. Arch Neurol 1999;56:172–177.
62. Butler MH, Hayashi A, Ohkoshi N, et al. Autoimmunity to gephyrin in stiff-man syndrome. Neuron 2000;26:307–312.
63. Vermeij FH, van Doorn PA, Busch HF. Improvement of stiff-man syndrome with vigabatrin. Lancet 1996;348:612.
64. Dalakas MC, Fujii M, Li M, et al. High-dose intravenous immune globulin for stiff-person syndrome. N Engl J Med 2001;345:1870–1876.
65. Schmierer K, Valdueza JM, Bender A, et al. Atypical stiff-person syndrome with spinal MRI findings, amphiphysin autoantibodies, and immunosuppression [see comments]. Neurology 1998;51:250–252.
66. Harada H, Hayashi A, Watanabe M, et al. A case of stiff-man syndrome with head retraction like reflex myoclonus and jerky myoclonus of bilateral lower extremities which responded well to removal of mediastinal carcinoma. Rinsho Shinkeigaku 1999;39:1025–1028.
67. Rosin L, DeCamilli P, Butler M, et al. Stiff-man syndrome in a woman with breast cancer: an uncommon central nervous system paraneoplastic syndrome. Neurology 1998;50:94–98.
68. Vernino S, Tuite P, Adler CH, et al. Paraneoplastic chorea associated with CRMP-5 neuronal antibody and lung carcinoma. Ann Neurol 2002;51:625–630.
69. Batchelor TT, Platten M, Palmer-Toy DE, et al. Chorea as a paraneoplastic complication of Hodgkin's disease. J Neurooncol 1998;36:185–190.
70. Kujawa KA, Niemi VR, Tomasi MA, et al. Ballistic-choreic movements as the presenting feature of renal cancer. Arch Neurol 2001;58:1133–1135.
71. Tremont-Lukats IW, Fuller GN, Ribalta T, et al. Paraneoplastic chorea: case study with autopsy confirmation. Neurooncol 2002;4:192–195.
72. Cervera R, Asherson RA, Font J, et al. Chorea in the antiphospholipid syndrome. Clinical, radiologic, and immunologic characteristics of 50 patients from our clinics and the recent literature. Medicine (Baltimore) 1997;76:203–212.
73. Cross SA, Salomao DR, Parisi JE, et al. Paraneoplastic autoimmune optic neuritis with retinitis defined by CRMP-5-IgG. Ann Neurol 2003;54:38–50.
74. Boeck K, Hofmann S, Klopfer M, et al. Melanoma-associated paraneoplastic retinopathy: case report and review of the literature. Br J Dermatol 1997;137:457–460.
75. Keltner JL, Thirkill CE, Yip PT. Clinical and immunologic characteristics of melanoma-associated retinopathy syndrome: eleven new cases and a review of 51 previously published cases. J Neuroophthalmol 2001;21:173–187.
76. Jacobson DM, Adamus G. Retinal anti-bipolar cell antibodies in a patient with paraneoplastic retinopathy and colon carcinoma. Am J Ophthalmol 2001;131:806–808.
77. Polans AS, Buczylko J, Crabb J, et al. A photoreceptor calcium binding protein is recognized by autoantibodies obtained from patients with cancer-associated retinopathy. J Cell Biol 1991;112:981–989.
78. Guy J, Aptsiauri N. Treatment of paraneoplastic visual loss with intravenous immunoglobulin: report of 3 cases. Arch Ophthalmol 1999;117:471–477.
79. Ohguro H, Ogawa K, Maeda T, et al. Retinal dysfunction in cancer-associated retinopathy is improved by Ca(2+) antagonist administration and dark adaptation. Invest Ophthalmol Vis Sci 2001;42:2589–2595.
80. Blumenthal D, Schochet S Jr, Gutmann L, et al. Small-cell carcinoma of the lung presenting with paraneoplastic peripheral nerve microvasculitis and optic neuropathy. Muscle Nerve 1998;21:1358–1359.
81. de la Sayette V, Bertran F, Honnorat J, et al. Paraneoplastic cerebellar syndrome and optic neuritis with anti-CV2 antibodies: clinical response to excision of the primary tumor. Arch Neurol 1998;55:405–408.
82. Luiz JE, Lee AG, Keltner JL, et al. Paraneoplastic optic neuropathy and autoantibody production in small-cell carcinoma of the lung. J Neuroophthalmol 1998;18:178–181.
83. Hoh ST, Teh M, Chew SJ. Paraneoplastic optic neuropathy in nasopharyngeal carcinoma—report of a case. Singapore Med J 1991;32:170–173.
84. Forsyth PA, Dalmau J, Graus F, et al. Motor neuron disease in cancer patients. Ann Neurol 1997;41:722–730.
85. Schold SC, Cho ES, Somasundaram M, et al. Subacute motor neuronopathy: a remote effect of lymphoma. Ann Neurol 1979;5:271–287.
86. Walton JN, Tomlinson BE, Pearce GW. Subacute "poliomyelitis" and Hodgkin's disease. J Neurol Sci 1968;6: 435–445.
87. Sadowski CH, Sachs E, Ochoa J. Postradiation motor neuron syndrome. Arch Neurol 1976;33:786–787.
88. Kristensen O, Melgard B, Schiodt AV. Radiation myelopathy of the lumbo-sacral spinal cord. Acta Neurol Scand 1977;56:217–222.
89. Rowland LP, Sherman WH, Latov N, et al. Amyotrophic lateral sclerosis and lymphoma: bone marrow examination and other diagnostic tests. Neurology 1992;42:1101–1102.
90. Forsyth PA, Dalmau J, Graus F, et al. Motor neuron syndromes in cancer patients. Ann Neurol 1997;41:722–730.

91. Rosenfeld MR, Posner JB. Paraneoplastic motor neuron disease. Adv Neurol 1991;56:445–459.
92. Norris FH, Engel WK. Carcinomatous amyotrophic lateral sclerosis. In: Brain WR, Norris FH, eds. The remote effects of cancer on the nervous system. New York: Grune and Stratton, 1965:24–34.
93. Evans BK, Fagan C, Arnold T, et al. Paraneoplastic motor neuron disease and renal cell carcinoma: improvement after nephrectomy. Neurology 1990;40:960–962.
94. Gritzman MC, Fritz VU, Perkins S, et al. Motor neuron disease associated with carcinoma. A report of 2 cases. S Afr Med J 1983;63:288–291.
95. Kloos L, Ang CW, Kruit W, et al. Paraneoplastic ophthalmoplegia and subacute motor axonal neuropathy associated with anti-GQ1b antibodies in a patient with malignant melanoma. J Neurol Neurosurg Psychiatry 2003;74: 507–509.
96. Berghs S, Ferracci F, Maksimova E, et al. Autoimmunity to beta IV spectrin in paraneoplastic lower motor neuron syndrome. Proc Natl Acad Sci USA 2001;98:6945–6950.
97. Denny-Brown D. Primary sensory neuropathy with muscular changes associated with carcinoma. J Neurol Neurosurg Psychiatry 1948;11:73–87.
98. Graus F, Ribalta T, Campo E, et al. Immunohistochemical analysis of the immune reaction in the nervous system in paraneoplastic encephalomyelitis. Neurology 1990;40: 219–222.
99. Horwich MS, Cho L, Porro RS, et al. Subacute sensory neuropathy: a remote effect of carcinoma. Ann Neurol 1977;2: 7–19.
100. Graus F, Bonaventura I, Uchuya M, et al. Indolent anti-Hu-associated paraneoplastic sensory neuropathy. Neurology 1994;44:2258–2261.
101. Molinuevo JL, Graus F, Serrano C, et al. Utility of anti-Hu antibodies in the diagnosis of paraneoplastic sensory neuropathy. Ann Neurol 1998;44:976–980.
102. Chalk CH, Lennon VA, Stevens JC, et al. Seronegativity for type 1 antineuronal nuclear antibodies ("anti-Hu") in subacute sensory neuronopathy patients without cancer. Neurology 1993;43:2209–2211.
103. Sillevis Smitt PAE, Posner JP. Paraneoplastic peripheral neuropathy. In: Hartung H-P, ed. Peripheral neuropathies, part I, vol 4. London: Bailliere Tindall, 1995:443–469.
104. Keime-Guibert F, Graus F, Broet P, et al. Clinical outcome of patients with anti-Hu-associated encephalomyelitis after treatment of the tumor. Neurology 1999;53:1719–1723.
105. Graus F, Dalmau J, Rene R, et al. Anti-Hu antibodies in patients with small-cell lung cancer: association with complete response to therapy and improved survival. J Clin Oncol 1997;15:2866–2872.
106. Croft PB, Wilkinson M. The incidence of carcinomatous neuromyopathy in patients with various types of carcinoma. Brain 1965;88:427–434.
107. Antoine JC, Honnorat J, Camdessanche JP, et al. Paraneoplastic anti-CV2 antibodies react with peripheral nerve and are associated with a mixed axonal and demyelinating peripheral neuropathy. Ann Neurol 2001; 49:214–221.
108. Camdessanche JP, Antoine JC, Honnorat J, et al. Paraneoplastic peripheral neuropathy associated with anti-Hu antibodies. A clinical and electrophysiological study of 20 patients. Brain 2002;125:166–175.
109. Kelly J Jr, Kyle RA, Miles JM, et al. Osteosclerotic myeloma and peripheral neuropathy. Neurology 1983;33:202–210.
110. Donofrio PD. Immunotherapy of idiopathic inflammatory neuropathies. Muscle Nerve 2003;28:273–292.
111. Kuwabara S, Hattori T, Shimoe Y, et al. Long term melphalan-prednisolone chemotherapy for POEMS syndrome. J Neurol Neurosurg Psychiatry 1997;63: 385–387.
112. Kyle RA. Clinical aspects of multiple myeloma and related disorders including amyloidosis. Pathol Biol (Paris) 1999;47:148–157.
113. Walsh JC. The neuropathy of multiple myeloma. An electrophysiological and histological study. Arch Neurol 1971;25: 404–414.
114. Ropper AH, Gorson KC. Neuropathies associated with paraproteinemia. N Engl J Med 1998;338:1601–1607.
115. Dimopoulos MA, Panayiotidis P, Moulopoulos LA, et al. Waldenström's macroglobulinemia: clinical features, complications, and management. J Clin Oncol 2000;18: 214–226.
116. Kyle RA, Treon SP, Alexanian R, et al. Prognostic markers and criteria to initiate therapy in Waldenström's macroglobulinemia: consensus panel recommendations from the Second International Workshop on Waldenström's Macroglobulinemia. Semin Oncol 2003;30:116–120.
117. Dalakas MC, Flaum MA, Rick M, et al. Treatment of polyneuropathy in Waldenström's macroglobulinemia: role of paraproteinemia and immunologic studies. Neurology 1983;33:1406–1410.
118. Renaud S, Gregor M, Fuhr P, et al. Rituximab in the treatment of polyneuropathy associated with anti-MAG antibodies. Muscle Nerve 2003;27:611–615.
119. Levine TD, Pestronk A. IgM antibody-related polyneuropathies: B-cell depletion chemotherapy using rituximab. Neurology 1999;52:1701–1704.
120. Vernino S, Low PA, Fealey RD, et al. Autoantibodies to ganglionic acetylcholine receptors in autoimmune autonomic neuropathies. N Engl J Med 2000;343:847–855.
121. O'Neill JH, Murray NM, Newsom-Davis J. The Lambert-Eaton myasthenic syndrome. A review of 50 cases. Brain 1988;111:577–596.
122. Lee HR, Lennon VA, Camilleri M, et al. Paraneoplastic gastrointestinal motor dysfunction: clinical and laboratory characteristics. Am J Gastroenterol 2001;96:373–379.
123. Low PA. Autonomic neuropathies. Curr Opin Neurol 2002;15:605–609.
124. Turner ML, Boland OM, Parker AC, et al. Subclinical autonomic dysfunction in patients with Hodgkin's disease and non-Hodgkin's lymphoma. Br J Haematol 1993;84: 623–626.
125. Calvet X, Martinez JM, Martinez M. Repeated neostigmine dosage as palliative treatment for chronic colonic pseudo-obstruction in a patient with autonomic paraneoplastic neuropathy. Am J Gastroenterol 2003;98:708–709.
126. Oh SJ, Dropcho EJ, Claussen GC. Anti-Hu-associated paraneoplastic sensory neuropathy responding to early aggressive immunotherapy: report of two cases and review of literature. Muscle Nerve 1997;20:1576–1582.

127. Matsumuro K, Izumo S, Umehara F, et al. Paraneoplastic vasculitic neuropathy: immunohistochemical studies on a biopsied nerve and post-mortem examination. J Intern Med 1994;236:225–230.
128. Hart IK, Maddison P, Newsom-Davis J, et al. Phenotypic variants of autoimmune peripheral nerve hyperexcitability. Brain 2002;125:1887–1895.
129. Auger RG. AAEM minimonograph #44: diseases associated with excess motor unit activity. Muscle Nerve 1994;17: 1250–1263.
130. Newsom-Davis J, Mills KR. Immunological associations of acquired neuromyotonia (Isaacs' syndrome). Report of five cases and literature review. Brain 1993;116:453–469.
131. Shillito P, Molenaar PC, Vincent A, et al. Acquired neuromyotonia: evidence for autoantibodies directed against K+ channels of peripheral nerves. Ann Neurol 1995;38: 714–722.
132. Buckley C, Oger J, Clover L, et al. Potassium channel antibodies in two patients with reversible limbic encephalitis. Ann Neurol 2001;50:73–78.
133. Elrington GM, Murray NM, Spiro SG, et al. Neurological paraneoplastic syndromes in patients with small cell lung cancer. A prospective survey of 150 patients. J Neurol Neurosurg Psychiatry 1991;54:764–767.
134. Hawley RJ, Cohen MH, Saini N, et al. The carcinomatous neuromyopathy of oat cell lung cancer. Ann Neurol 1980;7:65–72.
135. Motomura M, Johnston I, Lang B, et al. An improved diagnostic assay for Lambert-Eaton myasthenic syndrome. J Neurol Neurosurg Psychiatry 1995;58:85–87.
136. Rosenfeld MR, Wong E, Dalmau J, et al. Cloning and characterization of a Lambert-Eaton myasthenic syndrome antigen. Ann Neurol 1993;33:113–120.
137. Chalk CH, Murray NMF, Newsom-Davis J, et al. Response of the Lambert-Eaton myasthenic syndrome to treatment of associated small-cell lung carcinoma. Neurology 1990;40:1552–1556.
138. McEvoy KM, Windebank AJ, Daube JR, et al. 3,4-Diaminopyridine in the treatment of Lambert-Eaton myasthenic syndrome. N Engl J Med 1989;321:1567–1571.
139. Sanders DB, Massey JM, Sanders LL, et al. A randomized trial of 3,4-diaminopyridine in Lambert-Eaton myasthenic syndrome. Neurology 2000;54:603–607.
140. Newsom-Davis J, Murray NM. Plasma exchange and immunosuppressive drug treatment in the Lambert-Eaton myasthenic syndrome. Neurology 1984;34:480–485.
141. Bird SJ. Clinical and electrophysiologic improvement in Lambert-Eaton syndrome with intravenous immunoglobulin therapy. Neurology 1992;42:1422–1423.
142. Literature review of the usefulness of repetitive nerve stimulation and single fiber EMG in the electrodiagnostic evaluation of patients with suspected myasthenia gravis or Lambert-Eaton myasthenic syndrome. Muscle Nerve 2001;24:1239–1247.
143. Vincent A, Bowen J, Newsom-Davis J, et al. Seronegative generalised myasthenia gravis: clinical features, antibodies, and their targets. Lancet Neurol 2003;2:99–106.
144. Gautel M, Lakey A, Barlow DP, et al. Titin antibodies in myasthenia gravis: identification of a major immunogenic region of titin. Neurology 1993;43:1581–1585.
145. Hoch W, McConville J, Helms S, et al. Auto-antibodies to the receptor tyrosine kinase MuSK in patients with myasthenia gravis without acetylcholine receptor antibodies. Nat Med 2001;7:365–368.
146. Griggs RC, Mendell JR, Miller RG. Evaluation and treatment of myopathies. Philadelphia: FA Davis, 1995.
147. Buchbinder R, Forbes A, Hall S, et al. Incidence of malignant disease in biopsy-proven inflammatory myopathy. A population-based cohort study. Ann Intern Med 2001;134: 1087–1095.
148. Hill CL, Zhang Y, Sigurgeirsson B, et al. Frequency of specific cancer types in dermatomyositis and polymyositis: a population-based study. Lancet 2001;357:96–100.
149. Sigurgeirsson B, Lindelof B, Edhag O, et al. Risk of cancer in patients with dermatomyositis or polymyositis. A population-based study. N Engl J Med 1992;326:363–367.
150. Mastaglia FL, Garlepp MJ, Phillips BA, et al. Inflammatory myopathies: clinical, diagnostic and therapeutic aspects. Muscle Nerve 2003;27:407–425.
151. Targoff IN. Update on myositis-specific and myositis-associated autoantibodies. Curr Opin Rheumatol 2000;12: 475–481.
152. Vosskamper M, Korf B, Franke F, et al. Paraneoplastic necrotizing myopathy: a rare disorder to be differentiated from polymyositis. J Neurol 1989;236:489–490.
153. Levin MI, Mozaffar T, Al-Lozi MT, et al. Paraneoplastic necrotizing myopathy: clinical and pathological features. Neurology 1998;50:764–767.
154. Anderlini P, Buzaid AC, Legha SS. Acute rhabdomyolysis after concurrent administration of interleukin-2, interferon-alfa, and chemotherapy for metastatic melanoma. Cancer 1995;76:678–679.
155. Moertel CG, Kvols LK, Rubin J. A study of cyproheptadine in the treatment of metastatic carcinoid tumor and the malignant carcinoid syndrome. Cancer 1991;67:33–36.
156. Albrecht JT, Canada TW. Cachexia and anorexia in malignancy. Hematol Oncol Clin North Am 1996;10:791–800.
157. Verschuuren JJ, Perquin M, ten Velde G, et al. Anti-Hu antibody titre and brain metastases before and after treatment for small cell lung cancer. J Neurol Neurosurg Psychiatry 1999;67:353–357.
158. Furneaux HM, Rosenblum MK, Dalmau J, et al. Selective expression of Purkinje-cell antigens in tumor tissue from patients with paraneoplastic cerebellar degeneration. N Engl J Med 1990;322:1844–1851.
159. Jean WC, Dalmau J, Ho A, Posner JB. Analysis of the IgG subclass distribution and inflammatory infiltrates in patients with anti-Hu-associated paraneoplastic encephalomyelitis. Neurology 1994;44:140–147.
160. Bernal F, Graus F, Pifarre A, et al. Immunohistochemical analysis of anti-Hu-associated paraneoplastic encephalomyelitis. Acta Neuropathol (Berl) 2002;103:509–515.
161. Dalmau J, Furneaux HM, Rosenblum MK, et al. Detection of the anti-Hu antibody in specific regions of the nervous system and tumor from patients with paraneoplastic encephalomyelitis/sensory neuronopathy. Neurology 1991;41:1757–1764.
162. Verschuuren JJ, Rosenblum MK, Lieberman FS, et al. Complete absence of Purkinje cells in anti-Yo associated cerebellar degeneration. J Neuro Onc 1994;21:77.

163. Ridley A, Kennard C, Scholtz CL, et al. Omnipause neurons in two cases of opsoclonus associated with oat cell carcinoma of the lung. Brain 1987;110:1699–1709.
164. Darnell RB, DeAngelis LM. Regression of small-cell lung carcinoma in patients with paraneoplastic neuronal antibodies. Lancet 1993;341:21–22.
165. Byrne T, Mason WP, Posner JB, et al. Spontaneous neurological improvement in anti-Hu associated encephalomyelitis. J Neurol Neurosurg Psychiatry 1997;62:276–278.
166. Albert ML, Austin LM, Darnell RB. Detection and treatment of activated T cells in the cerebrospinal fluid of patients with paraneoplastic cerebellar degeneration. Ann Neurol 2000;47:9–17.
167. Albert ML, Darnell JC, Bender A, et al. Tumor-specific killer cells in paraneoplastic cerebellar degeneration. Nat Med 1998;4:1321–1324.
168. Tanaka M, Maruyama Y, Sugie M, et al. Cytotoxic T cell activity against peptides of Hu protein in anti-Hu syndrome. J Neurol Sci 2002;201:9–12.
169. Sillevis Smitt PAE, Manley GT, Posner JP. Immunization with the paraneoplastic encephalomyelitis antigen HuD does not cause neurologic disease in mice. Neurology 1995;45:1873–1878.
170. Benyahia B, Liblau R, Merle-Beral H, et al. Cell-mediated autoimmunity in paraneoplastic neurological syndromes with anti-Hu antibodies. Ann Neurol 1999;45:162–167.
171. Uchuya M, Fleury A, Graus F, et al. Lack of association between human leukocyte antigens and the anti-Hu syndrome in patients with small-cell lung cancer. Neurology 1998;50:565–566.
172. Wirtz PW, Willcox N, Roep BO, et al. HLA-B8 in patients with the Lambert-Eaton myasthenic syndrome reduces likelihood of associated small cell lung carcinoma. Ann N Y Acad Sci 2003;998:200–201.
173. Szabo A, Dalmau J, Manley G, et al. HuD, a paraneoplastic encephalomyelitis antigen, contains RNA-binding domains and is homologous to Elav and Sex-lethal. Cell 1991;67:325–333.
174. Fathallah-Shaykh H, Wolf S, Wong E, et al. Cloning of a leucine-zipper protein recognized by the sera of patients with antibody-associated paraneoplastic cerebellar degeneration. Proc Natl Acad Sci USA 1991;88:3451–3454.
175. Peterson K, Rosenblum MK, Kotanides H, et al. Paraneoplastic cerebellar degeneration. I. A clinical analysis of 55 anti-Yo antibody-positive patients. Neurology 1992;42:1931–1937.
176. Luque FA, Furneaux HM, Ferziger R, et al. Anti-Ri: an antibody associated with paraneoplastic opsoclonus and breast cancer. Ann Neurol 1991;29:241–251.
177. Buckanovich RJ, Posner JB, Darnell RB. Nova, the paraneoplastic Ri antigen, is homologous to an RNA-binding protein and is specifically expressed in the developing motor system. Neuron 1993;11:657–672.
178. Graus F, Dalmau J, Valldeoriola F, et al. Immunological characterization of a neuronal antibody (anti-Tr) associated with paraneoplastic cerebellar degeneration and Hodgkin disease. J Neuroimmunol 1997;74:55–61.
179. Graus F, Gultekin SH, Ferrer I, et al. Localization of the neuronal antigen recognized by anti-Tr antibodies from patients with paraneoplastic cerebellar degeneration and Hodgkin's disease in the rat nervous system. Acta Neuropathol (Berl) 1998;96:1–7.
180. Bataller L, Wade DF, Fuller GN, et al. Cerebellar degeneration and autoimmunity to zinc-finger proteins of the cerebellum. Neurology 2002;59:1985–1987.
181. Vernino S, Low PA, Lennon VA. Experimental autoimmune autonomic neuropathy. J Neurophysiol 2003;90:2053–2059.
182. Vernino S, Lennon VA. Ion channel and striational antibodies define a continuum of autoimmune neuromuscular hyperexcitability. Muscle Nerve 2002;26:702–707.
183. Nobile-Orazio E, Francomano E, Daverio R, et al. Anti-myelin-associated glycoprotein IgM antibody titers in neuropathy associated with macroglobulinemia. Ann Neurol 1989;26:543–550.
184. Braun PE, Frail DE, Latov N. Myelin-associated glycoprotein is the antigen for a monoclonal IgM in polyneuropathy. J Neurochem 1982;39:1261–1265.

CHAPTER 31

Neurologic Complications of Chemotherapy and Biologic Therapies

JULIE E. HAMMACK

The major strides in the treatment, and sometimes cure, of cancer in the last 50 years largely reflect the development and refinement of chemotherapeutic and biologic agents. These medications exert their antitumor effects at many different points in cell metabolism and reproduction, but share the common goal of reducing malignant cellular proliferation and/or producing cancer cell death. Although each agent has its own set of adverse effects, body tissues with a high rate of cell turnover (i.e., bone marrow, mucosal epithelium) are the most likely to be injured by chemotherapy agents. The central and peripheral nervous system contain cells with low proliferative index but nonetheless also can be adversely affected. The central nervous system (CNS) is protected by the blood–brain barrier that excludes most large and hydrophilic molecules. Most chemotherapy agents do not produce CNS toxicity unless instilled directly into the CNS or administered with an agent designed to disrupt the blood–brain barrier. Some concurrent therapies may increase the risk that a given drug will produce toxicity. Radiation therapy, for example, if given before or during treatment with methotrexate will increase the risk of developing methotrexate-induced leukoencephalopathy.

There are many instances in which antineoplastic drugs may produce nervous system toxicity indirectly. L-Asparaginase produces a coagulopathy that may lead to sagittal sinus thrombosis. Cisplatin-induced hypomagnesemia may produce seizures. Many chemotherapy agents produce thrombocytopenia, which may place the patient at risk for intracranial hemorrhage. Some agents require aggressive intravenous hydration, which may worsen cerebral edema in patients with brain tumors, or induce hyponatremia, which, in turn, may produce seizures. Many chemotherapy agents can produce hepatic, renal, or other organ dysfunction that may produce encephalopathy, seizures, or peripheral neuropathy.

The clinician caring for patients with cancer must be familiar with the central and peripheral nervous system effects of these agents and be able to distinguish them from the symptoms of metastatic tumor, opportunistic infection, paraneoplastic disease, metabolic disease, and the nervous system effects of other cancer treatments like radiation and surgery. This chapter is organized by class of drug. Tables 31-1 and 31-2 list the drugs grouped by common central neurotoxicities and Table 31-3 lists the chemotherapeutic and biologic therapies which most commonly produce peripheral neurotoxicity.

▶ ANTIMETABOLITES

Methotrexate

Methotrexate is an antimetabolite that inhibits DNA synthesis in the S-phase of the cell cycle. It inhibits the enzyme dihydrofolate reductase and thus prevents the conversion of folic acid into tetrahydrofolate. Tetrahydrofolate is necessary for purine and thymidylic acid production. Methotrexate is a common component of multiple chemotherapy regimens, particularly those for leukemia, lymphoma, and breast cancer. Methotrexate is highly ionized and relatively hydrophobic; therefore, only a small percentage crosses the blood–brain barrier. CNS toxicity is generally limited to those patients receiving high-dose intravenous methotrexate and those receiving methotrexate directly in the CNS. Peripheral nervous system toxicity

▶ **TABLE 31-1.** ADVERSE EFFECTS OF CHEMOTHERAPY

Seizures	Encephalopathy (Acute or Subacute)
Methotrexate	Methotrexate
Cisplatin	Cisplatin
Vinca alkaloids	Vinca alkaloids
Mechlorethamine	Mechlorethamine
Nitrosourea (IA or intracavitary administration)	Procarbazine
	Levamisole
	Ara-C
Chlorambucil (overdose only)	Fludarabine
	Gemcitabine
Hexamethylmelamine	Hydroxyurea
Cyclophosphamide	Pentostatin
Fluorouracil (5-FU)	Chlorambucil
Cytarabine (Ara-C)	Thiotepa (high dose)
Fludarabine	Ifosphamide
Gemcitabine	Hexamethymelamine
Pentostatin	Cyclophosphamide
Dacarbazine	Etoposide
Temozolomide	Paclitaxel
Ifosfamide	Docetaxel
Etoposide (VP16)	Pyrazoloactidine (PZA)
Paclitaxel	Doxorubicin (intrathecal only)
Docetaxel	Nitorimidazoles
Levamisole	Plicamycin
Metronidazole	Thalidomide
L-Asparaginase	Interferon
Interferon	Interleukin-2
Interleukin-2	Interleukin-3
Erythropoietin	Interleukin-6
Leuprolide	Interleukin-11
OKT3	Tumor necrosis factor-α (TNF-α)
	Tamoxifen
	Mitotane
	Corticosteroids
	OKT3
	L-Asparaginase

▶ **TABLE 31-2.** ADVERSE EFFECTS OF CHEMOTHERAPY

Headache	Encephalopathy (Chronic)
Methotrexate (intrathecal)	Methotrexate
Fluorouracil (5-FU)	Ara-C (intrathecal)
Cytarabine (Ara-C) (intrathecal)	5-FU + Levamisole
Cladribine	BCNU (intraarterial or high-dose IV)
Gemcitabine	Interferon
Hydroxyurea	Ifosfamide
Dacarbazine	Fludarabine
Temozolomide	Cisplatin (intraarterial)
Nitrosourea (BCNU) (intraarterial)	IL-2 (intrathecal)
Mechlorethamine	**Cerebrovascular Complications**
Procarbazine	Cisplatin
Thiotepa (intrathecal)	Doxorubicin (intraarterial)
Hexamethylmelamine	Mitomycin C
Retinoids	L-Asparaginase
Etoposide (VP16)	IL-2
Topotecan	Erythropoietin
Levamisole	Danazol
Mitomycin C	Estramustine
Plicamycin	
L-Asparaginase	**Visual System Abnormalities (visual loss)**
Thalidomide	Fludarabine
Interferon	Cisplatin (IA and high-dose IV)
Interleukin (IL)-2, IL-4, IL-3, IL-6, IL-11	BCNU (IA and high-dose IV)
Tumor necrosis factor-α (TNF-α)	Chlorambucil
Tamoxifen	Retinoids
Toremifene	Vinca alkaloids
Leuprolide	Paclitaxel
Goserelin	Interferon
Danazol	IL-2
Aromatase inhibitors	Tamoxifen
Octreotide	Mitotane
Mitotane	OKT3
OKT3	
Rituximab	
Trastuzumab	
Gemtuzumab ozogamicin	
Ibritumomab tiuxitan	
Cetuximab	
Imatinib mesylate	
Gefitinib, erlotinib	

► **TABLE 31-3.** COMMON CHEMOTHERAPY-INDUCED PERIPHERAL NEUROPATHIES

Vinca alkaloids	Sensorimotor axonal neuropathy (length-dependent) Autonomic neuropathy Acute inflammatory demyelinating polyneuropathy (AIDP)-like syndrome (rare) Cranial mononeuropathies
Platins	Sensory axonal neuronopathy Sensorineural hearing loss and vestibulopathy Sensorimotor and autonomic neuropathy (very rare)
Taxanes	Predominantly sensory axonal neuropathy Sensorimotor and autonomic neuropathy (rare) Facial nerve palsy
Suramin	Sensorimotor axonal neuropathy AIDP-like syndrome
Nitroimidazoles	Sensory axonal neuropathy
Thalidomide	Sensorimotor axonal neuropathy (sensory > motor)
Procarbazine	Sensorimotor axonal neuropathy
Cladribine	AIDP-like syndrome (rare)
Fludarabine	Sensorimotor axonal neuropathy (rare)
Etoposide (VP16)	Sensory axonal neuropathy
Ifosfamide	Sensorimotor axonal neuropathy
Hexamethylmelamine	Mild, predominantly sensory axonal neuropathy
Cytarabine (Ara-C)	Painful sensory axonal neuropathy (rare) Brachial plexopathy (rare)
Interferon	Inflammatory plexopathy AIDP-like syndrome
Interleukin (IL-2)	Inflammatory plexopathy
Tumor necrosis factor-α (TNF-α)	Focal mononeuropathies with isolated limb infusion

is not known to occur with methotrexate. CNS effects are best grouped into acute/subacute and late effects. Table 31-4 summarizes these effects.

Acute/Subacute Effects

Headache, stiff neck, and low-grade fever with cerebrospinal fluid (CSF) pleocytosis occur in approximately 10% of patients receiving intra-CSF administration of methotrexate, usually within a few hours of drug instillation. This chemical meningitis may be difficult to distinguish clinically from infectious meningitis. This chemical meningitis appears to be an idiosyncratic effect, which is unlikely to recur with subsequent administrations. The diluent used in the methotrexate solution may play a role in development. Patients receiving radiation concurrently with intrathecal methotrexate appear to be less likely to develop this syndrome. The occurrence of this adverse effect does not appear to predispose the patient to the late effects of methotrexate. Moreover, it is not definitely dose-related and it is usually self-limited. Methotrexate-induced chemical meningitis may be ameliorated or prevented by coadministration of corticosteroids.

► **TABLE 31-4.** ADVERSE EFFECTS OF METHOTREXATE (INTRA-CSF OR HIGH-DOSE IV)

Acute
Chemical meningitis
Headache (intra-CSF)
Diffuse encephalopathy
Transient focal neurologic deficits
Seizures
Transverse myelopathy (intra-CSF)
Subacute
Transverse myelopathy (intra-CSF)
Diffuse encephalopathy
Chronic
Leukoencephalopathy (dementia, seizures)
Mineralizing microangiopathy

CSF = cerebrospinal fluid.

There are reports of patients accidentally receiving many times the recommended dose without adverse effect,[1,2] as well as a report of a rapidly progressive fatal encephalopathy in a patient receiving an overdose of intrathecal methotrexate.[3] CSF drainage, ventriculolumbar perfusion, and the administration of carboxypeptidase-G2, an enzyme that hydrolyzes methotrexate into inactive metabolites, may be helpful in averting neurologic disaster.[4] Leucovorin does not penetrate the CNS to any appreciable degree, so is only useful in preventing peripheral methotrexate toxicity.

Yim and associates[5] reported three patient with transient hemiparesis and dysarthria 10 to 14 days after receiving intrathecal methotrexate. Magnetic resonance imaging (MRI) showed focal white matter abnormalities, but there was no additional evidence to support the authors' contention that this represented cerebral ischemia. All patients improved spontaneously after several days without additional treatment. Seizures are rare and self-limited after intra-CSF administration of methotrexate.[6] Figure 31-1 demonstrates a diffusion-weighted image of a patient who had received intrathecal methotrexate for treatment of acute lymphocytic leukemia (ALL). One week after treatment, the patient developed right hemiparesis, aphasia, and right homonymous hemianopia of gradual onset. The image suggests acute, multifocal ischemia, although the magnetic resonance (MR) angiogram and venogram were normal as was the echocardiogram. Coagulation profile revealed a positive lupus anticoagulant and anticardiolipin antibodies. The patient improved clinically, although was left with some residual deficits and the lesions persisted on a followup MRI 3 months later.

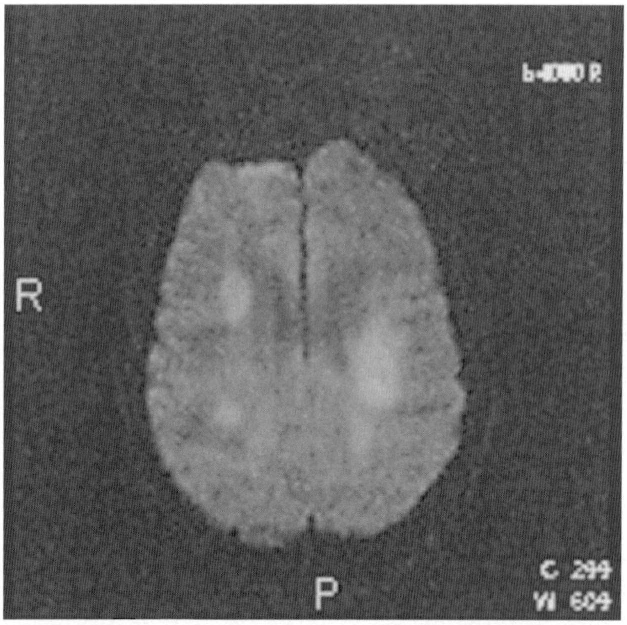

Figure 31-1. This 15-year-old with acute lymphocytic leukemia was receiving intrathecal methotrexate for CNS prophylaxis. One week after an injection, he gradually developed hemiparesis involving right face, arm, and leg, as well as global aphasia and right homonymous hemianopsia. Diffusion-weighted images demonstrated multiple sites of acutely restricted diffusion; magnetic resonance (MR) angiogram and venogram were normal. A cardiac embolic source was excluded. These lesions persisted on followup MRI 3 months later. Although the diffusion-weighted images are consistent with infarct, the lesions did not have a classic arterial distribution or acute mass effect. A direct cytotoxic effect of methotrexate has been hypothesized. (*Courtesy of Amrit Grewal, MD.*)

Transverse myelopathy, usually transient, may develop within hours to weeks of administration of intrathecal methotrexate.[7,8] Most of the reported cases of transverse myelopathy had received multiple prior doses of intrathecal methotrexate. MRI may show T_2 signal abnormalities with contrast enhancement.[9] Although little pathologic data are available, one case demonstrated vacuolar degeneration and necrosis without inflammation.[8]

An acute or subacute encephalopathy may result from moderate to high-dose methotrexate (3–12.5 g/m^2). This syndrome is characterized by somnolence and rarely focal or generalized seizures. Focal signs including hemiparesis, aphasia, dysarthria, sometimes with a stroke-like onset may be seen. Brain computerized tomography (CT) and MRI may be normal or show evidence of white matter abnormalities that typically resolve. When performed, angiography has been normal. Electroencephalography shows diffuse or sometimes focal slowing. There appears to be no correlation with serum or CSF levels of methotrexate. This syndrome occurs in 2.5% to 15% of patients receiving high-dose methotrexate. It can recur with subsequent doses. The mechanism is unknown. Complete recovery is usual, although a chronic leukoencephalopathy has been reported.

Late Effects

This describes toxicity that generally manifests 6 months or more after IV or intra-CSF administration. Most of the data are derived from retrospective studies of children with acute leukemia who received both IV and intrathecal methotrexate. A gradually progressive leukoencephalopathy with dementia, learning disorders and developmental delay (in children), gait disorders, and urinary incontinence are the most common symptoms. Brain radiation before or during methotrexate therapy increases the risk of this syndrome.[10] Both CT and MRI show diffuse white matter changes (Fig. 31-2). Cortical atrophy and ventricular enlargement are typical as are punctate areas of calcification in the basal ganglia and deep white matter. Even in asymptomatic patients who have received IV or intra-CSF methotrexate, similar, albeit less severe, white matter changes are typical.[11] Pathologically, this disorder is characterized by demyelination, sometimes with coagulative necrosis. Cortical U fibers are involved. Dystrophic calcification is seen in deep cerebral vessels. There is no treatment for this disorder. The administration of leucovorin does not prevent this disorder (or the acute and subacute effects of methotrexate).

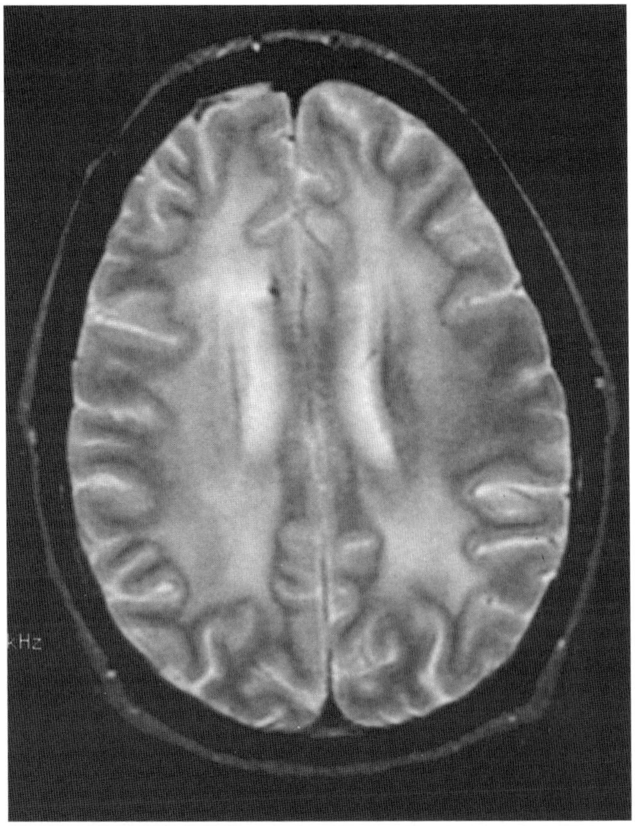

Figure 31-2. Methotrexate-induced leukoencephalopathy. Axial, T_2-weighted MRI of the head of a 30-year-old patient who had received multiple courses of IV and intra-Ommaya methotrexate for treatment of CNS lymphoma.

5-Fluorouracil

5-Fluorouracil (5-FU) is a synthetic, fluorinated, pyrimidine analogue of uracil that inhibits thymidylate synthetase and DNA synthesis. It also interferes with RNA function. It is used primarily in the treatment of gastrointestinal (GI), head and neck, and breast cancers. Peripheral nervous system toxicity is extremely rare, occurring in only 0.1% of patients receiving 5-FU.[12]

CNS toxicity is usually limited to patient receiving high IV dosages of the drug, and may be related more to peak plasma levels than to cumulative dosage. Toxicity is also more likely to occur in patients with deficiency of dihydropyrimidine dehydrogenase, an enzyme involved in 5-FU metabolism.[13]

An acute or subacute pancerebellar syndrome with ataxia of limb and gait, nystagmus, and dysarthria is the most common neurotoxicity associated with 5-FU.[14] It generally occurs during or shortly after infusion of 5-FU. Investigations including CT, MRI, and CSF, are normal, and the syndrome generally reverses completely after several days or weeks. Symptoms may recur if 5-FU is reinitiated. The clinical syndrome must be differentiated from vertebrobasilar ischemia, cerebellar metastases, paraneoplastic cerebellar disease, and other drug intoxications. Pathologic examination of the brains of patients with cerebellar toxicity from 5-FU generally reveals minimal if any abnormality.

Other CNS toxicity associated with 5-FU includes diffuse encephalopathy, headache, seizures, rarely optic neuropathy, and extrapyramidal syndromes.[15–17] Like the pancerebellar syndrome, the encephalopathy is more common when high dosages of 5-FU are administered.

Levamisole and 5-FU are commonly combined for the treatment of colon cancer. Levamisole was initially developed as an antihelminthic agent, but was later used as a chemotherapeutic agent because of its broad range of immunomodulatory functions. It also has been rarely associated with a variety of neurologic syndromes, including headache, encephalopathy, and seizures.[18–21] Orally administered levamisole causes demyelination in the central nervous system in dogs,[22] and a multifocal, inflammatory leukoencephalopathy has been reported in a single patient receiving levamisole alone for malignant melanoma.[23] Aseptic meningitis also has been reported as a rare adverse effect of treatment with levamisole.[24]

When combined with 5-FU, levamisole does not appear to increase the risk of 5-FU-induced cerebellopathy, but instead may produce a CNS inflammatory demyelinating disorder.[25–28] This disorder presents with subacute, multifocal central nervous system deficits, often weeks or months after discontinuing chemotherapy. MRI demonstrates multifocal white matter lesions, often with subtle enhancement (Fig. 31-3). CSF may demonstrate mild inflammatory changes, and oligoclonal bands may be present. Affected patients may respond to steroid therapy and the syndrome generally improves with or without steroids. The white matter abnormalities on MRI also resolve with time.[29]

Capecitabine

Capecitabine is an oral prodrug that is converted to 5-FU after metabolism in the liver. It is used in the treatment of colorectal, breast, and ovarian cancer. Despite its relationship to 5-FU, capecitabine has not been associated with significant central or peripheral neurotoxicity.

Cytosine Arabinoside

Cytosine arabinoside (Ara-C) is a pyrimidine analogue that is metabolized intracellularly to a compound that inhibits DNA polymerase. It is most commonly used in multiagent chemotherapy for leukemia and lymphoma. In addition to IV administration, it may be administered into the CSF for treatment of leptomeningeal malignancies. Ara-C toxicity is usually limited to the CNS, although

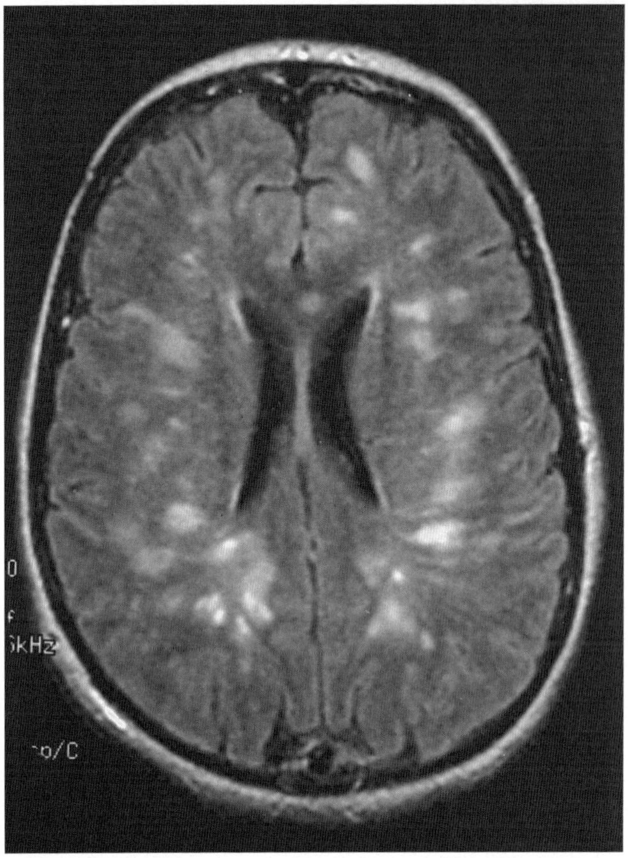

Figure 31-3. 5-FU and levamisole leukoencephalopathy: unenhanced axial fluid-attenuated inversion recovery (FLAIR) MRI of the head.

painful peripheral neuropathy and brachial plexopathy have been reported.[30,31]

Central neurotoxicity is usually associated with high-dose IV infusion (≥3 g/m² every 12 hours) for 4 to 6 days. The most common neurotoxicity is a subacute, pancerebellar syndrome, which generally develops during or within hours of completion of the high-dose infusion.[32] Occasionally encephalopathy, seizures, and coma may also occur after high-dose Ara-C infusion. The size of the individual dose may be more important than the cumulative dose, and patients with renal failure are more likely to develop this complication. Symptoms usually resolve after discontinuation of Ara-C. Cerebellar cortical atrophy and Purkinje cell loss has been seen on pathologic examination, as has rare leukoencephalopathy.[33,34] There is a single report of high-dose Ara-C producing transient parkinsonism.[35]

Intra-CSF administration of Ara-C may produce a benign, self-limited, chemical meningitis much like that described with methotrexate. It may recur with subsequent doses and is more common with the liposomal-encapsulated, sustained-release formulation (DepoCyt). Seizures and encephalopathy are rare complications. A subacute, occasionally necrotizing, myelopathy is a rare complication of intra-CSF Ara-C.[36] A fatal, "locked-in" syndrome has been described, occurring within a few hours of intrathecal administration.[37]

Fludarabine

Fludarabine phosphate is a synthetic purine nucleoside that inhibits DNA polymerase. It is used primarily in the treatment of refractory chronic lymphocytic leukemia (CLL). CNS toxicity predominates and appears to be dose-related. A nonspecific sensorimotor polyneuropathy has rarely been reported after the administration of fludarabine. The most common symptoms of fludarabine neurotoxicity involve the visual system. Symptoms generally consist of photophobia, and there is clinical evidence of either optic neuritis or cortical blindness.[38–40] Tremor, ataxia, myelopathy, and seizures have also been described. While most neurotoxicities occurred during treatment with fludarabine, some were delayed 1 to 9 months from the last dose of medication. The severe cases of neurotoxicity appear to be related to higher doses of fludarabine than those used currently. For example, more than 33% of patients receiving more than 96 mg/m² per day of IV fludarabine develop severe neurotoxicity, whereas less than 0.5% of patients receiving standard doses (<40 mg/m²/d) develop neurologic complications. In those patients with mild neurotoxicity, spontaneous improvement occurred once the drug was discontinued.

Brain MRI may show diffuse or multifocal white matter abnormalities on T_2 or fluid-attenuated inversion recovery (FLAIR) images. These do not enhance with gadolinium. CSF examination is usually normal. Pathologically, multifocal or diffuse demyelination with macrophage infiltration and necrosis has been reported. The abnormalities were most prominent in the occipital and parietal lobes.[39] The optic nerves, brainstem, and spinal cord have also been involved.

Cladribine

This purine nucleoside analogue inhibits DNA synthesis and ribonucleotide reductase. It is used in the treatment of leukemia and lymphoma. At the doses of cladribine currently in use, neurotoxicity appears to be relatively rare. With higher doses, nonspecific headache and ill-defined "weakness" have been reported. Rarely, myelopathy and a Guillain-Barré–like syndrome have been reported.[41]

Gemcitabine

Gemcitabine is a cell-cycle–specific pyrimidine analogue. It is cytotoxic to cells undergoing DNA synthesis (S-phase) and blocks the progression of cells through the G1/S-phase. It is used primarily in the treatment of pancreatic cancer, non–small cell lung cancer, and ovarian cancer. Neurologic toxicity is rare with this drug. Gemcitabine penetrates the blood–brain barrier in modest amounts. A reversible posterior leukoencephalopathy associated with headache and seizures has been described in a single patient receiving gemcitabine.[42] The coadministration of other drugs with peripheral neurotoxicity makes it difficult to determine whether gemcitabine itself produces peripheral neuropathy. Autonomic neuropathy has been reported in conjunction with gemcitabine.[43]

Hydroxyurea

Hydroxyurea's exact mechanism of action is unknown, but it is known to inhibit ribonucleotide reductase, thereby inhibiting DNA synthesis. Hydroxyurea is used primarily in the treatment of chronic hematologic malignancies and, more recently, in the treatment of inoperable meningiomas. Mild encephalopathy and headache have been reported,[44] but significant neurotoxicity appears to be rare.

Pentostatin

Pentostatin is a purine analogue that inhibits DNA synthesis. It is used primarily in the treatment of hairy cell leukemia. Somnolence, seizures, and coma have been reported in patients receiving high doses of the drug.[41] Neurotoxicity is dose related and is less common at the doses currently recommended.

▶ALKYLATING AGENTS

Cisplatin, Carboplatin

Cisplatin (CDDP) produces its antineoplastic effect by binding to DNA bases and producing interstrand and intrastrand cross-links. DNA synthesis and transcription is impaired and apoptosis results. Platinum analogues are used in combination to treat a number of malignancies, including sarcomas, testicular, ovarian, bladder, lung, brain, and head and neck malignancies. These drugs are also known to be radiosensitizers and may potentiate the benefits of radiation, as well as radiation-induced neurotoxicity. Carboplatin is a much less neurotoxic compound, but can produce the same spectrum of central and peripheral nervous system toxicities as CDDP.

Oxaliplatin, like carboplatin, is much less likely to produce peripheral neuropathy or other neurotoxicity. The most common acute side effect of oxaliplatin is a mild, transient, sensory polyneuropathy with neuronal hyperexcitability, manifesting as distal paresthesiae in the extremities, increased by cold exposure.[45] Transient Lhermitte phenomenon has also been described after administration of oxaliplatin.[46] As with cisplatin, these effects are cumulative and dose-dependent, and affect virtually all patients

▶ TABLE 31-5. ADVERSE NEUROLOGIC EFFECTS OF CISPLATIN

Intravenous	Intraarterial
Sensory axonal neuronopathy	Headache
Sensorineural hearing loss	Seizure
Vestibulopathy	Coma/diffuse encephalopathy
Lhermitte phenomenon	Leukoencephalopathy
Cerebral infarct	Cerebral edema
Seizure	Cerebral infarct
Diffuse encephalopathy	Cortical blindness
Optic neuritis (high dose)	Optic neuritis
Retinitis (high dose)	Retinitis

who receive doses greater than 540 mg/m^2. In more than 80% of patients who develop oxaliplatin neuropathy, the symptoms will resolve or regress within 4 to 6 months.[47]

The following discussion focuses primarily on CDDP, the most neurotoxic of the platinum analogues. Table 31-5 summarizes the most common central and peripheral nervous system toxicities of intravenous and intraarterial cisplatin.

Neurotoxicity is primarily expressed in the peripheral nervous system, as CDDP penetrates the blood–brain barrier to only a minor degree. After IV administration, high levels of CDDP have been demonstrated in the dorsal root ganglia and peripheral nerve. CDDP alters cell-cycle regulation and induces apoptosis in dorsal root ganglion cells.[48]

Sensory neuronopathy is the most common neurotoxicity associated with CDDP. The neuropathy predominantly affects large-fiber sensory axons.[49] It is characterized clinically by the onset of ascending distal paresthesias and dysesthesias. Although symptoms usually begin in the feet, eventually there is proximal spread and a "glove-and-stocking" distribution is noted in most patients. Clinical examination typically shows reduced vibration and joint position sense with lesser involvement of pain and temperature sensation. In severe cases, sensory ataxia and pseudoathetosis may result. There is no motor involvement, and autonomic dysfunction is rare with CDDP neuropathy.[50] Deep tendon reflexes are typically absent or markedly reduced. Symptoms of the peripheral neuropathy usually appear during the course of treatment with CDDP but may spontaneously worsen or first develop several months after discontinuing CDDP.[51] Pathologically there is length-dependent axonal loss in large myelinated fibers, with some secondary demyelination.

The incidence of CDDP-induced peripheral neuropathy is associated with repetitive CDDP dosing and is usually not apparent clinically until a cumulative dose of at least 200 to 350 mg/m^2 has been administered.[49,52,53] The signs and symptoms of CDDP neuropathy usually improve over time if the drug is discontinued. The painful dysesthesias typically abate spontaneously within 1 year of stopping CDDP, but may persist longer. The sensory deficits and reduced deep tendon reflexes may be permanent. Other than symptomatic care, there is no established treatment or preventive, although several compounds have been tried.[54,55] Transient Lhermitte phenomenon is a fairly common accompanying symptom, believed to result from degeneration in the central projecting sensory fibers of the dorsal root ganglia. Like the peripheral neuropathy, the incidence of Lhermitte phenomenon also appears to be dose related.

Ototoxicity is another common peripheral, dose-related effect of CDDP, which injures the hair cells in the organ of Corti.[56] A vestibulopathy may also occur. Other cranial neuropathies are rare but have been reported after the administration of IA CDDP.[57,58]

Table 31-5 summarizes the CNS toxicities associated with CDDP use. Seizures and diffuse encephalopathy are the most common and may result either from metabolic derangement caused by CDDP or as a direct effect of the drug. Hypomagnesemia occurs in up to 60% of patients receiving CDDP infusion and results from impaired magnesium reabsorption in the proximal renal tubule.[59] Hypomagnesemia may also produce encephalopathy, muscle weakness, and tetany in combination with secondary hypocalcemia. Hyponatremia may occur as a consequence of the syndrome of inappropriate antidiuretic hormone (SIADH),[60] excessive free water hydration during infusion of CDDP, or CDDP-induced emesis. Overhydration during CDDP infusion can produce cerebral edema, somnolence, seizures, and tonsillar herniation, particularly in those with preexisting space-occupying lesions in the brain.[61]

CDDP may produce encephalopathy as a direct effect of IV infusion, and this adverse effect is much more common after intraarterial injection. Generalized or focal seizures, cortical blindness, aphasia, and other focal deficits have been described after moderate to high-dose IV infusion, some with associated white matter changes on MRI.[62–65] While most of these effects occurred within a few hours of CDDP infusion, some were delayed by as many as 10 days from completion of treatment. In most cases, the symptoms resolved spontaneously and did not recur with subsequent CDDP treatment. Chronic leukoencephalopathy has been reported in a few patients receiving intraarterial CDDP.[57]

Ocular toxicity is particularly common after intraarterial infusion of CDDP. Optic neuropathy and retinopathy, sometimes with retinal infarcts, have been described after intraarterial administration.[66] The risk of this complication is lessened if the catheter is advanced beyond the origin of the ophthalmic artery. Recovery is usually spontaneous although some patients have permanent visual deficits. Retrobulbar neuritis and retinal toxicity have been described after administration of high-dose IV CDDP.[67–69]

Ischemic stroke and other vascular complications have been described after the administration of both IV and intraarterial CDDP, sometimes in combination with other chemotherapeutic agents.[70–72] Most of these infarcts occurred shortly after CDDP administration, although some were delayed. Angiography has shown branch vessel occlusions or has been normal. The mechanism of stroke in these cases is unknown, although hypomagnesemia-induced vasospasm, coagulopathy, and drug-induced endothelial injury have been invoked as possible mechanisms.

Dacarbazine

Dacarbazine (DTIC) acts both as an alkylating agent and as an inhibitor of DNA synthesis by hindering the incorporation of purine nucleosides. It is used in combination chemotherapy in the treatment of a variety of solid tumors, as well as lymphomas. Neurotoxicity appears to be extremely rare with dacarbazine. Neurologic effects, when they occur, are more likely to be secondary to coadministered chemotherapeutic agents.

Headache and general malaise are common, self-limited effects of dacarbazine therapy. There is a single case report of progressive dementia with cortical atrophy and focal neurologic deficit after two cycles of dacarbazine in a patient with metastatic melanoma.[73] The syndrome did not remit after the dacarbazine was discontinued. Seizures have been rarely reported in conjunction with dacarbazine use.[74]

Temozolomide

Temozolomide is an alkylating agent used primarily in the treatment of high-grade glioma and melanoma. No specific central or peripheral neurotoxicity has been reported with this drug. Headaches, seizures, and deterioration of preexisting neurologic deficits have been reported in some patient's receiving temozolomide, although these symptoms may have been caused by the patient's underlying disease and not the drug.[75,76] Transient neurologic deterioration has been reported in glioma patients at the commencement of treatment with temozolomide and has been postulated as a "tumor flare" syndrome.[77]

Nitrosoureas

Nitrosoureas are agents that alkylate DNA and RNA and include carmustine (BCNU), lomustine (CCNU), semustine (methyl-CCNU), fotemustine, and streptozotocin. All are highly lipid-soluble and penetrate the blood–brain barrier with CSF levels 15% to 30% of simultaneous plasma levels. They are most commonly used in the treatment of high-grade gliomas, melanoma, lymphoma, and islet cell tumors of the pancreas.

At conventional IV doses, CNS toxicity is rare and peripheral nervous system toxicity has not been reported. High-dose IV BCNU may produce optic neuropathy and leukoencephalopathy.[78,79]

Intraarterial BCNU, although rarely used now, at one time was a common therapy for high-grade glioma. There is a high incidence of retinal and cerebral toxicity with this method of drug administration. Intracarotid injection commonly produces ipsilateral eye and head pain immediately after injection. Optic neuropathy and retinal injury were common unless the catheter was advanced past the origin of the ophthalmic artery (supra-ophthalmic injection). A large percentage of patients given infra-ophthalmic injection were found to have electroretinographic (ERG) abnormalities after intraarterial injection of BCNU. Even contralateral eye ERGs were abnormal, suggesting a crossover effect from vascular collaterals.[80]

Necrotizing leukoencephalopathy was a common and sometimes fatal complication of intraarterial BCNU.[81,82] Focal or generalized seizures, coma, focal neurologic deficits, and ocular toxicity were common features of the disorder. Concurrent brain radiation therapy increases the risk of encephalopathy with intraarterial BCNU. The onset of symptoms may be delayed as long as 6 months from drug administration. CT and MRI of the head show significant edema and mass effect within the hemisphere ipsilateral to the BCNU injection, sometimes with evident gyral enhancement. Pathologic examination of the brains of patients who have died from this disorder demonstrates focal necrosis and mineralizing axonopathy in the affected hemisphere. Some patients had a necrotizing leukoencephalopathy similar to that seen as a delayed effect of radiation or methotrexate therapy.[82,83] Although the precise mechanism is unknown, a direct neurotoxic drug effect and endothelial injury are proposed mechanisms. The high risk of complications and the lack of survival benefit over that obtained with IV BCNU led to the eventual abandonment of intraarterial BCNU.

BCNU may also be implanted in wafer form directly into the brain tumor cavity. There does not appear to be a significant risk of increased neurotoxicity with this form of administration. Increased cerebral edema, seizures, and focal neurologic deficits have been reported. There is a 4% risk of brain infection with this mode of administration. Leukoencephalopathy has not been reported.

Mechlorethamine

Mechlorethamine is the original nitrogen mustard discovered in the development of biologic weapons during World War I. It continues to be an effective alkylating agent in the treatment of Hodgkin disease and other lymphomas. At standard IV dosages there is little risk of central neurotoxicity and peripheral neuropathy is not seen. With high-dose IV administration, as in preparation for bone marrow transplantation, encephalopathy, headache, and seizures have been reported within a few days of drug administration.[84] Spontaneous recovery is typical, although some patients are left with residual deficits. In the 1950s and 1960s, intracarotid mechlorethamine was used in the treatment of brain tumors and resulted in severe ipsilateral cerebral edema, uveitis, seizures, coma, focal neurologic deficits, and sometimes death.[85,86]

Estramustine

Estramustine is a nitrogen mustard linked to estradiol. It acts as an alkylating agent and also binds to tubulin and to microtubule-associated proteins, depolymerizes cytoplasmic microtubules, and thereby disrupts the nuclear matrix. Estramustine is primarily used in the treatment of refractory prostate cancer. Neurotoxicity is rare, although estramustine is associated with thrombotic microangiopathy and cerebral infarction.[87,88]

Busulfan

Busulfan in an alkylating agent that is not cell-cycle–specific. It interacts with cellular thiol groups and nucleic acids and produces cross-links between DNA molecules. It is a commonly used oral drug in the treatment of chronic myelogenous leukemia (CML) and is used intravenously in conditioning regimens for bone marrow transplantation. Busulfan crosses the blood–brain barrier rapidly with a CSF-to-plasma ratio of 1:1.

Generalized seizures have been reported in approximately 10% of patients receiving high-dose oral or IV busulfan, and are more common in adults than in children.[89] Busulfan-induced seizures are dose dependent, appear within 48 hours of drug administration, and may be prevented by the coadministration of anticonvulsants.[89] No other major neurotoxicity has been reported and long-term anticonvulsant therapy is generally not required.

Chlorambucil

Chlorambucil is an orally administered nitrogen mustard used primarily in the treatment of CLL and some lymphomas, often in conjunction with other chemotherapeutic agents. At standard dosages, neurotoxicity is extremely rare. Neurotoxicity associated with high-dose and overdose of chlorambucil has been reported. Seizures, delirium, and myoclonus occurred soon after drug ingestion.[90–92] Vision loss from retinopathy and optic nerve toxicity has been described after the administration of chlorambucil.[93,94]

Procarbazine

Procarbazine probably exerts its antineoplastic effect as an alkylating agent, although the exact mechanism of action is unknown. It is used primarily in the treatment of lymphoma and glioma, usually in combination with other chemotherapeutic agents. It was originally synthesized as an monoamine oxidase inhibitor (MAOI). Procarbazine is administered orally and crosses the blood–brain barrier readily. The drug itself has no antineoplastic activity, but its metabolites alkylate and methylate DNA.

Procarbazine is only administered orally, although at one time it was available in the intravenous formulation. IV procarbazine typically produced prolonged somnolence.[95] CNS effects are fairly common after high-dose oral therapy. These effects range from somnolence and depression to psychosis and obtundation.[96–98] These effects are generally self-limited and reversible. The drug may aggravate the sedative effects of other drugs including opioids, benzodiazepines, and neuroleptics. Hypertensive encephalopathy with headache and delirium are possible when procarbazine is used in conjunction with sympathomimetic agents or consumption of tyramine-containing products, because of the drug's weak MAOI activity. This rarely occurs in clinical practice, however.

Peripheral neuropathy is sometimes observed as a complication of procarbazine treatment.[99,100] When used in combination chemotherapy, peripheral neuropathy is more likely to be an effect of one of the other administered drugs, such as vincristine.

Thiotepa

Thiotepa is an alkylating agent related to nitrogen mustard. Thiotepa and its active metabolite TEPA are lipid-soluble, and readily cross the blood–brain barrier. It has been administered intravenously in the treatment of breast and ovarian tumors, as well as lymphoma. Thiotepa has been used as a component of an intensive chemotherapy regimen prior to autologous marrow transplantation for a variety of tumors. It may be used intrathecally for the treatment of leptomeningeal metastases and is directly instilled into the bladder for the treatment of superficial bladder cancer.

CNS toxicity after systemic administration is virtually unknown, although a diffuse, nonspecific encephalopathy may occur after high-dose IV administration.[24] Neurotoxicity is usually restricted to those patients receiving intra-CSF thiotepa for treatment of leptomeningeal metastases. A mild, reversible chemical meningitis is common in this setting. This syndrome is clinically identical to the chemical meningitis that may follow intra-CSF treatment with methotrexate and Ara-C. A transient or persistent myelopathy is a rare occurrence with intra-CSF thiotepa.[101] Demyelination of the posterior columns and dorsal roots was noted in these patients at postmortem examination. This effect appears to be idiosyncratic and not dose related.

Hexamethylmelamine

Hexamethylmelamine (altretamine) is an alkylating agent, although the mechanism of its antineoplastic activity is unknown. It is used primarily as a second-line agent in the treatment of ovarian cancer. Hexamethylmelamine crosses the blood–brain barrier in small amounts, although its metabolites readily enter the CNS. The most common CNS effects are headache, mild encephalopathy, and, rarely, seizures.[102,103] Ataxia, tremor, and parkinsonism have been reported.[104] These effects appear to be readily reversible when the drug is stopped. A mild, predominantly sensory, neuropathy occurs in approximately 30% of patients using this drug.[105]

Cyclophosphamide

Cyclophosphamide is an alkylating antineoplastic agent chemically related to the nitrogen mustards. It has a broad spectrum of activity against multiple solid tumors, including breast, lung, and ovarian tumors, as well as sarcomas. It is also used in combination chemotherapy for lymphomas and myeloma. Neurotoxicity is rare, although a mild, reversible encephalopathy with dizziness, blurred vision, and confusion is sometimes noted with high-dose IV infusions. A single case of seizure has been reported.[106]

Ifosfamide

Ifosfamide is an alkylating agent with structural similarities to cyclophosphamide and is used in multiagent regimens to treat a wide variety of solid and hematopoietic tumors. Although cyclophosphamide rarely produces neurotoxicity, ifosfamide produces CNS complications in as many as 20% to 40% of patients who receive high-dose ifosfamide therapy.[107–109] Fractionated IV doses over several days appears less likely to produce this effect than continued high-dose infusion or single large doses. Delirium, mutism, visual hallucinations, and seizures have been reported with ifosfamide.[110,111] Focal neurologic deficits, including cerebellar ataxia, facial nerve palsy, and aphasia, have been reported,[110] as has catatonia with bizarre affect.[112] These effects generally occur during or immediately after ifosfamide infusion. The electroencephalogram (EEG) typically shows diffuse, slow-wave activity, but usually no epileptiform activity.

The mechanism of these CNS effects is unknown, although the metabolite of ifosfamide, chloroacetaldehyde has been implicated. Chloroacetaldehyde shares structural similarity with metaldehyde, an epileptogenic derivative of ethanol. Treatment with benzodiazepines has been reported to produce immediate clinical and electrographic improvement in patients suffering ifosfamide neurotoxicity.[113] Methylene blue appears to reduce the incidence of ifosfamide-induced encephalopathy if it is given before ifosfamide, and may be helpful for symptomatic treatment once the encephalopathy has occurred.[114] Methylene blue prevents the formation of ifosfamide's centrally acting toxic aldehyde metabolites. A patient with ifosfamide-induced encephalopathy experienced improvement with IV thiamine.[115] Even without treatment, ifosfamide neurotoxicity is usually reversible once the drug is discontinued. This syndrome is rarely irreversible[116] or fatal.[117]

Ifosfamide infrequently produces peripheral neurotoxicity. A painful, length-dependent, sensorimotor, axonal neuropathy has been described.[118–120]

▶PLANT ALKALOIDS

Vinca Alkaloids

The vinca alkaloids include vincristine, vinblastine, vindesine, and vinorelbine. They are derived from the periwinkle plant and produce their antineoplastic effect by binding to tubulin and inhibiting microtubule formation in the mitotic spindle. Cell division is arrested in metaphase. These drugs have wide application in the treatment of leukemias, lymphomas, various carcinomas, sarcomas, and gliomas. Vincristine is the most commonly used drug in this group. The risk of neurotoxicity with the other vinca alkaloids appears to be less than that of vincristine.

A length-dependent, sensorimotor, axonal peripheral neuropathy is the most common neurologic complication with this group of drugs. The microtubular effects of vinca alkaloids disrupt axonal transport in the peripheral nervous system, leading to axonal degeneration. Some degree of peripheral neuropathy is present in the majority of patients receiving more than a few conventional doses of vincristine. The clinical spectrum ranges from an asymptomatic patient with absent or reduced ankle reflexes to one with painful paresthesias, bilateral foot drop, and autonomic dysfunction.[121,122] The risk of symptomatic peripheral neuropathy is dose-dependent and may be increased in elderly patients, in those who are poorly nourished, in those with preexisting neuropathies,[123,124] and in patients whose peripheral nerves are receiving concurrent radiation therapy.[125] Other neurotoxic chemotherapeutic agents and colony stimulating factors may increase the risk of developing vincristine neuropathy.[126,127]

Usually, the neuropathy is of gradual onset beginning with paresthesias in the feet and hands. Mild distal weakness may follow. Rarely, patients develop acute, fulminant symptoms and may present with a clinical picture similar to Guillain-Barré syndrome.[128] In most patients with mild to moderate peripheral neuropathy, the prognosis for recovery is quite good after the vinca alkaloid is discontinued,[129] although the ankle reflexes may never return.

Autonomic neuropathy with constipation, orthostatic hypotension, urinary retention, and erectile dysfunction[122,130,131] occurs in 20% to 60% of patients receiving vinca alkaloids. Cranial mononeuropathies are well described, particularly those involving the trigeminal and recurrent laryngeal nerves.[132,133] Ptosis, ophthalmoplegia, sensorineural hearing loss, and facial weakness have also been described in patients receiving vincristine.[134] Acute peripheral mononeuropathies occur rarely.[135]

Vinca alkaloids penetrate the blood–brain barrier poorly, and CNS effects are comparatively rare. On the rare occasion that vincristine has been administered intrathecally the effects were catastrophic, with ascending myelopathy, coma, and death.[136–139] Pathologic examination of the brain in such a patient has revealed diffuse necrosis in the brain and spinal cord in areas directly exposed to CSF.[138] Although CSF drainage and reperfusion have been attempted, no treatment is usually effective for this lethal treatment error.

Vinca alkaloids may produce SIADH, which, in turn, may cause encephalopathy and seizures. This effect is particularly common in patients receiving intensive hydration with their chemotherapy regimens.[140,141] Seizures have been reported with vincristine even in the absence of hyponatremia or other metabolic derangement.[142,143] One patient developed focal Jacksonian seizures shortly after a single injection of vincristine. Head CT and CSF examination showed no abnormalities, nor was any other metabolic derangement found.[143] Another leukemic patient developed generalized seizures during induction therapy with vincristine and prednisone. CT of the head revealed lucencies in the white matter. A brain biopsy revealed vacuolization and neurotubular dissociation on electron microscopy. When vincristine was discontinued, the encephalopathy and seizures resolved.[142]

Transient cortical blindness with clinical features very similar to those of posterior reversible leukoencephalopathy have been reported with vincristine, when used alone or in combination with other drugs.[144,145] Visual hallucinations have been reported in the absence of other signs or symptoms of neurologic dysfunction.[146] Transient ataxia, tremor, and parkinsonism have been rarely reported in conjunction with vincristine use.[147,148] A transient or permanent unilateral or bilateral optic neuropathy is a rare but reported complication of vincristine.[149–152] On pathologic examination some of these patients were noted to have loss of ganglion cells in the retina and selective loss of β-tubulin with the optic nerve.[151,152]

Etoposide and Teniposide

Both etoposide (VP16) and teniposide (VM-26) are semisynthetic derivatives of podophyllotoxin, an extract of the mandrake plant. Although the precise mechanism of action of these drugs is unknown, they are cell-cycle–specific, killing cells in G2 and S phases. Both etoposide and teniposide inhibit the enzyme topoisomerase II, producing single- and double-strand breaks in DNA and DNA/protein cross-links. Both drugs are used in the treatment of leukemias and lymphomas. Etoposide is widely used in combination chemotherapy for small cell lung cancer, germ cell tumors, and gliomas. Both drugs are highly protein bound and cross the blood–brain barrier very poorly. CNS and CSF levels are only a small fraction (0.3%–5%) of concurrent plasma levels.

CNS toxicity with either drug at standard doses is extremely rare. After large IV doses, severe headache, seizures, and encephalopathy have been reported with etoposide.[153] There is a single report of transient dystonia following the administration of etoposide for ALL.[154]

Peripheral neuropathy is a relatively rare complication of etoposide therapy, occurring in no more than 2% of patients receiving the drug.[155,156] Neuropathy is even less common with teniposide. The neuropathy with either drug is predominantly distal and sensory and usually resolves when the drug is stopped.

Taxanes

Paclitaxel and Docetaxel

Paclitaxel (Taxol) is a semisynthetic extract of the bark of the Western yew tree (*Taxus brevifolia*). The analogous drug docetaxel derives from needles of the European yew tree (*Taxus baccata*). Both of these drugs inhibit spindle formation producing mitotic arrest in dividing cells. They stabilize and produce polymerization of tubulin, promoting microtubule assembly and stable but malfunctioning microtubular structures.[157] Cancer cells are arrested in late G2 and M phases. These drugs also appear to act as radiosensitizers by synchronizing cellular arrest in the mitotic phase most sensitive to radiation.

Paclitaxel penetrates the blood–brain barrier very poorly and levels are not detectable in the CSF following IV administration. Very rarely, visual toxicity has been reported. Transient scintillating scotomas during paclitaxel infusion have been reported.[158] Some of these patients reported subjective visual loss. Visual evoked potentials were abnormal in some patients, but the ERGs were normal, suggesting localization to the optic nerve.[158,159] In most patients, the visual symptoms resolved when the drug was discontinued, although in a small number of patients the visual loss has been permanent. Generalized seizures and encephalopathy have been reported after paclitaxel administration.[160–163]

A symmetric, distal sensory, predominantly axonal, peripheral neuropathy is the most common neurologic complication of paclitaxel therapy. The neuropathy is dose dependent and is more likely to occur with higher cumulative doses and higher doses per cycle.[164] It occurs in more than 50% of patients receiving single doses over 250 mg/m^2 and cumulative dosages greater than 1000 mg/m^2 are invariably associated with development of sensorimotor, predominantly axonal neuropathy. An antecedent neuropathy appears to increase the risk of paclitaxel-induced neurotoxicity.[124,165] Sural nerve biopsy in patients with paclitaxel neuropathy shows axonal loss with secondary demyelination.[166]

Initial symptoms usually include painful paresthesias and sensory loss beginning in the feet, and may begin as soon as 48 hours after treatment. Large, sensory fiber dysfunction is more common than small fiber dysfunction. Loss of the ankle reflexes precedes generalized hyporeflexia. With more intensive dosing (>250 mg/m^2), distal motor weakness (usually mild) may develop. Apart from the optic nerves (see above), cranial nerves are usually not involved although bilateral facial nerve palsies have been reported.[167] Autonomic dysfunction with paralytic ileus and orthostatic hypotension have been rarely reported when paclitaxel was administered in the higher-dose range (170–250 mg/m^2).[168] Arthralgias and myalgias are very common during treatment with paclitaxel and a mild myopathy has been described.[165]

The peripheral nervous system effects of paclitaxel generally resolve spontaneously once the drug is discontinued. Deep tendon reflexes are often permanently reduced and some patients may experience persistent paresthesias which usually are not disabling. Symptomatic treatment with tricyclic antidepressants or gabapentin may be helpful in patients with paresthesias. Some preliminary data suggests that treatment with glutamine may prevent the development of paclitaxel-induced neuropathy,[169] although randomized, placebo-controlled trials are lacking.

Docetaxel (Taxotere) appears to be less neurotoxic than paclitaxel. It may produce a dose-dependent, predominantly sensory, axonal polyneuropathy similar to that of paclitaxel,[170] usually with cumulative doses greater than 600 mg/m^2.[171] Motor involvement is rare, as with paclitaxel.

Central nervous system toxicity is extremely rare with docetaxel, although transient encephalopathy and seizures have been reported.[172] Lhermitte phenomenon has been described in patients with docetaxel-induced peripheral neuropathy.[171,173]

Topoisomerase Inhibitors (Irinotecan, Topotecan, and Rubitecan)

These drugs share the ability to inhibit the enzyme topoisomerase I. Topoisomerase I relaxes torsional strain in DNA by producing reversible single strand breaks. Topotecan, irinotecan, and rubitecan bind the topoisomerase I–DNA complex and prevent religation of single-strand breaks. The cytotoxicity of topoisomerase inhibitors is a result of double-strand DNA damage occurring during DNA synthesis. Mammalian cells cannot effectively repair these double-strand breaks. These drugs are used to treat a variety of refractory solid tumors and some lymphomas and leukemias.

Topotecan has little or no neurotoxicity, although headache and lethargy have been reported during drug infusion.[174] Irinotecan is associated with nonspecific dizziness and insomnia during drug therapy. Several cases of dysarthria have been reported in conjunction with irinotecan administration.[175,176] One patient was receiving concomitant 5-FU, although the dysarthria only began during the irinotecan infusion.[175] Another patient developed dysarthria during infusion of monotherapy irinotecan.[177] In all cases, the dysarthria was short-lasting and resolved completely when the drug was discontinued. Rubitecan is a relatively new agent and no significant neurotoxicity has been associated with its use.

Pyrazoloacridine

Pyrazoloacridine (PZA) is a synthesized acridine derivative, which appears to be a dual inhibitor of the enzymes topoisomerase I and topoisomerase II, and diminishes the formation of topoisomerase–DNA adducts. In the experimental setting, it appears to have activity against a variety of solid tumors.

CNS neurotoxicity appears to be common and dose related.[178–180] Toxicities include irritability, anxiety, insomnia, nonspecific dizziness, delirium with hallucination, gait ataxia, and myoclonus. These adverse effects generally appear during or immediately after drug infusion and are transient and reversible. Some may be dose limiting.

►ANTINEOPLASTIC ANTIBIOTICS

Bleomycin

Bleomycin is an antibiotic that produces strand scission of DNA with single-strand breaks. It also inhibits DNA-directed RNA polymerase. Bleomycin is typically used in multiagent regimens for the treatment of lymphomas and germ cell tumors, as well as head and neck cancers. Neurotoxicity is rare with bleomycin; when it occurs, coadministered agents (i.e., cisplatin and vinca alkaloids) are more likely to be responsible. Encephalopathy, seizures, and visual disturbances have been reported,[181] but were more likely related to the other chemotherapeutic agents that the patient received. Cerebral infarction and peripheral neuropathy have been reported with bleomycin, but only when used in combination with other more neurotoxic agents.[182–184] making it difficult to implicate bleomycin as the responsible drug.

Doxorubicin, Daunorubicin

Both doxorubicin and daunorubicin are anthracycline antibiotics with antineoplastic activity against a broad spectrum of hematologic and solid tumors. They bind nucleic acids and disrupt the structure of DNA. Daunorubicin was discovered prior to doxorubicin and has no significant neurotoxicity.

Although doxorubicin produces pathologic changes in the dorsal root ganglia of laboratory animals, it is not known to produce peripheral neuropathy in humans. Doxorubicin does not cross the blood–brain barrier and is associated with no major central nervous system toxicity when administered intravenously. When administered intraarterially to treat brain tumors, doxorubicin produces cerebral infarcts and hemorrhagic necrosis.[185] Inadvertent intrathecal administration of doxorubicin or daunorubicin may produce an acute or subacute ascending myelopathy and encephalopathy that can be fatal.[186,187]

Cardiomyopathy with congestive heart failure and dysrhythmia may occur in a dose-dependent fashion in patients receiving doxorubicin. This, in turn, can predispose patients to embolic stroke.

Mitomycin C

Mitomycin C is an antineoplastic antibiotic that acts as an alkylating agent and inhibits DNA synthesis. It is used to treat adenocarcinomas of the breast, GI tract, and bladder. Neurotoxicity is rare, although there are reports of headache and CNS complications from mitomycin-induced disseminated intravascular coagulation and thrombotic microangiopathy.[188]

Mitoxantrone

Mitoxantrone is an antitumor antibiotic that intercalates into DNA causing strand breaks. It is also a potent inhibitor of topoisomerase II. Mitoxantrone has been used in the treatment of hormone refractory prostate cancer and non-lymphocytic leukemia.

Mitoxantrone is not associated with neurotoxicity when delivered systemically. However, when administered into the CSF it may produce a myeloradiculopathy.[189,190]

Nitroimidazoles (Misonidazole and Metronidazole)

Misonidazole and metronidazole are antimicrobial and antiprotozoal agents that are sometimes used in oncologic practice as radiosensitizers. These drugs are selective for hypoxic cells, impair nucleic acid synthesis, and produce DNA strand breakage.

Both drugs are highly toxic to the peripheral nerve and this effect is dose limiting in most patients.[191] The neuropathy is predominantly sensory and axonal in nature. It may remit or improve when misonidazole is discontinued. Sensorineural hearing loss has also been described.[192]

CNS toxicity of nitroimidazoles is relatively rare. As these drugs amplify the effects of radiation on tumor and normal tissue, they may theoretically increase the risk of radiation injury to neural tissues. This effect has never been definitively documented. Generalized seizures have been reported a few hours after the administration of large doses of metronidazole.[193] Diffuse encephalopathy has been occasionally noted, usually in patients who are dehydrated and severely debilitated, and who have received high doses of nitroimidazole.[194–196]

Plicamycin (Mithramycin)

Plicamycin is an antibiotic neoplastic agent used primarily in the treatment of hypercalcemia caused by malignancy. It is rarely used in the United States because of the high frequency of coagulopathy in association with this drug and the development of more effective, safer treatments for hypercalcemia. Drowsiness and headache are common adverse effects of plicamycin.

Suramin

Suramin is a polysulfonated naphthylurea antiparasitic agent that exerts its antitumor effects by blocking the activity of DNA primase and polymerase, and by inhibiting the activity of several growth factors. It is used primarily in the treatment of hormone-refractory prostate cancer, although it has been used experimentally in the treatment of other solid tumors. Peripheral neuropathy is an extremely common dose-related toxicity of suramin. The most common neuropathy is a length-dependent, axonal, sensorimotor polyneuropathy, which may occur in as many as 80% of patients, particularly in those receiving higher dosages of medication.[197] It typically presents with paresthesiae and mild distal leg weakness. The mechanism of this axonal neuropathy is thought to be an effect of suramin blocking nerve growth factor (NGF),[198] an effect on the nerve mitochondrial DNA,[199] and ceramide accumulation within the neuron leading to apoptotic cell death.[200]

Approximately 15% of patients develop a subacute demyelinating polyradiculoneuropathy resembling Guillain-Barré syndrome with bulbar and respiratory involvement during or shortly after treatment with suramin.[201,202] In these latter patients, nerve conduction studies show conduction block, CSF protein levels are elevated, and nerve biopsy shows demyelination with inflammatory changes. The demyelinating neuropathy occurs primarily in those patients with high peak serum concentrations of suramin,[202] and may be a result of an immunomodulatory effect of the drug. The demyelinating neuropathy typically remits with plasma exchange or intravenous immunoglobulin (IVIg) and with the discontinuance of suramin.

▶MISCELLANEOUS AGENTS

Retinoids

Tretinoin and alitretinoin are synthetic analogues of naturally occurring vitamin A (retinol); they induce cellular differentiation in some tumors, notably acute promyelocytic leukemia, and Kaposi sarcoma. These drugs have been used experimentally to treat a variety of solid tumors. Isotretinoin is used primarily in the treatment of cystic acne. Retinoids readily cross the blood–brain barrier. The most common neurologic side effect of these drugs is headache, which occurs in 50% to 80% of patients receiving higher dosages,[203–205] and is typically dose limiting. Most patients with retinoid-induced headache have no signs of raised intracranial pressure, although a small percentage of patients develop headache as a result of retinoid-induced pseudotumor cerebri.[206] These patients have the typical presentation of pseudotumor cerebri with headache and visual obscuration. It has been proposed that retinoids reduce CSF resorption at the level of the arachnoid granulations.[207] In all patients, with or without pseudotumor cerebri, the headache resolves after the retinoid is discontinued. If discontinuing the retinoid is impracticable, pseudotumor cerebri may respond to treatment with repeated lumbar puncture.[208]

Visual disturbances may occur in the absence of pseudotumor and include abnormal color vision and transient visual loss. Oculogyric crisis has been reported in conjunction with isotretinoin.[209] A single case of multiple mononeuropathies has been described in a patient with acute promyelocytic leukemia and disseminated intravascular coagulation (DIC) who was receiving tretinoin.[210] Ataxia has been rarely described after use of large amounts of topical tretinoin.[211] These effects are reversible when the drug is discontinued.

L-Asparaginase

L-Asparagine is an amino acid required for synthesis of many cellular proteins. Normal human cells contain the enzyme L-asparagine synthetase and can manufacture adequate quantities of L-asparagine. Some tumor cells lack sufficient L-asparagine synthetase to produce their own supply of the amino acid and must instead obtain it from the extracellular compartment. L-Asparaginase is a bacterial-derived enzyme that hydrolyzes L-asparagine to aspartic acid and ammonia. It depletes the extracellular supply of L-asparagine, thus "starving" tumor cells of L-asparagine and inhibiting protein synthesis in sensitive tumor cells. Fortunately, normal human cells contain within their cytoplasm high levels of L-asparagine synthetase, rendering L-asparaginase nontoxic to these cells. L-Asparaginase is used almost exclusively in the treatment of ALL, usually in combination with other antileukemic drugs. L-Asparagine is a very large protein that does not cross the blood–brain barrier to any significant degree; virtually none is detected in the CSF after IV administration. The drug is, however, associated with several unique forms of central neurotoxicity.

Diffuse encephalopathy, cerebral venous and dural sinus thrombosis with venous infarction, and cerebral hemorrhage are the most frequently noted CNS effects of L-asparaginase. The mechanism of diffuse encephalopathy from L-asparaginase is unclear, but appears to be dose related. The encephalopathy is acute or subacute and may result from hepatic toxicity and hyperammonemia.[212] In the early days of L-asparaginase use, high dosages were used. Encephalopathy developed in 33% to 60% of these patients within the first 24 hours of drug administration.[213,214] Symptoms ranged from mild lethargy and subtle personality change to coma and, rarely, death. Focal neurologic deficits (hemiparesis, hemianopia) were sometimes noted.[212] Seizures were relatively rare with this form of L-asparaginase toxicity, although EEGs were noted to be abnormal with diffuse slowing and triphasic waves,[215,216] the same electrographic abnormalities typically seen in hepatic encephalopathy from other causes. Some neurologically normal patients had slowing on EEG after the administration of L-asparaginase.[215] Very high serum ammonia levels were noted in most patients with L-asparaginase encephalopathy in whom it was checked.[215] The encephalopathy usually resolves a few days after stopping L-asparaginase. It appears to be much less common with the currently recommended lower dosages of L-asparaginase. Occasionally, this diffuse encephalopathy occurs after cumulative doses and even as a delayed phenomenon.

The cerebrovascular complications of L-asparaginase are potentially more serious, but, fortunately, less common.[217] L-Asparaginase depletes serum levels of hemostatic factors, including fibrinogen, antithrombin III, proteins C and S, and factors IX and X, as well as fibrinolytic enzymes (including plasminogen), in most patients. Serum prothrombin time (PT), partial thromboplastin time (PTT), and thrombin time typically rise during treatment, even in asymptomatic patients.[218] Fortunately, only a small percentage of patients develop ischemic or hemorrhagic complications.

The most common cerebrovascular complication of L-asparaginase is cerebral venous or dural sinus thrombosis with venous infarction and sometimes hemorrhage.[218–221] The first symptom of cerebral venous thrombosis is usually severe headache of acute or subacute onset. The headache has features of raised intracranial pressure: worse with reclining posture, aggravated by Valsalva maneuvers, and associated with vomiting and visual obscuration. Papilledema may be present. Seizures (generalized or partial) and reduced level of consciousness are common. Focal neurologic deficits may be present if venous infarction has occurred. Thrombosis in veins in other parts of the body may occur, although arterial thrombosis in the brain or elsewhere is rare with L-asparaginase.[217,222] In most patients, venous sinus thrombosis will occur during the course of treatment with L-asparaginase and only rarely will occur as a delayed phenomenon.

Brain CT and MRI may show venous infarction adjacent to the thrombosed vein or dural sinus. Hemorrhage may be seen as can diffuse cerebral edema. With superior sagittal sinus thrombosis, there is an absence of contrast in the sinus. On CT and MRI axial contrasted views, this is referred to as the "empty delta sign."[223] Brain MRI is the best diagnostic test when done in conjunction with magnetic resonance venogram (MRV). MRV will demonstrate lack of filling in the involved sinus (Fig. 31-4).

The appropriate initial therapy for this complication is to stop the L-asparaginase. Anticoagulation with heparin is appropriate if frank hemorrhage is absent. Fresh-frozen plasma may prevent extension of the thrombus.

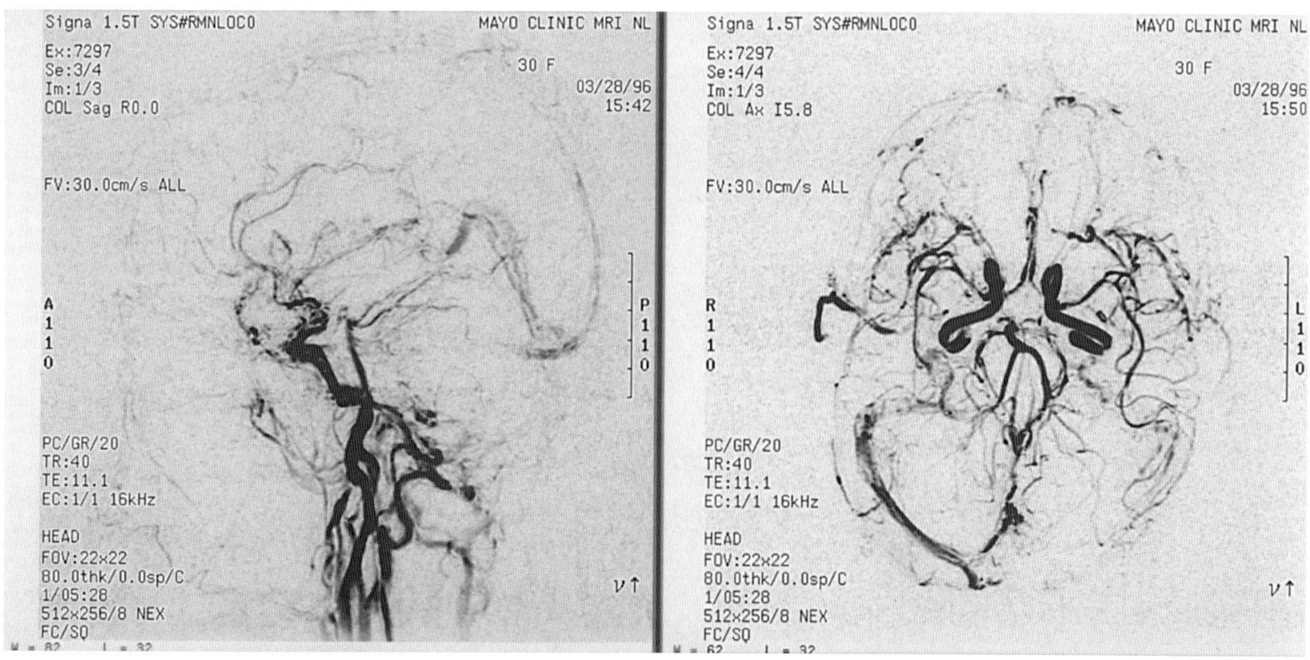

Figure 31-4. Venous sinus thrombosis in association with L-asparaginase. Magnetic resonance angiography/MRV demonstrating reduced flow in the superior sagittal and left lateral venous sinuses.

Corticosteroids and opioids are helpful symptomatic treatments for the headache and raised intracranial pressure. Most patients make a good recovery, even in the presence of intracerebral hemorrhage, without need for long term anticoagulation therapy.[224] Thrombosis may recur with subsequent courses of L-asparaginase.

Thalidomide

Thalidomide was originally used for its sedative properties. Later it was withdrawn from the market after it was found to produce limb agenesis (phocomelia) and other congenital anomalies in the fetuses of women taking the drug. Thalidomide has since been reintroduced as an immunomodulatory and antiangiogenesis agent to treat a variety of conditions, including malignancy. The drug is noted to have activity against myeloma, breast and prostate cancer, myeloma, Kaposi sarcoma, and glioblastoma multiforme.

Varying degrees of somnolence are extremely common with thalidomide use. Sedation is most prominent when therapy is first started and tends to subside with time.[225,226] Headache is an infrequent occurrence,[227] and seizures, when they occur, are primarily in patients with underlying epileptogenic brain disease.[228] Length-dependent, axonal, sensorimotor peripheral neuropathy occurs in a large percentage of patients, although the reported incidence varies widely in the literature.[229,230] It is not strictly dose related, but tends to occur earlier in patients receiving high-dose thalidomide than in those receiving lower doses. Clear correlation between the dose of thalidomide and the duration of therapy has not been unequivocally established.[231,232] Thalidomide neuropathy may be more likely to develop in those patients with preexisting peripheral neuropathy from other causes.[124] The neuropathy typically affects sensory more than motor function, and presents with painful acral paresthesias and sensory loss. Strength is usually preserved and deep tendon reflexes are reduced in the distal extremities. Thalidomide usually does not produce an autonomic neuropathy. Orthostatic hypotension and bradycardia are common, however, probably as a consequence of central sedative effects of the drug or activation of the vasovagal system. Nerve conduction studies show that sensory nerve action potentials (SNAPs) are reduced more than compound muscle action potentials (CMAPs). Sural nerve biopsy shows loss of predominantly large myelinated fibers with no inflammation.[229] The symptoms of neuropathy may improve when thalidomide is stopped, but sensory loss, hyporeflexia, and nerve conduction study abnormalities may be permanent.

Bacillus Calmette-Guérin

Bacillus Calmette-Guérin (BCG), a live-attenuated strain of *Mycobacterium bovis*, is most commonly used as a vaccine to promote active immunity to tuberculosis because of its immunologic similarity to *Mycobacterium tuberculosis*. BCG is also a potent stimulator of the host immune responses and is used as a biologic response modifier in the treatment of several tumors, including in situ carcinoma of the bladder, lymphoma, leukemia, melanoma, and breast and prostate cancer. For in situ carcinoma of the bladder, BCG is repeatedly instilled into the bladder over many months.

Although, BCG is an attenuated strain of *M. bovis*, it is capable of producing infection, particularly in those patients who are immunocompromised and those who are exposed to large amounts of BCG over prolonged periods. Pulmonary granulomas, miliary disease, and psoas abscess have resulted from *M. bovis* infection.[233–235] BCG has been reported to produce meningitis in three patients receiving intrathecal methotrexate in which BCG was a contaminant.[236] Rarely, *M. bovis* meningitis has been reported in patients receiving BCG vaccination.[237] We have seen a patient who developed an indolent, fatal *M. bovis* meningitis and psoas abscess after extensive therapy with intravesical BCG for bladder carcinoma in situ.

Interferons

Interferon (INF)-α, INF-β, and INF-γ are a diverse group of cytokines with cytotoxic, immunoregulatory, and antiviral activity. In oncologic practice, IFN-α has been used in the treatment of numerous hematologic malignancies including hairy-cell leukemia, CML, and several solid tumors, including melanoma, renal cell carcinoma, and Kaposi sarcoma. IFN-β and IFN-γ have not been employed in antineoplastic therapy and their toxicities are similar to those of IFN-α.

Flu-like symptoms with lethargy, myalgias, and low-grade fever occur within a few hours of IFN injection. CNS effects may include cognitive slowing, personality change, somnolence, and headache. Depression, mania, and other psychiatric effects are common with IFN therapy,[238] particularly in patients with preexisting psychiatric illness.[239] These neurologic and psychiatric effects appear to be dose related and are more common in elderly patients, in patients with preexisting brain lesions, and in patients who have undergone brain radiation.[240,241] Patients with primary and metastatic brain tumors often develop symptoms from increased cerebral edema following IFN administration. Otherwise unsuspected and asymptomatic brain lesions have been unmasked in cancer patients receiving IFN, many of whom developed diffuse encephalopathy.[240] Some patients with brain metastases who received IFN developed other unusual symptoms or signs, including parkinsonism, catatonia, akathisia, and visual hallucinations. Visual loss has been reported in patients receiving IFN-α and evidence of ischemic retinopathy may be detected, even in asymptomatic patients.[242–244] There have been several reports of children developing spastic diplegia during treatment with IFN.[245,246] Intraventricular administration of IFN has produced a severe encephalopathy with seizures and a prolonged vegetative state.[247,248]

With encephalopathy from systemically administered IFN, the EEG usually shows diffuse slow wave activity,[249] although epileptiform activity has been noted in a few patients.[250] No specific neuroimaging abnormalities have been described in IFN-induced encephalopathy, although some patients have been noted to have generalized cortical atrophy or nonspecific white matter changes.[240,251] Significant white matter signal changes have been noted in patients receiving intraventricular IFN for treatment of leptomeningeal tumor.[247]

In most patients, the neurologic and psychiatric effects resolve after the IFN is discontinued. In some patients, the neurologic and psychiatric sequelae persist,[251] or symptoms may recur if the patient is rechallenged with the drug.

The mechanism of IFN neurotoxicity is unknown. IFN may compete with naturally occurring neurotrophic hormones and brain opioids or may induce neurotoxic cytokines. Opioid antagonists and antidepressants have had some efficacy in preventing or treating IFN-induced encephalopathy and mood disorders.[252–255]

Peripheral nervous system toxicity is rare with IFN treatment. However, sensorineural hearing loss, peripheral neuropathy, and painless, reversible bilateral brachial plexopathy have been infrequently described.[256–258] Bauherz and associates[259] described a single patient with hairy-cell leukemia who developed bilateral oculomotor nerve palsies while receiving IFN-α. A Guillain-Barré–like syndrome has been reported after treatment with IFN-α for CML.[260] The neuropathies resolved after treatment was discontinued. Two patients who received IFN-α for treatment of malignancies developed myasthenia gravis during the course of their treatment.[261] In both cases, the symptoms of myasthenia gravis remitted after IFN therapy was discontinued, but each patient continued to have detectable acetylcholine receptor antibody several years later.

Interleukins

Interleukins (ILs), like interferons, are cytokines that have immunomodulatory and antineoplastic effects. They induce the transformation and proliferation of lymphocytes to cytolytic effector cells (lymphokine-activated killer [LAK] and natural killer [NK] cells). IL-4 and IL-2 are used as antineoplastic agents. IL-3, IL-6, and IL-11 are hematopoietic growth factors used in conjunction with chemotherapy to reduce hematologic toxicity. Their neurotoxicity is discussed under "Growth Factors" below. IL-2 is used most commonly to treat renal cell carcinoma and melanoma. It may be used alone or in combination with LAK cells. IL-4 is employed in the treatment of Hodgkin disease, non-Hodgkin lymphoma (NHL), and CLL.

IL-2 increases capillary permeability and may produce a "vascular leak" syndrome with peripheral edema, ascites, and pleural effusion. In patients with gliomas or metastatic brain tumors, IL-2 commonly produces increased peritumoral edema from increased vascular permeability.[262] This may be associated with somnolence, increased neurologic deficits, seizures, and headache. Cerebral water content increases in patients without intracranial metastases who have received IV IL-2,[262] although mental status changes were milder and more transient in these patients. Coma has been seen after IL-2 administration in patients without preexisting brain disease.[263,264] Most patients who develop IL-2 encephalopathy return to baseline a few weeks after IL-2 is discontinued.

Neuropsychiatric symptoms are extremely common after systemic administration of IL-2 with or without LAK cells.[265] These effects appear to be dose-related and are more common after prolonged courses of treatment with IL-2. These abnormalities include depression, delusions, hallucinations and evidence of cognitive impairment.

Rarely, patients receiving systemic IL-2 may develop focal neurologic deficits including monocular visual loss or homonymous quadrantanopia,[266] quadriparesis,[267] hemiparesis, aphasia, apraxia, and cortical blindness.[268] MRI may be normal or show multiple areas of cortical and subcortical T_2 signal abnormality.[267,268] In most of these patients, the neurologic deficits and MRI abnormalities resolved after IL-2 was discontinued. There is one report of a patient dying of multifocal cerebral venous thrombosis and acute subdural and subarachnoid hemorrhage after receiving IL-2 and granulocyte-macrophage colony-stimulating factor (GM-CSF) for treatment of renal cell carcinoma.[269] What role IL-2 may have played is speculative.

Peripheral nervous system toxicity is extremely rare. IL-2 has been reported to produce a reversible, painful brachial plexopathy with similarities to Parsonage-Turner syndrome.[270]

Progressive subcortical dementia with diffuse leukoencephalopathy after intraventricular administration of IL-2 for leptomeningeal tumor has been reported.[271] There is a report of a patient with a fatal diffuse leukoencephalopathy following IV treatment with IL-2.[272]

As with IFN, the mechanism of neurotoxicity is unknown. IL-2 is known to stimulate release of neuroendocrine hormones, including β-endorphin, corticotropin (ACTH), and cortisol.[273] IL-2 stimulates the production and release of tumor necrosis factor-α (TNF-α) and other cytokines, which may mediate the toxic effects on CNS neurons and glia.

IL-4 appears to have much less serious neurotoxicity than IL-2. Headache, lethargy, and fatigue are quite common and appear to be dose related.[274] Visual hallucinations may occur, but appear to be quite rare.[275]

Tumor Necrosis Factor-α

TNF-α (Tasonermin) is a cytokine with immunomodulatory and cytotoxic activity. It has been used to treat melanoma and sarcoma. Headache and fatigue are commonly associated with its use.[276] Focal peripheral neuropathies have been reported in patients receiving isolated limb perfusion of TNF-α.[277] The neuropathy was mild, predominantly sensory, and improved over time.

Growth Factors

These are drugs used in conjunction with chemotherapy to reduce hematologic toxicity. They include GM-CSF, erythropoietin, IL-3, IL-6, and IL-11.

Granulocyte-Macrophage Colony-Stimulating Factor

Transient headache, fatigue, nonspecific dizziness, mild confusion and paresthesias are common with GM-CSF and are not dose limiting. More serious nervous system effects are extremely rare. Bone pain is fairly common after the administration of GM-CSF and occasionally may be mistaken for bony metastases or radicular pain from epidural or leptomeningeal disease. There is a report of a patient on chronic interferon therapy for hepatitis C developing a fatal diffuse encephalopathy with gait disturbance after receiving several weeks of treatment with GM-CSF.[278] Autopsy revealed diffuse polyclonal lymphoid infiltrates throughout the CNS.

Erythropoietin

This is a synthetic glycoprotein that stimulates red cell production. Neurologic toxicity is very rare with this medication. Visual hallucinations have been reported with erythropoietin use.[279,280] Ischemic stroke may be more common in patients receiving erythropoietin because of the potential for polycythemia, hyperviscosity, and hypertension.[281] Cerebral venous thrombosis has been reported and attributed to erythropoietin-induced polycythemia.[282] Hypertension, headache, and seizures associated with a reversible posterior leukoencephalopathy have been reported in patients on dialysis receiving erythropoietin.[283]

Interleukin-3

IL-3 is a recombinant hematopoietic growth factor that improves neutrophil and platelet counts in patients with chemotherapy-induced bone marrow dysfunction and in myelodysplastic syndromes. Dose-dependent lethargy and headache, sometimes associated with nuchal rigidity, are relatively common in patients receiving this drug.[284,285]

Interleukin-6

IL-6 is a cytokine that hastens platelet recovery after chemotherapy. Nervous system toxicity is rare and usually limited to headache and fatigue at standard dosages. With higher doses, transient ataxia, hemiparesis, hallucinations, and delirium have been reported.[286]

Interleukin-11

IL-11 is a thrombopoietic growth factor that promotes the production of megakaryocyte progenitor cells. It is used primarily to increase the platelet count in patients receiving chemotherapy. Headache, fatigue, arthralgias, myalgias, and nonspecific dizziness occur in a sizable minority of patients receiving IL-11 at standard dosages.[287] Cerebral infarction was described in one patient while receiving IL-11.[288] A single patient receiving IL-11 for treatment of refractory idiopathic thrombocytopenic purpura developed a "systemic neuropathy" that apparently resolved after the IL-11 was discontinued.[289]

Hormonal Therapy

Tamoxifen

Tamoxifen citrate is a nonsteroidal estrogen receptor antagonist used most frequently in the treatment of estrogen receptor-positive breast cancer. Independent of its antiestrogen effects, tamoxifen inhibits and modulates protein kinase C, a key enzyme in transduction of various cellular responses to hormones, some growth factors, and neurotransmitters. Consequently, tamoxifen has been used experimentally in the treatment of gliomas, which are also solid tumors that lack estrogen receptors. Neurotoxicity is extremely rare. Visual system toxicity is the commonest and best described. Kaiser-Kupfer and Lippman first reported retinopathy and keratopathy in four women who had received large doses of tamoxifen for periods longer than 1 year.[290] The most common initial symptom of tamoxifen retinopathy is decreased visual acuity and central scotoma.[291] Retinal edema and pigmentary changes may be seen. ERGs are abnormal in some patients. Optic neuritis has also been noted in a few patients receiving tamoxifen.[292] The pathophysiology of tamoxifen-induced retinopathy and optic neuritis is unknown. Axonal degeneration in the nerve fiber layer and inner plexiform layer of the retina in one patient with high-dose tamoxifen-associated retinopathy has been reported.[293]

Although most patients who developed visual complications had received high cumulative doses of tamoxifen (>100 g) over prolonged periods of time, one patient with optic neuritis developed symptoms after only 3 weeks of low-dose therapy.[294] Other patients with retinopathy have received relatively low cumulative doses of tamoxifen.[295,296] In most cases, the visual symptoms resolved after the drug was discontinued.

Headache is a fairly frequent adverse effect in patients receiving tamoxifen, particularly in those patients with a previous history of migraine.[297] A reversible encephalopathy with prominent psychiatric manifestations[298] and cerebellar dysfunction[299] has been reported in association with tamoxifen use. Symptoms resolved within a few weeks of discontinuing the drug. Although tamoxifen increases the risk of vascular thrombosis, an excess risk of cerebrovascular thrombosis has not been firmly established.[300]

Toremifene

Toremifene is an antiestrogen agent with chemical similarities to tamoxifen. It is used primarily in the treatment of breast cancer. Headache, tremor, and vertigo are the most common neurologic effects of this drug.[301] Retinal and optic nerve toxicity have not been reported.

Leuprolide

Leuprolide is a gonadotrophin-releasing hormone analogue used primarily in the treatment of prostate cancer. Headache and nonspecific dizziness are the most common neurologic complications of leuprolide. At the initiation of therapy, leuprolide may transiently increase bone pain[302] by temporarily stimulating prostate tumor growth. Epidural cord compression may transiently worsen by the same mechanism.[303] Leuprolide is usually administered in conjunction with flutamide to reduce this risk. Pituitary apoplexy has occurred in patients receiving leuprolide with previously asymptomatic pituitary adenomas.[304–306] The mechanism is unknown but presumably relates to transient stimulation of gonadotrophic cells within the adenoma. A single patient with previous brain injury developed atypical absence seizures while receiving leuprolide, which resolved when leuprolide was discontinued.[307] Both an inflammatory and noninflammatory myopathy have been reported in conjunction with leuprolide use.[308,309] In both cases, drug withdrawal resulted in clinical remission.

Goserelin

Goserelin is a synthetic analogue of gonadotrophin-releasing hormone used primarily in the treatment of prostate cancer and in palliation of advanced breast cancer. Headache and fatigue are the most common neurologic effects. As with leuprolide, pituitary apoplexy has been reported in conjunction with goserelin use in patients with previously unsuspected pituitary macroadenomas.[310] Transient progression of prostate cancer has been observed in the first few weeks of treatment. This has produced epidural cord compression in a small percentage of patients.[311]

Danazol

Danazol is a synthetic steroid analogue with antigonadotrophic properties. It is used primarily in the treatment of metastatic breast cancer, endometrial cancer and the treatment of myelodysplastic syndromes. Benign headache, fatigue, and irritability are the most common neurologic adverse effects with this drug. Pseudotumor cerebri is associated both with administration of danazol and with its withdrawal.[312–314] In one case, cerebral vein thrombosis was noted.[312] Danazol may increase the risk of both arterial and venous thrombosis.[315] Several cases of cerebral vein thrombosis have been described,[312,316] as has arterial thrombosis.[317] Carpal tunnel syndrome is associated with danazol use.[313,318] A single case of rapidly reversible hearing loss has been described with danazol administration.[319] A single case of Guillain-Barré syndrome contemporaneous with danazol use for treatment of hereditary angioedema has been reported.[320] A relationship was postulated relating to danazol's effects on circulating immune complexes and complement.

Aromatase inhibitors (Anastrazole, Letrozole, Aminoglutethimide)

Anastrazole, letrozole, and aminoglutethimide are all aromatase inhibitors that inhibit steroid synthesis. All three drugs are employed in the treatment of breast cancer. Aminoglutethimide is also used in the treatment of Cushing syndrome, adrenal carcinoma, and prostate cancer. No serious peripheral or central nervous system toxicity has been reported with any of these drugs. Fatigue, headache, dizziness, and nonspecific paresthesias are fairly common adverse effects.

Octreotide

Octreotide is a long-acting somatostatin analogue used primarily in the treatment of gastrointestinal neuroendocrine tumors and acromegaly. Radiolabeled octreotide is sometimes useful in the diagnosis of neuroendocrine derived tumors. Headache, fatigue, insomnia, and vertigo are the most common neurologic effects of the drug.[321] Back pain and myalgias are also fairly common.

Mitotane

Mitotane has selective cytotoxic effects on the mitochondria of cells of the adrenal cortex. The precise mechanism of action is unknown, although the drug is known to block adrenal steroid 11-β-hydroxylation and reduces the production of adrenal corticosteroids. It is used in the treatment of tumors of carcinomas of the adrenal cortex.

Lethargy and headache are common adverse effects of mitotane. Less commonly, mitotane may produce cognitive slowing, ataxia, and language disorders.[322] Pigmentary retinopathy, optic neuritis, diplopia, and lens opacities also have been rarely reported.[323,324]

Corticosteroids

Corticosteroids are some of the most frequently prescribed medications in oncologic practice. They possess antiinflammatory, antiedema, antiemetic, analgesic, and appetite and mood-enhancing effects, making them indispensable in the treatment of cancer and treatment-related complications. Moreover, corticosteroids have an oncolytic effect in some tumors, particularly lymphoma, myeloma, and leukemia. All corticosteroids penetrate the blood–brain barrier well. In neuro-oncologic practice, dexamethasone and prednisone are used most frequently.

Corticosteroids are potent immunosuppressants and their use may predispose patients to a multitude of opportunistic infections. This adverse effect is not discussed further in this chapter.

Mild psychiatric disturbances are the most common CNS effect of corticosteroids and occur in as many as 50% of patients receiving these drugs, particularly at higher dosage levels.[325] Subtle elevation in mood is the most common effect, although hypomania and depression are also common. Severe psychiatric disorders including mania, psychosis, and major depression are rare, occurring in less than 5% of patients.[326] The incidence of these disorders is higher when larger doses of corticosteroid are used and in patients with preexisting psychiatric illness. Steroid-induced psychiatric disturbances resolve when the drug is tapered and discontinued.

Corticosteroids can produce a delirium characterized by a fluctuating level of awareness and global cognitive dysfunction. Visual hallucinations and delusions are common. The patient may become mute and withdrawn or vigorously combative. Other causes of delirium should be excluded. Corticosteroid-induced delirium resolves when the drug is discontinued. Treatment with antipsychotics may be indicated if the delirium is severe and if the corticosteroid cannot be discontinued. Rarely, withdrawal of the corticosteroid can produce transient agitation or delirium.

Insomnia is extremely common with corticosteroid use, both as a direct effect of the drug and as a result of the urinary frequency that commonly results from corticosteroid use. With higher doses, intractable hiccoughs, sometimes lasting days or weeks, are a bothersome side effect.[327] Chlorpromazine or nifedipine are sometimes effective therapy in this setting. Corticosteroids typically produce an action and static tremor identical to benign essential tremor. Moreover, corticosteroids aggravate a preexisting essential tremor.

A peculiar and very common effect noted with IV bolus doses of corticosteroid, particularly dexamethasone, is intense perineal burning and itching.[328] This effect last seconds to minutes during or immediately after the bolus infusion. It does not occur with oral administration or slow IV infusion. This side effect is entirely benign and not usually troublesome if the patient is forewarned.

Corticosteroids redistribute body fat from the extremities to the trunk, producing the “cushingoid habitus.” Fat may also accumulate in the mediastinum and epidural space. Epidural lipomatosis is usually asymptomatic and of no clinical significance. On rare occasion, it may produce a cauda equina syndrome or cord compression.[329,330] Spine and radicular pain may be present. Epidural lipomatosis is sometimes clinically mistaken for epidural tumor. Spine MRI demonstrates diffusely increased signal along the dorsal aspect of the spinal cord on T_2-weighted images. The epidural fat pad displaces the cord ventrally. Laminectomy with debulking of fat is rarely required, but is indicated in patients with symptomatic myelopathy. Epidural lipomatosis will eventually resolve once the corticosteroids are discontinued.

Corticosteroid-induced myopathy is a common adverse effect of treatment, developing in as many as 60% of patients receiving corticosteroids for more than a few weeks.[331] The risk of steroid myopathy is dependent on the dose and length of treatment. The myopathy typically presents with painless, predominantly proximal weakness. Dysphagia is extremely rare, and extraocular muscles and facial muscles are not affected. The myopathy will resolve when the corticosteroids are tapered.

Some patients experience symptoms when corticosteroids are tapered or discontinued. These symptoms include depression, myalgias, arthralgias (steroid pseudorheumatism) and headache. Pseudotumor cerebri is a rare consequence of steroid withdrawal.[332]

Monoclonal Antibodies

OKT3

OKT3, muromonab CD3, is a murine-derived, antilymphocyte, monoclonal antibody used primarily as an immunosuppressant agent in the prevention and treatment of graft-versus-host disease in patients who have received bone marrow transplants and organ allografts. It has been used experimentally in conjunction with IL-2 as an antineoplastic agent without great success.[333]

With initial doses, OKT3 produces a massive release of cytokines, including IL-2, IL-3, IL-6, and TNF, as a result of T-cell activation or lysis. Headache, fever, chills, and malaise characterize the accompanying clinical syndrome. The most frequently associated neurologic syndrome is a diffuse encephalopathy with headache, hallucinations, myoclonic jerks, focal or generalized seizures, and cortical blindness[334,335] often developing within a few hours of drug administration. Akinetic mutism and anomic aphasia have been reported in conjunction with the encephalopathy,[336] as have bilateral optic neuritis and transient sixth nerve palsies.[337] The mechanism appears to be an aseptic meningoencephalitis with breakdown of the blood–brain barrier. Brain MRI may be normal, reveal T_2 signal abnormalities in the subcortical white matter with cerebral edema, or show evidence of diffuse leptomeningeal enhancement (Fig. 31-5).[337,338] CSF examination typically demonstrates inflammatory changes with increased protein, normal glucose, and pleocytosis with a predominance of neutrophils. The clinical, CSF, and radiographic abnormalities usually

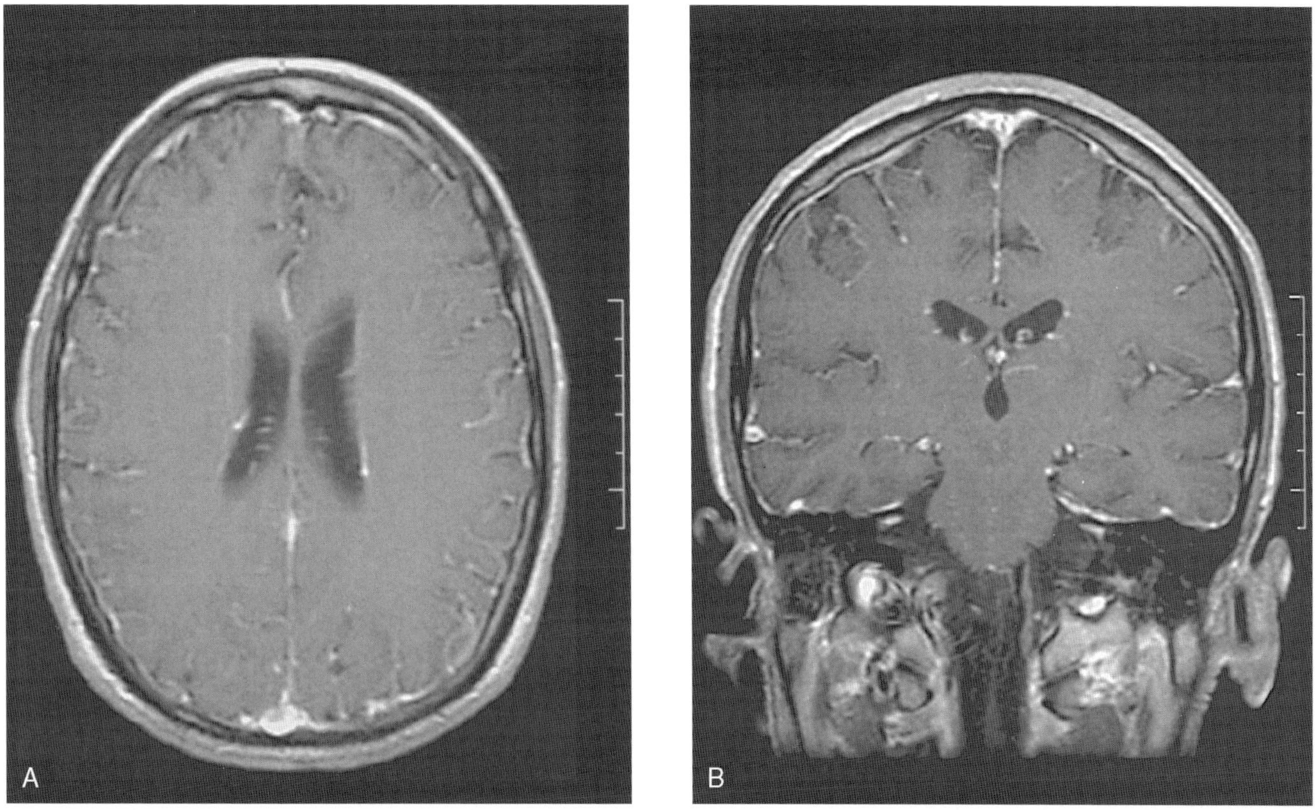

Figure 31-5. OKT3 aseptic meningitis. (A) Axial and (B) coronal T_1-weighted MRI with gadolinium, demonstrating diffuse leptomeningeal enhancement in a patient who had recently received OKT3.

resolve spontaneously within a few days of discontinuing OKT3. The syndrome may recur with readministration of OKT3.

Posttransplant lymphoproliferative disease and frank lymphoma involving the CNS may occur in patients receiving immunosuppressant therapy that includes OKT3.[339,340] This disorder is usually associated with latent Epstein-Barr viral infection and may resolve if the immunosuppressant is discontinued.

Rituximab

Rituximab (Rituxan) is a murine/human chimeric monoclonal antibody specific for the CD20 surface marker on B cells. It is used primarily in the treatment of non-Hodgkin lymphoma. Significant neurotoxicity is rare with rituximab, although headache, nonspecific dizziness, and paresthesias are fairly common during the first infusion.

Trastuzumab

Trastuzumab (Herceptin) is an anti–p185-HER2 monoclonal antibody used in the treatment of metastatic breast tumors that overexpress HER2 protein. Neurotoxicity is limited to mild headache and fatigue, although trastuzumab is often used in conjunction with other chemotherapeutic agents, including paclitaxel, which may have their own unique neurotoxicities.

Gemtuzumab Ozogamicin

Gemtuzumab ozogamicin (Mylotarg) consists is a recombinant anti-CD33 monoclonal antibody conjugated to calicheamicin, a cytotoxic antitumor antibiotic. It is used primarily in the treatment of CD33-positive acute myelogenous leukemia (AML). Headache and fatigue are the only significant neurotoxicities.

Ibritumomab Tiuxetan

Ibritumomab is a murine anti-CD20 monoclonal antibody. It is bound to the linker-chelator tiuxetan to form ibritumomab tiuxetan (Zevalin). This compound is chelated to yttrium-90 for radioimmunotherapy of non-Hodgkin lymphoma expressing CD20. As with most of the monoclonal antibody therapies, significant neurotoxicity has not been reported with ibritumomab.

Cetuximab

Cetuximab (Erbitux) is a chimeric antiepidermal growth factor receptor monoclonal antibody that targets the extracellular ligand-binding region. Cetuximab has been used in the treatment of colorectal cancer, head and neck cancers, and lung cancer. Neurotoxicity appears to be extremely rare. A single patient has been reported to have developed aseptic meningitis while receiving cetuximab.[341] Nonspecific dizziness, myalgias, and paresthesias are rare, but have been reported.[342]

Signal Transduction Inhibitors

Imatinib Mesylate

Imatinib mesylate (Gleevec, STI-571) is a selective tyrosine kinase inhibitor that blocks signaling by platelet-derived growth factor receptor kinase and bcr-abl tyrosine kinase, the constitutive abnormal tyrosine kinase created by the Philadelphia chromosome abnormality in CML. Imatinib is used to treat CML and malignant gastric stromal tumors, which express an activating c-kit mutation. Imatinib is under investigation for the treatment of a variety of solid tumors, including gliomas, breast, lung, and prostate cancers. Headache is the most common reported neurologic toxicity, occurring in approximately 25% of patients. Retinal hemorrhage, periorbital edema, papilledema, and other rare ocular effects have been reported.[343]

Gefitinib

Gefitinib (ZD-1839, Iressa) is a selective epidermal growth factor receptor–tyrosine kinase inhibitor. It is approved for the treatment of non–small cell lung cancer and is under investigation for treatment of a variety of solid tumors, including glioma. Significant neurotoxicity has not been reported with this drug. Headache and fatigue are relatively common, however.

Erlotinib

Erlotinib (OSI-774, Tarceva) is a selective inhibitor of epidermal growth factor receptor tyrosine kinase. It has been used in the treatment of solid tumors that overexpress epidermal growth factor receptor, including head and neck cancers, lung cancer, ovarian cancer, and high-grade gliomas. Approximately 25% of patients report mild headache within a few hours of the initial oral dose of medication.[344] This is not typically dose limiting and usually does not recur with subsequent doses.

▶ CONCLUSION

Central or peripheral neurotoxicity related to the use of chemotherapeutic and biologic agents is common, both as direct and indirect effects of these medications. These adverse sequelae may produce significant, lasting disability, even when the patient's underlying malignancy is cured or in remission. Moreover, neurotoxicity may be the dose-limiting factor in determining further antineoplastic treatment. It is therefore essential that the clinician caring for patients with cancer be familiar with the myriad neurologic adverse effects of these agents and be able to distinguish them from other potential neurologic problems associated with malignancy.

REFERENCES

1. Lampkin BC, Higgins GR, Hammond D. Absence of neurotoxicity following massive intrathecal administration of methotrexate. Case report. Cancer 1967;20(10):1780–1781.
2. Ettinger LJ, Freeman AI, Creaven PJ. Intrathecal methotrexate overdose without neurotoxicity: case report and literature review. Cancer 1978;41(4):1270–1273.
3. Ettinger LJ. Pharmacokinetics and biochemical effects of a fatal intrathecal methotrexate overdose. Cancer 1982;50(3):444–450.
4. Adamson PC, Balis FM, McCully CL, et al. Rescue of experimental intrathecal methotrexate overdose with carboxypeptidase-G2. J Clin Oncol 1991;9(4):670–674.
5. Yim YS, Mahoney DH Jr, Oshman DG. Hemiparesis and ischemic changes of the white matter after intrathecal therapy for children with acute lymphocytic leukemia. Cancer 1991;67(8):2058–2061.
6. Winick NJ, Bowman WP, Kamen BA, et al. Unexpected acute neurologic toxicity in the treatment of children with acute lymphoblastic leukemia. J Natl Cancer Inst 1992;84(4):252–256.
7. Luddy RE, Gilman PA. Paraplegia following intrathecal methotrexate. J Pediatr 1973;83(6):988–992.
8. Clark AW, Cohen SR, Nissenblatt MJ, et al. Paraplegia following intrathecal chemotherapy: neuropathologic findings and elevation of myelin basic protein. Cancer 1982;50(1):42–47.
9. McLean DR, Clink HM, Ernst P, et al. Myelopathy after intrathecal chemotherapy. A case report with unique magnetic resonance imaging changes. Cancer 1994;73(12):3037–3040.
10. Price RA, Jamieson PA. The central nervous system in childhood leukemia. II. Subacute leukoencephalopathy. Cancer 1975;35(2):306–318.
11. Matsumoto K, Takahashi S, Sato A, et al. Leukoencephalopathy in childhood hematopoietic neoplasm caused by moderate-dose methotrexate and prophylactic cranial radiotherapy—an MR analysis. Int J Radiat Oncol Biol Phys 1995;32(4):913–918.
12. Stein ME, Drumea K, Yarnitsky D, et al. A rare event of 5-fluorouracil-associated peripheral neuropathy: a report of two patients. Am J Clin Oncol 1998;21(3):248–249.
13. Takimoto CH, Lu ZH, Zhang R, et al. Severe neurotoxicity following 5-fluorouracil-based chemotherapy in a patient with dihydropyrimidine dehydrogenase deficiency. Clin Cancer Res 1996;2:477–481.
14. Boileau G, Piro AJ, Lahiri SR, et al. Cerebellar ataxia during 5-fluorouracil (NSC-19893) therapy. Cancer Chemother Rep 1971;55:595–598.
15. Greenwald ES. Organic mental changes with fluorouracil therapy. JAMA 1976;235:248–249.

16. Brashear A, Siemers E. Focal dystonia after chemotherapy: a case series. J Neurooncol 1997;34:163–167.
17. Adams JW, Bofenkamp TM, Kobrin J, et al. Recurrent acute toxic optic neuropathy secondary to 5-FU. Cancer Treat Rep 1984;68:565–566.
18. Parkinson DR, Cano PO, Jerry LM, et al. Complications of cancer immunotherapy with levamisole. Lancet 1977;1:1129–1132.
19. Symoens J, Veys E, Mielants M, et al. Adverse reactions to levamisole. Cancer Treat Rep 1978;62:1721–1730.
20. Clemens LE, Ansell BM, Bernstein RM, et al. A comparison of low dose levamisole and penicillamine in rheumatoid arthritis. Aust N Z J Med 1983;13:578–582.
21. Prieur AM, Buriot D, Lefur JM, et al. Possible toxicity of levamisole in children with rheumatoid arthritis. J Pediatr 1978;93:304–305.
22. Vandevelde M, Boring JG, Hoff EJ, et al. The effect of levamisole on the canine central nervous system. J Neuropathol Exp Neurol 1978;37(2):165–173.
23. Kimmel DW, Wijdicks EF, Rodriguez M. Multifocal inflammatory leukoencephalopathy associated with levamisole therapy. Neurology 1995;45(2):374–376.
24. Paleologos NS. Complications of chemotherapy. In: Biller J, ed. Iatrogenic neurology. Boston: Butterworth-Heinemann, 1998:439–460.
25. Yeo W, Tong MM, Chan YL. Multifocal cerebral demyelination secondary to fluorouracil and levamisole therapy. J Clin Oncol 1999;17(1):431–433.
26. Savarese DM, Gordon J, Smith TW, et al. Cerebral demyelination syndrome in a patient treated with 5-flurouracil and levamisole. Cancer 1996;77:387–394.
27. Fassas AB-T, Gattani AM, Morgello S. Cerebral demyelination with 5-fluoruracil and levamisole. Cancer Invest 1994; 13:379–383.
28. Chen TC, Hinton DR, Leichman L, et al. Multifocal inflammatory leukoencephalopathy associated with levamisole and 5-fluorouracil: case report. Neurosurgery 1994;35:1138–1143.
29. Hook CC, Kimmel DW, Kvols LK, et al. Multifocal inflammatory leukoencephalopathy with 5-fluorouracil and levamisole. Ann Neurol 1992;31(3):262–267.
30. Russell JA, Powles RL. Neuropathy due to cytosine arabinoside [letter]. Br Med J 1974;4(5945):652–653.
31. Scherokman B, Filling-Katz MR, Tell D. Brachial plexus neuropathy following high-dose cytarabine in acute monoblastic leukemia. Cancer Treat Rep 1985;69:1005–1006.
32. Grossman L, Baker MA, Sutton DMC, et al. Central nervous system toxicity of high-dose cytosine arabinoside. Med Pediatr Oncol 1983;11:246–250.
33. Winkelman MD, Hines JD. Cerebellar degeneration caused by high-dose cytosine arabinoside: a clinicopathological study. Ann Neurol 1983;14:520–527.
34. Hwang TL, Yung WKA, Lee Y-Y, et al. High dose Ara-C related leukoencephalopathy. J Neurooncol 1986;3:335–339.
35. Luque FA, Selhorst JB, Petrusks P. Parkinsonism induced by high-dose cytosine arabinoside. Move Disord 1987;2:219–222.
36. Dunton SF, Nitschke R, Spruce WE, et al. Progressive ascending paralysis following administration of intrathecal and intravenous cytosine arabinoside. A pediatric oncology group study. Cancer 1986;57:1083–1088.
37. Kleinschmidt-DeMasters BK, Yeh M. "Locked-in syndrome" after intrathecal cytosine arabinoside for malignant immunoblastic lymphoma. Cancer 1992;70:2504–2507.
38. Chun HG, Lelend-Jones BR, Caryk SM, et al. Central nervous system toxicity of fludarabine phosphate. Cancer Treat Rep 1986;70:1225–1228.
39. Spriggs DR, Stopa E, Mayer RJ, et al. Fludarabine phosphate (NSC 312878) infusions for the treatment of acute leukemia: phase I and neuropathological study. Cancer Res 1986;46:5953–5958.
40. Cohen RB, Abdallah JR, Gray JR, et al. Reversible neurologic toxicity in patients treated with standard-dose fludarabine phosphate for mycosis fungoides and chronic lymphocytic leukemia. Ann Intern Med 1983;118:392–393.
41. Cheson BD, Vena DA, Foss FM, et al. Neurotoxicity of purine analogs: a review. J Clin Oncol 1994;12(10):2216–2228.
42. Russell MT, Nassif AS, Cacayorin ED, et al. Gemcitabine-associated posterior leukoencephalopathy syndrome: MR imaging and MR spectroscopy findings. Magn Reson Imaging 2001;19:129–132.
43. Dormann AJ, Grunewald T, Wigginghaus B, et al. Gemcitabine-associated autonomic neuropathy. Lancet 1998;351(9103):644.
44. Barry M, Clarke S, Mulcahy F, et al. Hydroxyurea-induced neurotoxicity in HIV disease. AIDS 1999;13(12):1592–1594.
45. Grothey A. Oxaliplatin-safety profile: neurotoxicity. Semin Oncol 2003;30(4 Suppl 15):5–13.
46. Taieb S, Trillet-Lenoir V, Rambaud L, et al. Lhermitte sign and urinary retention: atypical presentation of oxaliplatin neurotoxicity in four patients. Cancer 2002;94(9):2434–2440.
47. Extra JM, Marty M, Brienza S, et al. Pharmacokinetics and safety profile of oxaliplatin. Semin Oncol 1998;25(2 Suppl 5):13–22.
48. Fischer SJ, McDonald ES, Gross L, et al. Alterations in cell cycle regulation underlie cisplatin-induced apoptosis of dorsal root ganglion neurons in vivo. Neurobiol Dis 2001;8(6):1027–1035.
49. Thompson SW, Davis LE, Kornfield M, et al. Cisplatin neuropathy: clinical, electrophysiologic, morphologic, and toxicologic studies. Cancer 1984;54:1269–1275.
50. Cohen SC, Mollman JE. Cisplatin-induced gastric paresis. J Neurooncol 1987;5(3):237–240.
51. Hovestadt A, Van der Burg MEL, Verbiest HBC, et al. The course of neuropathy after cessation of cisplatin treatment, combined with ORG 2766 or placebo. J Neurol 1992;239:143–146.
52. Cavaletti G, Marzorati L, Bogliun G, et al. Cisplatin-induced peripheral neurotoxicity is dependent on total-dose intensity and single-dose intensity. Cancer 1992;69:203–207.
53. LoMonaco M, Milone M, Batocchi AP, et al. Cisplatin neuropathy: clinical course and neurophysiological findings. J Neurol 1992;239(4):199–204.
54. Gradishar WJ, Stephenson P, Glover DJ, et al. A phase II trial of cisplatin plus WR-2721 (amifostine) for metastatic breast carcinoma: an Eastern Cooperative Oncology Group Study (E8188). Cancer 2001;92:2517–2522.

55. Roberts JA, Jenison EL, Kim K, et al. A randomized multicenter, double-blind, placebo-controlled, dose-finding study of ORG 2766 in the prevention or delay of cisplatin-induced neuropathies in women with ovarian cancer. Gynecol Oncol 1997;67:172–177.
56. Moroso MJ, Blair RL. A review of *cis*-platinum ototoxicity. J Otolaryngol 1983;12:365–369.
57. Newton HB, Page MA, Junck L, et al. Intra-arterial cisplatin for the treatment of malignant gliomas. J Neurooncol 1989;7:39–45.
58. Frustaci S, Barzan L, Comoretto R, et al. Local neurotoxicity after intra-arterial cisplatin in head and neck cancer. Cancer Treat Rep 1987;71:257–259.
59. Schilsky RL, Anderson T. Hypomagnesemia and renal magnesium wasting in patients receiving cisplatin. Ann Intern Med 1979;90:929–931.
60. Ritch PS. *Cis*-dichlorodiammineplatinum II-induced syndrome of inappropriate secretion of antidiuretic hormone. Cancer 1988;61:448–450.
61. Walker RW, Cairncross JG, Posner JB. Cerebral herniation in patients receiving cisplatin. J Neurooncol 1988;6:61–65.
62. Ito Y, Arahata Y, Goto Y, et al. Cisplatin neurotoxicity presenting as reversible posterior leukoencephalopathy syndrome. Am J Neuroradiol 1998;19;415–417.
63. Highley M, Meller ST, Pinkerton CR. Seizures and cortical dysfunction following high-dose cisplatin administration in children. Med Pediatr Oncol 1992;20:143–148.
64. Gorman DJ, Kefford R, Stuart-Harris R. Focal encephalopathy after cisplatin therapy. Med J Aust 1989;150:399–401.
65. Verschraegen C, Conrad CA, Hong WK. Subacute encephalopathic toxicity of cisplatin. Lung Cancer 1995;13(3):305–309.
66. Maise K, Walker RW, Gargan R, et al. Intra-arterial cisplatin-associated optic and otic toxicity. Arch Neurol 1992;49:83–86.
67. Ostrow S, Hahn D, Wiernik PH, et al. Ophthalmologic toxicity after cis-dichlorodiammineplatinum (II) therapy. Cancer Treat Rep 1978;62:1591–1594.
68. Wilding G, Caruso R, Lawrence TS, et al. Retinal toxicity after high-dose cisplatin therapy. J Clin Oncol 1985;3:1683–1689.
69. Katz BJ, Ward JH, Digre KB, et al. Persistent severe visual and electroretinographic abnormalities after intravenous cisplatin therapy. J Neuro-ophthalmol 2003;23(2):132–135.
70. Icli R, Karaogus H, Dincol D, et al. Severe vascular toxicity associated with cisplatin-based chemotherapy. Cancer 1993;72:587–593.
71. Licciardello JTW, Moane JL, Rudy CK, et al. Elevated plasma von Willebrand factor levels and arterial occlusive complications associated with cisplatin-based chemotherapy. Oncology 1985;42:296–300.
72. Samuels BL, Vogelzang NJ, Kennedy BJ. Severe vascular toxicity associated with vinblastine, bleomycin and cisplatin chemotherapy. Cancer Chemother Pharmacol 1987;19:253–256.
73. Paterson AH, McPherson TA. A possible neurologic complication of DTIC. Cancer Treat Rep 1977;61:105–106.
74. Gams RA, Carpenter JT. Central nervous system complications after combination treatment with Adriamycin (NSC-123127) and 5-(3,3-dimethyl-1-triazeno)imidazole-4-carboxamide (NSC-45388). Cancer Chemother Rep 1974;58(5 Pt 1):753–754.
75. Yung WK, Albright RE, Olson J, et al. A phase II study of temozolomide vs. procarbazine in patients with glioblastoma multiforme at first relapse. Br J Cancer 2000;83:588–593.
76. Estlin EJ, Lashford L, Ablett S, et al. Phase I study of temozolomide in paediatric patients with advanced cancer. Br J Cancer 1998;78(5):652–661.
77. Rosenthal MA, Ashley DL, Cher L. Temozolomide-induced flare in high-grade glioma: a new clinical entity. Intern Med J 2002;32(3):346–348.
78. Shingleton BJ, Bienfang DC, Albert DM, et al. Ocular toxicity associated with high-dose carmustine. Arch Ophthalmol 1982;100:1766–1772.
79. Schold SC, Fay JW. Central nervous system toxicity from high-dose BCNU treatment of systemic cancer. Neurology 1980;30:429.
80. Kupersmith MJ, Frohman LP, Choi IS, et al. Visual system toxicity following intra-arterial chemotherapy. Neurology 1988;38:284–289.
81. Foo SH, Choi IS, Berenstein A, et al. Supraophthlamic intracarotid administration of BCNU for malignant glioma. Neurology 1986;36:1437–1444.
82. Rosenblum MK, Delattre J-Y, Walker RW, et al. Fatal necrotizing encephalopathy complicating treatment of malignant gliomas with intra-arterial BCNU and irradiation: a pathological study. J Neurooncol 1989;7:269–281.
83. Kleinschmidt-Demaster BK, Geier JM. Pathology of high-dose intraarterial BCNU. Surg Neurol 1989;31:435–443.
84. Sullivan KM, Storb R, Shulman HM, et al. Immediate and delayed neurotoxicity after mechlorethamine preparation for bone marrow transplantation. Ann Intern Med 1982;97:182–189.
85. French JD, West PM, Von Amerongen FK, et al. Effects of intracarotid administration of nitrogen mustard. J Neurosurg 1952;9:378–389.
86. Owens G, Javid R, Tallon M, et al. Chemotherapy of primary gliomas of the brain. N Y State Med J 1964;64:1933–1937.
87. Hamilton A, Muggia F. Estramustine potentiates taxane in prostate and refractory breast cancers. Oncology (Huntingt) 2001;15(5 Suppl 7):40–43.
88. Halevy D, Radhakrishnan J, Markowitz G, et al. Thrombotic microangiopathies. Crit Care Clin 2002;18(2):309–320, vi.
89. Chan KW, Mullen CA, Worth LL, et al. Lorazepam for seizure prophylaxis during high-dose busulfan administration. Bone Marrow Transplant 2002;29(12):963–965.
90. Jourdan E, Topart D, Pinzani V, et al. Chlorambucil/prednisone-induced seizures in a patient with non-Hodgkin's lymphoma. Am J Hematol 2001;67(2):147.
91. Salloum E, Khan KK, Cooper DL. Chlorambucil-induced seizures. Cancer 1997;79(5):1009–1013.
92. Williams SA, Makker SP, Grupe WE. Seizures: a significant side effect of chlorambucil therapy in children. J Pediatr 1978;93(3):516–518.
93. Burns LJ. Ocular toxicities of chemotherapy. Semin Oncol 1992;19(5):492–500.
94. Yiannakis PH, Larner AJ. Visual failure and optic atrophy associated with chlorambucil therapy. BMJ 1993;306(6870):109.

95. Chabner BA, Sponzo R, Hummard S, et al. High-dose intermittent intravenous infusion of procarbazine (NSC-7777213). Cancer Chemother Rep 1973;57:361–363.
96. Carney MW, Ravindran A, Lewis DS. Manic psychosis associated with procarbazine. Br Med J (Clin Res Ed) 1982;284(6309):82–83.
97. Postma TJ, van Groeningen CJ, Witjes RJ, et al. Neurotoxicity of combination chemotherapy with procarbazine, CCNU and vincristine (PCV) for recurrent glioma. J Neurooncol 1998;38(1):69–75.
98. Stolinsky DC, Solomon J, Pugh RP, et al. Clinical experience with procarbazine in Hodgkin's disease, reticulum cell sarcoma, and lymphosarcoma. Cancer 1970;26(5): 984–990.
99. Weiss HD, Walker MD, Wiernik PH. Neurotoxicity of commonly used antineoplastic agents. N Engl J Med 1974;291(3): 127–133.
100. Spivack SD. Drugs 5 years later: procarbazine. Ann Intern Med 1974;81(6):795–800.
101. Gutin PH, Levi JA, Wiernik PH, et al. Treatment of malignant meningeal disease with intrathecal thiotepa: a phase II study. Cancer Treat Rep 1977;61(5):885–887.
102. Legha SS, Slavik M, Carter SK. Hexamethylmelamine. An evaluation of its role in the therapy of cancer. Cancer 1976;38:27–35.
103. Wharton JT, Rutledge F, Smith JP, et al. Hexamethylmelamine: an evaluation of its role in the treatment of ovarian cancer. Am J Obstet Gynecol 1979;133:833–844.
104. Bonomi PD, Mladineo J, Morrin B, et al. Phase II trial of hexamethylmelamine in ovarian carcinoma resistant to alkylating agents. Cancer Treat Rep 1979;63: 137–138.
105. Manetta A, MacNeill C, Lyter JA, et al. Hexamethylmelamine as a single second-line agent in ovarian cancer. Gynecol Oncol 1990;36:93–93.
106. Nagarajan R, Peters C, Orchard P, et al. Report of severe neurotoxicity with cyclophosphamide. J Pediatr Hematol Oncol 2000;22(6):544–546.
107. Nicolao P, Giometto B. Neurological toxicity of ifosfamide. Oncology 2003;65(Suppl 2):11–16.
108. Zalupski M, Baker LH. Ifosfamide. J Natl Cancer Inst 1988; 80(8):556–566.
109. Van Dyk JJ, Flakson HD, Van der Merwe AM, et al. Unexpected toxicity in patients treated with iphosphamide. Cancer Res 1972;32:921–924.
110. Pratt CB, Green AA, Horowitz ME, et al. Central nervous system toxicity following the treatment of pediatric patients with ifosfamide/mesna. J Clin Oncol 1986;4(8): 1253–1261.
111. DiMaggio JR, Brown R, Baile WF, et al. Hallucinations and ifosfamide-induced neurotoxicity. Cancer 1994;73(5): 1509–1514.
112. Cantwell BM, Harris AL. Ifosfamide/mesna and encephalopathy [letter]. Lancet 1985;1(8431):752.
113. Simonian NA, Gilliam FG, Chiappa KH. Ifosfamide causes a diazepam-sensitive encephalopathy. Neurology 1993; 43(12):2700–2702.
114. Turner AR, Duong CD, Good DJ. Methylene blue for the treatment and prophylaxis of ifosfamide-induced encephalopathy. Clin Oncol 2003;15(7):435–439.
115. Buesa JM, Garcia-Teijido P, Losa R, et al. Treatment of ifosfamide encephalopathy with intravenous thiamin. Clin Cancer Res 2003;9:4636–4637.
116. Watkin SW, Husband DJ, Green JA, et al. Ifosfamide encephalopathy: a reappraisal. Eur J Cancer Clin Oncol 1989;25(9):1303–1310.
117. Verdeguer A, Castel V, Esquembre C, et al. Fatal encephalopathy with ifosfamide/mesna. Pediatr Hematol Oncol 1989; 6(4):383–385.
118. Patel SR, Forman AD, Benjamin RS. High-dose ifosfamide-induced exacerbation of peripheral neuropathy. J Natl Cancer Inst 1994;86(4):305–306.
119. Fleming GF, Waggoner SE, Rotmensch J, et al. Absence of major peripheral neuropathy in a phase II trial of ifosfamide with vinorelbine in patients with ovarian cancer previously treated with platinum and paclitaxel. Am J Clin Oncol 2001;24(1):52–57.
120. Frisk P, Stalberg E, Stromberg B, et al. Painful peripheral neuropathy after treatment with high-dose ifosfamide. Med Pediatr Oncol 2001;37(4):379–382.
121. Casey EB, Jellife AM, Le Quesne PM, et al. Vincristine neuropathy. Clinical and electrophysiological observations. Brain 1973;96:69–86.
122. Pal PK. Clinical and electrophysiological studies in vincristine induced neuropathy. Electromyogr Clin Neurophysiol 1999;39:323–330.
123. Graf WD, Chane PF, Lensch MW, et al. Severe vincristine neuropathy in Charcot-Marie-Tooth disease type 1A. Cancer 1996;77:1356–1362.
124. Chaudhry V, Chaudhry M, Crawford TO, et al. Toxic neuropathy in patients with pre-existing neuropathy. Neurology 2003;60(2):337–340.
125. Cassady JR, Tonnesen GL, Wolfe LC, et al. Augmentation of vincristine neurotoxicity by irradiation of peripheral nerves. Cancer Treat Rep 1980;64:963–965.
126. Hildebrand J, Kenis Y. Additive toxicity of vincristine and other drugs for the peripheral nervous system. Acta Neurol Belg 1971;71:486–491.
127. Weintraub M, Adde MA, Venzon DJ, et al. Severe atypical neuropathy associated with administration of hematopoietic colony-stimulating factors and vincristine. J Clin Oncol 1996;14(3):935–940.
128. Moudgil SS, Riggs JE. Fulminant peripheral neuropathy with severe quadriparesis associated with vincristine therapy. Ann Pharmacother 2000;34:1136–1138.
129. Postma TJ, Benard BA, Huijgens PC, et al. Long-term effects of vincristine on the peripheral nervous system. J Neurooncol 1993;15(1):23–27.
130. Roca E, Bruera E, Politi PM, et al. Vinca alkaloid-induced cardiovascular autonomic neuropathy. Cancer Treat Rep 1985;69:149–151.
131. Hancock BW, Naysmith A. Vincristine-induced autonomic neuropathy. Br Med J 1975;3:207.
132. Delaney P. Vincristine-induced laryngeal nerve paralysis. Neurology 1982;32:1285–1288.
133. Rosenthal S, Kaufman S. Vincristine neurotoxicity. Ann Intern Med 1974;80(6):733–737.
134. Sandler SG, Tobin W, Henderson ES. Vincristine-induced neuropathy. A clinical study of fifty leukemic patients. Neurology 1969;19:367–374.

135. Levitt LP, Prager D. Mononeuropathy due to vincristine toxicity. Neurology 1975;25:894–895.
136. Shepherd DA, Steuber CP, Starling KA, et al. Accidental intrathecal administration of vincristine. Med Pediatr Oncol 1978;5(1):85–88.
137. Bleck TP, Jacobsen J. Prolonged survival following the inadvertent intrathecal administration of vincristine: clinical and electrophysiologic analyses. Clin Neuropharmacol 1991;14(5):457–462.
138. Williams ME, Walker AN, Bracikowski JP, et al. Ascending myeloencephalopathy due to intrathecal vincristine sulfate. A fatal chemotherapeutic error. Cancer 1983;51(11): 2041–2047.
139. Meggs WJ, Hoffman RS. Fatality resulting from intraventricular vincristine administration. J Toxicol Clin Toxicol 1998;6:36(3):243.
140. Robertson GL, Bhoopalam N, Zelkowitz LJ. Vincristine neurotoxicity and abnormal secretion of antidiuretic hormone. Arch Intern Med 1973;132(5):717–720.
141. Sorensen JB, Andersen MK, Hansen HH. Syndrome of inappropriate secretion of antidiuretic hormone (SIADH) in malignant disease. J Intern Med 1995;238(2):97–110.
142. Hurwitz RL, Mahoney DH Jr, Armstrong DL, et al. Reversible encephalopathy and seizures as a result of conventional vincristine administration. Med Pediatr Oncol 1988;16(3): 216–219.
143. Dallera F, Gamoletti R, Costa P. Unilateral seizures following vincristine intravenous injection. Tumori 1984;70(3): 243–244.
144. Edwards MJ, Walker R, Vinnicombe S, et al. Reversible posterior leukoencephalopathy syndrome following CHOP chemotherapy for diffuse large B-cell lymphoma. Ann Oncol 2001;12(9):1327–1329.
145. Byrd RL, Rohrbaugh TM, Raney RB Jr, Norris DG. Transient cortical blindness secondary to vincristine therapy in childhood malignancies. Cancer 1981;47(1):37–40.
146. Ghosh K, Sivakumaran M, Murphy P, et al. Visual hallucinations following treatment with vincristine. Clin Lab Haematol 1994;16(4):355–357.
147. Carpentieri U, Lockhart LH. Ataxia and athetosis as side effects of chemotherapy with vincristine in non-Hodgkin's lymphoma. Cancer Treat Rep 1978;62(4):561–562.
148. Boranic M, Raci F. A Parkinson-like syndrome as side effect of chemotherapy with vincristine and Adriamycin in a child with acute leukaemia. Biomedicine 1979;31(5):124–125.
149. Teichmann KD, Dabbagh N. Severe visual loss after a single dose of vincristine in a patient with spinal cord astrocytoma. J Ocul Pharmacol 1988;4(2):117–121.
150. Norton SW, Stockman JA 3rd. Unilateral optic neuropathy following vincristine chemotherapy. J Pediatr Ophthalmol Strabismus 1979;16(3):190–193.
151. Sanderson PA, Kuwabara T, Cogan DG. Optic neuropathy presumably caused by vincristine therapy. Am J Ophthalmol 1976;81(2):146–150.
152. Munier F, Perentes E, Herbort CP, et al. Selective loss of optic nerve beta-tubulin in vincristine-induced blindness. Am J Med 1992;93(2):232–234.
153. Leff RS, Thompson JM, Daly MB, et al. Acute neurologic dysfunction after high-dose etoposide therapy for malignant glioma. Cancer 1988;62(1):32–35.
154. Ascher DP, Delaney RA. Acute dystonia from etoposide. Drug Intell Clin Pharm 1988;22(1):41–42.
155. Imrie KR, Couture F, Turner CC, et al. Peripheral neuropathy following high-dose etoposide and autologous bone marrow transplantation. Bone Marrow Transplant 1994;13(1):77–79.
156. O'Dwyer PJ, Leyland-Jones B, Alonso MT, et al. Etoposide (VP-16–213). Current status of an active anticancer drug. N Engl J Med 1985;312(11):692–700.
157. Rowinsky EK, Donehower RC. Paclitaxel (Taxol) N Engl J Med 1995;332(15):1004–1014.
158. Capri G, Munzone E, Tarenzi E, et al. Optic nerve disturbances: a new form of paclitaxel neurotoxicity. J Natl Cancer Inst 1994;86(14):1099–1101.
159. Scaioli V, Caraceni A, Martini C, et al. Visual evoked potentials findings in course of paclitaxel doxorubicin combination chemotherapy. Report of a case. J Neurooncol 1995;25(3):221–225.
160. Perry JR, Warner E. Transient encephalopathy after paclitaxel (Taxol) infusion. Neurology 1996;46(6):1596–1599.
161. McGuire WP, Rowinsky EK, Rosenshein NB, et al. Taxol: a unique antineoplastic agent with significant activity in advanced ovarian epithelial neoplasms. Ann Intern Med 1989;111(4):273–279.
162. Brown T, Havlin K, Weiss G, et al. A phase I trial of Taxol given by a 6-hour intravenous infusion. J Clin Oncol 1991; 9(7):1261–1267.
163. Nieto Y, Cagnoni PJ, Bearman SI, et al. Acute encephalopathy: a new toxicity associated with high-dose paclitaxel. Clin Cancer Res 1999;5(3):501–506.
164. Postma TJ, Vermorken JB, Liefting AJ, et al. Paclitaxel-induced neuropathy. Ann Oncol 1995;6(5):489–494.
165. Rowinsky EK, Eisenhauer EA, Chaudhry V, et al. Clinical toxicities encountered with paclitaxel (Taxol). Semin Oncol 1993;20(4 Suppl 3):1–15.
166. Sahenk Z, Barohn R, New P, et al. Taxol neuropathy. Electrodiagnostic and sural nerve biopsy findings. Arch Neurol 1994;51(7):726–729.
167. Lee R, Oster M, Balmaceda C, et al. Bilateral facial nerve palsy secondary to the administration of high-dose paclitaxel. Ann Oncol 1999;10:1245–1247.
168. Jerian SM, Sarosy GA, Link CJ Jr, et al. Incapacitating autonomic neuropathy precipitated by Taxol. Gynecol Oncol 1993;51(2):277–280.
169. Vahdat L, Papadopoulos K, Lange D, et al. Reduction of paclitaxel-induced peripheral neuropathy with glutamine. Clin Cancer Res 2001;7(5):1192–1197.
170. New PZ, Jackson CE, Rinaldi D, et al. Peripheral neuropathy secondary to docetaxel (Taxotere). Neurology 1996;46(1): 108–111.
171. Hilkens PH, Verweij J, Vecht CJ, et al. Clinical characteristics of severe peripheral neuropathy induced by docetaxel (Taxotere). Ann Oncol 1997;8(2):187–190.
172. Polyzos A, Daskalopoulou E, Giannitsiotis E, et al. Transient encephalopathy followed by seizures after docetaxel infusion. Clin Drug Invest 1999;17(3):251–254.
173. Van den Bent MJ, Hilkens PH, Sillevis Smitt PA, et al. Lhermitte's sign following chemotherapy with docetaxel. Neurology 1998;50(2):563–564.

174. O'Brien S, Kantarjian H, Ellis A, et al. Topotecan in chronic lymphocytic leukemia. Cancer 1995;75:1104–1108.
175. Baz DV, Bofill JS, Nogueira JA. Irinotecan-induced dysarthria. J Natl Cancer Inst 2001;93(18):1419–1420.
176. Ceccaldi B, Kara F, Mommeja-Marin H, et al. Dysarthria during irinotecan administration. Rev Med Intern 2002;23(11): 950–951.
177. Seville Garcia I, Rueda A, Alba E. Irinotecan-induced central nervous system toxicity: a case report. J Natl Cancer Inst 1999;91(7):647.
178. Rowinsky EK, Noe DA, Grochow LB, et al. Phase I and pharmacologic studies of pyrazoloacridine, a novel DNA intercalating agent, on single-dosing and multiple-dosing schedules. J Clin Oncol 1995;13(8):1975–1984.
179. Pelley R, Ganapathi R, Wood L, et al. A phase II pharmacodynamic study of pyrazoloacridine in patients with metastatic colorectal cancer. Cancer Chemother Pharmacol 2000;46(3):251–254.
180. Zalupski MM, Philip PA, LoRusso P, et al. Phase II study of pyrazoloacridine in patients with advanced colorectal carcinoma. Cancer Chemother Pharmacol 1997;40(3):225–227.
181. Hitchins RN, Thomson DB. Encephalopathy following cisplatin, bleomycin and vinblastine therapy for nonseminomatous germ cell tumour of testis. Aust N Z J Med 1988;18(1):67–68.
182. Doll DC, Yarbro JW. Vascular toxicity associated with antineoplastic agents. Semin Oncol 1992;19(5):580–596.
183. Gerl A. Vascular toxicity associated with chemotherapy for testicular cancer. Anticancer Drugs 1994;5(6):607–614.
184. Santos AJ, Malheiros SM, Borges LR, et al. Ischemic stroke after chemotherapy with cisplatin, etoposide and bleomycin: case report. Arq Neuropsiquiatr 2003;61(1):129–133.
185. Neuwelt EA, Glasberg M, Frenkel E, et al. Neurotoxicity of chemotherapeutic agents after blood–brain barrier modification: neuropathological studies. Ann Neurol 1983;14(3): 316–324.
186. Arico M, Nespoli L, Porta F, et al. Severe acute encephalopathy following inadvertent intrathecal doxorubicin administration. Med Pediatr Oncol 1990;18(3):261–263.
187. Mortensen ME, Cecalupo AJ, Lo WD, et al. Inadvertent intrathecal injection of daunorubicin with fatal outcome. Med Pediatr Oncol 1992;20(3):249–253.
188. Pisoni R, Ruggenenti P, Remuzzi G. Drug-induced thrombotic microangiopathy: incidence, prevention and management. Drug Saf 2001;24:491–501.
189. Lakhani AK, Zuiable AG, Pollard CM, et al. Paraplegia after intrathecal mitoxantrone. Lancet 1986;2(8520):1393.
190. Siegal T, Melamed E, Sandbank U, et al. Early and delayed neurotoxicity of mitoxantrone and doxorubicin following subarachnoid injection. J Neurooncol 1988;6(2):135–140.
191. Melgaard B, Kohler O, Sand Hansen H, et al. Misonidazole neuropathy. A prospective study. J Neurooncol 1988;6(3): 227–230.
192. Abratt RP, Blackburn JD. Loss of hearing after misonidazole. Br J Radiol 1980;53(636):1208.
193. Frytak S, Moertel CH, Childs DS. Neurologic toxicity associated with high-dose metronidazole therapy. Ann Intern Med 1978;88(3):361–362.
194. Wasserman TH, Phillips TL, Johnson RJ, et al. Initial United States clinical and pharmacologic evaluation of misonidazole (Ro-07-0582), an hypoxic cell radiosensitizer. Int Radiat Oncol Biol Phys 1979;5(6):775–786.
195. Saunders ME, Dische S, Anderson P, et al. The neurotoxicity of misonidazole and its relationship to dose, half-life and concentration in the serum. Br J Cancer Suppl 1978;37(3): 268–270.
196. Kun LE, Ho KC, Moulder JE. Fatal misonidazole-induced encephalopathy: an RTOG case report. Cancer 1982;49(3): 423–426.
197. Chaudhry V, Eisenberger MA, Sinibaldi VJ, et al. A prospective study of suramin-induced peripheral neuropathy. Brain 1996;119(Pt 6):2039–2052.
198. Russell JW, Windebank AJ, Podratz JL. Role of nerve growth factor in suramin neurotoxicity studied in vitro. Ann Neurol 1994;36(2):221–228.
199. Peltier AC, Russell JW. Recent advances in drug-induced neuropathies. Curr Opin Neurol 2002;15(5):633–638.
200. Gill JS, Windebank AJ. Suramin induced ceramide accumulation leads to apoptotic cell death in dorsal root ganglion neurons. Cell Death Differ 1998;5(10):876–883.
201. Soliven B, Dhand UK, Kobayashi K, et al. Evaluation of neuropathy in patients on suramin treatment. Muscle Nerve 1997;20(1):83–91.
202. La Rocca RV, Meer J, Gilliatt RW, et al. Suramin-induced polyneuropathy. Neurology 1990;40(6):954–960.
203. Park SH, Gray WC, Hernandez I, et al. Phase I trial of all-trans retinoic acid in patients with treated head and neck squamous carcinoma. Clin Cancer Res 2000;6(3):847–854.
204. Kurie JM, Lee JS, Griffin T, et al. Phase I trial of 9-*cis* retinoic acid in adults with solid tumors. Clin Cancer Res 1996;2(2):287–293.
205. Windhorst DB, Nigra T. General clinical toxicology of oral retinoids. J Am Acad Dermatol 1982;6(4 Pt 2 Suppl):675–682.
206. Visani G, Manfroi S, Tosi P, et al. All-trans-retinoic acid and pseudotumor cerebri. Leuk Lymphoma 1996;23(5–6): 437–442.
207. Colucciello M. Pseudotumor cerebri induced by all-trans retinoic acid treatment of acute promyelocytic leukemia. Arch Ophthalmol 2003;121(7):1064–1065.
208. Naderi S, Nukala S, Marruenda F, et al. Pseudotumour cerebri in acute promyelocytic leukemia: improvement despite continued ATRA therapy. Ann Hematol 1999;78(7): 333–334.
209. Bigby M. Stern RS. Adverse reactions to isotretinoin. A report from the Adverse Drug Reaction Reporting System. J Am Acad Dermatol 1988;18(3):543–552.
210. Yamaji S, Kanamori H, Mishima A, et al. All-trans retinoic acid-induced multiple mononeuropathies. Am J Hematol 1999;60(4):311.
211. Bernstein AL, Leventhal-Rochon JL. Neurotoxicity related to the use of topical tretinoin (Retin-A). Ann Intern Med 1996;124(2):227–228.
212. Leonard JV, Kay JD. Acute encephalopathy and hyperammonaemia complicating treatment of acute lymphoblastic leukaemia with asparaginase. Lancet 1986;1(8473):162–163.
213. Haskell CM, Canellos GP, Leventhal BG, et al. L-Asparaginase: therapeutic and toxic effects in patients with neoplastic disease. N Engl J Med 1969;281(19):1028–1034.

214. Land VJ, Sutow WW, Fernbach DJ, et al. Toxicity of L-asparaginase in children with advanced leukemia. Cancer 1972;30(2):339–347.
215. Moure JM, Whitecar JP Jr, Bodey GP. Electroencephalogram changes secondary to asparaginase. Arch Neurol 1970; 23(4):365–368.
216. Pratt CB, Choi SI, Holton CP. Low-dosage asparaginase treatment of childhood acute lymphocytic leukemia. Am J Dis Child 1971;121(5):406–409.
217. Kucuk O, Kwaan HC, Gunnar W, et al. Thromboembolic complications associated with L-asparaginase therapy. Etiologic role of low antithrombin III and plasminogen levels and therapeutic correction by fresh frozen plasma. Cancer 1985;55(4):702–706.
218. Priest JR, Ramsay NK, Bennett AJ, et al. The effect of L-asparaginase on antithrombin, plasminogen, and plasma coagulation during therapy for acute lymphoblastic leukemia. J Pediatr 1982;100(6):990–995.
219. Cairo MS, Lazarus K, Gilmore RL, et al. Intracranial hemorrhage and focal seizures secondary to use of L-asparaginase during induction therapy of acute lymphocytic leukemia. J Pediatr 1980;97(5):829–833.
220. Alberts SR, Bretscher M, Wiltsie JC, et al. Thrombosis related to the use of L-asparaginase in adults with acute lymphoblastic leukemia: a need to consider coagulation monitoring and clotting factor replacement. Leuk Lymphoma 1999;32(5–6):489–496.
221. Kieslich M, Porto L, Lanfermann H, et al. Cerebrovascular complications of L-asparaginase in the therapy of acute lymphoblastic leukemia. J Pediat Hematol Oncol 2003; 25(6):484–487.
222. Gugliotta L, Mazzucconi MG, Leone G, et al. Incidence of thrombotic complications in adult patients with acute lymphoblastic leukaemia receiving L-asparaginase during induction therapy: a retrospective study. The GIMEMA Group. Eur J Haematol 1992;49(2):63–66.
223. Moots PL, Walker RW, Sze G, et al. Diagnosis of dural venous sinus thrombosis by magnetic resonance imaging. Ann Neurol 1987;22:431–432.
224. Feinberg WM, Swenson MR. Cerebrovascular complications of L-asparaginase therapy. Neurology 1988;38(1): 127–133.
225. Fanelli M, Sarmiento R, Gattuso D, et al. Thalidomide: a new anticancer drug? Expert Opin Investig Drugs 2003;12(7): 1211–1225.
226. Fine HA, Wen PY, Maher EA, et al. Phase II trial of thalidomide and carmustine for patients with recurrent high-grade gliomas. J Clin Oncol 2003;21(12):2299–2304.
227. Garcia-Albea E, Cabrera F, Tejeiro J, et al. Typical migraine and thalidomide. Med Clin 1993;100(14):557.
228. Clark TE, Edom N, Larson J, et al. Thalomid (Thalidomide) capsules: a review of the first 18 months of spontaneous postmarketing adverse event surveillance, including off-label prescribing. Drug Saf 2001;24(2):87–117.
229. Chaudhry V, Cornblath DR, Corse A, et al. Thalidomide-induced neuropathy. Neurology 2002;59(12):1872–1875.
230. Bastuji-Garin S, Ochonisky S, Bouche P, et al. Incidence and risk factors for thalidomide neuropathy: a prospective study of 135 dermatologic patients. J Invest Dermatol 2002;119(5): 1020–1026.
231. Fullerton PM, O'Sullivan DJ. Thalidomide neuropathy: a clinical, electrophysiological, and histological follow-up study. J Neurol Neurosurg Psychiatry 1968;31:543–551.
232. Calabrese L, Fleischer AB. Thalidomide. Current and potential clinical applications. Am J Med 2000;108:487–495.
233. Gupta RC, Lavengood R Jr, Smith JP. Miliary tuberculosis due to intravesical bacillus Calmette-Guérin therapy. Chest 1988;94(6):1296–1298.
234. Deresiewicz RL, Stone RM, Aster JC. Fatal disseminated mycobacterial infection following intravesical bacillus Calmette-Guérin. J Urol 1990;144(6):1331–1333; discussion 1333–1334.
235. Hakim S, Heaney JA, Heinz T, et al. Psoas abscess following intravesical bacillus Calmette-Guerin for bladder cancer: a case report. J Urol 1993;150(1):188–189.
236. Stone MM, Vannier AM, Storch SK, et al. Brief report: meningitis due to iatrogenic BCG infection in two immunocompromised children. N Engl J Med 1995;333(9):561–563.
237. Tardieu M, Truffot-Pernot C, Carriere JP, et al. Tuberculous meningitis due to BCG in two previously healthy children. Lancet 1988;1(8583):440–441.
238. Trask PC, Esper P, Riba M, Redman B. Psychiatric side effects of interferon therapy: prevalence, proposed mechanisms, and future directions. J Clin Oncol 2000;18(11): 2316–2326.
239. Hensley ML, Peterson B, Silver RT, et al. Risk factors for severe neuropsychiatric toxicity in patients receiving interferon alfa-2b and low-dose cytarabine for chronic myelogenous leukemia: analysis of Cancer and Leukemia Group B 9013. J Clin Oncol 2000;18(6):1301–1308.
240. Adams F, Fernandez F, Mavligit G. Interferon-induced organic mental disorders associated with unsuspected preexisting neurologic abnormalities. J Neurooncol 1988;6(4): 355–359.
241. Valentine AD, Meyers CA, Kling MA, et al. Mood and cognitive side effects of interferon-alpha therapy. Semin Oncol 1998;25(1 Suppl 1):39–47.
242. Guyer DR, Tiedeman J, Yannuzzi LA, et al. Interferon-associated retinopathy. Arch Ophthalmol 1993;111:350–356.
243. Esmaeli B, Koller C, Papadopoulos N, et al. Interferon-induced retinopathy in asymptomatic cancer patients. Ophthalmology 2001;108(5):858–860.
244. Neubauer AS, Hoops JP. Interferon-induced retinopathy in asymptomatic cancer patients. Ophthalmology 2002; 109(5):821–822.
245. Barlow CF, Priebe CJ, Mulliken JB, et al. Spastic diplegia as a complication of interferon Alfa-2a treatment of hemangiomas of infancy. J Pediatr 1998;132(3 Pt 1):527–530.
246. Vesikari T, Nuutila A, Cantell K. Neurologic sequelae following interferon therapy of juvenile laryngeal papilloma. Acta Paediatr Scand 1988;77(4):619–622.
247. Meyers CA, Obbens EAMT, Scheibel RS, et al. Neurotoxicity of intraventricularly administered alpha-interferon for leptomeningeal disease. Cancer 1991;68:88–92.
248. Herrlinger U, Weller M, Schabet M. New aspects of immunotherapy of leptomeningeal metastasis. J Neurooncol 1998;38(2–3):233–239.
249. Smedley H, Katrak M, Sikora K, et al. Neurological effects of recombinant human interferon. Br Med J (Clin Res Ed) 1983;286(6361):262–264.

250. Suter CC, Westmoreland BF, Sharbrough FW, et al. Electroencephalographic abnormalities in interferon encephalopathy: a preliminary report. Mayo Clin Proc 1984;59(12):847–850.
251. Meyers CA, Scheibel RS, Forman AD. Persistent neurotoxicity of systemically administered interferon-alpha. Neurology 1991;41(5):672–676.
252. Valentine AD, Meyers CA, Talpaz M. Treatment of neurotoxic side effects of interferon-alpha with naltrexone. Cancer Invest 1995;13(6):561–566.
253. Hauser P, Soler R, Reed S, Kane et al. Prophylactic treatment of depression induced by interferon-alpha. Psychosomatics 2000;41(5):439–441.
254. Levenson J, Fallon H. Fluoxetine treatment of depression caused by interferon-alpha. Am J Gastroenterol 1993;88:760–761.
255. Goldman LS. Successful treatment of interferon alfa-induced mood disorder with nortriptyline. Psychosomatics 1994;35(4):412–413.
256. Kanda Y, Shigeno K, Matsuo H, et al. Interferon-induced sudden hearing loss. Audiology 1995;34(2):98–102.
257. Mattson K, Niiranen A, Iivanainen M, et al. Neurotoxicity of interferon. Cancer Treat Rep 1983;67(10):958–961.
258. Bernsen PL, Wong Chung RE, Vingerhoets HM, et al. Bilateral neuralgic amyotrophy induced by interferon treatment. Arch Neurol 1988;45(4):449–451.
259. Bauherz G, Soeur M, Lustman F. Oculomotor nerve paralysis induced by alpha II-interferon. Acta Neurol Belg 1990;90(2):111–114.
260. Schwarzer A, Schulze E, Leiblein S, et al. Guillain Barre syndrome, a possible side effect of buffy coat transfusion and IFN alpha therapy in relapsed CML after bone marrow transplantation. Ann Oncol 1995;6(6):617.
261. Batocchi AP, Evoli A, Servidei S, et al. Myasthenia gravis during interferon alfa therapy. Neurology 1995;45(2):382–383.
262. Saris SC, Patronas NJ, Rosenberg SA, et al. The effect of intravenous interleukin-2 on brain water content. J Neurosurg 1989;71(2):169–174.
263. Meyers CA, Valentine AD. Neurological and psychiatric adverse effects of immunological therapy. CNS Drugs 1995;3:56–68.
264. Siegel JP, Puri RK. Interleukin-2 toxicity. J Clin Oncol 1991;9(4):694–704.
265. Denicoff KD, Rubinow DR, Papa MZ, et al. The neuropsychiatric effects of treatment with interleukin-2 and lymphokine-activated killer cells. Ann Intern Med 1987;107(3):293–300.
266. Bernard JT, Ameriso S, Kempf RA, et al. Transient focal neurologic deficits complicating interleukin-2 therapy. Neurology 1990;40:154–155.
267. Somers SS, Reynolds JV, Guillou PJ. Multifocal neurotoxicity during interleukin-2 therapy for malignant melanoma. Clin Oncol 1992;4:135–136.
268. Karp BI, Yang JC, Khorsand M, et al. Multiple cerebral lesions complicating therapy with interleukin-2. Neurology 1996;47(2):417–424.
269. Hotton KM, Khorsand M, Hank JA, et al. A phase Ib/II trial of granulocyte-macrophage-colony stimulating factor and interleukin-2 for renal cell carcinoma patients with pulmonary metastases: a case of fatal central nervous system thrombosis. Cancer 2000;88(8):1892–1901.
270. Loh FL, Herskovitz S, Berger AR, et al. Brachial plexopathy associated with interleukin-2 therapy. Neurology 1992;42(2):462–463.
271. Meyers CA, Yung WK. Delayed neurotoxicity of intraventricular interleukin-2: a case report. J Neurooncol 1993;15(3):265–267.
272. Vecht CJ, Keohane C, Menon RS, et al. Acute fatal leukoencephalopathy after interleukin-2 therapy. N Engl J Med 1990;323(16):1146–1147.
273. Denicoff KD, Durkin TM, Lotze MT, et al. The neuroendocrine effects of interleukin-2 treatment. J Clin Endocrinol Metab 1989;69(2):402–410.
274. Margolin K, Aronson FR, Sznol M, et al. Phase II studies of recombinant human interleukin-4 in advanced renal cancer and malignant melanoma. J Immunother 1994;15:147–153.
275. Gilleece MH, Scarffe JH, Ghosh A, et al. Recombinant human interleukin 4 (IL-4) given as daily subcutaneous injections- a phase I dose toxicity trial. Br J Cancer 1992;66:204–210.
276. Fraker DL, Alexander HR, Andrich M, et al. Treatment of patients with melanoma of the extremity using hyperthermic isolated limb perfusion with melphalan, tumor necrosis factor, and interferon gamma: results of a tumor necrosis factor dose-escalation study. J Clin Oncol 1996;14(2):479–489.
277. Drory VE, Lev D, Groozman GB, et al. Neurotoxicity of isolated limb perfusion with tumor necrosis factor. J Neurol Sci 1998;158(1):1–4.
278. Riggs JE, Mansmann PT, Cook LL, et al. Fulminant CNS perivascular lymphocytic proliferation: association with sargramostim, a hematopoietic growth factor. Clin Neuropharmacol 1999;22(5):288–291.
279. Steinberg H. Erythropoietin and visual hallucinations. N Engl J Med 1991;325:285.
280. Delanty N, Needell N. Erythropoietin and visual hallucinations in patients on dialysis. Psychosomatics 1998;39(1):83–85.
281. Kooistra MP, van Es A, Marx JJ, et al. Low-dose aspirin does not prevent thrombovascular accidents in low-risk haemodialysis patients during treatment with recombinant human erythropoietin. Nephrol Dial Transplant 1994;9(8):1115–1120.
282. Finelli PF, Carley MD. Cerebral venous thrombosis associated with epoetin alfa therapy. Arch Neurol 2000;57(2):260–262.
283. Delanty N, Vaughan C, Frucht S, et al. Erythropoietin-associated hypertensive posterior leukoencephalopathy. Neurology 1997;49:686–689.
284. Lindemann A, Ganser A, Herrmann F, et al. Biologic effects of recombinant human interleukin-3 in vivo. J Clin Oncol 1991;9:2120–2127.
285. Sunderland MC, Roodman GD. Interleukin-3. Its biology and potential uses in pediatric hematology/oncology. Am J Pediatr Hematol Oncol 1991;13:414–425.
286. Weber J, Gunn H, Yang J, et al. A phase I trial of intravenous interleukin-6 in patients with advanced cancer. J Immunother 1994;15:292–302.
287. Tepler I, Elias L, Smith JW II, et al. A randomized placebo-controlled trial of recombinant human interleukin-11 in

cancer patients with severe thrombocytopenia due to chemotherapy. Blood 1996;87:3607–3614.
288. Gordon MS, McCaskill-Stevens WJ, Battiato LA, et al. A phase I trial of recombinant human interleukin-11 (Neumega rhIL-11 growth factor) in women with breast cancer receiving chemotherapy. Blood 1996;87:3615–3624.
289. Bussel JB, Mukherjee R, Stone AJ. A pilot study of rhuIL-11 treatment of refractory ITP. Am J Hematol 2001;66(3):172–177.
290. Kaiser-Kupfer MI, Lippman ME. Tamoxifen retinopathy. Cancer Treat Rep 1978;62(3):315–320.
291. Nayfield SG, Gorin MB. Tamoxifen-associated eye disease. A review. J Clin Oncol 1996;14(3):1018–1026.
292. Pugesgaard T, Von Eyben FE. Bilateral optic neuritis evolved during tamoxifen treatment. Cancer 1986;58(2):383–386.
293. Kaiser-Kupfer MI, Kupfer C, Rodrigues MM. Tamoxifen retinopathy. A clinicopathologic report. Ophthalmology 1981;88(1):89–93.
294. Ashford AR, Donev I, Tiwari RP, et al. Reversible ocular toxicity related to tamoxifen therapy. Cancer 1988;61(1):33–35.
295. Pavlidis NA, Petris C, Briassoulis E, et al. Clear evidence that long-term, low-dose tamoxifen treatment can induce ocular toxicity. A prospective study of 63 patients. Cancer 1992;69(12):2961–2964.
296. Noureddin BN, Seoud M, Bashshur Z, et al. Ocular toxicity in low-dose tamoxifen: a prospective study. Eye 1999;13 (Pt 6):729–733.
297. Mathew P, Fung F. Recapitulation of menstrual migraine with tamoxifen. Lancet 1999;353(9151):467–468.
298. Ron IG, Inbar MJ, Barak Y, et al. Organic delusional syndrome associated with tamoxifen treatment. Cancer 1992;69(6):1415–1417.
299. Pluss JL, DiBella NJ. Reversible central nervous system dysfunction due to tamoxifen in a patient with breast cancer. Ann Intern Med 1984;101(5):652.
300. Saphner T, Tormey DC, Gray R. Venous and arterial thrombosis in patients who received adjuvant therapy for breast cancer. J Clin Oncol 1991;9(2):286–294.
301. Kohler PC, Hamm JT, Wiebe VJ, et al. Phase I study of the tolerance and pharmacokinetics of toremifene in patients with cancer. Breast Cancer Res Treat 1990;16(Suppl):S19–S26.
302. Waxman JH, Wass JAH, Hendry WF, et al. Treatment with gonadotrophin releasing hormone analogue in advanced prostatic cancer. Br Med J 1983;286;1309–1312.
303. Posner JB. Side effects of chemotherapy. In: Neurologic complications of cancer. Philadelphia: FA Davis, 1995:282–310.
304. Morsi SJ, Silverberg JD. Pituitary apoplexy after leuprolide administration for carcinoma of the prostate. Clin Endocrinol 1996;44:121–124.
305. Spengos K, Pavlopoulos C, Grivas A. Pituitary haemorrhage after leuprolide therapy for prostatic cancer, clinically imitating acute subarachnoidal haemorrhage. Cerebrovasc Dis 2002;14(3–4):272.
306. Engel G, Huston M, Oshima S, et al. Pituitary apoplexy after leuprolide injection for ovum donation. J Adolesc Health 2003;32(1):89–93.
307. Akaboshi S, Takeshita K. A case of atypical absence seizures induced by leuprolide acetate. Pediatr Neurol 2000;23(3):266–268.
308. Crayton H, Bohlmann T, Sufit R, et al. Drug induced polymyositis secondary to leuprolide acetate (Lupron) therapy for prostate carcinoma. Clin Exp Rheumatol 1991;9:525–528.
309. Van Gerpen JA, McKinley KL. Leuprolide-induced myopathy. J Am Geriatr Soc 2002;50(10):1746.
310. Eaton HJ, Phillips PJ, Hanieh A, et al. Rapid onset of pituitary apoplexy after goserelin implant for prostate cancer: need for heightened awareness. Intern Med J 2001;31(5):313–314.
311. Ahmann FR, Citrin DL, deHaan HA, et al. Zoladex: a sustained-release, monthly luteinizing hormone-releasing hormone analogue for the treatment of advanced prostate cancer. J Clin Oncol 1987;5(6):912–917.
312. Hamed LM, Glaser JS, Schatz NJ, et al. Pseudotumor cerebri induced by danazol. Am J Ophthalmol 1989;107(2):105–110.
313. Schmitz U, Honisch C, Zierz S. Pseudotumour cerebri and carpal tunnel syndrome associated with danazol therapy. J Neurol 1991;238(6):355.
314. Fanous M, Hamed LM, Margo CE. Pseudotumor cerebri associated with danazol withdrawal. JAMA 1991;266(9):1218–1219.
315. Alvarado RG, Liu JY, Zwolak RM. Danazol and limb-threatening arterial thrombosis: two case reports. J Vasc Surg 2001;34(6):1123–1126.
316. Satake R, Arakawa S, Hashimoto M, et al. Successful direct thrombolysis in a patient with extensive dural sinus thrombosis induced by danazol. Rinsho Shinkeigaku 1997;37(4):309–313.
317. Corno M, Vallar G, Scarlato G, et al. Danazol and internal carotid artery thrombosis. Eur Neurol 1989;29(4):235–237.
318. Sikka A, Kemmann E, Vrablik RM, et al. Carpal tunnel syndrome associated with danazol therapy. Am J Obstet Gynecol 1983;147(1):102–103.
319. Enyeart JJ, Price WA. Bilateral sensorineural hearing loss from danazol therapy. A case report. J Reprod Med 1984;29(5):351–353.
320. Hory B, Blanc D, Boillot A, et al. Guillain-Barré syndrome following danazol and corticosteroid therapy for hereditary angioedema. Am J Med 1985;79(1):111–114.
321. Jackson IM, Barnard LB, Lamberton P. Role of a long-acting somatostatin analogue (SMS 201–995) in the treatment of acromegaly. Am J Med 1986;81(6B):94–101.
322. Lanser JB, van Seters AP, Moolenaar AJ, et al. Neuropsychologic and neurologic side effects of mitotane and reversibility of symptoms. J Clin Oncol 1992;10(9):1504.
323. Hutter AM, Kayhoe DE. Adrenal cortical carcinoma, results of treatment with o,p'-DDD in 138 patients. Am J Med 1966;41:581–592.
324. Ng WT, Toohey MG, Mulhall L, et al. Pigmentary retinopathy, macular oedema, and abnormal ERG with mitotane treatment. Br J Ophthalmol 2003;87(4):500–501.
325. Stiefel FC, Breitbart WS, Holland JC. Corticosteroids in cancer: neuropsychiatric complications. Cancer Invest 1989;7(5):479–491.

326. Lewis DA, Smith RE. Steroid-induced psychiatric syndromes. A report of 14 cases and a review of the literature. J Affect Disord 1983;5(4):319–332.
327. Baethge BA, Lidsky MD. Intractable hiccups associated with high-dose intravenous methylprednisolone therapy. Ann Intern Med 1986;104(1):58–59.
328. Baharav E, Harpaz D, Mittelman M, et al. Dexamethasone-induced perineal irritation. N Engl J Med 1986;314(8): 515–516.
329. Lisai P, Doria C, Crissantu L, et al. Cauda equina syndrome secondary to idiopathic spinal epidural lipomatosis. Spine 2001;26(3):307–309.
330. Hierholzer J, Benndorf G, Lehmann T, et al. Epidural lipomatosis: case report and literature review. Neuroradiology 1996;38(4):343–348.
331. Batchelor TT, Taylor LP, Thaler HT, et al. Steroid myopathy in cancer patients. Neurology 1997;48(5):1234–1238.
332. Wall M. Idiopathic intracranial hypertension. Semin Ophthalmol 1995;10(3):251–259.
333. Buter J, Janssen RA, Martens A, et al. Phase I/II study of low-dose intravenous OKT3 and subcutaneous interleukin-2 in metastatic cancer. Eur J Cancer 1993;29A(15):2108–2113.
334. Thistlethwaite JR, Stuart JK, Mayes JT, et al. Complications and monitoring of OKT3 therapy. Am J Kidney Dis 1988; 11(2):112–119.
335. Capone PM, Cohen ME. Seizures and cerebritis associated with administration of OKT3. Pediatr Neurol 1991;7(4): 299–301.
336. Pittock SJ, Rabinstein AA, Edwards BS, et al. OKT3 neurotoxicity presenting as akinetic mutism. Transplantation 2003;75(7):1058–1060.
337. Marks WH, Perkal M, Bia M, et al. Aseptic meningitis and blindness complicating OKT3 therapy. Clin Transplant 1991;5:435–438.
338. Parizel PM, Snoeck HW, van den Hauwe L, et al. Cerebral complications of murine monoclonal CD3 antibody (OKT3): CT and MR findings. Am J Neuroradiol 1997;18(10): 1935–1938.
339. Berney T, Delis S, Kato T, et al. Successful treatment of posttransplant lymphoproliferative disease with prolonged rituximab treatment in intestinal transplant recipients. Transplantation 2002;74(7):1000–1006.
340. Miller WT Jr, Siegel SG, Montone KT. Posttransplantation lymphoproliferative disorder: changing manifestations of disease in a renal transplant population. Crit Rev Diagn Imaging 1997;38(6):569–585.
341. Baselga J, Pfister D, Cooper MR, et al. Phase I studies of anti-epidermal growth factor receptor chimeric antibody C225 alone and in combination with cisplatin. J Clin Oncol 2000;18(4):904–914.
342. Robert F, Ezekiel MP, Spencer SA, et al. Phase I study of anti-epidermal growth factor receptor antibody cetuximab in combination with radiation therapy in patients with advanced head and neck cancer. J Clin Oncol 2001; 19(13):3234–3243.
343. Fraunfelder FW, Solomon J, Druker BJ, et al. Ocular side-effects associated with imatinib mesylate (Gleevec). J Ocul Pharmacol Ther 2003;19(4):371–375.
344. Hidalgo M, Siu LL, Nemunaitis J, et al. Phase I and pharmacologic study of OSI-774, an epidermal growth factor receptor tyrosine kinase inhibitor, in patients with advanced solid malignancies. J Clin Oncol 2001;19(13):3267–3279.

CHAPTER 32

Neurologic Complications of Radiation Therapy

LAUREN E. ABREY / DENISE D. CORREA

The mechanisms by which radiation produces damage to the central and peripheral nervous system are controversial. Several risk factors have been identified, including volume of tissue irradiated, total dose, dose per fraction, duration of therapy, and radiation energy. Other contributing factors include age, preexisting neurologic or systemic diseases, genetic predisposition, and concomitant chemotherapy treatment.[1,2]

Vascular abnormalities and demyelination are the primary histologic changes associated with radiation injury.[3,4] *Several hypotheses have been proposed to explain radiation injury, but the exact cause of radiation damage remains to be elucidated.*

One hypothesis is that ionizing radiation may damage central nervous system (CNS) cells by causing DNA strand breaks, attacking RNA, lipids, and proteins, and stimulating apoptosis. Radiation-induced damage predominantly affects the white matter; a breakdown in the ability of O2A progenitors to reproduce and replace mature myelin-producing oligodendrocytes has been suggested as a potential mechanism.[5–7] *However, this theory has been questioned given evidence that loss of oligodendrocytes may account for early but not late-onset necrosis,*[8] *is not invariably associated with necrosis,*[9,10] *and that other demyelinating conditions are not often associated with necrosis.*[11]

A second hypothesis is that radiotherapy (RT) damages the vascular endothelium causing ischemia and necrosis of neural tissue. Vessel dilation and wall thickening, nuclear enlargement in endothelial cells after radiation, and a decrease in vessel density and endothelial cell loss have been described in support of this hypothesis.[1] *Although there is strong evidence for the role of vascular injury, necrosis without vascular damage has been reported,*[12] *and the degree of necrosis is often greater than expected for the amount of vascular damage.*[13]

The third hypothesis is that damaged glial cells release antigens that the immune system perceives as foreign, and an immune response produces vascular changes and necrosis.[14] *However, no direct evidence for this hypothesis has been found.*

Finally, the fourth hypothesis is based on animal studies that show that radiation interrupts cellular proliferation and kills dividing cells. The zone of subependymal cells at the atria of the lateral ventricles contains stem cells that can produce neurons and glia. Neurogenesis occurs both in the subventricular zone and in the subgranular zone of the dentate gyrus.[15] *Whole-brain radiation produces stem cell damage in rats and impairs regeneration of subependymal cells.*[16] *In adult rats, a 10-Gy dose produces apoptosis among the proliferating cells in the dentate gyrus of the hippocampus*[17] *and a decrease in stem cell differentiation into neurons in the hippocampus. Fractionated radiation (3 Gy) can arrest adult neurogenesis in the dentate gyrus of the hippocampus and is associated with a specific deficit in spatial memory.*[18] *These findings are relevant for the development of future therapeutic interventions that may target the protection or replacement of neural progenitor cells and treatment of microglial inflammation.*[15]

▶ RADIATION-INDUCED NEUROTOXICITY IN THE BRAIN

Radiation-induced injury to the CNS has been classified into three phases according to the time between administration of radiation therapy and onset of the injury.[3] These are described as acute, early delayed, and late-delayed (Table 32-1).

Acute Effects

Acute encephalopathy typically appears within days of initiation of radiotherapy. The most common symptoms are nausea and vomiting, headaches, drowsiness, and worsening of preexisting neurologic deficits.[19] Large doses of radiation per fraction (>300 cGy) delivered to large volumes of brain are the primary risk factor.[19] The pathogenesis most likely involves disruption of blood–brain barrier by ionizing radiation, with ensuing increased cerebral edema and intracranial pressure. Treatment with corticosteroids prior to initiation of radiation diminishes the disruption of the blood–brain barrier and prevents or limits most clinical symptoms.

Early Delayed Effects

This disorder occurs 2 weeks to 6 months following radiation and is reversible in most cases. Early delayed effects can manifest in various forms, depending on the dose and volume of brain radiated and the presence of underlying brain disease. Transitory demyelination related to blood–brain barrier disruption or injury to oligodendrocytes has been considered to explain the syndrome.[13]

Somnolence Syndrome

This disorder is most common in children after whole-brain radiation,[20,21] and in adults treated with accelerated fractionation.[22] The incidence of somnolence syndrome varies across studies,[22–24] possibly as a consequence of variables such as radiation dose, fractionation, and diagnostic criteria. The course of the syndrome is favorable, typically resolving between 2 weeks and 3 months. Corticosteroids have been found to ameliorate the symptoms or possibly prevent them if prescribed during RT.[24] The symptoms include drowsiness, lethargy, headache, nausea, and anorexia. Early delayed cognitive impairment reportedly affects primarily psychomotor speed, attention,

▶ **TABLE 32-1.** RADIATION INJURY OF THE BRAIN

Type	Onset	Symptoms	Pathology	Outcome
Acute	Hours to days	Nausea, headache, neurological signs	Disruption of blood–brain barrier, edema, increased intracranial pressure	Recovery
Early delayed	2–16 weeks	Somnolence, focal signs, encephalopathy, transitory cognitive dysfunction	Demyelination, edema	Recovery
Late-delayed	Months to years			
Necrosis		Focal signs, mild to moderate cognitive dysfunction	Necrosis	Responds to corticosteroids; surgery
Atrophy		Gait ataxia, incontinence, cognitive impairment	Demyelination, hydrocephalus	Modest response to shunting

and memory abilities, and typically occurs within 6 months of radiotherapy. Armstrong and associates[25] reported a decline in word retrieval after interference and delayed periods in adult patients with low-grade gliomas evaluated 3 months following focal radiotherapy; improvement was seen on a 6-month followup evaluation. Vigliani and associates[26] reported a transient reduction in reaction time on an attention task 6 months after radiation in 36% of glioma patients treated with focal radiation. Early delayed persistent or severe impairments are uncommon and do not predict the development of late-delayed cognitive dysfunction.[27]

Neurologic Deterioration

In patients with primary or metastatic brain tumors, the symptoms of early delayed encephalopathy can be similar to those associated with tumor progression. Headache, mental slowing, and worsening of preexisting neurologic focal deficits are commonly seen. This syndrome usually follows radiation treatment by about 2 months and resolves within 6 months[28]; corticosteroids can accelerate the recovery. Neuroimaging studies show increased surrounding edema and contrast enhancement, which makes it difficult to distinguish it from tumor recurrence. Positron emission tomography (PET) is often helpful in differentiating radiation necrosis from recurrent tumor, because radionecrosis is often characterized by hypometabolism and tumor growth by hypermetabolism.[31] However, a biopsy is the only procedure that can ascertain the diagnosis.

Focal Encephalopathy

This syndrome is seen following high-dose radiation to extracranial tumors for which the radiation field includes the brain. The symptoms develop within weeks after radiation and vary depending on the portion of the brain that is radiated. This is most common in ocular, pituitary, and head and neck tumors where radiation portals involve the brainstem; symptoms include ataxia, diplopia, dysarthria, nystagmus, and hearing loss. Patients typically recover within 6 to 8 weeks. Radiation-induced hearing impairment is very common in patients with brainstem gliomas irradiated conventionally, and some authors report treatment-related toxicity rates of 40% for skin reactions, otitis media and externa, nonspecific ear pain, tinnitus, and subjective hearing loss.[29]

Transient white matter hyperintensity consistent with demyelination may be detected on magnetic resonance imaging (MRI) scan. The pathogenesis is presumed to involve demyelination caused by temporary damage to oligodendroglia and subsequent breakdown of myelin sheaths[14]; loss of oligodendrocytes and abnormal giant astrocytes are also seen. Fractionated stereotactic conformal RT is associated with only mild toxicity. Schulz-Ertner and colleagues reported that only 6 of 41 patients showed onset of contrast enhancement after RT, which could be interpreted as a transient radiation-induced disruption of the blood–brain barrier.[30]

Late-Delayed Effects

These complications become apparent a few months to many years after treatment, and are often associated with irreversible damage to the CNS.[3] The extent and pattern of delayed radiation-induced brain injury usually vary according to the volume of radiated tissue, radiation dose, dose per fraction, disease, concomitant administration of chemotherapy, and age. The most common forms are radiation necrosis, atrophy, and cognitive impairment ranging from mild to severe.

Radiation Necrosis

Radiation necrosis usually follows radiation by 1 to 2 years, but can start as early as 3 months postradiotherapy.[31–33] A total external beam cranial radiation dose of 55 to 60 Gy, administered in fractions of 1.8 to 2 Gy per day, has been demonstrated to be the upper limit of what is considered a relatively safe dose. In most series, 60 Gy administered to the whole brain in 30 fractions is associated with the development of radiation necrosis in 5% to 15% of patients.[3,32] However, a 24% incidence of biopsy-proven necrosis has been reported in malignant glioma patients treated with radiation and chemotherapy.[34] Necrosis typically occurs near the tumor site after either focal or whole-brain radiation, suggesting that tissue damaged by tumor or edema may be more susceptible. However, extensive necrosis and white matter injury in areas distant from the tumor but within the irradiated field have been reported in a large series of autopsied cases.[35]

Clinical symptoms often involve new focal neurologic signs that mimic those of the brain tumor. Radionecrosis in the temporal lobes after radiation for nasopharyngeal tumors has been reported in a large series of patients.[36] In these patients, the inferior temporal lobe, inferior frontal lobe, and the brainstem are often in the path of the radiation beams. Microvascular damage from temporal lobe radiation can result in injury, particularly in the CA1 region of the hippocampus, and produce cognitive dysfunction.[37] Recent studies[38,39] have documented memory impairments in this population. Hemiparesis or behavioral changes may occur in patients treated for eye or maxillary tumors caused by radiation damage to the frontal or temporal lobes. Increased intracranial pressure with headache, lethargy, and papilledema may also occur.[40]

Computerized tomography (CT) scan often shows a hypodense area within the irradiated region and variable contrast enhancement. MRI shows predominantly white matter lesions appearing as T_1-weighted hypointensity and T_2-weighted hyperintensity, and enhancement is common (Fig. 32-1). Neither CT nor MRI scans can differentiate tumor recurrence from necrosis. Additional neuroimaging techniques may assist in assessing the nature of the lesion. PET studies[41,42] report high specificity, as radionecrosis is characterized by hypometabolism and tumor growth by hypermetabolism. Single-photon emission tomography (SPECT) shows a high thallium uptake in recurrent tumor and low thallium uptake in necrosis,[43] but its specificity has been questioned.[44,45] Magnetic resonance spectroscopy (MRS) studies show that tumors have increased choline and decreased N-acetylaspartate (NAA) compared with other tissues; this technique is used in combination with biopsy to increase diagnostic accuracy.[46] Recent studies suggest that several metabolic changes are associated with the effects of radiation, particularly a decrease in NAA in irradiated brain tissue.[47,48] Some studies have also described abnormal cellular metabolism in the white matter in regions remote from the radiated area.[49] However, current imaging modalities do not have adequate sensitivity or specificity to definitively distinguish between the tumor and radiation necrosis, and biopsy remains the only method that provides the definitive diagnosis.[50]

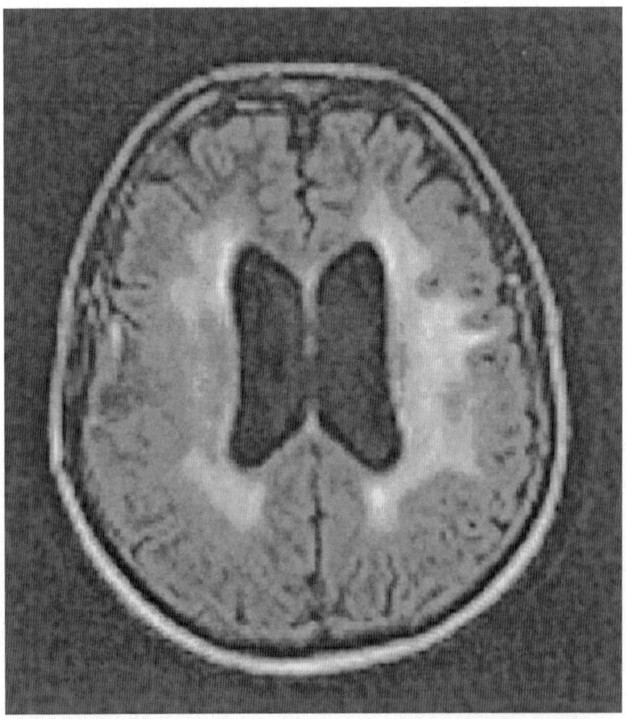

Figure 32-1. Axial fluid-attenuated inversion recovery (FLAIR) magnetic resonance image demonstrating leukoencephalopathy and ventriculomegaly in a 50-year-old male treated with a combination of high-dose methotrexate and whole-brain radiotherapy for primary CNS lymphoma.

Coagulative necrosis predominantly located in the white matter, with relative sparing of the cortex and deep gray matter, characterizes radiation-induced lesions. Blood vessels show hyalization of the vessel wall, thickening and fibroid necrosis associated with vascular hemorrhage, and thrombosis (Fig. 32-2).[13] These changes are often indistinguishable from the white matter damage produced by methotrexate (MTX). In less affected regions, demyelination is seen with loss of oligodendrocytes, axonal loss and swelling, dystrophic calcifications, fibrinoid necrosis, and perivascular infiltrates and mononuclear cells.

Treatment for radiation necrosis includes surgical resection of the necrotic tissue and corticosteroids; however, response to steroids tends to be transient. Anticoagulant and antiplatelet medications have been used to halt the progression of necrosis, based on the putative etiology of vascular changes associated with ischemia.[51] Hyperbaric oxygen has also been used to treat radiation necrosis.[52] However, to date there are no large-scale studies confirming the benefits of such treatments.

Cerebral Atrophy

Whole-brain radiotherapy may result in brain atrophy. In such cases MR scans show hyperintensity, most pronounced in the periventricular white matter, on the T_2-weighted image. These abnormalities are apparent approximately 1 year after radiation, tend to be progressive, and almost always follow whole-brain radiation. Very young children and the elderly are most susceptible. The pathogenesis of ventricular dilatation and cerebral atrophy is uncertain. In some patients radiation-induced arachnoiditis or obliteration of pacchionian granulations can lead to communicating hydrocephalus; loss of cerebral tissue because of direct radiation damage has also been implicated.[13] Although there is no treatment for cerebral atrophy at present, occasional patients may experience temporary benefit following ventriculoperitoneal shunting.

Endocrine Dysfunction

Radiation-induced endocrine dysfunction occurs after radiation to the pituitary and hypothalamus, or to the neck when the thyroid or parathyroid are within the radiation portal. Endocrine disorders may result from a hypothalamic–pituitary dysfunction induced by radiation for nasopharyngeal tumors,[53] low-grade gliomas,[54] and prophylactic radiation for acute lymphoblastic leukemia[55]; endocrine disorders are more frequent in patients who receive higher radiation doses.[56] Treatment with hormonal replacement therapy usually leads to improvement. Patients who have received a dose of 30 Gy or higher to the pituitary and/or hypothalamus should have an annual evaluation of anterior pituitary function by an endocrinologist.

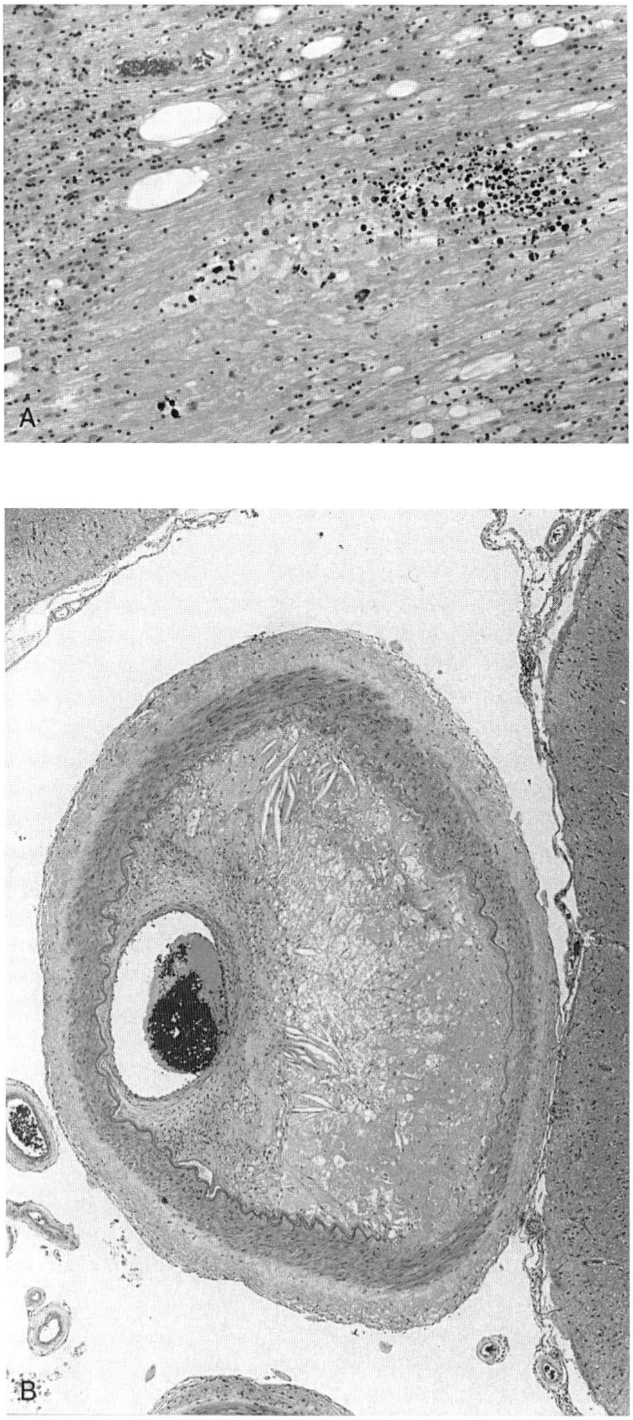

Figure 32-2 (PLATE 62). (A) Hematoxylin and eosin (H&E) stain of radiation-induced neurotoxicity demonstrating characteristic gliosis and spongiosis of the white matter with vacuolar change. (B) This panel demonstrates prominent atherosclerosis of the middle cerebral artery with thrombus in the vascular lumen.

Radiation-Induced Vasculopathy

Radiation can produce late-delayed damage to large blood vessels, which may have secondary effects on CNS function. The dose of radiation required to induce vascular lesions usually exceeds 50 Gy, but radiation type, fractionation, and portal also play a role. Lesions consist of stenosis or occlusions of the artery. Lesions of large intracranial and extracranial vessels can occur months to years after radiation, and the carotid artery is most vulnerable.[57] Several studies report carotid occlusion from atherosclerosis leading to focal seizures, transient ischemia, or cerebral infarction.[13] The lesions are similar to those induced by atherosclerosis, but the site of occlusion differs from its usual location in nonirradiated patients. Occlusion or stenosis of the supraclinoid portion of the internal carotid can be seen in children treated with cranial radiation, and such occlusions may lead to moyamoya disease.[58] This complication is most frequent in children treated for optic chiasm glioma, but may also occur with brainstem gliomas and craniopharyngiomas.[59] Treatment for large-vessel vasculopathy involves lowering serum cholesterol and carotid endarterectomy when indicated.[60]

Cognitive Dysfunction

A substantial number of brain tumor patients treated with radiation develop cognitive impairments that vary from mild to severe. It is currently considered the most frequent complication among long-term survivors.[1] Although the peak of neurocognitive abnormalities resulting from radiation treatment occurs approximately 6 months to 2 years after completion of radiotherapy[3] and is proportional to the percentage of patients with disease-free survival,[61] its incidence is unknown. In a large review of several studies, the incidence of severe cognitive impairment was at least 12.3%.[62] The variability in the documented frequency of radiation-induced cognitive deficits may be partially associated with the insensitivity of the methods of assessment that have been used,[61] duration of followup, and population discrepancies. Most studies have included only clinical observations, mental status examinations, or IQ measures. These variables have low sensitivity to detect cognitive impairment in this population.[63,64] In addition, the high incidence of tumor recurrence and short-term survival in patients with high-grade gliomas have often been considered confounding variables that have hampered the ability to quantify the frequency, onset, course, and causes of the delayed cognitive effects of radiotherapy.[62]

The pattern of neuropsychological impairments associated with the delayed effects of whole-brain radiotherapy and chemotherapy tends to be diffuse in nature,[65] relatively independent of tumor location, and deteriorate gradually over time.[66] In the studies that have included neuropsychological assessments of brain tumor patients treated with whole-brain radiation, cognitive domains that have been suggested to be particularly sensitive to radiation-induced cognitive dysfunction include attention, new learning and memory, and speed of cognitive processing.[67–69] Cognitive and emotional difficulties often have an impact on quality of life and interfere with the patient's ability to function at premorbid levels professionally and socially.[70,71] There is no recognized treatment for radiation-induced cognitive dysfunction, but some mild improvement in psychomotor speed and mood has been reported in patients treated with methylphenidate.[63]

Several contributing factors to the development of radiation-induced cognitive dysfunction have been identified. Its prevalence appears to increase with age, volume of brain irradiated, radiation dose and fraction size, and concomitant chemotherapy.[72] Patients age 60 years or older are at increased risk for delayed neurotoxicity.[10,25,73,74] Cognitive dysfunction is more common after whole-brain radiation.[75] Approximately 50% of patients with primary brain tumors treated with whole-brain radiation display cognitive impairments,[25,67] and figures range from 4% to 63% among patients treated with combined radiation and chemotherapy.[1] Followup studies of acute lymphoblastic lymphoma patients[76,77] treated with prophylactic whole-brain radiation have reported cognitive deficits involving attention, reading, arithmetic, and psychosocial functioning; however, these results have not been corroborated in adults with small cell lung cancer. Large daily fraction sizes are associated with a greater likelihood of developing neurotoxicity in patients with brain metastases treated with whole-brain radiation,[78] and memory impairment in low-grade glioma patients treated with focal radiation.[79]

Patients with low-grade tumors treated with radiation generally receive focal rather than whole-brain radiotherapy, in part as an attempt to avoid delayed neurotoxicity. However, even with local therapy, treated volumes are large considering that these tumors are infiltrative and often large at the time of diagnosis; radiation of a significant amount of surrounding healthy tissue is often difficult to avoid.[80] Most studies examining the effects of partial RT have been retrospective and revealed variable outcomes ranging from no morbidity to marked cognitive deficits. Differences in the sensitivity of the neuropsychological measures administered, the inclusion of patients with anaplastic and low-grade tumors,[25] and patients treated with partial and whole-brain RT[80] may account for some of the variability of the findings in the literature. In addition, the absence of baseline, pretreatment cognitive evaluations made it difficult to distinguish the specific effects of tumor versus treatment.

In a retrospective study, Taphoorn and colleagues[81] reported cognitive impairments in a small group of patients with low-grade tumors, but no significant differences were detected between patients who received focal radiation and those who had surgery or biopsy only. The authors concluded that cognitive deficits were tumor and not radiation-related. Similar findings were reported on a more recent retrospective study including 195 patients with low-grade tumors[79]; cognitive deficits were evident on measures of attention, psychomotor speed and memory, with no significant differences between patients who received partial-brain RT or no treatment. However, patients who received radiation fraction doses above 2 Gy displayed more impaired memory performance than did patients who received lower fractions. Age may have been a contributing factor given that patients in the large fraction group were also significantly older.

Armstrong and colleagues[25] prospectively studied a group of 20 patients with low-grade tumors treated with partial radiation (dose range: 54 to 63 Gy; fraction range: 1.8 to 2.0 Gy). A selective decrement in verbal memory retrieval was evident during the early delayed period postradiation (1.5–9 months) but patients improved subsequently; conversely, a pattern of pre-RT impairment and steady improvement in visual recall was evident over up to 1 year after RT. Verbal retrieval impairment was not associated with deficits in attention or working memory.[82] The long-term effects of radiation on cognition were examined on a subsequent study involving 26 patients with low-grade tumors.[83] A selective decline in learning and recall of visual information 5 years post-RT was detected despite continued improvement up to that point. Long-term improvements were noted on tests of attention, executive, and verbal recall abilities. The findings were found to suggest that partial radiation was not associated with significant delayed cognitive impairments in this population. Similarly, a recent study by Torres and colleagues[84] reported no evidence of cognitive decline in 15 patients with low-grade tumors treated with conformal fractionated partial-brain RT. Some of the limitations of these studies involve the inclusion of a small number of patients with various tumor types (adenoma, ependymoma) and locations (pituitary, pineal) who were treated with different radiation dosages (e.g., pituitary adenomas received less RT than other tumors).

The association between abnormalities in neuroimaging studies and the presence or severity of neuropsychological deficits is unclear,[71] with some, but not all, studies showing moderate correlations.[69,80,82,85] MRI scans show variable degrees of T_2-weighted hyperintensity in the white matter. In two studies, Johnson and colleagues[86,87] reported that approximately 60% of patients receiving prophylactic whole-brain cranial irradiation (with and without chemotherapy) for small cell lung cancer showed progressive impairment on a neuropsychological test battery over a period of 6 to 13 years. The degree of cognitive impairment correlated with radiation administered in high daily fractions and concurrent high-dose chemotherapy. A moderate correlation between periventricular white matter changes and neuropsychological test scores was also reported. A more recent study[88] provided further evidence of the sensitivity of cognitive evaluations to detect the presence of neurocognitive dysfunction in patients who received whole-brain prophylactic radiation. Dropcho[71] reported that approximately 30% to 50% of adults with malignant gliomas treated with whole-brain radiation had moderate to severe difficulties in attention and problem solving and were unable to return to their premorbid functional status. Radiographic changes included diffuse cortical atrophy and white matter abnormalities. Armstrong and colleagues[83] documented white matter atrophy as well as hyperintensity primarily around the tumor site and in the frontal, periventricular, and centrum semiovale white matter in 26 patients with low-grade tumors treated with partial radiation. White matter atrophy and hyperintensity progressed in at least half of the patients and peaked about 3 years after treatment. There were, however, no correlations between the slopes of cognitive decline and increasing radiographic changes. Earlier studies[89,90] also failed to detect significant correlations between white matter change and neurologic or performance status in brain tumor patients who received conformal radiation. Conversely, Postma and colleagues[80] reported moderate correlations between performance on tests of attention and information processing speed and white matter abnormalities on MRI, whereas memory performance correlated with cerebral atrophy in a small group of patients with low-grade tumors treated with focal radiation. Surma-aho and colleagues[85] examined long-term cognitive outcome in patients with low-grade gliomas who received partial radiotherapy or no treatment. The results revealed more severe leukoencephalopathy and memory impairment in patients who received radiation.

The incidence of radiation-induced dementia varies significantly in the literature,[58] possibly as a result of several confounding variables such as the inclusion of patients with progressive tumors and treated with higher whole-brain radiation doses than used currently.[72] Patients present with progressive memory, attention, and executive deficits and fatigue. Eventually patients develop gait ataxia, incontinence, depression, and apathy. Seizures, pyramidal and extrapyramidal signs, and tremor are also frequent developments.[1] Neuroimaging shows diffuse white matter lesions associated with cortical and subcortical atrophy and ventricular enlargement. There is no treatment for this condition. In some patients who display normal pressure hydrocephalus, ventriculoperitoneal shunting may provide temporary improvement in quality of life.[91] Death typically occurs within 48 months after the onset of the disorder.[78]

Combined Effects of Radiation and Chemotherapy

Combined treatment with radiation and chemotherapy may have a synergistic effect[58,92] and lower the brain tolerance for radiation.[93] Potential mechanisms by which chemotherapy may increase radiation neurotoxicity have been hypothesized. Chemotherapy agents may interfere with the same cellular structures as does radiation and may act as a radiosensitizer. Radiation may alter the distribution kinetics of chemotherapeutic agents in the CNS by increasing the permeability of the blood–brain barrier,[94] affecting the ability of arachnoid granulations or choroid plexus to clear the drug, or disrupting the ependymal barrier to allow drugs in the cerebrospinal fluid (CSF) to enter the cerebral white matter. Finally, radiation-induced cellular changes may allow greater amounts of the drug to enter nontumor cells or less drug to exit.[13]

The interactions between radiation and MTX are the most clearly demonstrated.[94,95] Risk factors for neurotoxicity include young or old age, leptomeningeal disease, timing of chemotherapy, and increasing dosages of radiation and MTX.[13] A 10% to 12% incidence of severe cognitive impairment has been reported in patients who received whole-brain radiation in combination with intravenous and intrathecal MTX, particularly in patients older than age 60 years who were treated for primary CNS lymphoma.[74] The administration of MTX after radiation enhances radiation-induced leukoencephalopathy. MRI shows periventricular white matter changes, and the pathologic changes include multifocal areas of coagulative necrosis in the deep white matter with loss of myelin, axonal swelling, fragmentation, and gliosis. Other chemotherapy agents that may produce CNS damage when combined with radiation are nitrosoureas, cytosine arabinoside, and vincristine[96]; however, the injury mechanisms are not so well understood.

►RADIOTHERAPY AND SPINAL CORD INJURY

Damage to the spinal cord is most often the result of RT administered for spinal cord tumors, Hodgkin disease, or tumors of the head and neck. There is no clinical or experimental evidence to suggest that RT is acutely damaging to the spinal cord even when delivered in fractions as large as 1000 cGy. However, postradiation myelopathy may occur either as a mild, transient early syndrome, or as an irreversible, progressive late event (Table 32-2). Delayed syndromes of motor neuron dysfunction and spinal cord hemorrhage are rarely observed.

Early Postradiotherapy Myelopathy

Early post-RT myelopathy is a relatively frequent clinical syndrome that occurs in as many as 15% of patients receiving mantle irradiation for Hodgkin disease. A large study of more than 1000 patients estimated an overall incidence of 3.6% in patients receiving RT to the cervical spine.[97] Higher total and per fraction doses of RT were associated with a high risk of developing this syndrome.

► **TABLE 32-2.** RADIATION INJURY OF THE SPINAL CORD

Type	Onset	Symptoms	Outcome
Early myelopathy	Weeks to months	Lhermitte sign	Resolution
Late myelopathy	Months to years	Brown-Sequard syndrome; paraplegia; spasticity	Progressive; irreversible
Motor neuron dysfunction	Up to 20 years	Flaccid leg weakness	Irreversible; may progress or plateau
Spinal cord hemorrhage	8–30 years	Acute back pain; weakness	Resolution

Patients become symptomatic within a few weeks to a few months of completing RT. Usually the syndrome is limited to Lhermitte sign, which is characterized by an electrical shock-like sensation induced by neck flexion. Patients will often describe this as brief, unpleasant sensations of numbness or tingling that shoot down the back and into their arms or legs. There is no associated MRI abnormality.[98] Most patients will have spontaneous resolution of symptoms and no treatment is indicated. There is no association between early post-RT myelopathy and progressive or late-delayed spinal cord injury.

This syndrome is felt to be the result of demyelination of the posterior columns; stretching of these fibers with neck flexion leads to a spontaneous discharge. While there is no histologic evidence to support this hypothesis, experimental studies in animals have shown loss of oligodendroglial cells and elevated levels of myelin basic protein in the CSF following RT.[99–101] Somatosensory-evoked potentials are delayed in some patients suggestive of a demyelinating process.[102]

Late Spinal Cord Injury

Progressive Myelopathy

A progressive, irreversible myelopathy is a relatively rare complication of spinal cord irradiation, occurring in less than 1% of patients treated with a dose of 5000 cGy or less. However, similar to early post-RT myelopathy, the incidence of this disorder increases with higher doses of RT, and as many as 5% of patients receiving a dose of 6000 cGy will develop a progressive myelopathy.[103] Other associated risk factors include older age, dose per fraction, re-irradiation, and prior chemotherapy.[104–106]

The clinical presentation features paresthesias and weakness in one leg with loss of pain and temperature sensation in the opposite leg, also known as Brown-Sequard syndrome. Pain may or may not be present and can be focal back or radicular pain. Occasional patients develop a transverse myelopathy with symmetric loss of motor and sensory function in both legs. Sphincter and diaphragmatic dysfunction may be present. Symptom onset is typically subacute and progressive starting months to years after treatment. Neurologic decline to quadra- or paraparesis with complete loss of all motor, sensory, and autonomic function can occur, but some patients will stabilize after an initial period of decline. There is no proven treatment for progressive RT-induced myelopathy. Steroids may result in temporary improvement. Individual patients have been reported to benefit from anticoagulation or hyperbaric oxygen treatment.[107,108]

Diagnostic studies are nonspecific. CSF is often normal, although CSF protein may be elevated. Early MRI findings may be normal, but there is often demonstrable cord edema and approximately 50% of cases will have some gadolinium enhancement. Late MRI findings include spinal cord atrophy and cyst formation.[109,110] Pathologically, there is evidence of demyelination and vascular injury. The posterior columns and lateral funiculi appear to be particularly prone to demyelination and focal necrosis. Vascular abnormalities include telangiectasia formation, fibrinoid necrosis, hyalinization, and perivascular fibrosis.[111]

Motor Neuron Dysfunction

Patients treated with pelvic or craniospinal RT have rarely been reported to develop a purely lower motor neuron syndrome as long as 20 or more years after treatment. Patients with testicular cancer account for most described cases. Clinically, there is a subacute onset of bilateral leg weakness with associated cramps, fasciculations and loss of reflexes. Associated sensory signs or sphincter changes are not seen, although this may be difficult to assess in some patients with chronic sphincter dysfunction on a mechanical basis. Evolution of this syndrome is variable; some patients stabilize whereas others have relentless progression resulting in paraplegia.

MRI scans are normal and CSF total protein may be slightly increased. Electrical diagnostic studies suggest damage to the proximal nerve roots with prolonged latency of F waves and preserved distal motor action potentials.[112] Autopsy of one patient with RT-induced motor neuron dysfunction found evidence of a radiation-induced vascular injury involving the spinal roots.[113]

Spinal Cord Hemorrhage

This is a very rare, and often very delayed, complication of radiotherapy, with cases described as occurring 8 to

30 years after treatment. Acute onset of leg weakness and back pain are the presenting features. MRI will demonstrate acute hemorrhage in the spinal cord in the absence of other lesions. Symptoms usually start to improve within several days and most reported patients have made a complete recovery. Because there is a risk of recurrent episodes of hemorrhage, and some have occurred in patients taking nonsteroidal antiinflammatory agents, patients should be advised to avoid aspirin and nonsteroidal antiinflammatory agents. Radiation-induced telangiectasias are believed to be responsible for this syndrome.

▶RADIATION INJURY OF THE BRACHIAL OR LUMBOSACRAL PLEXUS

The brachial plexus is exposed to radiation administered to the supraclavicular, infraclavicular, or axillary region. The tumors most frequently associated with radiotherapy to these regions include breast cancer, lung cancer, and Hodgkin disease. The clinical challenge is to distinguish a radiation-induced plexopathy (Table 32-3) from malignant infiltration of the brachial plexus by tumor (Table 32-4).

Acute Brachial Plexopathy

Acute development of a painful brachial plexopathy has been reported in patients receiving mantle RT for Hodgkin disease.[114,115] This syndrome is clinically indistinguishable from an idiopathic brachial plexopathy (Parsonage-Turner syndrome) and complete recovery is the rule. Onset of symptoms typically occurs within days to weeks of initiating RT, which can be completed safely.

Early Delayed Brachial Plexopathy

This relatively uncommon syndrome affects approximately 1% to 2% of patients irradiated for breast cancer.[116,117] Symptoms typically begin 4 to 5 months after completion of RT and are characterized by paresthesias in the hand and forearm with associated distal weakness and atrophy. Moderate pain provoked by movement of the shoulder or persistent aching in the axilla is reported in up to 60% of patients. Most patients have complete resolution of this syndrome over several months and there is no evidence that early delayed brachial plexopathy is a harbinger of progressive late-delayed plexopathy.

Late-Delayed Brachial Plexopathy

Delayed radiation-induced brachial plexopathy is a progressive syndrome characterized by painless weakness of proximal arm and shoulder girdle and paresthesias of the hand and forearm. Affected patients often have associated lymphedema and induration of the supraclavicular region. The prevalence of this late complication increases with prolonged survival, and a recent report of patients followed for more than 30 years after irradiation for breast cancer estimated that up to 75% of patients were affected.[118] This same study found that long-term survivors had a 5% risk of unilateral vocal cord paralysis; similarly, phrenic nerve paralysis with resultant diaphragmatic weakness has also been described.[119] Symptoms may begin as early as 1 year after RT, and progression to a pan-plexopathy with paralysis and atrophy of the entire arm is typical.

The presence or absence of pain is the critical distinguishing factor between the radiation-induced plexopathy (typically painless) and malignant infiltration of the plexus (usually associated with severe pain). The finding of myokymic discharges on electrophysiologic studies supports the diagnosis of radiation-induced plexopathy. MRI of the plexus can be useful if a mass lesion suggesting malignant infiltration is found; however, many of the radiologic findings are nonspecific.[120] PET evidence of hypermetabolism may also help to establish a diagnosis of malignant infiltration.[121] In select cases with mixed symptomatology and nondiagnostic evaluation, a biopsy should be considered to establish the diagnosis.

No effective treatment exists for radiation-induced plexopathy. A randomized phase II study of hyperbaric oxygen found no evidence of improvement in neurologic function, although there was an observed decrease in the degree of lymphedema in patients receiving hyperbaric oxygen.[122] Surgical exploration with neurolysis and transfer

▶ TABLE 32-3. RADIATION-INDUCED PLEXOPATHY

Type	Onset	Symptoms	Signs	Evolution
Acute	During RT	Painful	Weakness	Resolution; safe to complete RT
Early delayed	Months	Paresthesias; moderate pain	Distal weakness	Resolution
Late-delayed	Years	Paresthesias; painless	Proximal weakness; visible myokymia	Progressive

▶ **TABLE 32-4.** RADIATION-INDUCED VERSUS MALIGNANT PLEXOPATHY

Findings	RT	Tumor
Pain	Mild to absent	Severe
Horner syndrome	Infrequent	Common (>50%)
Dysesthesias	Common	Rare
Lymphedema	Common	Rare
Myokymia (EMG)	Present	Absent
MRI		
General	Diffuse thickening	Mass lesion
Gadolinium	Enhancement	Enhancement
T_1	Low signal intensity	Low signal intensity
T_2	Low signal intensity	High signal intensity
PET	Hypometabolic	Hypermetabolic

of a myocutaneous flap to revascularize the plexus has been reported to improve function in individual patients.[123] Two patients with radiation-induced plexopathy are reported to have improved with anticoagulation.[48]

Lumbosacral Plexopathy

Patterns of radiation-induced injury to the lumbosacral plexus are similar to although substantially less common than those seen in the brachial plexus. Radiation tolerance of the local peripheral nerves and lumbosacral plexus limits intraoperative radiotherapy of pelvic tumors.[124] Early delayed lumbosacral plexopathy is characterized by distal paresthesias and a normal examination; complete resolution over the course of several months is the rule. A slowly progressive late plexopathy can occur up to 30 years after RT. Erectile dysfunction will occur in up to 80% of patients treated for prostate cancer and is likely caused by vascular injury of the pudendal and penile arteries as opposed to injury of the sacral plexus.

▶RADIATION INJURY OF THE CRANIAL AND PERIPHERAL NERVES

Acute, often reversible, symptoms involving the olfactory, optic, or auditory nerves may develop during or shortly after the completion of radiotherapy. However, fewer than 1% of patients who receive RT encompassing the cranial nerves will go on to develop delayed cranial neuropathies as a result of radiation injury (Table 32-5). These complications are likely the result of direct axonal injury or damage to the Schwann cells; in contrast, in the neck, fibrosis of the connective tissue is often the mechanism of injury.

Olfactory Nerve (Cranial Nerve I)

During cranial irradiation many patients will report an unpleasant odor similar to ozone accompanying the actual radiation treatment.[125] This is believed to be the result of stimulation of olfactory nerve endings by the radiation. Radiation-induced taste disorders may complicate patient's perception of smell during and for an interval of several months after RT. Anosmia is a delayed complication. Most patients will have a demonstrable decrease in olfaction somewhere between 3 and 12 months after completing radiotherapy; however, this is often asymptomatic.[126,127]

Optic Nerve (Cranial Nerve II)

Radiotherapy has a wide range of potential impacts on vision. Glaucoma, cataracts, retinopathy, and optic neuropathy may all account for RT-induced visual loss. Patients receiving radiation may acutely report photopsias or visual sensations when the radiation beam is turned on. Radiation-induced optic neuropathy develops months to years after treatment and is characterized by the painless development of monocular or binocular blindness. A particularly high rate of optic neuropathy

▶ **TABLE 32-5.** RADIATION INJURY OF CRANIAL NERVES

Cranial Nerve	Acute	Delayed
I (olfactory)	Unpleasant odor	Anosmia
II (optic)	Photopsias	Visual loss
III, IV, and VI (oculomotor)	None	Neuromyotonia; rare isolated palsies
V (trigeminal)	None	Rare; exclude recurrent tumor
VII (facial)	Dysgeusia	Rare; exclude recurrent tumor
VIII (acoustic)	Tinnitus; high-frequency hearing loss	Otitis media; hearing loss
IX (glossopharyngeal)	None	None
X (vagus)	None	Vocal cord paralysis; Horner syndrome
XI (spinal accessory)	None	Shoulder droop; chronic pain
XII (hypoglossal)	None	Tongue paralysis

has been observed in patients treated with proton beam radiotherapy for clivus lesions.[128] Associated funduscopic changes include papilledema, telangiectasias, and hemorrhages. Retinal abnormalities include cotton wool spots, exudates, and arterial narrowing. Histologically, there is evidence of axonal loss, demyelination, gliosis, and vascular hyalinization. MRI may demonstrate initial enlargement and occasional enhancement of the optic nerves followed by atrophy.[129] MRI is also being used as a valuable tool to study the mechanism of radiation-induced optic neuropathy.[130] While the visual loss associated with radiation-induced optic neuropathy is typically permanent, individual patients have been reported to benefit from optic nerve sheath fenestration[131] and hyperbaric oxygen therapy.[132]

Oculomotor Nerves (Cranial Nerves III, IV, and VI)

Acute dysfunction of the oculomotor nerves during radiation is not observed. Even late complications are rare and typically occur in the setting of an optic neuropathy. Because of the association with optic neuropathy and visual loss it is possible that the true incidence is underreported. Transient ocular motor palsies are described following proton beam therapy to the pituitary; demyelination is the likely etiology.

Neuromyotonia is a late complication characterized by spontaneous spasm of the eye muscles. Patients may complain of intermittent diplopia, eye twitching or oscillopsia. The episodes are brief in duration and painless. The etiology of this phenomenon is thought to be spontaneous discharge of oculomotor nerves, and some patients have responded to treatment with membrane stabilizing anticonvulsants.[133]

Trigeminal Nerve (Cranial Nerve VI)

The trigeminal nerve is rarely reported to suffer either acute or delayed radiation-induced side effects. Therefore, the development of trigeminal neuropathy following radiation for head and neck cancer should raise the possibility of recurrent tumor invading along the nerve. Occasional patients will develop neuromyotonia involving the trigeminal nerve and may respond to anticonvulsants. When patients with trigeminal neuralgia are treated with radiosurgery, mild facial numbness may result.

Facial Nerve (Cranial Nerve VII)

Taste dysfunction is a common acute side effect reported during radiation that may linger for several months after treatment.[134] Treatment with zinc sulfate may benefit some patients.[135] Up to 50% of patients will have some permanent loss or change in taste; however, this is complicated as many cancer patients will have some change in taste prior to any treatment or related to chemotherapy.[136]

Radiosurgery for acoustic neuroma results in motor deficits in as many as 15% to 20% of patients. However, with dose fractionation, this risk is eliminated.[137,138] Consequently, patients who develop a motor deficit after fractionated radiation should be evaluated for recurrent tumor.

Acoustic Nerve (Cranial Nerve VIII)

Similar to vision, radiotherapy may impact auditory function in a variety of ways. Acute damage to the cochlea results in reversible tinnitus and high frequency hearing loss. Otitis media may result in hearing loss that develops shortly after the completion of radiotherapy and is often responsive to nasal vasoconstrictors; myringotomy is required in select patients. Delayed sensorineural hearing loss is predominantly attributed to injury of the inner ear, either the labyrinth or the organ of Corti with secondary atrophy of the eighth nerve.[139,140] Direct damage to the vestibular portion of the acoustic nerve is not described.

Glossopharyngeal Nerve (Cranial Nerve IX)

Neither acute nor delayed RT injury of the glossopharyngeal nerve has been reported; however, this nerve may be difficult to assess in isolation.

Vagus Nerve (Cranial Nerve X)

Damage to the vagus nerve with paralysis of the vocal cord and palate results in difficulty swallowing. Isolated damage of the recurrent laryngeal nerve, a branch of the vagus, may cause a vocal cord paralysis with a normal palate; patients present with hoarseness and aspiration. Horner syndrome from injury to the sympathetic fibers may be seen in association with other lower cranial neuropathies or in isolation. Acute radiation injury of the vagus nerve has not been reported.

Spinal Accessory Nerve (Cranial Nerve XI)

Injury of the spinal accessory nerve may result in shoulder droop and chronic arm pain. It is important to distinguish this on clinical exam from other causes of limited range of motion and pain following RT, including frozen shoulder, radiation-induced brachial plexopathy, and recurrent tumor.

Hypoglossal Nerve (Cranial Nerve XII)

The hypoglossal nerve is the most commonly affected lower cranial nerve. Unilateral tongue paralysis developing several years after RT is often asymptomatic; patients may complain of food being caught between their teeth and cheek. Bilateral tongue paralysis results in disabling dysarthria and swallowing difficulty.[141] Tongue atrophy with fatty infiltration or edema may be visible on MRI.[142]

Peripheral Nerves

Late radiation injury to peripheral nerves is rare. However, with prolonged patient survival following radiotherapy, it is clear that the incidence of complications involving muscles and nerves increases. Large volumes and dose per fraction are likely to increase the risk of peripheral nerve injury, and patients receiving intraoperative radiotherapy or high-dose brachytherapy may be at increased risk.

▶RADIATION-INDUCED TUMORS

Radiotherapy has been reported as a cause of meningiomas, gliomas, schwannomas, and peripheral nerve sheath tumors. Evidence supporting a causal relationship between radiotherapy and the development of a second malignancy include histology differing from the original tumor, second tumor that develops within the prior radiotherapy port, and significant time (years to decades) elapsed since radiotherapy. Biopsy is critical to establish the diagnosis.

Of particular interest is the observation of second tumors after treatment with radiosurgery. Although this treatment modality only recently became widespread, several authors have reported cases of glioblastoma, meningioma and malignant schwannoma developing after stereotactic radiosurgery. These cases have developed with somewhat shorter latency (6 years) than tumors reported after standard fractionation schedules.[143,144]

A recent review of the literature found 116 reported cases of radiotherapy-induced glioma.[145] On average, patients had received a dose of 32 Gy to the brain and secondary gliomas developed a median of 9.6 years after treatment. The largest subgroup of patients were young adult survivors of acute lymphoblastic leukemia (Fig. 32-3). A pathologic study of radiation-induced malignant gliomas found that they had a similar pattern of molecular genetic alterations as malignant gliomas arising de novo.[146] However, no mutations were identified in phosphatase tensin homologue (PTEN), a commonly altered tumor suppressor gene in glioblastoma multiforme, and no activating point mutations of the K-ras protooncogene or base-pair deletions of tumor suppressor genes were noted, both common findings in other radiation-induced tumors. Similarly, attempts to evaluate the outcome of patients with radiation-induced gliomas suggest that their outcomes are similar to patients with spontaneous tumors. The therapeutic options offered to these patients should be standard therapies.[147]

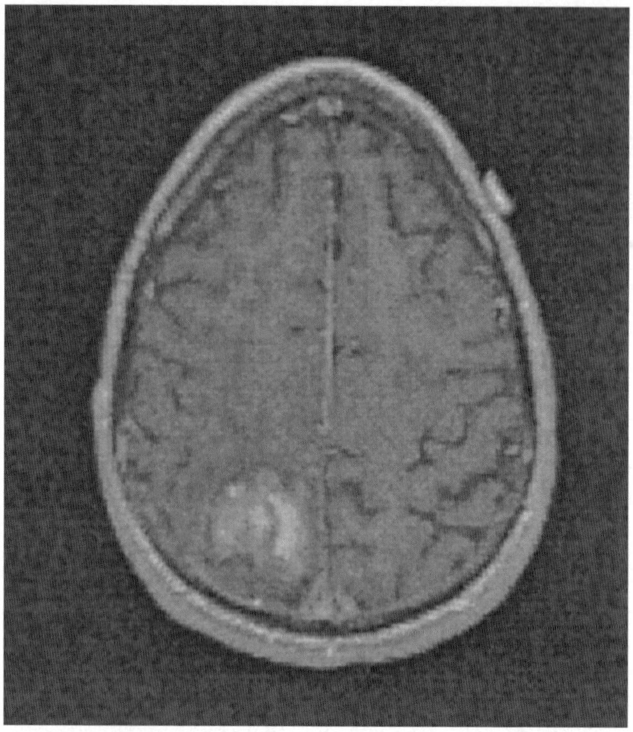

Figure 32-3. Axial, T_1-weighted, gadolinium-enhanced MRI of an anaplastic astrocytoma in a 24-year-old male treated for and cured of acute lymphoblastic leukemia 10 years earlier.

Meningiomas have been reported after both high and low doses of cranial irradiation. Children who received low-dose radiotherapy to treat tinea capitis in Israel during the 1950s developed both benign and malignant meningiomas with a median latency of more than four decades.[148] After higher doses of radiotherapy, meningiomas are five times more likely to occur than are gliomas, and patients treated for acute lymphoblastic leukemia comprise 40% of patients reported with RT-induced meningioma.[144] Half of the observed cases of meningioma as a second neoplasm in survivors of childhood malignancy occurred in patients previously treated for acute lymphocytic leukemia.[149] There are mixed reports as to the natural history of RT-induced meningiomas; some authors report a higher-than-expected rate of recurrence and a greater proportion of atypical or malignant tumors, wheras other series do not support this observation.[144,148,150] One cytogenetic study of six radiation-induced meningiomas identified an abnormality on 1p13 in all cases.[151]

Patients with retinoblastoma have a 24-fold increased risk of developing a benign or malignant tumor of the brain or meninges and significant excess mortality as a result of these secondary tumors (Fig. 32-4).[152,153] It is likely that the germ line mutation associated with the development of retinoblastoma enhances the inborn

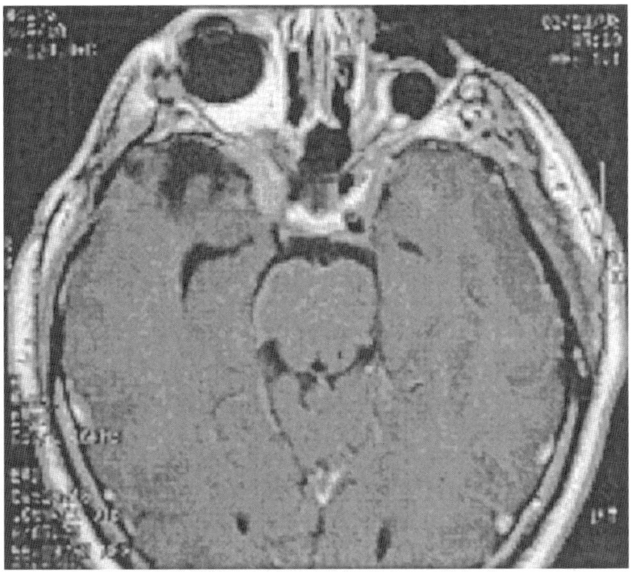

Figure 32-4. Axial, T_1-weighted, gadolinium-enhanced MRI of a recurrent cavernous sinus meningioma (arrow) in a 34-year-old survivor of childhood retinoblastoma that was treated with radiotherapy.

susceptibility to develop a second malignancy after exposure to radiotherapy.

Peripheral nerve sheath tumors typically follow radiotherapy of the brachial, cervical, or lumbar plexus in patients with Hodgkin lymphoma, breast cancer, and abdominal or pelvic tumors. Surgical exploration is critical to make the diagnosis and aggressive surgical resection is the most effective therapy. Patients with neurofibromatosis type 1 have an increased risk of developing tumors of the peripheral nerve sheath and comprise as many as one-third of reported cases.[154]

REFERENCES

1. Behin A, Delattre J-Y. Neurologic sequelae of radiotherapy on the nervous system. In: Schiff D, Wen PY, eds. Cancer neurology in clinical practice. Totowa, NJ: Humana Press, 2003:173–191.
2. New P. Radiation injury to the nervous system. Curr Opin Neurol 2001;14:725–734.
3. Sheline G, Wara WM, Smith V. Therapeutic irradiation and brain injury. Int J Radiat Oncol Biol Physics 1980;6: 1215–1228.
4. Van der Koegel A. Radiation-induced damage in the central nervous system: an interpretation of target cell response. Br J Cancer 1986;53:207–217.
5. Van der Maazen RWM, Berhagen I, Kleiboer BJ, et al. Radiosensitivity of glial progenitor cells of the perinatal and adult rat optic nerve studied by an in vitro clonogenic assay. Radiother Oncol 1991;20:258–264.
6. Van der Maazen RWM, Kleiboer BJ, Berhagen I, et al. Irradiation in vitro discriminates between different O-2A progenitor cell subpopulations in the perinatal central nervous system of rats. Radiat Res 1991;128:64–72.
7. Van der Maazen RWM, Kleiboer BJ, Berhagen I, et al. Repair capacity of adult rat glial progenitor cells determined by an in vitro clonogenic assay after in vitro or in vivo fractionated irradiation. Int J Radiat Biol 1993;63:661–666.
8. Hornsey S, Myers R, Coultas PG, et al. Turnover of proliferative cells in the spinal cord after X irradiation and its relation to time-dependent repair of radiation damage. Br J Radiol 1981;54:1081–1085.
9. Fike JR, Cann CE, Turowski K, et al. Radiation dose response of normal brain. Int J Radiat Oncol Biol Phys 1988;14:63–70.
10. Asai A, Matsutani M, Kohno T, et al. Subacute brain atrophy after radiation therapy for malignant brain tumor. Cancer 1989;63:1962–1974.
11. Tofilon PJ, Fike JR. The radio response of the central nervous system: a dynamic process. Radiat Res 2000;153:357–370.
12. Schultheiss TE, Kun LE, Ang KK, et al. Radiation response of the central nervous system. Int J Radiat Oncol Biol Phys 1995;31:1093–1112.
13. Posner JB. Side effects of radiation therapy. In: Posner JB, ed. Neurologic complications of cancer. Philadelphia: FA Davis, 1995:311–337.
14. Lampert PW, Davis RL. Delayed effects of radiation on the human central nervous system; "early" and "late" delayed reactions. Neurology 1964;14:912–917.
15. Monje ML, Palmer TD. Radiation injury and neurogenesis. Curr Opin Neurol 2003;16:129–134.
16. Tada E, Yang C, Gobbel GT, et al. Long-term impairment of subependymal repopulation following damage by ionizing irradiation. Exp Neurol 1999;160:66–77.
17. Peissner W, Kocher M, Treuer H, et al. Ionizing radiation-induced apoptosis of proliferating stem cells in the dentate gyrus of the adult rat hippocampus. Mol Brain Res 1999;71:61–68.
18. Madsen TM, Kristjansen PE, Bolwig TG, et al. Arrested neuronal proliferation and impaired hippocampal function following fractionated brain irradiation in the adult rat. Neuroscience 2003;119:635–642.
19. Young DF, Posner JB, Chu F, et al. Rapid-course radiation therapy of cerebral metastases: results and complications. Cancer 1974;34:1069–1076.
20. Berg RA, Ch'ien LT, Lancaster W, et al. Neuropsychological sequelae of postradiation somnolence syndrome. J Dev Behav Pediatr 1983;4:103–107.
21. Littman P, Rosenstock J, Gale G, et al. The somnolence syndrome in leukemic children following reduced daily dose fractions of cranial radiation. Int J Radiat Oncol Biol Phys 1984;10:1851–1853.
22. Faithfull S, Brada M. Somnolence syndrome in adults following cranial irradiation for primary brain tumors. Clin Oncol 1998;10:250–254.
23. Ch'ien LT, Aur RJ, Stagner S, et al. Long-term neurological implications of somnolence syndrome in children with acute lymphocytic leukemia. Ann Neurol 1980;8:273–277.

24. Mandell LR, Walker RW, Steinherz P, et al. Reduced incidence of the somnolence syndrome in leukemic children with steroid coverage during prophylactic cranial radiation therapy. Results of a pilot study. Cancer 1989;63: 1975–1978.
25. Armstrong, CL, Corn, BW, Ruffer, JE, et al. Radiotherapeutic effects on brain function: double dissociation of memory systems. Neuropsychiatry Neuropsychol Behav Neurol 2000;13: 101–111.
26. Vigliani MC, Sichez N, Poisson M, et al. A prospective study of cognitive functions following conventional radiotherapy for supratentorial gliomas in young adults: 4-year results. Int J Rad Oncol Biol Phys 1996;35:527–533.
27. Chak LY, Zatz LM, Wasserstein P, et al. Neurologic dysfunction in patients treated for small cell carcinoma of the lung: a clinical and radiological study. Int J Radiat Oncol Biol Phys 1986;12:385–389.
28. Shrieve DC, Wara WM, Edwards MS, et al. Hyperfractionated radiation therapy for gliomas of the brainstem in children and in adults. Int J Radiat Oncol Biol Phys 1992;24:599–610.
29. Schulz-Ertner D, Debus J, Lohr F, et al. Fractionated stereotactic conformal radiation therapy of brainstem gliomas: outcomes and prognostic factors. Radiother Oncol 2000; 57:215–223.
30. Watne K, Hager B, Heier M, et al. Reversible edema and necrosis after irradiation of the brain. Diagnostic procedures and clinical manifestations. Acta Oncol 1990;29:891–895.
31. Langleben DD, Segall GM. PET in differentiation of recurrent brain tumor from radiation injury. J Nucl Med 2000;41: 1861–1867.
32. Marks JE, Wong J. The risk of cerebral radionecrosis in relation to dose, time and fractionation. A follow-up study. Prog Exp Tumor Res 1985;29:210–218.
33. Morris JG, Grattan-Smith P, Panegyres PK, et al. Delayed cerebral radiation necrosis. Q J Med 1994;87:119–129.
34. Kumar AJ, Leeds NE, Fuller GN, et al. Malignant gliomas: MR imaging spectrum of radiation therapy- and chemotherapy-induced necrosis of the brain after treatment. Radiology 2000;217:377–384.
35. Mahaley MS, Vogel FS, Burger P, et al. Neuropathology of tissues from patients treated by the Brain Tumor Study Group. Natl Cancer Inst Monogr 1977;46:77–82.
36. Lee AW, Law SC, Ng SH, et al. Retrospective analysis of nasopharyngeal carcinoma treated during 1976–1985: late complications following megavoltage irradiation. Br J Radiol 1992;65:918–928.
37. Abayomi OK. Pathogenesis of cognitive decline following therapeutic irradiation for head and neck tumors. Acta Oncol 2002;41:346–351.
38. Cheung M, Chan AS, Law SC, et al. Cognitive function of patients with nasopharyngeal carcinoma with and without temporal lobe radionecrosis. Arch Neurol 2000;57: 1347–1352.
39. Lam LC, Leung SF, Chan YL. Progress of memory function after radiation therapy in patients with nasopharyngeal carcinoma. J Neuropsychiatry Clin Neurosci 2003;15: 90–97.
40. Rottenberg DA, Chernik NL, Deck MD, et al. Cerebral necrosis following radiotherapy of extracranial neoplasms. Ann Neurol 1977;1:339–357.
41. Thompson TP, Lunsford LD, Kondziolka D. Distinguishing recurrent tumor and radiation necrosis with positron emission tomography versus stereotactic biopsy. Stereotact Funct Neurosurg 1999;73:9–14.
42. Chao ST, Suh JH, Raja S, et al. The sensitivity and specificity of FDG PET in distinguishing recurrent brain tumor from radionecrosis in patients treated with stereotactic radiosurgery. Int J Cancer 2001;96:191–197.
43. Kline JL, Noto RB, Glantz M. Single-photon emission CT in the evaluation of recurrent brain tumor in patients treated with gamma knife radiosurgery or conventional radiation therapy. Am J Neuroradiol 1996;17: 1681–1686.
44. Moody EB, Hodes JE, Walsh JW, et al. Thallium-avid cerebral radiation necrosis. Clin Nucl Med 1994;19:611–613.
45. Yoshii Y, Moritake T, Suzuki K, et al. Cerebral radiation necrosis with accumulation of thallium 201 on single-photon emission CT. Am J Neuroradiol 1996;17: 1773–1776.
46. Lin A, Blum LS, Mamelak AN. Efficacy of proton magnetic resonance spectroscopy in clinical decision making for patients with suspected malignant brain tumors. J Neuroocol 1999;45:69–81.
47. Chong, VFH, Rumpel H, Fan, YF, et al. Temporal lobe changes following radiation therapy: imaging and proton MR spectroscopy findings. Eur Radiol 2001;11:317–324.
48. Usenius T, Usenius JP, Tenhunen M, et al. Radiation-induced changes in human brain metabolites as studied by 1H nuclear magnetic resonance spectroscopy in vivo. Int J Radiat Oncol Biol Phys 1995;33:719–724.
49. Virta A, Patronas N, Raman R, et al. Spectroscopy imaging of radiation-induced effects in the white matter of glioma patients. Magn Res Imaging 2000;18:851–857.
50. Forsyth PA, Kelly PJ, Cascino TL, et al. Radiation necrosis or glioma recurrence: is computer-assisted stereotactic biopsy useful? J Neurosurg 1995;82:436–444.
51. Glantz MJ, Burger PC, Friedman AH, et al. Treatment of radiation-induced nervous system injury with heparin and warfarin. Neurology 1994;44:2020–2027.
52. Chuba PJ, Aronin P, Bhambhani K, et al. Hyperbaric oxygen therapy for radiation-induced brain injury in children. Cancer 1997;80:2005–2012.
53. Woo E, Lam K, Yu YL, et al. Temporal lobe and hypothalamic-pituitary dysfunctions after radiotherapy for nasopharyngeal carcinoma: a distinct clinical syndrome. J Neurol Neurosurg Psychiatry 1988;51:1302–1307.
54. Taphoorn MJ, Heimans JJ, van der Veen EA, et al. Endocrine functions in long-term survivors of low-grade supratentorial glioma treated with radiation therapy. J Neurooncol 1995; 25:97–102.
55. Pasqualini T, McCalla J, Berg S, et al. Subtle primary hypothyroidism in patients treated for acute lymphoblastic leukemia. Acta Endocrinol (Copenh) 1991;124:375–380.
56. Clayton PE, Shalet SM. Dose dependency of time of onset of radiation-induced growth hormone deficiency. J Pediatr 1991;118:226–228.
57. Bitzer M, Topka H. Progressive cerebral occlusive disease after radiation therapy. Stroke 1995;26:131–136.
58. Murros KE, Toole JF. The effect of radiation on carotid arteries. A review article. Arch Neurol 1989;46:449–455.

59. Kestle JR, Hoffman HJ, Mock AR. Moyamoya phenomenon after radiation for optic glioma. J Neurosurg 1993;79: 32–35.
60. Loftus CM, Biller J, Hart MN, et al. Management of radiation-induced accelerated carotid atherosclerosis. Arch Neurol 1987;44:711–714.
61. DeAngelis, LM, Yahalom J, Thaler HT, et al. Combined modality therapy for primary CNS lymphoma. J Clin Oncol 1992;10:635–643.
62. Crossen, JR, Garwood D, Glatstein E, et al. Neurobehavioral sequelae of cranial irradiation in adults: a review of radiation-induced encephalopathy. J Clin Oncol 1994; 12:627–642.
63. Weitzner MA, Meyers CA. Cognitive functioning and quality of life in malignant glioma patients: a review of the literature. Psychooncology 1997;6:169–177.
64. Meyers CA, Wefel JS. The use of the mini-mental state examination to assess cognitive functioning in cancer trials: no ifs, ands, buts, or sensitivity. J Clin Oncol 2003;21:3557–3558.
65. Brouwers P, Poplack D. Memory and learning sequelae in long-term survivors of acute lymphoblastic leukemia: association with attention deficits. Am J Pediatr Hematol Oncol 1990;12:174–181.
66. Duffey P, Chari G, Cartlidge NEF, et al. Progressive deterioration of intellect and motor function occurring several decades after cranial irradiation. Arch Neurol 1996;53: 814–818.
67. Archibald YM, Lunn D, Ruttan LA, et al. Cognitive functioning in long-term survivors of high-grade glioma. J Neurosurg 1994;80:247–253.
68. Hochberg FH, Slotnick B. Neuropsychologic impairment in astrocytoma survivors. Neurology 1980;30:172–177.
69. Scheibel RS, Meyers CA, Levin VA. Cognitive dysfunction following surgery for intracerebral glioma: influence of histopathology, lesion location, and treatment. J Neurooncol 1996;30:61–69.
70. Correa DD, DeAngelis LM, Shi W, et al. Cognitive functions in survivors of primary central nervous system lymphoma. Neurology 2004;62(4):548–255.
71. Dropcho E. Central nervous system injury by therapeutic irradiation. Neurol Clin 1991;9:969–988.
72. Seiler C, Armstrong CL. Proceedings of the conference on the effects of radiotherapy on the brain and on behavior through the life span, San Juan, Puerto Rico, December 6–8, 2002. Med Pediatr Oncol 2003;41:460–466.
73. Imperato JP, Paleologos NA, Vick NA. Effects of treatment on long-term survivors with malignant astrocytomas. Ann Neurol 1990;28:818–822.
74. Abrey, LE, DeAngelis, LM, Yahalom J. Long-term survival in primary CNS lymphoma. J Clin Oncol 1998;16: 859–863.
75. Gregor A, Cull A, Traynor E, et al. Neuropsychometric evaluation of long-term survivors of adult brain tumours: relationship with tumour and treatment parameters. Radiother Oncol 1996;41:55–59.
76. Kramer JH, Crowe AB, Larson DA, et al. Neuropsychological sequelae of medulloblastoma in adults. Int J Radiat Oncol Biol Phys 1997;38:21–26.
77. Cetingul N, Aydinok Y, Kantar M, et al. Neuropsychologic sequelae in the long-term survivors of childhood acute lymphoblastic leukemia. Pediatr Hematol Oncol 1999;16: 213–220.
78. DeAngelis LM, Delattre JY, Posner JB. Radiation-induced dementia in patients cured of brain metastases. Neurology 1989;39:789–796.
79. Klein M, Heimans, JJ, Aaronson, NK, et al. Effect of radiotherapy and other treatment-related factors on mid-term to long-term cognitive sequelae in low-grade gliomas: a comparative study. Lancet 2002;360:1361–1368.
80. Postma TJ, Klein M, Verstappen CCP, et al. Radiotherapy-induced cerebral abnormalities in patients with low-grade glioma. Neurology 2002;59:121–123.
81. Taphoorn MJ, Schiphorst AK, Snoek FJ, et al. Cognitive functions and quality of life in patients with low-grade gliomas: the impact of radiotherapy. Ann Neurol 1994;36: 48–54.
82. Armstrong CL, Stern CH, Corn BW. Memory performance used to detect radiation effects on cognitive functioning. Appl Neuropsychol 2001;8:129–139.
83. Armstrong, CL, Hunter, JV, Ledakis, GE, et al. Late cognitive and radiographic changes related to radiotherapy. Neurology 2002;59:40–48.
84. Torres IJ, Mundt AJ, Sweeney PJ, et al. A longitudinal neuropsychological study of partial brain radiation in adults with brain tumors. Neurology 2003;60:1113–1118.
85. Surma-aho O, Niemela M, Vikki J, et al. Adverse long-term effects of brain radiotherapy in adult low-grade glioma patients. Neurology 2001;56:1285–1290.
86. Johnson, BE, Becker B, Goff, WB, et al. Neurologic, neuropsychologic, and computed cranial tomography scan abnormalities in 2- to 10-year survivors of small-cell lung cancer. J Clin Oncol 1985;8:1659–1667.
87. Johnson, BE, Patronas N, Hayes W, et al. Neurologic, computed cranial tomographic and magnetic resonance imaging abnormalities in patients with small-cell lung cancer: further follow-up of 6- to 13-year survivors. J Clin Oncol 1990;8:48–56.
88. Cull A, Gregor A, Hopwood P, et al. Neurological and cognitive impairment in long-term survivors of small cell lung cancer. Eur J Cancer 1994;30:1067–1074.
89. Corn BW, Yousem, DM, Scott CB, et al. White matter changes are correlated significantly with radiation dose. Cancer 1994;74:2828–2835.
90. Tsuruda, JS, Kortman, KE, Bradley WG, et al. Radiation effects in the white matter: MR evaluation. Am J Neuroradiol 1987;8:431–437.
91. Thiessen B, DeAngelis LM. Hydrocephalus in radiation leukoencephalopathy: results of ventriculoperitoneal shunting. Arch Neurol 1998;55:705–710.
92. Keime-Guibert F, Napolitano M, Delattre JY. Neurological complications of radiotherapy and chemotherapy. J Neurol 1998;245:695–708.
93. Leibel SA, Sheline GE. Radiation therapy for neoplasms of the brain. J Neurosurg 1987;66:1–22.
94. Storm AJ, van der Kogel AJ, Nooter K. Effect of X-irradiation on the pharmacokinetics of methotrexate in rats: alteration of the blood-brain barrier. Eur J Cancer Clin Oncol 1985;21: 759–764.
95. Geyer JR, Taylor EM, Milstein JM, et al. Radiation, methotrexate, and white matter necrosis: laboratory evidence for

neural radioprotection with preirradiation methotrexate. Int J Radiat Oncol Biol Phys 1988;15:373–375.
96. DeAngelis LM, Shapiro WR. Drug/radiation interactions and central nervous system injury. In: Gutin PH, Leibel SA, Sheline GE, eds. Radiation injury to the nervous system. New York: Raven Press, 1991;361–382.
97. Fein DA, Marcus RB Jr, Parsons JT, et al. Lhermitte's sign: incidence and treatment variables influencing risk after irradiation of the cervical spinal cord. Int J Radiat Oncol Biol Phys 1993;27:1029–1033.
98. Esik O, Csere T, Stefanits K, et al. A review on radiogenic Lhermitte's sign. Pathol Oncol Res 2003;9:115–120.
99. Li YQ, Jay V, Wong CS. Oligodendrocytes in the adult rat spinal cord undergo radiation-induced apoptosis. Cancer Res 1996;56:5417–5422.
100. Chiang CS, Mason KA, Withers HR, et al. Alteration in myelin-associated proteins following spinal cord irradiation in guinea pigs. Int J Radiat Oncol Biol Phys 1992;24: 929–937.
101. Atkinson S, Li YQ, Wong CS. Changes in oligodendrocytes and myelin gene expression after radiation in the rodent spinal cord. Int J Radiat Oncol Biol Phys 2003;57:1093–1100.
102. Dorfman LJ, Donaldson SS, Gupta PR, et al. Electrophysiologic evidence of subclinical injury to the posterior columns of the human spinal cord after therapeutic radiation. Cancer 1982;50:2815–2819.
103. Schultheiss TE, Stephens LC. Invited review: permanent radiation myelopathy. Br J Radiol 1992;65:737–753.
104. Rampling R, Symonds P. Radiation myelopathy. Curr Opin Neurol 1998;11:627–632.
105. Raney B, Tefft M, Heyn R, et al. Ascending myelitis after intensive chemotherapy and radiation therapy in children with cranial parameningeal sarcoma. Cancer 1992;69: 1498–1506.
106. Chao MW, Wirth A, Ryan G, et al. Radiation myelopathy following transplantation and radiotherapy for non-Hodgkin's lymphoma. Int J Radiat Oncol Biol Phys 1998;41:1057–1061.
107. Liu CY, Yim BT, Wozniak AJ. Anticoagulation therapy for radiation-induced myelopathy. Ann Pharmacother 2001; 35:188–191.
108. Angibaud G, Ducasse JL, Baille G, et al. Potential value of hyperbaric oxygenation in the treatment of post-radiation myelopathies. Rev Neurol 1995;151:661–666.
109. Wang PY, Shen WC, Jan JS. Serial MRI changes in radiation myelopathy. Neuroradiology 1995;37:374–377.
110. Michikawa M, Wada Y, Sano M, et al. Radiation myelopathy: significance of gadolinium-DTPA enhancement in the diagnosis. Neuroradiol 1991;33:286–289.
111. Okada S, Okeda R. Pathology of radiation myelopathy. Neuropathology 2001;21:247–265.
112. Lalu T, Mercier B, Birouk N, et al. Pure motor neuropathy after radiation therapy: 6 cases. Rev Neurol 1998; 154:40–44.
113. Bowen J, Gregory R, Squier M, et al. The post-irradiation lower motor neuron syndrome neuronopathy or radiculopathy? Brain 1996;119:1429–1439.
114. Churn M, Clough V, Slater A. Early onset of bilateral brachial plexopathy during mantle radiotherapy for Hodgkin's disease. Clin Oncol 2000;12:289–291.
115. Malow BA, Dawson DM. Neuralgic amyotrophy in association with radiation therapy for Hodgkin's disease. Neurology 1991;41:440–441.
116. Salner AL, Botnick LE, Herzog AG, et al. Reversible brachial plexopathy following primary radiation therapy for breast cancer. Cancer Treat Rep 1981;65:797–802.
117. Pierce SM, Recht A, Lingos TI, et al. Long-term radiation complications following conservative surgery (CS) and radiation therapy (RT) in patients with early stage breast cancer. Int J Radiat Oncol Biol Phys 1992;23:915–923.
118. Johansson S, Svensson H, Denekamp J. Timescale of evolution of late radiation injury after postoperative radiotherapy of breast cancer patients. Int J Radiat Oncol Biol Phys 2000;48:745–750.
119. Brander PE, Jarvinen V, Lohela P, et al. Bilateral diaphragmatic weakness: a late complication of radiotherapy. Thorax 1997;52:829–831.
120. Wittenberg KH, Adkins MC. MR imaging of nontraumatic brachial plexopathies: frequency and spectrum of findings. Radiographics 2001;20:1023–1032.
121. Ahmad A, Barrington S, Maisey M, et al. Use of positron emission tomography in evaluation of brachial plexopathy in breast cancer patients. Br J Cancer 1999;79: 478–482.
122. Pritchard J, Anand P, Broome J, et al. Double-blind randomized phase II study of hyperbaric oxygen in patients with radiation-induced brachial plexopathy. Radiother Oncol 2001;58:279–286.
123. Lu L, Gong X, Liu Z, Wang D, et al. Diagnosis and operative treatment of radiation-induced brachial plexopathy. Chin J Traumatol 2002;5:329–332.
124. Kinsella TJ, DeLuca AM, Barnes M, et al. Threshold dose for peripheral neuropathy following intraoperative radiotherapy (IORT) in a large animal model. Int J Radiat Oncol Biol Phys 1991;20:697–701.
125. Sagar SM, Thomas RJ, Loverock LT, et al. Olfactory sensations produced by high-energy photon irradiation of the olfactory receptor mucosa in humans. Int J Radiat Oncol Biol Phys 1991;20:771–776.
126. Ho WK, Kwong DL, Wei WI, et al. Change in olfaction after radiotherapy for nasopharyngeal cancer—a prospective study. Am J Otolaryngol 2002;23:209–214.
127. Hua MS, Chen ST, Tang LM, et al. Olfactory function in patients with nasopharyngeal carcinoma following radiotherapy. Brain Inj 1999;13:905–915.
128. Bowyer J, Natha S, Marsh I, et al. Visual complications of proton beam therapy for clival chordoma. Eye 2003;17: 318–323.
129. Piquemal R, Cottier JP, Arsene S, et al. Radiation-induced optic neuropathy 4 years after radiation: report of a case followed up with MRI. Neuroradiology 1998;40: 439–441.
130. Ryu S, Brown SL, Kolozsvary A, et al. Noninvasive detection of radiation-induced optic neuropathy by manganese-enhanced MRI. Radiat Res 2002;157:500–505.
131. Mohamed IG, Roa W, Fulton D, et al. Optic nerve sheath fenestration for a reversible optic neuropathy in radiation oncology. Am J Clin Oncol 2000;23:401–405.
132. Borruat FX, Schatz NJ, Glaser JS, et al. Visual recovery from radiation-induced optic neuropathy. The role of

hyperbaric oxygen therapy. J Clin Neuroophthalmol 1993; 13:98–101.

133. Yee RD, Purvin VA. Ocular neuromyotonia: three case reports with eye movement recordings. J Neuroophthalmol 1998;18:1–8.

134. Vissink A, Jansma J, Spijkervet FK, et al. Oral sequelae of head and neck radiotherapy. Crit Rev Oral Biol Med 2003;14:199–212.

135. Ripamonti C, Zecca E, Brunelli C, et al. A randomized, controlled clinical trial to evaluate the effects of zinc sulfate on cancer patients with taste alterations caused by head and neck irradiation. Cancer 1998;82: 1938–1945.

136. Ripamonti C, Fulfaro F. Taste alterations in cancer patients. J Pain Symptom Manage 1998;16:349–351.

137. Kalapurakal JA, Silverman CL, Akhtar N, et al. Improved trigeminal and facial nerve tolerance following fractionated stereotactic radiotherapy for large acoustic neuromas. Br J Radiol 1999;72:1202–1207.

138. Fuss M, Salter BJ, Sadeghi A, et al. Fractionated stereotactic intensity-modulated radiotherapy (FS-IMRT) for small acoustic neuromas. Med Dosim 2002;27:147–154.

139. Johannesen TB, Rasmussen K, Winther FO, et al. Late radiation effects on hearing, vestibular function, and taste in brain tumor patients. Int J Radiat Oncol Biol Phys 2002;53:86–90.

140. Honore HB, Bentzen SM, Moller K, et al. Sensorineural hearing loss after radiotherapy for nasopharyngeal carcinoma: individualized risk estimation. Radiother Oncol 2002;65:9–16.

141. Johnston EF, Hammond AJ, Cairncross JG. Bilateral hypoglossal palsies: a late complication of curative radiotherapy. Can J Neurol Sci 1989;16:198–199.

142. King AD, Ahuja A, Leung SF, et al. MR features of the denervated tongue in radiation induced neuropathy. Br J Radiol 1999;72:349–353.

143. Loeffler JS, Niemierko A, Chapman PH. Second tumors after radiosurgery: tip of the iceberg or a bump in the road? Neurosurgery 2003;52:1436–1440.

144. Salvati M, Cervoni L, Puzzilli F, et al. High-dose radiation-induced meningiomas. Surg Neurol 1997;47:435–441.

145. Salvati M, Frati A, Russo N, et al. Radiation-induced gliomas: report of 10 cases and review of the literature. Surg Neurol 2003;60:60–67.

146. Brat DJ, James CD, Jedlicka AE, et al. Molecular genetic alterations in radiation-induced astrocytomas. Am J Pathol 1999;154:1431–1438.

147. Maluf FC, DeAngelis LM, Raizer JJ, et al. High-grade gliomas in patients with prior systemic malignancies. Cancer 2002; 94:3219–3224.

148. Pollak L, Walach N, Gur R, et al. Meningiomas after radiotherapy for tinea capitis—still no history. Tumori 1998;84:65–68.

149. Gold DG, Neglia JP, Dusenbery KE. Second neoplasms after megavoltage radiation for pediatric tumors. Cancer 2003;97:2588–2596.

150. Musa BS, Pople IK, Cummins BH. Intracranial meningiomas following irradiation—a growing problem? Br J Neurosurg 1995;9:629–637.

151. Zattara-Cannoni H, Roll P, Figarella-Branger D, et al. Cytogenetic study of six cases of radiation-induced meningiomas. Cancer Genet Cytogenet 2001;15;126:81–84.

152. Eng C, Li FP, Abramson DH, Ellsworth RM, et al. Mortality from second tumors among long-term survivors of retinoblastoma. J Natl Cancer Inst 1993;85:1121–1128.

153. Schulz CJ, Riddle MP, Valdimirsdottir HB, et al. Impact on survivors of retinoblastoma when informed of study results on risk of second cancers. Med Pediatr Oncol 2003;41:36–43.

154. Foley KM, Woodruff JM, Ellis FT, et al. Radiation-induced malignant and atypical peripheral nerve sheath tumors. Ann Neurol 1980;7:311–318.

INDEX

NOTE: Page numbers followed by *t* refer to tables; page numbers followed by *f* refer to figures.

A

Acoustic nerve (CN VIII), radiation injury to, 721
Acoustic neuroma, 465–466, 465*f*
Acoustic schwannomas, 240, 241*f*
Acute brachial plexopathy, 719
Acute necrotizing myopathy, 668
Adapter proteins, 21
ADC (apparent diffusion coefficient), 76
Adenocarcinoma, 455–456
Adjuvant chemotherapy, 166
Adrenocorticotropic-secreting adenomas, 389–390, 390*f*
Alcohol and brain cancer, 7
Alkylating agents, 23–24, 23*t*
  CNS penetration of, 617*t*
  neurologic complications of
    busulfan, 687
    carboplatin, 685–686
    chlorambucil, 687
    cisplatin, 685–686, 685*t*
    cyclophosphamide, 688
    dacarbazine, 686
    estramustine, 687
    hexamethylmelamine, 688
    ifosfamide, 688–689
    mechlorethamine, 687
    nitrosoureas, 686–687
    procarbazine, 687–688
    temozolomide, 686
    thiotepa, 688
  treatment of malignant gliomas, 23–24, 23*t*
Altered mental status, 38
Aminoglutethimide, neurologic complications of, 697
Analgesics, 193*t*
Anaplastic astrocytoma, 84–87, 86*f*, 271*f*
  imaging, 57*t*
Anaplastic ependymoma, 98–99
Anaplastic gangliogliomas, 103
Anaplastic glioma, imaging, 74*f*
Anaplastic (malignant) meningiomas, 109*f*, 110
Anaplastic oligoastrocytoma, 97, 97*f*
Anaplastic oligodendroglioma, 95–96, 96*f*
Anastrazole, neurologic complications of, 697
Angiography, 41
Anterior skull base/anterior fossa lesions (crista galli, cribriform plate, orbital roof, planum sphenoidale)
  clinical presentation, 448
  diagnoses and management
    adenocarcinoma, 455–456
    brown tumor of skull base, 459
    chondrosarcoma and chordoma, 449–450
    encephalocele, 458
    esthesioneuroblastoma, 449, 450*f*
    fibrosarcoma, 451
    fibrous histiocytoma, 450–451
    giant cell tumor, 451
    hemangiopericytoma, 454–455
    inverted papilloma, 456–457
    juvenile neuroangiofibroma, 452, 452*f*
    malignant salivary and lacrimal gland lesions, 457
    meningioma, 452–454, 453*f*
    mucocele, 458
    mucosal melanoma, 456, 457*f*
    nasal glioma, 459
    nasopharyngeal carcinoma, 456
    neuroendocrine carcinoma, 457–458
    neurofibroma, 451–452
    orbital lesions, 458, 458*f*
    osteochondroma, 451
    osteoclastoma, 451
    osteogenic sarcoma, 451
    osteoma, 451
    plasmacytoma, 451, 452*f*
    rhabdomyosarcoma, 450
    sinonasal undifferentiated carcinoma, 457, 458*f*
    squamous cell carcinoma, 455–456
  evaluation, 448–449
Anthracyclines, CNS penetration of, 617*t*
Antiepileptic drugs, 48–49
Antimetabolites
  CNS penetration of, 617*t*
  neurologic complications of
    capecitabine, 683
    cladribine, 684
    cytosine arabinoside, 683–684
    5-fluoruracil, 683, 684*f*
    fludarabine, 684
    gemcitabine, 684–685
    hydroxyurea, 685
    methotrexate
      acute/subacute effects, 681–682, 682*f*
      late effects, 682, 683*f*
      overview, 680–681, 681*t*
    pentostatin, 685
Antineoplastic antibiotics, neurologic complications of
  bleomycin, 691
  daunorubicin, 691
  doxorubicin, 691
  mitomycin C, 691
  mitoxantrone, 691
  nitroimidazoles (misonidazole, metronidazole), 691
  plicamycin (mithramycin), 692
  suramin, 692
Anxiety, 191–192
APC gene, 420–421
Apoptosis, 25*t*
Apparent diffusion coefficient (ADC), 76
Approach to patient
  multiple brain lesions
    overview, 48, 48*t*, 49*f*
    supportive care
      antiepileptic drugs, 48–49
      corticosteroids, 49, 50*f*
      prophylactic therapy for venous thromboembolic disease (VTED), 49
      psychosocial support, 49–50
  overview, 43

Approach to patient (*Cont.*):
  single brain lesion
    diagnosis
      enhancing lesions
        benign conditions, 46–47
        brain metastasis, 44–45, 46*f*
        gliomas, 43–44, 45*f*
        primary central nervous system lymphoma (PCNSL), 45–46
      nonenhancing lesions, 47, 47*f*–48*f*
      staging, 47–48
    overview, 40*t*, 43, 44*f*, 44*t*–45*t*
Aromatase inhibitors (anastrazole, letrozole, aminoglutethimide), neurologic complications of, 697
Assessment bias, 228
Astroblastoma, 303
Astrocytic tumors
  anaplastic astrocytoma, 85–87, 86*f*
  astrocytoma. *See* Astrocytoma
  diffuse infiltrating astrocytomas, 84
  giant cell glioblastoma, 88, 89*f*–90*f*
  glioblastoma multiforme, 87, 87*f*–89*f*
  gliosarcoma, 88
  molecular genetics of diffuse astrocytomas, 88–89
  neuroimaging
    CT, 56
    MRI, 56, 58, 59*f*–62*f*
    overview, 56, 57*t*–58*t*
  overview, 84
  special categories
    overview, 89–90
    pilocytic astrocytoma, 90–91, 91*f*
    pleomorphic xanthoastrocytoma, 91–93, 92*f*
    subependymal giant cell astrocytoma, 93–94, 93*f*
Astrocytoma, 84–85, 86*f*. *See also* Astrocytic tumors
  anaplastic, 85–87, 86*f*
  diffuse, 84, 88–89
  high-grade. *See* High-grade astrocytomas
  histology and molecular genetics, 3–4
  low-grade. *See* Low-grade astrocytomas
  therapeutic management and outcomes
    chemotherapy, 515
    overview, 84, 512, 513*f*–514*f*
    prognostic factors, 512–513, 515
    radiation therapy, 515
    surgery, 515
Atypical meningiomas, 109–110
Atypical teratoid/rhabdoid tumor, 107, 107*f*
Audiometry, 43
Autonomy, respect for, 194

B

Bacillus Calmette-Guérin, neurologic complications of, 694
Beneficence, 194
β-catenin, 420–421
Biologic therapies, neurologic complications of. *See* Neurologic complications of chemotherapy and biologic therapies
Bleomycin, neurologic complications of, 691
Blinding/masking of treatment in clinical trials
  overview, 228
  pertinent issues, 228
Blood–brain barrier, manipulating permeability of, 28–29, 171, 361
Bolus-tracking MRI, 74
Bourneville disease, 242–243, 242*t*, 244*f*–245*f*, 245–246
Brachial or lumbosacral plexus, radiation injury of
  acute brachial plexopathy, 719
  early delayed brachial plexopathy, 719
  late delayed brachial plexopathy, 719–720
  lumbosacral plexopathy, 720
  overview, 719, 719*t*–720*t*
Brachytherapy, 133, 155, 278–279
Bragg peak, 145
Brain
  metastases to, 44–45, 46*f*
    biology, 554–555, 555*t*
    chemotherapy, 571–573
    clinical presentation and symptomatic treatment, 559–560
    definitive therapy
      chemotherapy, 571–573
      focused therapies, 562–563
      focused therapies and adjuvant whole-brain radiation therapy, 570–571, 571*t*
      miscellaneous adjuvant therapies, 573–574
      overview, 560
      radiosurgery, 567–570, 567*f*
      surgery for multiple metastases, 565–566
      surgery for single metastases
        breast primaries, 564, 564*f*
        gastrointestinal primaries, 565
        genitourinary primaries, 565
        gynecologic primaries, 565
        lung primaries, 564
        melanoma, 564–565
        overview, 563–564
        surgical technique, 566–567
        whole-brain radiation therapy, 560–562, 561*f*
    diagnosis, 557–558, 558*f*
    epidemiology, 553–554
    overview, 553, 575
    pathology and distribution, 555–557, 556*f*–557*f*
    steps in metastatic cascade, 555*t*
    treatment algorithm for patients with cerebral metastases, 574–575
  primary tumors. *See* Primary tumors; Specific tumors
  radiation-induced neurotoxicity in
    acute effects, 712
    combined effects of radiation and chemotherapy, 717–718, 717*f*
    early delayed effects
      focal encephalopathy, 713
      neurologic deterioration, 713
      overview, 712
      somnolence syndrome, 712–713
    late delayed effects
      cerebral atrophy, 714
      cognitive dysfunction, 715–717
      endocrine dysfunction, 714–715
      overview, 713
      radiation necrosis, 713–714, 714*f*–715*f*
    overview, 712, 712*t*
Brainstem auditory-evoked potentials (BSAEPs), 42
Brainstem tumors, 340
  focal neurologic symptoms and signs, 39
  gliomas
    diagnosis
      management, 335
      neuroimaging, 334
      pathology, 335
      pathophysiology, 335
    neuroimaging
      CT, 69
      MRI, 69, 70*f*, 71
      overview, 58t, 69
    overview, 333, 340
    specific subtypes
      brainstem tumors, 340
      cervicomedullary tumors, 338, 339*f*
      diffuse infiltrating pontine glioma, 335–337, 336*f*
      dorsal exophytic brainstem tumors, 337–338, 338*f*
      intrinsic tectal gliomas, 338–340, 339*f*
      neurofibromatosis type I, 340
    symptoms, 333–334, 334*t*
Brain–tumor barrier, manipulating permeability of, 171

Breast metastasis to brain, surgery for, 564, 564*f*
Bremsstrahlung, 144
Brown-Roberts-Wells base ring and localizer, 132*f*
Brown tumor of skull base, 459
BSAEPs (Brainstem auditory-evoked potentials), 42
Busulfan, neurologic complications of, 687

C
Cachectic myopathy, 668
Café-au-lait macules, 236, 236*t*
Cancer stem cells, 169
Capecitabine, neurologic complications of, 683
Carboplatin
  CNS penetration of, 617*t*
  neurologic complications of, 685–686
Carmustin, CNS penetration of, 617*t*
Carotid body tumors, 474–475
Cauda equina tumors, 503
Cavernoma, 470
Cavernous sinus/middle fossa lesions (squamous temporal bone, greater sphenoid wing, lower parietal bone, tegmen, petrous temporal bone)
  diagnosis and management
    cholesteatoma, 463
    cholesterol granuloma, 463
    chordoma/chondrosarcoma, 463
    dermoid cyst, 462
    epidermoid cyst, 462
    general management considerations, 460–461
    hemangioma, 462
    meningioma, 462–463, 462*f*
    neurofibroma, 461–462
    nonneoplastic temporal bone and middle fossa mass, 463–464
    schwannoma, 461, 461*f*
    temporal bone adenomatous lesions, 463
  evaluation, 460
  presentation, 459–460
CCND1 (cyclin D1) oncogene, 387–388, 387*t*
CDK4 (cyclin-dependent kinase 4) gene, 25–26, 25*t*
CDKN2A gene (cyclin-dependent kinase N2A), 312, 320
Cell-cycle inhibitors
  cell cycle phases distal to G1/S checkpoint, 26
  G1/S checkpoint, 25–26, 25*t*
  overview, 24, 24*t*
Cell-cycle specificity of chemotherapy agents, 165, 165*f*
Cell division, 19
Cell kill, 164
Cell of origin, 261
Cell phones and brain cancer, 6–7
Cell surface growth factor receptors
  overview, 19
  platelet-derived growth factor receptor inhibitors (PDGFR), 21
  targeting epidermal growth factor receptor (EGFR), 19–21, 20*t*
Cellular ependymomas, 98
Central nervous system (CNS)
  leukemic or lymphomatous meningitis
    leptomeningeal metastases from solid tumors, 622
    overview, 621–622
    palliative therapy, 622
  paraneoplasia
    cancer- and melanoma-assciated retinopathy
      antineuronal odies, 661
      diagnostic evaluation, 660–661
      differential diagnosis, 661
      overview, 660
      treatment and prognosis, 661
      underlying tumor, 660
    chorea
      antineuronal antibodies, 660
      diagnostic evaluation, 660
      differential diagnosis, 660
      overview, 660
      treatment and prognosis, 660
      underlying tumor, 660
    encephalomyelitis, 656–658
      antineuronal antibodies, 658
      diagnostic evaluation, 658
      differential diagnosis, 658
      treatment and prognosis, 658
      underlying tumor, 658
    limbic encephalitis
      antineuronal antibodies, 656
      diagnostic evaluation, 656
      differential diagnosis, 656
      overview, 656, 657*f*
      treatment and prognosis, 656
      underlying tumor, 656
    opsoclonus–myoclonus
      antineuronal antibodies, 658–659
      diagnostic evaluation, 658
      differential diagnosis, 659
      overview, 658
      treatment and prognosis, 659
      underlying tumor, 658
    optic neuritis
      antineuronal antibodies, 661
      overview, 661
      treatment and prognosis, 661
      underlying tumor, 661
    stiff-person syndrome (SPS)
      antineuronal antibodies, 659
      diagnostic evaluation, 659
      differential diagnosis, 660
      overview, 659
      treatment and prognosis, 660
      underlying tumor, 659
    subacute cerebellar ataxia
      antineuronal antibodies, 650, 655, 655*f*
      diagnostic evaluation, 650
      differential diagnosis, 655
      overview, 650
      treatment and prognosis, 655–656
      underlying tumor, 650
    subacute motor neuronopathies/motor neuron disease
      characteristic associations of motor neuron syndromes with typical tumor, 661–662
      improvement following treatment of tumor, 662
      overview, 661
      paraneoplastic antibodies, 662
Central neurocytoma, 100, 102–103, 102*f*
Cerebellar tumors, 39
  pilocytic astrocytomas, 302–303, 303*f*
Cerebellopontine angle tumors, differential diagnosis of, 45*t*
Cerebrospinal fluid (CSF) analysis, 42–43
Cervicomedullary tumors, 338, 339*f*
Cetuximab (Erbitux), neurologic complications of, 699–700
C-fos, 388
Chemotherapy
  astrocytoma, 515
  barriers to drug delivery, overcoming
    intraarterial chemotherapy, 171
    intracerebrospinal fluid chemotherapy, 171–172
    manipulating permeability of blood–brain and brain–tumor barriers, 171
    wafers/implants, 172
  for brain metastases, 571–573
  chondrosarcoma, 522
  ependymomas, 177, 439–440, 517
  factors influencing delivery to brain, 169–170, 170*t*
  germinomas, 493
  high-grade astrocytomas
    chemotherapy at tumor recurrence, 281
    multiagent regimens, 280
    newer chemotherapeutic agents, 281, 282*t*
    overall benefit, 280
    overview, 279

Chemotherapy
  high-grade astrocytomas (*Cont.*):
    prediction of response and prognosis, 280–281, 280*t*
    single-agent regimens, 279–280
    symptomatic treatments, 281–282
  leptomeningeal metastases
    high-dose systemic, 618
    intrathecal, 618–621, 618*f*–619*f*, 619*t*–621*t*
    overview, 617–618, 617*t*
  low-grade fibrillary astrocytoma, 300–302, 301*f*
  meningioma, 519
  neurologic complications. *See* Neurologic complications of chemotherapy and biologic therapies
  neuropsychological sequelae, 208
  nongerminoma germ cell tumors, 494–495
  oligodendroglioma and mixed gliomas
    adjuvant therapy, 327
    first-line chemotherapy in recurrent oligodendroglial tumors, 322, 322*t*, 323*f*–325*f*, 324
    high-dose chemotherapy with autologous bone marrow rescue, 326–327
    recurrent oligodendroglial tumors, 322, 322*t*
    second-line chemotherapy, 324–326, 325*t*
      following first-line PCV or temozolomide, 326, 326*t*
    upfront chemotherapy in low-grade oligodendroglial tumors, 327–328, 328*f*
    upfront chemotherapy in newly diagnosed anaplastic oligodendroglioma, 327
  overview, 163
  pilocytic astrocytoma, 302
  primary CNS lymphoma, 360
  primary meningeal neoplasms, 377
  primary spinal tumors, 512
  primitive neuroectodermal tumors (PNETs), 173
  principles of
    adjuvant chemotherapy, 166
    basic concepts, 163
    cancer stem cells, 169
    cell-cycle specificity of chemotherapy agents, 165, 165*f*
    cell kill, 164
    clinical trials, 165–166
    combination therapy, 166–167
    dose intensity, 167
    drug resistance, 164–165, 164*f*
    Gompertzian growth curves, 163–164, 164*f*
    in-vitro drug sensitivity testing, 169
    mechanisms of drug resistance and strategies to overcome them
      DNA repair enzymes, 168–169
      multidrug resistance, 168
      overview, 167–168, 168*t*
    tumor burden, 163
  steroids, 170–171
  by tumor type
    central nervous system germ cell tumors, 173–174
    ependymomas, 177
    high-grade gliomas, 174–175, 175*t*
    low-grade gliomas, 175–177, 176*f*
    meningiomas, 177
    oligodendrogliomas, 177
    overview, 172, 172*t*–173*t*
    primary central nervous system lymphomas, 172–173
    primitive neuroectodermal tumors, 173
  vertebral metastases with epidural extension, 592–593
Chlorambucil, neurologic complications of, 687
Cholesteatoma, 463
Cholesterol granuloma, 463
Chondrosarcoma, 449–450, 463, 467–469, 468*f*
  therapeutic management and outcomes
    chemotherapy, 522
    overview, 521
    radiation therapy, 522
    surgery, 522
Chordoma, 449–450, 463, 469–470, 469*f*
  histology and molecular genetics, 5
  therapeutic management and outcomes
    outcomes, 521
    overview, 521
    prognostic factors, 521
    treatment, 521
Chorea
  antineuronal antibodies, 660
  diagnostic evaluation, 660
  differential diagnosis, 660
  overview, 660
  treatment and prognosis, 660
  underlying tumor, 660
Choroid plexus tumors
  papilloma, 472
  pathology, 443
Chromosome instability, 12
Cilengitide, 175*t*
Cisplatin
  CNS penetration of, 617*t*
  neurologic complications of, 685–686, 685*t*
Cladribine, neurologic complications of, 684
Clear-cell ependymomas, 98
Clear-cell meningiomas, 518*f*–519*f*
Clinical trial design
  basic concepts and definitions
    basic concepts
      clinical study team, 218
      consent form, 217
      data monitoring committee, 218
      site principal investigator, 218
      trial oversight, 217
    definitions, 217
  essential elements of clinical trial design
    choosing end points for neuro-oncology trials, 220
    clinical versus surrogate end points, 219–220
    event-time variables
      choosing end points, 222–223, 223*f*
      progression-free survival, 222
      survival, 222
      time to progression, 222
    overview, 218
    patient/subject selection
      broad versus restrictive eligibility criteria, 224
      overview, 223
      prognostic variables in brain tumors, 223–224, 224*f*
    placebo control, 229
    primary variables, 223
    randomization and stratification
      overview, 226
      randomization procedures, 227
        stratified randomization, 227–228
        unstratified randomization, 227
      treatment assignment issues, 226–227
    response or regression rates
      definition, 220
      factors affecting response rates, 221–222, 221*f*
      imaging issues, 220–221
    scientific rationale, 219
    significance of question, 219
    statistical designs
      overview, 224
      phase I designs, 224–225
      phase II designs, 225
      phase III designs
        multifactor designs, 225–226
        overview, 225
        single-factor designs, 225
    study goals, 219

treatment blinding/masking
overview, 228
pertinent issues, 228
feasibility assessment, 231
overview, 217, 231–232
sample size calculations
calculating sample sizes, 230–231
importance of appropriate sample sizes
overview, 229
key concepts, 229
overview, 229
types of clinical trials, 218
C-myc oncogene, 387*t*, 388
Combination therapy, 166–167
Complications of cancer, indirect
neurologic complications of chemotherapy and biologic therapies. *See* Neurologic complications of chemotherapy and biologic therapies
neurologic complications of radiation therapy. *See* Neurologic complications of radiation therapy
paraneoplasia. *See* Paraneoplasia
Compton effect, 144
Computed tomography (CT), basic concepts of, 40, 54
Congenital teratomas, 483
Consent form (clinical trials), 217
Conus medullaris, tumors of, 503
Convection approaches to improving targeting of therapeutic agents to tumor, 29–30
Cortical tumors, focal neurologic symptoms and signs of, 38–39
Corticosteroids, 49, 50*f*
neurologic complications of, 697–698
primary CNS lymphoma, 359
supportive care, 49, 50*f*, 186–187
vertebral metastases with epidural extension, 593–594
Corticotropin-secreting adenomas
clinical presentation and diagnosis, 397–398
therapy, 398
Cowden syndrome, 100
Cranial nerves, radiation injury of
acoustic nerve (CN VIII), 721
facial nerve (CN VII), 721
glossopharyngeal nerve (CN IX), 721
hypoglossal nerve (CN XII), 722
oculomotor nerves (CN III, IV, VI), 721
olfactory nerve (CN I), 720–721
optic nerve (CN II), 721
overview, 720, 720*t*
spinal accessory nerve (CN XI), 722
trigeminal nerve (CN V), 721
vagus nerve (CN X), 721–722
Cranial nerves and skull base, primary tumors of
anterior skull base/anterior fossa lesions (crista galli, cribriform plate, orbital roof, planum sphenoidale)
clinical presentation, 448
diagnoses and management
adenocarcinoma, 455–456
brown tumor of skull base, 459
chondrosarcoma and chordoma, 449–450
encephalocele, 458
esthesioneuroblastoma, 449, 450*f*
fibrosarcoma, 451
fibrous histiocytoma, 450–451
giant cell tumor, 451
hemangiopericytoma, 454–455
inverted papilloma, 456–457
juvenile neuroangiofibroma, 452, 452*f*
malignant salivary and lacrimal gland lesions, 457
meningioma, 452–454, 453*f*
mucocele, 458
mucosal melanoma, 456, 457*f*
nasal glioma, 459
nasopharyngeal carcinoma, 456
neuroendocrine carcinoma, 457–458
neurofibroma, 451–452
orbital lesions, 458, 458*f*
osteochondroma, 451
osteoclastoma, 451
osteogenic sarcoma, 451
osteoma, 451
plasmacytoma, 451, 452*f*
rhabdomyosarcoma, 450
sinonasal undifferentiated carcinoma, 457, 458*f*
squamous cell carcinoma, 455–456
evaluation, 448–449
cavernous sinus/middle fossa lesions (squamous temporal bone, greater sphenoid wing, lower parietal bone, tegmen, petrous temporal bone)
diagnosis and management
cholesteatoma, 463
cholesterol granuloma, 463
chordoma/chondrosarcoma, 463
dermoid cyst, 462
epidermoid cyst, 462
general management considerations, 460–461
hemangioma, 462
meningioma, 462–463, 462*f*
neurofibroma, 461–462
nonneoplastic temporal bone and middle fossa mass, 463–464
schwannoma, 461, 461*f*
temporal bone adenomatous lesions, 463
evaluation, 460
presentation, 459–460
extracranial lesions
diagnoses and management
benign and malignant nerve sheath tumors of head and neck, 475
carotid body tumor and malignant carotid body tumor, 474–475
evaluation, 474
outcome, 475
presentation, 474
overview, 39, 110–111, 447–448, 475
posterior fossa/clival (posterior temporal bone, occipital bone, clivus)
diagnoses and management
acoustic neuroma, 465–466, 465*f*
cavernoma, 470
chondrosarcoma, 467–469, 468*f*
chordoma, 469–470, 469*f*
choroid plexus papilloma, 472
craniopharyngioma, 473–474
dermoid cyst, 472
epidermoid cyst, 471–472, 471*f*
epithelial cyst, 470–471
facial nerve schwannomas, 467, 468*f*
lipoma, 470
meningioma, 466–467, 467*f*
nerve sheath tumor of jugular foramen, 472
overview, 464–465
paragangliomas, 472–473, 473*f*
teratoma, 470
evaluation, 464
presentation, 464
sellar/parasellar, 459, 459*f*
Craniopharyngioma, 401–402, 403*f*, 404, 473–474
imaging, 58*t*, 69*f*
neuroimaging
CT, 69
MRI, 69, 69*f*
overview, 68–69
CSF (cerebrospinal fluid) analysis, 42–43
CT (computed tomography), basic concepts of, 40, 54
CyberKnife, 159, 159*f*
Cyclophosphamide
CNS penetration of, 617*t*
neurologic complications of, 688
Cytarabine
CNS penetration of, 617*t*
intrathecal, 619*t*–621*t*, 620–621
Cytosine arabinoside, neurologic complications of, 683–684

D

Dacarbazine, neurologic complications of, 686
Dactinomycin, CNS penetration of, 617*t*
DAL-1 tumor suppressor protein, 370–371
Danazol, neurologic complications of, 697
Data monitoring committees (DMCs), 217–218
Daunorubicin, neurologic complications of, 691
Depression, 189–190, 190*t*–191*t*, 209–210
Dermatomyositis/polymyositis/inclusion body myositis
  associated antibodies, 668
  diagnostic evaluation, 668
  overview, 667
  treatment and prognosis, 668
  underlying tumor, 668
Dermoid cyst, 462, 472
Desmoids, 542
Desmoplastic infantile ganglioglioma (DIG), 304
Desmoplastic medulloblastoma, 105
Dexamethasone
  CNS penetration of, 617*t*
  vertebral metastases, 592
DFMO (difluoromethylornithine), 175*t*
Diet and brain cancer, 7
  high-grade astrocytomas, 260–261
Diffuse infiltrating astrocytomas, 84
Diffuse infiltrating pontine glioma, 335–337, 336*f*
Diffusion magnetic resonance
  overview, 74, 76, 77*f*
  tumor delineation, 76
  tumor grading, 76
  tumor invasion assessment, 76, 78
Diffusion-weighted imaging (DWI), 74, 76, 77*f*
Difluoromethylornithine (DFMO), 175*t*
DIG (desmoplastic infantile ganglioglioma), 304
DNA repair enzymes, 168–169
DNA replication, 19
DNT (dysembryoplastic neuroepithelial tumor), 103–104, 104*f*, 304–305
Docetaxel, neurologic complications of, 690
Dorsal exophytic brainstem tumors, 337–338, 338*f*
Dose intensity, chemotherapy, 167
Down syndrome, 10
Doxorubicin, neurologic complications of, 691
Drug resistance, 164–165, 164*f*
Dural and skull-based metastases, 623
DWI (diffusion-weighted imaging), 74, 76, 77*f*
Dynamic contrast-enhanced (DCE) MRI, 74, 75*f*
Dysembryoplastic neuroepithelial tumor (DNT), 103–104, 104*f*, 304–305
Dysphagia and swallowing disorders, 188–189
Dysplastic gangliocytoma of the cerebellum, 100, 101*f*

E

Effector molecules, targeting
  angiogenesis mediators, 28
  overview, 19, 26, 27*t*
  proteinases and integrins as mediators of tumor invasiveness
    integrins in tumor motility, 27–28
    proteinases, 26–27, 27*t*
EGF (epidermal growth factor), 371
EGFR (epidermal growth factor receptor), 19–21, 20*t*, 266, 371
EGFR gene, 88–89, 93, 312, 320
Electroencephalography, 42
Electromagnetic fields and brain cancer, 6, 260
Embryonal tumors
  atypical teratoid/rhabdoid tumor, 107, 107*f*
  medulloblastomas
    description, 105–106, 105*f*–106*f*
    molecular genetics, 106
  overview, 104
Encephalocele, 458
Encephalomyelitis, 656–658
  antineuronal antibodies, 658
  diagnostic evaluation, 658
  differential diagnosis, 658
  treatment and prognosis, 658
  underlying tumor, 658
Endocrine evaluation, 43
End points for neuro-oncology trials
  choosing, 219–220, 222–223, 223*f*
  clinical versus surrogate end points, 219–220
Enhancing lesions
  benign conditions, 46–47
  brain metastasis, 44–45, 46*f*
  gliomas, 43–44, 45*f*
  primary central nervous system lymphoma (PCNSL), 45–46
EORTC (European Organization of Research and Treatment of Cancer) QLQ-C30, 203
Ependymal tumors
  anaplastic ependymoma, 98–99
  ependymomas. *See* Ependymomas
  molecular genetics, 100
  myxopapillary ependymoma, 99
  subependymoma, 99–100
Ependymomas, 98, 98*f*–99*f*. *See also* Ependymal tumors
  clinical manifestations, 433, 434*t*
  diagnostic evaluation and imaging characteristics, 433–434, 434*t*, 435*f*–437*f*, 437
  epidemiology, 432
  histology and molecular genetics, 5
  imaging, 57*t*, 66*f*
  molecular biology and cytogenetics, 433
  neuroimaging
    CT, 65
    MRI, 65, 66*f*
    overview, 65
  overview, 431–432
  pathology, 432–433
  prognosis, 440–441, 440*t*–441*t*
  therapeutic management and outcomes
    chemotherapy, 517
    overview, 515, 516*f*
    pathology, 515, 517
    prognostic factors, 517
    radiation therapy, 517
    surgery, 517
  treatment
    adjuvant therapy
      chemotherapy, 177, 439–440
      radiotherapy, 438–439
    surgery
      infratentorial ependymomas, 437–438
      management of hydrocephalus, 438
      overview, 437
      supratentorial ependymomas, 438
Epidemiology of brain cancer
  etiology and risk factors of brain tumors
    cell phones, 6–7
    diet
      alcohol, 7
      N-nitroso compounds, 7
      vitamins, 7
    drugs and medications, 9
    electromagnetic fields, 6
    industry and occupation, 8–9
    ionizing radiation, 5–6
    smoking, 7–8
    viruses, 9
  genetic susceptibility to brain tumors
    chromosome instability, 12
    familial aggregation, 10
    hereditary syndromes, 10–11, 10*t*
    metabolic polymorphisms, 11
    mutagen sensitivity, 11–12
    overview, 9–10

histology and molecular genetics of brain tumors
astrocytomas, 3–4
chordomas, 5
ependymomas, 5
ganglioglioma, 5
medulloblastomas, 5
meningiomas, 5
oligodendrogliomas, 4
overview, 3, 4*f*
schwannomas (neurilemomas), 5
overview, 3, 12
Epidermal growth factor (EGF), 371
Epidermal growth factor receptor (EGFR), 19–21, 20*t*, 266, 371
Epidermoid cyst, 460–462, 471–472, 471*f*
Epipodophyllotoxins, CNS penetration of, 617*t*
Epithelial cyst, 470–471
E1 protein, 31
Equivalence trial, 230
ER-α
pituitary adenomas and sellar lesions, 388
Erlotinib (Tarceva), neurologic complications of, 700
ERM (ezrin, radixin, and moesin) proteins, 235, 235*f*
Erythropoietin, neurologic complications of, 696
Esthesioneuroblastoma, 449, 450*f*
Estramustine, neurologic complications of, 687
Ethics, supportive care and, 194–196
Etoposide, neurologic complications of, 689–690
European Organization of Research and Treatment of Cancer (EORTC) QLQ-C30, 203
Event-time variables
choosing end points, 222–223, 223*f*
progression-free survival, 222
survival, 222
time to progression, 222
Evoked potentials, 42
Extracranial lesions
diagnoses and management
benign and malignant nerve sheath tumors of head and neck, 475
carotid body tumor and malignant carotid body tumor, 474–475
evaluation, 474
outcome, 475
presentation, 474

F

Facial nerve (CN VII)
radiation injury to, 721
schwannomas, 467, 468*f*
FACT (Functional Assessment of Cancer Therapy) with brain disease-specific subscale, 203
False localizing signs, 39
Familial aggregation, 10
Familial cancer syndromes, 10–11
Familial polyposis, 10*t*
Feasibility assessment (clinical trials), 231
FERM domain, 235, 235*f*
Fibrosarcoma, 451
Fibrous histiocytoma, 450–451
5-Fluorouracil
CNS penetration of, 617*t*
neurologic complications of, 683, 684*f*
Fludarabine, neurologic complications of, 684
Focal neurologic symptoms and signs
brainstem tumors, 39
cortical tumors, 38–39
pineal region and third ventricular tumors, 39
Focused therapies for brain metastases, 562–563
with adjuvant whole-brain radiation therapy, 570–571, 571*t*
Formaldehyde, cancer incidence and, 8–9
Frameless stereotaxy, 128*f*
Functional Assessment of Cancer Therapy (FACT) with brain disease-specific subscale, 203

G

Gamma Knife, 156–157, 157*f*–158*f*
Gangliocytoma, 100, 101*f*
neuroimaging
CT, 65
MRI, 66
overview, 65
Ganglioglioma, 57*t*, 103, 304
histology and molecular genetics, 5
neuroimaging
CT, 65
MRI, 66, 67*f*
overview, 65
Ganglion cyst, 542
Gardner syndrome, 10*t*
Gastric acid inhibitors, 187
Gastrointestinal metastasis to brain, surgery for, 565
Gefitinib (Iressa), 175*t*
neurologic complications of, 700
Gemcitabine, 622
neurologic complications of, 684–685
Gemtuzumab ozogamicin (Mylotarg), neurologic complications of, 699
Genitourinary metastasis to brain, surgery for, 565
Germ cell tumors
pathology, 443
young infants, 483
Germinomas
long-term survival, 495
surgical management, 490
Giant cell glioblastoma, 88, 89*f*–90*f*
Giant cell tumor, 451
Glioblastoma multiforme, 84, 87, 87*f*–89*f*
imaging, 57*t*, 62*f*, 126*f*
Gliomas, 43–44, 45*f*
astrocytic tumors
anaplastic astrocytoma, 85–87, 86*f*
astrocytoma. *See* Astrocytoma
diffuse infiltrating astrocytomas, 84
giant cell glioblastoma, 88, 89*f*–90*f*
glioblastoma multiforme, 87, 87*f*–89*f*
gliosarcoma, 88
molecular genetics of diffuse astrocytomas, 88–89
overview, 84
special categories
overview, 89–90
pilocytic astrocytoma, 90–91, 91*f*
pleomorphic xanthoastrocytoma, 91–93, 92*f*
subependymal giant cell astrocytoma, 93–94, 93*f*
brainstem
diagnosis
management, 335
neuroimaging, 334
pathology, 335
pathophysiology, 335
overview, 333, 340
specific subtypes
brainstem tumors, 340
cervicomedullary tumors, 338, 339*f*
diffuse infiltrating pontine glioma, 335–337, 336*f*
dorsal exophytic brainstem tumors, 337–338, 338*f*
intrinsic tectal gliomas, 338–340, 339*f*
neurofibromatosis type I, 340
symptoms, 333–334, 334*t*
ependymal tumors
anaplastic ependymoma, 98–99
ependymoma, 98, 98*f*–99*f*
molecular genetics, 100
myxopapillary ependymoma, 99
subependymoma, 99–100
oligodendroglial tumors
anaplastic oligoastrocytoma, 97, 97*f*
anaplastic oligodendroglioma, 95–96, 96*f*
mixed oligoastrocytoma, 96–97, 97*f*
molecular genetics, 97
oligodendroglioma, 94–95, 94*f*–95*f*
overview, 84, 85*t*

Gliomas (*Cont.*):
pathology, 441
single brain lesion, 43–44, 45*f*
Gliomatosis cerebri, 305, 305*f*
Gliosarcoma, 88
Glossopharyngeal nerve (CN IX), radiation injury to, 721
Glycoprotein adenomas, 390–391, 391*f*
GM-CSF (granulocyte-macrophage colony-stimulating factor), neurologic complications of, 696
Gompertzian growth curves, 163–164, 164*f*
G1/S checkpoint, 25–26, 25*t*
Gorlin syndrome, 247, 249, 249*t*, 250*f*, 420
Goserelin, neurologic complications of, 697
Granulocyte-macrophage colony-stimulating factor (GM-CSF), neurologic complications of, 696
Growing teratoma syndrome, surgical management of, 491
Growth factor pathways, high-grade astrocytomas and
epidermal growth factor receptor (EGRF), 266
overview, 265
platelet-derived growth factor (PDGF), 265
Growth factor receptor signaling and downstream effectors, high-grade astrocytomas and
overview, 266, 267*f*
P13K/AKT/PTEN, 266
Ras, 266
Growth factors, neurologic complications of
erythropoietin, 696
granulocyte-macrophage colony-stimulating factor (GM-CSF), 696
interleukin-3, 696
interleukin-6, 696
interleukin-11, 696
Growth hormone-secreting adenomas, 389, 390*f*
clinical presentation and diagnosis, 396
therapy, 396–397
Growth-regulatory pathways in tumor cells, 17, 18*f*, 19
Gsp (stimulatory guanine nucleotide-binding protein) oncogene, 387, 387*t*
Guanosine triphosphatase (GTPase)-activating proteins (GAPs), 234–235, 234*f*
Gynecologic metastasis to brain, surgery for, 565

H

Headaches, 37
Hemangioblastoma
imaging, 58*t*
neuroimaging
CT, 71
MRI, 71, 71*f*
overview, 71
therapeutic management and outcomes
outcomes, 523
overview, 522–523, 522*f*
prognostic factors, 523
treatment, 523
Hemangiopericytoma, 110, 111*f*, 377, 454–455
Hematopoietic system tumors
primary central nervous system lymphoma, 113–114, 113*f*
Hereditary syndromes, 10–11, 10*t*
Hexamethylmelamine, neurologic complications of, 688
High-grade astrocytomas
chemotherapy
chemotherapy at tumor recurrence, 281
multiagent regimens, 280
newer chemotherapeutic agents, 281, 282*t*
overall benefit, 280
overview, 279
prediction of response and prognosis, 280–281, 280*t*
single-agent regimens, 279–280
symptomatic treatments, 281–282
clinical presentation
diagnostic evaluation
definitive diagnosis, 275, 276*t*
radiographic imaging, 274–275, 274*f*–275*f*, 275*t*
presenting signs and symptoms
brainstem and cerebrospinal fluid involvement, 273–274
cognitive dysfunction, 273
duration and onset of symptoms, 273
focal symptoms, 273
generalized symptoms, 273
overview, 273, 273*t*
seizures, 273
epidemiology
causative and risk factors, 259–260
environmental factors
diet and other factors, 260–261
electromagnetic fields and cellular telephones, 260
ionizing radiation, 260
genetic predisposition
Li-Fraumeni syndrome, 260
neurofibromatosis types 1 and 2, 260
Ollier disease, 260
overview, 260
Turcot syndrome, 260
incidence, 259
genetics and molecular biology
cell of origin, 261
growth factor pathways
epidermal growth factor receptor (EGRF), 266
overview, 265
platelet-derived growth factor (PDGF), 265
growth factor receptor signaling and downstream effectors
overview, 266, 267*f*
P13K/AKT/PTEN, 266
Ras, 266
key genetic and molecular pathways in high-grade astrocytomas
overview, 262
p53 pathway, 262–263, 264*f*
Rb pathway, 264–265, 265*f*
molecular alterations associated with primary and secondary glioblastoma, 261–262
molecular and genetic changes associated with astrocytoma progression, 262, 263*f*
molecular classification and markers of prognosis, 267–268
overview, 261
targeted and individualized therapy, 268
vascular endothelial growth factor and angiogenesis (VEGF), 266–267
histopathology of high-grade astrocytic tumors
classification and grading, 268–270
glioblastoma histopathology, 270, 272*f*, 273
histopathology, 270, 271*f*
overview, 249
terminal care, 282
treatment of anaplastic astrocytomas and glioblastoma
interstitial brachytherapy, 278–279
overview, 275–276, 276*f*
role of radiation, 277–278, 279*f*
role of surgical resection, 276–277
stereotactic radiosurgery, 278
surgical resection for tumor recurrence, 277
High-grade gliomas, chemotherapy for, 174–175, 175*t*
HIV+ primary CNS lymphoma, 361

Hormonal therapy, neurologic complications of
aromatase inhibitors (anastrazole, letrozole, aminoglutethimide), 697
danazol, 697
goserelin, 697
leuprolide, 697
mitotane, 697
octreotide, 697
tamoxifen, 696–697
toremifene, 697
Hospice care and end of life, 193–194
H-ras oncogene, 387*t*, 388
Hydrocephalus, management of, 438
Hydroxyurea, neurologic complications of, 685
Hypoglossal nerve (CN XII), radiation injury to, 722

I

Ibritumomab tiuxetan (Zevalin), neurologic complications of, 699
Ifosfamide
CNS penetration of, 617*t*
neurologic complications of, 688–689
IGF (insulin-like growth factors) I and II, 371
Ilocytic astrocytoma, chemotherapy for, 302
Imatinib mesylate (Gleevec), 175*t*
neurologic complications of, 700
IMRT (intensity-modulated radiation therapy), 152, 154*f*
Indirect complications of cancer
neurologic complications of chemotherapy and biologic therapies. *See* Neurologic complications of chemotherapy and biologic therapies
neurologic complications of radiation therapy. *See* Neurologic complications of radiation therapy
paraneoplasia. *See* Paraneoplasia
Industry and brain cancer, 8–9
Infratentorial ependymomas, 437–438
Insulin-like growth factors (IGF)-I and -II, 371
Integrins, 27–28, 27*t*
Intensity-modulated radiation therapy (IMRT), 152, 154*f*
Intent to treat (ITT) sample, 231
Interferons, neurologic complications of, 694–695
Interleukins, neurologic complications of, 695–696
Interstitial brachytherapy, 278–279
Interstitial chemotherapy, 29
Intraarterial chemotherapy, 171
Intracellular second messenger components
overview, 21
protein kinase C inhibitors, 22
targeting Ras with farnesyltransferase inhibitors, 22
Intracerebrospinal fluid chemotherapy, 171–172
Intracranial germ cell tumors
chemotherapy
germinomas, 493
nongerminoma germ cell tumors (NGGCT), 494–495
overview, 486*t*, 493
diagnostic evaluation
histologic diagnosis
pineal region tumors
miscellaneous nongerm cell pineal region tumors, 487–488
overview, 486–487
pineal parenchymal tumors, 487
suprasellar tumors, 486
neuroimaging, 484, 486
overview, 485*t*–486*t*
tumor staging
overview, 486*t*
radiologic staging and cerebrospinal fluid cytology, 488–489
tumor markers, 488, 488*t*
epidemiology and known influences on tumor, 482
genetics and molecular biology
tumor cytogenetics, 482–483
tumor pathogenesis, 482
neuropathology, 489–490, 489*f*
overview, 481
prognosis
long-term survival of germinomas, 495
long-term survival of nongerminoma germ cell tumors, 495
tumor-related morbidity and therapy-related sequelae
neurocognitive sequelae, 495
neuroendocrine sequelae, 495–496
overview, 495
secondary neoplasms, 496
radiation therapy
germinomas, 491–492
nongerminoma germ cell tumors, 492–493
overview, 486*t*
specific clinical presentations
congenital teratomas, 483
germ cell tumors in young infants, 483
overview, 483
pineal region germ cell tumors in older children and adults, 483, 484*f*
suprasellar germ cell tumors in older children and adults, 483
surgical management
general considerations, 490
germinomas, 490
growing teratoma syndrome, 491
nongerminoma germ cell tumors, 490–491
overview, 485*t*–486*t*
second-look surgery, 491
Intradural extramedullary tumors, 507
Intradural spinal metastases
intradural extramedullary metastases, 599–600, 600*f*
intramedullary metastases, 600–602, 601*f*
overview, 599, 600*f*–601*f*
Intramedullary tumors, 503, 507–508
Intraocular lymphoma, 352–353, 352*f*–353*f*
Intrathecal chemotherapy, for leptomeningeal metastases, 618–621, 618*f*–619*f*, 619*t*–621*t*
Intraventricular tumors
clinical manifestations, 441
ependymomas. *See* Ependymomas
imaging, 441
overview, 441
pathology
choroid plexus tumors, 443
germ cell tumors, 443
gliomas, 441
neurocytomas, 442*f*, 443
oligodendrogliomas, 443
overview, 441
pineal region tumors, 443
subependymomas, 443
Intrinsic tectal gliomas, 338–340, 339*f*
Inverted papilloma, 456–457
In-vitro drug sensitivity testing, 169
Ionizing radiation, 5–6, 144, 260
Irinotecan
CNS penetration of, 617*t*
neurologic complications of, 690–691
ITT (intent to treat) sample, 231

J

Juvenile neuroangiofibroma, 452, 452*f*

K

Karnofsky Performance Status (KPS), 202

L

Laboratory diagnosis
audiometry, 43
cerebrospinal fluid analysis, 42–43

Laboratory diagnosis (*Cont.*):
  electroencephalography, 42
  endocrine evaluation, 43
  evoked potentials, 42
  perimetry, 42
Lambert-Eaton myasthenic syndrome
  antineuronal antibodies, 666
  diagnostic evaluation, 666, 666*f*
  differential diagnosis, 667
  overview, 666
  treatment and prognosis, 667
  underlying tumor, 666
Large cell/anaplastic medulloblastoma, 106
L-asparaginase
  CNS penetration of, 617*t*
  neurologic complications of, 692–694, 693*f*
Late delayed brachial plexopathy, 719–720
Leksell Gamma Knife, 156–157, 157*f*–158*f*
Leptomeningeal and dural/skull metastases
  dural and skull-based metastases, 623
  future directions, 623
  leptomeningeal metastases
    clinical presentation
      overview, 609, 610*t*
      signs and symptoms of cerebral hemisphere involvement, 610–611
      signs and symptoms of cranial nerve involvement, 610
      signs and symptoms of spinal cord involvement, 610
    diagnosis
      cerebrospinal fluid examination, 611–612, 611*t*–612*t*
      overview, 610–611
      radiographic evaluation
        CSF flow studies, 615
        MRI, 613–615, 613*f*–615*f*
        overview, 612–613
    incidence and prognosis
      leptomeningeal metastases from leukemias and lymphomas, 608–609
      leptomeningeal metastases from solid tumor, 608, 608*t*
      overview, 607–608
    overview, 607
    pathogenesis, 609
    treatment
      chemotherapy
        high-dose systemic, 618
        intrathecal, 618–621, 618*f*–619*f*, 619*t*–621*t*
        overview, 617–618, 617*t*
      CNS leukemic or lymphomatous meningitis
        leptomemingeal metastases from solid tumors, 622
        overview, 621–622
        palliative therapy, 622
      investigational agents for treatment of leptomeningeal metastases
        gemcitabine, 622
        mafosfamide, 622–623
        miscellaneous strategies, 623
        overview, 622
        topotecan, 622
      overview, 616, 616*t*
      radiotherapy
        adults, 616
        adverse effects, 617
        children, 616–617
  overview, 607, 623
Leskell Gamma Knife, 568
Letrozole, neurologic complications of, 697
Leuprolide, neurologic complications of, 697
Lhermite-Duclos disease, 100
Li-Fraumeni syndrome, 10–11
  high-grade astrocytomas and, 260
Limbic encephalitis
  antineuronal antibodies, 656
  diagnostic evaluation, 656
  differential diagnosis, 656
  overview, 656, 657*f*
  treatment and prognosis, 656
  underlying tumor, 656
Linear accelerator (LINAC) based radiosurgery, 157, 568
Lipoma, 470, 542
Low-grade astrocytomas
  chemotherapy
    low-grade fibrillary astrocytoma, 300–302, 301*f*
    pilocytic astrocytoma, 302
  epidemiology, 290
  future directions, 305–306
  genetics and molecular biology, 290–291
  less common low-grade astrocytomas
    astroblastoma, 303
    cerebellar pilocytic astrocytomas, 302–303, 303*f*
    desmoplastic infantile ganglioglioma (DIG), 304
    dysembryoplastic neuroepithelial tumor (DNT), 304–305
    ganglioglioma, 304
    gliomatosis cerebri, 305, 305*f*
    pleomorphic xanthoastrocytoma, 303–304
    subependymal giant cell astrocytoma, 304
  natural history, 294–295
  overview, 289, 305–306
  pathology, 292–293, 293*t*
  presenting clinical signs and symptoms, 293–294
  prognostic features
    overview, 295
    patient-related
      age, 295
      performance status, 295–296
      seizures, 296
      sex, 295
    tumor-related
      cyst formation, 295
      flow cytometry, 295
      molecular genetic markers, 295
      MRI and CT, 295
      proliferative markers, 295
      tumor characteristics, 295
  radiologic features
    CT and MRI, 291–292, 291*f*–292*f*
    magnetic resonance spectroscopy, 292
    overview, 291, 291*t*
    PET, 292
  radiotherapy, 297–300, 298*f*, 300*f*
  recurrence, 302, 302*f*
  surgical management, 296–297
    pilocytic astrocytomas, 297
Low-grade gliomas, chemotherapy for, 175–177, 176*f*
Lumbosacral plexopathy, 720
Lumbosacral plexus
  metastases
    clinical setting, 638
    clinical signs, 638–639, 638*t*
    differential diagnosis, 639–640
    electrophysiologic diagnosis, 639
    imaging, 639, 640*f*
    overview, 637–638
    surgical exploration, 639
    treatment/prognosis, 640–641
  radiation injury of. *See* Brachial or lumbosacral plexus, radiation injury of
Lung metastasis to brain, surgery for, 564

M

Mafosfamide, 622–623
Magnetic resonance imaging (MRI), basic concepts of, 40–41, 54–55
Magnetic resonance spectroscopy (MRS), 72–73, 74*f*, 279*f*
Malignant peripheral nerve sheath tumor, 112, 542–543, 543*f*
Malignant salivary and lacrimal gland lesions, 457
Marimastat, 175*t*

Masking of treatment in clinical trials
overview, 228
pertinent issues, 228
Mdm2 gene, 482
Mechlorethamine, neurologic complications of, 687
Medulloblastoma
analyses of gene expression, 419–420
cell of origin, 419
clinical diagnosis, 416
histology and molecular genetics, 5
imaging diagnosis, 57*t*, 62, 64, 64*f*, 416–417, 417*f*–419*f*
karotypic abnormalities, 419
miscellaneous growth factor pathways, 421–422
molecular biology, 420–421
nonsurgical therapy, 423–424
outcome, 424–425, 425*t*
overview, 416
pathologic diagnosis, 417, 419
recurrent, 424
surgical treatment
associated hydrocephalus, 422
resection, 422–423
Medullomyoblastoma, 106
Melanocytic tumors, 377–378
Melanoma metastasis to brain, surgery for, 564–565
Melanotic medulloblastoma, 106
Meningeal tumors
hemangiopericytoma, 110, 111*f*
meningiomas
anaplastic (malignant) meningiomas, 110
atypical meningiomas, 109–110
meningioma. *See* Meningioma
molecular genetics, 110
overview, 107–108, 108*f*, 109*t*
sarcomas, 377
solitary fibrous tumor, 110
Meningioma, 108–109, 109*f*, 452–454, 453*f*, 462–463, 462*f*, 466–467, 467*f*. *See also* Meningeal tumors
chemotherapy, 177
histology and molecular genetics of brain tumors, 5
neuroimaging, 57*t*, 68*f*
CT, 67
MRI, 67–68, 68*f*
overview, 66–67
therapeutic management and outcomes
chemotherapy, 519
overview, 517–518, 518*f*–519*f*
radiation therapy, 519
surgery, 518–519
MEN-1 (multiple endocrine neoplasia-1) tumor suppressor gene, 387*t*, 388
MERLIN/Schwannomin protein, 546
Metabolic polymorphisms, 11
Metastatic brachial plexopathy
clinical setting, 630–633, 631*f*
Pancoast tumors, 631–632, 632*f*
diagnosis
differential diagnosis, 635–636, 636*t*
electrophysiology, 633
imaging
metastatic brachial plexopathy, 633, 634*f*, 635
Pancoast tumor, 633, 634*f*
surgery, 635
treatment/prognosis, 636–637
Pancoast tumors, 636
Metastatic disease
brain. *See* Brain, metastases to
leptomeningeal and dural/skull metastases. *See* Leptomeningeal and dural/skull metastases
peripheral nervous system. *See* Peripheral nervous system, tumors, metastases
spine. *See* Spinal metastases
Methotrexate
CNS penetration of, 617*t*
intrathecal, 619–620, 619*t*
neurologic complications of
acute/subacute effects, 681–682, 682*f*
late effects, 682, 683*f*
overview, 680–681, 681*t*
Metronidazole, neurologic complications of, 691
MG (myasthenia gravis). *See* Myasthenia gravis (MG)
Middle fossa lesions. *See* Cavernous sinus/middle fossa lesions
Misonidazole, neurologic complications of, 691
Mitomycin C, neurologic complications of, 691
Mitotane, neurologic complications of, 697
Mitoxantrone, neurologic complications of, 691
Mixed neuronal-glial tumors
dysembryoplastic neuroepithelial tumor (DNT), 103–104, 104*f*
ganglioglioma and malignant ganglioglioma, 103
Mixed oligoastrocytoma, 96–97, 97*f*
MLC (multileaf collimator), 152, 153*f*
Monoclonal antibodies, neurologic complications of
cetuximab (Erbitux), 699–700
gemtuzumab ozogamicin (Mylotarg), 699
ibritumomab tiuxetan (Zevalin), 699
OKT3, 698–699, 699*f*
rituximab (Rituxan), 699
trastuzumab (Herceptin), 699
Mood, 209
MRI (magnetic resonance imaging), basic concepts of, 40–41, 54–55
MRS (magnetic resonance spectroscopy), 72–73, 74*f*, 279*f*
Mucocele, 458
Mucosal melanoma, 456, 457*f*
Multidrug resistance, 168
Multifactor statistical designs, 225–226
Multileaf collimator (MLC), 152, 153*f*
Multiple brain lesions
approach to patient
overview, 48, 48*t*, 49*f*
supportive care
antiepileptic drugs, 48–49
corticosteroids, 49, 50*f*
prophylactic therapy for venous thromboembolic disease (VTED), 49
psychosocial support, 49–50
differential diagnosis, 48*t*
supportive care
antiepileptic drugs, 48–49
corticosteroids, 49, 50*f*
prophylactic therapy for venous thromboembolic disease (VTED), 49
psychosocial support, 49–50
Multiple endocrine neoplasia-1 (MEN-1) tumor suppressor gene, 387*t*, 388
Multiple metastases, surgery for, 565–566
Multiple myeloma, 664
Mutagen sensitivity, 11–12
Myasthenia gravis (MG)
antineuronal antibodies, 667
diagnostic evaluation, 667
differential diagnosis, 667
overview, 667
treatment and prognosis, 667
underlying tumor, 667
Myxopapillary ependymoma, 99

N

Nasal glioma, 459
Nasopharyngeal carcinoma, 456
Nemangioma, 462
Nerve sheath tumors, 112, 464–465, 472, 475, 542–543, 543*f*
Neurocytomas, 442*f*, 443
Neuroendocrine carcinoma, 457–458
Neuroepithelial tumors
embryonal tumors. *See* Embryonal tumors
gliomas
astrocytic tumors
anaplastic astrocytoma, 85–87, 86*f*
astrocytoma. *See* Astrocytoma
diffuse infiltrating astrocytomas, 84

Neuroepithelial tumors
gliomas
astrocytic tumors (*Cont.*):
giant cell glioblastoma, 88, 89*f*–90*f*
glioblastoma multiforme, 87, 87*f*–89*f*
gliosarcoma, 88
molecular genetics of diffuse astrocytomas, 88–89
special categories
overview, 89–90
pilocytic astrocytoma, 90–91, 91*f*
pleomorphic xanthoastrocytoma, 91–93, 92*f*
subependymal giant cell astrocytoma, 93–94, 93*f*
ependymal tumors
anaplastic ependymoma, 98–99
ependymoma, 98, 98*f*–99*f*
molecular genetics, 100
myxopapillary ependymoma, 99
subependymoma, 99–100
oligodendroglial tumors
anaplastic oligoastrocytoma, 97, 97*f*
anaplastic oligodendroglioma, 95–96, 96*f*
mixed oligoastrocytoma, 96–97, 97*f*
molecular genetics, 97
oligodendroglioma, 94–95, 94*f*–95*f*
overview, 84, 85*t*
histological classification, 85*t*
neuronal and mixed neuronal-glial tumors. *See* Neuronal and mixed neuronal-glial tumors
Neurofibroma, 111–112, 111*f*, 451–452, 461–462, 541, 541*f*
Neurofibromatosis type 1, 340, 544–546, 546*f*
Neurofibromatosis type 2, 546
Neurofibromatosis types 1 (von Recklinghausen disease) and 2
high-grade astrocytomas and, 260
nevoid basal cell carcinoma syndrome (Gorlin syndrome), 247, 249, 249*t*, 250*f*
overview, 10*t*, 234–236, 234*f*–235*f*
tuberous sclerosis complex (Bourneville disease), 242–243, 242*t*, 244*f*–245*f*, 245–246
type 1, 236–237, 236*t*, 238*f*, 239–240, 340, 544–546, 546*f*
type 2, 240–242, 240*t*, 241*f*, 546
von Hipple-Lindau (VHL) disease, 246–247, 247*t*, 248*f*
Neuroimaging
approach to patient, 55–56
astrocytic tumors
CT, 56
MRI, 56, 58, 59*f*–62*f*
overview, 56, 57*t*–58*t*
basic concepts
CT, 54
MRI, 54–55
overview, 54, 54*t*
PET, 55
SPECT, 55
brainstem glioma
CT, 69
MRI, 69, 70*f*, 71
overview, 69
comparison of techniques, 54*t*
craniopharyngioma
CT, 69
MRI, 69, 69*f*
overview, 68–69
ependymoma
CT, 65
MRI, 65, 66*f*
overview, 65
gangliocytoma
CT, 65
MRI, 66
overview, 65
ganglioglioma
CT, 65
MRI, 66, 67*f*
overview, 65
hemangioblastoma
CT, 71
MRI, 71, 71*f*
overview, 71
medical image storage and retrieval, 53–54
medulloblastoma
CT, 64
MRI, 64, 64*f*
overview, 62, 64
meningioma
CT, 67
MRI, 67–68, 68*f*
overview, 66–67
oligodendroglioma
CT, 61–62
general imaging findings, 60–61
MRI, 62
overview, 58
PET, 62, 63*f*
overview, 53, 57*t*–58*t*
primary CNS lymphoma (PCNSL)
CT, 72
MRI, 72, 73*f*
overview, 72
special imaging studies
diffusion magnetic resonance
overview, 74, 76, 77*f*
tumor delineation, 76
tumor grading, 76
tumor invasion assessment, 76, 78
magnetic resonance spectroscopy (MRS), 72–73, 74*f*
perfusion magnetic resonance, 74, 75*f*
Neurologic complications of chemotherapy and biologic therapies
alkylating agents
busulfan, 687
carboplatin, 685–686
chlorambucil, 687
cisplatin, 685–686, 685*t*
cyclophosphamide, 688
dacarbazine, 686
estramustine, 687
hexamethylmelamine, 688
ifosfamide, 688–689
mechlorethamine, 687
nitrosoureas, 686–687
procarbazine, 687–688
temozolomide, 686
thiotepa, 688
antimetabolites
capecitabine, 683
cladribine, 684
cytosine arabinoside, 683–684
5-fluoruracil, 683, 684*f*
fludarabine, 684
gemcitabine, 684–685
hydroxyurea, 685
methotrexate
acute/subacute effects, 681–682, 682*f*
late effects, 682, 683*f*
overview, 680–681, 681*t*
pentostatin, 685
antineoplastic antibiotics
bleomycin, 691
daunorubicin, 691
doxorubicin, 691
mitomycin C, 691
mitoxantrone, 691
nitroimidazoles (misonidazole, metronidazole), 691
plicamycin (mithramycin), 692
suramin, 692
miscellaneous agents
bacillus Calmette-Guérin, 694
corticosteroids, 697–698
growth factors
erythropoietin, 696
granulocyte-macrophage colony-stimulating factor (GM-CSF), 696
interleukin-3, 696
interleukin-6, 696
interleukin-11, 696

hormonal therapy
aromatase inhibitors (anastrazole, letrozole, aminoglutethimide), 697
danazol, 697
goserelin, 697
leuprolide, 697
mitotane, 697
octreotide, 697
tamoxifen, 696–697
toremifene, 697
interferons, 694–695
interleukins, 695
L-asparaginase, 692–694, 693*f*
monoclonal antibodies
cetuximab (Erbitux), 699–700
gemtuzumab ozogamicin (Mylotarg), 699
ibritumomab tiuxetan (Zevalin), 699
OKT3, 698–699, 699*f*
rituximab (Rituxan), 699
trastuzumab (Herceptin), 699
retinoids, 692
signal transduction inhibitors
erlotinib (Tarceva), 700
gefitinib (Iressa), 700
imatinib mesylate (Gleevec), 700
thalidomide, 694
tumor necrosis factor-α, 696
overview, 679, 680*t*–681*t*, 700
plant alkaloids
etoposide, 689–690
pyrazoloacridine, 691
taxanes
docetaxel, 690
paclitaxel, 690
teniposide, 689–690
topoisomerase inhibitors
irinotecan, 690–691
rubitecan, 690–691
topotecan, 690–691
vinca alkaloids, 689
Neurologic complications of radiation therapy
overview, 711–712
radiation-induced neurotoxicity in the brain
acute effects, 712
combined effects of radiation and chemotherapy, 717–718, 717*f*
early delayed effects
focal encephalopathy, 713
neurologic deterioration, 713
overview, 712
somnolence syndrome, 712–713
late delayed effects
cerebral atrophy, 714
cognitive dysfunction, 715–717
endocrine dysfunction, 714–715
overview, 713
radiation necrosis, 713–714, 714*f*–715*f*
overview, 712, 712*t*
radiation-induced tumors, 722–723, 722*f*–723*f*
radiation injury of brachial or lumbosacral plexus
acute brachial plexopathy, 719
early delayed brachial plexopathy, 719
late delayed brachial plexopathy, 719–720
lumbosacral plexopathy, 720
overview, 719, 719*t*–720*t*
radiation injury of cranial and peripheral nerves
acoustic nerve (CN VIII), 721
facial nerve (CN VII), 721
glossopharyngeal nerve (CN IX), 721
hypoglossal nerve (CN XII), 722
oculomotor nerves (CN III, IV, VI), 721
olfactory nerve (CN I), 720–721
optic nerve (CN II), 721
overview, 720, 720*t*
peripheral nerves, 722
spinal accessory nerve (CN XI), 722
trigeminal nerve (CN V), 721
vagus nerve (CN X), 721–722
radiotherapy and spinal cord injury
early postradiotherapy myelopathy, 718
late spinal cord injury
motor neuron dysfunction, 719
progressive myelopathy, 718
spinal cord hemorrhage, 719
overview, 718, 718*t*
Neuromuscular junction and muscle paraneoplasia
acute necrotizing myopathy, 668
cachectic myopathy, 668
dermatomyositis/polymyositis/inclusion body myositis
associated antibodies, 668
diagnostic evaluation, 668
overview, 667
treatment and prognosis, 668
underlying tumor, 668
Lambert-Eaton myasthenic syndrome
antineuronal antibodies, 666
diagnostic evaluation, 666, 666*f*
differential diagnosis, 667
overview, 666
treatment and prognosis, 667
underlying tumor, 666
myasthenia gravis (MG)
antineuronal antibodies, 667
diagnostic evaluation, 667
differential diagnosis, 667
overview, 667
treatment and prognosis, 667
underlying tumor, 667
paraneoplastic carcinoid myopathy, 668
Neuromyotonia
antineuronal antibodies, 665
diagnostic evaluation, 665
differential diagnosis, 665–666
overview, 665
treatment and prognosis, 665
underlying tumor, 665
Neuronal and mixed neuronal-glial tumors
central neurocytoma, 100, 102–103, 102*f*
gangliocytoma and dysplastic gangliocytoma of the cerebellum, 100, 101*f*
mixed neuronal-glial tumors
dysembryoplastic neuroepithelial tumor (DNT), 103–104, 104*f*
ganglioglioma and malignant ganglioglioma, 103
neuronal tumors, 100
Neuronal tumors, 100
Neuropathology
cranial and peripheral nerve tumors
malignant peripheral nerve sheath tumor, 112, 542–543, 543*f*
neurofibroma, 111–112, 111*f*
overview, 110–111
schwannoma, 111, 112*f*
general considerations
classification and grading, 81–82
overview, 81
prognostic features, 82
hematopoietic system tumors
primary central nervous system lymphoma, 113–114, 113*f*
intraoperative diagnosis and handling of surgical specimen, 82, 83*f*
meningeal tumors. *See* Meningeal tumors
molecular genetics, 112–113
overview, 81
primary CNS tumors
neuroepithelial tumors. *See* Neuroepithelial tumors
overview, 84
tissue evaluation, general approach to, 83–84
Neuropsychological issues
future directions
expand survivorship research in neuro-oncology, 211–212
overview, 211

Neuropsychological issues
  future directions (*Cont.*):
    promote patient-oriented outcomes research in neuro-oncology, 211
  neurocognitive prognosis and quality of life
    depression, 210
    neurocognition, 210
    quality of life, 210
  neuropsychological sequelae
    effect of patient age, 208
    effects of edema, 207
    effects of surgery and tumor location, 207
    influence of chemotherapy, 208
    influence of radiation, 207–208
    overview, 206–207
    treatment of neurocognitive sequelae, 208
  overview, 201
  psychiatric sequelae
    depression, 209
    mood, 209
    overview, 209
    pain, 209
  quality of life
    assessment
      European Organization of Research and Treatment of Cancer (EORTC) QLQ-C30, 203
      Functional Assessment of Cancer Therapy (FACT) with brain disease-specific subscale, 203
      Karnofsky Performance Status (KPS), 202
      overview, 202
      Short Form Health Survey (SF-36), 202–203
    measure of neurocognition and neurocognitive dysfunction, 205–206
      overview, 205
      quality of life assessment considerations, 206
    neuropsychology and, 203–205, 204*f*
    overview, 202
Neurothekeomas, 542
Nevoid basal cell carcinoma syndrome, 10*t*, 247, 249, 249*t*, 250*f*, 420
NF1 gene, 112, 234–235, 545
NF2 gene, 112, 235, 242, 546
NGGCTs (nongerminoma germ cell tumors). *See* Nongerminoma germ cell tumors (NGGCTs)
Nitroimidazoles (misonidazole, metronidazole), neurologic complications of, 691
Nitrosoureas, neurologic complications of, 686–687
N-nitroso compounds and brain cancer, 7
Nonenhancing lesions, 47, 47*f*–48*f*
Nonfunctioning adenomas
  clinical presentation and diagnosis, 393–394
  therapy, 394–395, 394*t*
Nongerminoma germ cell tumors (NGGCTs)
  chemotherapy, 494–495
  long-term survival of, 495
  radiation therapy, 492–493
  surgical management, 490–491
Nonmaleficence, 195
Nonneoplastic temporal bone and middle fossa mass, 463–464
Null cell adenomas, 391

O

Observational trials, 218
Occupation and brain cancer, 8–9
Octreotide, neurologic complications of, 697
Oculomotor nerves (CN III, IV, VI), radiation injury to, 721
OKT3, neurologic complications of, 698–699, 699*f*
Olfactory nerve (CN I), radiation injury to, 720–721
Oligodendroglial tumors
  anaplastic oligoastrocytoma, 97, 97*f*
  anaplastic oligodendroglioma, 95–96, 96*f*
  mixed oligoastrocytoma, 96–97, 97*f*
  molecular genetics, 97
  oligodendroglioma. *See* Oligodendroglioma and mixed gliomas
Oligodendroglioma and mixed gliomas, 94–95, 94*f*–95*f*
  clinical presentation, 313
  epidemiology, 312
  future directions, 328
  genetics and molecular biology, 4
    genetic lesions in oligodendroglioma, 312
  molecular biology, 312–313
  genotyping of oligodendroglioma, 315–316
  histology, 4
  histopathology
    differential diagnosis, 318
    grading, 317–318
    histopathologic features, 317
    mixed oligoastrocytomas and oligodendrogliomas containing glial fibrillary acidic protein (GFAP)-positive cells, 318
    overview, 316–317, 316*f*
  neuroimaging, 57*t*, 63*f*, 313–315, 314*f*–315*f*
    CT, 61–62
    general imaging findings, 60–61
    MRI, 62
    overview, 58
    PET, 62, 63*f*
  overview, 311, 328
  prognosis
    genotype and, 320–321
    in the "pregenetic" era, 318–320, 319*f*–320*f*
  treatment
    chemotherapy, 177
      adjuvant chemotherapy, 327
      first-line chemotherapy in recurrent oligodendroglial tumors, 322, 322*t*, 323*f*–325*f*, 324
      high-dose chemotherapy with autologous bone marrow rescue, 326–327
      recurrent oligodendroglial tumors, 322, 322*t*
      second-line chemotherapy, 324–326, 325*t*
        following first-line PCV or temozolomide, 326, 326*t*
      upfront chemotherapy in low-grade oligodendroglial tumors, 327–328, 328*f*
      upfront chemotherapy in newly diagnosed anaplastic oligodendroglioma, 327
    low-grade glioma/oligodendroglioma, 321
    overview, 321
    radiotherapy, 321–322
    surgical management, 321
Ollier disease, high-grade astrocytomas and, 260
Opsoclonus–myoclonus
  antineuronal antibodies, 658–659
  diagnostic evaluation, 658
  differential diagnosis, 659
  overview, 658
  treatment and prognosis, 659
  underlying tumor, 658
Optic nerve (CN II), radiation injury to, 721
Optic neuritis
  antineuronal antibodies, 661
  overview, 661
  treatment and prognosis, 661
  underlying tumor, 661
Optic pathway glioma, 237
Orbital lesions, 458, 458*f*
Osteochondroma, 451
Osteoclastoma, 451
Osteogenic sarcoma, 451

Osteoma, 451
Osteosclerotic myeloma, 664

P

Paclitaxel, neurologic complications of, 690
Pain
  control, 192–193, 193*t*
  prevalence of, 209
Palisaded, encapsulated neuromas, 542
Pancoast tumors, 544, 631–632, 632*f*, 633, 634*f*
Papillary ependymomas, 98
Papilledema, 38, 38*t*
Paragangliomas, 472–473, 473*f*
Paraneoplasia
  autoantibodies, 651*t*–654*t*, 668–669, 669*t*
  diagnostic evaluation, 669–670, 670*f*
  neuropathology, 670–671
  overview, 649, 650*t*–651*t*
  pathogenesis, 671
  specific clinical presentations
    central nervous system
      cancer- and melanoma-associated retinopathy
        diagnostic evaluation, 660–661
        differential diagnosis, 661
        overview, 660
        treatment and prognosis, 661
        underlying tumor, 660
      cancer- and melanoma-associated retinopathy
        antineuronal antibodies, 661
      chorea
        antineuronal antibodies, 660
        diagnostic evaluation, 660
        differential diagnosis, 660
        overview, 660
        treatment and prognosis, 660
        underlying tumor, 660
      encephalomyelitis, 656–658
        antineuronal antibodies, 658
        diagnostic evaluation, 658
        differential diagnosis, 658
        treatment and prognosis, 658
        underlying tumor, 658
      limbic encephalitis
        antineuronal antibodies, 656
        diagnostic evaluation, 656
        differential diagnosis, 656
        overview, 656, 657*f*
        treatment and prognosis, 656
        underlying tumor, 656
      opsoclonus–myoclonus
        antineuronal antibodies, 658–659
        diagnostic evaluation, 658
        differential diagnosis, 659
        overview, 658
        treatment and prognosis, 659
        underlying tumor, 658
      optic neuritis
        antineuronal antibodies, 661
        overview, 661
        treatment and prognosis, 661
        underlying tumor, 661
      stiff-person syndrome (SPS)
        antineuronal antibodies, 659
        diagnostic evaluation, 659
        differential diagnosis, 660
        overview, 659
        treatment and prognosis, 660
        underlying tumor, 659
      subacute cerebellar ataxia
        antineuronal antibodies, 650, 655, 655*f*
        diagnostic evaluation, 650
        differential diagnosis, 655
        overview, 650
        treatment and prognosis, 655–656
        underlying tumor, 650
      subacute motor neuronopathies/motor neuron disease
        characteristic associations of motor neuron syndromes with typical tumor, 661–662
        improvement following treatment of tumor, 662
        overview, 661
        paraneoplastic antibodies, 662
    neuromuscular junction and muscle
      acute necrotizing myopathy, 668
      cachectic myopathy, 668
      dermatomyositis/polymyositis/inclusion body myositis
        associated antibodies, 668
        diagnostic evaluation, 668
        overview, 667
        treatment and prognosis, 668
        underlying tumor, 668
      Lambert-Eaton myasthenic syndrome
        antineuronal antibodies, 666
        diagnostic evaluation, 666, 666*f*
        differential diagnosis, 667
        overview, 666
        treatment and prognosis, 667
        underlying tumor, 666
      myasthenia gravis (MG)
        antineuronal antibodies, 667
        diagnostic evaluation, 667
        differential diagnosis, 667
        overview, 667
        treatment and prognosis, 667
        underlying tumor, 667
      paraneoplastic carcinoid myopathy, 668
    overview, 650, 651*t*–654*t*
    peripheral nervous system
      multiple myeloma, 664
      neuromyotonia
        antineuronal antibodies, 665
        diagnostic evaluation, 665
        differential diagnosis, 665–666
        overview, 665
        treatment and prognosis, 665
        underlying tumor, 665
      osteosclerotic myeloma, 664
      sensorimotor neuropathy
        associated tumors, 663
        associated with M proteins, 663–664
        differential diagnosis, 663
        overview, 663
        paraneoplastic antibodies, 663
      subacute autonomic neuropathy
        antineuronal antibodies, 664–665
        differential diagnosis, 665
        overview, 664
        treatment and prognosis, 665
        underlying tumor, 664
      subacute sensory neuronopathy
        antineuronal antibodies, 662–663
        diagnostic evaluation, 662
        differential diagnosis, 663
        overview, 662
        treatment and prognosis, 663
        underlying tumor, 662
      vasculitis of nerve and muscle
        antineuronal antibodies, 665
        diagnostic evaluation, 665
        overview, 665
        treatment and prognosis, 665
        underlying tumor, 665
      Waldenström macroglobulinemia 664
  syndromes, 650*t*–651*t*
  treatment and prognosis, 671, 672*t*
Paraneoplastic carcinoid myopathy, 668
Paraneoplastic cerebellar degeneration (PCD), 650. *See also* Subacute cerebellar ataxia
Particulate radiation, 144–145
Patient, approach to. *See* Approach to patient
Patient/subject selection for clinical trials
  broad versus restrictive eligibility criteria, 224
  overview, 223
  prognostic variables in brain tumors, 223–224, 224*f*

PCNSL (primary central nervous system lymphoma). *See* Primary CNS lymphoma (PCNSL)
PDGF (platelet-derived growth factor), 21, 265, 371
Pentostatin, neurologic complications of, 685
Perfusion magnetic resonance, 74, 75*f*
Perimetry, 42
Perineuromas, 542
Peripheral nervous system
  paraneoplasia
    multiple myeloma, 664
    neuromyotonia
      antineuronal antibodies, 665
      diagnostic evaluation, 665
      differential diagnosis, 665–666
      overview, 665
      treatment and prognosis, 665
      underlying tumor, 665
    osteosclerotic myeloma, 664
    sensorimotor neuropathy
      associated tumors, 663
      associated with M proteins, 663–664
      differential diagnosis, 663
      overview, 663
      paraneoplastic antibodies, 663
    subacute autonomic neuropathy
      antineuronal antibodies, 664–665
      differential diagnosis, 665
      overview, 664
      treatment and prognosis, 665
      underlying tumor, 664
    subacute sensory neuronopathy
      antineuronal antibodies, 662–663
      diagnostic evaluation, 662
      differential diagnosis, 663
      overview, 662
      treatment and prognosis, 663
      underlying tumor, 662
    vasculitis of nerve and muscle
      antineuronal antibodies, 665
      diagnostic evaluation, 665
      overview, 665
      treatment and prognosis, 665
      underlying tumor, 665
    Waldenström macroglobulinemia, 664
  radiation injury to, 722
  tumors, 110–113, 534–535, 536*t*, 537, 538*f*, 540*f*, 542–543, 543*f*. *See also* Spinal root and peripheral nerve tumors
    clinical presentation, 112, 535, 536*t*
    metastases
      lumbosacral plexus
        clinical setting, 638
        clinical signs, 638–639, 638*t*
        differential diagnosis, 639–640
        electrophysiologic diagnosis, 639
        imaging, 639, 640*f*
        overview, 637–638
        surgical exploration, 639
        treatment/prognosis, 640–641
      metastatic brachial plexopathy
        clinical setting, 630–633, 631*f*
          Pancoast tumors, 631–632, 632*f*
        diagnosis
          differential diagnosis, 635–636, 636*t*
          electrophysiology, 633
          imaging, 633, 634*f*, 635
          surgery, 635
        imaging
          Pancoast tumor, 633, 634*f*
        treatment/prognosis, 636–637
          Pancoast tumors, 636
      overview, 629
      pathophysiology of metastatic neuropathy, 629–630, 630*f*
      peripheral neuropathy
        biopsy, 642, 643*f*
        clinical setting, 641
        clinical signs, 641
        diagnosis, 641
        electrophysiology, 641
        imaging, 642, 642*f*
        treatment/prognosis, 642–643
    molecular genetics, 112–113
    overview, 110–111
Per protocol (PP) subsample, 231
PET (positron emission tomography), basic concepts of, 41–42, 55
p53 oncogene, 25*t*, 31, 88–89, 93, 100, 262–263, 264*f*, 290, 312, 387*t*, 388, 482
Phakomatoses
  genetic testing in routine clinical practice, 252
  molecular genetics and role of mouse models
    neurofibromatosis, 250–251
    overview, 250
    tuberous sclerosis complex, 251
  neurofibromatosis types 1 (von Recklinghausen disease) and 2
    nevoid basal cell carcinoma syndrome (Gorlin syndrome), 247, 249, 249*t*, 250*f*
    overview, 234–236, 234*f*–235*f*
    tuberous sclerosis complex (Bourneville disease), 242–243, 242*t*, 244*f*–245*f*, 245–246
    type 1, 236–237, 236*t*, 238*f*, 239–240
    type 2, 240–242, 240*t*, 241*f*
    von Hipple-Lindau (VHL) disease, 246–247, 247*t*, 248*f*
  overview, 233, 234*t*
Phase I trials, 218, 224–225
Phase II trials, 218, 225
Phase III trials, 218
  multifactor designs, 225–226
  single-factor designs, 225
Phase IV trials, 218
Phosphatase tensin homologue (PTEN) gene, 25*t*, 266, 312, 320
Photoelectric effect, 144
Photons, 144
Pilocytic astrocytoma, 90–91, 91*f*
  imaging, 57*t*, 59*f*
Pilot trials, 218
Pineal region tumors, 39, 483, 484*f*
  approach to patient with, 485*t*–486*t*
  differential diagnosis, 44*t*
  histologic diagnosis
    miscellaneous nongerm cell pineal region tumors, 487–488
    overview, 486–487
    pineal parenchymal tumors, 487
  pathology, 443
Pit-1, 388
Pituitary adenomas and sellar lesions
  clinical diagnosis and management
    corticotropin-secreting adenomas
      clinical presentation and diagnosis, 397–398
      therapy, 398
    growth hormone-secreting adenomas
      clinical presentation and diagnosis, 396
      therapy, 396–397
    nonfunctioning adenomas
      clinical presentation and diagnosis, 393–394
      therapy, 394–395, 394*t*
    overview, 393
    prolactinomas
      clinical presentation and diagnosis, 395
      therapy, 395–396
    surgery, 399, 399*f*–400*f*
    thyroid-stimulating hormone-secreting adenomas
      clinical presentation and diagnosis, 398–399
      therapy, 399
  future prospects, 404–405
  imaging, 391–393, 392*f*
  miscellaneous pathologic entities
    craniopharyngioma, 401–402, 403*f*, 404
    pituitary apoplexy, 400–401, 400*f*
    pituitary carcinoma, 401
    Rathke cleft cysts, 404, 404*f*

normal anatomy and neuroimaging of sellar region, 382, 382*f*–386*f*, 384–385
overview, 381, 404–405
pathogenesis
autocrine/paracrine stimulation, growth factors, cytokines, 388–389
c-fos, 388
c-myc, 388
ER-α, 388
oncogenes, 387–388
overview, 386, 387*t*
Pit-1, 388
tumor suppressor genes, 388
pathology
adrenocorticotropic-secreting adenomas, 389–390, 390*f*
glycoprotein adenomas, 390–391, 391*f*
growth hormone-secreting adenomas, 389, 390*f*
null cell adenomas, 391
overview, 389
prolactin-secreting adenomas, 389
pituitary adenomas
classification, 385–386, 387*t*
sellar/parasellar lesions, 459, 459*f*
Pituitary apoplexy, 400–401, 400*f*
Pituitary carcinoma, 401
Pituitary region tumors, differential diagnosis of, 45*t*
Pituitary tumor-transforming gene (PTTG), 387*t*, 388
P13K/AKT/PTEN, 266
Placebo control, 229
Plant alkaloids
CNS penetration of, 617*t*
neurologic complications of
etoposide, 689–690
pyrazoloacridine, 691
taxanes
docetaxel, 690
paclitaxel, 690
teniposide, 689–690
topoisomerase inhibitors
irinotecan, 690–691
rubitecan, 690–691
topotecan, 690–691
vinca alkaloids, 689
Plasmacytoma, 451, 452*f*
Platelet-derived growth factor (PDGF), 21, 265, 371
Pleomorphic xanthoastrocytoma, 91–93, 92*f*, 303–304
imaging, 57*t*, 59*f*
Plexiform neurofibromas, 237, 238*f*
Plicamycin (mithramycin), neurologic complications of, 692
PNETs (primitive neuroectodermal tumors). *See* Primitive neuroectodermal tumors (PNETs)
Positron emission tomography (PET), basic concepts of, 41–42
Posterior fossa/clival lesions (posterior temporal bone, occipital bone, clivus)
diagnoses and management
acoustic neuroma, 465–466, 465*f*
cavernoma, 470
chondrosarcoma, 467–469, 468*f*
chordoma, 469–470, 469*f*
choroid plexus papilloma, 472
craniopharyngioma, 473–474
dermoid cyst, 472
differential diagnosis, 44*t*
epidermoid cyst, 471–472, 471*f*
epithelial cyst, 470–471
facial nerve schwannomas, 467, 468*f*
lipoma, 470
meningioma, 466–467, 467*f*
nerve sheath tumor of jugular foramen, 472
overview, 464–465
paragangliomas, 472–473, 473*f*
teratoma, 470
evaluation, 464
presentation, 464
P21-Ras, 545, 546*f*
Prednisolone, CNS penetration of, 617*t*
Presentation
altered mental status, 38
cerebellar tumors, 39
cranial nerves, 39
differential diagnosis, 39–40, 40*t*
false localizing signs, 39
focal neurologic symptoms and signs
brainstem tumors, 39
cortical tumors, 38–39
pineal region and third ventricular tumors, 39
headaches, 37
overview, 37
papilledema, 38, 38*t*
radiologic diagnosis
angiography, 41
CT, 40
MRI, 40–41
PET, 41–42
skull x-rays, 40
SPECT, 42
ultrasonography, 42
seizures, 38
Primary CNS lymphoma (PCNSL), 45–46, 113–114, 113*f*
basic science that informs pathogenesis, 347–349
chemotherapy, 172–173
clinical features
intraocular lymphoma, 352–353, 352*f*–353*f*
overview, 351–352, 352*t*
PCNSL associated with profound immunodeficiency, 353–354
secondary forms, 354–355, 354*f*
epidemiology
antigen discovery, 346–347
etiology, 344, 345*t*
"host factors," 345–346
immunocompetence, 347
incidence, 344, 345*f*
infectious agents, 346, 346*t*
neuroimaging, 58*t*, 73*f*
CT, 72
HIV-PCNSL and CNS-PTLD, 356*f*–357*f*, 357–358
MRI, 72, 73*f*
overview, 72, 355–356, 355*f*–356*f*
"sentinel lesions," 256–357
overview, 343–344
pathology, 349–351, 349*f*–350*f*, 350*t*–351*t*
single brain lesion, 45–46
treatment
autologous stem cell transplant, 360–361
blood–brain barrier disruption therapy, 361
chemotherapy, 360
CNS posttransplantation lymphoproliferative disease, 361
corticosteroids, 359
evolution of, 358*t*
HIV+ primary CNS lymphoma, 361
immunosuppressed forms of primary CNS lymphoma, 361
overview, 358–359, 358*t*, 359*f*
prophylaxis, 362
radiation therapy, 359–360
radiosurgery, 360
salvage therapies
recurrent disease, 362
"secondary" and "orphan" forms, 361–362
surgery, 359
Primary meningeal neoplasms
chemotherapy, 377
diagnostic evaluation, 372, 374
epidemiology and known influences on tumor, 369–370
genetics and molecular biology
genetics, 370–371
growth factors and receptors, 371
miscellaneous meningeal neoplasms
hemangiopericytomas, 377
melanocytic tumors, 377–378
meningeal sarcomas, 377

Primary meningeal neoplasms (*Cont.*):
natural history, 374–375
neuropathology, 374, 374*t*, 375*f*
overview, 369, 370*f*, 378
radiation, 376–377
specific clinical presentations, 371, 372*f*–373*f*
surgical management, 375–376, 376*t*
Primary sarcoma, therapeutic management and outcomes of, 522
Primary spinal tumors. *See also* Spinal root and peripheral nerve tumors
anatomy, clinical presentation, neurologic diagnosis
by location
cauda equina, 503
conus medullaris, 503
intramedullary, 503
by sign or symptom, 503–504
epidemiology, 501, 502*f*, 502*t*, 503
neurodiagnostic tests
neuroimaging, 504
nonneoplastic lesions mimicking spinal cord tumors, 505
tumor and cerebrospinal fluid markers, 504–505
overview, 501, 524
pathology, 503
therapeutic management, general principles of
chemotherapy, 512
radiation therapy
complications, 511–512
definitions of treatment volumes and reporting of dose, 508, 509*t*
overview, 508
selecting doses, 511, 511*t*
tolerance of spinal cord and lumbosacral nerve roots, 511
toxicity scoring, 512
treatment techniques, 509–511, 509*t*, 510*f*
surgery
complications, 508
intradural extramedullary tumors, 507
intramedullary tumors, 507–508
outcomes, 506*t*
overview, 505, 506*t*
surgical planning, 505, 507
therapeutic management and outcomes, by histology
astrocytoma
chemotherapy, 515
overview, 512, 513*f*–514*f*
prognostic factors, 512–513, 515
radiation therapy, 515
surgery, 515
chondrosarcoma
chemotherapy, 522
overview, 521
radiation therapy, 522
surgery, 522
chordoma
outcomes, 521
overview, 521
prognostic factors, 521
treatment, 521
ependymoma
chemotherapy, 517
overview, 515, 516*f*
pathology, 515, 517
prognostic factors, 517
radiation therapy, 517
surgery, 517
hemangioblastoma
outcomes, 523
overview, 522–523, 522*f*
prognostic factors, 523
treatment, 523
meningioma
chemotherapy, 519
overview, 517–518, 518*f*–519*f*
radiation therapy, 519
surgery, 518–519
miscellaneous tumors, 523–524
primary sarcoma
outcomes, 522
overview, 522
treatment, 522
schwannoma, 519, 520*f*, 521
vertebral hemangioma
overview, 523
radiation therapy, 523
surgery, 523
Primary tumors. *See also* Specific tumors
approach to patient. *See* Approach to patient
chemotherapy. *See* Chemotherapy
clinical trial design. *See* Clinical trial design
epidemiology. *See* Epidemiology of brain cancer
laboratory diagnosis. *See* Laboratory diagnosis
neuroimaging. *See* Neuroimaging
neuropathology. *See* Neuropathology
neuropsychological issues. *See* Neuropsychological issues
phakomatoses. *See* Phakomatoses
presentation. *See* Presentation
radiotherapy and radiosurgery, principles of. *See* Radiotherapy and radiosurgery
supportive care. *See* Supportive care
surgical management. *See* Surgical management
translational applications of molecular biology in neuro-oncology. *See* Translational applications of molecular biology in neuro-oncology
Primitive neuroectodermal tumors (PNETs)
chemotherapy, 173
medulloblastoma
analyses of gene expression, 419–420
cell of origin, 419
clinical diagnosis, 416
imaging diagnosis, 416–417, 417*f*–419*f*
karotypic abnormalities, 419
miscellaneous growth factor pathways, 421–422
molecular biology, 420–421
nonsurgical therapy, 423–424
outcome, 424–425, 425*t*
overview, 416
pathologic diagnosis, 417, 419
recurrent, 424
surgical treatment
associated hydrocephalus, 422
resection, 422–423
overview, 415
supratentorial PNETs, 425–426
Procarbazine, neurologic complications of, 687–688
Prognostic variables in brain tumors, 223–224
Progression-free survival, 222
Prolactinomas
clinical presentation and diagnosis, 395
therapy, 395–396
Proteinases, 26–27, 27*t*
Proteolysis, overactive, 30
Pseudotumor of peripheral nerve, 542
P16 gene, 25–26, 25*t*
Psychiatric issues, 189–192, 190*t*–191*t*
Psychological bias, 228
Psychosocial support, 49–50
PTCH gene, 249, 420
PTEN (phosphatase tensin homologue) gene, 25*t*, 266, 312, 320
PTTG (pituitary tumor-transforming gene), 387*t*, 388
Pyrazoloacridine, neurologic complications of, 691

Q
Quality of life, 210
assessment
European Organization of Research and Treatment of Cancer (EORTC) QLQ-C30, 203

Functional Assessment of Cancer Therapy (FACT) with brain disease-specific subscale, 203
Karnofsky Performance Status (KPS), 202
overview, 202
Short Form Health Survey (SF-36), 202–203
measure of neurocognition and neurocognitive dysfunction, 205–206
overview, 205
quality of life assessment considerations, 206
neuropsychology and, 203–205, 204*f*
overview, 202

R

Radiation-induced plexopathy, 544
Radiation necrosis, 713–714, 714*f*–715*f*
Radiotherapy and radiosurgery
astrocytoma, 515
biologic properties of radiation
cell death caused by radiation, 145–146
overview, 145
radiation tolerance of normal CNS tissues, 147–148, 147*f*–150*f*, 149*t*
therapeutic ratio, 146–147, 146*f*
brain metastases, radiosurgery for, 567–570, 567*f*
chondrosarcoma, 522
clinical applications, overview of
brachytherapy, 155
immobilization and simulation, 149, 151–155, 151*f*–154*f*
overview, 148–149
patient assessment, 149
treatment delivery, 155
ependymoma, 438–439, 517
germinomas, 491–492
high-grade astrocytomas, 277–278, 279*f*
leptomeningeal metastases
adults, 616
adverse effects, 617
children, 616–617
low-grade astrocytomas, 297–300, 298*f*, 300*f*
meningioma, 519
neurologic complications of. *See* Neurologic complications of radiation therapy
neuropsychological sequelae, 207–208
nongerminoma germ cell tumors, 492–493
oligodendroglioma and mixed gliomas, 321–322
overview, 143, 144*f*, 159, 486*t*
physical properties of radiation
particulate radiation, 144–145
radiation measurements, 145
primary CNS lymphoma, 359–360
primary meningeal neoplasms, 376–377
primary spinal tumors
complications, 511–512
definitions of treatment volumes and reporting of dose, 508, 509*t*
overview, 508
selecting doses, 511, 511*t*
tolerance of spinal cord and lumbosacral nerve roots, 511
toxicity scoring, 512
treatment techniques, 509–511, 509*t*, 510*f*
radiosurgical instruments
CyberKnife, 159, 159*f*
Gamma Knife, 156–157, 157*f*–158*f*
linear accelerator (LINAC) based radiosurgery, 157
stereotactic radiosurgery, 155–156, 156*f*–157*f*
vertebral hemangioma, 523
vertebral metastases, 583–584
with epidural extension, 594–595, 595*t*, 598
Randomization and stratification in clinical trials
overview, 226
randomization procedures, 227
stratified randomization, 227–228
unstratified randomization, 227
treatment assignment issues, 226–227
Ras, 30, 234, 234*f*, 266
Rathke cleft cysts, 404, 404*f*
Rb (retinoblastoma protein) gene, 25–26, 25*t*, 31, 264–265, 265*f*
Receptor protein tyrosine kinase (RPTK), gliomas and, 19, 20*t*
Research studies. *See* Clinical trial design
Response or regression rates in clinical trials
definition, 220
factors affecting response rates, 221–222, 221*f*
imaging issues, 220–221
Retinoids, neurologic complications of, 692
Retinopathy, cancer- and melanoma-associated
antineuronal odies, 661
diagnostic evaluation, 660–661
differential diagnosis, 661
overview, 660
treatment and prognosis, 661
underlying tumor, 660
Rhabdomyosarcoma, 450
Rituximab (Rituxan), neurologic complications of, 699
RPTK (receptor protein tyrosine kinase), gliomas and, 19, 20*t*
Rubitecan, neurologic complications of, 690–691

S

Sample size calculations for clinical trials
calculating sample sizes, 230–231
importance of appropriate sample sizes
overview, 229
key concepts, 229
overview, 229
Schwannoma, 111, 112*f*, 240, 241*f*, 461, 461*f*, 541, 541*f*
histology and molecular genetics, 5
therapeutic management and outcomes, 519, 520*f*, 521
Schwannomatosis, 547
Scientific rationale for clinical trials, 219
Seizures, 38
anticonvulsant therapy, 184–186, 185*t*
Sellar lesions. *See* Pituitary adenomas and sellar lesions
Sensorimotor neuropathy
associated tumors, 663
associated with M proteins, 663–664
differential diagnosis, 663
overview, 663
paraneoplastic antibodies, 663
Short Form Health Survey (SF-36), 202–203
Signal transduction, 17, 18*f*, 19, 20*t*
Signal transduction inhibitors, neurologic complications of
erlotinib (Tarceva), 700
gefitinib (Iressa), 700
imatinib mesylate (Gleevec), 700
Significance (clinical trials), 219, 229
Single brain lesion
diagnosis
enhancing lesions
benign conditions, 46–47
brain metastasis, 44–45, 46*f*
gliomas, 43–44, 45*f*
primary central nervous system lymphoma (PCNSL), 45–46
nonenhancing lesions, 47, 47*f*–48*f*
staging, 47–48
differential diagnosis, 40*t*
overview, 40*t*, 43, 44*f*, 44*t*–45*t*
Single-factor statistical designs, 225
Single metastases, surgery for
breast primaries, 564, 564*f*
gastrointestinal primaries, 565
genitourinary primaries, 565

Single metastases, surgery for (*Cont.*):
  gynecologic primaries, 565
  lung primaries, 564
  melanoma, 564–565
  overview, 563–564
Single-photon emission computed tomography (SPECT), basic concepts of, 42, 55
Sinonasal undifferentiated carcinoma, 457, 458*f*
6-Mercaptopurine, CNS penetration of, 617*t*
Smear preparations, 83*f*
Smoking and brain cancer, 7–8
Somnolence syndrome, 712–713
Specific tumors
  brainstem gliomas. *See* Brainstem tumors, gliomas
  ependymomas and intraventricular tumors. *See* Ependymomas; Intraventricular tumors
  high-grade astrocytomas. *See* High-grade astrocytomas
  intracranial germ cell tumors. *See* Intracranial germ cell tumors
  low-grade astrocytomas. *See* Low-grade astrocytomas
  oligodendroglioma and mixed gliomas. *See* Oligodendroglioma and mixed gliomas
  pituitary adenomas and sellar lesions. *See* Pituitary adenomas and sellar lesions
  primary central nervous system lymphoma. *See* Primary CNS lymphoma
  primary meningeal neoplasms. *See* Primary meningeal neoplasms
  primary spinal tumors. *See* Primary spinal tumors
  primary tumors of cranial nerves and skull base. *See* Cranial nerves and skull base, primary tumors of
  primitive neuroectodermal tumors (PNETs). *See* Primitive neuroectodermal tumors (PNETs)
  spinal root and peripheral nerve tumors. *See* Spinal root and peripheral nerve tumors
SPECT (single-photon emission computed tomography), basic concepts of, 42, 55
Spinal accessory nerve (CN XI), radiation injury to, 722
Spinal cord compression, 587, 591, 599
Spinal cord injury and radiotherapy
  early postradiotherapy myelopathy, 718
  late spinal cord injury
    motor neuron dysfunction, 719
    progressive myelopathy, 718
    spinal cord hemorrhage, 719
  overview, 718, 718*t*
Spinal metastases
  intradural metastases
    intradural extramedullary metastases, 599–600, 600*f*
    intramedullary metastases, 600–602, 601*f*
    overview, 599, 600*f*–601*f*
  overview, 581
  vertebral metastases
    clinical and imaging criteria for spinal stability in neoplastic disease, 581–583, 582*f*–583*f*
    overview, 581, 582*t*
    treatment
      biomechanically stable vertebral metastases
        biophosphonates, 584
        overview, 583
        radiation therapy, 583–584
      metastases with biomechanical potential or overt instability, 584, 584*f*
    vertebral compression fracture in cancer patients, 584–586, 585*f*, 585*t*
      treatment, 585–586
  vertebral metastases with epidural extension
    factors influencing recovery of function
      administration of high-dose dexamethasone, 592
      pretreatment neurologic status, 591–592
      progression rate of symptoms, 592
      tumor biology and cell type, 591
    frequency, 586–587, 587*f*
    location
      epidural tumor in relation to spinal cord and yield of diagnostic imaging, 587–588, 589*f*
      level of spinal cord compression, 587
    management
      complications
        radiotherapy, 598
        surgery, 598–599, 599*t*
      nonspecific pharmacotherapy
        analgesia, 594
        corticosteroids, 593–594
      overview, 592, 593*f*, 593*t*
      radiation therapy, 594–595, 595*t*
      recurrent epidural spinal cord compression, 599
      specific chemotherapy, 592–593
      surgery
        approach, 597–598, 597*t*, 598*f*
        indications, 596–597
        overview, 595–596, 596*t*
    overview, 586, 599
    pathophysiology, 588, 590–591, 590*f*
    survival and spinal cord compression, 591
    symptoms and signs, 588
Spinal root and peripheral nerve tumors
  classification, 533–534, 534*t*
  clinical presentation
    peripheral nerve tumors, 535, 536*t*
    spinal root tumors, 534–535
  malignant tumors of peripheral nerve
    intraneural metastasis, 544
    malignant peripheral nerve sheath tumor, 112, 542–543, 543*f*
    Pancoast tumor, 544
    primary lymphoma of peripheral nerve, 544
    radiation-induced plexopathy, 544
  management pearls
    peripheral nerve tumors, 539–540
    spinal root tumors, 537–539
  metastases. *See* Peripheral nervous system, tumors, metastases; Spinal metastases
  overview, 533, 547
  predisposition syndromes
    neurofibromatosis type 1, 544–546, 546*f*
    neurofibromatosis type 2, 546
    schwannomatosis, 547
  preoperative investigations
    peripheral nerve tumors, 535, 537, 538*f*, 540*f*
    spinal root tumors, 535, 536*f*–537*f*
  special considerations
    desmoids, 542
    ganglion cyst, 542
    lipoma, 542
    neurofibromas, 541, 541*f*
    neurothekeomas, 542
    palisaded, encapsulated neuromas, 542
    perineuromas, 542
    pseudotumor of peripheral nerve, 542
    schwannomas, 541, 541*f*
Spinal tumors. *See* Primary spinal tumors; Spinal metastases; Spinal root and peripheral nerve tumors
Squamous cell carcinoma, 455–456
Statistical designs
  overview, 224
  phase I designs, 224–225
  phase II designs, 225
  phase III designs
    multifactor designs, 225–226
    overview, 225
    single-factor designs, 225

Stereotactic biopsy, 132*f*
Stereotactic radiosurgery, 155–156, 156*f*–157*f*
  high-grade astrocytomas, 278
  meningiomas, 376
Stereotactic radiotherapy
  meningiomas, 376
Steroids, 170–171
Stiff-person syndrome
  antineuronal antibodies, 659
  diagnostic evaluation, 659
  differential diagnosis, 660
  overview, 659
  treatment and prognosis, 660
  underlying tumor, 659
Stratification, 227
Stratified randomization, 227–228
Subacute autonomic neuropathy
  antineuronal antibodies, 664–665
  differential diagnosis, 665
  overview, 664
  treatment and prognosis, 665
  underlying tumor, 664
Subacute cerebellar ataxia
  antineuronal antibodies, 650, 655, 655*f*
  diagnostic evaluation, 650
  differential diagnosis, 655
  overview, 650
  treatment and prognosis, 655–656
  underlying tumor, 650
Subacute motor neuronopathies/motor neuron disease
  characteristic associations of motor neuron syndromes with typical tumor, 661–662
  improvement following treatment of tumor, 662
  overview, 661
  paraneoplastic antibodies, 662
Subacute sensory neuronopathy
  antineuronal antibodies, 662–663
  diagnostic evaluation, 662
  differential diagnosis, 663
  overview, 662
  treatment and prognosis, 663
  underlying tumor, 662
Subependymal giant cell astrocytoma, 93–94, 93*f*, 304
  imaging, 57*t*, 59*f*
Subependymoma, 99–100
  pathology, 443
Suicidal ideation, 190
Supportive care
  corticosteroids, 186–187
  dysphagia and swallowing disorders, 188–189
  ethics, 194–196
  gastric acid inhibitors, 187
  hospice care and end of life, 193–194
  multiple brain lesions
    antiepileptic drugs, 48–49
    corticosteroids, 49, 50*f*
    prophylactic therapy for venous thromboembolic disease (VTED), 49
    psychosocial support, 49–50
  overview, 183–184, 196
  pain control, 192–193, 193*t*
  psychiatric issues, 189–192, 190*t*–191*t*
  seizures and anticonvulsant therapy, 184–186, 185*t*
  thromboembolic complications and anticoagulation, 187–188
Suprasellar tumors, 483
  approach to patient with, 485*t*–486*t*
  histologic diagnosis, 486
Supratentorial ependymomas, 438
Supratentorial PNETs, 106, 425–426
Supratentorial tumors, 43*t*
Suramin, neurologic complications of, 692
Surgical management
  craniotomy for brain tumor
    complications
      avoidance
        awake technique, 130–131, 130*f*
        functional MRI, 128–130, 129*f*
        overview, 127
        surgical navigation, 127–128, 128*f*
      description, 126–127
    postoperative care, 124–126
    procedure, 124, 125*f*
  future directions, 138–139
  goals, 122*t*
  indications for surgery
    cytoreduction
      description, 122, 123*f*
      improvement in duration or quality of life, 123–124
      improvement in symptoms and signs, 123
    diagnosis, 121
  low-grade glioma, 134, 134*f*–135*f*, 136, 136*t*
  miscellaneous interventions in glioma patients
    brachytherapy, 133
    cerebrospinal fluid access, 133
    cerebrospinal fluid diversion, 132–133
    intratumoral chemotherapy, 133–134
  noninvasive tissue diagnosis, 131–132
  overview, 121, 122*t*
  pediatric gliomas, 136–137
  recurrent gliomas, 137–138, 137*f*–138*f*
  stereotactic brain tumor biopsy, 131, 132*f*
Survival (clinical trials), 222
Swallowing disorders, 188–189
Synthetic rubber industry, cancer incidence and, 8

T

Tamoxifen, neurologic complications of, 696–697
Tanycytic ependymomas, 98
Tarceva, 175*t*
Taxanes, neurologic complications of
  docetaxel, 690
  paclitaxel, 690
Temozolomide
  neurologic complications of, 686
  for treatment of oligodendroglioma, 324–325, 325*t*
Temporal bone adenomatous lesions, 463
Teniposide, neurologic complications of, 689–690
Teratoma, 470
TGF-α (transforming growth factor-α), 371
Thalidomide, neurologic complications of, 694
Therapeutic ratio, 146–147, 146*f*
Thiotepa
  CNS penetration of, 617*t*
  intrathecal, 621
  neurologic complications of, 688
Thromboembolic complications and anticoagulation, 187–188
Thyroid-stimulating hormone-secreting adenomas
  clinical presentation and diagnosis, 398–399
  therapy, 399
Time to progression, 222
Topoisomerase inhibitors
  CNS penetration of, 617*t*
  neurologic complications of
    irinotecan, 690–691
    rubitecan, 690–691
    topotecan, 690–691
Topotecan, 622
  CNS penetration of, 617*t*
  neurologic complications of, 690–691
Toremifene, neurologic complications of, 697
TP53 (tumor suppressor gene p53), 88–89, 93, 100, 262–263, 264*f*, 290, 312, 387*t*, 388, 482
Transforming growth factor-α (TGF-α), 371
Translational applications of molecular biology in neuro-oncology
Translational applications of molecular biology in neuro-oncology
  components of signal transduction pathways as chemotherapeutic targets
    cell surface growth factor receptors
      overview, 19

Translational applications of molecular biology in neuro-oncology
components of signal transduction pathways as chemotherapeutic targets
cell surface growth factor receptors (*Cont.*):
platelet-derived growth factor receptor inhibitors (PDGFR), 21
targeting epidermal growth factor receptor (EGFR), 19–21, 20*t*
intracellular second messenger components
overview, 21
protein kinase C inhibitors, 22
targeting Ras with farnesyltransferase inhibitors, 22
overview, 20*t*
drugs that directly damage DNA or impair DNA replication
alkylating agents, 23–24, 23*t*
cell-cycle inhibitors
cell cycle phases distal to G1/S checkpoint, 26
G1/S checkpoint, 25–26, 25*t*
overview, 24, 24*t*
overview, 22–23
effector molecules, targeting
angiogenesis mediators, 28
overview, 26, 27*t*
proteinases and integrins as mediators of tumor invasiveness
integrins in tumor motility, 27–28
proteinases, 26–27
growth-regulatory pathways in tumor cells, 17, 18*f*, 19
improving targeting of therapeutic agents to tumor
direct administration of chemotherapy into brain parenchyma—interstitial therapy, 29
functional targeting of therapeutic agent to tumor cell
low activity of tumor suppressors as targets, 30–31
overactive proteolysis, 30
overactive Ras, 30
overview, 30
increasing amount of drug delivered to tumor—agents that increase permeability of blood–brain barrier, 28–29
increasing drug distribution in brain—convection approaches, 29–30
overview, 28
overview, 17, 31
Trastuzumab (Herceptin), neurologic complications of, 699
Treatment management bias, 228
Trigeminal nerve (CN V), radiation injury to, 721
Truth telling
TSC2 gene region, 94
Tuberin–hamartin protein complex (THC), 242–243, 244*f*
Tuberous sclerosis complex (Bourneville disease), 93–94, 242–243, 242*t*, 244*f*–245*f*, 245–246
Tumor burden, 163
Tumor necrosis factor-α, neurologic complications of, 696
Tumors. *See* Metastatic disease; Primary tumors; Specific tumors
Tumor suppressor genes, 25, 25*t*, 387*t*, 388
p53 (TP53), 88–89, 93, 100, 262–263, 264*f*, 290, 312, 387*t*, 388, 482
Turcot syndrome, 10*t*, 420
high-grade astrocytomas and, 260

U

Ultrasonography, basic concepts of, 42
Unstratified randomization, 227

V

Vagus nerve (CN X), radiation injury to, 721–722
Vascular endothelial growth factor (VEGF), 266–267, 371
Vasculitis of nerve and muscle
antineuronal antibodies, 665
diagnostic evaluation, 665
overview, 665
treatment and prognosis, 665
underlying tumor, 665
Vertebral hemangioma, therapeutic management and outcomes of, 523
Vertebral metastases
clinical and imaging criteria for spinal stability in neoplastic disease, 581–583, 582*f*–583*f*
with epidural extension
factors influencing recovery of function
administration of high-dose dexamethasone, 592
pretreatment neurologic status, 591–592
progression rate of symptoms, 592
tumor biology and cell type, 591
frequency, 586–587, 587*f*
location
epidural tumor in relation to spinal cord and yield of diagnostic imaging, 587–588, 589*f*
level of spinal cord compression, 587
management
complications
radiotherapy, 598
surgery, 598–599, 599*t*
nonspecific pharmacotherapy
analgesia, 594
corticosteroids, 593–594
overview, 592, 593*f*, 593*t*
radiation therapy, 594–595, 595*t*
recurrent epidural spinal cord compression, 599
specific chemotherapy, 592–593
surgery
approach, 597–598, 597*t*, 598*f*
indications, 596–597
overview, 595–596, 596*t*
overview, 586, 599
pathophysiology, 588, 590–591, 590*f*
survival and spinal cord compression, 591
symptoms and signs, 588
overview, 581, 582*t*
treatment
biomechanically stable vertebral metastases
biophosphonates, 584
overview, 583
radiation therapy, 583–584
metastases with biomechanical potential or overt instability, 584, 584*f*
vertebral compression fracture in cancer patients, 584–586, 585*f*, 585*t*
treatment, 585–586
Vinca alkaloids
CNS penetration of, 617*t*
neurologic complications of, 689
Vinyl chloride, cancer incidence and, 8
Viruses, 9, 30
Vitamins and brain cancer, 7
Von Hipple-Lindau (VHL) disease, 246–247, 247*t*, 248*f*
Von Recklinghausen disease (neurofibromatosis type 1). *See* Neurofibromatosis types 1 (von Recklinghausen disease) and 2

W

Wafers/implants, 172
Waldenström macroglobulinemia, 664
Whole-brain radiation therapy, 560–562, 561*f*

Z

Zarnestra, 175*t*